NEURO-ONCOLOGY COMPENDIUM FOR THE BOARDS AND CLINICAL PRACTICE

NEURO-ONCOLOGY COMPENDIUM FOR THE BOARDS AND CLINICAL PRACTICE

EDITED BY

Maciej M. Mrugala, MD, PhD, MPH, FAAN

MAYO CLINIC
PHOENIX, AZ, USA

Na Tosha N. Gatson, MD, PhD, FAAN

BANNER MD ANDERSON CANCER CENTER
PHOENIX, AZ, USA
GEISINGER COMMONWEALTH SCHOOL OF MEDICINE
SCRANTON, PA, USA

Sylvia C. Kurz, MD, PhD

EBERHARD KARLS UNIVERSITY
TÜBINGEN, GERMANY

Kathryn S. Nevel, MD

INDIANA UNIVERSITY SCHOOL OF MEDICINE
INDIANAPOLIS, IN, USA

Jennifer L. Clarke, MD, MPH

UNIVERSITY OF CALIFORNIA
SAN FRANCISCO, CA, USA

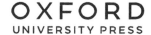

OXFORD
UNIVERSITY PRESS

OXFORD
UNIVERSITY PRESS

Oxford University Press is a department of the University of Oxford. It furthers
the University's objective of excellence in research, scholarship, and education
by publishing worldwide. Oxford is a registered trade mark of Oxford University
Press in the UK and certain other countries.

Published in the United States of America by Oxford University Press
198 Madison Avenue, New York, NY 10016, United States of America.

© Oxford University Press 2023

CIP data is on file at the Library of Congress
ISBN 978–0–19–757377–8

DOI: 10.1093/med/9780197573778.001.0001

Printed by Integrated Books International, United States of America

DEDICATIONS

The years 2020–2021 were particularly difficult for the medical community due to the global pandemic. Hats off to the providers who maintained excellent care of their patients and helped to usher innovations using telemedicine and distance learning. This book is dedicated to those on the frontline (physicians, advanced care providers, nurses, aides, technicians, and others) and those acting behind the scenes (laboratory medicine, maintenance, housekeeping, food services, and more). Finally, to all the healthcare workers who continuously go to great lengths to take the best care of patients. Together, we elevate and educate in medicine.

IN MEMORIAM

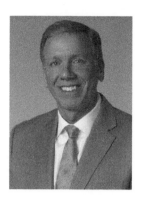

Gordon A. Watson, MD, PhD, co-author of the Rare Tumors chapter, was a beloved Associate Professor and Vice Chair for Clinical Affairs for the Department of Radiation Oncology at Indiana University. He was among the most popular and busiest physicians in the department and the Indiana University Melvin and Bren Simon Comprehensive Cancer Center. Due to his vast wisdom and well-known desire to help, his input was always sought after for the most challenging of clinical cases. He was an outstanding physician in every way imaginable, who is dearly missed by his colleagues, patients, family, and friends.

CONTENTS

FOREWORD

This slim volume manages to be both comprehensive and succinct at the same time—a welcome combination. The editors compiled a list of stellar authors, and employed a standard structure for each chapter, making this book easy to read and the information highly accessible. The book fills a critical need for those seeking rapid and current information to care for patients with a neuro-oncologic problem. The focus is on primary intracranial tumors, but the authors also cover CNS metastases, and other neuro-oncologic topics such as paraneoplastic syndromes. They review the core diagnostic methods and summarize their clinical relevance; the vivid images of MRI scans and pathology throughout the book are especially informative. The latest therapeutic studies are summarized in a clear fashion along with the potential benefits and toxicities of each therapeutic modality. For those seeking information to prepare for an oncology or neuro-oncology Board certification examination, they will find the key points of each chapter highlighted throughout the text, followed by flash cards and multiple-choice questions for future referral and test practice. The editors and authors are to be congratulated on this highly practical compilation of data; it is a "must have" for anyone who cares for neuro-oncologic patients.

Lisa M. DeAngelis, MD
Physician-in-Chief and Chief Medical Officer
Memorial Sloan Kettering Cancer Center
New York, NY, USA

Within the growing field of Neuro-Oncology, heavy-volume textbooks or detailed review articles do not meet the need for rapidly accessible and up-to-date practice-related information. This comprehensive, well-structured and good–to-read volume allows the newcomer to swiftly achieve an overview and the more advanced practitioner to recapitulate important facts, i.e. on recent trials, for which main efficacy outcomes and unwanted effects are summarized.

The present book by a group of experienced practitioners from all important subspecialties feeding into Neuro-Oncology covers many different aspects of modern Neuro-Oncology with the focus on primary Central Nervous System (CNS) tumors, CNS metastases, and neurological complications of cancer. Each chapter is structured in a standard way, allowing for recapitulating diagnostic challenges, clinical courses, and standard treatments including clinical trial updates. The book follows a high educational standard and fosters learning, self-testing as well as preparation for board certification in Neuro-Oncology for learners around the globe. The editors and authors are to be congratulated on this highly scholarly and useful volume, which certainly will help to inform care for patients with neuro-oncologic disease.

Wolfgang Wick, MD
Chairman, Neurology Clinic, University of Heidelberg
Neuro-Oncology Program Chair, National Center for Tumor
Diseases, Heidelberg and German Cancer Research Center
Heidelberg, Germany

PREFACE

THE NEURO-ONCOLOGY COMPENDIUM

It is with great joy that we deliver this textbook to our readers. This work would not have been possible without the tremendous dedication of the contributing authors, the Oxford University Press staff, and our team of editors. We started this journey several years ago when the five of us identified gaps in the neuro-oncology curriculum for test takers and those who sought an up-to-date clinical reference guide. Our field changes rapidly, leaving gaps in the neuro-oncology library for books that would provide a high-yield overview of the various facets of our sub-specialty. This work is designed to not only address the board exam requirements but also provide practical knowledge for those who take care of patient population. We were fortunate that some of the top talents from across the world were enthusiastic to contribute to this project. A tremendous thanks is owed to the contributing authors, who spent countless hours making sure the content of their chapters was filled with relevant information and laid out to maximize retention and recall of the information for the boards and daily clinical practice. We hope this textbook will become a staple educational offering and will be widely used by all who wish to enhance their knowledge in neuro-oncology.

On a personal note, working on this book brought us immense joy, allowed for excellent networking, and solidified our friendships for the years to come. We are very grateful for this opportunity! We wish you an enjoyable read, success on the board exams, and satisfaction in your clinical practices. We would appreciate your feedback and remain open to new and continued collaborations for future editions of the Neuro-Oncology Compendium.

The Editors
Maciej M. Mrugala
Na Tosha N. Gatson
Sylvia C. Kurz
Kathryn S. Nevel
Jennifer L. Clarke

ACKNOWLEDGMENTS

We would like to acknowledge the patients and their caregivers who allowed us to share in their care and for their participation in clinical trials or other research that led to advancements in our field. Words of gratitude go to scientists and academicians who led the research projects described in this book. We would also like to acknowledge donors and funding agencies for their contribution to the science presented in this book. Finally, we would like to thank the Society for Neuro-Oncology for supporting our original idea for this work and Craig Panner and Oxford University Press team for taking our project on.

CONTRIBUTORS

Haroon Ahmad, MD
University of Maryland, School of Medicine
Baltimore, MD, USA

Iyad Alnahhas, MD
Thomas Jefferson University
Philadelphia, PA, USA

Nikolaos Andreatos, MD
Mayo Clinic
Rochester, MN, USA

Ashok R. Asthagiri, MD
University of Virginia
Charlottesville, VA, USA

Amir Azadi, MD
Honor Health Neuroscience
Scottsdale, AZ, USA

Molly Havard Blau, MD, MS
University of Washington
Seattle, WA, USA

Maria L. Boccia, PhD, LM
Baylor University Robbins College of Health and Human Sciences
Waco, TX, USA

Adrienne A. Boire, MD, PhD
Memorial Sloan Kettering Cancer Center
New York, NY, USA

Cameron Brimley, MD
Geisinger Health
Danville, PA, USA

Alyssa Callela, PA-C
Geisinger Health
Danville, PA, USA

Jennifer L. Clarke, MD, MPH
University of California
San Francisco, CA, USA

Andrew R. Conger, MD, MS
Geisinger Health
Danville, PA, USA

Scott L. Coven, DO, MPH
Riley Hospital for Children at IU Health
Indianapolis, IN, USA

Kara L. Curley, PA-C
Mayo Clinic
Phoenix, AZ, USA

Logan S. DeWitt, DO
Indiana University School of Medicine
Indianapolis, IN, USA

Radhika Dhamija, MD
Mayo Clinic
Phoenix, AZ, USA

Richard S. Dowd, MD, MS
Tufts Medical Center
Boston, MA, USA

Reginald Fong, MD
Geisinger Health
Danville, PA, USA

Ekokobe Fonkem, DO
Medical College of Wisconsin
Milwaukee, WC, USA

Morgan Freret, MD, PhD
Memorial Sloan Kettering Cancer Center
New York, NY, USA

Shobhit Kumar Garg, MD, FRCR
William Harvey Hospital,
East Kent Hospitals University Foundation Trust
Ashford, Kent, UK

Na Tosha N. Gatson, MD, PhD, FAAN
Banner MD Anderson Cancer Center
Phoenix, AZ, USA
Geisinger Commonwealth School of Medicine
Scranton, PA, USA

Pierre Giglio, MD
The Ohio State University
Columbus, OH, USA

Michael Glantz, MD
Penn State College of Medicine - Milton S. Hershey
    Medical Center
Hershey, PA, USA

Andrew J. Gogos, MBBS, FRACS
St Vincents Hospital Melbourne
Fitzroy, AU

David Gritsch, MD
Mass General Brigham
Boston, MA, USA

Simon Gritsch, MD, PhD
Mass General Brigham
Boston, MA, USA

Lia M. Halasz, MD
University of Washington
Seattle, WA, USA

Shawn L. Hervey-Jumper, MD
University of California San Francisco
San Francisco, CA, USA

Joseph M. Hoxworth, MD
Mayo Clinic
Phoenix, AZ, USA

Maya Hrachova, DO
University of Oklahoma
Oklahoma City, OK, USA

Valeria Internò, MD
University of Bari
Bari, Italy

Rajan Jain, MD
New York University Grossman School of Medicine
New York, NY, USA

George I. Jallo, MD
Johns Hopkins All Children's Hospital
St. Petersburg, FL, USA

Thomas J. Kaley, MD
Memorial Sloan Kettering Cancer Center
New York, NY, USA

Matthias Karajannis, MD, MS
Memorial Sloan Kettering Cancer Center
New York, NY, USA

John M. Kindler, MD
Indiana University School of Medicine
Indianapolis, IN, USA

Peter Kobalka, MD
Ohio State University
Columbus, OH, USA

Ibrahim Kulac, MD
Koç University School of Medicine
Istanbul, Turkey

Sylvia C. Kurz, MD, PhD
Eberhard Karls University
Tübingen, Germany

Erika N. Leese, PA-C
Geisinger Health
Danville, PA, USA

Mary Jane Lim-Fat, MD, MSc
Sunnybrook Health Sciences
Toronto, ON, Canada

Rimas V. Lukas, MD
Northwestern University
Chicago, IL, USA

Alireza Mansouri, MD, MSc, FRCSC
Penn State Health
Hershey, PA, USA

Aaron Mochizuki, DO
Cincinnati Children's Hospital Medical Center
Cincinnati, OH, USA

Jamal Mohamud, DO
Indiana University School of Medicine
Indianapolis, IN, USA

Ramin A. Morshed, MD
University of California San Francisco
San Francisco, CA, USA

Maciej M. Mrugala, MD, PhD, MPH, FAAN
Mayo Clinic
Phoenix, AZ, USA

Lakshmi Nayak, MD
Dana-Farber Cancer Institute, Harvard Medical School
Boston, MA, USA

Matthew T. Neal, MD, MBA
Mayo Clinic
Phoenix, AZ, USA

Kathryn S. Nevel, MD
Indiana University School of Medicine
Indianapolis, IN, USA

Theodore Nicolaides, MD
Caris Life Sciences
New York, NY, USA

Mohammad Hassan A. Noureldine, MD, MSc
University of South Florida
Tampa, FL, USA

Samanthalee C. S. Obiorah, BSc
Warren Alpert Medical School of Brown University
Providence, RI, USA

Shirley Ong, MD
The Ohio State University Wexner Medical Center
Columbus, OH, USA

Sonia Partap, MD
Stanford University & Lucile Packard
Children's Hospital
Palo Alto, CA, USA

David M. Peereboom, MD
Cleveland Clinic
Cleveland, OH, US

Melike Pekmezci, MD
University of California
San Francisco, CA, USA

Katherine B. Peters, MD, PhD, FAAN
Duke University School of Medicine
Durham, NC, USA

Sheetal Phadnis, MD
University of Alabama
Birmingham, AL, USA

Scott R. Plotkin, MD, PhD
Massachusetts General Hospital
Boston, MA, USA

Vinay K. Puduvalli, MD
UT MD Anderson Cancer Center
Houston, TX, USA

Appaji Rayi, MD
Charleston Area Medical Center Health System
Charleston, WV, USA

Alexander Ropper, MD
Baylor College of Medicine
Houston, TX, USA

Roberta Rudà, MD
University of Turin
Turin, Italy

Sameer Farouk Sait, MBBS
Memorial Sloan Kettering Cancer Center
New York, NY, USA

David Schiff, MD
University of Virginia Health System
Charlottesville, VA, USA

Nir Shimony, MD
St. Jude Children's Hospital
Memphis, TN, USA
Johns Hopkins University SoM
Baltimore, MD, USA

Kevin Shiue, MD
Indiana University School of Medicine
Indianapolis, IN, USA

Wayne Slone, MD
Ohio State University
Columbus, OH, USA

Riccardo Soffietti, MD, PhD
University Hospital of Turin
Turin, Italy

Kun-Wei Song, MD
Massachusetts General Hospital / Dana-Farber Cancer Institute
Boston, MA, USA

Ramya Tadipatri, MD
Banner MD Anderson Cancer Center
Gilbert, AZ, USA

Hirokazu Takami, MD, PhD
University of Tokyo
Tokyo, Japan

Kerianne R. Taylor, RN
Banner MD Anderson Cancer Center
Phoenix, AZ, USA

Steven A. Toms, MD, MPH
Brown University / Lifespan Health System
Providence, RI, USA

Cristina Valencia-Sanchez, MD, PhD
Mayo Clinic
Scottsdale, AZ, USA

Terrence Verla, MD
Baylor College of Medicine
Houston, TX, USA

Gordon A. Watson[†], MD, PhD
Indiana University School of Medicine
Indianapolis, IN, USA

Jessica A. Wilcox, MD
Memorial Sloan Kettering Cancer Center
New York, NY, USA

Terri L. Woodard, MD, MPH
Baylor University College of Medicine
Houston, TX, USA
UT MD Anderson Cancer Center
Houston, TX, USA

[†] Deceased

PART I. | NEURO-ONCOLOGY OVERVIEW

1 | NEUROPATHOLOGY PRIMER

IBRAHIM KULAC AND MELIKE PEKMEZCI

INTRODUCTION

Tumors of the central nervous system (CNS) have been traditionally classified based on their histomorphologic features and by presumed cell of origin. Histologic grading has been across tumor entities, and each tumor is assigned to a grade as part of the nomenclature. Histologic grading is only one of the prognostic criteria, and a tumor with low histologic grade may behave aggressively depending on the location, patient's performance status, radiographic features, proliferation index, and, more recently, genetic changes.

The revised fourth edition (2016) of the World Health Organization (WHO) classification introduced a combined histologic and molecular classification (integrated diagnosis), which dramatically changed the nomenclature.[2] But this updated classification and grading scheme has already become insufficient, given our rapidly growing understanding of molecular features and numerous new techniques including methylation profiling. For this purpose, a group of experts gathered to create cIMPACT-NOW (Consortium to Inform Molecular and Practical Approaches to CNS Tumor Taxonomy—Not Official WHO), which has already published multiple update reports, and many of these updates are expected to be incorporated into the imminent fifth edition of the WHO classification (2021).[3] Important changes in the upcoming classification include designation of WHO grade using Arabic numerals, rather than Roman numerals (which practice we have adopted for this volume) and reserving the term "glioblastoma" for isocitrate dehydrogenase (IDH)-wildtype diffuse astrocytomas with histologic or molecular features of grade 4, while all IDH-mutant astrocytomas will be diagnosed as such with accompanying histologic grade (2–4). In this chapter we cover the most common CNS tumors in a fairly detailed manner and briefly touch base with the relatively rare ones using the current diagnostic criteria and terminology, some of which may change in the near future.

Editors' Note: This book is being published just as the new 2021 World Health Organization (WHO) classification of CNS tumors is being released.[1] While this chapter is largely based on the 2016 classification, significant impending changes are noted where appropriate.[4] For the most up-to date information, please see: WHO Classification of Tumours; 5th Edition. Central Nervous System Tumours. Edited by the WHO Classification of Tumours Editorial Board. International Agency for Research on Cancer 2021.

GLIAL TUMORS

CNS glial tumors are a diverse group of neoplasms originating from the supportive cellular elements of CNS. Glial tumors can be classified as diffuse (infiltrative) or solid glial tumors by their growth pattern.

Glial tumors can be classified as diffuse (infiltrative) or solid by their growth pattern.

DIFFUSE GLIAL TUMORS

The mainstay of the classification of adult diffuse gliomas is the presence of *IDH1/IDH2* mutations, which is associated with concerted CpG island methylation at many gene loci (G-CIMP phenotype) and with better outcome.

Diffuse gliomas (Chapter 4) have an infiltrative growth pattern, in which neoplastic glial cells diffusely infiltrate into the existing neuropil structures of the gray and white matter without a sharp border between the tumor and the adjacent parenchyma. Earlier classifications of diffuse gliomas relied only on the morphologic features; however, the 2016 WHO classification of diffuse glial tumors has had a major update, including the addition of certain genetic alterations to the diagnostic criteria, thus providing an integrated diagnosis.[2] Currently, the mainstay of the classification is the presence of *IDH1/IDH2* mutations, which is associated with concerted CpG island methylation at many gene loci (G-CIMP phenotype) and with better outcome. Furthermore, regardless of the morphologic features, tumors with IDH mutation and 1p/19q co-deletion are categorized as oligodendroglioma, while the rest are diagnosed as astrocytoma. While this classification addresses many important issues and provides an increased level of objectivity, its application to pediatric diffuse gliomas has been somewhat limited. Pediatric-type diffuse gliomas rarely harbor IDH mutations, and their molecular features overlap significantly with solid glial and glioneuronal tumors. Those with oligodendroglial morphology often harbor *FGFR1* alterations, and astrocytomas often show *MYB/MYBL1* rearrangements.[5] And, unlike adult counterparts, pediatric high-grade gliomas frequently harbor H3 G34 mutations, and infantile gliomas are frequently associated with *NTRK*, *ALK*, or *ROS* fusions.[6–8] The upcoming WHO classification will incorporate molecular alterations of pediatric-type diffuse gliomas and address the role of molecular alterations in grading of diffuse gliomas.

> Pediatric type diffuse gliomas rarely harbor IDH mutations, and their molecular features overlap significantly with solid glial and glioneuronal tumors.

DIFFUSE ASTROCYTOMA, IDH-MUTANT, WHO GRADE 2

Diffuse astrocytomas are composed of moderately pleomorphic cells with hyperchromatic, oval to round nuclei with irregular nuclear contours interspersed in the parenchyma where neurons or axonal fibers are visible between tumor cells (see Figure 1.1A). Cellularity may vary but often it is moderately increased compared to normal parenchyma. Mitoses are absent or rare. Necrosis or microvascular proliferation is not seen. By definition, these tumors have a mutation in either *IDH1* or *IDH2*, and the most common mutation is the R132H mutation in *IDH1*.[9] Concurrent mutations in *ATRX* and *TP53* are typical features of IDH-mutant diffuse astrocytomas.[10] Immunohistochemistry (IHC) is almost always very helpful for diagnosis. Antibody against IDH1 R132H mutant protein shows diffuse cytoplasmic positivity in majority of the tumors, as seen in Figure 1.1B, although it is negative in tumors with non-canonical IDH mutations. Therefore, sequencing for other *IDH1* and *IDH2* mutations may be necessary. Loss of nuclear ATRX expression by IHC suggests presence of an *ATRX* mutation and can be used to strongly argue against an oligodendroglioma. While strong and diffuse p53 nuclear staining is suggestive of a *TP53* mutation, the sensitivity and specificity as well as the ideal cutoff value of p53 staining are still debated. Tumor cells are variably positive with GFAP, OLIG2, SOX10, and MAP2, none of which is specific for the diagnosis. Neurofilament protein is useful to identify the entrapped axonal fibers, confirming the infiltrative growth pattern.

ANAPLASTIC ASTROCYTOMA, IDH-MUTANT, WHO GRADE 3

Anaplastic astrocytomas either arise from a grade 2 diffuse astrocytoma or, more frequently, are diagnosed de novo. Histomorphological features are somewhat similar to diffuse astrocytoma, IDH-mutant, WHO grade 2, but they tend to have more prominent cytologic atypia, increased cellularity, and elevated mitotic activity. Necrosis and microvascular proliferation are not seen. Increased number of mitoses is the key characteristic feature of anaplastic astrocytoma, IDH-mutant, WHO grade 3; however, no strict cutoff is set for the number of mitosis for the diagnosis, and mitotic activity should be assessed in the context of specimen size. Molecular characteristics of these tumors are also similar to their grade 2 counterpart, including mutations in *IDH1* or *IDH2*, *ATRX*, and *TP53* genes, but with more frequent copy number alterations. There is ongoing debate about the utility of the current grading system since some studies showed no significant difference in prognosis between histologic grade 2 and 3 astrocytomas while others did so.[11–13] Future studies may refine mitotic thresholds and may identify additional genetic alterations associated with more aggressive clinical behavior to establish better grading criteria.

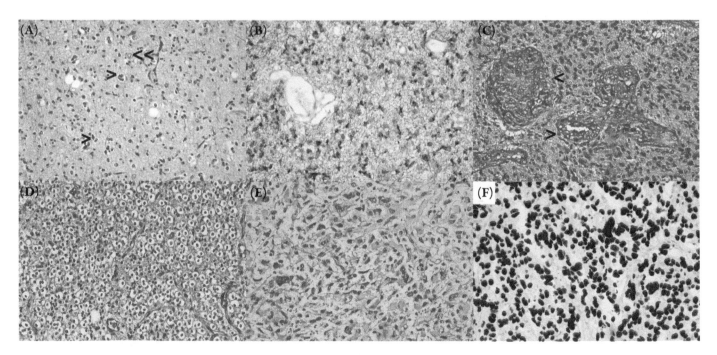

Figure 1.1 *Infiltrating glial tumors. (A) Diffuse astrocytoma, WHO grade 2: Note atypical tumor cells with irregular nuclear borders (>) diffusely infiltrating to background cortex evidenced by entrapped cortical neurons (>>), Hematoxylin & eosin (H&E). (B) Immunohistochemistry for isocitrate dehydrogenase (IDH)-1 R132H mutant protein. (C) Glioblastoma, WHO grade 4: Note multilayered endothelial cells referred to as microvascular proliferation (>), H&E. (D) Oligodendroglioma, IDH-mutant and 1p/19q-co-deleted, WHO grade 2: Note fine, chicken-wire vasculature and perinuclear halos giving cells a fried-egg appearance, H&E. (E) Diffuse midline glioma, H3 K27M-mutant, WHO grade 4: Note that the absence of microvascular proliferation or necrosis does not preclude the designation of WHO grade 4, H&E. (F) Immunohistochemistry for H3 K27M mutant protein in diffuse midline glioma.*

Glioblastoma, IDH-Mutant, WHO Grade 4

IDH mutant glioblastoma comprises approximately 10% of all glioblastomas and either arises from a preexisting low-grade astrocytoma or develops de novo. These tumors are composed of pleomorphic cells with increased mitotic activity and contain microvascular proliferation and/or areas of necrosis, often palisading necrosis (see Figure 1.1C). Presence of an IDH mutation can be demonstrated by IDH1 R132H IHC in most cases.[14] ATRX loss and p53 positivity are also common findings similar to other IDH-mutant astrocytomas. *IDH1* and *IDH2* sequencing should be performed for IDH1 R132H IHC-negative glioblastomas if there is a history of a lower grade glioma or if a patient is younger than 55 years at the time of diagnosis and additional IHC studies suggest strong association with an IDH mutation (i.e., ATRX loss).

While the morphologic features of IDH-mutant and IDH-wildtype glioblastomas are essentially identical, their molecular features and clinical outcomes are significantly different.[15,16] Recent studies demonstrated that homozygous deletion of *CDKN2A/B* in IDH-mutant diffuse gliomas without microvascular proliferation or necrosis is associated with a disease course at least as adverse as a histologically defined IDH-mutant glioblastoma.[17] Based on a recent consensus paper, there is a consideration to change the grading scheme of IDH-mutant diffuse gliomas, including assigning grade 4 to tumors with *CDKN2A/B* loss regardless of presence of microvascular proliferation or necrosis, and limiting the term "glioblastoma" to IDH-wildtype tumors,[18] so that these tumors will instead be named astrocytoma, IDH-mutant, WHO grade 4.

Glioblastoma, IDH-Wildtype, WHO Grade 4

The vast majority of high-grade gliomas in older adults are IDH-wildtype glioblastomas (Chapter 3). They are characterized by highly atypical, pleomorphic cells with frequent mitoses, necrosis, and/or microvascular proliferation, similar to their IDH-mutant counterparts (see Figure 1.1C). Chromosome 7p gain in combination with 10q loss is the most frequent chromosomal alteration in glioblastoma. Frequent molecular alterations include *TERT* promoter mutation, *CDKN2A/B* homozygous deletion, *EGFR* amplification, *PTEN* truncating mutations, and other alterations in *p53/MDM2*, *CDKN2A/RB1*, and receptor tyrosine kinase pathways.[19] MGMT (O6-methylguanine-DNA methyltransferase) promoter methylation, which is predictive of response to alkylating agents such as temozolomide, is seen in a subset of glioblastomas; however, it is more common in IDH-mutant glioblastomas that have a G-CIMP phenotype.[20]

> IDH-wildtype glioblastomas are characterized by highly atypical, pleomorphic cells with frequent mitoses, necrosis, and/or microvascular proliferation.

There are a number of histomorphologic variants, some of which are associated with unique molecular alterations or clinical behavior. *Giant cell glioblastoma* is predominantly composed of highly atypical, multinucleated or mononuclear giant cells and harbors frequent *TP53* mutations. *Small cell glioblastoma* is relatively monomorphic, with bland morphology mimicking a low-grade glioma but harbors frequent

EGFR amplification and other genetic features of glioblastoma. Epithelioid glioblastoma has a dominant population of closely packed epithelioid, sometimes rhabdoid cells; shows significant morphologic and molecular overlap with anaplastic pleomorphic xanthoastrocytoma (PXA); and nearly half of them harbor BRAF V600E mutation. Gliosarcoma is another well-recognized morphological variant that has areas resembling various sarcomas, most often undifferentiated sarcoma, previously referred as *fibrosarcoma*. Similar to IDH-mutant glioblastoma, tumor cells are positive for glial markers (GFAP, OLIG2, SOX10). IHC for IDH1 R132H is negative. Nuclear ATRX expression is retained. Ki67 proliferation index is high.

> Gliosarcoma is another well-recognized morphological variant that has areas resembling various sarcomas, most often undifferentiated sarcoma, previously referred as *fibrosarcoma*.

Oligodendroglioma, IDH-Mutant, 1p/19q Co-Deleted, WHO Grade 2

The classic morphologic features of oligodendroglioma includes an infiltrative tumor composed of cells with round nuclei with a crisp, fine chromatin structure on a background of delicate, chicken-wire vasculature. Due to the processing steps in routine histopathology, the cytoplasm looks clear, which gives the cells a classic fried egg appearance on hematoxylin and eosin (H&E)-stained sections, as seen in Figure 1.1D. So-called secondary structures represent accentuation of the tumor cells around neurons (perineuronal satellitosis) and blood vessels and in subpial regions. Microcalcifications and myxoid degeneration is common. Tumor cells with eccentric, eosinophilic cytoplasm are referred to as *minigemistocytes*, which can be quite numerous. Occasional mitoses can be seen, but the tumors do not show a brisk mitotic activity.

> The classic morphologic features of oligodendroglioma includes an infiltrative tumor composed of cells with round nuclei with a crisp, fine chromatin structure on a background of delicate, chicken-wire vasculature.

By definition, all oligodendrogliomas are IDH-mutant; therefore, IDH1 R132H stain is positive in almost all cases. Cases with histomorphologic features of an oligodendroglioma but negative IDH1 R132H stain should be further tested for non-canonical IDH mutations by sequencing. Similarly, all oligodendrogliomas harbor co-deletion of entire chromosome arms of 1p and 19q, which can be shown by fluorescence in-situ hybridization (FISH), array comparative genomic hybridization (aCGH) or next-generation sequencing, although sensitivity and specificity may vary.[2] Frequent alterations include mutations in *FUBP1* and *CIC* genes, located on chromosomes 1p and 19q, respectively. Oligodendrogliomas frequently harbor *TERT* promoter mutations and are *ATRX*-wildtype; therefore, they show retained ATRX nuclear staining by IHC.[10] Likewise, diffuse strong p53 staining is not expected as *TP53* mutations are not common in oligodendrogliomas. Tumor cells are usually positive with OLIG2, SOX10, and MAP2, none of which is specific for the diagnosis. GFAP staining is usually limited and more often seen in minigemistocytes or occasional tumors with astrocytic morphology.

ANAPLASTIC OLIGODENDROGLIOMA, IDH-MUTANT, 1P/19Q CO-DELETED, WHO GRADE 3

Anaplastic oligodendroglioma arises either de novo or by progression of a grade 2 oligodendroglioma. Anaplastic oligodendroglioma can be defined as a tumor with high cellularity, brisk mitotic activity (>6 mitosis per 10 high-power field [HPF]), and/or microvascular proliferation and/or necrosis that shows the classic molecular oligodendroglioma signature (IDH mutation and 1p/19q co-deletion). Anaplastic oligodendrogliomas are prominently more cellular than grade 2 oligodendrogliomas but may still show classic oligodendroglioma morphology with round nuclei, perinuclear halos, and chicken-wire vasculature. The highest grade assigned for a tumor of oligodendroglial lineage is grade 3, per WHO 2016.[2] Molecular features of anaplastic oligodendroglioma are similar to grade 2 oligodendroglioma, with increased copy number alterations and more frequent *CDKN2A* loss. In addition to defining molecular alterations (IDH mutation and 1p/19q codeletion), anaplastic oligodendrogliomas also typically harbor *TERT* promoter mutations.

DIFFUSE MIDLINE GLIOMA, H3 K27M-MUTANT, WHO GRADE 4

As the name specifies, diffuse midline glioma, H3 K27M-mutant (Chapter 18), is an infiltrative glioma, typically of astrocytic morphology, involving midline structures such as thalamus, basal ganglia, and spinal cord, which harbors a K27M mutation involving histone H3.3 (*H3F3A*) or H3.1 (*HIST1H3B/C*) genes. Tumors often consist of monomorphic, small glial cells and frequently exhibit features of high-grade glioma, as seen in Figure 1.1E.[21] However, paucicellular tumors without mitoses, necrosis, or microvascular proliferation are not uncommon. Regardless of the histologic features, these tumors are assigned WHO grade 4. Additional molecular alterations include frequent mutations in *TP53*, *PTEN*, *ATM*, *PPM1D*, and *CHEK2*.[22,23] *ACVR1* mutations and *FRGR1* rearrangements seem to correlate with the type of histone mutation and tumor location.[24] These tumors are diffusely positive for H3K27M antibody that reacts with both mutant protein products of either H3.1 or H3.3 genes, as seen in Figure 1.1F.[25] Mutation leads to inhibition of PRC2 complex, resulting decreased levels of trimethylation at the lysine 27 mark of histone 3 (H3K27me3), which can also be detected by IHC.

> Regardless of the histologic features, diffuse midline glioma, H3 K27M mutant, is assigned WHO grade 4.

DIFFUSE HEMISPHERIC GLIOMA, H3 G34-MUTANT

H3 G34-mutant gliomas (Chapter 18) are defined by their molecular alteration but show variable histology.[26,27] It is not yet accepted as a distinct entity by the WHO 2016 classification, but it is often seen in cerebral hemispheres of young adults. Most commonly, they have a biphasic appearance, with a glial component characterized by a fibrillary background and atypical, pleomorphic cells, and areas of embryonal features

which sometimes may be the dominant feature. Because of the embryonal features, in the past, these tumors were diagnosed as glioblastoma, with primitive neuronal features, or as a CNS embryonal tumor. They are almost always high grade and often have morphological hallmarks of a high-grade glial tumor such as microvascular proliferation and/or palisading necrosis which is very helpful for the correct diagnosis. A GFAP-positive, OLIG2-negative hemispheric tumor with loss of nuclear ATRX staining and diffuse p53 staining in the absence of IDH mutations is highly suggestive of a H3 G34 mutation.

DIFFUSE ASTROCYTIC GLIOMA, IDH-WILDTYPE

Although diffuse astrocytoma, IDH-wildtype, WHO grade 2 and anaplastic astrocytoma, IDH-wildtype, WHO grade 3 have been included in the 2016 WHO classification, they have been referred to as "provisional entities." It is well-documented that IDH-wildtype astrocytomas have significantly worse outcome than IDH-mutant astrocytomas, and some tumors show a disease course similar to IDH-wildtype glioblastomas. Multiple studies showed that this group may include diffuse gliomas with distinct molecular alterations other than IDH mutations, such as H3 K27M or H3 G34R mutations, and these tumors should now be diagnosed as such. Recent cIMPACT-NOW updates have recommended additional molecular testing to identify these tumors, which are expected to behave aggressively, and the group uses the terminology "diffuse astrocytic glioma, IDH-wildtype with molecular features of glioblastoma WHO grade 4."[19] Molecular features suggesting aggressive behavior in this setting includes *EGFR* amplification, *TERT* promoter mutation, and gain of chromosome 7q with concurrent loss of chromosome 10p.

> Molecular features suggesting aggressive behavior in IDH-wildtype astrocytoma include *EGFR* amplification, *TERT* promoter mutation, and gain of chromosome 7q with concurrent loss of chromosome 10p.

ASTROCYTOMA, NOT OTHERWISE SPECIFIED (NOS) AND OLIGODENDROGLIOMA, NOS

These tumors have the morphological features of an astrocytoma or an oligodendroglioma but the molecular workup needed for definitive integrated diagnosis cannot be completed. In this setting, the WHO 2016 classification recommends that pathologists use these diagnostic categories. Although the diagnostic categories for oligoastrocytoma and anaplastic oligoastrocytoma, NOS, still exist in the WHO guidelines, these categories should only be used when further testing will not or cannot be completed.[28] Histologic features, corresponding molecular alterations and integrated diagnosis pathways in diffuse adult and pediatric gliomas are summarized in Figures 1.2 and 1.3.

SOLID GLIAL TUMORS

PILOCYTIC ASTROCYTOMA, WHO GRADE 1

Pilocytic astrocytoma is the most common glioma in children but can also be seen in adults of all ages. Although clinical and radiological features of pilocytic astrocytomas are

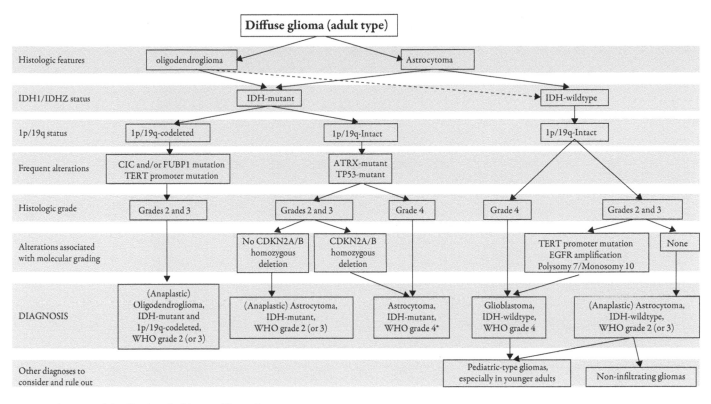

Figure 1.2 *Summary of classification of adult type diffuse gliomas.*

often pathognomonic for the diagnosis, histomorphology can be challenging since they have a wide range of tissue patterns. Most commonly pilocytic astrocytomas have a biphasic growth pattern with relatively compact areas composed

of bipolar glial cells with long, hair-like (piloid) processes and loosely arranged microcystic areas composed of bland, glial cells with small nuclei and short, cobweb-like processes in a variably myxoid background (see Figure 1.4A). Rosenthal

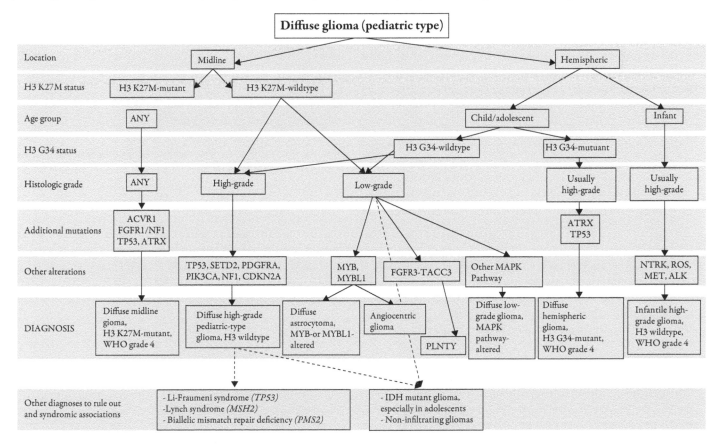

Figure 1.3 *Summary of classification of pediatric type diffuse gliomas.*

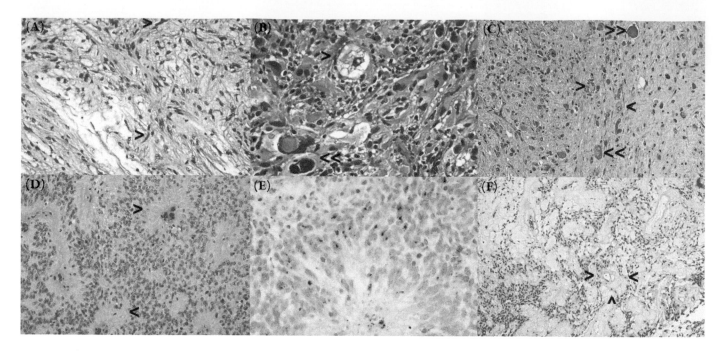

Figure 1.4 *Solid glial, glioneuronal, and ependymal tumors. (All except panel E are hematoxylin & eosin [H&E] stained sections.) (A) Pilocytic astrocytoma, WHO grade 1: Note bland bipolar cells, microcystic background, and Rosenthal fibers (>). (B) Pleomorphic xanthoastrocytoma, WHO grade 2: Note mixture of spindle cells, large atypical cells with smudgy irregular nuclei (>), and large cells with foamy (xanthomatous) cytoplasm (>>). (C) Ganglioglioma, WHO grade 1: Note large, dysmorphic ganglion cells (>) in the background of bland spindled glial cells and numerous eosinophilic granular bodies (>>). (D) Ependymoma, WHO grade 2: Note perivascular fibrillary anucleate zones, referred to as perivascular pseudorosettes (>). (E) Epithelial membrane antigen (EMA) immunohistochemical stain shows dot-like paranuclear staining in ependymomas. (F) Myxopapillary ependymoma, WHO grade 1: Note papillary structures containing a central vessel with mucoid degeneration surrounded by small ependymal cells (>) in the myxoid background.*

fibers (intracytoplasmic, thick, and long eosinophilic fibers) are often seen in compact areas, and eosinophilic granular bodies (EGBs) are prominent in microcystic areas. Atypical cells with naked nuclei can be seen, especially at the periphery of the lesion, raising the differential diagnosis of a diffuse astrocytoma. Oligodendroglioma-like cytomorphology can be prominent in other cases. Tumors may show degenerative atypia as well as multinucleated cells.

> Most commonly pilocytic astrocytomas have a biphasic growth pattern with relatively compact areas composed of bipolar glial cells with long, hair-like (piloid) processes and loosely arranged microcystic areas composed of bland, glial cells with small nuclei and short, cobweb-like processes in a variably myxoid background.

Pilocytic astrocytomas are highly vascular and may show complex glomeruloid vascular structures, especially lining the tumoral cyst walls. Necrosis can be focal or extensive and is usually an infarct type as opposed to a palisading type; therefore, this should not be interpreted as an alarming finding. Likewise, mitosis can be seen and may be quite frequent. While the clinical significance is not fully established, mitotic counts in excess of 4 mitoses per 10 HPFs associated with palisading necrosis may indicate a potential for more aggressive behavior, and these tumors are referred to as *anaplastic pilocytic astrocytoma*, without an officially designated WHO grade.

Pilocytic astrocytomas typically harbor alterations activating the mitogen-activated protein (MAP) kinase pathway, most frequent of which is a tandem duplication of *BRAF* resulting *KIAA1549-BRAF* fusion.[29] Other typical alterations include *BRAF* V600E, *KRAS*, and *NF1* mutations, and *FGFR1* and *RAF1* fusions. Presence of additional alterations such as *CDKN2A/B* homozygous deletion, *ATRX* mutation, or *TERT* promoter mutation seems to be associated with more aggressive behavior.[30]

Tumor cells are positive for GFAP, OLIG2, S100, and SOX10. Synaptophysin often shows weak cytoplasmic staining, and this should not be interpreted as infiltrative growth pattern or evidence for a neuronal component. Neurofilament is useful to demonstrate well-demarcated, solid growth pattern with scarce entrapped axons at the periphery. However, it should be kept in mind that rare examples, especially in cerebellum, may show an extensive infiltrative pattern. Because these tumors do not harbor IDH mutations, IDH1 R132H stain is expected to be negative. Although Ki67 proliferation index is typically low (<5%), some cases may reveal a quite high index.

PILOMYXOID ASTROCYTOMA
Pilomyxoid astrocytoma (PMA) is considered a variant of pilocytic astrocytoma, with additional, somewhat characteristic features. These tumors tend to localize in the thalamic or hypothalamic region and are seen in earlier ages compared to pilocytic astrocytomas.[31,32] PMAs are solid tumors composed of monomorphous, bipolar cells with fusiform nuclei and long glial processes in a homogenous myxoid background. Tumor

cells are typically arranged around blood vessels, forming pseudorosettes. Immunohistochemical and molecular features are almost identical to pilocytic astrocytomas, with frequent MAP kinase pathway alterations.[33] Current literature emphasizes a worse prognosis for PMAs compared to pilocytic astrocytomas; however, a definite grade has not been assigned.

PLEOMORPHIC XANTHOASTROCYTOMA, WHO GRADE 2

Pleomorphic xanthoastrocytoma (Chapter 10) is a well-circumscribed glial neoplasm with a frequent cystic component and is typically located superficially with leptomeningeal extension. It is characterized by large, often multinucleated cells with abundant foamy cytoplasm (referred as *xanthomatous cells*), which may show variable nuclear atypia, and a frequent spindle cell component with abundant pericellular reticulin (see Figure 1.4B). EGBs and perivascular lymphocytic infiltrate are frequent, but not specific for diagnosis. These tumors are categorized as WHO grade 2 with mitotic activity of less than 5 mitoses per 10 HPFs by definition. Necrosis is not a common finding, but its presence is not sufficient for a WHO grade 3 designation.

Typical molecular alterations include *BRAF* V600E mutation and concurrent *CDKN2A* homozygous deletion, which are present in more than half of the cases. Noncanonical *BRAF* mutations, *BRAF* and *RAF1* fusions, and complex chromosomal copy number changes have been also reported.[34] Tumor cells are positive for glial (GFAP, OLIG2) and occasional neuronal (MAP2, synaptophysin) markers. CD34 is also commonly positive in PXAs. BRAF V600E mutation can be demonstrated with a mutation-specific antibody using IHC. There is correlation with *CDKN2A* homozygous deletion and loss of p16 IHC expression, which can be useful in the diagnostic workup of these cases.

> Typical molecular alterations in PXA include *BRAF* V600E mutation and concurrent *CDKN2A* homozygous deletion.

ANAPLASTIC PLEOMORPHIC XANTHOASTROCYTOMA, WHO GRADE 3

Anaplastic PXA shares morphologic similarities with PXA, WHO grade 2, but, by definition, anaplastic PXA has a mitotic rate of 5 or more mitoses per 10 HPFs. While necrosis is common, its significance in the absence of mitotic activity is unclear. Molecular features also overlap with PXA and include combination of *CDKN2A* homozygous deletion with *BRAF* or *RAF1* alterations. Recent studies suggested that anaplastic transformation may be due to accumulation of additional copy number changes and/or *TERT* gene alterations (amplification or promoter mutation).[35]

SUBEPENDYMAL GIANT CELL ASTROCYTOMA, WHO GRADE 1

Subependymal giant cell astrocytoma (SEGA) is a benign tumor arising in the wall of the lateral ventricle, composed of large, ganglion/gemistocyte-like cells and variable amounts of spindle cells arranged in sweeping fascicles. Considerable pleomorphism and multinucleated giant cells are common and have no impact on prognosis. Vascular-rich stroma with

calcifications is also a common finding. Although a significant number of mitoses can be evident, this does not have an impact on the grade or outcome. Tumor cells are positive for GFAP and S100 and may show focal expression of neuronal markers such as NeuN. SEGAs are seen in the setting of tuberous sclerosis and show biallelic inactivation of *TSC1* or *TSC2* genes.

> SEGAs are seen in the setting of tuberous sclerosis and show biallelic inactivation of *TSC1* or *TSC2* genes.

NEURONAL AND GLIONEURONAL TUMORS

GANGLIOGLIOMA, WHO GRADE 1

Gangliogliomas (Chapter 10) are glioneuronal neoplasms composed of dysplastic ganglion cells (clustering, cytomegaly, binucleation, abnormal Nissl substance) intermixed with neoplastic glial cells with variable morphology resembling fibrillary astrocytomas, oligodendrogliomas, or pilocytic astrocytomas and are WHO grade 1 by definition (see Figure 1.4C). Anaplastic gangliogliomas (WHO grade 3) usually have increased cellularity and mitoses, necrosis, and microvascular proliferation.[36]

The glial component stains with glial markers (GFAP, OLIG2, SOX10). The dysplastic ganglion cells are positive with synaptophysin, show variable staining with NeuN, and show abnormal perikaryonic staining with neurofilament. They harbor solitary alterations activating MAP kinase pathways (*BRAF* p.V600E mutation and other mutations and fusions in *BRAF*, *FGFR1*, and *FGFR2* genes).[37,38] BRAF V600E mutation-specific stain can be helpful in the diagnosis.[39] Additional genetic alterations (homozygous deletion of *CDKN2A* and *DMBT1*, gain/amplification of *CDK4*) are associated with anaplasia.[40]

DYSEMBRYOPLASTIC NEUROEPITHELIAL TUMOR, WHO GRADE 1

Dysembryoplastic neuroepithelial tumor (DNET) is a low-grade glioneuronal tumor with nodular growth and is typically composed of axonal bundles perpendicular to pial surface (columns) lined by oligodendrocyte-like bland cells embedded in a mucoid matrix, which contains scattered "floating neurons."[41] Reported molecular alterations vary between studies and include *FGFR1* kinase domain tandem duplications or missense mutations in more than 80% and *BRAF* p.V600E mutations in 30% of cases.[38,42]

OTHER NEURONAL AND GLIONEURONAL TUMORS

Multinodular and vacuolating neuronal tumor (MVNT) is a low-grade neuronal neoplasm with prominent nodules composed of small to medium-sized neuronal cells demonstrating prominent intracytoplasmic and stromal vacuolation.[43] The tumor cells are positive with some glial and neuronal markers (OLIG2, synaptophysin) but negative with others (GFAP,

NeuN) and show nearby CD34-positive ramified processes. They harbor solitary alterations in the MAP kinase pathway (*MAP2K1* or non-canonical *BRAF* mutations, *FGFR2* fusion).[44]

Papillary glioneuronal tumor (PGNT) is a low-grade biphasic neoplasm composed of flat to cuboidal astrocytes lining around hyalinized vessels and intervening collections of round, oligodendrocyte-like neurocytes and occasional ganglion cells.[45,46] Astrocytes are positive for GFAP, and neurocytes are positive with synaptophysin and occasionally with OLIG2. A majority of cases harbor *SLC44A1-PRKCA* fusion.[47]

> A majority of papillary glioneuronal tumors harbor *SLC44A1-PRKCA* fusion.

Rosette-forming glioneuronal tumor (RGNT) is a low-grade biphasic neoplasm composed of round, uniform neurocytes forming neurocytic rosettes and/or perivascular pseudorosettes[48] intermixed with a pilocytic astrocytoma-like component. The neuronal component is positive with MAP2 and occasionally with NeuN, while the glial component is positive with GFAP and S100. Synaptophysin highlights the neuropil in the center of the rosettes. *FGFR1* mutations co-occurring with either *PIK3CA* or *NF1* define RGNT.[49]

Diffuse leptomeningeal glioneuronal tumor (Chapter 10) is characterized by widespread leptomeningeal growth despite low-grade morphology and is composed of monomorphic, oligodendrocyte-like cells with uniform round nuclei, frequently associated with desmoplasia or myxoid background.[50] Tumor cells are positive with OLIG2, MAP2, and S100, and some cases are positive with GFAP or synaptophysin. Tumor shows recurrent *KIAA1549-BRAF* fusion (similar to pilocytic astrocytomas) in addition to 1p deletion or, less often, 1p/19q co-deletion.[51]

·*Central neurocytoma* is an intraventricular neuronal neoplasm composed of uniform round cells with fine chromatin embedded in the fine neuropil. Homer Wright rosettes are rare. Synaptophysin is diffusely positive, and glial markers are essentially negative. They contain numerous copy number alterations, including *MYCN* gain, but do not harbor 1p/19q co-deletion.

EPENDYMAL TUMORS

EPENDYMOMA, WHO GRADE 2

Ependymomas (Chapter 6) are circumscribed gliomas composed of monomorphic cells with oval nuclei radially arranged around blood vessels with fine fibrillary processes in between (perivascular pseudorosettes) or arranged around a central lumen forming tubular canals (true ependymal rosettes), as seen in Figure 1.4D. Less common morphologic forms include tanycytic (bland spindle-shaped glial cells resembling pilocytic astrocytoma), clear cell, and papillary ependymoma. Ependymomas are WHO grade 2 by definition, although their clinical behavior varies by patient age and tumor location.[52] Some features, such as increased mitotic activity, palisading necrosis, and microvascular proliferation, are associated with

anaplasia (grade 3), but grading criteria are not well-established due to inconsistent association with outcome.[53]

Ependymomas are positive with GFAP, especially in pseudorosettes, and show dot-like paranuclear staining with EMA (Figure 1.4D).[54] OLIG2 and SOX10 are typically negative. Several studies showed distinct molecular subgroups among ependymal neoplasms that show significant association with anatomic location.[52] Supratentorial ependymomas may show loss of chromosome 9, associated with homozygous deletion of *CDKN2A*. In addition, they carry fusion genes either involving *RELA* or *YAP1*.[52,55] L1CAM IHC can be used as a surrogate marker for *RELA* fusion in ependymomas but should not be used for diagnosis of ependymoma since it is positive in other tumor types.[55] Posterior fossa ependymomas have a very low mutation rate but harbor either gains or losses of whole chromosomes or chromosome arms (posterior fossa B, PFB) or have few copy number changes (PFA).[56] These groups correlate with subgroups identified by methylation profiling, and loss of H3 K27me3 staining can be used as a surrogate marker for PFA ependymomas, which show global DNA hypomethylation.[57,58] Spinal cord ependymomas harbor frequent deletions and translocations of chromosome 22q, some of which are associated with *NF2* gene mutations, especially in patients with neurofibromatosis 2 (NF2) syndrome.[59] More recently, spinal cord ependymomas with *MYCN* amplification, which show aggressive behavior, have been reported.[60]

> Spinal cord ependymomas harbor frequent deletions and translocations of chromosome 22q, some of which are associated with *NF2* gene mutations, especially in patients with NF2 syndrome.

SUBEPENDYMOMA, WHO GRADE 1

Subependymomas (Chapter 6) are slow-growing glial neoplasms with exophytic growth toward the ventricle, composed of clusters of bland uniform cells in a dense fibrillary matrix of glial processes. They are variably GFAP-positive, but usually do not show staining with EMA.[61] They do not harbor any recurrent mutations, and only posterior fossa subependymomas seem to harbor copy number alterations, specifically involving chromosome 6.[52]

MYXOPAPILLARY EPENDYMOMA

Myxopapillary ependymomas (Chapter 6) are glial tumors exclusively located in the region of conus medullaris, cauda equina, and filum terminale; they are composed of elongate tumor cells with fibrillary processes arranged around hyalinized vessels (papillary) and variable amounts of myxoid matrix, as seen in Figure 1.4F. They are currently considered WHO grade 1; however, given their relatively frequent rate of recurrence, which is not significantly different from ependymoma, the upcoming WHO update will likely designate these tumors as WHO grade 2. Furthermore, increased mitoses and Ki-67 proliferation index and the presence of microvascular proliferation and spontaneous necrosis have been associated with aggressive behavior.[62] They are typically positive with GFAP and S100 and frequently show staining with AE1/AE3 keratin. Occasional cases have overlapping features with classical ependymomas. They do not harbor any recurrent mutations, but they frequently have a polyploid genome and form a distinct cluster by methylation profiling.[52,63]

EMBRYONAL TUMORS

MEDULLOBLASTOMA, WHO GRADE 4

Medulloblastomas (Chapter 10) are the most common CNS embryonal tumors, arising in the cerebellum or dorsal brainstem. They are classified into four groups by histopathologic or molecular features.[2,64] There are significant associations between the histologic and molecular variants; however, an integrated diagnosis combining both provides optimal prognostic information.[65,66] The classic histologic variant, which is the most common one, can be seen in all molecular subtypes and is composed of tightly packed, small, round, primitive neuronal cells with high mitotic count and may show Homer Wright rosettes, as seen in Figure 1.5A. The desmoplastic/nodular variant, which always shows activation of the sonic hedgehog (SHH) pathway, contains pale nodules of variably differentiated neuronal cells that are reticulin-free and surrounded by densely packed undifferentiated, highly proliferative cells with abundant pericellular reticulin (see Figure 1.5B). Those with even more

prominent, expanded nodules containing neurocytic differentiation are designated *medulloblastoma with extensive nodularity* (MBEN) variant. The large cell/anaplastic histologic variant is characterized by undifferentiated cells with marked nuclear pleomorphism, prominent nucleoli, cell wrapping, and increased mitoses and apoptosis (Figure 1.5C). All medulloblastomas show staining with synaptophysin, but staining can be limited to the nodules in desmoplastic/nodular variant.

> Medulloblastomas are the most common CNS embryonal tumors, arising in the cerebellum or dorsal brainstem.

Molecular classification is based on transcriptome or methylation profiling and includes four main groups.[64,66-69] Wingless (WNT)-activated medulloblastomas almost always show classic histology and often harbor *CTNNB1* mutation and/or monosomy 6. WNT-activated tumors show YAP1, LEF1, and nuclear beta-catenin expression, which can be used as surrogate markers.[70] SHH-activated medulloblastomas include all desmoplastic/nodular and MBEN variants but can also show classic and anaplastic large cell morphology. They harbor mutations in *PTCH1*, *SUFU*, *SMO*, or amplification of *GLI2*, *MYCN*, and *SHH*. Medulloblastomas associated with hereditary tumor syndromes, such as Gorlin and Li-Fraumeni, are always SHH-activated. SHH-activated medulloblastomas with additional *TP53* mutations have worse clinical outcome and

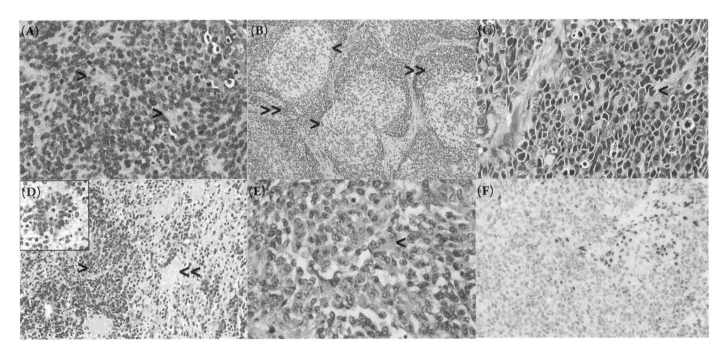

Figure 1.5 Embryonal tumors. (All except panel F are hematoxylin & eosin [H&E] stained sections.)
(A) Medulloblastoma, classic histologic type, WHO grade 4: Note fine neuropil surrounded by immature neuronal cells (>), referred to as neuroblastic rosettes (Homer Wright). (B) Desmoplastic/nodular medulloblastoma, WHO grade 4: Note pale nodular islands of embryonal cells and neuropil (>), surrounded by small, immature cells (>>) which have extensive perivascular reticulin (stain not shown). (C) Large cell/anaplastic medulloblastoma, WHO grade 4: Note increased cytologic atypia, cell-cell wrapping (>), and abundant apoptosis. (D) Embryonal tumor with multilayered rosettes, C19MC-altered, WHO grade 4: Note mixed areas of immature embryonal cells (>) and areas of abundant pale-pink neuropil (>>). Inset demonstrates the characteristic multilayered rosette, which is not required for diagnosis because this entity is defined by the presence of a microRNA cluster at chromosome 19q13. (E) Atypical teratoid/rhabdoid tumor, WHO grade 4: Note immature cells, some of which have eccentric eosinophilic cytoplasm containing globular inclusions (>). (F) Immunohistochemistry shows loss of INI1 in tumor cells (retained in endothelial cells) consistent with the presence of SMARCB1 alteration defining AT/RT.

are considered a subtype separate from *TP53*-wildtype SHH-activated medulloblastomas.[71] SHH-activated medulloblastomas are positive for YAP1 and GAB1 stains. Non-WNT/non-SHH medulloblastomas are classic or large cell/anaplastic subtypes and are comprised of two distinct groups by methylome profiles. Group 3 tumors typically have *MYCN* amplification, and group 4 tumors typically have isochromosome 17q.

EMBRYONAL TUMOR WITH MULTILAYERED ROSETTES, C19MC-ALTERED, WHO GRADE 4

Embryonal tumor with multilayered rosettes (ETMR) represents a wide spectrum of tumors with shared histologic feature of multilayered rosettes and molecular alteration of amplification of a microRNA cluster at chromosome 19q13, designated as C19MC.[72] Histologic variants used to be different entities in prior WHO classifications and include "embryonal tumor with abundant neuropil and true rosettes" with biphasic areas of small embryonal cells arranged in multilayered rosettes intermixed with paucicellular, mature neuropil-like areas containing neurocytic and ganglion cells (Figure 1.5D); "medulloepithelioma" with tubular and trabecular structures formed by a pseudostratified epithelium with a limiting membrane and without cilia recapitulating the primitive neural tube; and "ependymoblastoma" with sheets of poorly differentiated cells occasionally forming multilayered true rosettes with a central lumen. Small embryonal cells may be positive with EMA and cytokeratins but are typically negative for neuronal and glial markers. Neuropil-rich areas, on the other hand, are positive with synaptophysin. LIN28 protein expression can be used as a surrogate marker for C19MC alteration; however, its presence is not specific and would require additional confirmatory tests.[73]

ATYPICAL TERATOID/RHABDOID TUMOR, WHO GRADE 4

Atypical teratoid/rhabdoid tumor (AT/RT) is a malignant embryonal tumor with inactivation of *SMARCB1* (*INI1*) or rarely of *SMARCA4* (*BRG1*) and contains variable amounts of poorly differentiated small embryonal cells, rhabdoid cells with eccentric nuclei and globular eosinophilic cytoplasmic inclusions, and spindle cells (Figure 1.5E).[74–76] Large areas of necrosis and hemorrhage are common. They show variable staining with various IHC stains, including EMA, SMA, GFAP, cytokeratin, and synaptophysin, but their defining feature is the loss of nuclear expression of INI1 or BRG1 corresponding to the genetic alterations (Figure 1.5F).[77]

The defining feature of AT/RTs is the loss of nuclear expression of INI1 or BRG1.

CENTRAL NERVOUS SYSTEM EMBRYONAL TUMOR, NOS

Other extracerebellar CNS embryonal tumors without distinct genetic alterations of AT/RT and ETMR exist and used to be called CNS-primitive neuroectodermal tumor (PNET), which is now an antiquated term. More recent studies identified recurrent molecular alterations within this group, leading to reclassification of some of the tumors as high-grade gliomas (i.e., diffuse hemispheric glioma with H3 G34R mutation) or as more specific embryonal tumors, such as those with frequent *BCOR* exon 15 internal tandem duplication, *FOXR2* gene activation, *MN1* activation, and *CIC* alterations.[28,78,79]

MENINGIOMA

Meningiomas (Chapter 5), which are the most common neoplasms involving the meninges, originate from the arachnoid cap cells and carry diverse phenotypes between mesenchymal and epithelioid differentiation. They frequently present as dural-based tumors involving the convexity, skull base, and spine, and they occasionally involve Virchow-Robin spaces, presenting as intraparenchymal lesions, or they originate from tela choroidea at the base of the choroid plexus, presenting as intraventricular lesions.

Macroscopically, most meningiomas present as well-circumscribed, firm lesions with a broad-based dural attachment. Typical histologic features of meningioma include bland, epithelioid-to-spindled cells with oval nuclei and nuclear pseudoinclusions, arranged in nests, whorls, or fascicles and associated with concentric psammomatous calcifications as seen in Figure 1.6A.

Typical histologic features of meningioma include bland, epithelioid-to-spindled cells with oval nuclei and nuclear pseudoinclusions, arranged in nests, whorls, or fascicles and associated with concentric psammomatous calcifications.

Meningiomas are histologically graded as benign (grade 1), atypical (grade 2), and anaplastic (grade 3, malignant) based on the histologic variant, mitotic activity, presence of brain invasion (see Figure 1.6B), and other morphologic features.[2] Clear cell and chordoid histologic variants, tumors with mitotic activity of 4 mitoses or greater per 10 HPFs, and/or brain invasion, and/or those demonstrating three of five histologic features (hypercellularity, loss of architecture, small-cell change, macronucleoli, and spontaneous necrosis) are classified as atypical meningioma, WHO grade 2.[80] Predominantly rhabdoid or papillary histologic variants, tumors with overt malignant morphology resembling a sarcoma or carcinoma, and/or those with mitotic activity of 20 or more mitoses per 10 HPFs are graded as anaplastic meningioma, WHO grade 3.

Meningiomas have numerous histologic variants due to the diverse morphologic appearances, only some of which are associated with certain clinical or radiological features or outcome. *Meningothelial meningioma* shows nests of epithelioid cells with indistinct cytoplasmic borders (also known as syncytial growth pattern), while *fibrous meningioma* shows spindle cells arranged in storiform or fascicular pattern in a collagen-rich stroma. *Transitional meningioma*, which is the most common

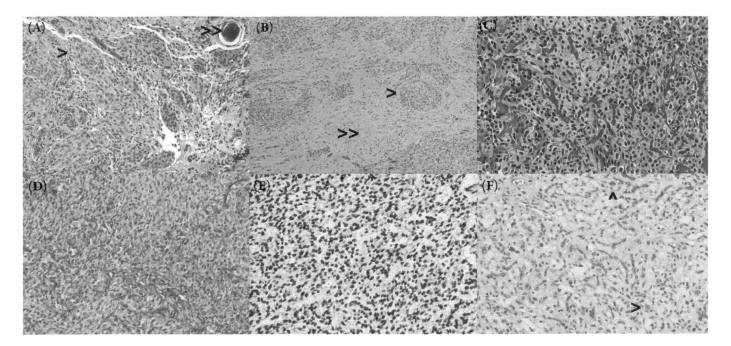

Figure 1.6 Meningothelial and non-meningeal mesenchymal tumors. (All except panel E are hematoxylin & eosin [H&E] stained sections.) (A) Meningioma, meningothelial pattern, WHO grade 1: Note whorls (>) and psammomatous calcification (>>). (B) Atypical meningioma, brain-invasive, WHO grade 2: Note nests of meningioma (>) surrounded by fibrillary neuropil of the brain parenchyma (>>). (C) Rhabdoid meningioma, WHO grade 3; Note epithelioid cells with eccentric nuclei and eosinophilic cytoplasmic inclusions. (D) Solitary fibrous tumor: Note bland spindled to epithelioid cells in the background of variably thick collagen fibers. (E) STAT6 immunohistochemistry in solitary fibrous tumor: Nuclear staining is a surrogate marker for NAB2-STAT6 fusion, which is the defining molecular alteration in this entity. (F) Hemangioblastoma: Note numerous capillaries lined by non-tumorous endothelial cells. Neoplastic cells (>) are those with foamy cytoplasm with irregular, dark nuclei, also referred to as stromal cells.

histologic variant, displays a mixture of meningothelial and fibrous morphology. Psammomatous calcifications can be seen in any variant, but it predominates in *psammomatous meningioma*. *Microcystic meningioma* shows microcystic spaces in the background, giving a cobweb-like appearance to the tumor. In angiomatous meningioma, vascular channels constitute a majority of the tumor, with predominantly small, capillary-like vessels and occasional large hyalinized vessels. Microcystic and *angiomatous* variants are frequently seen together and are associated with significant peritumoral edema. *Secretory meningioma* shows prominent epithelial differentiation, including intracytoplasmic gland-like lumina containing eosinophilic globules, which are positive with cytokeratins and CEA. These also are associated with peritumoral edema out of proportion to tumor size. *Lymphoplasmacyte-rich meningioma* is a rare variant associated with prominent chronic inflammatory cell infiltrate and is considered to be a meningothelial hyperplasia rather than a true meningioma variant by some authors, given its association with monoclonal gammopathies and occasional spontaneous regression.[81]

Four meningioma variants are associated with worse outcome and are designated with a higher grade when they predominate in the tumor. These include clear cell and chordoid meningiomas, which are WHO grade 2, and rhabdoid and papillary meningiomas, which are WHO grade 3.[82–86] *Clear cell meningioma* is composed of polygonal, epithelioid cells with abundant clear cytoplasm on H&E stains, which is in fact filled with glycogen, which shows strong staining on periodic acid-Schiff (PAS) stain.[82] Prominent perivascular and stroma hyalinization leads to characteristic ropy collagen

in the background. *Chordoid meningioma* is composed of epithelioid cells with foamy cytoplasm arranged in cords and trabeculae in a myxoid, mucin-rich matrix which stains with PAS, mucicarmine, and Alcian blue.[84] *Papillary meningioma* is composed of epithelioid cells arranged around a fibrovascular core, which may be partially due to the clinging of otherwise discohesive cells to the vessels.[85] *Rhabdoid meningioma* is composed of discohesive epithelioid cells with eccentric nuclei and eosinophilic, paranuclear, globular inclusions, as seen in Figure 1.6C.[86] In many of these variants, other high-grade features such as increased mitotic activity are also present. When these variants present as a minor component without accompanying high-grade features, they seem to have comparable outcomes with other meningioma variants and may not qualify for a higher grade designation.[83,87]

Meningiomas typically stain with epithelial membrane antigen (EMA) and somatostatin receptor 2a (SSTR2a).[88] They are essentially negative for cytokeratins (except secretory variant), glial stains (GFAP, OLIG2), and neural crest markers (S100, SOX10). The Ki67 proliferation index can be used to identify those with increased proliferation, although labeling index is not a grading criterion. Prognostic value of increased Ki-67 is unclear, although recent meta-analysis suggests 4% as a potential cutoff.[89] Progesterone receptor (PR) expression varies among meningiomas, often with an inverse correlation with Ki67 proliferation index. PR expression is often decreased or lost in atypical and anaplastic meningiomas, but its independent role for prognostication is unclear. Loss of H3K27me3 has been described as a negative prognostic marker in a small subset of adult meningiomas.

> Meningiomas typically stain with epithelial membrane antigen (EMA) and somatostatin receptor 2a (SSTR2a).

In addition to the well-known inactivating alterations in *NF2*, several other gene mutations are involved in meningiomagenesis including *AKT1*, *TRAF7*, *KLF4*, *SMO*, *SUFU*, *POLR2A*, *PIK3CA*, *BAP1*, *SMARCB1*, and *SMARCE1*.[90] Overall, *NF2* mutations are associated with male gender, convexity and spinal cord locations, and increased recurrence rates as well as multiple meningiomas in the setting of NF2. The vast majority of secretory meningiomas harbor mutations in *KLF4* with or without *TRAF7* mutations.[91] *SMARCE1* mutations are associated with clear cell variant and have been reported in hereditary tumors.[92] *BAP1* mutations or deletions are identified in some meningiomas and may be seen in association with the recently described BAP1 tumor predisposition syndrome defined by germline *BAP1* mutations.[93] In addition to the driver mutations, a subset of meningiomas harbor *TERT* promoter mutations, and these seem to correlate with poor outcome independent of histologic grade.[94] Moreover, methylation profiling has been proposed as a robust method for identifying those tumors with worse outcome, and these data show some overlap with decreased H3K27me3 positivity in high-risk meningiomas.[95,96]

> *NF2* mutations in meningiomas are associated with male gender, convexity and spinal cord locations, and increased recurrence rates.

MESENCHYMAL, NON-MENINGOTHELIAL TUMORS

SOLITARY FIBROUS TUMOR

Solitary fibrous tumor, which is the most common non-meningothelial neoplasm involving the meninges, is a fibroblastic mesenchymal neoplasm frequently involving falx cerebri and tentorium cerebelli. It represents a spectrum of neoplasms ranging from low grade to frankly anaplastic, and they show two major histologic patterns.[97] Given the morphologic differences, solitary fibrous tumor and hemangiopericytoma were considered to be different entities up until the 2016 WHO classification of CNS tumors, but identification of a shared molecular driver (NAB2/STAT6 fusion) led to a unified diagnosis.

> Solitary fibrous tumor and hemangiopericytoma were considered to be different entities up until the 2016 WHO classification of CNS tumors, but identification of a shared molecular driver (NAB2/STAT6 fusion) led to a unified diagnosis.

Tumors with solitary fibrous tumor histologic pattern show low to moderate cellularity, slit-like vessels with thin walls and bland endothelial cells, and abundant eosinophilic collagen between spindle-shaped tumor cells that are arranged in a "patternless pattern," as seen in Figure 1.6D. Tumors with hemangiopericytoma histologic pattern show high cellularity, epithelioid cells with round to oval nuclei arranged in a jumbled pattern in the background of delicate, branching vessels also referred as "staghorn." Soft-tissue SFTs are graded as SFT or malignant SFT based on the mitotic activity, while proposed grading systems for CNS SFTs include grade 1 tumors with low mitotic count (<5 mitoses per 10 HPFs), grade 2 (increased mitotic count without necrosis), and grade 3 (increased mitoses with associated necrosis).[98,99]

The defining molecular alteration in all SFTs regardless of the histologic pattern is the presence of *NAB2-STAT6* gene fusion, which leads to the translocation of STAT6 protein to the nucleus (see Figure 1.6E).[100] Different fusion types involving different exons of both genes are identified, and the exon 6-exon 16/17 fusion seem to be more frequent among tumors with an HPC histologic pattern and higher-grade tumors than the exon 4-exon 2 fusion. Approximately 30% of the tumors harbor additional *TERT* promoter mutations, which is associated with poor prognosis in soft-tissue tumors but not in CNS tumors.[99,101]

All SFTs show diffuse nuclear staining with STAT6 IHC. Those with SFT histologic pattern are diffusely positive with CD34 and show pericellular collagen IV staining, while those with HPC histologic pattern have limited to absent staining with these markers.

HEMANGIOBLASTOMA, WHO GRADE 1

Hemangioblastoma is a low-grade, well-circumscribed, highly vascular tumor composed of stromal cells of uncertain histogenesis, which have discrete cell borders, abundant vacuolated cytoplasm filled with lipid, and variably pleomorphic hyperchromatic nuclei, as seen in Figure 1.6F. The most common locations for hemangioblastomas include the cerebellum and brainstem. Tumor cells are positive with S100, inhibin-A, and occasionally with GFAP.[102] Vascular markers such as CD34 and CD31 are positive in the endothelial cells, which may predominate the lesion but are negative in tumor cells. Due to increased pseudohypoxic signaling, tumor is also positive with hypoxia markers such as GLUT1 and carbonic anhydrase IX. Approximately 10% of cases are seen in the setting of von Hippel-Lindau syndrome associated with germline *VHL* mutations, which are more likely to be multiple and/or disseminated.[103] Sporadic tumors carry inactivating mutations in the *VHL* gene or activating mutations in the *HIF2A* gene.

> The most common locations for hemangioblastomas include the cerebellum and brainstem.

OTHER MESENCHYMAL TUMORS

In principle, the CNS can be involved by any type of mesenchymal neoplasm similar to those seen in soft tissue and bone and share similar histologic findings. Primary mesenchymal tumors are quite rare and, when present, mostly involve dura. They essentially share the same morphologic features, IHC staining patterns, and molecular alterations with their soft-tissue and bone counterparts, which is beyond the scope of this chapter.

TUMORS OF THE CRANIAL AND PARASPINAL NERVES

SCHWANNOMA, WHO GRADE 1

Schwannomas are benign, typically encapsulated nerve sheath tumors composed entirely of well-differentiated Schwann cells with oval to elongate, somewhat wavy nuclei with tapered ends.[2] Typical biphasic architecture includes compact, cellular areas (Antoni A) and less cellular, loosely textured areas (Antoni B). Antoni A areas may show intersecting fascicles and occasional nuclear palisades (Verocay bodies), as seen in Figure 1.7A. Thick-walled hyalinized vessels and subcapsular inflammatory cells are commonly seen. Significant degenerative atypia with large irregular nuclei and smudgy chromatin, referred to as *ancient changes*, may be seen and should not be interpreted as signs of malignancy. Cellular schwannomas are entirely composed of Antoni A areas with intersecting fascicles which may raise the differential diagnosis of malignant peripheral nerve sheath tumor (MPNST).

> The typical biphasic architecture of a schwannoma includes compact, cellular areas (Antoni A) and less cellular, loosely textured areas (Antoni B).

Schwannomas are diffusely positive with antibodies against S100 and SOX10 and are negative with melanocytic markers such as Melan-A and HMB-45. Schwannomas show extensive pericellular collagen IV and reticulin staining and are largely devoid of entrapped neurofilament-positive axons. A majority of schwannomas harbor inactivating mutations in *NF2* gene, and many *NF2*-wildtype tumors show loss of chromosome 22q, where *NF2* is located. Bilateral vestibular schwannomas are associated with NF2 syndrome with germline NF2 alterations, and multiple non-vestibular schwannomas are associated with familial schwannomatosis (Chapter 27), which may show germline *SMARCB1* mutations.[104,105] Loss-of-function

mutations in *LZTR1* gene are another type of germline alteration leading to multiple schwannomas, with overlapping features between NF2 and schwannomatosis.

> Multiple non-vestibular schwannomas are associated with familial schwannomatosis, which may show germline *SMARCB1* mutation.

NEUROFIBROMA, WHO GRADE 1

Neurofibromas are benign, well-demarcated, often intraneural nerve sheath tumors composed of well-differentiated Schwann cells in the background of fibroblasts and variably myxoid to collagenous stroma. Tumor cells have elongated, wavy nuclei and scant cytoplasm (see Figure 1.7B). Those affecting multiple fascicles, giving a beaded gross and microscopic appearance, are called *plexiform neurofibromas.* Increased cellularity, monomorphic cytology, scattered mitotic figures, and nuclear atypia raise concern for premalignant changes, which may be diagnosed as atypical neurofibroma, which is extremely difficult to differentiate from low-grade MPNST. Especially in the setting of NF1 (Chapter 27), clinical outcome of tumors with these worrisome features beyond neurofibroma but short of diagnosis of overt malignancy may vary. An alternate terminology of "atypical neurofibromatous neoplasm of uncertain biologic potential" (ANNUBP) has been proposed for these tumors.[106]

Neurofibromas are positive with S100 and SOX10, but, due to the abundance of background fibroblasts, stains do not look as diffuse as they do in schwannomas. There is an extensive fibroblastic network in the background, which can be highlighted by CD34 staining. Neurofilament stain highlights entrapped axons, unlike schwannomas. Neurofibromas demonstrate inactivation of the *NF1* gene encoding neurofibromin protein. Multiple and plexiform neurofibromas are associated with germline inactivation of *NF1* in the setting of NF1 syndrome. They often lack additional alterations, but the histologic and molecular changes can be considered as a spectrum from benign neurofibromas to MPNSTs. Atypical neurofibromas show frequent *CDKN2A/B* deletions, associated with loss of p16 staining.[107]

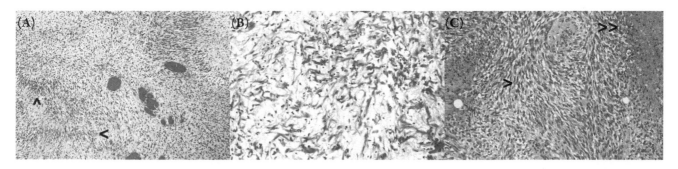

Figure 1.7 Peripheral nerve sheath tumors. (All are hematoxylin & eosin [H&E] stained sections.)
(A) Schwannoma: Note a biphasic tumor with cellular (Antoni A) and hypocellular (Antoni B) areas. Nuclear palisades, typically seen in Antoni A areas, are referred to as Verocay bodies (>). (B) Neurofibroma: Note hyperchromatic wavy nuclei in the background of fragmented collagen. (C) Malignant peripheral nerve sheath tumor: Note intersecting fascicles of hyperchromatic spindle cells (>) associated with increased mitotic activity and geographic areas of necrosis (>>).

MALIGNANT PERIPHERAL NERVE SHEATH TUMORS

MPNSTs are malignant neoplasms with Schwann or perineurial cell differentiation, which can be sporadic or associated with NF1 syndrome (Chapter 27), in which case they often arise from a preexisting plexiform neurofibroma. Many MPNSTs show tightly packed, hyperchromatic cells with spindle-shaped nuclei with tapered ends arranged in intersecting fascicles or in a herringbone pattern, as seen in Figure 1.7C. Increased mitotic activity and geographic necrosis are common. MPNSTs may show divergent differentiation toward a variety mesenchymal tissues, most common of which is rhabdomyosarcomatous differentiation (malignant triton tumor). MPNSTs have also been rarely noted to have divergent differentiation toward glandular elements. Rare MPNSTs show focal or diffuse epithelioid morphology with rhabdoid cells. These "epithelioid MPNSTs" are typically not associated with NF1 and seem to have better outcome than classic sporadic MPNSTs.

> MPNSTs are malignant neoplasms with Schwann or perineurial cell differentiation, which can be sporadic or associated with NF1 syndrome, in which case they often arise from a preexisting plexiform neurofibroma.

MPNSTs show S100 and/or SOX10 staining in only 50–70% of cases, and they are usually focal and patchy.[108] While this pattern can be helpful in the diagnosis of MPNST versus a benign nerve sheath tumor, it is not useful in differentiating a high-grade MPNST from other sarcomas (i.e., synovial sarcoma, undifferentiated pleomorphic sarcoma). Most MPNSTs show loss of p16 stain (CDKN2A/B deletion) and increased staining with p53 (TP53 mutation). A majority of MPNSTs harbor mutations in components of PCR2 complex (SUZ12 and EED) leading to loss of H3K27me3, which can be demonstrated by IHC.[109–111] Epithelioid MPNST are diffusely S100 positive and show recurrent SMARCB1 alterations leading to loss of INI1 expression.[112]

MALIGNANT MELANOTIC SCHWANNIAN TUMOR

Malignant melanocytic schwannian tumor (MMST) is a rare, darkly pigmented neoplasm composed of spindle cells arranged in fascicles carrying cytoplasmic melanosomes.[2] Due to their architectural overlap with schwannoma, they used to be referred as "melanotic schwannoma," a terminology not representative of its aggressive clinical behavior. They are frequently associated with psammomatous calcifications, especially in the setting of typical genetic alterations.[113,114]

MMST shows diffuse staining with neural crest (S100, SOX10) and melanocytic markers (HMB-45, Melan-A). Pericellular collagen IV staining is often present, which resembles schwannoma more than melanocytoma or melanoma. Recent molecular studies show inactivating PRKAR1A mutations in MMSTs, associated with loss of cytoplasmic PRKAR1A staining, which can be used for diagnosis. Germline PRKAR1A alterations are associated with Carney complex.[113,114]

PRIMARY MELANOCYTIC TUMORS OF THE CNS

Primary melanocytic tumors are those diffuse or localized tumors arising from the leptomeningeal melanocytes. Localized tumors are often seen in the meninges of the spinal cord and less likely in posterior fossa. Intraparenchymal lesions are more likely to be metastases rather than primary tumors. Histologic features show a wide spectrum ranging from bland, heavily pigmented melanocytes without mitotic activity arranged in nests in melanocytomas to highly pleomorphic cells with frequent mitoses and necrosis in malignant melanoma.[115] However, many tumors show overlapping features along the spectrum, and the grading criteria are not well-established. Tumors with borderline features but not fulfilling the criteria for melanoma are referred to as *intermediate-grade melanocytic neoplasms*.

All primary melanocytic tumors show staining with melanocytic markers including S100, SOX10, Melan-A, HMB-45, and MART1. These markers may be essential for diagnosis, especially in malignant tumors devoid of melanin pigment. Molecular features are similar to uveal nevi and melanomas with frequent, mutually exclusive GNAQ or GNA11 mutations. Additional mutations seen in uveal melanomas, including EIF1AX, SF3B1, and BAP1, are reported in some tumors, along with copy number alterations including monosomy 3 and gain of 6p and 8q.[116–118] Not only do histologic grade and molecular features not always correlate, but there is prominent overlap in their outcome. Presence of BRAF, KRAS, NF1, and TERT promoter mutations and a UV mutational signature should raise concern for metastasis rather than a primary meningeal neoplasm.

TUMORS OF THE PINEAL REGION

Pineal gland neoplasms comprise a heterogeneous group of tumors including germ cell tumors (50–75%), pineal parenchymal tumors (Chapter 10) (PPT; 14–30%), papillary tumor of the pineal region (PTPR), and, rarely, gliomas and other tumors.

PPTs represent a spectrum ranging from well-differentiated, WHO grade 1 pineocytoma, composed of uniform round cells forming pineocytomatous rosettes and/or ganglion cells to PPT with intermediate differentiation (PPTID) to poorly differentiated, WHO grade 4 pineoblastoma, which is an embryonal tumor composed of small immature cells arranged in sheets or forming Homer Wright and, less commonly, Flexner-Wintersteiner rosettes.[2] PPTs also show a range of staining with neuronal IHC markers where pineocytomas are positive with synaptophysin and neurofilament, and pineoblastomas have variable synaptophysin and essentially negative neurofilament staining.[119,120] PPTIDs harbor small in-frame insertions involving KBTBD4.[121] Pineoblastomas contain multiple subgroups associated with RB1, DICER1, DROSHA, and DGCR8 alterations or MYC overexpression.[121]

PTPR is a neuroepithelial tumor derived from ependymal cells of the subcommissural organ and is characterized by combination of papillary and solid areas and cytokeratin positivity.[122] It is negative for neurofilament but may show staining with other neuronal markers such as synaptophysin and MAP2. The most frequent alteration in PTPR is the loss of chromosome 10 with or without *PTEN* gene alterations.[121,122]

TUMORS OF THE SELLAR REGION

PITUITARY ADENOMA

Pituitary adenoma (Chapter 7) is a neoplastic proliferation of anterior pituitary hormone–producing cells, and histologic features range from tubular or papillary structures to sheets of epithelial cells with variably eosinophilic or amphophilic cytoplasm based on the cell type.[123,124] IHC for hormones, hormone subunits, and transcription factors is used to classify pituitary adenomas into seven main subtypes: somatotroph, lactotroph, thyrotroph, corticotroph, gonadotroph, null cell (hormone-negative and transcription factor–negative), and plurihormonal. Clinically non-functioning (silent) pituitary adenomas are only rarely truly null cell, which requires all hormone and transcription factor stains to be negative. Mitotic count as well as the Ki-67 proliferation index have some prognostic role. Stains for SSTR2A may be helpful to determine response to somatostatin analogues.[125]

PITUICYTOMA, SPINDLE CELL ONCOCYTOMA, AND GRANULAR CELL TUMOR

The tumors of the posterior hypophysis include a group of neoplasms that are accepted as a spectrum by some authors due to overlapping histologic features and IHC profiles.[126,127] All are positive with S100, vimentin, and TTF1, with variable staining with GFAP and EMA.[128] Pituicytoma (Chapter 7) is composed of compact fascicles or storiform arrangements of bipolar spindle cells.[129] Spindle cell oncocytoma (Chapter 7) is composed of spindled or epithelioid cells with eosinophilic cytoplasm, filled with mitochondria, which can be highlighted by anti-mitochondrial stains. Granular cell tumor (Chapter 7) is composed of epithelioid cells with abundant eosinophilic, granular cytoplasm filled with phagolysosomes, which can be highlighted by CD68.[130]

CRANIOPHARYNGIOMA, WHO GRADE 1

Craniopharyngioma (Chapter 7) is a low-grade epithelial neoplasm of the sellar region presumably derived from embryonic remnants of the Rathke pouch. *Adamantinomatous craniopharyngioma* is composed of compact sheets and anastomosing trabeculae of squamous epithelium with peripheral palisading, stellate reticulin, and wet keratin and harbors frequent CTNNB1 alterations, which can be demonstrated by nuclear beta-catenin staining.[131] *Papillary craniopharyngioma* is composed of non-keratinizing epithelium and fibrovascular cores resembling squamous papilloma and harbors *BRAF V600E* mutation in 95% of cases.[131,132]

> *Papillary craniopharyngioma* is composed of non-keratinizing epithelium and fibrovascular cores resembling squamous papilloma and harbors *BRAF V600E* mutation in 95% of cases.

METASTASIS TO CNS

Essentially any tumor type can metastasize to the CNS (Chapter 12), but those with high propensity to do so include lung, breast, melanoma, gastrointestinal, and renal cell carcinoma. Most are well-demarcated from the adjacent brain parenchyma, but lymphomas, small-cell carcinoma, and melanoma may show a more infiltrative growth pattern. Histologic features and immunohistochemical profiles are diverse and often resemble the primary tumor.[133] Molecular testing can be useful in very poorly differentiated tumors with unknown origin or to identify prognostic and predictive biomarkers such as *HER2* in breast carcinoma; *EGFR*, *ALK*, and *ROS1* in pulmonary adenocarcinoma; or *BRAF V600E* in melanoma. In addition, PD-L1 expression (as evaluated by immunohistochemistry) and overall mutational burden (as evaluated by next-generation sequencing methods) are important predictors for immunotherapy response for various tumors, including pulmonary adenocarcinoma and melanoma.

> Tumor types with a high propensity to metastasize to the CNS include lung, breast, melanoma, gastrointestinal, and renal cell carcinoma.

TABLE 1.1 Molecular Alterations of Primary CNS Neoplasms

CENTRAL NERVOUS SYSTEM NEOPLASMS—1

	KEY MOLECULAR ALTERATION(S)	ADDITIONAL MOLECULAR ALTERATION(S)
DIFFUSE GLIOMAS		
Adult-type		
Astrocytoma, IDH-mutant	*IDH1/2, ATRX,* and *TP53* mutations	*CDKN2A/B* deletion*
Oligodendroglioma, IDH-mutant and 1p/19q-co-deleted	*IDH1/2* mutation and 1p/19q co-deletion	*TERT* promoter, *CIC* and *FUBP1* mutations
Glioblastoma, IDH-wildtype	*TERT* promoter mutation, *EGFR* amplification, 10p loss, 7q gain	*TP53* mutation, *FGFR3-TACC3* fusion
Pediatric-type diffuse high grade		
Diffuse midline glioma, H3 K27-altered	*H3F3A* or *HIST1H3B/C* p.K27M mutation	*TP53, PTEN, ATM, PPM1D,* and *CHEK2*
Diffuse hemispheric glioma, H3 G34-mutant	*H3F3A* p.G34 mutation	*TP53* and *ATRX* mutation, *PDGFRA* amplification
Diffuse pediatric high-grade glioma, H3-*wt*	*TP53, SETD2, PDGFRA, PIK3CA, NF1*	*CDKN2A/B* deletion*
Infant-type hemispheric glioma	Fusions involving *NTRK1/2/3, ALK, ROS1* or *MET* at the 3' end	
Pediatric-type diffuse low grade		
Diffuse astrocytoma, MYB or MYBL1-altered	*MYB, MYBL1* alterations	
Angiocentric glioma	*MYB-QKI* fusion	
Polymorphous low-grade neuroepithelial tumor of the young	*FGFR3-TACC3* and *FGFR2-KIAA1598* fusions, *BRAF* p.V600E mutation	
Diffuse low-grade glioma, MAPK pathway-altered	*BRAF* p.V600E, *BRAF* fusion, *NF1*	
CIRCUMSCRIBED ASTROCYTIC GLIOMAS		
Pilocytic astrocytoma	*KIAA1549-BRAF* fusion, *NF1* mutation	*BRAF* p.V600E, *KRAS* mut; *RAF1, FGFR1* fusions; *ATRX*; *CDKN2A/B* deletion* *TERT* promoter* mut
Pleomorphic xanthoastrocytoma	*BRAF* p.V600E mutation *CDKN2A/B* deletion	*TERT* amplification or promoter mutation*
Subependymal giant cell astrocytoma	*TSC1, TSC2*	
Chordoid glioma	*PRKCA* p.D463H fusion	
Astroblastoma, MN1-altered	*MN1-BEND2* or *MN1-CXXC5* fusions	
NEURONAL AND GLIONEURONAL TUMORS		
Ganglioglioma	*BRAF* p.V600E mutation	Non-V600 *BRAF* mutations, other MAPK pathway alterations
Desmoplastic infantile astrocytoma and ganglioglioma	*BRAF* mutations	
Dysembryoplastic neuroepithelial tumor	*FGFR1* tyrosine kinase domain mutation and duplication	*BRAF* p.V600E
Papillary glioneuronal tumor	*SLC44A1-PRKCA* fusion	
Rosette forming glioneuronal tumor	*FGFR1* mutations	*PIK3CA, NF1* mutations
Myxoid glioneuronal tumor	*PDGFRA* K385 mutations	

TABLE 1.1 Continued

CENTRAL NERVOUS SYSTEM NEOPLASMS—1

	KEY MOLECULAR ALTERATION(S)	ADDITIONAL MOLECULAR ALTERATION(S)
Diffuse leptomeningeal glioneuronal tumor	*KIAA1549-BRAF* fusion and 1p deletion	
Multinodular and vacuolating neuronal tumor	*MAP2K1* mutations	Non-V600 *BRAF* mutations
Dysplastic cerebellar gangliocytoma (Lhermitte-Duclos disease)	*PTEN* mutation	
Central neurocytoma	No known recurrent alterations	
Extraventricular neurocytoma	*FGFR1-TACC1* fusion	Other *FGFR1* alterations

CENTRAL NERVOUS SYSTEM NEOPLASMS—2

	KEY MOLECULAR ALTERATION(S)	ADDITIONAL MOLECULAR ALTERATION(S)
EPENDYMAL TUMORS		
Supratentorial ependymoma, C11orf95 fusion positive	*C11orf95-RELA* fusion	*CDKN2A* deletion*
Supratentorial ependymoma, YAP1 fusion positive	*YAP1* fusion	
Posterior fossa ependymoma, Group PFA	Hypermethylation of CpG islands; global DNA hypomethylation	Gain of 1q*
Posterior fossa ependymoma, Group PFB	-	Multiple chromosomal copy number abnormalities including loss of 22q and 6, and trisomy 18
Spinal ependymoma	*NF2* mutation/deletion	
Spinal ependymoma, MYCN-amplified	*MYCN* amplification	
Myxopapillary ependymoma	Unique DNA methylation profile	
Subependymoma	–	Loss of chromosome 19; partial loss of chromosome 6
EMBRYONAL TUMORS		
Medulloblastoma		
Medulloblastoma, WNT-activated	*CTNNB1* mutation, monosomy 6	
Medulloblastoma, SHH-activated and TP53-wildtype	*PTCH1, SUFU, SMO* mutations Amplification of *GLI2, MYCN* and *SHH*	Loss of 9q, loss of 10q
Medulloblastoma, SHH-activated and TP53-mutant	*PTCH1, SUFU, SMO* mutations Amplification of *GLI2, MYCN,* and *SHH* *TP53 mutation*	
Medulloblastoma, non-WNT/non-SHH	*MYCC, MYCN* amplification	
Other CNS embyonal tumors		
Atypical teratoid/rhabdoid tumor	*SMARCB1, SMARCA4* mutations	
Cribriform neuroepithelial tumor	*SMARCB1* mutations	
Embryonal tumor with multilayered rosettes	Amplification of *C19MC*	
CNS neuroblastoma, FOXR2 activated	*FOXR2* rearrangements	Gain of 1q
CNS tumor with BCOR internal tandem duplication	*BCOR* in-frame internal tandem duplication	

TABLE 1.1 Continued

CENTRAL NERVOUS SYSTEM NEOPLASMS—2

	KEY MOLECULAR ALTERATION(S)	ADDITIONAL MOLECULAR ALTERATION(S)
CHOROID PLEXUS TUMORS		
Choroid plexus papilloma	-	Hyperploidy with whole chromosomal gains
Atypical choroid plexus papilloma	-	Hyperploidy
Choroid plexus carcinoma	*TP53* mutation	Aneuploidy, hypodiploidy
PINEAL TUMORS		
Pineocytoma	-	
Pineal parenchymal tumor with intermediate differentiation	Small in-frame insertions of *KBTBD4*	
Pineoblastoma	*DICER1, DROSHA, DGCR8, RB1* alterations	*MYCN* gain or amplification
Papillary tumor of the pineal region		Monosomy 10, polysomy 4 and 9
Desmoplastic myxoid tumor, SMARCB1-mutant	*SMARCB1* mutations	
SELLAR TUMORS		
Papillary craniopharyngioma	*BRAF* p.V600E mutation	
Adamantinomatous craniopharyngioma	*CTNNB1* mutations	
Pituicytoma, granular cell tumor, spindle cell oncocytoma	-	
Pituitary adenoma/neuroendocrine tumor	-	*GNAS, USP8* mutations
Pituitary blastoma	*DICER1* alterations	
MENINGIOMA		
Meningioma, overall	*NF2* mutation, monosomy 22q; *AKT1, KLF4, SMO, PIK3CA, TRAF7* mutations	*TERT* promoter mutation*, *CDKN2A* deletion*
Clear cell meningioma	*SMARCE1* mutation	
Papillary meningioma	*PBRM1* mutation	
Rhabdoid meningioma	*BAP1* mutation	
SOLITARY FIBROUS TUMOR		
Solitary fibrous tumor grades 1, 2, and 3	*NAB2-STAT6* fusion	TERT promoter mutation
Meningeal melanocytic tumors		
Melanocytoma, borderline, melanoma	*GNAQ* or *GNA11* mutations	*BAP1, SF3B1, EIF1AX* mutations
CRANIAL AND PARASPINAL NERVE TUMORS		
Schwannoma	*NF2* mutation, monosomy 22q	*LZTR1* mutation
Epithelioid schwannoma	*SMARCB1* mutation	
Neurofibroma	*NF1* mutation/inactivation	*CDKN2A/CDKN2B* deletion
Malignant peripheral nerve sheath tumor	*SUZ12, EED* mutations, bi-allelic NF1 inactivation	*EGFR, PDGFRA, MET* amplification; copy number changes
Epithelioid MPNST	*SMARCB1* inactivation	
Malignant melanotic nerve sheath tumor	*PRKAR1A* mutation/inactivation	

* These alterations are suggestive of a higher tumor grade when present in addition to the key alterations for a given tumor type.

How are diffuse glial tumors with infiltrative growth pattern classified?	Using an integrated approach combining morphologic features with molecular alterations
What are molecular hallmarks of oligodendroglioma?	*IDH1* or *IDH2* mutations and 1p/19q-codeletion
What are three other common mutations seen in oligodendrogliomas?	Oligodendrogliomas frequently harbor *TERT* promoter mutations, as well as mutations in *FUBP1* and *CIC* genes on chromosomes 1p and 19q, respectively
What histologic criteria lead to classification of an oligodendroglioma as grade 3?	Increased mitoses, microvascular proliferation, or necrosis
What are three common molecular alterations seen in IDH-mutant astrocytomas, and which one carries worsened prognosis?	IDH-mutant astrocytomas frequently harbor *ATRX* and *TP53* mutations. Presence of *CDKN2A* homozygous deletion is associated with worse prognosis and therefore higher grade.
What are five common molecular hallmarks of IDH-wildtype glioblastoma?	*EGFR* amplification *PTEN* truncating mutation *TERT* promoter mutation *CDKN2A/B* homozygous deletion Polysomy 7 and monosomy 10
What grade are diffuse gliomas involving the midline structures and harboring mutations involving lysine 27 (K27) of histone 3 genes (*H3F3A* or *HIST13B/C*)?	Grade 4, regardless of histological appearance
What morphologic features do pilocytic astrocytoma cells commonly contain, and what gene fusion do they frequently harbor?	Piloid (hair-like) processes, microcystic areas, and Rosenthal fibers *KIAA1549-BRAF* fusion

Describe the two cell types frequently seen in pleomorphic xanthoastrocytomas	Pleomorphic xanthoastrocytomas frequently contain large, multinucleated cells with foamy cytoplasm and spindle cells with abundant pericellular reticulin
Describe the two molecular abnormalities frequently seen in pleomorphic xantho-astrocytomas	*BRAF V600E* mutation and concurrent *CDKN2A* loss
Describe the molecular abnormalities frequently seen in gangliogliomas	*BRAF V600E* mutation or other MAP kinase pathway alterations
What are the four histologic classifications of medulloblastomas?	Classic Desmoplastic/nodular Extensive nodularity Large cell/anaplastic
What are the three molecular classifications of medulloblastomas?	SHH-activated WNT-activated Non-WNT/non-SHH-activated
What molecular alterations do atypical teratoid/rhabdoid tumors harbor?	*SMARCB1* and (very rarely) *SMARCA4* alterations
What molecular alteration do embryonal tumors with multilayered rosettes harbor?	Amplification of microRNA cluster at chromosome 19 (C19MC)
What are two common morphologic features of meningiomas?	Whorls and psammomatous calcifications
What morphologic features define an atypical meningioma, WHO grade 2?	Increased mitotic activity (4–19 mitoses per 10 high power fields), brain invasion, and/or three of five minor morphologic criteria

What two types of meningioma are automatically considered grade 2?	Clear cell or chordoid histologic variants
What morphologic features define an anaplastic meningioma, WHO grade 3?	Overt malignant morphology and/or extensive mitotic activity (≥20 per 10 high power fields)
What two types of meningioma are automatically considered grade 3?	Rhabdoid or papillary histologic variants
What morphologic features define a solitary fibrous tumor?	Bland spindle cells in a collagen-rich background or jumbled epithelioid cells associated with thin-walled, branching vessels
What molecular feature defines a solitary fibrous tumor?	*NAB2-STAT6* fusion, which can be recognized with STAT6 nuclear staining

QUESTIONS

1. A 7-year-old boy presented with a solid-cystic cerebellar mass, and histopathological evaluation revealed a well-demarcated tumor composed of bland spindle cells in a compact fibrillary background intermixed with loose, myxoid areas. Linear, glomeruloid vascular structures and hyalinized vessels are seen. No mitosis or necrosis is observed. What is the most common likely genetic alteration in this tumor?
   a. *IDH1* mutation
   b. *TERT* promoter mutation
   c. *BRAF* fusion
   d. *EGFR* amplification
   e. 1p/19q co-deletion

2. A 58-year-old woman presented with an intra-axial, ring-enhancing tumor with central necrosis involving the left frontal lobe. She had magnetic resonance imaging (MRI) 3 years ago and did not have any visible lesions. What is the most probable diagnosis of this tumor?
   a. Ganglioglioma, WHO grade 1
   b. Ependymoma, WHO grade 2
   c. Pilocytic astrocytoma, WHO grade 1
   d. Glioblastoma, IDH wildtype, WHO grade 4
   e. Subependymal giant cell astrocytoma

3. An IDH-wildtype diffuse astrocytic neoplasm should be further tested for specific molecular alteration for appropriate grading. Which of the following is a molecular feature that assigns grade 4 to an IDH-wildtype diffuse astrocytic tumor even in the absence of necrosis or microvascular proliferation?
   a. *EWSR* fusion
   b. *EGFR* amplification
   c. *MET* mutation
   d. *MYC* amplification
   e. *TP53* deletion

4. A 6-year-old girl presented with visual loss and was found to have on optic nerve mass. A physical examination revealed multiple palpable lesions on extremities and trunk as well as pigmented skin lesions. What is the most probable diagnosis of the mass in optic nerve and the associated tumor syndrome in this patient?
   a. Subependymal giant cell astrocytoma: tuberous sclerosis
   b. Schwannoma: neurofibromatosis type 2
   c. Pilocytic astrocytoma: neurofibromatosis type 1
   d. Ependymoma: Turcot syndrome type 1
   e. Anaplastic oligodendrioglioma: Ehlers Danlos syndrome

5. A 35-year-old man presented with a non-enhancing mass in left temporal lobe. A stereotactic biopsy was performed and revealed scattered atypical cells with large, hyperchromatic nuclei infiltrating white and gray matter. Mitotic figures were not seen. Tumor cells were negative for IDH1 R132H by immunohistochemistry (IHC), positive for OLIG2, GFAP, and p53. ATRX expression was lost in tumor nuclei. What should be the immediate next step for further workup for this tumor?
   a. Fluorescence in-situ hybridization for 1p/19q codeletion
   b. Sequencing IDH1 and IDH2 genes
   c. Next-generation sequencing for epidermal growth factor receptor (EGFR) amplification
   d. Real-time polymerase chain reaction (PCR) for EGFR mutation
   e. Immunohistochemistry for p16 staining

6. A 37-year-old woman presented with a non-enhancing mass in right frontal lobe, and histopathologic examination showed an infiltrating glial neoplasm composed of a mixture of round cells with fine chromatin and atypical cells with naked, elongate, and hyperchromatic nuclei. Mitotic figures, microvascular proliferation, and necrosis are not identified. Upon immunohistochemical stains and molecular tests, a diagnosis of oligodendroglioma, IDH-mutant and 1p/19q-co-deleted, WHO grade 2 was rendered. Which one of these results is expected for this tumor?
   a. *BRAF-KIAA1549* fusion
   b. *PTEN* deep deletion
   c. *TERT* promoter mutation
   d. *ATRX* mutation
   e. *EGFR* amplification

7. Which one of the tumors described here corresponds to WHO grade 2?
   a. Infiltrating hemispheric glioma without microvascular proliferation or necrosis, harboring *IDH1* and *TERT* promoter hotspot mutations
   b. Infiltrating thalamic glioma without microvascular proliferation or necrosis, harboring H3 K27M mutation
   c. Infiltrating hemispheric glioma without microvascular proliferation or necrosis, harboring *EGFR* amplification and *TERT* promoter mutation
   d. Circumscribed hemispheric glioma without microvascular proliferation or necrosis, harboring *BRAF-KIAA1549* fusion
   e. Infiltrating hemispheric glioma with numerous mitoses and microvascular proliferation, harboring *IDH1* mutation and 1p/19q co-deletion

8. A 15-month-old girl was found to have a cerebellar mass, which was diagnosed as "medulloblastoma, desmoplastic/nodular histologic type, WHO grade 4" on histopathologic examination. What is the most likely molecular subgroup of this medulloblastoma?
   a. WNT-activated
   b. SHH-activated and *TP53*-mutant
   c. SHH-activated and *TP53*-wildtype
   d. Non-WNT/non-SHH, group 3
   e. Non-WNT/non-SHH, group 4

9. A 40-year-old man presented with new-onset seizures and was found to have a dural-based circumscribed tumor involving left parietal-temporal convexity. Histopathologic examination revealed a hypercellular neoplasm composed

of epithelioid cells arranged in a patternless pattern in the background of thin-walled, branching vessels. Immunohistochemical stains for EMA, S100, and GFAP are negative and show nuclear staining for STAT6 and INI1. What is the most likely diagnosis?

a. Epithelioid sarcoma
b. Rhabdoid meningioma
c. Fibrous meningioma
d. Solitary fibrous tumor
e. Hemangioblastoma

10. A 64-year-old man presented with a paraspinal mass, and histopathologic examination showed a hypercellular neoplasm composed of elongate cells tightly packed in intersecting fascicles. Immunohistochemical stains are focally positive for S100 and negative for desmin, cytokeratin, Melan-A, and CD34. Immunohistochemistry for trimethylated lysine 27 of Histone 3 shows loss of nuclear staining. What is the most likely underlying genetic alteration for this tumor?

a. *H3F3A (H3.3)* mutation
b. *SUZ12* mutation
c. *NF2* mutation
d. *SMARCB1* mutation
e. *BAP1* mutation

11. A 10-month-old boy presented with a posterior fossa mass, and histopathologic examination revealed poorly differentiated small cells with scant cytoplasm and hyperchromatic nuclei admixed with epithelioid cells with eccentric nuclei and globular cytoplasmic inclusions. Tumor cells show polyphenotypic staining, including patchy staining with synaptophysin, cytokeratin, smooth muscle actin, and GFAP. What is the most common molecular alteration in this neoplasm?

a. *PTCH1* mutation
b. *H3F3A* mutation
c. *BRAF* mutation
d. *SMARCB1* mutation
e. *TP53* mutation

12. A 45-year-old woman presented with headaches and was found to have a dural-based neoplasm involving the falx cerebri, associated with significant edema and mass effect. Histopathologic examination of the resected tumor demonstrated variably sized nests of epithelioid meningothelial cells. Round, intracytoplasmic inclusions, highlighted by PAS stain, were present throughout the tumor. Mitoses were rare, and the tumor was graded as WHO grade 1. What is the most likely meningioma subtype in this patient?

a. Chordoid meningioma
b. Clear cell meningioma
c. Papillary meningioma
d. Rhabdoid meningioma
e. Secretory meningioma

13. A 38-year-old man presents with an intradural extramedullary mass involving T6 spinal cord. Histopathologic examination revealed epithelioid cells with round nuclei and prominent nucleoli arranged singly and in nests. Mitotic figures were easy to identify. Immunohistochemical stains showed positive nuclear staining with SOX10 and MART1. Which one of the following results should suggest a metastasis over a primary meningeal neoplasm?

a. Presence of necrosis
b. Diffuse staining with Melan-A immunohistochemistry
c. Presence of *TERT* promoter mutation
d. Presence of *GNAQ* mutation
e. Presence of *PRKAR1A* mutation

14. A 36-year-old man presents with an intramedullary tumor involving T2 associated with syrinx. Biopsy of the tumor showed fibrillary acellular zones around vessels, surrounded by uniform cells with round nuclei. Tumor cells show cytoplasmic GFAP and dot-like EMA staining. The patient had a history of schwannoma resected from the left cerebellopontine angle 5 years ago. What is the most likely genetic alteration in this tumor?

a. *NF1* mutation
b. *NF2* mutation
c. *SMARCB1* mutation
d. *SMARCA4* mutation
e. *TP53* mutation

15. A 24-year-old man presented with seizures and was found to have a circumscribed, solid, and cystic right temporal lobe mass. Histopathological examination revealed scattered large cells with prominent nucleoli, abundant amphiphilic cytoplasm with Nissl substance in the background of uniform small cells with elongate nuclei, and long fibrillary processes associated with eosinophilic granular bodies. Large cells stain with synaptophysin and small cells stain with GFAP. Immunohistochemical stain against BRAF V600E mutant protein is also positive. What is the most likely diagnosis?

a. Oligodendroglioma, IDH-mutant and 1p/19q-co-deleted, WHO grade 2
b. Pilocytic astrocytoma, WHO grade 1
c. Ganglioglioma, WHO grade 1
d. Diffuse astrocytoma, IDH-wildtype, WHO grade 2
e. Central neurocytoma, WHO grade 2

ANSWERS

1. c
2. d
3. b
4. c
5. b
6. c
7. a
8. c
9. d
10. b
11. d
12. e
13. c
14. b
15. c

REFERENCES

1. Louis DN, Perry A, Wesseling P, et al. The 2021 WHO Classification of Tumors of the Central Nervous System: a summary. *Neuro-Oncology.* 2021;23(8):1231–1251. https://doi.org/10.1093/neuonc/noab106

2. Louis DN, Ohgaki H, Wiestler OD, Cavenee WK, World Health Organization, International Agency for Research on Cancer. *WHO Classification of Tumours of the Central Nervous System.* 4th ed. rev. Lyon: International Agency for Research on Cancer; 2016.

3. Louis DN, Aldape K, Brat DJ, et al. Announcing cIMPACT-NOW: The Consortium to Inform Molecular and Practical Approaches to CNS Tumor Taxonomy. *Acta Neuropathol.* 2017;133(1):1–3.

4. WHO Classification of Tumours; 5th Edition. Central Nervous System Tumours. Edited by the WHO Classification of Tumours Editorial Board. International Agency for Research on Cancer 2021.

5. Qaddoumi I, Orisme W, Wen J, et al. Genetic alterations in uncommon low-grade neuroepithelial tumors: BRAF, FGFR1, and MYB mutations occur at high frequency and align with morphology. *Acta Neuropathol.* 2016;131(6):833–845.

6. Gilani A, Donson A, Davies KD, et al. Targetable molecular alterations in congenital glioblastoma. *J Neurooncol.* 2020;146(2):247–252.

7. Guerreiro Stucklin AS, Ryall S, Fukuoka K, et al. Alterations in ALK/ROS1/NTRK/MET drive a group of infantile hemispheric gliomas. *Nat Commun.* 2019;10(1):4343.

8. Johnson A, Severson E, Gay L, et al. Comprehensive genomic profiling of 282 pediatric low- and high-grade gliomas reveals genomic drivers, tumor mutational burden, and hypermutation signatures. *Oncologist.* 2017;22(12):1478–1490.

9. Lopez GY, Van Ziffle J, Onodera C, et al. The genetic landscape of gliomas arising after therapeutic radiation. *Acta Neuropathol.* 2019;137(1):139–150.

10. Cancer Genome Atlas Research N, Brat DJ, Verhaak RG, et al. Comprehensive, integrative genomic analysis of diffuse lower-grade gliomas. *N Engl J Med.* 2015;372(26):2481–2498.

11. Reuss DE, Mamatjan Y, Schrimpf D, et al. IDH mutant diffuse and anaplastic astrocytomas have similar age at presentation and little difference in survival: A grading problem for WHO. *Acta Neuropathol.* 2015;129(6):867–873.

12. Pekmezci M, Rice T, Molinaro AM, et al. Adult infiltrating gliomas with WHO 2016 integrated diagnosis: Additional prognostic roles of ATRX and TERT. *Acta Neuropathol.* 2017;133(6):1001–1016.

13. Olar A, Wani KM, Alfaro-Munoz KD, et al. IDH mutation status and role of WHO grade and mitotic index in overall survival in grade II-III diffuse gliomas. *Acta Neuropathol.* 2015;129(4):585–596.

14. Brennan CW, Verhaak RG, McKenna A, et al. The somatic genomic landscape of glioblastoma. *Cell.* 2013;155(2):462–477.

15. Nobusawa S, Watanabe T, Kleihues P, Ohgaki H. IDH1 mutations as molecular signature and predictive factor of secondary glioblastomas. *Clin Cancer Res.* 2009;15(19):6002–6007.

16. Yan H, Parsons DW, Jin G, et al. IDH1 and IDH2 mutations in gliomas. *N Engl J Med.* 2009;360(8):765–773.

17. Shirahata M, Ono T, Stichel D, et al. Novel, improved grading system(s) for IDH-mutant astrocytic gliomas. *Acta Neuropathol.* 2018;136(1):153–166.

18. Brat DJ, Aldape K, Colman H, et al. cIMPACT-NOW update 5: Recommended grading criteria and terminologies for IDH-mutant astrocytomas. *Acta Neuropathol.* 2020;139(3):603–608.

19. Brat DJ, Aldape K, Colman H, et al. cIMPACT-NOW update 3: Recommended diagnostic criteria for "Diffuse astrocytic glioma, IDH-wildtype, with molecular features of glioblastoma, WHO grade IV." *Acta Neuropathol.* 2018;136(5):805–810.

20. Hegi ME, Diserens AC, Gorlia T, et al. MGMT gene silencing and benefit from temozolomide in glioblastoma. *N Engl J Med.* 2005;352(10):997–1003.

21. Solomon DA, Wood MD, Tihan T, et al. Diffuse midline gliomas with histone H3-K27M mutation: A series of 47 cases assessing the spectrum of morphologic variation and associated genetic alterations. *Brain Pathol.* 2016;26(5):569–580.

22. Porkholm M, Raunio A, Vainionpaa R, et al. Molecular alterations in pediatric brainstem gliomas. *Pediatr Blood Cancer.* 2018;65(1):e26751.

23. Wu G, Diaz AK, Paugh BS, et al. The genomic landscape of diffuse intrinsic pontine glioma and pediatric non-brainstem high-grade glioma. *Nat Genet.* 2014;46(5):444–450.

24. Fontebasso AM, Papillon-Cavanagh S, Schwartzentruber J, et al. Recurrent somatic mutations in ACVR1 in pediatric midline high-grade astrocytoma. *Nat Genet.* 2014;46(5):462–466.

25. Venneti S, Santi M, Felicella MM, et al. A sensitive and specific histopathologic prognostic marker for H3F3A K27M mutant pediatric glioblastomas. *Acta Neuropathol.* 2014;128(5):743–753.

26. Korshunov A, Capper D, Reuss D, et al. Histologically distinct neuroepithelial tumors with histone 3 G34 mutation are molecularly similar and comprise a single nosologic entity. *Acta Neuropathol.* 2016;131(1):137–146.

27. Gessi M, Gielen GH, Hammes J, et al. H3.3 G34R mutations in pediatric primitive neuroectodermal tumors of central nervous system (CNS-PNET) and pediatric glioblastomas: Possible diagnostic and therapeutic implications? *J Neurooncol.* 2013;112(1):67–72.

28. Louis DN, Wesseling P, Paulus W, et al. cIMPACT-NOW update 1: Not Otherwise Specified (NOS) and Not Elsewhere Classified (NEC). *Acta Neuropathol.* 2018;135(3):481–484.

29. Pfister S, Janzarik WG, Remke M, et al. BRAF gene duplication constitutes a mechanism of MAPK pathway activation in low-grade astrocytomas. *J Clin Invest.* 2008;118(5):1739–1749.

30. Rodriguez FJ, Brosnan-Cashman JA, Allen SJ, et al. Alternative lengthening of telomeres, ATRX loss and H3-K27M mutations in histologically defined pilocytic astrocytoma with anaplasia. *Brain Pathol.* 2019;29(1):126–140.

31. Chikai K, Ohnishi A, Kato T, et al. Clinico-pathological features of pilomyxoid astrocytoma of the optic pathway. *Acta Neuropathol.* 2004;108(2):109–114.

32. Johnson MW, Eberhart CG, Perry A, et al. Spectrum of pilomyxoid astrocytomas: Intermediate pilomyxoid tumors. *Am J Surg Pathol.* 2010;34(12):1783–1791.

33. Kulac I, Tihan T. Pilomyxoid astrocytomas: A short review. *Brain Tumor Pathol.* 2019;36(2):52–55.

34. Vaubel RA, Caron AA, Yamada S, et al. Recurrent copy number alterations in low-grade and anaplastic pleomorphic xanthoastrocytoma with and without BRAF V600E mutation. *Brain Pathol.* 2018;28(2):172–182.

35. Phillips JJ, Gong H, Chen K, et al. The genetic landscape of anaplastic pleomorphic xanthoastrocytoma. *Brain Pathol.* 2019;29(1):85–96.

36. Luyken C, Blumcke I, Fimmers R, Urbach H, Wiestler OD, Schramm J. Supratentorial gangliogliomas: Histopathologic grading and tumor recurrence in 184 patients with a median follow-up of 8 years. *Cancer.* 2004;101(1):146–155.

37. Pekmezci M, Villanueva-Meyer JE, Goode B, et al. The genetic landscape of ganglioglioma. *Acta Neuropathol Commun.* 2018;6(1):47.

38. Chappe C, Padovani L, Scavarda D, et al. Dysembryoplastic neuroepithelial tumors share with pleomorphic xanthoastrocytomas and gangliogliomas BRAF(V600E) mutation and expression. *Brain Pathol.* 2013;23(5):574–583.

39. Koelsche C, Wohrer A, Jeibmann A, et al. Mutant BRAF V600E protein in ganglioglioma is predominantly expressed by neuronal tumor cells. *Acta Neuropathol.* 2013;125(6):891–900.

40. Hoischen A, Ehrler M, Fassunke J, et al. Comprehensive characterization of genomic aberrations in gangliogliomas by CGH, array-based CGH and interphase FISH. *Brain Pathol.* 2008;18(3):326–337.

41. Thom M, Toma A, An S, et al. One hundred and one dysembryoplastic neuroepithelial tumors: An adult epilepsy series with immunohistochemical, molecular genetic, and clinical correlations and a review of the literature. *J Neuropathol Exp Neurol.* 2011;70(10):859–878.

42. Qaddoumi I, Orisme W, Wen J, et al. Genetic alterations in uncommon low-grade neuroepithelial tumors: BRAF, FGFR1, and MYB mutations occur at high frequency and align with morphology. *Acta Neuropathologica.* 2016;131(6):833–845.

43. Huse JT, Edgar M, Halliday J, Mikolaenko I, Lavi E, Rosenblum MK. Multinodular and vacuolating neuronal tumors of the cerebrum: 10 cases of a distinctive seizure-associated lesion. *Brain Pathol.* 2013;23(5):515–524.

44. Pekmezci M, Stevers M, Phillips JJ, et al. Multinodular and vacuolating neuronal tumor of the cerebrum is a clonal neoplasm defined by genetic alterations that activate the MAP kinase signaling pathway. *Acta Neuropathol.* 2018;135(3):485–488.

45. Li D, Wang JM, Li GL, et al. Clinical, radiological, and pathological features of 16 papillary glioneuronal tumors. *Acta Neurochir (Wien).* 2014;156(4):627–639.

46. Komori T, Scheithauer BW, Anthony DC, et al. Papillary glioneuronal tumor: A new variant of mixed neuronal-glial neoplasm. *Am J Surg Pathol.* 1998;22(10):1171–1183.

47. Bridge JA, Liu XQ, Sumegi J, et al. Identification of a novel, recurrent SLC44A1-PRKCA fusion in papillary glioneuronal tumor. *Brain Pathol.* 2013;23(2):121–128.

48. Yang C, Fang J, Li G, et al. Histopathological, molecular, clinical and radiological characterization of rosette-forming glioneuronal tumor in the central nervous system. *Oncotarget.* 2017;8(65):109175–109190.

49. Sievers P, Appay R, Schrimpf D, et al. Rosette-forming glioneuronal tumors share a distinct DNA methylation profile and mutations in FGFR1, with recurrent co-mutation of PIK3CA and NF1. *Acta Neuropathol.* 2019;138(3):497–504.

50. Rodriguez FJ, Perry A, Rosenblum MK, et al. Disseminated oligodendroglial-like leptomeningeal tumor of childhood: A distinctive clinicopathologic entity. *Acta Neuropathol*. 2012;124(5):627–641.

51. Rodriguez FJ, Schniederjan MJ, Nicolaides T, et al. High rate of concurrent BRAF-KIAA1549 gene fusion and 1p deletion in disseminated oligodendroglioma-like leptomeningeal neoplasms (DOLN). *Acta Neuropathol*. 2015;129(4):609–610.

52. Pajtler KW, Witt H, Sill M, et al. Molecular classification of ependymal tumors across all CNS compartments, histopathological grades, and age groups. *Cancer Cell*. 2015;27(5):728–743.

53. Tihan T, Zhou T, Holmes E, et al. The prognostic value of histological grading of posterior fossa ependymomas in children: A Children's Oncology Group study and a review of prognostic factors. *Mod Pathol*. 2008;21(2):165–177.

54. Kawano N, Yasui Y, Utsuki S, et al. Light microscopic demonstration of the microlumen of ependymoma: A study of the usefulness of antigen retrieval for epithelial membrane antigen (EMA) immunostaining. *Brain Tumor Pathol*. 2004;21(1):17–21.

55. Parker M, Mohankumar KM, Punchihewa C, et al. C11orf95-RELA fusions drive oncogenic NF-kappaB signalling in ependymoma. *Nature*. 2014;506(7489):451–455.

56. Witt H, Mack SC, Ryzhova M, et al. Delineation of two clinically and molecularly distinct subgroups of posterior fossa ependymoma. *Cancer Cell*. 2011;20(2):143–157.

57. Bayliss J, Mukherjee P, Lu C, et al. Lowered H3K27me3 and DNA hypomethylation define poorly prognostic pediatric posterior fossa ependymomas. *Sci Transl Med*. 2016;8(366):366ra161.

58. Panwalkar P, Clark J, Ramaswamy V, et al. Immunohistochemical analysis of H3K27me3 demonstrates global reduction in group-A childhood posterior fossa ependymoma and is a powerful predictor of outcome. *Acta Neuropathol*. 2017;134(5):705–714.

59. Ebert C, von Haken M, Meyer-Puttlitz B, et al. Molecular genetic analysis of ependymal tumors. NF2 mutations and chromosome 22q loss occur preferentially in intramedullary spinal ependymomas. *Am J Pathol*. 1999;155(2):627–632.

60. Swanson AA, Raghunathan A, Jenkins RB, et al. Spinal cord ependymomas with MYCN amplification show aggressive clinical behavior. *J Neuropathol Exp Neurol*. 2019;78(9):791–797.

61. You H, Kim YI, Im SY, et al. Immunohistochemical study of central neurocytoma, subependymoma, and subependymal giant cell astrocytoma. *J Neurooncol*. 2005;74(1):1–8.

62. Lee JC, Sharifai N, Dahiya S, et al. Clinicopathologic features of anaplastic myxopapillary ependymomas. *Brain Pathol*. 2019;29(1):75–84.

63. Mack SC, Agnihotri S, Bertrand KC, et al. Spinal myxopapillary ependymomas demonstrate a Warburg phenotype. *Clin Cancer Res*. 2015;21(16):3750–3758.

64. Taylor MD, Northcott PA, Korshunov A, et al. Molecular subgroups of medulloblastoma: The current consensus. *Acta Neuropathol*. 2012;123(4):465–472.

65. Pietsch T, Schmidt R, Remke M, et al. Prognostic significance of clinical, histopathological, and molecular characteristics of medulloblastomas in the prospective HIT2000 multicenter clinical trial cohort. *Acta Neuropathol*. 2014;128(1):137–149.

66. Ellison DW, Dalton J, Kocak M, et al. Medulloblastoma: Clinicopathological correlates of SHH, WNT, and non-SHH/WNT molecular subgroups. *Acta Neuropathol*. 2011;121(3):381–396.

67. Cho YJ, Tsherniak A, Tamayo P, et al. Integrative genomic analysis of medulloblastoma identifies a molecular subgroup that drives poor clinical outcome. *J Clin Oncol*. 2011;29(11):1424–1430.

68. Kool M, Korshunov A, Remke M, et al. Molecular subgroups of medulloblastoma: An international meta-analysis of transcriptome, genetic aberrations, and clinical data of WNT, SHH, Group 3, and Group 4 medulloblastomas. *Acta Neuropathol*. 2012;123(4):473–484.

69. Northcott PA, Buchhalter I, Morrissy AS, et al. The whole-genome landscape of medulloblastoma subtypes. *Nature*. 2017;547(7663):311–317.

70. Ellison DW, Onilude OE, Lindsey JC, et al. beta-Catenin status predicts a favorable outcome in childhood medulloblastoma: The United Kingdom Children's Cancer Study Group Brain Tumour Committee. *J Clin Oncol*. 2005;23(31):7951–7957.

71. Waszak SM, Northcott PA, Buchhalter I, et al. Spectrum and prevalence of genetic predisposition in medulloblastoma: A retrospective genetic study and prospective validation in a clinical trial cohort. *Lancet Oncol*. 2018;19(6):785–798.

72. Korshunov A, Sturm D, Ryzhova M, et al. Embryonal tumor with abundant neuropil and true rosettes (ETANTR), ependymoblastoma, and medulloepithelioma share molecular similarity and comprise a single clinicopathological entity. *Acta Neuropathol*. 2014;128(2):279–289.

73. Spence T, Sin-Chan P, Picard D, et al. CNS-PNETs with C19MC amplification and/or LIN28 expression comprise a distinct histogenetic diagnostic and therapeutic entity. *Acta Neuropathol*. 2014;128(2):291–303.

74. Versteege I, Sevenet N, Lange J, et al. Truncating mutations of hSNF5/INI1 in aggressive paediatric cancer. *Nature*. 1998;394(6689):203–206.

75. Bookhout C, Bouldin TW, Ellison DW. Atypical teratoid/rhabdoid tumor with retained INI1 (SMARCB1) expression and loss of BRG1 (SMARCA4). *Neuropathology*. 2018;38(3):305–308.

76. Johann PD, Erkek S, Zapatka M, et al. Atypical teratoid/rhabdoid tumors are comprised of three epigenetic subgroups with distinct enhancer landscapes. *Cancer Cell*. 2016;29(3):379–393.

77. Al-Hussaini M, Dissi N, Souki C, Amayiri N. Atypical teratoid/ rhabdoid tumor, an immunohistochemical study of potential diagnostic and prognostic markers. *Neuropathology*. 2016;36(1):17–26.

78. Sturm D, Orr BA, Toprak UH, et al. New brain tumor entities emerge from molecular classification of CNS-PNETs. *Cell*. 2016;164(5):1060–1072.

79. Hwang EI, Kool M, Burger PC, et al. Extensive molecular and clinical heterogeneity in patients with histologically diagnosed CNS-PNET treated as a single entity: A report from the Children's Oncology Group Randomized ACNS0332 Trial. *J Clin Oncol*. 2018;65(1):JCO2017764720.

80. Perry A, Stafford SL, Scheithauer BW, Suman VJ, Lohse CM. Meningioma grading: An analysis of histologic parameters. *Am J Surg Pathol*. 1997;21(12):1455–1465.

81. Bruno MC, Ginguene C, Santangelo M, et al. Lymphoplasmacyte rich meningioma: A case report and review of the literature. *J Neurosurg Sci*. 2004;48(3):117–124; discussion 124.

82. Zorludemir S, Scheithauer BW, Hirose T, Van Houten C, Miller G, Meyer FB. Clear cell meningioma: A clinicopathologic study of a potentially aggressive variant of meningioma. *Am J Surg Pathol*. 1995;19(5):493–505.

83. Lin JW, Lu CH, Lin WC, et al. A clinicopathological study of the significance of the proportion of choroid morphology in chordoid meningioma. *J Clin Neurosci*. 2012;19(6):836–843.

84. Couce ME, Aker FV, Scheithauer BW. Chordoid meningioma: A clinicopathologic study of 42 cases. *Am J Surg Pathol*. 2000;24(7):899–905.

85. Wang XQ, Chen H, Zhao L, et al. Intracranial papillary meningioma: A clinicopathologic study of 30 cases at a single institution. *Neurosurgery*. 2013;73(5):777–790; discussion 789.

86. Perry A, Scheithauer BW, Stafford SL, Abell-Aleff PC, Meyer FB. "Rhabdoid" meningioma: An aggressive variant. *Am J Surg Pathol*. 1998;22(12):1482–1490.

87. Vaubel RA, Chen SG, Raleigh DR, et al. Meningiomas with rhabdoid features lacking other histologic features of malignancy: A study of 44 cases and review of the literature. *J Neuropathol Exp Neurol*. 2016;75(1):44–52.

88. Menke JR, Raleigh DR, Gown AM, et al. Somatostatin receptor 2a is a more sensitive diagnostic marker of meningioma than epithelial membrane antigen. *Acta Neuropathol*. 2015;130(3):441–443.

89. Liu N, Song SY, Jiang JB, et al. The prognostic role of Ki-67/MIB-1 in meningioma: A systematic review with meta-analysis. *Medicine (Baltimore)*. 2020;99(9):e18644.

90. Youngblood MW, Duran D, Montejo JD, et al. Correlations between genomic subgroup and clinical features in a cohort of more than 3000 meningiomas. *J Neurosurg*. 2019:1–10.

91. Reuss DE, Piro RM, Jones DT, et al. Secretory meningiomas are defined by combined KLF4 K409Q and TRAF7 mutations. *Acta Neuropathol*. 2013;125(3):351–358.

92. Tauziede-Espariat A, Parfait B, Besnard A, et al. Loss of SMARCE1 expression is a specific diagnostic marker of clear cell meningioma: A comprehensive immunophenotypical and molecular analysis. *Brain Pathol*. 2018;28(4):466–474.

93. Shankar GM, Abedalthagafi M, Vaubel RA, et al. Germline and somatic BAP1 mutations in high-grade rhabdoid meningiomas. *Neuro Oncol*. 2017;19(4):535–545.

94. Mirian C, Duun-Henriksen AK, Juratli T, et al. Poor prognosis associated with TERT gene alterations in meningioma is independent of the WHO classification: An individual patient data meta-analysis. *J Neurol Neurosurg Psychiatry*. 2020;91(4):378–387.

95. Sahm F, Schrimpf D, Stichel D, et al. DNA methylation-based classification and grading system for meningioma: A multicentre, retrospective analysis. *Lancet Oncol*. 2017;18(5):682–694.

96. Katz LM, Hielscher T, Liechty B, et al. Loss of histone H3K27me3 identifies a subset of meningiomas with increased risk of recurrence. *Acta Neuropathol*. 2018;135(6):955–963.

97. Barthelmess S, Geddert H, Boltze C, et al. Solitary fibrous tumors/hemangiopericytomas with different variants of the NAB2-STAT6 gene fusion

are characterized by specific histomorphology and distinct clinicopathological features. *Am J Pathol.* 2014;184(4):1209–1218.

98. Macagno N, Vogels R, Appay R, et al. Grading of meningeal solitary fibrous tumors/hemangiopericytomas: Analysis of the prognostic value of the Marseille Grading System in a cohort of 132 patients. *Brain Pathol.* 2019;29(1):18–27.

99. Fritchie K, Jensch K, Moskalev EA, et al. The impact of histopathology and NAB-STAT6 fusion subtype in classification and grading of meningeal solitary fibrous tumor/hemangiopericytoma. *Acta Neuropathol.* 2019;137(2):307–319.

100. Chmielecki J, Crago AM, Rosenberg M, et al. Whole-exome sequencing identifies a recurrent NAB2-STAT6 fusion in solitary fibrous tumors. *Nat Genet.* 2013;45(2):131–132.

101. Vogels R, Macagno N, Griewank K, et al. Prognostic significance of NAB2-STAT6 fusion variants and TERT promotor mutations in solitary fibrous tumors/hemangiopericytomas of the CNS: Not (yet) clear. *Acta Neuropathol.* 2019;137(4):679–682.

102. Jung SM, Kuo TT. Immunoreactivity of CD10 and inhibin alpha in differentiating hemangioblastoma of central nervous system from metastatic clear cell renal cell carcinoma. *Mod Pathol.* 2005;18(6):788–794.

103. Shankar GM, Taylor-Weiner A, Lelic N, et al. Sporadic hemangioblastomas are characterized by cryptic VHL inactivation. *Acta Neuropathol Commun.* 2014;2:167.

104. Smith MJ, Bowers NL, Banks C, et al. A deep intronic SMARCB1 variant associated with schwannomatosis. *Clin Genet.* 2020;97(2):376–377.

105. Caltabiano R, Magro G, Polizzi A, et al. A mosaic pattern of INI1/SMARCB1 protein expression distinguishes Schwannomatosis and NF2-associated peripheral schwannomas from solitary peripheral schwannomas and NF2-associated vestibular schwannomas. *Childs Nerv Syst.* 2017;33(6):933–940.

106. Miettinen MM, Antonescu CR, Fletcher CDM, et al. Histopathologic evaluation of atypical neurofibromatous tumors and their transformation into malignant peripheral nerve sheath tumor in patients with neurofibromatosis 1-a consensus overview. *Hum Pathol.* 2017;67:1–10.

107. Rhodes SD, He Y, Smith A, et al. Cdkn2a (Arf) loss drives NF1-associated atypical neurofibroma and malignant transformation. *Hum Mol Genet.* 2019;28(16):2752–2762.

108. Pekmezci M, Reuss DE, Hirbe AC, et al. Morphologic and immunohistochemical features of malignant peripheral nerve sheath tumors and cellular schwannomas. *Mod Pathol.* 2015;28(2):187–200.

109. Pekmezci M, Cuevas-Ocampo AK, Perry A, Horvai AE. Significance of H3K27me3 loss in the diagnosis of malignant peripheral nerve sheath tumors. *Mod Pathol.* 2017;30(12):1710–1719.

110. Schaefer IM, Fletcher CD, Hornick JL. Loss of H3K27 trimethylation distinguishes malignant peripheral nerve sheath tumors from histologic mimics. *Mod Pathol.* 2016;29(1):4–13.

111. Rohrich M, Koelsche C, Schrimpf D, et al. Methylation-based classification of benign and malignant peripheral nerve sheath tumors. *Acta Neuropathol.* 2016;131(6):877–887.

112. Schaefer IM, Dong F, Garcia EP, et al. Recurrent SMARCB1 inactivation in epithelioid malignant peripheral nerve sheath tumors. *Am J Surg Pathol.* 2019;43(6):835–843.

113. Torres-Mora J, Dry S, Li X, et al. Malignant melanotic schwannian tumor: A clinicopathologic, immunohistochemical, and gene expression profiling study of 40 cases, with a proposal for the reclassification of "melanotic schwannoma." *Am J Surg Pathol.* 2014;38(1):94–105.

114. Shields LB, Glassman SD, Raque GH, Shields CB. Malignant psammomatous melanotic schwannoma of the spine: A component of Carney complex. *Surg Neurol Int.* 2011;2:136.

115. Brat DJ, Giannini C, Scheithauer BW, Burger PC. Primary melanocytic neoplasms of the central nervous systems. *Am J Surg Pathol.* 1999;23(7):745–754.

116. Kusters-Vandevelde HV, Creytens D, van Engen-van Grunsven AC, et al. SF3B1 and EIF1AX mutations occur in primary leptomeningeal melanocytic neoplasms; yet another similarity to uveal melanomas. *Acta Neuropathol Commun.* 2016;4:5.

117. van de Nes J, Gessi M, Sucker A, et al. Targeted next generation sequencing reveals unique mutation profile of primary melanocytic tumors of the central nervous system. *J Neurooncol.* 2016;127(3):435–444.

118. Koelsche C, Hovestadt V, Jones DT, et al. Melanotic tumors of the nervous system are characterized by distinct mutational, chromosomal and epigenomic profiles. *Brain Pathol.* 2015;25(2):202–208.

119. Chatterjee D, Lath K, Singla N, Kumar N, Radotra BD. Pathologic prognostic factors of pineal parenchymal tumor of intermediate differentiation. *Appl Immunohistochem Mol Morphol.* 2019;27(3):210–215.

120. Jouvet A, Saint-Pierre G, Fauchon F, et al. Pineal parenchymal tumors: A correlation of histological features with prognosis in 66 cases. *Brain Pathol.* 2000;10(1):49–60.

121. Pfaff E, Aichmuller C, Sill M, et al. Molecular subgrouping of primary pineal parenchymal tumors reveals distinct subtypes correlated with clinical parameters and genetic alterations. *Acta Neuropathol.* 2020;139(2):243–257.

122. Fevre Montange M, Vasiljevic A, Champier J, Jouvet A. Papillary tumor of the pineal region: Histopathological characterization and review of the literature. *Neurochirurgie.* 2015;61(2-3):138–142.

123. Nishioka H, Inoshita N, Mete O, et al. The complementary role of transcription factors in the accurate diagnosis of clinically nonfunctioning pituitary adenomas. *Endocr Pathol.* 2015;26(4):349–355.

124. Trouillas J, Roy P, Sturm N, et al. A new prognostic clinicopathological classification of pituitary adenomas: A multicentric case-control study of 410 patients with 8 years post-operative follow-up. *Acta Neuropathol.* 2013;126(1):123–135.

125. Chinezu L, Vasiljevic A, Jouanneau E, et al. Expression of somatostatin receptors, SSTR2A and SSTR5, in 108 endocrine pituitary tumors using immunohistochemical detection with new specific monoclonal antibodies. *Hum Pathol.* 2014;45(1):71–77.

126. Shibuya M. Welcoming the new WHO classification of pituitary tumors 2017: Revolution in TTF-1-positive posterior pituitary tumors. *Brain Tumor Pathol.* 2018;35(2):62–70.

127. Guerrero-Perez F, Vidal N, Marengo AP, et al. Posterior pituitary tumours: The spectrum of a unique entity. A clinical and histological study of a large case series. *Endocrine.* 2019;63(1):36–43.

128. Cole TS, Potla S, Sarris CE, et al. Rare thyroid transcription factor 1-positive tumors of the sellar region: Barrow Neurological Institute retrospective case series. *World Neurosurg.* 2019;129:e294–e302.

129. Viaene AN, Lee EB, Rosenbaum JN, et al. Histologic, immunohistochemical, and molecular features of pituicytomas and atypical pituicytomas. *Acta Neuropathol Commun.* 2019;7(1):69.

130. Cohen-Gadol AA, Pichelmann MA, Link MJ, et al. Granular cell tumor of the sellar and suprasellar region: Clinicopathologic study of 11 cases and literature review. *Mayo Clin Proc.* 2003;78(5):567–573.

131. Esheba GE, Hassan AA. Comparative immunohistochemical expression of beta-catenin, EGFR, ErbB2, and p63 in adamantinomatous and papillary craniopharyngiomas. *J Egypt Natl Canc Inst.* 2015;27(3):139–145.

132. Brastianos PK, Taylor-Weiner A, Manley PE, et al. Exome sequencing identifies BRAF mutations in papillary craniopharyngiomas. *Nat Genet.* 2014;46(2):161–165.

133. Pekmezci M, Perry A. Neuropathology of brain metastases. *Surg Neurol Int.* 2013;4(Suppl 4):S245–255.

2 | IMAGING OF CENTRAL NERVOUS SYSTEM TUMORS

SHOBHIT KUMAR GARG AND RAJAN JAIN

INTRODUCTION

Imaging has played an increasing role in the diagnosis and management of central nervous system (CNS) tumors. However, with the paradigm shift toward using molecular markers to guide tumor classification, prognosis, and management, there has been a demand for radiologic and genomic correlation. This has led to a blossoming of the field of radio-genomics, and, over the past decades, various imaging phenotypes identified using conventional and advanced imaging techniques have been shown to correlate with tumor genotypes.[1] It is important for neuroradiologists and neuro-oncologists to identify these imaging phenotypes in order to anticipate tumor genomics, especially to facilitate management or when biopsy and pathologic examination is delayed or not possible. In this chapter, we review conventional and advanced magnetic resonance imaging (MRI) phenotypes of CNS tumors and the role of imaging in identifying molecular markers preoperatively, specifically in gliomas. We also review some of the pearls and pitfalls of surveillance imaging to assess treatment-related changes.

BRAIN TUMOR IMAGING PROTOCOLS

MRI is the current gold standard for imaging of CNS tumors, with a wide array of conventional and advanced sequences now available to detect and characterize brain tumors as well as aid in treatment planning. Brain tumor MR protocols typically include T1, T2, fluid-attenuated inversion recovery (FLAIR), diffusion, T2*, and post-contrast sequences. In addition, advanced imaging sequences like perfusion, spectroscopy, functional MRI (fMRI), and diffusion tensor imaging (DTI) are also part of many standard brain tumor MRI protocols. The role of positron emission tomography (PET) and hybrid MR-PET in brain tumor imaging is evolving rapidly. Imaging in brain tumors aims towards determining the tumor location, extent, and type, guiding surgical approaches, planning treatment, delineating tumor from functionally important neuronal tissue, and assessing the treatment response.[2] Computed tomography (CT) and MRI are widely used for primary diagnosis of brain tumors. CT and MRI reveal mostly anatomical information on the tumor, whereas MR spectroscopy and PET give important information on the metabolic state and molecular events within the tumor.[2]

PRIMARY CNS TUMORS AND THEIR IMAGING FEATURES

GLIOMAS

Diffusely infiltrating gliomas (astrocytomas and oligodendrogliomas) have been grouped together in the 2016 World Health Organization (WHO) classification. They are now subdivided into isocitrate dehydrogenase (IDH)-mutant, IDH-wildtype, and NOS (if IDH status is unavailable) categories and based on presence or absence of 1p19q co-deletion. The majority of WHO grade 2 and 3 diffuse gliomas are IDH-mutant and have a favorable prognosis compared to IDH-wildtype gliomas.[3,4]

IMAGING FEATURES AND RADIOGENOMICS IN GLIOMAS

Gliomas have a variable appearance on MRI, but usually are T2-hyperintense lesions with associated mass effect. Low-grade tumors (WHO grade 1–2) are less likely to demonstrate contrast enhancement or may feature an enhancing mural nodule (Figure 2.1). Meanwhile higher-grade tumors (WHO grade 3–4) may demonstrate heterogeneous enhancement, usually with extensive surrounding infiltrative FLAIR hyperintense signal (Figure 2.2 and 2.3). These general features on initial imaging historically allowed for a broad radiologic diagnosis of glioma, with precise subclassification left to neuropathologists after detailed tissue and genomic analysis. However, a number of imaging findings are now known to further predict molecular subtype and allow for a more precise preoperative imaging diagnosis. This can allow radiologists to avoid vague terminology such as "primary glioma," "low-grade tumor," or "high-grade neoplasm." We review a number of imaging features of tumors that can be useful in correctly classifying gliomas, including location, signal, enhancement, and morphology. We also discuss advanced MRI techniques that add value in glioma diagnosis.

RADIOGENOMICS USING CONVENTIONAL MRI

TISSUE SIGNAL, MORPHOLOGY, AND ENHANCEMENT

Contrast-enhanced imaging continues to prove its value during the new genomic era. Compared to IDH-wildtype

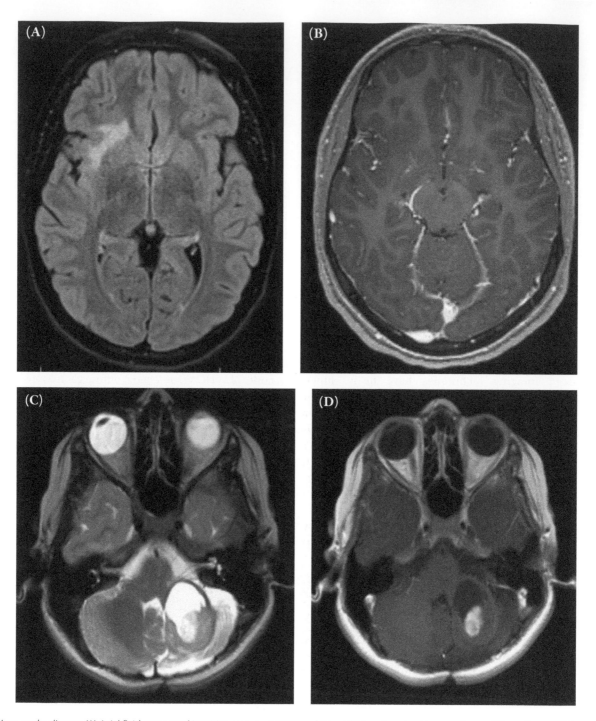

Figure 2.1 *Low-grade gliomas. (A) Axial fluid-attenuated inversion recovery (FLAIR) and (B) axial T1 post-contrast images show a diffuse glioma WHO grade 2 appearing as a poorly defined, hyperintense, non-enhancing lesion involving the right external capsule. (C) Axial T2 and (D) axial T1 post-contrast images show a BRAF-mutated juvenile pilocytic astrocytoma WHO grade 1 in the left cerebellar hemisphere, showing a cystic lesion with enhancing mural nodule.*

gliomas, most IDH-mutant gliomas demonstrate less overall contrast enhancement and more non-enhancing solid components. On the other hand, higher grade IDH-wildtype gliomas often demonstrate peripheral ring enhancement with central necrotic or cystic components (Figure 2.3).[5]

Some studies have reported that nodular enhancement is more commonly found in methylated O6-methylguanine-DNA-methyltransferase (MGMT) promoter tumors, while rim enhancement is more commonly seen in unmethylated tumors.[6] However, it is difficult to distinguish MGMT

promoter methylation status on imaging because of multiple overlapping imaging features.

Imaging signal characteristics can also be used to help predict tumor genotype radiologically. 1p/19q co-deleted tumors often have indistinct tumor margins and commonly contain calcifications, which appear as low signal foci, best seen on susceptibility-weighted images (SWI) and hyperdense foci on CT images (Figure 2.4).[7–9] It is important to identify 1p/19q co-deleted tumors as these are now considered essentially synonymous with oligodendrogliomas and are associated with

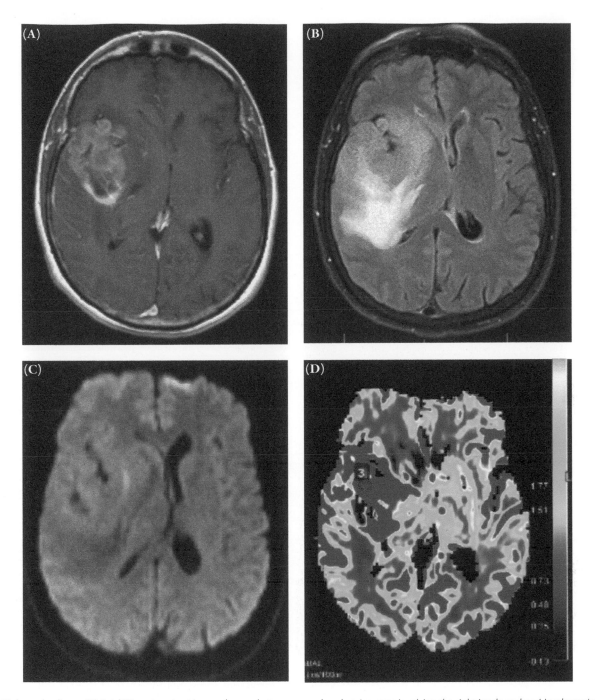

Figure 2.2 High-grade glioma. (A) Axial T1 post-contrast image shows a heterogeneously enhancing mass involving the right insula and peri-insular region. (B) Axial fluid-attenuated inversion recovery (FLAIR) image shows extensive surrounding hyperintense signal. (C) Axial diffusion image shows a small focus of restricted diffusion along the medial margin of the enhancing lesion (arrow). (D) Axial perfusion shows markedly elevated rCBV in the lesion.

slow progressive growth and better prognosis (Figure 2.5). On the contrary, IDH-wildtype gliomas show a very rapid growth consistent with a highly aggressive tumor biology.

> 1p/19q co-deleted tumors often have indistinct tumor margins and commonly contain calcifications, which appear as low signal foci, best seen on susceptibility-weighted images (SWI) and hyperdense foci on CT images.

Helpful in the differentiation between 1p/19q co-deleted and non–co-deleted tumors is the recently discovered T2–FLAIR mismatch sign. This sign has been shown in a study to have 100% specificity in the differentiation between these tumor genotypes; however, sensitivity is limited.[10] T2–FLAIR mismatch sign is defined by two distinct MRI features: (1) complete or near-complete and homogenous hyperintense signal on T2-weighted images and (2) relatively hypointense signal on T2-weighted FLAIR sequence except for a hyperintense peripheral rim (Figure 2.6).[10] The high diagnostic specificity of the sign has been validated in multiple studies and is currently used in neuroradiology and neuro-oncology clinical practice.[6,11–14]

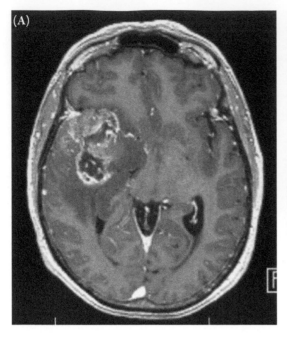 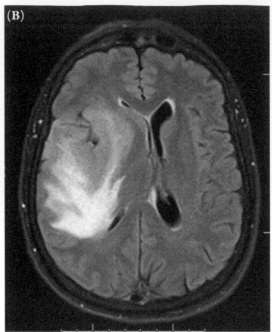

Figure 2.3 Glioblastoma multiforme. Isocitrate dehydrogenase (IDH)-wildtype (WHO grade 4). (A) Axial T1 post-contrast image shows thick irregular peripheral enhancement with central necrosis in a insular/peri-insular mass. (B) Axial fluid-attenuated inversion recovery (FLAIR) image shows extensive surrounding infiltrative hyperintense signal.

T2–FLAIR mismatch sign is defined by two distinct MRI features: (1) complete or near-complete and homogenous hyperintense signal on T2-weighted images and (2) relatively hypointense signal on T2-weighted FLAIR sequence except for a hyperintense peripheral rim.

TUMOR LOCATION

Lesion location is also important in the radiogenomics of gliomas. IDH-mutant gliomas, including high-grade and low-grade tumors, have been found to most commonly involve a single lobe, usually the frontal lobe.[15,16] IDH-wildtype gliomas more commonly involve multiple lobes, reflecting their infiltrative nature, and can involve any lobe. 1p19q co-deleted tumors are commonly found in the frontal, parietal, or occipital lobes.[17,18] 1p19q non–co-deleted tumors are more likely to involve the temporal and insular lobes.

BRAF alteration is often seen in lower grade gliomas in the pediatric population, such as most pilocytic astrocytomas. H3K27M mutation is seen in higher grade diffuse gliomas. BRAF alteration is associated with superficial or cortical location, whereas H3K27M-mutant tumors are more infiltrative and found in midline structures such as the thalamus, brainstem, and spinal cord (Figure 2.7).

DIFFUSION WEIGHTED IMAGING

Diffusion weighted imaging (DWI) measures the amount of motion of free water protons in the tissue. Highly cellular tumors allow for a lesser degree of free proton movement, which is represented by lower apparent diffusion coefficient (ADC) values and high signal on DWI. This is also known as *reduced* or *restricted diffusion*. Wu et al. showed that IDH-wildtype tumors demonstrate areas of lower ADC values compared to IDH-mutant tumors.[19] Low ADC values also correlated with poorer survival.

RADIOGENOMICS USING ADVANCED MRI TECHNIQUES

MR SPECTROSCOPY

MR spectroscopy was one of the first advanced imaging techniques that was found to identify presence of the IDH mutation with high specificity through detection of 2-hydroxyglutarate (2-HG), which is abundant in these gliomas.[20] Unfortunately, this has not translated to practical clinical utility due to difficulty in differentiating the spectral peak of 2-HG from those of normally found metabolites, such as glutamate and glutamine, using readily available MR spectroscopy technology.

PERFUSION IMAGING

IDH-wildtype tumors are more pro-angiogenic compared to IDH-mutant tumors. This has been detectable using perfusion imaging due to the resulting differential microvascular density between the tumors. IDH-wildtype gliomas will typically show higher cerebral blood flow as a result, as described in multiple studies.[21,22] Arterial spin labeling (ASL) allows perfusion imaging without the use of intravenous contrast and has also demonstrated significantly elevated absolute blood flow and relative blood flow in IDH-wildtype tumors compared to IDH-mutant tumors.[23]

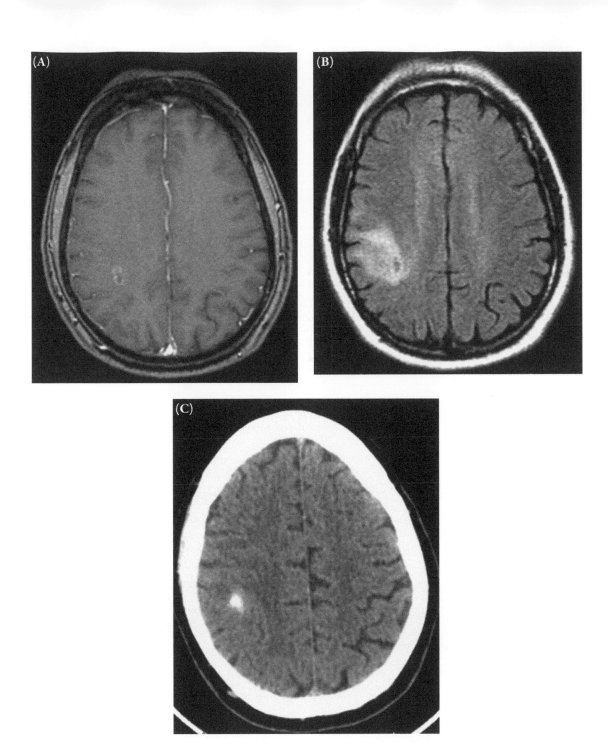

Figure 2.4 Oligodendroglioma 1p/19q co-deleted (A). Axial T1 post-contrast image shows enhancement along the margin of the calcified focus. (B) Axial fluid-attenuated inversion recovery (FLAIR) image shows a hyperintense lesion with indistinct tumor margins. (C) Axial CT image shows calcification in the lesion appearing as hyperdense focus.

CHARACTERISTIC MRI APPEARANCE OF SPECIFIC GLIOMA SUBTYPES

Oligodendrogliomas are WHO grade 2 or grade 3 diffuse infiltrating glial tumors which characteristically demonstrate a mutation of the IDH-gene family and 1p/19q co-deletion.[2] Oligodendrogliomas typically are located in the frontal lobes and have typical MRI features like indistinct tumor margins, heterogeneous signal intensity, and calcifications (Figure 2.4). They appear hypointense on T1 weighted and hyperintense to grey matter on T2 weighted images. Nearly 50% show variable contrast enhancement. There is typically no restriction of diffusion, and vasogenic edema is not prominent. Perfusion imaging has been used for differentiating grade 2 from grade 3 oligodendrogliomas. Tumors with rCBV higher than 1.75 are associated with higher grade and more rapid tumor progression.[24] MR spectroscopy shows moderately elevated Cho and decreased NAA without a lactate peak. On PET, the metabolic activity of the oligodendroglioma correlates with its histological grade.

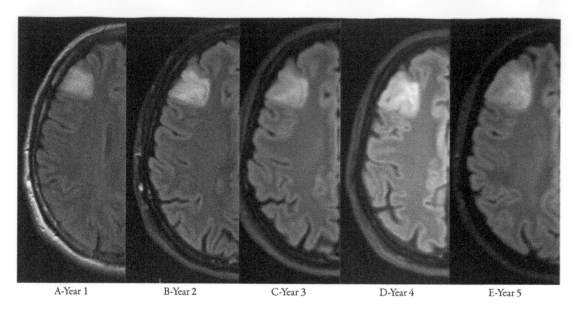

| A-Year 1 | B-Year 2 | C-Year 3 | D-Year 4 | E-Year 5 |

Figure 2.5 Isocitrate dehydrogenase (IDH)-mutant 1p/19q co-deleted oligodendroglioma WHO grade 2 (Year 1, 2, 3, 4, 5). Serial images show slow progressive growth of this lesion.

Oligodendrogliomas appear hypointense on T1, hyperintense to gray matter on T2W images, and nearly 50% show variable contrast enhancement.

Diffuse low-grade astrocytomas are WHO grade 2 infiltrative tumors of the brain. They are usually well-marginated lesions that are isointense to hypointense on T1W images, homogeneously hyperintense on T2W images (Figure 2.1A), and may show the "T2-FLAIR mismatch sign" (Figure 2.6). These tumors usually do not show restriction of diffusion, and no enhancement is seen on post-contrast imaging (Figure 2.1B). There is typically no increase in relative cerebral blood volume (rCBV) on perfusion-weighted imaging.

Diffuse low-grade astrocytomas are usually well-marginated lesions that are isointense to hypointense on T1W images, homogeneously hyperintense on T2W images, and may show the "T2-FLAIR mismatch sign" (Figure 2.6).

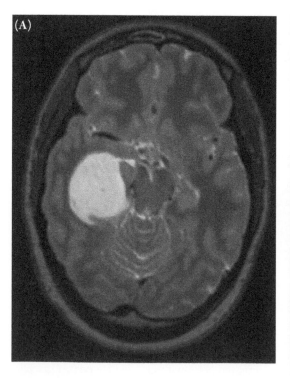
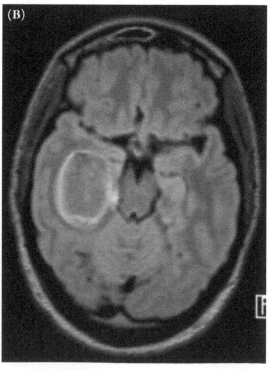

Figure 2.6 (A) Axial T2 and (B) axial fluid-attenuated inversion recovery (FLAIR) images showing a isocitrate dehydrogenase (IDH) mutant glioma with T2-FLAIR mismatch sign.

Anaplastic astrocytomas are WHO grade 3 tumors that show imaging appearance somewhat similar to WHO grade 2 diffuse low-grade astrocytomas, but anaplastic astrocytomas are often more heterogeneous on T2W images with more frequent enhancement and prominent vasogenic edema. Necrosis is usually absent. These tumors may show elevated rCBV on perfusion imaging. In WHO grade 2 and 3 astrocytomas, presence of the T2–FLAIR mismatch sign represents a highly specific imaging biomarker for the IDH-mutant, 1p/19q non–co-deleted molecular subtype (Figure 2.6).[10]

Glioblastomas are poorly differentiated WHO grade 4 tumors. They are the most common primary malignant brain tumors in adults. In the 2016 WHO classification, glioblastomas are divided into (1) glioblastoma IDH-wildtype (seen in about 90% of cases), usually primary glioblastomas that develop *de novo* in elderly patients, without clinical or histologic evidence of any precursor lesion; (2) glioblastoma, IDH-mutant (about 10% of cases), usually secondary glioblastomas that arise from a preexisting low-grade diffuse astrocytoma in younger patients and are almost always MGMT hypermethylated[25]; and (3) glioblastoma, NOS which is used for tumors in which full IDH evaluation cannot be performed.[3] Secondary IDH-mutant glioblastomas are less aggressive and carry a somewhat better prognosis than primary glioblastomas. Glioblastomas tend to infiltrate along white matter tracts and can invade the corpus callosum to cross the midline in a butterfly pattern (Figure 2.7). There can be diffuse involvement of more than two lobes in a "gliomatosis cerebri" pattern, although this entity is no longer included in the 2016 and 2021 WHO classifications. Glioblastomas can also be multifocal or multicentric. On imaging, glioblastomas are large, T1 isointense to hypointense, T2 hyperintense infiltrating tumors with a thick irregular enhancing wall, central necrosis, hemorrhage, neovascularity, and marked surrounding edema (Figure 2.3).

> On imaging, glioblastomas are large, T1 isointense to hypointense, T2 hyperintense infiltrating tumors with thick irregular enhancing wall, central necrosis, hemorrhage, neovascularity, and marked surrounding edema.

The solid-enhancing components of the tumor characteristically show restricted diffusion (ADC values are lower in IDH-wildtype tumors compared to IDH-mutant tumors). Necrotic glioblastomas can show an incomplete, irregular, hypointense rim on SWI which is frequently found at the inner aspect of the contrast-enhancing rim due to random deposition of hemorrhagic products at the edge of the necrotic cavity.[26] In glioblastomas and IDH-wildtype tumors, MR perfusion shows elevated blood flow and increased rCBV as compared to IDH-mutant tumors. MR spectroscopy shows elevated choline, decreased NAA, decreased myoinositol, and a lipid/lactate peak due to necrosis. PET shows increased FDG uptake, greater than gray matter.

> In glioblastomas and IDH-wildtype tumors, MR perfusion shows elevated blood flow and increased rCBV as compared to IDH-mutant tumors.

Diffuse midline glioma, H3 K27M-mutant is a newly defined entity in the 2016 WHO classification of CNS tumors[3] and is categorized as an aggressive WHO grade 4 tumor. In children, this tumor often represents the molecular-pathological correlate to the radiographically defined entity of diffuse intrinsic pontine gliomas (DIPG), which usually appears as a T2-hyperintense non-enhancing mass lesion expanding the pons, with displacement of the basilar artery flow void and flattening of the floor of the fourth ventricle (Figure 2.8). Minimal patchy enhancement may sometimes be seen, and, occasionally, there is mild restriction of diffusion. Leptomeningeal spread is more common than in other glioma subtypes. In addition, H3 K27M *diffuse midline glioma* can also be encountered in adolescents and young adults; it has a predilection for midline structures of the brain, including the thalamus, midbrain, brainstem, and spinal cord.[27]

ASSESSING TREATMENT RESPONSE IN HIGH-GRADE GLIOMAS

The growing variety of treatment options for high-grade gliomas (WHO grade 3–4) have resulted in increasingly varying imaging manifestations of treatment-related changes. Certain treatment modalities or drugs such as radiation therapy or bevacizumab (anti-vascular endothelial growth factor [VEGF]) are known for causing characteristic imaging changes that may mimic either true progression of disease or treatment (pseudo-)response.

PROGRESSION AND PSEUDOPROGRESSION

Tumor progression can be characterized on imaging by increasing size of tumor components, increasing amount or intensity of enhancement, or increased mass effect. However,

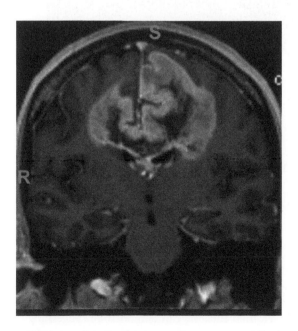

Figure 2.7 Glioblastoma invading the corpus callosum to cross midline in a butterfly pattern.

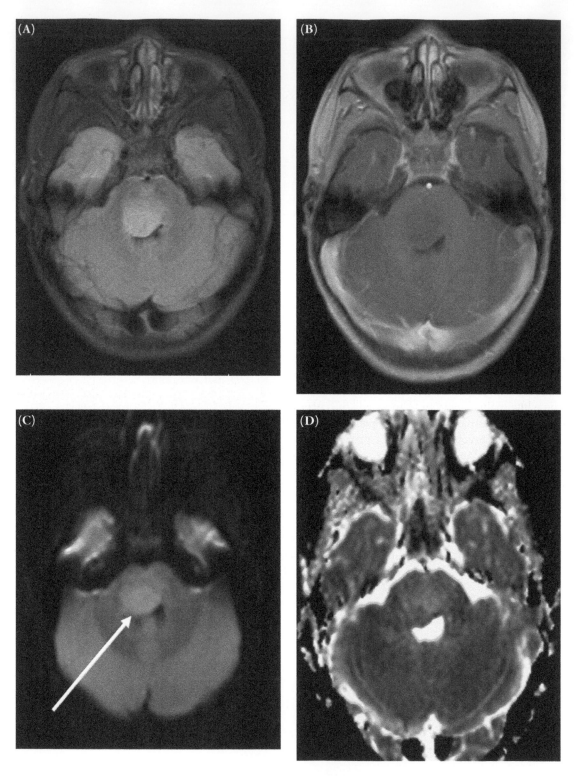

Figure 2.8 Diffuse midline glioma, H3 K27M-mutant. (A) Axial fluid-attenuated inversion recovery (FLAIR) and (B) axial T1 post-contrast images show a hyperintense non-enhancing mass lesion expanding the pons and causing flattening of the floor of the fourth ventricle. (C and D) Axial diffusion and apparent diffusion coefficient (ADC) images show an area of restricted diffusion and low ADC in the posterior aspect of the lesion.

these conventional MRI features do not always correspond with histopathologically proven tumor progression.

> Pseudoprogression can occur in about 20–30% of glioma patients who have undergone temozolomide and radiation treatment.

An entity known as *pseudoprogression* can occur in about 20–30% of glioma patients who have undergone temozolomide and radiation treatment. These patients often demonstrate stability of clinical signs and symptoms at the time of follow-up. However, their imaging can demonstrate concerning findings such as increasing size of enhancing components of the tumor and/or increased mass effect that appear similar to imaging

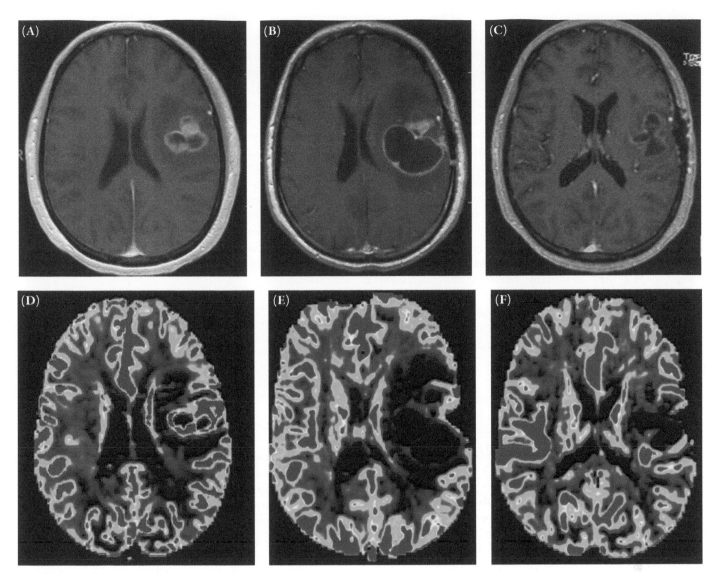

Figure 2.9 Pseudoprogression. (A and B) Serial axial T1 post-contrast images show increase in size of the enhancing solid cystic tumor 2 months after starting chemoradiation. However, corresponding perfusion images (D and E) show decreased rCBV on a 2-month follow-up scan, indicating pseudoprogression. (C and F) Four-month follow-up scan shows reduction in size of enhancing tumor with low rCBV.

findings seen in true tumor progression. The pathophysiological mechanism for pseudoprogression is thought to be breakdown of the blood–brain barrier secondary to treatment-associated tissue necrosis, resulting in increased edema and more contrast extravasation.[28,29]

Advanced imaging modalities can help to differentiate between true progression and pseudoprogression. Unlike in true tumor progression, MRI perfusion maps often show a *decreased* or *stable* rCBV compared to the pre-treatment values (Figure 2.9).[30] It has also been shown that DWI can show higher ADC values within these lesions; in other words, the lesions of pseudoprogression demonstrate relatively less restricted diffusion compared to true progression.[31,32]

In pseudoprogression, imaging can demonstrate concerning findings such as increasing size of enhancing components of lesion and/or increased mass effect that appear similar to imaging findings seen in true tumor progression.

Unlike in true tumor progression, MRI perfusion maps often show a *decreased* or *stable* rCBV compared to the pre-treatment values.

Tumor pseudoprogression is associated with longer survival, and imaging findings likely reflect the strong response to the received therapy. Studies have also shown that tumors with hypermethylated MGMT promoter status have up to 91% incidence of pseudoprogression, possibly reflecting the increased sensitivity of these tumors to chemoradiation.[33] It is therefore important to identify pseudoprogression and differentiate it from true progression as it supports continuation of an efficacious treatment regimen.

TREATMENT RESPONSE AND PSEUDORESPONSE

Treatment response can be characterized by decreasing size and amount of tumor enhancement after initiation of therapy.

Correctly identifying treatment response is important in affirming the choice of treatment regimen. However, the pitfall of pseudoresponse must be considered whenever imaging suggests treatment response.

Pseudoresponse can mimic the conventional MRI findings of treatment response, when in reality the glioma is stable or has even progressed. This entity is seen most commonly after therapy with anti-angiogenic drugs such as bevacizumab, which act to inhibit VEGF. VEGF promotes neovascularity as well as increased capillary leakage in gliomas.[34,35]

Imaging findings in pseudoresponse may reveal an apparent decrease in the enhancing component of the tumor, but close examination of T2-weighted or FLAIR images will reveal that the tumor has either not changed or has grown. Some studies have demonstrated improvement of edema surrounding tumor in many patients undergoing anti-VEGF therapy, but they eventually demonstrate progression of hyperintense non-enhancing tumor, best represented on FLAIR sequences.[36,37] MR perfusion may also reveal that the areas of apparent decreased enhancement still demonstrate relatively high rCBV.[38,39] Follow-up imaging is essential to confirm the true status of the tumor.

> Imaging findings in pseudoresponse may reveal the apparent decrease in enhancing component of the tumor, but close examination of T2-weighted or FLAIR images will reveal that the tumor has either not changed or has grown.

Imaging as a diagnostic or surveillance tool is integral to the management of brain tumors. Conventional MRI is still the workhorse of neuro-oncologic imaging, although some of the advanced imaging techniques such as DWI and perfusion-weighted imaging have also become essential considering the complex imaging appearance noted following therapy of these infiltrative tumors. Neuro-oncologists treating these patients are usually very well versed with common imaging patterns seen with these tumors, both before and after treatment. Nevertheless, focused discussions in multidisciplinary tumor boards of the clinical and molecular tumor characteristics and their correlation with imaging findings definitely influences and enhances clinical decision-making in a significant number of these patients.

RESPONSE ASSESSMENT IN NEURO-ONCOLOGY (RANO) CRITERIA

Response assessment in neuro-oncology (RANO) criteria are being used in neuro-oncology to assess treatment response in high-grade gliomas. These criteria address many limitations of the previously used Macdonald criteria by including definitions for disease progression and measurable disease and allowance of up to five target lesions. RANO criteria address problems in tumor measurement posed by pseudoprogression and pseudoresponse. In addition, the RANO criteria also include the presence of significant T2/FLAIR hyperintense non-enhancing disease in their definition of progression.[40]

RANO criteria define response to treatment based on imaging (MRI) and clinical features and recognizes the entities of complete response, partial response, stable disease, and progression of disease.

In addition, the RANO criteria provide guidance in regards to "measurable" and "non-measurable" lesions. Measurable disease comprises those enhancing lesions with clearly defined margins and two perpendicular diameters of at least 10 mm, visible on two or more axial slices preferably more than 5 mm thick, with no interslice gap. Cystic cavities should not be measured.

Complete response is defined as disappearance of all enhancing disease (measurable and non-measurable) sustained for at least 4 weeks with stable or improved non-enhancing FLAIR/T2W lesions and no new lesions. This should be without corticosteroids in patients who are clinically stable or improving.

> Measurable disease comprises of enhancing lesions with clearly defined margins and two perpendicular diameters of at least 10 mm, visible on two or more axial slices preferably more than 5 mm thick with no interslice gap. Cystic cavities should not be measured.

Partial response is defined as 50% or more reduction in all measurable enhancing lesions, no progression of non-measurable disease, stable or improved non-enhancing FLAIR/T2W lesions, and no new lesions. This should be with similar or reduced corticosteroid doses (compared to baseline) in patients who are clinically stable or improving.

Stable disease is one that does not qualify for complete response, partial response, or progression and features stable non-enhancing FLAIR/T2W lesions, stable or reduced corticosteroids (compared to baseline), and clinical stability.

Progression is defined as 25% or more increase in enhancing lesions, significant increase in non-enhancing FLAIR/T2W lesions, or development of any new lesions with clinical deterioration (that is not attributable to other non-tumor causes or reduction in steroids).

Beyond the RANO criteria for high-grade glioma, the RANO working group has also proposed response criteria for low-grade gliomas that are similar to those for high-grade gliomas but that measure tumor lesions based on T2/FLAIR rather than contrast enhancement as these tumors rarely enhance after gadolinium administration. In addition, because responses are often relatively modest, minor response criteria that are characterized by a decrease in T2/FLAIR tumor of 25–50% was introduced for low-grade gliomas.[40]

> The RANO working group has also proposed response criteria for low-grade gliomas that are similar to that for high-grade gliomas but that measure lesions based on T2/FLAIR.

Furthermore, the *immunotherapy response assessment for neuro-oncology* (iRANO) criteria have been developed to address the challenges of emerging novel immunotherapy for high-grade gliomas. iRANO criteria are based on guidance for determination of tumor progression outlined by the immune-related response criteria (irRC) and the RANO working group.[41] Among patients who demonstrate imaging findings meeting RANO criteria for progressive disease within 6 months of initiating immunotherapy including the development of new lesions, confirmation of radiographic progression with another 3-month follow-up imaging is recommended before progression of disease can be determined, provided the patient does not have new or worsening neurologic deficits.[41]

IMAGING OF SPECIFIC TUMOR SUBTYPES

CIRCUMSCRIBED GLIAL TUMORS

Pilocytic astrocytoma (PA) is a WHO grade 1 circumscribed glial tumor. It is the most common primary brain tumor in children, accounting for 15% of all pediatric brain tumors.[42] The cerebellum is the most common location. On imaging, the typical pilocytic astrocytoma appears as a cystic mass lesion with an intensely enhancing mural nodule (Figure 2.1C,D). Pilocytic astrocytomas can also present as an infiltrating lesion along the optic pathway,[43] causing enlargement of the optic nerve. Optic nerve pilocytic astrocytomas can often be seen in patients with neurofibromatosis type 1 (NF1).

> On imaging, the typical pilocytic astrocytoma appears as a cystic mass lesion with an intensely enhancing mural nodule.

Pilomyxoid astrocytoma is an uncommon, aggressive neoplasm that was previously considered a "juvenile" variant of PA. However, it is now recognized as a distinct entity with unique clinical characteristics and histological appearance. These tumors usually present in young children. The hypothalamus/optic chiasm is the most common location.[44] On imaging, they are usually bulky masses in a suprasellar location, which can show hemorrhage and cerebrospinal fluid (CSF) dissemination.

Subependymal giant cell astrocytomas (SEGAs) are WHO grade 1 tumors usually associated with tuberous sclerosis (TS). These tumors typically appear as subependymal masses extending into the ventricles that enlarge over time (on serial imaging). They are often located near the foramen of Monro. They frequently show intense enhancement and calcifications.

Pleomorphic xanthoastrocytomas (PXA) are rare WHO grade 2 tumors, typically seen in children and young adults. Anaplastic pleomorphic xanthoastrocytoma (WHO grade 3) has been added to the 2016 CNS WHO classification as a distinct entity.[3] These are superficially located solid-cystic tumors with a predilection for the temporal lobe. They typically have an enhancing solid component and a cystic component that appears hyperintense to CSF on FLAIR images due to its high protein content. Often, there is little or no surrounding edema. These tumors commonly involve the overlying leptomeninges[45] (Figure 2.10).

> Pleomorphic xanthoastrocytomas typically have an enhancing solid component and a cystic component that appears hyperintense to CSF on FLAIR images due to its high protein content. Often, there is little or no surrounding edema. These tumors commonly involve the overlying leptomeninges.

EPENDYMAL TUMORS

Ependymomas comprise low-grade (WHO grade 2) tumors and histologically aggressive anaplastic ependymomas (WHO grade 3). Recently, there has been a shift toward molecular markers to subdivide ependymomas in order to predict treatment response and prognosis. These molecular subgroups correlate with location on imaging.[42] The more common infratentorial ependymomas are either posterior fossa A (lateral) or posterior fossa B (midline) subgroups. Ependymoma, RELA fusion-positive, and ependymoma, YAP1 fusion-positive, are new tumor entities in the 2016 WHO classification that are characterized by supratentorial location. It is estimated that 40% of ependymomas are supratentorial and 60% are infratentorial in location.[46] Posterior fossa ependymomas are more common in children and present as T1 iso- to hypointense, T2 hyperintense, heterogeneously enhancing intraventricular masses filling the fourth ventricle and extending through the foramina of Luschka and Magendie (Figure 2.11). They may show necrosis, calcifications (50%), cystic changes (50%), and hemorrhage. Solid components may show restricted diffusion, especially in anaplastic tumors. Due to their location, these lesions can cause obstructive hydrocephalus. CSF seeding can commonly be seen; therefore imaging of the entire neuroaxis is recommended as part of the workup.[47]

Subependymomas are well-circumscribed, slow-growing, WHO grade 1 tumors that are considered benign entities and usually found in middle-aged and older adults. The fourth ventricle is the most common location, and they usually appear as small, T2 hyperintense, non-enhancing intraventricular lesions without any surrounding edema. Cystic changes and calcifications may be seen.[48]

CHOROID PLEXUS TUMORS

Choroid plexus tumors are papillary neoplasms derived from the choroid plexus epithelium and comprise benign choroid plexus papillomas and choroid plexus carcinomas. *Choroid plexus papilloma* (CPP) is a WHO grade 1 tumor that is commonly seen in children under 5 years of age.[49] On imaging, CPP typically appears as a lobulated contrast-enhancing intraventricular mass that is commonly seen at the trigone of the lateral ventricle and can be associated with hydrocephalus. It enhances in a "frondlike" pattern. Calcifications can be seen in 25% of cases.[49] There is also an

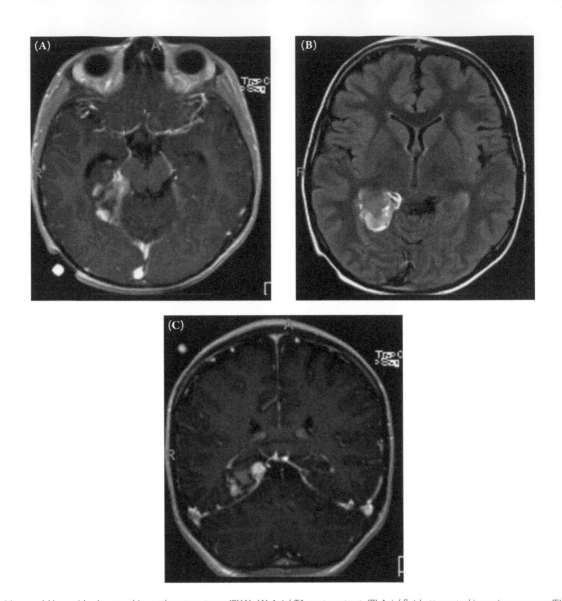

Figure 2.10 A 14-year-old boy with pleomorphic xanthoastrocytoma (PXA). (A) Axial T1 post-contrast, (B) Axial fluid-attenuated inversion recovery (FLAIR) and (C) coronal T1 post-contrast images show a heterogeneous enhancing right temporal lesion along the right tentorium with dural involvement. There is little or no surrounding edema.

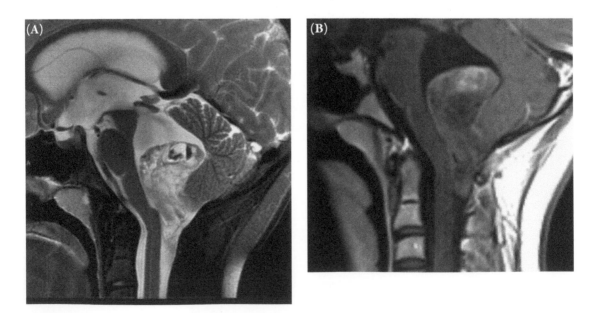

Figure 2.11 An 18-year-old man with ependymoma. (A) Sagittal T2 and (B) sagittal T1 post-contrast images show a T2 hyperintense, heterogeneous, enhancing intraventricular mass filling the fourth ventricle and extending through the foramen of Magendie.

increased risk for CSF seeding. While it is difficult to differentiate choroid plexus papilloma from carcinoma on imaging, imaging features of increased tumor heterogeneity, brain invasion, and CSF seeding are more in favor of choroid plexus carcinomas.[50]

NEURONAL, NEUROEPITHELIAL, AND MIXED NEURONAL–GLIAL TUMORS

These are WHO grade 1 or grade 2 tumors that are often associated with seizures. These tumors are less aggressive and have a favorable prognosis compared to most other glial tumors.[51]

Dysembryoplastic neuroepithelial tumor (DNET) is a slow-growing tumor with predilection for the cortex in the temporal and frontal lobes of children and young adults presenting with complex partial seizures. These lesions are often associated with cortical dysplasia.[52] On imaging, these tumors are characterized as well-circumscribed, T1 hypointense, T2 hyperintense lesions with multicystic or septated "bubbly" appearance (Figure 2.12). Contrast enhancement is uncommon and seen in only one-third of cases.[53] These lesions can show a "hyperintense ring sign" on FLAIR images.[54] While calcification may be seen, there is typically no surrounding edema, and there is no restriction of diffusion.

Gangliogliomas are low-grade tumors commonly seen in young patients with temporal lobe epilepsy. On imaging, these tumors can either appear as a solid mass or a cystic lesion with an enhancing mural nodule. There is typically very little edema or mass effect. Calcification can be seen in up to 30% cases.[55] The solid component often shows a variable degree of enhancement in approximately 50% cases. The cystic component can show variable signal due to variable degrees of proteinaceous or hemorrhagic contents.[56]

Gangliocytomas are uncommon and benign tumors, most often seen in children presenting with epilepsy. On imaging, there is usually an enhancing-solid cortical lesion without any perilesional edema. It may show calcification and cystic change.[55]

Dysplastic cerebellar gangliocytoma (also called *Lhermitte-Duclos disease*; LDD) is a benign hamartomatous cerebellar lesion characterized by overgrowth of the cerebellar cortex. It has a typical striated imaging appearance, which has also been described as "laminated" or "corduroy." The striated appearance is due to alternating isointense and hypointense signals on T1 weighted images.[57] Enhancement is rare. This lesion may show T2 shine-through on diffusion.

> Dysplastic cerebellar gangliocytoma has a typical striated imaging appearance, which has also been described as "laminated" or "corduroy."

Central neurocytoma is a WHO grade 2 intraventricular tumor, most commonly seen in young adults. It usually appears as a heterogeneous lobulated mass with numerous cystic areas, most commonly located in the lateral ventricle and with attachment to the septum pellucidum. It may show calcification, hemorrhage, and prominent flow voids. These lesions show moderate heterogeneous enhancement, and the solid component typically shows restricted diffusion. Obstructive hydrocephalus is fairly common.[58]

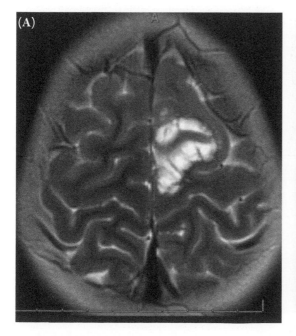 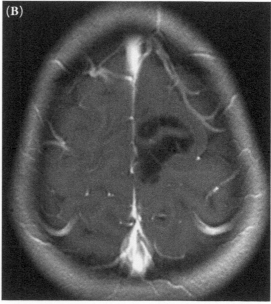

Figure 2.12 A 7-year-old boy fell at school; imaging shows an incidentally found lesion: dysembryoplastic neuroepithelial tumor (DNET). (A) Axial T2 image shows hyperintense lesion with multicystic/septated "bubbly" appearance. (B) Axial T1 post-contrast image shows absence of enhancement in the lesion.

Diffuse leptomeningeal glioneuronal tumor is a newly recognized entity in the 2016 WHO classification. These tumors appear as thick nodular leptomeningeal enhancement along the basal cisterns and surface of brain and spinal cord in children and adolescents presenting with hydrocephalus. Another peculiar and specific neuroradiological finding in these tumors is the presence of numerous small cysts scattered over the surface of the cerebellum, brainstem, spinal cord, medial temporal lobes, and inferior frontal lobes.[59] It is difficult to differentiate this tumor from other causes of leptomeningeal enhancement on imaging, and the differential diagnosis includes tubercular meningitis, leptomeningeal carcinomatosis, and leptomeningeal seeding from other primary CNS tumors.

It is difficult to differentiate diffuse leptomeningeal glioneuronal tumor from other causes of leptomeningeal enhancement on imaging and the differential diagnosis includes tubercular meningitis, leptomeningeal carcinomatosis, and leptomeningeal seeding from other primary CNS tumors.

MULTINODULAR AND VACUOLATING NEURONAL TUMOR

Multinodular and vacuolating neuronal tumor (MVNT) is a newly recognized architectural appearance in the 2016 WHO classification that may be related to ganglion cell tumors.[3] Patients with MVNT may be asymptomatic or can present with seizures or headaches.[60] MVNT has distinct radiological features and appears as a cluster of tiny, T2 hyperintense nodular lesions along deep cortical ribbon and superficial subcortical white matter following a gyral contour.[61] There is no associated edema or mass effect. These lesions do not suppress on FLAIR images, do not show any diffusion restriction, and there is no enhancement (Figure 2.13). MVNT is a probable

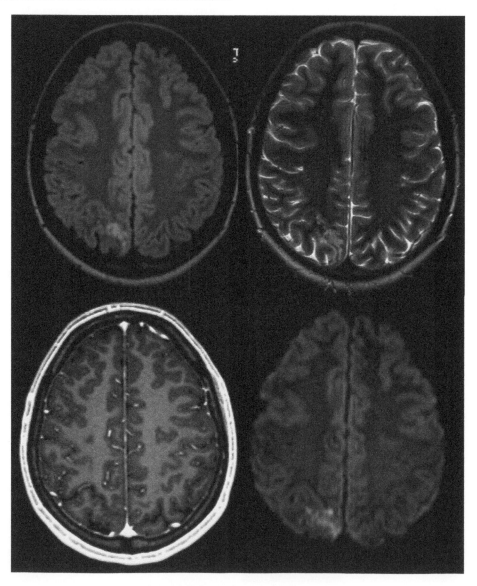

Figure 2.13 *Multinodular and vacuolating neuronal tumor (MVNT). Axial fluid-attenuated inversion recovery (FLAIR), axial T2, axial post-contrast T1, and axial diffusion images show a cluster of tiny T2 hyperintense nodular lesions in the right parietal subcortical white matter that do not suppress on FLAIR images and do not show any enhancement.*

low-grade epilepsy-associated lesion in patients of all ages, with a benign and stable course as it constitutes a curable cause of focal epilepsy.[62]

PINEAL PARENCHYMAL TUMORS

Pineal parenchymal tumors include low-grade pineocytoma, pineal parenchymal tumor of intermediate differentiation (PPTID), and the highly malignant pineoblastoma.[63] These intrinsic pineal tumors need to be differentiated from other tumors that can arise in the pineal region, especially germinoma, which is the most common tumor in pineal region. In contrast to pineal parenchymal tumors like pineocytoma or pineoblastoma, which characteristically "disperse" calcification peripherally, germ cell tumors tend to engulf the calcification.[64]

> Pineoblastomas appear as large pineal masses with intermediate signal intensity on T1 and T2 sequences and heterogeneous enhancement. They can invade the adjacent brain parenchyma and often show calcification, cystic change, necrosis, and restricted diffusion.

Pineoblastomas are malignant WHO grade 4 tumors that most often occur in children. These typically appear as large pineal masses with intermediate signal intensity on T1 and T2 sequences and heterogeneous enhancement. They can invade the adjacent brain parenchyma and often show calcification, cystic change, necrosis, and restricted diffusion. These tumors have a high risk for leptomeningeal seeding (45%), and imaging of the entire neuroaxis is typically recommended.[65]

PPTIDs are rare WHO grade 2 or grade 3 tumors. PPTIDs are lobulated, vascular pineal region masses that can extend into adjacent structures such as the ventricles or thalami. They are usually hyperdense on CT due to high cellularity. On MRI, PPTIDs appear as T1 hypointense, T2 hyperintense heterogeneously enhancing masses. They are likely to be larger, more heterogeneous, and more locally invasive than pineocytomas. Subarachnoid and spinal seeding is less likely compared to pineoblastomas.[66]

> On MRI, PPTIDs appear as T1 hypointense, T2 hyperintense heterogeneously enhancing masses. They are likely to be larger, more heterogeneous, and more locally invasive than pineocytomas.

Pineocytomas are WHO grade 1 tumors, commonly seen in adults from the third to sixth decades. They are small, well-circumscribed, solid enhancing tumors. Cystic change is common.

Pineal cysts are thin-walled simple cysts that are commonly seen in the pineal region as incidental findings. However, large size, presence of a thick and irregular cystic wall, or enhancing-solid components in a pineal cyst should raise suspicion of a pineal tumor.

EMBRYONAL TUMORS

Medulloblastoma (WHO grade 4) is the most common pediatric malignant brain tumor. Medulloblastoma is no longer thought of as a single entity. The 2016 WHO classification of CNS tumors has divided medulloblastomas into four distinct molecular subgroups with overlapping clinical, histological, and imaging features.[67] These subgroups are WNT, SHH, Group 3, and Group 4.[3] On imaging, typical medulloblastoma is a well-defined midline mass arising from the cerebellar vermis. They are usually hyperdense on CT. On MRI, medulloblastomas are hypointense on T1, iso- to hyperintense on T2/FLAIR, show restricted diffusion, and have marked heterogeneous enhancement with surrounding edema (Figure 2.14). These tumors may appear heterogeneous due to calcification, necrosis, and cystic changes. Commonly, there is associated hydrocephalus.

> Typically, medulloblastomas appear as a well-defined midline mass arising from the cerebellar vermis. They are usually hyperdense on CT. On MRI, medulloblastomas are hypointense on T1, iso- to hyperintense on T2/FLAIR, show restricted diffusion, and have marked heterogeneous enhancement with surrounding edema.

The molecular subgroup of medulloblastomas can be predicted on the basis of their location on imaging. WNT subgroup lesions have the best prognosis and are usually located in the cerebellar peduncle. In contrast, group 3, group 4, and some SHH subgroup tumors are commonly seen in the midline cerebellar vermis. In adults, SHH subgroup medulloblastomas can also be located laterally in the cerebellar hemispheres. MR spectroscopy typically shows elevated choline peak, reduced NAA and creatine, and, occasionally, elevated lipid and lactate peaks, which is a characteristic sign for neuroectodermal tumors but not necessarily specific for medulloblastoma.[68] CSF seeding is common at presentation, therefore contrast-enhanced imaging of the entire neuraxis is recommended.

Embryonal tumor with multilayered rosettes (ETMR) is a new entity in the 2016 WHO classification. ETMR usually occurs in children younger than 4 years and is more common in girls.[69] They are more commonly seen in the supratentorial compartment. On imaging, ETMR usually presents as a large tumor with frequent calcifications, little to no edema, absent or weak contrast enhancement, intratumoral veins, restricted diffusion, and low cerebral blood flow.[70]

Atypical teratoid/rhabdoid tumor (ATRT) is a malignant WHO grade 4 tumor that usually occurs in very young children. It can be infratentorial or supratentorial; however, the cerebellum is the most common location. It appears as a rapidly progressive, large, heterogeneous invasive mass lesion with necrosis, cyst formation, hemorrhage, and restricted diffusion. CSF seeding may be seen. These tumors can resemble medulloblastomas on imaging, however, ATRT presents at a younger age than medulloblastoma, and intratumoral hemorrhage is relatively more common in ATRT.[71]

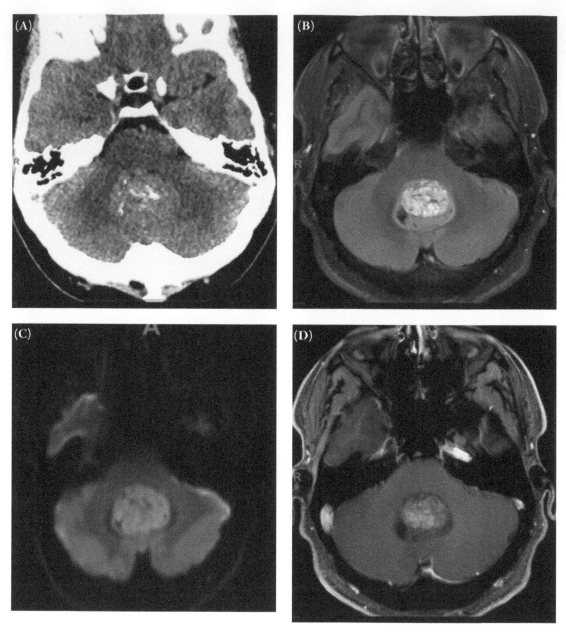

Figure 2.14 *A 31-year-old man with medulloblastoma. (A) Axial CT image shows a hyperdense mass with calcifications in the midline cerebellar vermis. (B) Axial fluid-attenuated inversion recovery (FLAIR) shows a hyperintense vermian mass projecting into the fourth ventricle. (C) Axial diffusion image shows restricted diffusion due to high cellularity of the lesion. (D) Axial T1 post-contrast image shows marked enhancement.*

MENINGIOMAS

Meningiomas are the most common benign intracranial tumors. While the vast majority represents benign (WHO grade 1) tumors, there are histological variants which show more aggressive biological behavior.[72] Atypical meningiomas (WHO grade 2) account for up to 30% and anaplastic or malignant meningiomas (WHO grade 3) account for nearly 1% of meningiomas.[73] Presence of brain invasion on histology is now considered a diagnostic criterion for higher-grade meningiomas.[3] Meningiomas are extra-axial mass lesions with a broad-based dural attachment. They are usually hyperdense on CT and can show calcification in 20–30% cases. There may be associated bony changes like hyperostosis (Figure 2.15).

On MRI, meningiomas are usually hypo- to isointense on T1, iso- to hyperintense on T2W images. They frequently show restricted diffusion and intense homogeneous enhancement with a characteristic dural tail. Approximately 15% of benign meningiomas appear as multiple tumors and demonstrate features such as tumor necrosis, cystic change, hemorrhage, and fatty infiltration.[74] Peritumoral brain edema may be seen, but this does not reliably distinguish between benign and atypical/anaplastic meningiomas. MR spectroscopy shows choline and alanine peaks with reduced NAA. Elevated alanine is relatively specific for meningioma but can be difficult to identify. Perfusion imaging shows high relative cerebral blood flow (rCBF) and rCBV.

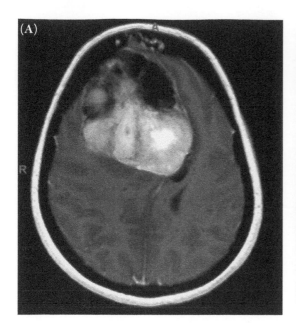 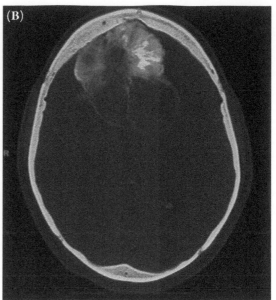

Figure 2.15 Meningioma. (A) Axial T1 post-contrast image shows a contrast-enhancing right frontal parafalcine extra-axial mass lesion with mass effect and midline shift. (B) Axial CT image shows calcification in the mass and associated hyperostosis in the right frontal bone.

On MRI, meningiomas are usually hypo- to isointense on T1, iso- to hyperintense on T2W images. They frequently show restricted diffusion and intense homogeneous enhancement with a characteristic dural tail.

MESENCHYMAL, NON-MENINGOTHELIAL TUMORS

Solitary fibrous tumors are grouped together with *hemangiopericytomas* in the 2016 WHO classification.[3] Solitary fibrous tumors of the dura are WHO grade 1 tumors, whereas hemangiopericytomas are WHO grade 2 or grade 3 (anaplastic) tumors. Solitary fibrous tumors occur in middle-aged individuals. They are usually hyperdense on CT and may show calcifications and erosion of the adjacent bone. These tumors show isointense signal on T1, iso- to hypointense signal on T2, and heterogeneous enhancement. They can show areas of restricted diffusion.[75,76] Hemangiopericytomas are seen in younger adults (30–50 years) and usually appear as large, lobulated, vividly enhancing, heterogeneous locally invasive extra-axial dural masses that can cause bone destruction.[76]

HEMANGIOBLASTOMA

Hemangioblastomas are WHO grade 1 tumors of vascular origin, and the majority is seen in the posterior fossa in adults. They have an association with von Hippel Lindau (vHL) disease but can also occur sporadically. On imaging, hemangioblastomas typically appear as solid enhancing mural nodules with an adjacent non-enhancing peripheral cyst. They can also be purely solid tumors. The most common appearance is that of a well-defined cystic lesion with an intensely enhancing solid mural nodule. Characteristically, there is no enhancement in the cyst wall. Peripheral serpentine flow voids may be seen in the cyst.[77]

CNS LYMPHOMA

Primary CNS lymphoma (PCNSL) by definition is limited to the brain, leptomeninges, eyes, and rarely the spinal cord, without evidence of systemic disease at primary diagnosis.[78] It is usually seen in patients older than 50 years and can be sporadic or associated with HIV and an immunocompromised state. PCNSL often has a characteristic imaging appearance due to its hypercellularity, high nuclear-to-cytoplasmic ratio, disruption of the blood–brain barrier, and predilection for the periventricular and superficial regions.[79] Lesions are usually hyperdense on CT. On MRI, PCNSL typically presents as single or multiple, relatively T2- hypointense lesions showing restricted diffusion and marked enhancement in the periventricular location (along the ependymal surface of the ventricles) or in the corpus callosum (Figure 2.16). MR spectroscopy shows markedly reduced NAA, large choline peak, elevated choline-to-creatine ratio, and lipid and lactate peaks. Lipid peak in the absence of necrosis seems to be the most specific finding in PCNSL.[80] MR perfusion shows mild increase in rCBV. PET shows increased FDG uptake. Of note, the imaging appearance of lymphoma can change significantly after administration of steroids, with reduction in contrast enhancement and edema.

Lymphoma lesions are usually hyperdense on CT. On MRI, PCNSL typically presents as single or multiple, relatively T2- hypointense lesions showing restricted diffusion and marked enhancement in the periventricular location (along the ependymal surface of the ventricles) or in the corpus callosum.

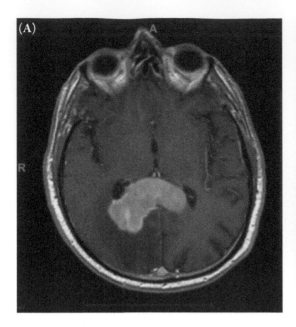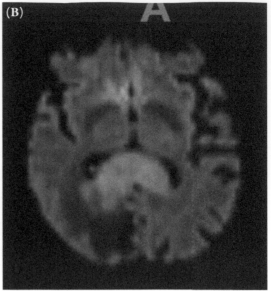

Figure 2.16 A 78-year-old woman with lymphoma. (A) Axial T1 post-contrast image shows an intensely enhancing mass lesion in the splenium of corpus callosum. (B) Axial diffusion image shows restricted diffusion in the mass due to high cellularity.

Secondary CNS lymphoma is more common than primary CNS lymphoma, and leptomeningeal involvement is much more common than parenchymal lesions. Contrast- enhanced MRI frequently shows leptomeningeal or cranial nerve enhancement, superficial cerebral lesions, and communicating hydrocephalus.[79]

CHRONIC LYMPHOCYTIC INFLAMMATION WITH PONTINE PERIVASCULAR ENHANCEMENT RESPONSIVE TO STEROIDS (CLIPPERS)

CLIPPERS is an uncommon disorder characterized by infiltration of the brain by inflammatory cells, predominantly T-cell lymphocytes. It has a predilection for the pons, with variable extension into adjacent structures such as the cerebellum, medulla oblongata, and midbrain. CLIPPERS has a fairly characteristic pattern of punctate and/or curvilinear enhancement "peppering" the pons with or without spread into the adjacent structures on contrast MRI (Figure 2.17), highly suggestive of a perivascular distribution.[81] Lesions usually cause no mass effect and minimal or no vasogenic edema.[82] This syndrome usually shows a prompt and significant response to steroid-based immunosuppression, with both radiological improvement and clinical response. CLIPPERS can be a differential diagnosis for diffuse intrinsic pontine glioma (DIPG) and lymphoma on imaging in some cases.

GERMINOMA

Germinomas are germ cell tumors that commonly occur in midline structures in young patients. The pineal gland is the most common location, followed by the suprasellar region.

They are hyperdense on non-contrast CT and can show central calcification. They appear isointense on T1, iso- to hyperintense on T2, and typically show intense enhancement (Figure 2.18). They may show cystic changes, hemorrhage, calcification, and edema due to involvement of the adjacent brain.[83] These lesions often show restricted diffusion due to high cellularity. Dissemination by CSF and invasion of the adjacent brain structures is common.[84]

TUMORS OF THE SELLAR REGION

Pituitary macroadenoma is the most common suprasellar mass in adults. They are larger than 10 mm in size and can present with compression of the optic chiasm and/or with endocrine disturbances. On MR imaging, they are characterized as sellar-suprasellar masses associated with intermediate signal intensity, moderate enhancement, with a "waist" at the diaphragma sellae or a "figure of eight" appearance.[85,86] The sella typically appears enlarged, and these tumors can invade the cavernous sinuses. Tumor necrosis and hemorrhage may be seen, and this can present with an acute clinical syndrome called *pituitary apoplexy*. They can be radiographically differentiated from meningiomas, which show stronger enhancement and cause narrowing of the flow void and encasement of the internal carotid artery (ICA). In case of a meningioma, the pituitary gland may be identified separately from the mass.[87]

Craniopharyngiomas are WHO grade 1 sellar-suprasellar tumors which are usually seen in children between 5 and 15 years of age. They are subdivided into the adamantinomatous subtype, which presents as a cystic mass in children and is more common than the papillary subtype, which presents as a solid mass in older adults (Figure 2.19). On imaging, they can appear as large multiloculated cystic lesions with small enhancing solid components. Calcification is seen in up to

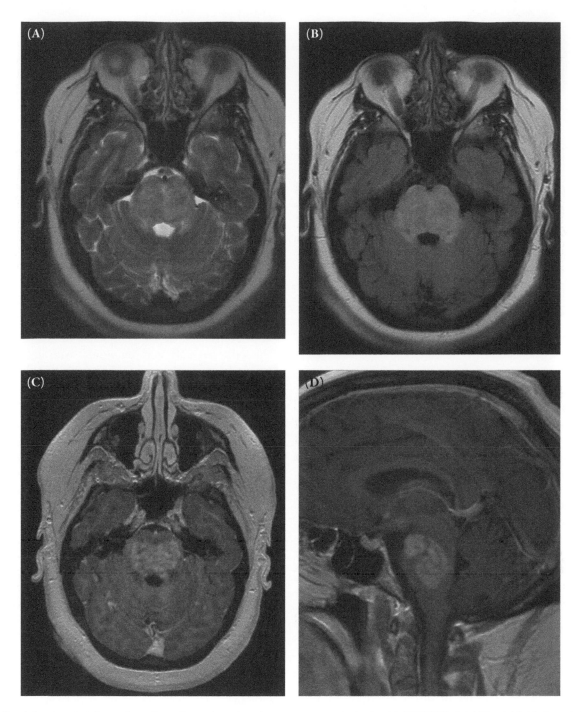

Figure 2.17 Chronic lymphocytic inflammation with pontine perivascular enhancement responsive to steroids (CLIPPERS). Axial T2, axial fluid-attenuated inversion recovery (FLAIR), post-contrast axial and sagittal T1 W images show diffuse T2 and FLAIR hyperintense signal in pons with patchy and curvilinear enhancement "peppering" the pons without any significant mass effect.

90% of pediatric craniopharyngiomas.[88] The cystic component can show isointense to hyperintense signal on T1 due to pro-teinaceous "motor oil" contents.

BRAIN METASTASES

Imaging of brain metastases is challenging due to difficulties in reliably differentiating metastases from potential mimics such as primary brain tumors and infection, detecting small metastases,

and differentiating treatment response from tumor recurrence and progression. MRI remains the modality of choice to identify brain metastases and monitor their response to treatment.[89] On standard imaging, metastatic lesions are usually well-defined enhancing lesions located at the gray–white matter junction, with a disproportionate amount of vasogenic edema. They can show nodular or ring enhancement. Calcification and hemor-rhage may be seen in metastatic lesions from certain primary tumors. T1 hyperintensity can be seen in hemorrhagic and mel-anoma metastases. Larger metastases tend to become necrotic

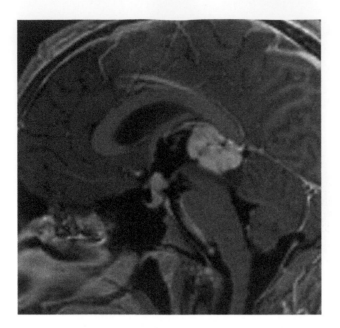

Figure 2.18 A 15-year-old girl with germinoma. Sagittal T1 post-contrast image shows intensely enhancing midline masses in the pineal and suprasellar regions.

centrally and may appear cystic. Tiny superficial nodular cortical metastatic lesions are sometimes only detected on contrast enhanced scans. Delayed sequences may show additional lesions. Advanced imaging, including perfusion, diffusion, and MR spectroscopy of peritumoral regions, may help differentiate primary from metastatic disease. MR spectroscopy of metastatic lesions typically shows reduced NAA and an intratumoral choline peak with no choline elevation in the peritumoral edema. This differentiates metastases from glioblastomas on MR spectroscopy. MR perfusion and amino acid PET are proving valuable adjuvants to standard imaging in distinguishing radiation necrosis from treatment effect. Standardization and validation of these biomarkers are ongoing endeavors.[89]

LEPTOMENINGEAL METASTASES

Leptomeningeal metastases can be seen in many primary CNS tumors due to involvement of subarachnoid CSF space by malignant cells as a result of direct extension or drop metastases. Leptomeningeal metastases can also occur due to hematogenous spread from distant tumors like breast, lung, melanoma, gastrointestinal, and hematological malignancies. Leptomeningeal metastases appears as diffuse continuous leptomeningeal enhancement on post-contrast MRI (Figure 2.20). FLAIR images may show abnormal hyperintense signal within the sulci. Contrast-enhanced FLAIR imaging has superior sensitivity to contrast-enhanced T1-weighted MR imaging in detecting leptomeningeal metastases.[90]

PSEUDOTUMORS AND TUMOR MIMICS

Intracranial inflammatory pseudotumors (IIPs) are non-neoplastic "mass-like" lesions which could be infectious, inflammatory, or reactive and reparative processes. Inflammatory pseudotumors are characterized histologically by the presence of acute and chronic inflammatory cells with a predominance of lymphocytes, variable fibrous response, and prominent fibrocollagenous stroma. If their etiology is unknown, IIPs are designated as "idiopathic," although a growing number of these lesions now have known causes such as chronic dural sinus thrombosis, inflammatory myofibroblastic tumor, and IgG4-related disease.[51]

Idiopathic IIP can present as hypertrophic pachymeningitis, which can appear as T2 hypointense dural thickening along the posterior falx and tentorium with intense peripheral enhancement around a central non-enhancing area, an appearance that has been described as the "Eiffel by night" sign.[91]

In addition to idiopathic IIP, the differential diagnosis of a non-invasive dural-based mass includes *en plaque* meningioma, dural metastases, neurosarcoidosis, and tuberculosis.[51]

> Idiopathic IIP can present as hypertrophic pachymeningitis, which can appear as T2 hypointense dural thickening along the posterior falx and tentorium with intense peripheral enhancement around a central non-enhancing area, an appearance that has been described as the "Eiffel by night" sign.

However, idiopathic inflammatory pseudotumors can also invade bone, meninges, and dural venous sinuses as well as brain parenchyma. On imaging, invasive IIPs can appear as dural-based soft-tissue mass lesions with adjacent bone destruction. It can behave aggressively and may simulate a malignant neoplasm.

Inflammatory myofibroblastic tumor (also called *plasma cell granuloma*) is now recognized as distinct pathologic entity. It is a myofibroblastic neoplasm that is rare in the CNS. On imaging, there is T1 isointense, T2 hypointense, intensely enhancing focal mass-like dural thickening. Invasion of adjacent brain can be seen in 10% cases.[51]

Other *tumor-like inflammatory lesions* (tumor mimics) in the brain include tumefactive demyelination, tumefactive vasculitis, tumefactive cerebral amyloid angiopathy–related inflammation (CAA-I), thrombosed vascular malformation, textiloma, and calcifying pseudoneoplasm of the neuroaxis (CAPNON).

Open rim enhancement can help in differentiating tumefactive demyelination from a neoplasm.[92] These lesions show low rCBV on perfusion maps compared to high-grade gliomas[93] (Figure 2.21).

Thrombosed vascular malformation will usually show tortuous vessels, thrombosed venous sinus, edema, variable hemorrhage, and minimal enhancement.

On imaging, CAA-I (also called *amyloidoma*) can present as patchy or confluent T2/FLAIR hyperintense lesions with prominent vasogenic edema and absent contrast enhancement.[94] T2*-weighted gradient-recalled echo (T2*-GRE) or SWI demonstrate extensive cortical microbleeds, lobar macrobleeds, and marginal siderosis. CAA-I can be misinterpreted as CNS neoplasm due to absence of T2*-GRE

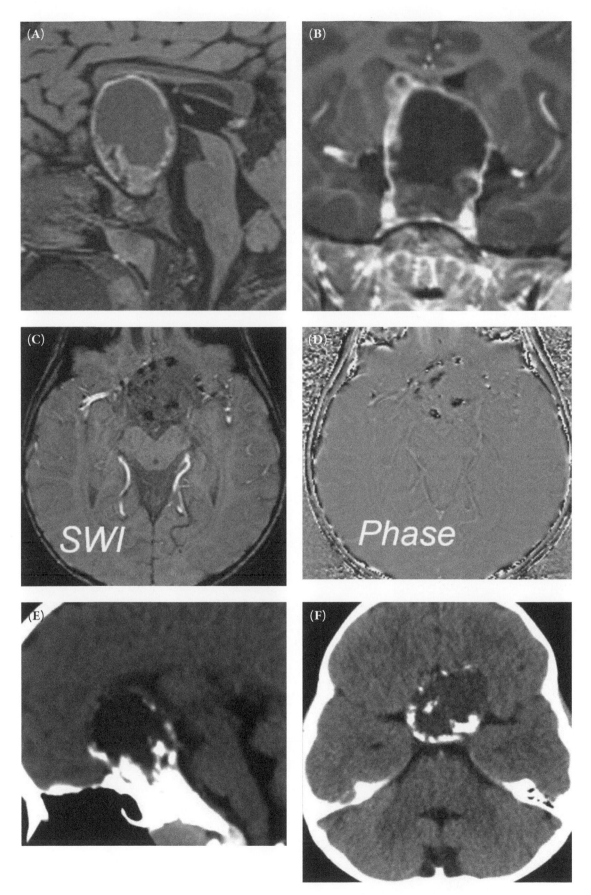

Figure 2.19 Craniopharyngioma, adamantinomatous type. (A) Sagittal fluid-attenuated inversion recovery (FLAIR) and (B) coronal T1 post-contrast images show a suprasellar cystic mass lesion with a small enhancing solid component. (C) Axial SWI. (D) Axial phase image. (E) Axial CT and (F) sagittal CT images show peripheral calcification in the lesion.

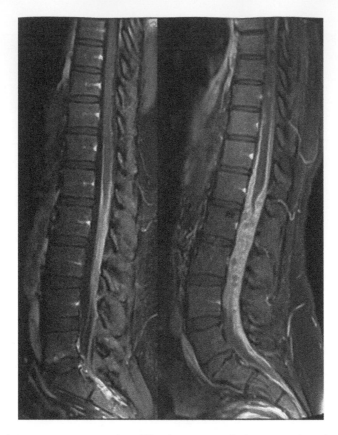

Figure 2.20 *Melanoma metastasis. Sagittal T1 post-contrast images show diffuse leptomeningeal enhancement along the conus and cauda equina nerve roots due to leptomeningeal metastases.*

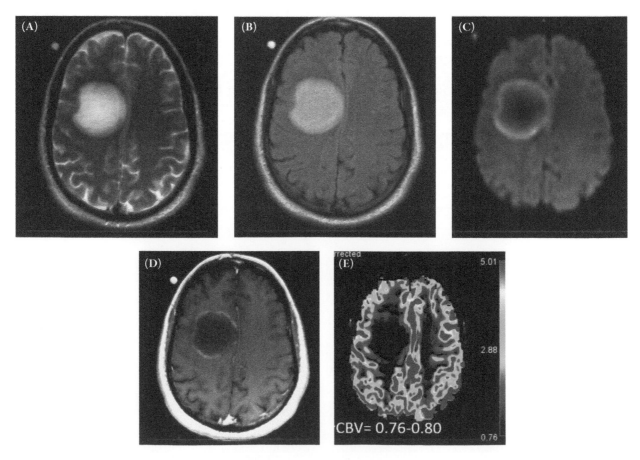

Figure 2.21 *Tumefactive demyelination. (A) Axial T2 and (B) axial fluid-attenuated inversion recovery (FLAIR) images show a hyperintense mass lesion in the right frontal lobe. (C) Axial diffusion image shows restricted diffusion along the margin of the lesion. (D) Axial T1 post-contrast image shows open rim enhancement in this lesion. (E) Axial perfusion map shows very low rCBV in the lesion.*

sequences on initial imaging.[86] Rarely, cerebral microbleeds can be absent in CAA-I.[95]

A textiloma is characterized as a mass from retained surgical elements. It is iso- to hypointense on T2.[51] It can show variable degrees of associated edema and enhancement.

CAPNON or "brain rocks" can usually be seen in meninges or cerebral sulci (may appear intraparenchymal). On CT, these are discrete calcified masses with variable amounts of associated edema. On MRI, these lesions appear isointense on T1, hypointense on T2 with little mass effect, variable perilesional edema, and variable enhancement.[51] When considering the differential for calcifying intra- or extra-axial lesions, the uniform T1 and T2 hypointensity without solid enhancement is a key distinguishing feature. Calcified lesions with heterogeneous T2 signal intensity or T2 hyperintensity are more likely to be a calcified neoplasm and inconsistent with CAPNON. Calcified lesions with the typical popcorn "T2 hyperintensity" and hemosiderin ring are more consistent with cavernous malformation and also distinguish themselves from CAPNON.[96]

Can imaging inform molecular tumor characteristics?

Yes, there is growing interest in radiogenomics, as conventional and advanced imaging technology have been shown to correlate with certain molecular tumor characteristics

What is a commonly observed difference in the MRI appearance of IDH-wildtype or IDH-mutant gliomas, respectively?

Most IDH-mutant gliomas demonstrate less overall contrast enhancement

How may MRI be able to differentiate between MGMT methylated and MGMT unmethylated gliomas?

Nodular enhancement is more common in MGMT hypermethylated tumors, while rim enhancement is more commonly seen in MGMT unmethylated tumors

What is the typical appearance of 1p19q co-deleted gliomas (oligodendrogliomas)?

1p/19q co-deleted tumors often have indistinct tumor margins and contain calcifications

What is a radiogenomic biomarker for IDH-mutant and 1p19q intact gliomas?

The T2–FLAIR mismatch sign represents a highly specific imaging biomarker for IDH-mutant, 1p/19q intact low-grade gliomas

What is the typical predilection for tumor location of IDH-mutant versus IDH-mutant gliomas?

IDH-mutant gliomas commonly involve a single lobe, usually the frontal lobe. IDH-wildtype gliomas typically involve multiple lobes

How can diffusion-weighted imaging be useful in the differentiation of IDH-wildtype and IDH-mutant gliomas?

IDH-wildtype tumors typically demonstrate areas of lower ADC values compared to IDH-mutant tumors

What is the value of MR spectroscopy in IDH-mutant gliomas?

Detection of a characteristic 2-hydroxyglutarate (2-HG) peak on MR spectroscopy was found to be highly specific for IDH-mutant gliomas. This has not yet been translated into routine clinical practice

How is perfusion-weighted imaging utilized to describe IDH-wildtype versus IDH-mutant gliomas?

Perfusion imaging typically demonstrates higher elevation in blood volume in IDH-wildtype gliomas when compared to IDH-mutant gliomas

How is perfusion-weighted imaging utilized to differentiate between disease progression and pseudoprogression in glioblastoma patients who have received treatment with radiation and chemotherapy?	In the case of tumor progression, the area of increased enhancement often correlates with high blood volume, while lower blood volume values are observed in the case of pseudoprogression
What imaging appearance is associated with tumors characterized by a BRAF alteration?	BRAF alterations are commonly seen in lower grade gliomas in pediatric patients (e.g., pilocytic astrocytomas). These tumors are associated with a superficial or cortical location
What is the characteristic imaging appearance of H3K27M-mutant gliomas?	H3K27M-mutant tumors appear as infiltrative tumors and typically involve midline structures such as the thalamus, brainstem, and spinal cord
What is the typical imaging appearance of the various medulloblastoma subgroups?	Based on their molecular subtype, medulloblastomas may appear in characteristic supra- versus infratentorial locations within the brain, respectively

1. Which of the following tumor entity is not a part of the 2016 WHO classification of CNS tumors?
   a. Diffuse midline glioma
   b. Epithelioid glioblastoma
   c. Gliomatosis cerebri
   d. Medulloblastoma-WNT

2. Which of the following tumors is associated with tuberous sclerosis?
   a. Subependymal giant cell astrocytoma
   b. Optic nerve glioma
   c. Hemangioblastoma
   d. Medulloblastoma

3. Which molecular subtype of medulloblastoma is most likely to arise in the cerebellar peduncle?
   a. Group 3
   b. Group 4
   c. WNT
   d. SHH

4. Which of the following tumors is the least likely cause of CSF seeding/dissemination?
   a. Pineoblastoma
   b. Craniopharyngioma
   c. Ependymoma
   d. Medulloblastoma

5. Which of these statements is false about diffuse midline gliomas?
   a. Some of them were previously called diffuse intrinsic pontine gliomas (DIPG).
   b. They are H3 K27M-mutant.
   c. They are WHO grade 4 tumors.
   d. They usually show diffuse intense enhancement.

6. Which of these statements is false about primary CNS lymphoma (PCNSL)?
   a. They are usually hypodense on CT.
   b. They show restricted diffusion.
   c. Lipid peak may be seen on MR spectroscopy.
   d. Periventricular location is common.

7. Which of these tumors is usually seen in young children?
   a. Glioblastoma
   b. Primary CNS lymphoma
   c. Embryonal tumors with multilayered rosettes (ETMR)
   d. Meningioma

8. Which of these tumors is usually nonenhancing?
   a. Subependymoma
   b. Primary CNS lymphoma
   c. Medulloblastoma
   d. Hemangiopericytoma

9. Which of these tumors typically show IDH mutation and 1p/19q co-deletion?
   a. Ependymoma
   b. Oligodendroglioma
   c. Diffuse midline glioma
   d. Gangliocytoma

10. Which of these tumors commonly show multicystic bubbly appearance on T2W MRI?
    a. Solitary fibrous tumor
    b. Oligodendroglioma
    c. Dysembryoplastic neuroepithelial tumor (DNET)
    d. Germinoma

11. Which of these tumors commonly presents as an intraventricular mass attached to the wall of lateral ventricle or septum pellucidum with numerous intratumoral cystic areas?
    a. Ependymoma
    b. Choroid plexus papilloma
    c. Central neurocytoma
    d. Germinoma

12. "Which of these tumor shows a "laminated" or "corduroy" appearance?
    a. Medulloblastoma
    b. Dysplastic cerebellar gangliocytoma (Lhermitte-Duclos disease; LDD)
    c. Atypical teratoid/rhabdoid tumor (ATRT)
    d. Ependymoma

13. Which of these tumors is associated with bony hyperostosis?
    a. Meningioma
    b. Glioblastoma
    c. Pilocytic astrocytoma
    d. Craniopharyngioma

14. Which is the most common pineal region tumor?
    a. Pineoblastoma
    b. Pineocytoma
    c. Pineal parenchymal tumor with intermediate differentiation
    d. Germinoma

15. Which of these statements is false about pseudoprogression?
    a. Pseudoprogression is associated with longer survival.
    b. Studies have shown that tumors with hypermethylated MGMT promoter status have up to 91% incidence of pseudoprogression.
    c. MRI perfusion maps commonly show increase in relative cerebral blood volume (rCBV) in pseudoprogression compared to the pre-treatment values.
    d. Imaging can demonstrate increasing size of enhancing components of the tumor.

ANSWERS

1. c
2. a
3. c
4. b
5. d
6. a
7. c
8. a
9. b
10. c
11. c
12. b
13. a
14. d
15. c

REFERENCES

1. Smits M, van den Bent MJ. Imaging correlates of adult glioma genotypes. *Radiology*. 2017;284(2):316–331.
2. Jacobs AH, Kracht LW, Gossmann A, et al. Imaging in neurooncology. *NeuroRx*. 2005;2(2):333–347.
3. Louis DN, Perry A, Reifenberger G, et al. The 2016 World Health Organization Classification of Tumors of the Central Nervous System: A summary. *Acta Neuropathol*. 2016;131(6):803–820.
4. Louis DN, Ohgaki H, Wiestler OD et al. *World Health Organization Histological Classification of Tumors of the Central Nervous System*. 4th ed. rev. Paris: International Agency for Research on Cancer; 2016.
5. Carrillo JA, Lai A, Nghiemphu PL, et al. Relationship between tumor enhancement, edema, IDH1 mutational status, MGMT promoter methylation, and survival in glioblastoma. *AJNR Am J Neuroradiol*. 2012;33(7):1349–1355.
6. Drabycz S, Roldan G, de Robles P, et al. An analysis of image texture, tumor location, and MGMT promoter methylation in glioblastoma using magnetic resonance imaging. *Neuroimage*. 2010;49(2):1398–1405.
7. Kim JW, Park CK, Park SH, et al. Relationship between radiological characteristics and combined 1p and 19q deletion in World Health Organization grade III oligodendroglial tumours. *J Neurol Neurosurg Psychiatry*. 2011;82(2):224–227.
8. Megyesi JF, Kachur E, Lee DH, et al. Imaging correlates of molecular signatures in oligodendrogliomas. *Clin Cancer Res*. 2004;10(13):4303–4306.
9. Jenkinson MD, du Plessis DG, Smith TS, et al. Histological growth patterns and genotype in oligodendroglial tumours: Correlation with MRI features. *Brain*. 2006;129(Pt 7):1884–1891.
10. Patel SH, Poisson LM, Brat DJ, et al. T2-FLAIR mismatch, an imaging biomarker for IDH and 1p/19q status in lower-grade gliomas: A TCGA/TCIA project. *Clin Cancer Res*. 2017;23(20):6078–6085.
11. Broen MPG, Smits M, Wijnenga MMJ, et al. The T2-FLAIR mismatch sign as an imaging marker for non-enhancing IDH-mutant, 1p/19q-intact lower-grade glioma: A validation study. *Neuro Oncol*. 2018;20(10):1393–9.
12. Juratli TA, Tummala SS, Riedl A, et al. Radiographic assessment of contrast enhancement and T2/FLAIR mismatch sign in lower grade gliomas: Correlation with molecular groups. *J Neurooncol*. 2019;141(2):327–335.
13. Lasocki A, Gaillard F, Gorelik A, et al. MRI features can predict 1p/19q status in intracranial gliomas. *AJNR Am J Neuroradiol*. 2018;39(4):687–692.
14. Johnson DR, Kaufmann TJ, Patel SH, et al. There is an exception to every rule-T2-FLAIR mismatch sign in gliomas. *Neuroradiology*. 2019;61(2):225–227.
15. Wang Y, Zhang T, Li S, et al. Anatomical localization of isocitrate dehydrogenase 1 mutation: A voxel-based radiographic study of 146 low-grade gliomas. *Eur J Neurol*. 2015;22(2):348–354.
16. Qi S, Yu L, Li H, et al. Isocitrate dehydrogenase mutation is associated with tumor location and magnetic resonance imaging characteristics in astrocytic neoplasms. *Oncol Lett*. 2014;7(6):1895–1902.
17. Sherman JH, Prevedello DM, Shah L, et al. MR imaging characteristics of oligodendroglial tumors with assessment of 1p/19q deletion status. *Acta Neurochir (Wien)*. 2010;152(11):1827–1834.
18. Kim JW, Park CK, Park SH, et al. Relationship between radiological characteristics and combined 1p and 19q deletion in World Health Organization grade III oligodendroglial tumours. *J Neurol Neurosurg Psychiatry*. 2011;82(2):224–227.
19. Wu CC, Jain R, Radmanesh A, et al. Predicting genotype and survival in glioma using standard clinical mr imaging apparent diffusion coefficient images: A pilot study from the Cancer Genome Atlas. *AJNR Am J Neuroradiol*. 2018;39(10):1814–1820.
20. Choi C, Ganji SK, DeBerardinis RJ, et al. 2-hydroxyglutarate detection by magnetic resonance spectroscopy in IDH-mutated patients with gliomas. *Nat Med*. 2012;18(4):624–629.
21. Kickingereder P, Sahm F, Radbruch A, et al. IDH mutation status is associated with a distinct hypoxia/angiogenesis transcriptome signature which is non-invasively predictable with rCBV imaging in human glioma. *Sci Rep*. 2015;5:16238.
22. Tan W, Xiong J, Huang W, et al. Noninvasively detecting Isocitrate dehydrogenase 1 gene status in astrocytoma by dynamic susceptibility contrast MRI. *J Magn Reson Imaging*. 2017;45(2):492–499.
23. Yamashita K, Hiwatashi A, Togao O, et al. MR imaging-based analysis of glioblastoma multiforme: Estimation of IDH1 mutation status. *AJNR Am J Neuroradiol*. 2016;37(1):58–65.
24. Law M, Yang S, Wang H, et al. Glioma grading: Sensitivity, specificity, and predictive values of perfusion MR imaging and proton MR spectroscopic imaging compared with conventional MR imaging. *AJNR Am J Neuroradiol*. 2003;24(10):1989–98.
25. Mulholland S, Pearson DM, Hamoudi RA, et al. MGMT CpG island is invariably methylated in adult astrocytic and oligodendroglial tumors with IDH1 or IDH2 mutations. *Int J Cancer*. 2011;131(5):1104–1113.
26. Toh CH, Wei KC, Chang CN, et al. Differentiation of pyogenic brain abscesses from necrotic glioblastomas with use of susceptibility-weighted imaging. *AJNR Am J Neuroradiol*. 2012;33(8):1534–1538.
27. Solomon DA, Wood MD, Tihan T, et al. Diffuse midline gliomas with histone H3-K27M mutation: A series of 47 cases assessing the spectrum of morphologic variation and associated genetic alterations. *Brain Pathol*. 2016;26(5):569–580.
28. Chamberlain MC, Glantz MJ, Chalmers L, et al. Early necrosis following concurrent Temodar and radiotherapy in patients with glioblastoma. *J Neuro-Oncol*. 2007;82(1):81–83.
29. Taal W, Brandsma D, de Bruin HG, et al. Incidence of early pseudoprogression in a cohort of malignant glioma patients treated with chemoirradiation with temozolomide. *Cancer*. 2008;113(2):405–410.
30. Shin KE, Ahn KJ, Choi HS, et al. DCE and DSC MR perfusion imaging in the differentiation of recurrent tumour from treatment-related changes in patients with glioma. *Clin Radiol*. 2014;69(6):e264–e272.
31. Lee WJ, Choi SH, Park CK, et al. Diffusion-weighted MR imaging for the differentiation of true progression from pseudoprogression following concomitant radiotherapy with temozolomide in patients with newly diagnosed high-grade gliomas. *Acad Radiol*. 2012;19(11):1353–1361.
32. Chu HH, Choi SH., Ryoo I, et al. Differentiation of true progression from pseudoprogression in glioblastoma treated with radiation therapy and concomitant temozolomide: Comparison study of standard and high-b-value diffusion-weighted imaging. *Radiology*. 2013;269(3):831–840.
33. Brandes AA, Franceschi E, Tosoni A, et al. MGMT promoter methylation status can predict the incidence and outcome of pseudoprogression after concomitant radiochemotherapy in newly diagnosed glioblastoma patients. *J Clin Oncol*. 2008;26(13):2192–2197.
34. Brandsma D, van den Bent MJ. Pseudoprogression and pseudoresponse in the treatment of gliomas. *Curr Opin Neurol*. 2009;22(6):633–638.
35. Clarke JL, Chang S. Pseudoprogression and pseudoresponse: Challenges in brain tumor imaging. *Curr Neurol Neurosci Rep*. 2009;9(3):241–246.
36. Batchelor TT, Sorensen AG, di Tomaso E, et al. AZD2171, a pan-VEGF receptor tyrosine kinase inhibitor, normalizes tumor vasculature and alleviates edema in glioblastoma patients. *Cancer Cell*. 2007;11(1):83–95.
37. Norden AD, Young GS., Setayesh K, et al. Bevacizumab for recurrent malignant gliomas: Efficacy, toxicity, and patterns of recurrence. *Neurology*. 2008;70(10):779–787.
38. Stadlbauer A, Pichler P, Karl M, et al. Quantification of serial changes in cerebral blood volume and metabolism in patients with recurrent glioblastoma undergoing antiangiogenic therapy. *Eur J Radiol*. 2015;84(6):1128–1136.
39. Essock-Burns E, Lupo JM, Cha S, et al. Assessment of perfusion MRI-derived parameters in evaluating and predicting response to antiangiogenic therapy in patients with newly diagnosed glioblastoma. *Neuro-oncology*. 2010;13(1):119–131.
40. Wen PY, Chang SM, Van den Bent MJ, et al. Response assessment in neuro-oncology clinical trials. *J Clin Oncol*. 2017;35(21):2439–2449.

41. Okada H, Weller M, Huang R, et al. Immunotherapy response assessment in neuro-oncology: A report of the RANO working group. *Lancet Oncol.* 2015 Nov;16(15):e534–e542.

42. AlRayahi J, Zapotocky M, Ramaswamy V, et al. Pediatric brain tumor genetics: What radiologists need to know. *Radiographics.* 2018;38(7):2102–2122.

43. Gaudino S, Martucci M, Russo R, et al. MR imaging of brain pilocytic astrocytoma: Beyond the stereotype of benign astrocytoma. *Child Nerv Syst.* 2017;33:35–54.

44. Komotar RJ, Mocco J, Carson BS et al. Pilomyxoid astrocytoma: A review. *MedGenMed.* 2004;6 (4):42.

45. Kahramancetin N, Tihan T. Aggressive behavior and anaplasia in pleomorphic xanthoastrocytoma: A plea for a revision of the current WHO classification. *CNS Oncol.* 2013;2(6):523–530.

46. Spoto GP, Press GA, Hesselink JR, et al. Intracranial ependymoma and subependymoma: MR manifestations. *AJR Am J Roentgenol* 1990;154:837–845.

47. Cachia D, Johnson DR, Kaufmann TJ, et al. Case-based review: Ependymomas in adults. *Neurooncol Pract.* 2018;5(3):142–153. doi:10.1093/nop/npy026

48. Koral K, Kedzierski RM, Gimi B et al. Subependymoma of the cerebellopontine angle and prepontine cistern in a 15-year-old adolescent boy. *AJNR Am J Neuroradiol.* 2008;29(1):190–191.

49. Kornienko VN, Pronin IN. *Diagnostic Neuroradiology.* New York: Springer Verlag; 2009:412.

50. Johnson MD, Atkinson JB. *Central Nervous System Tumors, Modern Surgical Pathology.* 2nd ed. New York: W. B. Saunders; 2009:1984–2038.

51. Osborn A, Hedlund G, Salzman K. *Osborn's Brain Imaging, Pathology and Anatom.* 2nd ed. Elsevier; 2018.

52. Koeller KK, Henry JM. From the archives of the AFIP: Superficial gliomas: Radiologic-pathologic correlation. Armed Forces Institute of Pathology. *Radiographics.* 2001;21(6):1533–1556.

53. Fernandez C, Girard N, Paz Paredes A, et al. The usefulness of MR imaging in the diagnosis of dysembryoplastic neuroepithelial tumor in children: A study of 14 cases. *AJNR Am J Neuroradiol.* 2003;24(5):829–834.

54. Parmar H, Hawkins C, Ozelame R, et al. Fluid-attenuated inversion recovery ring sign as a marker of dysembryoplastic neuroepithelial tumors. *J Comput Assist Tomogr.* May-Jun 2007;31(3):348–353.

55. Shin JH, Lee HK, Khang SK, et al. Neuronal tumors of the central nervous system: Radiologic findings and pathologic correlation. *RadioGraphics.* 2002;22(5):1177–1189.

56. Park SH, Kim E, Son EI. Cerebellar ganglioglioma. *J Korean Neurosurg Soc.* 2008;43(3):165–168.

57. Casperson BK, Anaya-Baez V, Kirzinger SS, et al. Coexisting MS and Lhermitte-Duclos disease. *J Radiol Case Rep.* 2010;4(8):1–6.

58. Chen CL, Shen CC, Wang J, Lu CH, Lee HT. Central neurocytoma: A clinical, radiological and pathological study of nine cases. *Clin Neurol Neurosurg.* 2008;110(2):129–136.

59. Gardiman MP, Fassan M, Orvieto E, et al. Diffuse leptomeningeal glioneuronal tumors: A new entity? *Brain Pathol.* 2010;20(2):361–366.

60. Pekmezci M, Stevers M, Phillips JJ, et al. Multinodular and vacuolating neuronal tumor of the cerebrum is a clonal neoplasm defined by genetic alterations that activate the MAP kinase signaling pathway. *Acta Neuropathol.* 2018;135(3):485–488.

61. Nunes RH, Hsu CC, da Rocha AJ, et al. Multinodular and vacuolating neuronal tumor of the cerebrum: A new "leave me alone" lesion with a characteristic imaging pattern. *Am J Neuroradiol.*Oct 2017;38(10):1899–1904.

62. Nunes Dias L, Candela-Cantó S, Jou C, et al. Multinodular and vacuolating neuronal tumor associated with focal cortical dysplasia in a child with refractory epilepsy: A case report and brief review of literature. *Childs Nerv Syst.* 2020;36:1557–1561. https://doi.org/10.1007/s00381-019-04496-3

63. Smith A, Rushing E, Smirniotopoulos J. Lesions of the pineal region: Radiologic pathologic correlation. *Radiographics.* 2010;30(7):2001–2020.

64. Valle MMD, Jesus OD. Pineal gland cancer (updated 2021 Aug 30). In: StatPearls [Internet]. Treasure Island (FL): StatPearls Publishing; 2021 Jan. https://www.ncbi.nlm.nih.gov/books/NBK560567/

65. Chang SM, Lillis-Hearne PK, Larson DA, et al. Pineoblastoma in adults. *Neurosurgery.* 1995;37:383–390, discussion 390–391.

66. Yoon DJ, Park J, Lezama LM, Heller GD. Pineal parenchymal tumour of intermediate differentiation: A rare differential diagnosis of pineal region tumours. *BJR Case Rep.* 2016;2(4):20150371.

67. Kool M, Korshunov A, Remke M, et al. Molecular subgroups of medulloblastoma: An international meta-analysis of transcriptome, genetic aberrations, and clinical data of WNT, SHH, Group 3, and Group 4 medulloblastomas. *Acta Neuropathol.* 2012;123(4):473–484.

68. Barkovich AJ. *Pediatric Neuroimaging.* 3rd ed. Philadelphia: Lippincott Williams & Wilkins; 2000.

69. Kram DE, Henderson JJ, Baig M, et al. Embryonal tumors of the central nervous system in children: The era of targeted therapeutics. *Bioengineering (Basel).* 2018;5(4):78. doi:10.3390/bioengineering5040078

70. Dangouloff-Ros V, Tauziède-Espariat A, Roux CJ, et al. CT and multimodal MR imaging features of embryonal tumors with multilayered rosettes in children. *Am J Neuroradiol.* 2019;40(4):732–736.

71. Koral K, Gargan L, Bowers DC, et al. Imaging characteristics of atypical teratoid-rhabdoid tumor in children compared with medulloblastoma. *Am J Roentgenol.* 2008;190(3):809–814.

72. Perry A, Gutmann DH, Reifenberger G. Molecular pathogenesis of meningiomas. *J Neurooncol.* 2004 Nov;70(2):183–202.

73. Backer-Grøndahl T, Moen BH, Torp SH. The histopathological spectrum of human meningiomas. *Int J Clin Exp Pathol.* 2012;5(3):231–242.

74. Russell EJ, George AE, Kricheff II, et al. Atypical computed tomography features of intracranial meningioma: Radiological-pathological correlation in a series of 131 consecutive cases. *Radiology.* 1980;135(3):673–682.

75. Chourmouzi D, Potsi S, Moumtzouoglou A, et al. Dural lesions mimicking meningiomas: A pictorial essay. *World J Radiol.* 2012;4(3):75–82.

76. Lyndon D, Lansley JA, Evanson J, Krishnan AS. Dural masses: Meningiomas and their mimics. *Insights Imaging.* 2019;10(1):11.

77. Ho VB, Smirniotopoulos JG, Murphy FM, et al. Radiologic-pathologic correlation: Hemangioblastoma. *Am J Neuroradiol.* Sep 1992;13(5):1343–1352.

78. Jahnke K, Schilling A, Heidenreich J, et al. Radiologic morphology of low-grade primary central nervous system lymphoma in immunocompetent patients. *Am J Neuroradiol.* Nov 2005;26(10):2446–2454.

79. Haldorsen IS, Espeland A, Larsson EM. Central nervous system lymphoma: Characteristic findings on traditional and advanced imaging. *Am J Neuroradiol.* 2011;32(6):984–992.

80. Chiavazza C, Pellerino A, Ferrio F, et al. Primary CNS lymphomas: Challenges in diagnosis and monitoring. *Biomed Res Int.* 2018;2018:2. Article ID: 3606970.

81. Pittock SJ, Debruyne J, Krecke KN, et al. Chronic lymphocytic inflammation with pontine perivascular enhancement responsive to steroids (CLIPPERS). *Brain.* 2010;133(9):2626–2634.

82. Dudesek A, Rimmele F, Tesar A, et al. CLIPPERS: Chronic lymphocytic inflammation with pontine perivascular enhancement responsive to steroids. Review of an increasingly recognized entity within the spectrum of inflammatory central nervous system disorders. *Clin. Exp. Immunol.* 2014;175(3):385–396.

83. Solomou AG. Magnetic resonance imaging of pineal tumors and drop metastases: A review approach. *Rare Tumors.* 2017;9(3):6715.

84. Osorio DS, Allen JC. Management of CNS germinoma. *CNS Oncol.* 2015;4(4):273–279.

85. Pisaneschi M, Kapoor G. Imaging the sella and parasellar region. *Neuroimaging Clin N Am.* 2005;15(1):203–219.

86. Gupta K, Sahni S, Saggar K, et al. Evaluation of clinical and magnetic resonance imaging profile of pituitary macroadenoma: A prospective study. *J Nat Sci Biol Med.* 2018;9(1):34–38.

87. Abele TA, Yetkin ZF, Raisanen JM, et al. Non-pituitary origin sellar tumours mimicking pituitary macroadenomas: Pictorial review. *Clin Radiol.* 2012;67:821–827.

88. Lee IH, Zan E, Bell WR, et al. Craniopharyngiomas: Radiological differentiation of two types. *J Korean Neurosurg Soc.* 2016;59(5):466–470.

89. Pope WB. Brain metastases: Neuroimaging. *Handb Clin Neurol.* 2018;149:89–112.

90. Singh SK, Leeds N E, Ginsberg LE. MR imaging of leptomeningeal metastases: Comparison of three sequences. *Am J Neuroradiol.* 2002;23(5):817–821.

91. Thomas B, Thamburaj K, Kesavadas C. "Eiffel-by-night": A new MR sign demonstrating reactivation in idiopathic hypertrophic pachymeningitis. *Neuroradiol J.* 2007;20(2):194–195.

92. Masdeu JC, Quinto C, Olivera C, et al. Open-ring imaging sign: Highly specific for atypical brain demyelination. *Neurology.* 2000 Apr 11;54(7):1427–1433.

93. Parks N, Bhan V, Shankar J. Perfusion imaging of tumefactive demyelinating lesions compared to high grade gliomas. *Can J Neurol Sci.* 2016;43(2):316–318.

94. Ronsin S, Deiana G, Geraldo AF, et al. Pseudotumoral presentation of cerebral amyloid angiopathy-related inflammation. *Neurology.* 2016;86(10):912–919.

95. Liang JW, Zhang W, Sarlin J, et al. Case of cerebral amyloid angiopathy-related inflammation: Is the absence of cerebral microbleeds a good prognostic sign? *J Stroke Cerebrovasc Dis.* 2015;4(2):319–322.

96. Aiken AH, Akgun H, Tihan T, et al. Calcifying pseudoneoplasms of the neuraxis: CT, MR imaging, and histologic features. *Am J Neuroradiol.* 2009;30(6):1256–1260.

PART II. | ADULT NEURO-ONCOLOGY

3 | GLIOBLASTOMA

RIMAS V. LUKAS

INTRODUCTION

Glioblastoma (GBM) is a malignant brain tumor, the care of which comprises a central component of most neuro-oncology clinical practices. In parallel, it is the disease in neuro-oncology on which the greatest research efforts are focused. This chapter covers GBM from the clinical perspective, devoting much of the content to the surgical, radiation, and medical management of these tumors.

EPIDEMIOLOGY

Primary brain tumors represent only a subset of central nervous system (CNS) tumors. CNS metastases are more common than tumors which arise primarily in the CNS. Among primary brain tumors, infiltrating gliomas comprise a substantial portion. More than half of all infiltrating gliomas are GBM. Among all primary CNS tumors, GBM compose 14.7%.[1] The incidence of specific molecular subtypes of these tumors is less certain at the population level. It is estimated that isocitrate dehydrogenase (*IDH*) wildtype (wt) comprise approximately 90% of GBM.

Majority of glioblastomas are *IDH* wildtype.

A number of demographic factors correlate with the incidence of GBM. A higher incidence is noted in men, with a ratio of 1.58:1. Incidence is higher in Caucasians than African Americans and Asians.[1] It also notably increases with advancing age, with the median age at diagnosis being 65 years.[1] These tumors are quite rare in the pediatric population, and the underlying biology of the disease in that population differs from that in adults. A complete understanding of incidence at the global level is limited by a lack of national registries. In turn, our epidemiologic knowledge is based heavily on data from Western nations. At least within the United States, the incidence of GBM has been stable outside of the expected increase commensurate with the aging of the population.[2]

The majority of GBM are deemed to be sporadic. A limited number are thought to develop due to prior ionizing radiation exposure.[3,4] This is preceded by a lag of years to decades between exposure and tumor diagnosis. Unlike radiation-induced meningioma, at this time a molecular signature

does not exist for radiation-induced GBM. In addition to the post-radiation population, a higher incidence of GBM is also seen in a number of rare inheritable cancer predisposition syndromes including neurofibromatosis type 1, Li-Fraumeni, and Lynch syndrome. GBMs associated with these syndromes or secondary to radiation, however, comprise only a small proportion of the overall GBM population. Genome-wide association studies (GWAS) have demonstrated potential candidate susceptibility genes for glioma.[5] These, however, require further validation. In contrast to these risk factors for GBM, the presence of some allergies appears to be protective with respect to GBM incidence.[2,6] This may be secondary to more robust immuno-surveillance. While studies using various methodologies have presented conflicting results, at this time there is no definitive evidence of a causal relationship between cellular phone use and GBM incidence.[7] In addition, at this time there are no known interventions that prevent development of GBM.

While most of the GBMs are sporadic, several predisposition syndromes have been described.

CLINICAL PRESENTATION

Patients with GBM often present with the subacute onset of neurological symptoms. These may reflect either the specific neuroanatomic locations involved or non-localizable symptoms related to increased intracranial pressure. Ischemic lesions such as strokes have distinct borders between infarcted and non-infarcted tissue and a relatively limited penumbra of suboptimally functioning tissue. In contrast, GBM are non-circumscribed lesions with areas of non-functioning brain and normally functioning brain, with a substantial area of imperfectly functioning brain comprising the majority of the lesion in most cases. The severity of the neurologic dysfunction often waxes and wanes over the course of a day or week. Numerous factors including systemic illnesses (such as urinary tract infections and upper respiratory infections), electrolyte imbalances, seizure activity, and postictal dysfunction can influence this.

Seizures may be the initial presenting symptom of GBM but are more common in lower-grade gliomas. Prevalence of seizures throughout the course of disease is somewhat unclear (approximately one-third to two-thirds of patients)[8] as these events are not always accurately recorded. The incidence of seizure at time of diagnosis is highest in *IDH* mutated tumors[9] making seizures as a presenting symptom more common in lower-grade infiltrating gliomas (both oligodendrogliomas and astrocytomas) compared to GBM. Also reassuringly, there is a lower likelihood of medically refractory seizures.[10] Perioperative utilization of anti-epileptic drugs (AEDs) is highly variable, but there is no recommendation for routine prophylactic use of AEDs.[11] The decision-making regarding perioperative ED management is often driven by the neurosurgery team. Preferred anti-epileptic drugs for GBM patients share a number of common properties. These include: no/limited drug-drug interactions, limited myelotoxicity, limited hepatotoxicity, limited risk of hyponatremia, and limited risk of severe rash. Examples of preferred medications include levetiracetam, lacosamide, and brivaracetam. These and other non–enzyme inducing anti-epileptics are often favored because of the lack of potential drug-drug interactions. This is of particular importance with respect to systemic cancer treatments such as chemotherapy or targeted therapies whose levels may be altered by enzyme-inducing agents. Earlier reports suggestive of improved survival outcomes in GBM with some specific AEDs such as valproic acid have not held up to scrutiny.[12]

In contrast to the localizable symptoms just described, non-localizable symptoms are most frequently secondary to increased intracranial pressure. Symptoms of elevated intracranial pressure are not specific for brain tumors but can be seen across a variety of etiologies. These symptoms include positional headaches which are frequently present upon first awakening. They are often accompanied by nausea and/or vomiting, somnolence, and diplopia due to compression of cranial nerve VI at the skull base impairing abduction of the eyes. Funduscopic examination may reveal papilledema. Presentation with either the localizable or non-localizable symptomatology described often leads to imaging of the CNS.

GBM patients frequently present to acute care settings for their symptoms. Some of these emergency room visits and hospitalizations may be avoidable.[13] As disease progresses, decreased mobility, dysphagia, cognitive impairment, and increased somnolence are seen. Many of these symptoms are secondary to brainstem involvement in progressed disease, which appears to be the etiology of death in the majority of GBM patients in contemporary clinical practice.[14] Similar to patients with such symptoms due to other etiologies, end-stage GBM patients are at risk for aspiration, pneumonia, skin ulceration, bacteremia, and pulmonary emboli. In addition to traditional outcome measures of overall survival (OS) and progression-free survival (PFS), there is a growing understanding of the importance of a range of symptoms including fatigue, distress, and cognitive impairment and how they affect quality of life in this patient population.[15] These are increasingly being utilized as outcome measures in trials of therapeutic interventions for GBM. Many institutions are including up-front referral to palliative medicine/supportive medicine to aid in the treatment of symptoms and establish goals of care.

DIAGNOSTIC EVALUATION AND RESPONSE ASSESSMENT

Often, a non-contrast head computed tomography (CT) may be performed in the initial evaluation of patients presenting with new neurological symptoms. CT scanning can quickly evaluate for catastrophic acute abnormalities and may reveal findings of less acute pathologies such as brain tumors as well. For these reasons, the emergency department is often the milieu in which this imaging modality is utilized. CT scanning may also be utilized when magnetic resonance imaging (MRI) scanning is not feasible.

MRI with and without contrast, however, is superior to CT in detecting radiographic abnormalities concerning for tumor. MRI can also more clearly delineate what can and should be addressed with therapeutic modalities such as surgery, radiation, and tumor-treating fields (TTFields). Gadolinium contrast dye often demonstrates robust heterogenous enhancement in high-grade gliomas such as GBM (Figure 3.1). This likely reflects the neovascularization and imperfection of the blood–brain barrier (BBB) noted on the histopathology.

In addition to the diagnostic value of brain MRI, it is also the primary means for radiographically assessing progression of disease. Some clinicians add perfusion-weighted imaging sequences to the MRI to better discern treatment related changes from true progression in enhancing tumors, but this has not been defined as the standard recommendation for surveillance imaging. The Response Assessment in Neuro-Oncology (RANO) criteria are the most frequently utilized imaging assessment in GBM trials, although this has not been prospectively validated.[16] RANO utilizes the cross-sectional area of the enhancing lesion as the primary measurement endpoint. Progression of disease is defined as a 25% or greater increase in this or the development of a new lesion. A substantial increase in the fluid-attenuated inversion recovery (FLAIR) signal abnormality can also be used to define progression of disease. Partial response is defined as a 50% or greater decrease, and complete response is defined as the resolution of all enhancement. All of these features are assessed within the context of stable or decreasing steroid doses and stable or improving clinical status. Per RANO, it is recommended that patients within the first 12 weeks post-radiotherapy (RT) not be deemed to have progressed disease (unless there are new lesions outside of the RT field) for the purposes of clinical trials because of the high potential for pseudoprogression during this time frame.

> Interpretation of brain imaging in GBM patients within the first 12 weeks post-radiotherapy must be done with caution as abnormal changes seen might represent pseudoprogression rather than true disease progression.

ADVANCED IMAGING

A number of advanced imaging techniques have been and continue to be investigated in the evaluation of gliomas. Efforts have been made to provide diagnostic insight including molecular

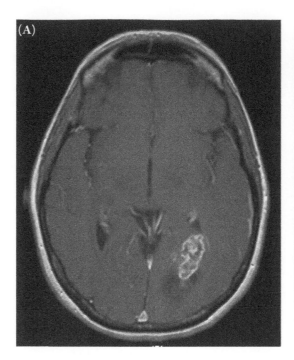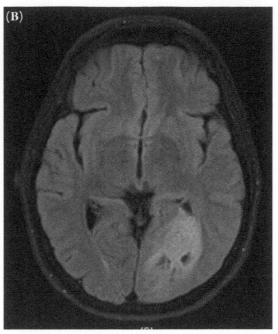

Figure 3.1 MRI of the brain. T1 with contrast (A) and fluid-attenuated inversion recovery (FLAIR). (B) showing typical enhancing pattern seen in glioblastoma with associated peri-tumoral edema.

subclassification prior to histologic diagnosis, evaluate more definitively extent of tumor, and evaluate for progressed disease. This has led to tremendous growth within the field of radiomics.[17] A range of imaging advanced modalities have been utilized.[18] These have included MRI, positron emission tomography (PET), and artificial intelligence (AI) to efficiently process the enormous amount of data generated via these imaging studies. At this time none of these techniques is universally employed across all institutions, and they are not a component of the standard of care.

PATHOLOGY

Based on its heterogenous histologic appearance, GBM had initially been termed as "glioblastoma multiforme" by Cushing and Bailey. It represented a primary tumor thought to arise from a precursor cell they termed a "bipolar spongioblast."[19] While "multiforme" is no longer a part of the nomenclature, the histologic heterogeneity across single tumors still holds true. The molecular heterogeneity may be even more varied, contributing to the difficulty of adequately treating this malignancy. These tumors consist of astrocytic-appearing tumor cells infiltrating diffusely through the brain parenchyma. They have areas of necrosis, often pseudopallisading in appearance, and/or areas of endothelial proliferation, somewhat glomeruloid in configuration.

While the classification systems have evolved since Bailey and Cushing's text, the reliance on histology remained paramount until the recent past. The 2016 World Health Organization (WHO) classification of CNS tumors incorporated molecular characteristics as integral features defining subtypes of infiltrating gliomas.[20] GBM were divided into two

distinct tumor types, both still grade 4, based on the mutational status of the *IDH* genes. The overwhelming majority of GBM lack mutations in *IDH* (*IDH*wt) and are representative of primary GBM, which are thought to develop quickly and progress rapidly. They harbor the other molecular aberrancies classically associated with GBM, including epidermal growth factor receptor (*EGFR*) amplification and mutation as well as phosphatase and tensin homolog (*PTEN*) loss and telomerase reverse transcriptase (*TERT*) promoter mutation. Since the 2016 WHO classification, it has been acknowledged that infiltrating gliomas deemed lower grade (2 or 3) with the same molecular features follow a natural history similar to GBM *IDH*wt and should be viewed as such.[21] It is anticipated that these changes will take greater hold over time in both routine clinical practice as well as in the clinical investigations in patients with these tumors. In environments in which the resources are available, there is substantial additive value in the detailed molecular characterization of glial tumors[22,23] (see Chapter 1, for additional details).

The second tumor type that still holds the name glioblastoma is GBM, *IDH* mutated. These tumors comprise what has long been viewed as secondary GBMs, which arise from lower-grade infiltrating astrocytomas. Approximately 10% of GBMs are *IDH* mutated. These tumors should be viewed as distinct from GBM, *IDH*wt and future iterations of the WHO classification system may not include the "glioblastoma" in their nomenclature.[24] Suggestion has been made to rename these tumors "astrocytoma *IDH* mutant WHO grade 4."[24] Consideration has been proposed to further subdivide this category based on the presence or absence of homozygous deletion of cyclin-dependent kinase inhibitor 2A/B (CDKN2A/B). Presence of this deletion is associated with shorter survival.[24] In the contemporary era clinical management of the

IDHwt and *IDH*-mutated GBM remain similar, although outcomes are superior in the *IDH*-mutated variant. In summary, in the upcoming 2021 edition of the WHO classification of CNS tumors, *IDH*-mutant astrocytomas are grouped into a separate category reflecting their less aggressive clinical course compared to wildtype tumors. In addition, in lieu of Roman numerals, the new classification will use Arabic numerals to designate the grade. Tumors showing "significant" mitotic activity will be designated grade 3. It is now recommended that grade 3 tumors undergo testing for homozygous CDKN2A/B deletions, given the prognostic implications (see earlier discussion). Using these recommendations, tumors with homozygous CDKN2A/B deletions or microvascular proliferation and/or necrosis should be classified as astrocytoma, *IDH*-mutant, WHO grade 4, and no longer as glioblastoma.[24]

PROGNOSIS

A number of factors influence outcomes in patients with GBM. These can broadly be divided into factors intrinsic to the tumor, intrinsic to the patient, and dependent on the therapeutic management.

Tumor-specific molecular characteristics have a substantial influence on outcomes. As discussed, these tumors are now conceptualized as distinct entities based on their *IDH* mutational status, with the *IDH*wt tumors demonstrating worse outcomes. Even when *IDH*-mutated astrocytoma transform phenotypically into GBM, these secondary GBM exhibit better survival. GBM *IDH*-mutated have a median OS of 31 months compared to the de novo *IDH* wildtype GBM with a median OS of 15 months (p = .002).[25] While not a component of the WHO classification system, the methylation status of the promoter for the methylguanine methyl transferase (*MGMT*) gene is a commonly assessed prognostic and predictive biomarker. The *MGMT* promoter is methylated in approximately 45% of GBM and, when present, is prognostically favorable and predicts greater benefit from temozolomide (TMZ) chemotherapy.[26] We discuss its predictive value in the "Therapeutic Management" section of this chapter. Numerous other molecular biomarkers have been associated with OS[27] but they remain beyond the scope of this chapter. In addition to these biomarkers, radiographically easily assessed features can also influence prognosis. Unsurprisingly, larger tumor size at time of diagnosis appears to be associated with inferior outcomes.[28]

Various patient intrinsic factors have been shown to be related to outcome. A patient's performance status, a measure of their overall functionality, associates with survival, with more functional patients faring better. This has held true across numerous studies. In contemporary neuro-oncology practice, the Karnofsky performance status (KPS) scale is the most frequently used performance status measure.[29] Because this was developed more than 70 years ago to quantify functional impairment in lung cancer patients treated with nitrogen mustard and not neuro-oncology patients, it imperfectly correlates with clinical assessments in contemporary neuro-oncologic practice. A contemporary metric to quantify neurologic functioning, the Neurologic Assessment in Neuro-Oncology

(NANO) scale, has been developed,[30] but its prognostic value has yet to be validated. Another patient-intrinsic factor, patient age, has also been shown to be strongly associated with survival across multiple studies. This is in part, but not exclusively, driven by increased medical comorbidities with increasing age and increased incidence of *IDH*wt GBM (in comparison to *IDH*-mutated) in the older population. Gender may also impact survival, with women having improved OS compared to men.[31] The details of this require further investigation.

Finally, therapeutic interventions impact outcome, with aggressive therapeutic approaches being associated with improved survival. These are discussed in greater detail in the following section.

THERAPEUTIC MANAGEMENT

Management of both *IDH*wt and *IDH*-mutated GBM is discussed here. In many neuro-oncology practices, management of *IDH*wt astrocytoma (grade 2) and anaplastic astrocytoma (AA, grade 3) follows a paradigm similar to that of GBM. Clinical management of *IDH*-mutated astrocytoma and AA may differ somewhat and will not be covered in this chapter. The treatment of newly diagnosed GBM is well established.[32,33] For progressed GBM, it is less clearly defined.[33]

SURGERY

Surgery plays a role is establishing a diagnosis as well as in providing therapeutic benefit in GBM. With respect to its diagnostic role this can be achieved either via a biopsy or a craniotomy with more extensive resection. As the importance of molecular characterization increases[22,23] there is growing value in obtaining adequate tissue to perform all of the neuropathological evaluations of interest on the specimen. Current practice at many institutions involves an attempt at gross total resection (GTR) of enhancing tumor without perioperative complications causing any new deficits as these are associated with worse outcomes[34] and lower likelihood of receiving RT and chemotherapy.[35]

GTR of enhancing tumor is associated with a diminished risk of early tumor growth prior to the initiation of radiation. In turn it is also associated with improved OS and PFS.[36,37] There is also suggestion that postoperative residual non-enhancing tumor is unfavorable.[38] This non-enhancing tissue consists predominantly of non-neoplastic tissue with a small percentage of neoplastic cells interspersed. This presence of tumor cells has led some to suggest that there may be value in supra-total resection of GBM.[39–41] While the limited data appear to support this hypothesis, this has not yet become the standard clinical practice at most centers. Reports of even more aggressive approaches from the pre-CT era involving total hemispherectomies noted no meaningful benefits.[42,43]

GTR is one of the key prognostic factors in newly diagnosed GBM.

The role for surgical resection for progressive disease is less clearly defined. There are retrospective studies, impacted by selection bias, supporting the role of extensive surgical resection for progressive disease.[44–47] A number of patient-specific factors influence this clinical decision-making. These include whether the progressive tumor growth is symptomatic and whether resection will help alleviate the symptoms. Other factors include, but are not limited to, tumor size, location, patient's performance status, medical comorbidities, prior lines of therapy, and plans for postsurgical treatments. Re-resection of progressive GBM should only be considered as part of a comprehensive management plan which may include the pre- or postoperative utilization of other treatment modalities. This may be within the context of a clinical trial or outside of that framework. At times, biopsy is utilized as a means to clarify if radiographic findings are representative of recurrent disease or treatment effect. Often, a combination of both can be seen. Decision-making regarding the role for biopsy for possible progressive disease is patient-specific.

A number of techniques have been utilized to improve on the extent of resection for GBM. These include advances in imaging, direct tumor visualization, and neurophysiologic studies. MRI-based imaging techniques can include preoperative assessment with diffusion tensor imaging (DTI) sequences to more clearly delineate the relationship between white matter tracts and the tumor burden that may be resected. This is sometimes paired with functional MRI (fMRI), which can help provide an understanding of which specific anatomic structures play a role in specific tasks, in turn helping plan resection. This is typically not viewed as a substitute for intraoperative neurophysiologic studies, but instead as a tool to augment real-time neurophysiologic evaluation. The utilization of such intraoperative electrocorticography (ECoG) can be beneficial for the neurosurgeon as they attempt to maximize the extent of resection while limiting the morbidity of postoperative neurological dysfunction. PET has been undergoing investigation as means of better defining the extent of infiltrating tumor. While the success of widely available fluorodeoxyglucose (FDG) PET has been limited in this regard, the use of a variety of amino acid PET tracers has demonstrated promise. Amino acid PET, however, is limited by the need for a cyclotron to produce the tracers for the imaging study. In turn, this technique has limited its scalability. Imaging has not only been used for preoperative planning and postoperative assessment of extent of resection, but also for intraoperative assessment of extent of resection. Both head CT and brain MRI have been used in this regard. In large tumors there may be intraoperative shift of structures which decreases the reliability of the intraoperative navigation tools. In turn, reimaging during surgery may help the surgeon understand the extent of residual tumor, allowing them to adjust their operative plan in real time. The value of this is limited to a select subset of patients. Intraoperative imaging is not available in all centers and does increase the time of the operative case. While it may be associated with improved extent of resection it has not been shown to improve survival. Finally, another technique to facilitate the extent of resection is the use of an intravenously administered fluorescing dye, which allows the surgeon to visualize tumor in normal-appearing brain parenchyma intraoperatively when exposed to ultraviolet light. 5-aminolevulinic acid (5-ALA) has been investigated in a phase III trial and was associated with an increased extent of resection but no significant improvement in OS.[48] These techniques can be used in combination, and the decision-making regarding which technique(s) to employ in the surgical management of GBM patients is typically driven by the neurosurgeon.

Finally, surgery can be utilized as a means to deliver a therapeutic directly to the region of tumor. One example of this is the use of small wafers impregnated with bischloroethyl nitrosourea (BCNU; carmustine, Gliadel), used to line the tumor resection cavity during surgery. These are currently approved by the US Food and Drug Administration (FDA) for newly diagnosed and progressed GBM. Their use in clinical practice is somewhat limited. The BCNU from the wafers diffuses into the surrounding tissue to treat tumor adjacent to the resection cavity while avoiding the toxicity of systemically delivered nitrosourea. The lack of systemic toxicity is traded for some additional local toxicity, specifically increased risk of cerebrospinal fluid (CSF) leak (5% vs. 0.8%) and increased risk of intracranial hypertension (9.1% vs. 1.7%).[49] Additionally, the wafers are associated with some difficulty in interpreting imaging studies. This has led to many clinical trials listing them as an exclusion criterion. However, over the past number of years this may be decreasing in occurrence. When initially studied in a randomized placebo-controlled trial (wafers with BCNU vs. wafers without BCNU; $n = 222$) in recurrent high-grade gliomas, two-thirds of whom had GBM, there was a nonsignificant trend toward improved survival (hazard ratio [HR] 0.83; 95% confidence interval [CI] 0.63–1.10; p = .19). When limited to GBM patients and after adjusting for multiple prognostic factors, the findings became significant.[50] A subsequent phase III trial ($n = 240$) in newly diagnosed high-grade gliomas (GBM as well as anaplastic astrocytoma, oligoastrocytoma, and oligodendroglioma) compared surgical resection with Gliadel followed by focal RT to 55-60 Gy versus surgery with placebo wafer implantation followed by the same RT regimen. The Gliadel arm demonstrated improved OS compared to the control arm (13.9 months vs. 11.6 months; however, PFS was similar in both groups (5.9 months).[49] Molecular characteristics including *IDH* and *MGMT* status were not reported. Postoperative systemic chemotherapy was not employed as this was prior to the TMZ-era.

Other therapeutic agents that can be delivered surgically include forms of *brachytherapy*, a means for delivering radiation locally. Similar to the BCNU-impregnated wafers, a different wafer impregnated with radioactive cesium-131 (GammaTile) can line the resection cavity, delivering treatment prior to initiation of the next therapeutic agent. Although FDA approved, published data regarding efficacy are scant. Another FDA-approved method for brachytherapy involves implantation of an implantable balloon catheter that can be filled with iodine-125.[51] Unlike with systemic therapies, the prospective clinical investigations are less robust. This may be a factor in the less enthusiastic uptake of the use of these therapeutics and their lack of inclusion in any standard treatment algorithms. For additional information regarding these treatment options, please see Chapter 22.

RADIATION

The role of RT for the management of GBM has been long established. While brachytherapy was briefly discussed, the overwhelming majority of RT is delivered via an external beam. It is typically delivered in small daily fractions (routinely Monday through Friday) to a total cumulative dose of 60 Gy administered over approximately 6 weeks. In general, this is fairly well-tolerated, with the most frequently encountered side effects being fatigue and alopecia. Both of these often begin partway through the RT course and continue through much of the post-RT time period prior to adjuvant therapy. Typically, RT is delivered concurrently with TMZ chemotherapy, as described in the EORTC/NCIC trial.[52] It is not clear that there is any true radiosensitizing value of the concomitant regimen. There have been no studies comparing concurrent chemoradiation to sequential radiation and TMZ for up-front treatment of newly diagnosed GBM. When studied specifically in anaplastic astrocytoma (grade 3) in a prospective phase III trial (CATNON) which includes *IDH*-wildtype and *IDH*-mutated tumors concurrent RT/TMZ appears to lack benefit in these tumors.[53] Final outcome results for this ongoing trial are awaited. It is reasonable that if these results hold up as data mature these findings may be applicable to patients with GBM. Even if this proves the case, however, it is uncertain that it would alter routine clinical practice as there are no published randomized studies which definitively demonstrate that one regimen (with concurrent TMZ vs. without) is superior to another. Thus far, other radiosensitizing approaches have not proved efficacious, although this remains an area of continued investigation.[54]

The optimal dosing of RT has been evaluated and continues to undergo investigation. A phase I cooperative group study (RTOG 9803) demonstrated the feasibility of RT dose-escalation with concurrent alkylating chemotherapy (in this case carmustine) in newly diagnosed GBM.[55] Tolerability of higher RT doses had also subsequently been demonstrated in a phase I trial with TMZ.[56] The randomized phase II NRG oncology cooperative group study BN001 (NCT02179086) is comparing standard-dose RT (60 Gy) to dose-escalated RT (75 Gy). There are distinct cohorts using photons or protons to treat these patients. The primary endpoint of the trial is OS. This study is limited to patients with enhancing tumors with diameters less than 5 cm due to concerns regarding toxicity with dose-escalation for larger tumors. While this trial may not be generalizable to larger tumors, it will help clarify if there is a role for higher-dose RT in GBM. The preliminary results for patients treated in the photon cohorts did not demonstrate survival benefit of dose escalation of RT.[57]

Photons are the primary means of delivering RT to GBM. Photons deliver their energy as they traverse the tumor as well as surrounding non-tumor tissue. While the maximum dose is delivered to the tumor, other tissues receive radiation as well. Protons, which have mass and which deliver their maximum energy where they stop within the tumor, can be used to limit the exit dose of radiation and in turn avoid treatment of other tissues. This has theoretical benefit with respect to toxicity, particularly long-term toxicity. In turn, there are special circumstances where use of proton therapy can be considered in GBM. However, this is not routine practice as there is no definitive data demonstrating improved efficacy or decreased toxicity with protons over photons.

The role of RT for progressed GBM is not clearly defined. Numerous trials utilizing a variety of dosing schedules have evaluated re-RT in this patient population. No consensus exists regarding if, when, and how it should optimally be applied. Common themes include consideration in patients with a longer interval since prior RT, shorter courses (when compared to up-front RT), and consideration of concurrent bevacizumab.[58] (See also Chapter 20.)

CHEMOTHERAPY

Chemotherapy, specifically the alkylating agent TMZ, was definitively shown to improve survival in patients with GBM in the pivotal EORTC 26981/22981; NCIC CE3 phase III trial.[52] This study compared RT alone against RT with concomitant TMZ followed by six cycles of TMZ. Median OS was 14.6 months in the investigational arm compared to 12.1 months in the control arm.[52] The 2-year survival was respectively 26.5% and 10.4%,[52] and the 5-year survival was 9.8% and 1.9%, a fivefold improvement.[59] Thus far, the only validated predictive biomarker established for GBM is the methylation status of the promoter for the *MGMT* gene. *MGMT* promoter methylation silences the gene, leading to a lack of the suicide enzyme MGMT, which binds to methyl adducts on the O6-guanine position of DNA. In short, positive methylation status results in the inability to repair the damage done by alkylating TMZ therapy. Lack of the repair mechanism for this specific type of DNA damage within the tumor leads to increased efficacy of TMZ. Patients with newly diagnosed GBM with *MGMT* promoter methylation fared better (OS 21.7 months) as compared to patients with MGMT unmethylated tumor status (15.3 months) when both were treated with TMZ.[26]

> *MGMT* methylation is a critically important predictive biomarker in GBM and is clinically useful for treatment decision-making.

The TMZ is typically administered daily (for 42 consecutive days) during RT at a dose of 75 mg/m²/day. This is followed by a 4–6 week break after the completion of chemoradiation with TMZ, at which point another brain MRI is performed as the baseline for comparison of response assessment.

Approximately one-third of patients have evidence of pseudoprogression. The incidence is almost twice as much in *MGMT* methylated tumors as compared to unmethylated.[60] This is a radiographic phenomenon in which there is an increase in enhancement within the RT field but which does not represent true tumor progression (see discussion in the diagnostic section). The concurrent phase of treatment is then followed by the adjuvant phase, in which patients receive a 5-day course of TMZ on a 28-day cycle. The dosing in the pivotal trial began the first cycle at 150 mg/m²/day and then advanced to 200 mg/m²/day for subsequent cycles if well tolerated. Many neuro-oncologists in the contemporary era will begin the first cycle at 200 mg/m²/day. Frequently encountered side effects include constipation and nausea/vomiting. Almost all patients require some type of stool softener/laxative regimen as well as anti-emetics because constipation and nausea are common side effects of TMZ. Ondansetron is a frequently used agent that is typically effective in controlling the nausea. With respect to hematologic toxicities, the most frequently encountered are thrombocytopenia and lymphopenia. During the concurrent RT/TMZ phase the incidence of grade III/IV thrombocytopenia has been reported a approximately 8% and during the adjuvant phase at 10–12%.[33] Clinicians will often transfuse patients with GBM at higher platelet counts when compared to other malignancies due to concerns regarding the risk of intracranial hemorrhage. TMZ may also decrease white blood cell (WBC) counts, in particular the lymphocytes. Prolonged lymphopenia can be seen with TMZ.[61] Decreasing lymphocyte counts, specifically CD4+ cells are associated with shorter survival.[62] When lymphocyte counts are low, patients are at greater risk of developing pneumocystic pneumonia (PCP), caused by the *Pneumocystis jirovecii*. Sulfamethoxazole-trimethoprim, dapsone, or pentamidine inhalation are often used for PCP prophylaxis. Use of these prophylactic agents up-front or with proven lymphopenia is debated and generally left to physician choice. Details regarding PCP prophylaxis vary between practitioners. Another extremely infrequent toxicity with the use of alkylating chemotherapies in general, including TMZ, is the increased risk of developing secondary treatment-related hematologic disorders such as acute myelodysplastic leukemia (t-AML) and myelodysplastic syndrome (t-MDS). The exact risk of developing these is incompletely understood, in part due to the limited number of long-term survivors with GBM and the lack of population-based data on the incidence of t-AML/t-MDS.[63] While there is theoretical concern regarding a dose–risk relationship, this has not been demonstrated in primary CNS tumors.

Optimal dosing of TMZ has been studied in a number of clinical trials. The largest such evaluation was in the RTOG 0525 phase III trial (n = 833) which compared standard dose (150–200 mg/m² for 5/28 days) adjuvant TMZ to dose-dense (75 mg/m² for 21/28 days) TMZ for 6–12 cycles. There was no difference in OS (16.6 months vs. 14.9 months, p = .63) or PFS (5.5 months vs. 6.7 months, p = .06). When evaluated by *MGMT* promoter methylation status, the lack of benefit persisted. While the dose-dense regimen was relatively well tolerated there was a higher incidence of grade 3–4 toxicities, predominantly those associated with myelosuppression.[64]

Thrombocytopenia and lymphopenia are commonly seen complications in patients with GBM treated with temozolomide.

In turn, the TMZ regimen described in the EORTC 26981/22981; NCIC CE3 trial is most widely used. Questions regarding the optimal duration of adjuvant TMZ persist. There have been no adequately powered comparisons of 6 versus more (often 12) cycles of adjuvant TMZ. A number of retrospective analyses have been performed which suggest no additional benefit in survival associated with more than 6 cycles.[65] Preliminary results of a small underpowered randomized trial are suggestive of no benefit from additional cycles.[66] There have been numerous attempts at improving the efficacy of TMZ, often by impairing mechanisms of DNA repair. Thus far, these approaches have not proved adequately successful. One promising approach based on preclinical studies utilizing patient-derived xenograft (PDX) models combines TMZ with the poly (ADP ribose) polymerase (PARP) inhibitor veliparib.[67] The results of the ongoing cooperative group phase II/III trial (A071102) in newly diagnosed *MGMT* promoter methylated GBM are eagerly awaited. Novel approaches to decrease systemic toxicity have also been evaluated. One such approach used gene therapy with mutant *MGMT* hematopoietic stem/progenitor cells to limit TMZ-induced myelotoxicity allowing for the potential administration of higher dose TMZ.[68,69] Another approach to augment therapeutic efficacy in the newly diagnosed *MGMT* promoter methylated GBM population is the addition of a second alkylator, cyclonexyl-chloroethyl-nitrosourea (CCNU), to the TMZ. This was studied in the small phase III CeTeG/NOA-09 trial (n = 144) in which the standard TMZ regimen was compared to TMZ (100–200 mg/m², days 2–6 of 6-week cycle) with CCNU (100 mg/m², day 1 of 6-week cycle) for both the concurrent-RT and adjuvant phases of treatment. OS was improved in the investigational arm (48.1 months vs. 31.4 months, p = .0492). The investigational regimen proved surprisingly tolerable.[70] The results are based on a limited number of patients with improved survival.[71] While this treatment regimen has entered into practice, it has not been widely adopted as the standard of care. Summary of larger, more important studies conducted in GBM can be found in Table 3.1.

Due to inferior outcomes in elderly patients and greater difficulty tolerating treatments, there have been a number investigations into de-escalation of therapeutic intensity in this patient population.[72] This has led to a number of acceptable management approaches in this patient population ranging from very short-course RT alone (5 fractions) to standard full-course treatment with surgery, RT/TMZ, followed by TMZ/TTFields. The decision-making regarding this weighs a number of factors, often with the greatest weight placed on performance status. One frequently utilized approach involves shorter course RT (3 weeks to 40 Gy) with concurrent TMZ followed by adjuvant TMZ as studied in the NCIC CTG CE.6/EORTC 26062-22061/TROG 08.02 phase III trial. This study demonstrated improved survival when compared to short-course RT alone.[73] We do not have direct comparisons to full-course RT/TMZ followed by TMZ or full-course RT/TMZ followed by TMZ/TTFields. In turn, numerous regimens are deemed valid, and the decision-making is typically on a patient-specific basis. In some patients with MGMT promoter methylated tumors, TMZ monotherapy is considered; in others who

TABLE 3.1 Summary of selected studies in high-grade glioma patients

TRIAL DESIGNATION	AUTHOR	YEAR	PHASE	N	AGE	STUDY DESIGN	OVERALL SURVIVAL (OS)	PROGRESSION-FREE SURVIVAL (PFS)
	Walker et al.	1978	3	222	6–79	HGG patients BCNU/ RT + BCNU vs. BCNU vs. RT vs. Supportive care	34.5 weeks vs. 18.5 weeks vs. 35 weeks vs. 14 weeks	
	Westphal et al.	2003	3	240	18–65	HGG patients BCNU-wafers + RT vs. Placebo-wafers + RT	13.9 mo vs. 11.6 mo in HGG patients 13.5 mo Vs. 11.4 mo in GBM subgroup	5.9 mo vs. 5.9 mo in HGG patients
EORTC22981/ 26981 NCIC CE.3	Stupp et al.	2005	3	573	18–71	RT/TMZ + TMZ vs. RT	14.6 mo vs. 12.1 mo	6.9 mo vs. 5.1 mo
	Keime-Guibert et al.	2007		85	≥70	RT/supportive care vs. Supportive care	29.1 weeks vs. 16.9 weeks	14.9 weeks vs. 5.4 weeks
RTOG 0525	Gilbert et al.	2013	3	833	≥18	RT/TMZ + TMZ (150–200 mg/m²/day for 5/28 days) vs. RT/TMZ + TMZ (75 mg/m²/day for 21/28 days)	16.6 mo vs. 14.9 mo	5.5 mo vs. 6.7 mo
RTOG 0825	Gilbert et al.	2014	3	637	≥18	RT/TMZ/bev + TMZ/bev vs. RT/TMZ + TMZ	15.7 mo vs. 16.1 mo	10.7 mo vs. 7.3 mo
AVAglio	Chinot et al.	2014	3	921	≥18	RT/TMZ/bev + TMZ/bev vs. RT/TMZ + TMZ	16.8 mo vs. 16.7 mo	10.6 mo vs. 6.2 mo
CENTRIC EORTC 26071-22072	Stupp et al.	2014	3	545	≥18	MGMT methylated RT/TMZ/cilengitide + TMZ/ cilengitide vs. RT/TMZ + TMZ	26.3 mo vs. 26.3 mo	10.6 mo vs. 7.9 mo
GLARIUS	Herrlinger et al.	2016	2	182		RT/bev + bev/ CPT11 vs. RT/TMZ + TMZ	16.6 mo vs. 17.5 mo	9.7 mo vs. 5.99 mo
ACT-IV	Weller et al.	2017	3	745	≥18	Enrolled after completion of RT/TMZ TMZ/rindopepimut vs. TMZ	21.1 mo vs. 20.0 mo	8.0 mo vs. 7.4 mo

TABLE 3.1 Continued

TRIAL DESIGNATION	AUTHOR	YEAR	PHASE	N	AGE	STUDY DESIGN	OVERALL SURVIVAL (OS)	PROGRESSION-FREE SURVIVAL (PFS)
EF-14	Stupp et al.	2017	3	695	≥18	Enrolled after completion of RT/TMZ TMZ/TTF vs. TMZ	20.9 mo vs. 16.0 mo	6.7 mo vs. 4.0 mo
CCTG CE.6, EORTC 26062-22061, TROG 08.02	Perry at al.	2017	3	562	≥65	Short-course RT/ TMZ + TMZ vs. short-course RT	9.3 mo vs. 7.6 mo	5.3 mo vs. 3.9 mo
CeTeG/NOA-09	Herrlinger et al.	2018	3	141	18–70	MGMT methylated RT/TMZ + TMZ vs. RT/CCNU/TMZ + CCNU/TMZ	31.4 mo vs. 48.1 mo	16.7 mo vs. 16.7 mo

Adapted from Lukas RV et al.[32]

OS, median overall survival; PFS, median progression free survival; RR, response rate; NNA, not available; RT, radiation therapy; TMZ, temozolomide; bev, bevacizumab; BCNU-wafers, carmustine wafer (Gliadel); HGG, high-grade glioma including glioblastoma; GBM, glioblastoma; CPT11, irinotecan; TTF, tumor-treating fields.

may not be good candidates for systemic chemotherapy (including those with MGMT promoter unmethylated tumors) RT alone can be used.[72] For summary of studies examining hypofractionation, see Table 3.2. (Please see Chapter 30 for additional information regarding treatment of elderly patients.)

> Treatment options for elderly patients with GBM may differ from the standard of care for the younger population.

For progressed GBM, there is no single systemic therapy regimen that all patients should receive. A number of regimens have been investigated.[33] In contemporary practice, patients are often treated with CCNU (lomustine). CCNU is an oral chemotherapy typically dose once every 6 weeks (100–110 mg/m^2). It has the potential to cause pronounced prolonged myelosuppression. As with TMZ, platelets and lymphocytes are most often affected. In the phase III EORTC 26101 trial CCNU was associated with median OS of 8.6 months but a median PFS of only 1.5 months.[74]

For patients with symptomatic cerebral edema, the anti-vascular endothelial growth factor (VEGF) antibody bevacizumab may decrease cerebral edema, improve symptoms, and improve the radiographic imaging. While a very favorable radiographic response rate and PFS were demonstrated in a number of phase II trials for progressed GBM,[75,76] these findings are driven primarily by the mechanism of BBB normalization and not via direct tumor cytotoxicity. There is no definitive evidence that bevacizumab prolongs OS in patients with GBM. In clinical practice bevacizumab may be added to CCNU for symptom improvement. In that setting the dose of CCNU is usually decreased to 90 mg/m^2.[74] Numerous additional systemic therapies are undergoing investigation for these patients. One that has demonstrated favorable outcomes

TABLE 3.2 Selected studies examining hypofractionated radiotherapy in glioma

AUTHOR	MINIMUM AGE (Y)	FRACTIONAL DOSE	TOTAL DOSE	DURATION	CONCURRENT CHEMOTHERAPY	MEDIAN SURVIVAL
Baumann et al. (1994)	65 (or KPS≤ 50)	3 Gy	30 Gy	10 days	No	6 months
Roa et al. (2004)	60	2.67 Gy	40 Gy	15 days	No	5.6 months
Malmstrom et al. (2012)	60	3.4 Gy	34 Gy	10 days	No	7.5 months
Roa et al. (2015)	65 (or KPS 50–70)	5 Gy	25 Gy	5 days	No	7.9 months
Perry et al. (2017)	65	2.67 Gy	40 Gy	15 days	Yes	9.3 months

Adapted from Lukas RV et al.[32]

KPS, Karnofsky Performance Status.

when compare to CCNU is the multi-tyrosine kinase inhibitor regorafenib.[77] Additional investigation is required before this is widely adopted in clinical practice.

ALTERNATING ELECTRICAL FIELD THERAPY

Alternating electrical fields have been shown to impair tumor cell division and facilitate tumor cell death when delivered at a moderate frequency and low intensity.[78,79] This mechanism of action has been developed into a therapeutic approach termed "tumor-treating fields." When utilized for the treatment of glioblastoma the electrical fields are delivered at 200 kHz with an intensity of approximately 1–3+ volts at the tumor site. Field intensity delivered to tumor cells, as well as the orientation of the tumor cells within the field, appear to be factors influencing efficacy.[80]

TTFields first received FDA approval for recurrent GBM based on the results of the randomized phase III EF-11 trial and the modality holds a Category 1 treatment recommendation for newly diagnosed GBM according to the National Comprehensive Cancer Network (NCCN). In this study patients were treated with TTField monotherapy versus physicians' choice systemic therapy. Thirty-one percent of the control arm patients received bevacizumab and 25% received nitrosoureas. While there was no improvement in OS (6.6 months TTFields, 6.0 months control arm, p = .27) or PFS (2.2 months TTFields, 2.1 months control arm) the comparable efficacy and superior toxicity profile led to FDA approval. Some patients treated with TTField monotherapy were noted to have radiographic responses supporting biologic activity of this therapeutic approach. Often these responses were delayed.[81] When moved to the newly diagnosed setting, the addition of TTFields was demonstrated to improve outcomes, leading to its FDA approval for this indication in 2015. The phase III EF-14 trial enrolled newly diagnosed GBM patients after the completion of RT with concurrent TMZ but prior to the adjuvant phase of therapy. Patients were randomized to either 6 cycles of TMZ monotherapy or TMZ + TTFields. The study was not placebo-controlled in that no sham device was utilized in the control arm. Lack of a sham device in the control allows for clearer assessment of TTField toxicity because the majority of side effects appear to be directly related to the application of the arrays to the scalp. In the EF-14 trial an improvement in the primary endpoint of PFS (6.7 months vs. 4.0 months; HR 0.63; p < .001) was seen. OS, a secondary endpoint, also demonstrated significant improvement (20.9 months vs. 16.0 months; HR 0.63; p <. 001). Exploratory endpoints also favored the addition of TTFields. Survival at 2 years (43% vs. 31%) and out to 5 years (13% vs. 5%) was superior in the TTField arm. Post hoc subgroup analyses demonstrated improved OS and PFS regardless of *MGMT* promoter methylation status, age, gender, performance status, and extent of resection.[82] Formal health-related quality of life evaluations demonstrated comparable outcomes in both treatment arms.[83]

The primary toxicity is cutaneous, with approximately half of newly diagnosed patients experiencing low-grade (CTC toxicity criteria grade 1 and 2) skin toxicity. In most cases this improves or resolves with a brief break from utilization of TTFields. Some patients benefit from the application of topical steroids or antibiotics. A limited subset require more aggressive intervention to manage these toxicities.[84,85]

PROGRESSIVE GBM

As noted earlier, the management of recurrent GBM is not well codified[33] and is often made on a patient-specific basis. It is impossible to make a blanket recommendation which encompasses therapeutic management of all patients with progressive GBM. There are, however, a number of viable options. These can be organized into two overlapping frameworks, one based on therapeutic modality, the other on a clinical trial versus off-trial framework. We have discussed the role of each modality in progressed disease in the respective sections and acknowledge that each individual modality may be part of a larger comprehensive plan. Consideration of clinical trials for these patients is also important to note because adequately effective therapies are lacking.

For focal tumors in resectable locations, particularly if removal of tumor mass will improve or alleviate symptoms, surgical resection can be considered as a component of a comprehensive therapeutic plan.

HISTONE-MUTATED GLIOBLASTOMA

In addition to the tumors described, there is a growing understanding of a variety of high-grade infiltrating astrocytic tumors with histone mutations. Some of these would still be categorized as glioblastoma in the current WHO classification system. It is possible that in the future they may be divided into distinct categories dictated by their biology and natural history. The most frequently encountered and best studied infiltrating astrocytoma with histone mutation is the one which harbors the H3K27M mutation on the gene encoding histone 3 (H3).[86,87] This leads to an amino acid substitution, which impairs epigenetic regulation. This mutation is associated with tumor involving midline CNS structures and is most seen most often in the pediatric population, highlighting the interaction between genomic and epigenetic abnormalities within the context of the neuroanatomic microenvironment and the host. The predominant tumor cell population resembles oligodendroglial precursor cells.[88] This tumor subtype is discussed in detail in Chapter 14. In addition, other less common histone mutations, such as the G34R on H3, are found in infiltrating astrocytomas, which differ in their neuroanatomic location and natural history from the H3K27M tumors.

H3K27M-mutated high-grade gliomas in adults follow an aggressive natural history. In adult patients, they skew toward presence in younger adults and are most frequently encountered in the thalamus and spinal cord, unlike the pontine location most often seen in the pediatric population. These tumors also appear to be less aggressive than their pediatric counterparts and lie between classic *IDH*wt glioblastoma and *IDH*-mutated grade 4 astrocytoma, with a median survival of more than 27 months.[89] The G34R-mutated tumors are most often lobar, particularly temporal or parietal, in location. The OS in these patients is superior to glioblastoma IDHwt and H3K27M mutated high-grade gliomas.[90] Therapies addressing the underlying biology of the diseases are under active investigation. It is hoped that this will impact our therapeutic management of these patients in the future.

CONCLUSION

GBM is a malignant tumor now better defined by its molecular characteristics. A multidisciplinary approach is central to its optimal management. For newly diagnosed patients, surgical resection is typically followed by concurrent RT/TMZ followed by TMZ and often the addition of TTFields. While this multimodality therapeutic approach has been associated with improved OS as well as benefits in other clinically relevant parameters there is still need for ideally transformative advance in the management of this disease. Whenever possible, a clinical trial should be offered to the patient. Elderly patients with newly diagnosed GBM frequently require a more customized approach based on their age, performance status, comorbidities, and the molecular characteristics of the tumor. There are several different options for patients with recurrent disease, but outcomes are generally poor. New forms of aggressive gliomas with histone mutations are being recognized and characterized.

What percentage of infiltrating gliomas are GBMs?	50%
Most GBMs are *IDH* wildtype or IDH mutated?	*IDH* wildtype
What histological features are hallmarks of GBM?	Microvascular proliferation and necrosis
On brain MRI, GBM typically appears as	Heterogeneously enhancing lesion, sometimes with central necrosis
Positive prognostic factors for a patient with GBM include:	1. Younger age 2. Gross total resection 3. IDH mutation 4. MGMT methylation 5. Good performance status
What is the standard of care for newly diagnosed GBM?	Maximal safe resection followed by radiotherapy with concomitant and adjuvant TMZ plus/minus TTFields
Reasonable choices for older patients with GBM include:	1. Hypofractionated radiotherapy (RT) alone 2. Hypofractionated radiotherapy with concomitant and adjuvant TMZ 3. Conventional radiotherapy and chemotherapy (Stupp protocol) 4. TMZ alone in patients with MGMT promoter methylation
What adverse effect does TMZ frequently cause?	Lymphopenia and thrombocytopenia
What do RANO criteria recommend within the first 12 weeks post-RT?	Progressive disease is not declared (unless there are new lesions outside of the RT field) for the purposes of clinical trials because of the high potential for pseudoprogression during this time frame

Genetic predisposition syndromes associated with GBM include	Neurofibromatosis type 1, Li- Fraumeni, and Lynch syndromes
Potential treatment options for recurrent GBM may include:	1. Clinical trial 2. Re-resection or re-irradiation 3. Carmustine wafer 4. Lomustine 5. Bevacizumab
In what anatomical locations are H3K27M-mutated high-grade gliomas found in adults?	They are typically located in the thalamus or spinal cord and are very aggressive
MGMT **promoter methylation is associated with better outcomes in patients treated with what agents?**	Alkylating agents such as temozolomide
Tumors involving midline CNS structures may harbor what mutation?	H3K27M

QUESTIONS

1. Glioblastoma (GBM)
   a. Comprises 35% of all primary central nervous system (CNS) tumors
   b. Is the most common primary CNS tumor
   c. Comprises 15% of all primary CNS tumors
   d. Comprises 90% of infiltrating gliomas

2. The following is true of the Response Assessment n Neuro-Oncology (RANO) criteria for assessing GBM:
   a. Progressive disease is defined as a 10% increase in volume of the enhancing lesion.
   b. Progressive disease is defined as a 25% or greater increase in cross-sectional area of the enhancing lesion.
   c. Partial response is defined as a 25% or greater decrease in cross-sectional area of the enhancing lesion.
   d. Response assessments are independent of the steroid dosing.

3. The EF-14 trial demonstrated that the addition of tumor-treating fields (TTFields) to adjuvant temozolomide (TMZ) was associated with
   a. A doubling of median overall survival (OS)
   b. A more than doubling of 5-year survival
   c. A shorter progression-free survival
   d. A decrease in health-related quality of life

4. The most frequently encountered toxicity with TTFields is
   a. Low-grade (grade 1–2) skin toxicity
   b. High-grade (grade 3–4) skin toxicity
   c. An electric-like sensation
   d. A heat sensation

5. The blood count most frequently decreased with the utilization of temozolomide (TMZ) is
   a. Erythrocyte
   b. Neutrophil
   c. Eosinophil
   d. Platelet

6. For young patients with newly diagnosed GBM, radiation is classically administered
   a. To 40 Gy over 3 weeks
   b. To 60 Gy over 6 weeks
   c. To 75 Gy over 6 weeks
   d. To 60 Gy over 6 weeks with an 15–24 Gy SRS boost

7. For elderly patients with newly diagnosed GBM, which of the following regimens has been demonstrated to be superior to short-course radiation (40 Gy) monotherapy in a randomized trial?
   a. Radiation (40 Gy) + nivolumab
   b. Radiation (60 Gy) + with concurrent TMZ + adjuvant TMZ + adjuvant TTFields
   c. Radiation (60 Gy) with concurrent TMZ + adjuvant TMZ
   d. Radiation (40 Gy) with concurrent TMZ + adjuvant TMZ

8. In the pivotal phase III EF-11 trial, subjects in in the control arm received the following treatments:
   a. 10% of patients received nitrosoureas.
   b. 15% of patients received bevacizumab.
   c. 40% of patients received regorafenib.
   d. 25% of patients received nitrosoureas.

9. The use of intraoperative 5-aminolevulinic acid (5-ALA) is associated with
   a. A moderate risk of thrombocytopenia
   b. A high risk of venous thromboembolism
   c. An improvement in overall survival when compared to placebo
   d. An improvement in radiographically determined extent of resection

10. In the landmark study of *IDH* mutational status impact on prognosis by Yan et al. (2009), the median overall survival was
    a. 9 months in GBM *IDH* wildtype and 18 months in GBM *IDH*-mutated
    b. 12 months in GBM *IDH* wildtype and 24 months in GBM-*IDH* mutated
    c. 15 months in GBM *IDH* wildtype and 31 months in GBM-*IDH* mutated
    d. 24 months in GBM *IDH* wildtype and 38 months in GBM-*IDH* mutated

11. The following therapeutic modality is *not* approved by the FDA for the treatment of newly diagnosed GBM:
    a. Bevacizumab
    b. Temozolomide
    c. BCNU-impregnated wafers
    d. Tumor-treating fields

12. In the EORTC 26981/22981; NCIC CE3 phase III trial that established the benefit of TMZ in newly diagnosed GBM, the 2-year survival in patients treated with TMZ compared to those not treated with TMZ was
    a. 90% vs. 10%
    b. 75% vs. 25%
    c. 25% vs. 10%
    d. 10% vs. 5%

13. The use of a dose-dense (75 mg/m² for 21/28 days in the adjuvant phase) regimen of TMZ when compared to "standard" dose TMZ (150–200 mg/m² for 5/28 days in the adjuvant phase) is associated with
    a. Improved overall survival
    b. Improved response rates
    c. Improved tolerability
    d. Increased rate of grade 3/4 toxicities

14. The following criteria are utilized to standardize imaging assessments in clinical trials for GBM:
    a. Response Assessment in Neuro-Oncology (RANO)
    b. Neurological Assessment in Neuro-Oncology (NANO)
    c. MacDonald criteria
    d. Karnofsky Performance Status (KPS)

15. New postoperative deficits after surgical resection for GBM are associated with
    a. Improved outcomes with regards to survival
    b. Decreased likelihood of receiving radiation and/or chemotherapy
    c. No effect on survival outcomes
    d. Improved quality of life

ANSWERS

1. c
2. b
3. b
4. a
5. d
6. b
7. d
8. d
9. d
10. c
11. a
12. c
13. d
14. a
15. b

REFERENCES

1. Ostrum QT, Gittleman H, Truitt G, et al. CBTRUS statistical report: Primary brain and other central nervous system tumors diagnosed in the United States in 2011–2015. *Neuro Oncol.* 2018;20(Suppl 4):iv1–iv86.
2. Ostrum QT, Bauchet L, Davis FG, et al. The epidemiology of glioma in adults: A "state of the science" review. *Neuro Oncol.* 2014;16:896–913.
3. Elsamadicy AA, Babu R, Kirkpatrick JP, Adamson DC. Radiation-induced malignant gliomas: A current re-view. *World Neurosurg.* 2015;83:530–542.
4. Neglia JP, Robison LL, Stovall M, et al. New primary neoplasms of the central nervous system in survivors of childhood cancer: A report from the Childhood Cancer Survivor Study. *J Natl Cancer Inst.* 2006;98:1528–1537.
5. Atkins I, Kinnersley B, Ostrum QT, et al. Transcriptome-wide association study identifies new candidate susceptibility genes for glioma. *Cancer Res.* 2019;79(8):2065–2071.
6. Amirian ES, Zhou R, Wrensch MR, et al. Approaching a scientific consensus on the association between al-lergies and glioma risk: A report from the Glioma International Case-Control Study. *Cancer Epidemiol Biomarkers Prev.* 2016;25:282–290.
7. Karipidis Elwood M, Benke G, Sanagou M, Tjong L, Croft RJ. Mobile phone use and incidence of brain tumor histological types, grading or anatomical location: A population-based ecological study. *BMJ Open.* 2018;8(12):e024489.
8. Kerkhof M, Vecht CJ. Seizure characteristics and prognostic factors of gliomas. *Epilepsia.* 2013;54(Suppl 9):12–17.
9. Chen H, Judkins J, Thomas C, et al. Mutant IDH1 and seizures in patients with glioma. *Neurology.* 2017;88(19):1805–1813.
10. Berntsson SG, Merrell RT, Amirian ES, et al. Glioma-related seizures in relation to histopathological subtypes: A report from the glioma international case-control study. *J Neurooncol.* 2018;265(6):1432–1442.
11. Youngerman BE, Joiner EF, Wang X, et al. Patterns of seizure prophylaxis after oncologic neurosurgery. *J Neurooncol.* 2020;146(1):171–180.
12. Happold C, Gorlia T, Chinot O, et al. Does valproic acid or levetiracetam improve survival in glioblastoma? A pooled analysis of prospective clinical trials in newly diagnosed glioblastoma. *J Clin Oncol.* 2016;34(7):731–739.
13. Wasilewski A, Serventi J, Kamalyan L, Wychowski T, Mohile NA. Acute care in glioblastoma: The burden and the consequences. *Neurooncol Pract.* 2017;4(4):248–254.
14. Drumm MR, Dixit KS, Grimm S, et al. Extensive brainstem infiltration, not mass effect, is a common feature of end-stage cerebral glioblastomas. *Neuro Oncol.* 2020;22(4):470–479.
15. Amidei C. Symptom based interventions to promote quality survivorship. *Neuro Oncol.* 2019;20(Suppl 7):vi27–vi39.
16. Wen PY, Macdonald DR, Reardon DA, et al. Updated response assessment criteria for high-grade gliomas: Response assessment in neuro-oncology working group. *Neuro Oncol.* 2010;28(11):1963–1972.
17. Chaddad A, Kucharczyk MA, Daniel P, et al. Radiomics in glioblastoma: Current status and challenges facing clinical implementation. *Front Oncol.* 2019;9:374.
18. Nandu H, Wen PY, Huang RY. Imaging in neuro-oncology. *Ther Adv Neurol Disord.* 2018;11:1756286418759865
19. Bailey P, Cushing H. *A Classification of the Tumors of the Glioma Group on a Histogenetic Basis with a Correlated Study of Prognosis.* Philadelphia: Lippincott; 1926.
20. Louis DN, Perry A, Reifenberger G, et al. The 2016 World Health organization classification of tumors of the central nervous system: A summary. *Acta Neuropathol* 2016;131:803–820.
21. Brat DJ, Aldape K, Colman H, et al. cIMPACT-NOW update 3: Recommended diagnostic criteria for "diffuse astrocytic glioma, IDH-wildtype, with molecular features of glioblastoma, WHO grade IV". *Acta Neuropathol.* 2018;136:805–810.
22. Molinaro AM, Taylor JW, Wiencke JK, Wrensch MR. Genetic and molecular epidemiology of adult diffuse glioma. *Nat Rev Neurol.* 2019;15:405–417.
23. Horbinski C, Ligon KL, Brastianos P, et al. The medical necessity of advanced molecular testing in the diagnosis and treatment of brain tumor patients. *Neuro Oncol.* 2019;21(12):1498–1508.
24. Brat DJ, Aldape K, Colman H, et al. cIMPACT-NOW update 5: Recommended grading criteria and terminologies for IDH-mutant astrocytomas. *Acta Neuropathol.* 2020;139(3):603–608.
25. Yan H, Parsons DW, Jin G, et al. IDH1 and IDH2 mutations in gliomas. *N Engl J Med.* 2009;360(8):765–773.
26. Hegi ME, Diserens AC, Gorlia T, et al. MGMT gene silencing and benefit from temozolomide in glioblastoma. *N Engl J Med.* 2005;352:997–1003.
27. Aquilanti E, Miller J, Santagata S, et al. Updates in prognostic markers for gliomas. *Neuro Oncol.* 2019;20(Suppl 7):vii17–vii26.
28. Leu S, Boulay JL, Thommen S, et al. Pre-operative two-dimensional size of glioblastoma is associated with patient survival. *World Neurosurg.* 2018;115:e448–e463.
29. Karnofsky DA, Ableman WH, Craver LF, Burchenal JH. Cancer. The use of nitrogen mustards in the palliative treatment of carcinoma with particular reference to bronchogenic carcinoma. *Cancer.* 1948;1(4):634–656.
30. Nayak L, DeAngelis LM, Brandes AA, et al. The Neurologic Assessment in Neuro-Oncology (NANO) scale: A tool to assess neurologic function for integration into the Response Assessment in Neuro-Oncology (RANO) criteria. *Neuro Oncol.* 207;19(5):625–635.
31. Gittleman H, Ostrum QT, Stetson LC, et al. Sex is an important prognostic factor for glioblastoma but not for non-glioblastoma. *Neuro Oncol Pract.* 2019;6(6):451–462.
32. Lukas RV, Wainwright DA, Ladomersky E, Sachdev S, Sonabend AM, Stupp R. Newly diagnosed glioblastoma: A review on clinical management. *Oncology (Williston Park).* 2019;33(3):91–100.
33. Lukas RV, Mrugala MM. Pivotal therapeutic trials for infiltrating gliomas and how they affect clinical practice. *Neuro Oncol Pract.* 2017;4(4):209–219.
34. Rahman M, Abbatematteo J, De Leo EK, et al. The effects of new or worsened postoperative neurological deficits on survival of patients with glioblastoma. *J Neurosurg.* 2017;127(1):123–131.
35. Gulati S, Jakola AS, Nerland US, Weber C, Solheim O. The risk of getting worse: Surgically acquired deficits, perioperative complications, and functional outcomes after primary resection of glioblastoma. *World Neurosurg.* 2011;76(6):572–579.
36. Villanueva-Meyer JE, Han SJ, Cha S, Butowski NA. Early tumor growth between initial resection and radiotherapy of glioblastoma: Incidence and impact on clinical outcomes. *J Neurooncol.* 2017;134(1):213–219.

37. Ellingson BM, Abrey LE, Nelson SJ, et al. Validation of postoperative residual contrast-enhancing tumor volume as an independent prognostic factor for overall survival in newly diagnosed glioblastoma. *Neuro Oncol.* 2018;20(9):1240–1250.

38. Kotrotsou A, Elakkad A, Sun J, et al. Multi-center study finds postoperative residual non-enhancing component of glioblastoma as a new determinant of patient outcome. *J Neurooncol.* 2018;139(1):125–133.

39. Duffau H. Is supratotal resection of glioblastoma in noneloquent areas possible? *World Neurosurg.* 2014;82(1-2):e101–e103.

40. Esquenazi Y, Friedman E, Liu Z, et al. The survival advantage of "supratotal" resection of glioblastoma using selective cortical mapping and the subpial technique. *Neurosurgery.* 2017;81(2):275–288.

41. Incekara F, Koene S, Vincent AJPE, et al. Association between supratotal glioblastoma resection and patient survival: A systematic review and meta-analysis. *World Neurosurg.* 2019;127:617–624.e2.

42. Hillier Jr WF. Total left cerebral hemispherectomy for malignant glioma. *Neurology.* 1954;4(9):718–721.

43. Smith A, Burklund CW. Dominant hemispherectomy: Preliminary report on neuopsychological sequelae. *Science.* 1966;153(3741):1280–1282.

44. Farina Nunez MT, Franco P, Cipriani D, et al. Resection of recurrent glioblastoma multiforme in elderly patients: A pseudo-randomized analysis revealed clinical benefit. *J Neurooncol.* 2020;146(2):381–387.

45. Sanai N, Polley MY, McDermott MW, et al. An extent of resection threshold for newly diagnosed glioblastoma. *J Neurosurg.* 2011;115(1):3–8.

46. Laws ER, Parney IF, Huang W, et al. Survival following surgery and prognostic factors for recently diagnosed malignant glioma: Data from the Glioma Outcomes Project. *J Neurosurg.* 2003;99(3):467–473.

47. Lacroix M, Abi-Said D, Fourney DR, et al. A multivariate analysis of 416 patients with glioblastoma multiforme: Prognosis, extent of resection, and survival. *J Neurosurg.* 2001;95(2):190–198.

48. Stummer W, Pichlmeier U, Meinel T, et al. Fluorescence-guided surgery with 5 amino-levulinic acid for resection of malignant glioma: A randomised controlled muliticentre phase III trial. *Lancet Oncol.* 2006;7(5):392–401.

49. Westphal M, Hilt DC, Bortey E, et al. A phase 3 trial of local chemotherapy with biodegradable carmustine (BCNU) wafers (Gliadel) in patients with primary malignant glioma. *Neuro Oncol.* 2003;5(2):79–88.

50. Brem H, Piantadosi S, Burger PC, et al. Placebo-controlled trial of safety and efficacy of intraoperative controlled delivery by biodegradable polymers of chemotherapy for recurrent gliomas. The Polymer-brain Tumor Treatment Group. *Lancet.* 1995;345(8956):1008–1012.

51. Wernicke AG, Scherr DL, Schwartz TH, et al. Feasibility and safety of GliaSite brachytherapy in treatment of CNS tumors following neurosurgical resection. *J Cancer Res Ther.* 2010;6(1):65–74.

52. Stupp R, Mason WP, van den Bent MJ, et al. Radiotherapy plus concomitant and adjuvant temozolomide for glioblastoma. *N Engl J Med.* 2005;352:987–996.

53. Van den Bent MJ, Errige S, Vogelbaum MA, et al. PL3.3. Second interim and first molecular analysis of the EORTC randomized phase III intergroup CATNON trial on concurrent and adjuvant temozolomide in anaplastic glioma without 1p/19q codeletion. *Neuro Oncol.* 2019;21(Suppl_3):ii3.

54. Bindra RS, Chalmers AJ, Evans S, Dewhirst M. GBM radiosensitization: Dead in the water . . . or just the beginning? *J Neurooncol.* 2017;134(3):513–521.

55. Tsien C, Moughan J, Michalski JM, et al. Phase I three-dimensional conformal radiation dose escalation study in newly diagnosed glioblastoma: Radiation Therapy Oncology Group Trial 98-03. *Int J Radiat Oncol Biol Phys.* 2009;73(3):699–708.

56. Truc G, Bernier V, Mirjolet C, et al. A phase I dose escalation study using simultaneous integrated-boost IMRT with temozolomide in patients with unifocal glioblastoma. *Cancer Radiother.* 2016;20(3):193–198.

57. Gondi V, Pugh S, Tsien C, et al. Radiotherapy (RT) dose-intensification (DI) using intensity-modulated RT (IMRT) versus standard dose (SD) RT with temozolomide (TMZ) in newly diagnosed glioblastoma (GBM): Preliminary results of NRG Oncology BN001. *Int J Radiat Oncol Biol Phys.* 2020;108(3):S22–S23.

58. Kazmi F, Soon YY, Leong YH, Koh WY, Vellayapan B. Re-irradiation for recurrent glioblastoma (GBM): A systematic review and meta-analysis. *J Neurooncol.* 2019;142(1):79–90.

59. Stupp R, Hegi ME, Mason WP, et al. Effects of radiotherapy with concomitant and adjuvant temozolomide versus radiotherapy alone on survival in glioblastoma in a randomised phase III study: 5-year analysis of the EORTC-NCIC trial. *Lancet Oncol.* 2009;10(5):459–466.

60. Brandes AA, Franceschi E, Tosoni A, et al. MGMT promoter methylation status can predict the incidence and outcome of pseudoprogression and concomitant chemoradiotherapy in newly diagnosed glioblastoma patients. *J Clin Oncol.* 2008;26(13):2192–2197.

61. Campian JL, Piotrowski AF, Ye X, et al. Serial changes in lymphocyte subsets in patients with newly diagnosed high grade astrocytomas treated with standard radiation and temozolomide. *J Neurooncol.* 2017;135(2):343–351.

62. Grossman SA, Ye X, Lesser G, et al. Immunosuppression in patients with high-grade gliomas treated with radiation and temozolomide. *Clin Cancer Res.* 2011;17(16):5473–5480.

63. Baehring JM, Marks PW. Treatment-related myelodysplasia in patients with primary brain tumors. *Neuro Oncol.* 2012;14(5):529–540.

64. Gilbert MR, Wang M, Aldape KD, et al. Dose-dense temozolomide for newly diagnosed glioblastoma: A randomized phase III clinical trial. *J Clin Oncol.* 2013;31(32):4085–4091.

65. Blumenthal DT, Gorlia T, Gilbert MR, et al. Is more better? The impact of extended adjuvant temozolomide in newly diagnosed glioblastoma: A secondary analysis of EORTC and NRG oncology/RTOG. *Neuro Oncol.* 2017;19:1119–1126.

66. Balana C, Barroso CM, Del Barco Berron S, et al. Randomized phase IIb clinical trial of continuation or non-continuation with six cycles of temozolomide after the first six cycles of standard first-line treatment in patients with glioblastoma: A Spanish research group in neuro-oncology (GEINO) trial. *J Clin Oncol.* 2019;37(15 Suppl):2001.

67. Gupta SK, Mladek AC, Carlson BL, et al. Discordant in vitro and in vivo chemopotentiating effects of the PARP inhibitor veliparib in temozolomide-sensitive versus –resistant glioblastoma multiforme xenografts. *Clin Cancer Res.* 2014;20(14):3730–3741.

68. Adair JE, Beard BC, Trobridge GD, et al. Extended survival of glioblastoma patients after chemoprotective HSC gene therapy. *Sci Transl Med.* 2012;4(133):133ra57.

69. Adair JE, Johnston SK, Mrugala MM, et al. Gene therapy enhances chemotherapy tolerance and efficacy in glioblastoma patients. *J Clin Invest.* 2014;124(9):4082–492.

70. Herrlinger U, Tzaridis T, Mack F, et al. Phase III trial of CCNU/temozolomide (TMZ) combination therapy vs. standard TMZ therapy for newly diagnosed MGMT- methylated glioblastoma patients: The randomized, open-label CeTeG/NOA-09 trial. *Lancet* 2019;393:678–688.

71. Stupp R, Lukas RV, Hegi ME. Improving survival in molecularly selected glioblastoma. *Lancet* 2019;393:615–617.

72. Young JS, Chmura SJ, Wainwright DA, Yamini B, Peters KB, Lukas RV. Management of glioblastoma in elderly patients. *J Neurol Sci.* 2017;380:250–255.

73. Perry JR, Laperriere N, O'Callaghan CJ, et al. Short-course radiation plus temozolomide. *N Engl J Med.* 2017;376:1027–1037.

74. Wick W, Gorlia T, Bendszus M, et al. Lomustine and bevacizumab in progressive glioblastoma. *New Engl J Med.* 2017;377(20):1954–1963.

75. Friedman HS, Prados MD, Wen PY, et al. Bevacizumab alone and in combination with irinotecan in recurrent glioblastoma. *J Clin Oncol.* 2009;27(28):4733–4740.

76. Kreisl TN, Kim L, Moore K, et al. Phase II trial of single-agent bevacizumab followed by bevacizumab plus irinotecan at tumor progression in recurrent glioblastoma. *J Clin Oncol.* 2009;27(5):740–745.

77. Lombardi G, De Salvo GL, Brandes AA, et al. Regorafenib compared with lomustine in patients with relapsed glioblastoma (REGOMA): A multicentre, open-label, randomised, controlled, phase 2 trial. *Lancet Oncol.* 2019;20(1):110–119.

78. Kirson ED, Gurvich Z, Schneiderman R, et al. Disruption of cancer cell replication by alternating electrical fields. *Cancer Res.* 2004;64:3288–3295.

79. Kirson ED, Dblay V, Tovarys F, et al. Alternating electrical fields arrest cell proliferation in animal tumor models and human brain tumors. *Proc Natl Acad Sci USA.* 2007;104:10152–10157.

80. Korshoej AR, Thielscher A. Estimating the intensity and anisotropy of tumor treating fields jsing singular value decomposition. Toward a more comprehensive estimation of anti-tumor efficacy. *Conf Proc IEEE Eng Med Biol Soc.* 2018:4897–4900.

81. Stupp R, Wong ET, Kanner AA, et al. Novo-TTF100A versus physicians' choice chemotherapy in recurrent glioblastoma: A randomized phase III trial of a novel treatment modality. *Eur J Cancer.* 2012;48(14):2192–2202.

82. Stupp R, Taillibert S, Kanner A, et al. Effect of tumor-treating fields plus maintenance temozolomide vs maintenance temozolomide alone on survival in patients with glioblastoma: A randomized clinical trial. *JAMA.* 2017;318:2306–2316.

83. Taphoorn MJB, Dirven L, Kanner AA, et al. Influence of treatment with tumor-treating fields on health-related quality of life of patients with newly diagnosed glioblastoma: A secondary analysis of a randomized clinical trial. *Lancet Oncol.* 2018;4(4):495–504.

84. Lacouture ME, Davis ME, Elzinga G, et al. Characterization and management of dermatologic adverse events with the NovoTTF-100A system, a novel anti-mitosis electric field device for the treatment of recurrent glioblastoma. *Semin Oncol.* 2014;41(Suppl 4):S1–14.

85. Lukas RV, Ratermann KL, Wong ET, Villano JL. Skin toxicities associated with tumor treating fields: Case based review. *J Neurooncol*. 2017;135(3):593–599.

86. Schwartzentruber J, Korshunov A, Liu XY, et al. Driver mutations in histone H3.3 and chromatin remodeling genes in paediatric glioblastoma. *Nature*. 2012;482(7384):226–231.

87. Buczkowicz P, Hoeman C, Rakopoulos P, et al. Genomic analysis of diffuse intrinsic pontine gliomas identifies three molecular subgroups and recurrent activating ACVR1 mutations. *Nature Genetics*. 2014;46:451–456.

88. Filbin MG, Tirosh I, Hovestadt V, et al. Developmental and oncogenic programs in H3K27M gliomas dissected by single-cell RNA-seq. *Science*. 2018;360(6386):331–335.

89. Schulte JD, Buerki RA, Lapointe S, et al. Clinical, radiologic, and genetic characteristics of histone H3 K27M mutant diffuse midline gliomas in adults. *Neurooncol Adv*. 2020;2(1):vdaa142.

90. Sturm D, Witt H, Hovestadt V, et al. Hotspot mutations in H3F3A and IDH1 define distinct epigenetic and biological subgroups of glioblastoma. *Cancer Cell*. 2012;22(4):425–437.

4 | DIFFUSE GLIOMAS (WHO GRADE 2–3)

HAROON AHMAD AND DAVID SCHIFF

INTRODUCTION

Choosing treatment of grade 2 and 3 diffuse gliomas can be more challenging than their grade 4 counterparts. An oncologist treating a glioblastoma (GBM) can follow a well-accepted treatment regimen, whereas patients with lower grade gliomas will take their care team through multiple difficult treatment decisions. Many of these crossroads are faced without consensus guidelines, let alone Level 1 evidence to support them.

Some blame for lack of consensus can be placed on the nature of lower grade gliomas themselves: longer overall survival (OS), relative rarity, and multiple distinct phenotypes. For example, a randomized prospective trial would ideally resolve the debate of using procarbazine, lomustine, and vincristine (PCV) versus temozolomide (TMZ) in the treatment of oligodendrogliomas. Such a trial is under way, but years may pass before accrual is complete and data mature.[1]

Much of what we know about these malignancies has developed over just the past 5–10 years. The significance of the isocitrate dehydrogenase (IDH) mutation was discovered in 2010, and the resultant classification paradigm shift just occurred in 2016. Prior studies have lost some significance, lacking analyses of now-known critical glioma subtypes.

Still, the treatment of patients with lower grade gliomas can be rewarding. A neuro-oncologist with a robust understanding of available data can glean recommendations for each individual situation. The longer OS lends to long-lasting, meaningful relationships with patients and their families.

Here, we review the available evidence in the diagnosis, management, and future direction of lower grade glioma treatment. This chapter is a clinically focused management guide, with intermixed pearls for the neuro-oncology certification exam. Pediatric, spinal cord, grade 4, and circumscribed gliomas are not discussed in this chapter.

For clarity, in glioma literature "low-grade" glioma specifically refers to grade 2 gliomas. "Anaplastic glioma" is synonymous with a grade 3 tumor. "High-grade" glioma could mean a grade 3 or 4 glioma (GBM). "Lower grade" glioma is sometimes used to refer to grade 2 and 3 gliomas (i.e., not GBMs). In this chapter we specify tumor grade whenever possible.

EPIDEMIOLOGY

Primary brain and other central nervous system (CNS) gliomas accounted for an annual average of 22,456 cases from 2012 to 2016, according to data from the Central Brain Tumor Registry of the United States (CBTRUS) 2019 report.[2] Glial tumors are far less common than tumors of the meninges or pituitary, comprising just 23.2% of primary CNS tumors. When focusing only on malignant primary brain tumors, the proportion of glial tumors jumps to 71.2%, the majority of which are GBM (48.3%). The most common non-GBM subtypes were malignant glioma, not-otherwise-specified (NOS) (7.5%), diffuse astrocytoma (7.3%), anaplastic astrocytoma (6.8%), ependymal tumors (6.7%), and oligodendrogliomas (5.3%).[2]

Analyzing World Health Organization (WHO) classified grade 2 and 3 diffuse gliomas, there was an annual case rate of 4,420 (excluding malignant glioma, NOS) comprising 5.3% of all primary CNS tumors. The total annual incidence rate was 1.35 (per 100,000 per year), comprised of diffuse astrocytoma (0.46), anaplastic astrocytoma (0.42), oligodendroglioma (0.23), anaplastic oligodendroglioma (0.11), and oligoastrocytic tumors (0.13). This illustrates the difficulty in developing lower grade glioma clinical trials: the total annual incidence for all subtypes is less than one-half of the annual GBM incidence (3.22). It should be noted that the data from the 2019 CBTRUS report are not parsed directly by WHO grade, rather ICD-O-3 codes, although confirmed WHO gradings were provided when available. For example, 87.9% of coded oligodendrogliomas were confirmed WHO grade 2, while 88.7% of coded anaplastic oligodenrogliomas were confirmed grade 3.[2]

> Developing and executing clinical trials for patients with lower grade gliomas is challenging due to the rarity of these tumors. The total incidence for all lower grade glioma subtypes is less than one-half of the annual incidence of GBM.

The average age of diagnosis for patients with grade 2 gliomas is younger than those with grade 3 gliomas. Astrocytomas most commonly present in patients between 30 and 40 years of age and oligodendrogliomas, slightly older, between 40 and 45 years.[2,3] New diagnoses of grade 3 tumors are most common in the 40–60 year age range, still slightly younger than patients with GBM.[4] Younger patients are not unaffected: adolescents and young adults (age 15–39 years) comprised an annual average of 1,385 cases of lower grade glioma, with total incidence of 1.31.[2]

> The average age of diagnosis is younger for patients with grade 2 gliomas than for those with grade 3 gliomas.

There is a higher incidence of all glioma subtypes in males. The incidence rate ratios for males to female patients was 1.29, 1.25, and 1.39 for non-GBM astrocytomas, oligodendrogliomas, and oligoastrocytic tumors, respectively.[2] There is a racial predilection for the development of all glial tumors. Incidence rates for astrocytic tumors (including GBM) were approximately two times greater in Caucasians than in African Americans. Incidence of oligodendroglioma was approximately 2.28 times greater in Caucasians.[2]

> All glioma subtypes are more common in males than females.

Few cases of lower grade gliomas have familial or genetic links. There are known cancer syndromes that can predispose to the development of these malignancies, including neurofibromatosis 1 and 2, Li-Fraumeni syndrome, Turcot syndrome, and Lynch syndrome. Certain polymorphisms have also been shown to increase the risk of developing gliomas, such as CCDC26 on chromosome 8.[5] However, the vast majority of patients (>95%) develop sporadic gliomas.[4]

> Given the low incidence of genetically predisposed gliomas, there are no recommendations for genetic screening in patients with diffuse gliomas.

The only known environmental risk factor for the development of these tumors is ionizing radiation. This refers to deliberate delivery of high doses of radiation, as in the treatment for hematologic malignancies. Cell phone use, other radiation exposure, toxins, and diet have never been definitively linked to glioma development.

PRESENTATION

Patients with lower grade gliomas can present with a variety of symptoms and in various settings. The most common presentation for all glial tumors is seizures, but it is most common in low-grade gliomas. Seizures at presentation have prevalence rates of 85%, 69%, and 49% in patients with grade 2, 3, and 4 gliomas, respectively.[6] It is postulated that the slower growth of low-grade tumors invades, rather than destroys, neural circuits. Patients with low-grade oligodendroglioma have an even higher risk of epilepsy given their predilection for these

tumors to invade the cortex. IDH mutations have also been shown to predispose to seizures and could be a factor in these trends.[7] Patients presenting with seizures tended to be younger, correlating with lower grade tumors.[8]

> The most common presentation for all glial tumors is seizures, but it is most common in lower grade gliomas.

Given the ubiquity of neuro-imaging available in modern age, more lesions are being found "incidentally" as a part of headache, dizziness, or trauma workup. No data are available on whether incidentally found lesions tend to longer OS.

Higher grade gliomas also most commonly present with seizures, but there is a higher incidence of presenting with fixed neurologic deficits. These may include fixed numbness, aphasia, or hemiparesis. This is believed to be due to the destructive nature of the rapidly growing lesions, in comparison to low-grade gliomas. Patients also more frequently present with cognitive deficits, which is a negative prognostic factor.[8] Presenting with a seizure portends better prognosis in higher grade gliomas, but interestingly is not solely explained by earlier diagnosis.[9]

Other presenting signs are common but less specific to gliomas. A retrospective study of all brain tumor types over a 10-year-period found that focal neurologic deficits (59.5%), mental status change (24.9%), headache (14.6%), seizures (14.1%), trauma (7.8%), and nausea/vomiting (4.4%) were the most common presenting signs of brain tumors.[10] Gliomas made up 50% of that sample size.

DIAGNOSIS

Brain magnetic resonance imaging (MRI) enhanced with gadolinium contrast is the standard for assessing a suspected brain tumor. For grade 2 gliomas, 95% occur supratentorially and are roughly equally split between the frontal and temporal lobes.[3] Astrocytic tumors tend to dwell in the white matter, while oligodendrogliomas often invade the cortex. On computed tomography (CT) scans, low-grade gliomas are hypodense and exhibit mild mass effect in the form of gyral edema and sulcal effacement. Calcifications are evident in about 20% of low-grade gliomas, particularly in oligodendrogliomas, and are best visualized on the CT scan. On MRI, the lesions are hyperintense on the T2 fluid attenuation inversion recovery (T2/FLAIR) sequence with isointensity on the T1 sequence. The classic radiographic description is a non-enhancing mass on contrast-enhanced T1 sequences. However, some low-grade gliomas can exhibit patchy enhancement, and many high-grade gliomas can be non-enhancing, as illustrated in Figure 4.1. A recent retrospective review identified that 27.9% of non-enhancing gliomas are in fact high grade.[11] The susceptibility weighted imaging (SWI) MRI sequence may also illustrate calcifications for slow-growing lesions.

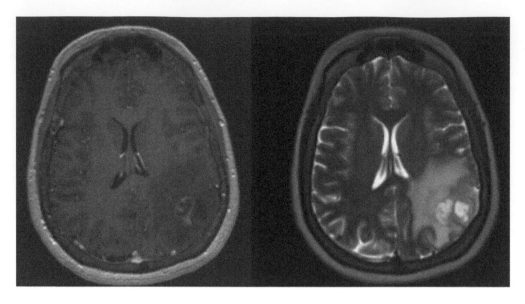

Figure 4.1 *Grade 3 oligodendroglioma. A left parieto-occipital grade 3 oligodendroglioma is shown with T1 gadolinium-enhanced sequence on the left and T2 sequence on the right. The lesion expresses classic contrast enhancement and surrounding vasogenic edema of a grade 3 glioma.*

Some low-grade gliomas can exhibit patchy enhancement and many high-grade gliomas can be non-enhancing.

Grade 3 gliomas also present most commonly in the supratentorium. The imaging hallmark is the alteration of the blood–brain barrier leading to contrast enhancement (see Figure 4.2). This can vary from patchy contrast enhancement within a tumor bed to fully ring-enhancing lesions. They typically exhibit more surrounding vasogenic edema with mass effect. This can manifest as midline shift or, less commonly, herniation. Signal on the SWI sequence can represent areas

of intratumoral or surrounding hemorrhage rather than calcification. Restricted diffusion on diffusion-weighted imaging (DWI) can represent hypercellularity, infarctions, or both. It is difficult to predict whether a tumor will be a grade 3 or 4 glioma based on imaging alone.

It is difficult to predict whether a tumor will be a grade 3 or 4 glioma based on imaging alone.

Though contrast-enhanced brain MRIs are the gold standard of imaging; MRI perfusion sequencing, positron

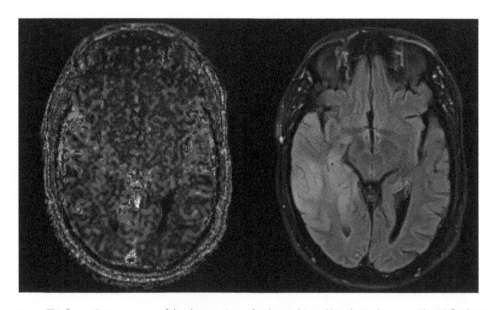

Figure 4.2 *Grade 2 astrocytoma. This figure illustrates some of the shortcomings of radiographic and histologic diagnosis. The T2/fluid-attenuated inversion recovery (FLAIR) sequence on the right shows an expansile mass without contrast enhancement (contrast-enhanced sequences not shown). On the left, there is no associated increased blood volume on perfusion sequencing. The lesion was resected and diagnosed a WHO grade 2 isocitrate dehydrogenase (IDH)-wildtype (WT) astrocytoma. However, molecular analysis later showed TERT promotor mutation, reclassifying the tumor to molecular GBM. The patient had early recurrence during adjuvant temozolomide (TMZ) cycles.*

tomography (PET), and magnetic resonance spectroscopy may have roles in glioma diagnosis and recurrence. Perfusion and PET imaging demonstrate relative increased metabolic activity in a brain region by assessing increased blood volume or fluoro-deoxyglucose uptake, respectively. Spectroscopic imaging shows increased choline peak and reduced N-acetyl aspartate peaks for active tumors. These are particularly helpful post-radiation therapy when assessing progression, pseudoprogression, or radiation necrosis effect.

The field of radiomics is advancing and already assists in predicting glioma subtypes based on imaging. For example, a 2017 study showed mismatch in hyperintensity on T2/FLAIR and conventional T2 MRI sequences is highly specific for IDH-mutant astrocytomas.[12]

PATHOLOGY

Traditionally, tumors were diagnosed based on their microscopic appearance on hematoxylin and eosin (H&E) staining (Figure 4.3). The subjective assessment of cell morphology diagnosed a tumor as astrocytic or oligodendroglial-appearing. Hence, the now-defunct diagnosis of oligoastrocytoma was possible. It was demonstrated that pathologic diagnoses for a given sample varied even within academic centers.[13] Tumor grading is still determined by extent of mitosis, vascular proliferation, necrosis, and nuclear atypia.

The shift to molecular diagnoses began in the early 2000s. The significance of the deletion of the short arm of chromosome 1 and the long arm of chromosome 19 (1p/19q

co-deletion) was established in the late 1990s and is now the defining characteristic of oligodendrogliomas. Following discovery of the IDH mutation in 2008, the correlation between better prognoses in IDH-mutated tumors became evident and was believed to be related to the 2-hydroxyglutarate (2-HG) effect on gene expression.[14,15] Interestingly, 2-HG has also been found to promote epileptogenesis, which supports the previously discussed finding that lower grade tumors are more often associated with epilepsy.[16] Transcription factor p53 (TP53) gene mutation was found to be oncogenic in astrocytomas in the early 2000s.[17] Transcriptional regulator ATRX mutations are found associated with IDH-mutant gliomas. The mutation (commonly referred to as "loss of ATRX") is only seen in 1p/19q intact gliomas, aiding in diagnosis of IDH-mutant astrocytomas.[18]

With the WHO 2016 classification change, non-GBM glial tumors are classified by their molecular profile using IDH mutation, 1p/19q co-deletion. For simplification purposes, IDH mutations are always present with 1p/19 co-deletion. TP53 promotes astrocytic oncogenesis, so is not seen with 1p/19q codeletion. Resultantly, six main lower grade glioma subtypes exist: grade 2 oligodendroglioma, grade 2 IDH-mutant astrocytoma, grade 2 IDH-wildtype (IDH-WT) astrocytoma, grade 3 oligodendroglioma, grade 3 IDH-mutant astrocytoma, and grade 3 IDH-WT astrocytoma. A simplified version of the classification scheme is included in Figure 4.3.

> Six main lower grade glioma subtypes exist: grade 2 oligodendroglioma, grade 2 IDH-mutant astrocytoma,

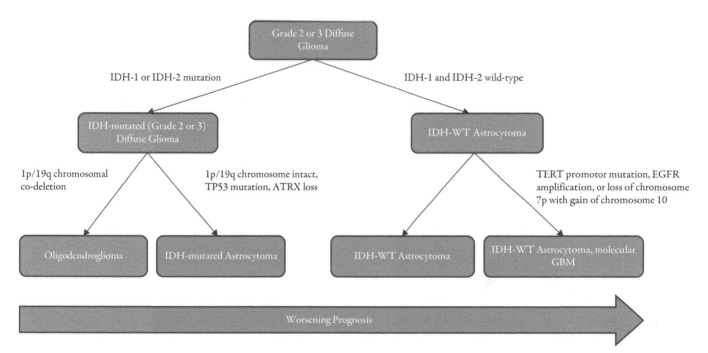

Figure 4.3 *Simplified molecular characterization of lower grade gliomas*

This represents a general scheme, as not all molecular findings are required for diagnosis, ex. IDH-2 mutations are not routinely assessed. Additionally, not-otherwise-specified (NOS) diagnoses are removed for simplicity. IDH, isocitrate dehydrogenase; WT, wildtype; ATRX, transcriptional regulator ATRX; GBM, glioblastoma; TP53, tumor promoter p53; EGFR, epidermal growth factor receptor.

grade 2 IDH-wildtype (IDH-WT) astrocytoma, grade 3 oligodendroglioma, grade 3 IDH-mutant astrocytoma, and grade 3 IDH-WT astrocytoma.

Grade 2 tumors are defined as having low mitotic activity on histopathology. The IDH-WT grade 2 astrocytoma is uncommon because the wildtype IDH leads to a more aggressive tumor usually presenting as grade 3. The IDH-mutated grade 2 gliomas are subdivided into oligodendroglioma if harboring the 1p/19q co-deletion and astrocytoma if those chromosomes are intact. TP53 mutation is present only in astrocytomas.

For grade 3 tumors, the co-deletion similarly defines oligodendroglioma versus astrocytoma. The IDH-WT phenotype is more common in grade 3 astrocytomas and prognosticates aggressive tumors. Grade 3 IDH-mutant astrocytomas are more aggressive than their grade 2 counterparts but are a very distinct phenotype from the IDH-WT anaplastic astrocytomas.

As the field advances, more molecular subtypes are gaining clinical relevancy.[19] Molecular GBMs harbor certain profiles that are often present in histologically classic GBM, such as the telomerase reverse transcriptase (TERT) promoter gene mutation, epidermal growth factor receptor (EGFR) gene amplification, or loss of chromosome 7p with gain of chromosome 10q. These molecular equivalents of GBM confer a lower than expected survival than grade 3 astrocytomas and behave very similarly to histologically classic GBMs.[20]

Finally, the clinical role of O6-methylguanine-methyltransferase (MGMT) promoter hypermethylation in GBMs is well established as a prognostic and predictive marker[21] but is less commonly applied in lower grade gliomas. Opinions are mixed on its value in lower grade gliomas. In itself, MGMT has prognostic and predictive value but is highly correlated with IDH status.[22,23]

TREATMENT

The treatment of grade 2 and grade 3 gliomas is less delineated than for their more aggressive counterpart. In fact, the closer a tumor is to the GBM phenotype, the easier the decision to use the maximal available up-front therapy. Patients with "lower risk" tumors require careful consideration. Evidence does support the use of combined chemoradiation in terms of efficacy over a sequential approach, but toxicity is factored into decision making.

SURGERY

The need for surgery is consistent across all glioma subtypes, in that a tissue diagnosis is required before treatment can be initiated. For patients with obvious high-grade lesions, mass effect, or neurologic deficits, the recommendation for surgery is straightforward. In other cases, such as patients with incidentally found lesions or well-controlled secondary epilepsy, some

neuro-oncologists prefer a watch-and-wait method. However, we now know that a significant portion of high-grade gliomas can be non-enhancing, so tissue diagnosis is critical even when all evidence points toward a low-grade glioma.[11]

A significant portion of high-grade gliomas can be non-enhancing, so tissue diagnosis is critical even when all evidence (radiographic, clinical) points toward a low-grade glioma.

There is no Level 1 evidence to support resection over biopsy, but it has been shown repeatedly that maximal total resection correlates to improved 5-year survival rate.[24–27] One study showed that survival benefit is lost when controlling for confounders, but it predates the trials supporting maximal resection.[28]

The role of re-resection at tumor recurrence is less well supported. Resection of recurrence provides symptom relief and improves progression-free survival (PFS), but the evidence to assess improved OS is mixed.[29] Re-resection is helpful from a diagnostic perspective, especially in cases of tumors transforming to a higher grade or in differentiating between progression and pseudoprogression. For such diagnoses, the more tissue obtained, the better. Muragaki et al. showed that resections are definitively more sensitive, as a biopsy could potentially miss higher-grade components within the tumor heterogeneity.[30]

Although maximal safe resection is a positive prognostic factor, glioma resection causing new neurologic deficits has been shown to lessen OS.[31] Advancing technology in neurosurgery helps mitigate those risks as techniques such as functional MRI, awake craniotomy, and intraoperative mapping are becoming more widely available. A recent study found improved OS and neuro-cognitive outcomes for patients with high-grade gliomas who underwent awake surgery.[32]

RADIATION THERAPY

Radiation therapy (RT) predates most modern glioma chemotherapy and is still a mainstay in treatment regimens. Though whole-brain RT, stereotactic radiosurgery, and even brachytherapy have been tried in glioma therapy, focal fractionated external beam photon RT remains the standard for up-front therapy. Proton radiotherapy is becoming more popular, although its efficacy compared to photon radiotherapy has not been established.

For grade 2 gliomas, the standard dose is 50–54 Gy divided in fractions over 5–6 weeks. Its efficacy has been well established as compared to higher doses.[33,34] For these low-grade tumors, the question becomes whether the RT should be given at diagnosis or later. Because these patients are typically younger with longer OS, the risk of developing cognitive deficits with radiation must be considered. Measurable cognitive deficits have been demonstrated in long-term glioma survivors having received RT.[35] Additionally, RT can complicate the assessment of radiographic progression due to progressive white matter changes. This was more of a concern before the development of the Response Assessment in Neuro-Oncology (RANO) criteria were established.[36] A phase III European study of early versus late RT in low-grade gliomas showed equal OS but improved PFS in patients treated earlier.[37] Hence, the decision is often based on patient preference.

> As patients with low-grade gliomas are typically younger with longer OS, the risk of developing cognitive deficits with radiation must be considered.

Grade 3 tumors require early high-dose RT due to their aggressive nature.[38–40] The dose for grade 3 and grade 4 tumors is 60 Gy, again fractionated over 5–6 weeks.

Some retrospective data suggest that patients with oligodendrogliomas are more susceptible to radiation necrosis, particularly at doses greater than 54 Gy.[41,42] This correlation has not been demonstrated in a prospective setting and is not incorporated into treatment guidelines as of yet. It suggests that grade 3 oligodendrogliomas be treated with lower radiation doses, especially given their chemosensitivity.

For astrocytic tumors, TMZ is typically given with the fractionated radiation therapy akin to standard glioblastoma therapy, but with little supporting evidence. Radiosensitizers have been studied in multiple glioma trials but have not been shown to have significant efficacy and are not used.

For disease recurrence, the role of re-irradiation is not well established. Small recurrent tumors are considered for repeat radiation if a patient has good functional status. Stereotactic radiosurgery is more commonly used in this setting. Brachytherapy had shown benefit in some observational studies but is associated with high risk of radiation necrosis.[43]

CHEMOTHERAPY

TMZ and PCV are the chemotherapeutics indicated for the upfront treatment of gliomas. Though now believed to be about equal in efficacy, PCV is supported by many of the older clinical trials. The logistics and side-effect profile for TMZ are more palatable and thus TMZ is slowly supplanting PCV. Currently, for "high-risk" grade 2 gliomas, the National Comprehensive Cancer Network (NCCN) guidelines recommend RT with PCV (category 1, high level of evidence), RT with TMZ, or observation in very select neurologically stable "lower-risk" patients (category 2A).[44] High-risk features include patients older than 40 years or those with subtotal resections.

For grade 2 gliomas, the role of chemotherapy has been extensively studied. Early studies aimed to compare the efficacy of chemotherapy against radiation therapy. The EORTC 22033 study compared RT to TMZ head to head and showed about equal efficacy in terms of PFS in low-grade oligodendroglioma. However, PFS was better in the RT cohort for all astrocytic tumors.[45] Another landmark study, RTOG 9802, compared RT with PCV against RT alone in patients with high-risk diffuse grade 2 gliomas. "High-risk" in this study was defined as patients with advanced age with any extent of resection or patients younger than 40 years with less than gross

total resection. Though initial results showed no significant difference in the two cohorts, long-term follow-up has shown improved OS in patients who also received PCV.[46] This was especially pronounced in patients with IDH-mutant tumors, although not all patients had these data available. It is accepted that patients with low-grade gliomas benefit in survival by receiving both RT and chemotherapy. Patients who are initially observed or receive either one of the therapies inevitably will require further treatment with the other. There is some speculation that initial treatment with chemotherapy alone can lead to tumor mutation and resistance down the road, as evidenced by preclinical and observational studies.[47] This has gained traction in both concern (TMZ inducing transformation to a higher grade glioma) and promise (targeted or immunotherapy to treat these phenotypes). However, neither have been clearly demonstrated on a clinical level.[48]

For grade 3 astrocytic tumors with IDH-WT phenotypes, the NCCN recommendation is to treat with some form of chemotherapy following RT: adjuvant TMZ with or without concomitant TMZ, or adjuvant PCV. Clinical practice is largely extrapolated from GBM management, and the Stupp protocol with TMZ is often used.[49] The early data from the EORTC 26053-22054 (CATNON) study presented in 2019 questioned the efficacy of chemotherapy in IDH-WT patients.[50] There was no benefit observed of concurrent or adjuvant TMZ in anaplastic astrocytoma IDH-WT. This is not an unprecedented finding: long-term results from phase III studies assessing RT versus RT and PCV in anaplastic gliomas showed no benefit from the addition of PCV to radiation in non–co-deleted tumors.[51] Another phase III study showed only marginal benefit in non–co-deleted tumors.[52] For grade 3 astrocytic tumors with IDH mutation, data from the CATNON trial support TMZ use in the adjuvant setting.[53] A planned second interim analysis of the CATNON trial revealed that concomitant TMZ with RT did not add a significant survival benefit to patients in grade 3 astrocytic tumors with IDH mutations.[53]

> Data from the CATNON trial support TMZ use in the adjuvant setting for patients with grade 3 astrocytoma tumors.

Grade 3 oligodendrogliomas have been proved more chemosensitive than astrocytomas, and there is clear indication for the use of chemotherapy.[51,52,55] The choice between PCV and TMZ remains contentious among neuro-oncologists. TMZ is again less toxic and logistically simpler, but trials demonstrating the chemosensitivity of oligodendrogliomas used PCV. A study assessing the sequence of RT and chemotherapy in anaplastic gliomas showed no difference in using chemotherapy initially or after RT. A subgroup analysis demonstrated efficacy of PCV over TMZ in 1p/19q co-deleted tumors.[56,57] However, this study was not powered to make that comparison. The pending CODEL study will help address this issue as it is assessing RT and TMZ versus RT and PCV in anaplastic oligodendrogliomas.[1,58]

Chemotherapy at the time of recurrence has limited efficacy. Bevacizumab, lomustine, TMZ, or combination therapy are commonly used. No single agent or regimen has been shown to be superior, especially in improving OS. The choice of therapy is individualized to a patients' prior chemotherapy history, size of tumor or mass effect, and goals of care. Molecular profiling can be obtained at the time of recurrence to attempt genome-directed therapies. Mutation-directed tyrosine kinase inhibitors (TKIs) have been beneficial in other solid tumor malignancies, but their benefit has not translated to the neuro-oncology world. Clinical trials should be explored at the time of recurrence.

> Chemotherapy at the time of recurrence has limited efficacy. Bevacizumab, lomustine, TMZ, or combination therapy are commonly used.

PROGNOSIS

Diffuse gliomas of all grades are malignancies. Patients should be made aware that gliomas are treatable but not curable. Some patients are confused by the term "tumor" rather than "cancer" or "malignancy."

While grade 2 gliomas usually have an indolent course after initial therapy, they will eventually recur. The OS is estimated at 10–20 years for grade 2 oligodendrogliomas,[46,51,52] 10–12 years for grade 2 IDH-mutant astrocytomas, and 1.5–3 years for grade 2 IDH-WT astrocytomas.[2,59,60] As can be gleaned from these clinical trial data, the presence of an IDH mutation is one of the strongest prognostic factors.[15,61] The 1p/19q co-deletion defining oligodendrogliomas is also both prognostic and predictive.[51,59] Other positive prognostic factors are younger patient age (<40), maximal tumor resection (>90%), performance status, and initial presentation with seizures.[3] Poor prognostic factors include older age, presentation with a fixed neurologic deficit, involvement of corpus callosum or contralateral hemisphere, and tumors larger than 5 cm in diameter.[62] Many of these prognostic factors were identified prior to advances in molecular neuro-oncology so it is unclear if the factors still have relevance. MGMT promoter hypermethylation has an uncertain role in the prognostication of low-grade gliomas.

> As can be gleaned from clinical trial data, the presence of an IDH mutation is one of the strongest prognostic factors.

Grade 3 gliomas are often more aggressive from the onset and often recur within months to a few years. Grade 3 astrocytomas have survival of 8–10 years for IDH-mutated tumors and 1.5–3 years for IDH-WT.[2,59] Grade 3 oligodendrogliomas have median survivals of about 14 years.[51] Many of the same prognostic factors for grade 2 hold true for grade 3 tumors. MGMT hypermethylation is assessed more commonly in these higher grade tumors and does carry prognostic value,[22] though it is not relied on as heavily in management of patients with GBM. It is clear that tumor molecular markers are critical factors in patient prognosis. Some have even questioned the utility of using mitotic index to grade IDH-mutated tumors.[63]

It is vital to inform patients of the nature of these tumors and honestly answer their questions about prognosis. However, they should be encouraged not to dwell on the figures as each patient is an individual case. Some hope can be provided to patients that the field of neuro-oncology continues to advance, as evidenced by the improved 3-year survival for GBM patients over recent years.[64] The data from the CATNON study also show improved survival in IDH-mutant astrocytomas treated with TMZ.[50] Patients and families should also be advised that available internet survival data are often dated because it lumps together multiple glioma subtypes. Since the identification of IDH and 1p/19q co-deletion, prognostication has become more accurate.

CONCLUSION

Patients with lower grade gliomas represent a challenging population to treat, even in comparison to patients with GBM. Given their younger age of onset and longer expected survival, factors such as chemoradiation toxicity must strongly be taken into consideration. Every effort must be made to avoid treating patients with superfluous regimens. As clinical trial data continue to mature, it is prudent for a neuro-oncologist to remain abreast of available evidence when tailoring treatment regimens to a patient's specific tumor molecular profile.

What is the epidemiology for grade 2 and 3 gliomas?	Annual incidence rate of 1.35 per 100,000 Median age at diagnoses is 30–40 years for WHO grade 2 tumors, 40–60 years for grade 3 More common in males
What is the only known environmental risk factor for diffuse gliomas?	Ionizing radiation
What grade of gliomas is more likely to present with fixed neurologic deficits?	Higher
Low-grade gliomas most commonly show what after contrast administration on MRI?	No enhancement, though approximately 30% of non-enhancing gliomas are in fact high-grade
Pathologic diagnosis of astrocytomas and oligodendrogliomas is based on these molecular markers:	IDH mutation and 1p19q co-deletion status
Differentiation between grade 2 and 3 gliomas (astrocytomas and oligodendrogliomas) is based on this histopathological feature:	Mitotic index
What is the standard radiation dose in grade 3 gliomas?	60 Gy
What is the most commonly used chemotherapy in lower grade gliomas?	Temozolomide
Adjuvant therapy after surgery with what two treatments prolongs survival in patients with low-grade gliomas?	Radiation and chemotherapy
Positive prognostic factors for patients with diffuse gliomas include:	Lower tumor grade, presence of IDH mutation, presence of 1p/19q co-deletion, younger patient age, maximal tumor resection (>90%), performance status, and initial presentation with seizures

1. The molecular analysis of a resected glioma reveals high mitotic index, IDH-1 mutation, and intact 1p/19q chromosomes. What is the pathologic diagnosis?
   a. WHO grade 2, IDH-1 mutated astrocytoma
   b. WHO grade 2, oligodendroglioma
   c. WHO grade 3, IDH-1 mutated astrocytoma
   d. WHO grade 3, oligodendroglioma

2. Which of the following is a positive prognostic factor in a patient with newly diagnosed glioma?
   a. Age older than 40 at diagnosis
   b. Biopsy only for tissue diagnosis
   c. Initial presentation with seizure
   d. Initial presentation with cognitive impairment

3. Which of the following glioma findings is not associated with the diagnosis of "molecular equivalent of glioblastoma?"
   a. TERT promoter gene mutation
   b. EGFR amplification
   c. Absence of MGMT promoter methylation
   d. Chromosome 7p gain, 10q loss

4. Current practice guidelines recommend WHO grade 3, IDH-1 mutated astrocytomas be treated with
   a. Maximal resective surgery, high-dose RT, concomitant TMZ, adjuvant TMZ
   b. Maximal resective surgery, low-dose RT, concomitant TMZ, adjuvant TMZ
   c. Maximal resective surgery, high-dose RT
   d. Maximal resective surgery, low-dose RT

5. The current CODEL study aims to assess
   a. The role of radiation therapy in treatment of oligodendrogliomas
   b. The role of radiation therapy in treatment of astrocytomas
   c. The role of TMZ versus PCV in treatment of oligodendrogliomas
   d. The role of TMZ versus PCV in treatment of astrocytomas

6. What is the most common location for WHO grade 2 gliomas?
   a. Supratentorial
   b. Infratentorial
   c. Brainstem
   d. Spinal cord

7. What is (are) the most common utility of susceptibility weighted imaging (SWI) sequence on MRI for gliomas?
   a. Assessing for calcifications in low-grade gliomas
   b. Assessing for intratumoral hemorrhage in high-grade gliomas

   c. Both a and b
   d. None of the above

8. Which of the following tumors is statistically most likely to cause epilepsy?
   a. Frontal lobe glioblastoma
   b. Frontal lobe grade 2 oligodendroglioma
   c. Brainstem glioma
   d. Occipital lobe IDH-WT astrocytoma

9. Which of the following radiation therapy regimens could be recommended for a newly diagnosed WHO grade 2 astrocytoma?
   a. Stereotactic radiosurgery
   b. Whole brain radiation therapy
   c. Intensity-modulated radiation therapy (IMRT) 60.0 Gy
   d. IMRT 50.4 Gy

10. Which of the following glioma subtypes was eliminated from the WHO 2016 classification scheme?
    a. Grade 2 astrocytoma
    b. Grade 2 oligodendroglioma
    c. Grade 2 oligoastrocytoma
    d. Glioblastoma, IDH-mutant

11. Which of the following tumor markers could be seen together in a glioma diagnosis?
    a. TP53 mutation and 1p/19q codeletion
    b. IDH WT and 1p/19qcodeletion
    c. ATRX loss and 1p/19q codeletion
    d. IDH WT and TERT promoter mutation

12. A diffuse glioma could be any of the following grades, *except*
    a. Grade 1
    b. Grade 2
    c. Grade 3
    d. Grade 4

13. Which of the following factors would have the largest impact on prognosticating a patient's overall survival after new glioma diagnosis?
    a. IDH mutation status
    b. Extent of resection
    c. Completion of chemotherapy cycles
    d. Total dose given for radiation therapy

14. Which of the following familial syndromes would not be expected to increase risk for glioma development?
    a. Li-Fraumeni
    b. Neurofibromatosis, type 1
    c. Multiple endocrine neoplasia (MEN) type 2a
    d. Lynch syndrome

15. Which of the following can be considered an established risk factor to developing a glioma?
    a. Receiving ionizing radiation as a child for hematologic malignancy
    b. Living next to a nuclear power plant during childhood
    c. Poor diet regimen
    d. Positive Epstein-Barr virus (EBV) titer

ANSWERS

1. c
2. c
3. c
4. a
5. c
6. a
7. c
8. b
9. d
10. c
11. d
12. a
13. a
14. c
15. a

REFERENCES

1. Jaeckle KA, Ballman KV, van den Bent M, et al. CODEL: Phase III study of RT, RT + Temozolomide (TMZ), or TMZ for newly-diagnosed 1p/19q Codeleted Oligodendroglioma. Analysis from the initial study design. *Neuro-Oncology.* 2021;23(3):457–467.
2. Ostrom QT, Cioffi G, Gittleman H, et al. CBTRUS statistical report: Primary brain and other central nervous system tumors diagnosed in the United States in 2012–2016. *Neuro-oncology.* 2019;21(Suppl 5):v1–v100.
3. Schiff D. Low-grade gliomas. *Continuum.* 2017;23(6):1564–1579.
4. Nayak L, Reardon DA. High-grade gliomas. *Continuum.* 2017;23(6):1548–1563.
5. Rice T, Lachance DH, Molinaro AM, et al. Understanding inherited genetic risk of adult glioma: A review. *Neuro-oncology Pract.* 2016;3(1):10–16.
6. Lote K, Stenwig AE, Skullerud K, Hirschberg H. Prevalence and prognostic significance of epilepsy in patients with gliomas. *Eur J Cancer (Oxf 1990).* 1998;34(1):98–102.
7. Chen H, Judkins J, Thomas C, et al. Mutant IDH1 and seizures in patients with glioma. *Neurology.* 2017;88(19):1805–1813.
8. Posti JP, Bori M, Kauko T, et al. Presenting symptoms of glioma in adults. *Acta Neurologica Scandi.* 2015;131(2):88–93.
9. Berendsen S, Varkila M, Kroonen J, et al. Prognostic relevance of epilepsy at presentation in glioblastoma patients. *Neuro-Oncology.* 2016;18(5):700–706.
10. Comelli I, Lippi G, Campana V, Servadei F, Cervellin G. Clinical presentation and epidemiology of brain tumors firstly diagnosed in adults in the Emergency Department: A 10-year, single center retrospective study. *Ann Translat Med.* 2017;5(13):269.
11. Eichberg DG, Di L, Morell AA, et al. Incidence of high grade gliomas presenting as radiographically non-enhancing lesions: Experience in 111 surgically treated non-enhancing gliomas with tissue diagnosis. *J Neuro-Oncology.* 2020;147(3):671–679.
12. Patel SH, Poisson LM, Brat DJ, et al. T2–FLAIR mismatch, an imaging biomarker for IDH and 1p/19q status in lower-grade gliomas: A TCGA/TCIA Project. *Clin Cancer Res.* 2017;23(20):6078–6085.
13. van den Bent MJ. Interobserver variation of the histopathological diagnosis in clinical trials on glioma: A clinician's perspective. *Acta Neuropathologica.* 2010;120(3):297–304.
14. Balss J, Meyer J, Mueller W, Korshunov A, et al. Analysis of the IDH1 codon 132 mutation in brain tumors. *Acta Neuropathologica.* 2008;116(6):597–602.
15. Yan H, Parsons DW, Jin G, et al. IDH1 and IDH2 mutations in gliomas. *N Engl J Med.* 2009;360(8):765–773.
16. Liang R, Fan Y, Wang X, et al. The significance of IDH1 mutations in tumor-associated seizure in 60 Chinese patients with low-grade gliomas. *Sci World J.* 2013;2013:403942.
17. Zhang Y, Dube C, Gibert M, Jr., et al. The p53 pathway in glioblastoma. *Cancers.* 2018 Sep 1;10(9):297.
18. Nandakumar P, Mansouri A, Das S. The role of ATRX in glioma biology. *Front Oncol.* 2017;7:236–236.
19. Bourne TD, Schiff D. Update on molecular findings, management and outcome in low-grade gliomas. *Nature Rev Neurol.* 2010;6(12):695–701.
20. Brat DJ, Aldape K, Colman H, et al. cIMPACT-NOW update 3: Recommended diagnostic criteria for "Diffuse astrocytic glioma, IDH-wildtype, with molecular features of glioblastoma, WHO grade IV." *Acta Neuropathologica.* 2018;136(5):805–810.
21. Hegi ME, Diserens A-C, Gorlia T, et al. MGMT gene silencing and benefit from temozolomide in glioblastoma. *N Engl J Med.* 2005;352(10):997–1003.
22. van den Bent MJ, Erdem-Eraslan L, Idbaih A, et al. MGMT-STP27 methylation status as predictive marker for response to PCV in anaplastic oligodendrogliomas and oligoastrocytomas: A report from EORTC study 26951. *Clin Cancer Res.* 2013;19(19):5513–5522.
23. Dubbink HJ, Atmodimedjo PN, Kros JM, et al. Molecular classification of anaplastic oligodendroglioma using next-generation sequencing: A report of the prospective randomized EORTC Brain Tumor Group 26951 phase III trial. *Neuro-Oncology.* 2016;18(3):388–400.
24. Jakola AS, Skjulsvik AJ, Myrmel KS, et al. Surgical resection versus watchful waiting in low-grade gliomas. *Ann Oncol.* 2017;28(8):1942–1948.
25. Smith JS, Chang EF, Lamborn KR, et al. Role of extent of resection in the long-term outcome of low-grade hemispheric gliomas. *J Clin Oncol.* 2008;26(8):1338–1345.
26. McGirt MJ, Chaichana KL, Attenello FJ, et al. Extent of surgical resection is independently associated with survival in patients with hemispheric infiltrating low-grade gliomas. *Neurosurgery.* 2008;63(4):700-707; author reply 707–708.
27. Hervey-Jumper SL, Berger MS. Role of surgical resection in low- and high-grade gliomas. *Curr Treat Options Neurol.* 2014;16(4):284.
28. Pignatti F, van den Bent M, Curran D, et al. Prognostic factors for survival in adult patients with cerebral low-grade glioma. *J Clin Oncol.* 2002;20(8):2076–2084.
29. Birk HS, Han SJ, Butowski NA. Treatment options for recurrent high-grade gliomas. *CNS oncology.* 2017;6(1):61–70.
30. Muragaki Y, Chernov M, Maruyama T, et al. Low-grade glioma on stereotactic biopsy: How often is the diagnosis accurate? *Minimally Invasive Neurosurg.* 2008;51(5):275–279.
31. Rahman M, Abbatematteo J, De Leo EK, et al. The effects of new or worsened postoperative neurological deficits on survival of patients with glioblastoma. *J Neurosurg.* 2017;127(1):123–131.
32. Zigiotto L, Annicchiarico L, Corsini F, et al. Effects of supra-total resection in neurocognitive and oncological outcome of high-grade gliomas comparing asleep and awake surgery. *J Neuro-Oncol.* 2020 May;148(1):97–108.
33. Shaw E, Arusell R, Scheithauer B, et al. Prospective randomized trial of low- versus high-dose radiation therapy in adults with supratentorial low-grade glioma: Initial report of a North Central Cancer Treatment Group/Radiation Therapy Oncology Group/Eastern Cooperative Oncology Group study. *J Clin Oncol.* 2002;20(9):2267–2276.
34. Karim AB, Maat B, Hatlevoll R, et al. A randomized trial on dose-response in radiation therapy of low-grade cerebral glioma: European Organization for Research and Treatment of Cancer (EORTC) Study 22844. *Intl J Radiat Oncol Biol Physics.* 1996;36(3):549–556.
35. Douw L, Klein M, Fagel SS, et al. Cognitive and radiological effects of radiotherapy in patients with low-grade glioma: Long-term follow-up. *Lancet Neurol.* 2009;8(9):810–818.
36. van den Bent MJ, Wefel JS, Schiff D, et al. Response assessment in neuro-oncology (a report of the RANO group): Assessment of outcome in trials of diffuse low-grade gliomas. *Lancet Oncol.* 2011;12(6):583–593.
37. van den Bent MJ, Afra D, de Witte O, et al. Long-term efficacy of early versus delayed radiotherapy for low-grade astrocytoma and oligodendroglioma in adults: The EORTC 22845 randomised trial. *Lancet.* 2005;366(9490):985–990.
38. Walker MD, Strike TA, Sheline GE. An analysis of dose-effect relationship in the radiotherapy of malignant gliomas. *Intl J Radiat Oncol Biol Physics.* 1979;5(10):1725-1731.

39. Chang CH, Horton J, Schoenfeld D, et al. Comparison of postoperative radiotherapy and combined postoperative radiotherapy and chemotherapy in the multidisciplinary management of malignant gliomas: A joint Radiation Therapy Oncology Group and Eastern Cooperative Oncology Group study. *Cancer.* 1983;52(6):997–1007.

40. Nelson DF, Diener-West M, Horton J, et al. Combined modality approach to treatment of malignant gliomas: Re-evaluation of RTOG 7401/ECOG 1374 with long-term follow-up: A joint study of the Radiation Therapy Oncology Group and the Eastern Cooperative Oncology Group. *NCI Monographs.* 1988(6):279–284.

41. Acharya S, Robinson CG, Michalski JM, et al. Association of 1p/19q codeletion and radiation necrosis in adult cranial gliomas after proton or photon therapy. *Intl J Radiat Oncol Biol Physics.* 2018;101(2):334–343.

42. Ahmad H, Martin D, Patel SH, et al. Oligodendroglioma confers higher risk of radiation necrosis. *J Neuro-Oncol.* 2019;145(2):309–319.

43. Scharfen CO, Sneed PK, Wara WM, et al. High activity iodine-125 interstitial implant for gliomas. *Intl J Radiat Oncol Biol Physics.* 1992;24(4):583–591.

44. National Comprehensive Cancer Network I. NCCN Clinical Practice Guidelines in Oncology (NCCN Guildelines). *NCCN Evidence Blocks.* 2019(Version 1.2019).

45. Baumert BG, Hegi ME, van den Bent MJ, et al. Temozolomide chemotherapy versus radiotherapy in high-risk low-grade glioma (EORTC 22033-26033): A randomised, open-label, phase 3 intergroup study. *Lancet Oncol.* 2016;17(11):1521–1532.

46. Buckner JC, Shaw EG, Pugh SL, et al. Radiation plus procarbazine, CCNU, and vincristine in low-grade glioma. *N Engl J Med.* 2016;374(14):1344–1355.

47. Daniel P, Sabri S, Chaddad A, et al. Temozolomide induced hypermutation in glioma: Evolutionary mechanisms and therapeutic opportunities. *Front Oncol.* 2019;9:41–41.

48. Ahmad H, Fadul CE, Schiff D, Purow B. Checkpoint inhibitor failure in hypermutated and mismatch repair-mutated recurrent high-grade gliomas. *Neuro-Oncology Pract.* 2019;6(6):424–427.

49. Stupp R, Mason WP, van den Bent MJ, et al. Radiotherapy plus concomitant and adjuvant temozolomide for glioblastoma. *N Engl J Med.* 2005;352(10):987–996.

50. Bent MJVD, Erridge S, Vogelbaum MA, et al. Second interim and first molecular analysis of the EORTC randomized phase III intergroup CATNON trial on concurrent and adjuvant temozolomide in anaplastic glioma without 1p/19q codeletion. *J Clin Oncol.* 2019;37(15 Suppl):2000.

51. Cairncross G, Wang M, Shaw E, et al. Phase III trial of chemoradiotherapy for anaplastic oligodendroglioma: Long-term results of RTOG 9402. *J Clin Oncol.* 2013;31(3):337–343.

52. van den Bent MJ, Brandes AA, Taphoorn MJ, et al. Adjuvant procarbazine, lomustine, and vincristine chemotherapy in newly diagnosed anaplastic oligodendroglioma: Long-term follow-up of EORTC brain tumor group study 26951. *J Clin Oncol.* 2013;31(3):344–350.

53. van den Bent MJ, Baumert B, Erridge SC, et al. Interim results from the CATNON trial (EORTC study 26053-22054) of treatment with concurrent and adjuvant temozolomide for 1p/19q non-co-deleted anaplastic glioma: A phase 3, randomised, open-label intergroup study. *Lancet.* 2017;390(10103):1645–1653.

54. van den Bent MJ, Tesileanu C, Wick W, et al. Adjuvant and concurrent temozolomide for 1p/19q non-co-deleted anaplastic glioma (CATNON;EORTC study 26053-22054): second interim analysis of a randomised, open-label, phase 3 study. *Lancet Oncol.* 2021;22(6):813–823.

55. van den Bent MJ, Carpentier AF, Brandes AA, et al. Adjuvant procarbazine, lomustine, and vincristine improves progression-free survival but not overall survival in newly diagnosed anaplastic oligodendrogliomas and oligoastrocytomas: A randomized European Organisation for Research and Treatment of Cancer phase III trial. *J Clin Oncol.* 2006;24(18):2715–2722.

56. Wick W, Hartmann C, Engel C, et al. NOA-04 randomized phase III trial of sequential radiochemotherapy of anaplastic glioma with procarbazine, lomustine, and vincristine or temozolomide. *J Clin Oncol.* 2009;27(35):5874–5880.

57. Wick W, Roth P, Hartmann C, et al. Long-term analysis of the NOA-04 randomized phase III trial of sequential radiochemotherapy of anaplastic glioma with PCV or temozolomide. *Neuro-Oncology.* 2016;18(11):1529–1537.

58. Jaeckle K, Vogelbaum M, Ballman K, et al. CODEL (Alliance-N0577; EORTC-26081/22086; NRG-1071; NCIC-CEC-2): Phase III randomized study of RT vs. RT+TMZ vs. TMZ for newly diagnosed 1p/19q-codeleted anaplastic oligodendroglial tumors: Analysis of patients treated on the original protocol design (PL02.005). *Neurology.* 2016;86(16 Supplement):PL02.005.

59. Louis DN, Perry A, Reifenberger G, et al. The 2016 World Health Organization Classification of Tumors of the Central Nervous System: A summary. *Acta Neuropathologica.* 2016;131(6):803–820.

60. Ohgaki H, Kleihues P. Population-based studies on incidence, survival rates, and genetic alterations in astrocytic and oligodendroglial gliomas. *J Neuropathol Exp Neurol.* 2005;64(6):479–489.

61. Gorlia T, Wu W, Wang M, et al. New validated prognostic models and prognostic calculators in patients with low-grade gliomas diagnosed by central pathology review: A pooled analysis of EORTC/RTOG/NCCTG phase III clinical trials. *Neuro-Oncology.* 2013;15(11):1568–1579.

62. Gorlia T, Delattre JY, Brandes AA, et al. New clinical, pathological and molecular prognostic models and calculators in patients with locally diagnosed anaplastic oligodendroglioma or oligoastrocytoma: A prognostic factor analysis of European Organisation for Research and Treatment of Cancer Brain Tumour Group Study 26951. *Eur J Cancer(Oxf 1990).* 2013;49(16):3477–3485.

63. Olar A, Wani KM, Alfaro-Munoz KD, et al. IDH mutation status and role of WHO grade and mitotic index in overall survival in grade II-III diffuse gliomas. *Acta Neuropathologica.* 2015;129(4):585–596.

64. Zreik J, Moinuddin FM, Yolcu YU, et al. Improved 3-year survival rates for glioblastoma multiforme are associated with trends in treatment: Analysis of the national cancer database from 2004 to 2013. *J Neuro-Oncology.* 2020 May;148(1):69–79.

5 | MENINGIOMA

THOMAS J. KALEY

INTRODUCTION

Meningiomas are the most common primary brain tumor in adults and encompass a wide spectrum of illness varying from the incidentally found presumed meningioma to the multiply recurrent radiation- and surgery-refractory malignant meningioma. As neuroimaging has increased in availability and computed tomography (CT) and magnetic resonance imaging (MRI) are performed for a multitude of various neurologic symptoms, meningiomas are by far the most likely primary brain tumor physicians will encounter in practice. Although the majority of meningiomas are "benign," they may enlarge and/or cause neurologic dysfunction and even substantial morbidity depending on location within the brain or rate of growth (Figure 5.1). Surgery is typically the first-line consideration for treatment, but not all meningiomas are amenable to complete resection, and some will recur and require further therapy, especially the higher grade meningiomas. Therefore, a thorough understanding of these tumors and the preferred management algorithms is imperative to the best management of these patients.

EPIDEMIOLOGY

The Central Brain Tumor Registry of the United States estimates an annual incidence of approximately 20,000 new meningioma cases, representing approximately one-third of all primary brain tumors and more than half of all non-malignant brain tumors.[1,2]

> The annual incidence of new meningioma cases is estimated to be approximately 20,000, representing approximately one-third of all primary brain tumors and over half of all non-malignant brain tumors.

These tumors very rarely occur in children, and incidence increases with advancing age, with the highest incidence in adults, especially those older than 65 years. Meningiomas have a clear female predominance, occurring approximately twice as often in women as in men.[3] The overwhelming majority of meningiomas encountered in clinical practice have no clearly identified risk factor contributing to their development. Infrequently, meningiomas may occur as part of a neurogenetic syndrome such as neurofibromatosis type 2 (NF2). These meningiomas are often multiple and occur along with vestibular schwannomas. The incidence of NF2-related meningiomas may be higher than appreciated due to the unknown incidence of genetic mosaicism.

The only clearly demonstrated risk factor for sporadic meningiomas is prior exposure to ionizing radiation involving the head and neck region.[4] Patients may present with meningiomas in adulthood after having received prior cranial radiation for childhood malignancies such as leukemia or medulloblastoma, although they may also occur after radiation for various head and neck malignancies.[5,6] Unfortunately, these radiation-induced meningiomas tend to have a much more aggressive clinical course. Historically, scalp radiation for tinea capitis and older dental x-rays have demonstrated an association with meningiomas, however scalp radiation for fungal infections is no longer performed and newer, more refined dental x-rays likely do not carry an increased risk.[7]

> The only clearly demonstrated risk factor for sporadic meningiomas is prior exposure to ionizing radiation involving the head and neck region. Unfortunately, these radiation-induced meningiomas tend to have a much more aggressive clinical course.

Additional risk factors for meningiomas are less certain. Head trauma has been postulated as a potential risk factor, although not proved to be so.[8] Breast cancer has been suggested as a potential risk factor as well, although this is likely more complicated.[9] Meningiomas often express hormone (progesterone or estrogen) receptors, and therefore the breast cancer correlation may simply be a shared hormonal association. Similarly, some meningiomas may grow during pregnancy due to hormonal stimulation. Probably the most controversial current risk factor is the use of cellular phones; however, to date there is no clear convincing data to support cell phone use as a risk factor for meningioma.

PATHOPHYSIOLOGY

Meningiomas are primary central nervous system (CNS) tumors arising from neoplastic meningothelial arachnoid cap cells along the coverings of the brain. Histologically, the key

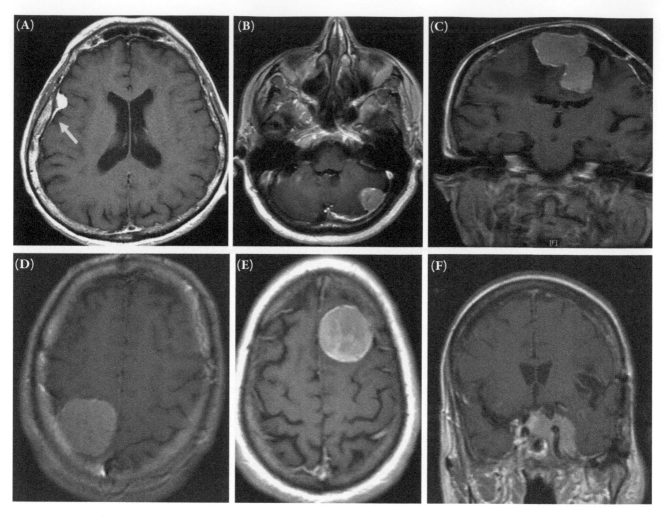

Figure 5.1 Meningiomas encompass a heterogenous presentation on imaging. (A) Small incidental meningioma with arrow highlighting the "dural tail." (B) Small incidental posterior fossa meningioma. (C) Larger symptomatic meningioma with peritumoral edema. (D) Large asymptomatic meningioma. (E) Large symptomatic meningioma. (F) Unresectable symptomatic cavernous sinus meningioma.

features for the diagnosis of meningioma are the identification of "whorls" (which references the pattern of tumor cells) and "psammoma bodies" (calcium deposits).[1] Meningiomas are classified into three grades with many various subtypes (Table 5.1). The World Health Organization (WHO) grade 1 meningiomas (approximately 80%) are most commonly referred to as the "benign" meningioma, and these tend to have the best prognosis. As the grade increases to WHO grade 2 (20%) and 3 (<3%), there is a proportionate increase in the overall aggressivity of the meningioma, with WHO grade 3 meningiomas representing the most aggressive subtype which are typically eventually refractory to all treatments.

The pathogenesis of meningiomas is largely unknown. As recent attempts to identify genetic and molecular characteristics of cancers as a whole have been successful in a wide variety of diseases, no such success has yet occurred with meningiomas. The most common genetic abnormality in sporadic meningiomas is an inactivating alteration of the *NF2* gene, either through chromosomal loss or point mutations. The *NF2* gene codes for the protein merlin, but scientists have not yet identified the exact mechanism of action of these genetic mutations, and multiple

hypotheses exist. Furthermore, there is no clear anticancer therapy that specifically targets *NF2* alterations.

> The most common genetic abnormality in sporadic meningiomas is an inactivating alteration of the *NF2* gene, either through chromosomal loss or point mutations.

Additional mutations have been discovered in meningioma, and initially there was much excitement after the identification of mutations in *AKT* and *SMO* in a small subset of meningiomas.[10,11] The major enthusiasm about these mutations was that the specific mutations identified were well-described oncogenic hot-spot mutations with pre-existing targeted therapies designed to inhibit those specific alterations. Although these mutations may play a therapeutic role in a very small subset of meningiomas, it has since become clear that these mutations do not occur in the majority of the meningiomas that require additional therapy and have the more aggressive clinical course. Therefore, the likely benefit of targeting these alterations is currently undetermined.

TABLE 5.1 World Health Organization (WHO) classification of meningiomas

WHO grade 1 meningioma	Angiomatous
	Fibrous
	Lymphoplasmacyte-rich
	Meningothelial
	Metaplastic
	Microcystic
	Psammomatous
	Secretory
	Transitional
WHO grade 2 meningioma	Clear cell
	Chordoid
	Atypical
	Increased mitotic activity (≥4 mitoses per 10 high-powered fields)
	or
	Brain invasion
	or
	At least three of the following features:
	Increased cellularity
	Small cells with a high nuclear to cytoplasmic ratio
	Prominent nucleoli
	Patternless or sheet like growth
	Necrosis
WHO grade 3 meningioma	Rhabdoid
	Papillary
	Anaplastic (malignant)
	Increased mitotic activity (≥20 mitoses per 10 high-powered fields) *and/or* malignant characteristics:
	Loss of usual meningioma growth patterns
	Infiltration of underlying brain
	Abundant mitoses with atypical forms
	Multifocal necrosis

CLINICAL PRESENTATION AND DIAGNOSIS

Like most brain tumors, the clinical presentation of meningiomas typically falls into two categories: either location-specific symptoms or general non-specific symptoms. However, for many newly diagnosed meningiomas there are no symptoms at all, and the tumors are discovered incidentally when imaging is performed for an alternate reason.

Location-specific symptoms may occur due to local compression of one particular area of brain causing dysfunction of the underlying brain tissue, with symptoms consistent with the area of brain affected. For example, meningiomas compressing the optic nerve may cause vision loss, whereas meningiomas occurring in the cerebellopontine angle may cause hearing loss. Additionally, if allowed to grow to a large enough size, a meningioma may cause the typically non-specific symptoms of a space-occupying lesion such as headache, nausea/vomiting, and/or hydrocephalus. Regardless of where they occur in the brain, supratentorial meningiomas may also cause seizures (the most common symptom) owing to the extraparenchymal location of the tumor and local compression of the nearby cortex.

The diagnosis of a meningioma can usually be suspected on radiographic grounds. Typically, a meningioma is first identified on either a CT or MRI scan. Although meningiomas have a rather stereotypical appearance of a homogenously enhancing mass with a clear linear extension into the dura called the "dural tail" (Figure 5.1A), this is not a definitive diagnosis because there are some much rarer entities that appear similar on imaging, such as hemangiopericytomas, dural metastases, or hypertrophic pachymeningitis. These differential diagnoses may be suspected in rare cases given the clinical context (i.e., the patient with a known active malignancy may be suspected to have dural metastases), however only histologic sampling can definitely diagnose any of these specific disorders.

> Although meningiomas have a rather stereotypical appearance of a homogenously enhancing mass with a clear linear extension into the dura called the "dural tail" (Figure 5.1A), this is not a definitive diagnosis because there are some much rarer entities that appear similar on imaging, such as hemangiopericytomas, dural metastases, or hypertrophic pachymeningitis.

Current standard imaging does have limitations. One of the major limitations of current standard imaging is the inability of CT or MRI to differentiate between grades or subtypes of meningiomas and identify which meningiomas are more likely to behave in a more aggressive manner. Another major limitation is in evaluation of the extent of resection of a meningioma, as both CT and MRI are inadequate at defining the extent of resection, which is graded according to the Simpson grade. As a result, many treatment decisions are instead made based on more standard neuro-oncologic language (gross total resection [GTR] and subtotal resection [STR]).

COMPUTED TOMOGRAPHY

Meningiomas have a consistent appearance on CT scan, as demonstrated in Figure 5.2A. On non-contrast images, meningiomas appear as either hyperdense or isodense, with the hyperdensity resulting largely from calcification, which, when present, may be an indicator of more indolent growth and a more benign process. On post-contrast images, meningiomas typically brightly and homogenously enhance as a result of their high vascularity.

MAGNETIC RESONANCE IMAGING

MRI produces similar imaging characteristics of meningiomas, although with better delineation of tumor versus neighboring structures. Therefore, unless there is a contraindication, MRI should be pursued upon identification of a meningioma on CT. Contrast enhanced T1-weighted sequences are best to visualize meningiomas, where they appear as brightly and homogenously enhancing masses. T2 or fluid-attenuated inversion recovery (FLAIR) sequences may be helpful in the identification of peritumoral edema, which is not typically seen in the benign or small/incidental meningiomas and, if observed, may influence the decision to treat a meningioma sooner rather than simply observing with a follow-up scan.

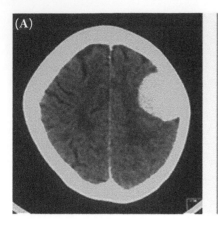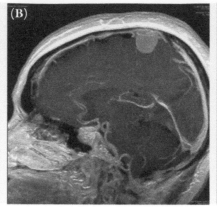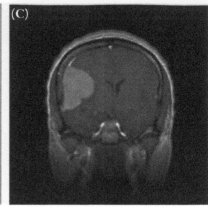

Figure 5.2 *Demonstration of radiographic appearance of meningiomas on (A) CT and (B and C) contrast-enhanced T1-weighted MRI sequences.*

ADVANCED IMAGING

Rarely is advanced imaging required in the diagnosis of a meningioma, as typically the standard imaging characteristics in conjunction with the clinical picture are adequate to make the decision whether or not to treat initially or to observe. One issue where advanced imaging would be beneficial is in the distinction between grades of meningioma, although no such modality has been validated to date. Positron emission tomography (PET) scans using tracers targeting the somatostatin receptors (SSTRs) are potentially helpful as nearly all meningiomas express SSTRs. However, therapies targeting these receptors have been ineffective in the clinical studies available to date, therefore, the true value of these PET scans can be debated.[12] However, PET scans using SSTR-targeting tracers may provide some benefit in differentiating recurrent tumor from radiation necrosis in the treated population as PET scans targeting the SSTRs are typically very "hot" in the case of active meningioma.

MANAGEMENT AND PROGNOSIS

NEWLY DIAGNOSED MENINGIOMA

After the identification of a presumed meningioma on radiographic imaging, the decision of whether or not to treat is not always clear. Even though meningiomas are the most common primary brain tumor, there is still a paucity of randomized trial data on both treatment comparisons and clinical outcomes. However, physicians can assess a number of clinical and radiographic characteristics to make a treatment decision. One of the most important factors is the clinical context leading to meningioma identification: incidentally found versus symptomatic. An incidentally found meningioma can often be observed with serial imaging, whereas a symptomatic meningioma may warrant treatment. Second, the overall size of the meningioma should be factored in, and a "soft" guideline of larger or smaller than 3 cm is typically used to decide between intervention or observation, respectively.[13] Even if the initial decision is to observe, subsequent growth should influence the subsequent treatment decision. Imaging characteristics such as substantial peritumoral edema may lead to an earlier intervention. Last, one must consider the age of the patient and other medical comorbidities prior to making a decision of whether or not to

treat. Overall, the decision to intervene on newly diagnosed meningioma is made on a case-by-case basis: those tumors that are symptomatic, larger in size, demonstrate growth, and occur in younger healthy individuals are more likely to be intervened upon earlier in the disease course. On the other hand, meningiomas that are incidentally found, smaller in size, stable on serial imaging, and/or occur in older individuals with other medical comorbidities are more likely to be observed.

> Overall, the decision to intervene on newly diagnosed meningioma is made on a case-by-case basis: those tumors that are symptomatic, larger in size, demonstrate growth, and occur in younger healthy individuals are more likely to be intervened upon earlier in the disease course.

However, not all factors must be present. For example, a small incidental meningioma in a young healthy patient would still typically be observed, and a larger, even slowly growing, meningioma in a much older patient may still be observed as well. Once a decision for treatment has been made, the primary treatment of a meningioma is neurosurgical, with the goal of maximum surgical resection with minimal surgical morbidity. If surgical resection is not feasible due to either tumor location or patient characteristics (i.e., age and medical comorbidities), radiation

TABLE 5.2 Postoperative recommendations for meningiomas by grade

WHO grade 1 meningioma	Gross total resection	Postoperative radiation generally not recommended
	Subtotal resection	Postoperative radiation considered if residual symptomatic meningioma
WHO grade 2 meningioma	Gross total resection	Benefit of postoperative radiation is unknown and remains highly controversial
	Subtotal resection	Postoperative radiation recommended
WHO grade 3 meningioma	Any extent of resection	Postoperative radiation recommended

is typically considered as a primary treatment. Radiation is considered postoperatively in some patients if there is residual symptomatic tumor or based on histological characteristics and tumor grade (Table 5.2). Radiation is typically administered as either external beam radiation therapy (EBRT) or stereotactic radiosurgery (SRS). EBRT utilizes standard radiation techniques to deliver a lower daily dose of radiation over many doses (fractions). SRS delivers a much higher dose of radiation in a fewer number of fractions (usually 1–3 fractions). There have not been any comparative randomized trials of EBRT versus SRS for the treatment of meningioma but both have demonstrated efficacy and are likely comparable. The decision to employ one method over the other must take into account the location of the tumor and the potential for toxicity to nearby structures, the overall health and well-being of the patient, and expertise of the treating clinician. Last, chemotherapy is rarely used in the up-front initial management of a meningioma.

If surgical resection is selected as the initial therapy, radiation (either EBRT or SRS) is occasionally considered postoperatively as part of the initial treatment plan (Table 5.2). If pathologic examination demonstrates a WHO grade 1 meningioma, then postoperative radiation is rarely administered but can be considered in cases where there is residual symptomatic tumor or possibly other individual patient circumstances. At the opposite end of the spectrum, if pathology reveals a WHO grade 3 meningioma, then, irrespective of the extent of resection, postoperative radiation is most often recommended.

> If pathology reveals a WHO grade 3 meningioma, then, irrespective of the extent of resection, postoperative radiation is most often recommended.

The more challenging situation occurs if pathology reveals a WHO grade 2 meningioma, where the extent of resection becomes the single most important factor. For a STR WHO grade 2 meningioma, postoperative radiation is usually administered unless there are individual patient circumstances suggesting otherwise. But the most controversial situation arises when a meningioma is found to be a GTR WHO grade 2 meningioma. In this particular circumstance, it is not clear whether postoperative radiation is beneficial or not. There are ongoing trials trying to answer this question, where patients in this circumstance are randomized to receive radiation or observation postoperatively.

> For a STR WHO grade 2 meningioma, postoperative radiation is usually administered unless there are individual patient circumstances suggesting otherwise.

RECURRENT MENINGIOMA

Unfortunately, even with best initial management, many meningiomas will still recur, with higher rates of recurrence occurring in meningiomas of higher WHO grade (Table 5.3).[14]

WHO grade 1 meningiomas are typically considered benign and "cured" once treated. However, a large literature review

TABLE 5.3 Recurrence rates for meningiomas by grade

MENINGIOMA GRADE	EXTENT OF RESECTION	5-YEAR RECURRENCE RATE
WHO grade 1 meningioma	Gross total resection	7–25%
	Subtotal resection	27–47%
WHO grade 2 meningioma	Gross total resection	50%
	Subtotal resection	>>>50%
WHO grade 3 meningioma	Any extent of resection	80–100%

From Rogers et al.[14]

effort by the Response Assessment in Neuro-Oncology (RANO) Meningioma group identified that this may not always be the case. Even with GTR, the 5-year recurrence rates ranged from 7% to 25% and even higher in patients after STR. As seen in Table 5.3, the recurrence rates increase with higher grade. For a STR WHO grade 3 meningioma, the 5-year recurrence rate is approximately 100%. Patients requiring therapy for meningioma recurrence often receive either surgery or radiation (sometimes a second course) or chemotherapy. Unfortunately, patients with surgery- and radiation-refractory meningiomas who are treated with chemotherapy have much higher recurrence rates, and these patients tend to have a very aggressive disease course. The same RANO group analyzed the literature in these patients and found that the 6-month progression-free survival rate for patients treated with chemotherapy for recurrence after surgery and radiation ranged from approximately 0% to 25%.[15]

CHEMOTHERAPY FOR MENINGIOMA

Although many chemotherapies (including other medical therapies such as targeted therapies, hormonal modulators, and conventional cytotoxic therapies) have been investigated for the treatment of meningiomas, there is still a tremendous unmet medical need for the treatment of recurrent meningioma and, in particular, for the surgery- and radiation-refractory subset of patients. Additionally, chemotherapy could be beneficial for patients for whom surgery or radiation are not feasible and/or not recommended for individual patient reasons.

> There is still a tremendous unmet medical need for the treatment of recurrent meningioma, in particular for the surgery- and radiation-refractory subset of patients.

Due to the overall rarity of this subset of patients, large randomized comparative trials simply do not exist to guide management. The mainstay of chemotherapy has been with agents designed to interfere with angiogenesis either through receptor blockade (sunitinib) or ligand sequestration (bevacizumab).[16,17] Both of these therapies have shown modest efficacy in stabilizing these tumors and are included in the National Comprehensive Cancer Network (NCCN) guidelines

TABLE 5.4 Current National Comprehensive Cancer Network (NCCN) recommendations for chemotherapy regimens for recurrent meningiomas

NCCN GUIDANCE	REGIMEN
Preferred	Sunitinib Bevacizumab Bevacizumab + everolimus
May be suitable in special circumstances	SSTR2-targeted agents

(Table 5.4) for management of meningiomas.[13] However, better therapies are clearly needed, and clinical trials using immunotherapy or SSTR2-targeting approaches are under way. Patients should be encouraged to participate in a clinical trial evaluating chemotherapy options if one is available.

Patients should be encouraged to participate in a clinical trial evaluating chemotherapy options if one is available.

CONCLUSION

In summary, although meningiomas are the most common primary brain tumor, they present in a very heterogenous manner and the optimal management strategy varies depending on several different factors as detailed earlier. A comprehensive understanding of the presentation, imaging characteristics, natural history, and treatment options is essential to the optimal management of these patients. For patients whose disease recurs despite prior surgery and radiation, the disease course can be very aggressive and better systemic treatment options are desperately needed.

FLASHCARD

What fraction of primary brain tumors are meningiomas, and what fraction of non-malignant brain tumors are meningiomas?	One-third and more than one-half
What is the relationship between age and incidence of meningioma?	Incidence increases with age, especially in patients >65 years
What is the only validated risk factor for development of a meningioma?	Ionizing radiation
From what cell type are meningiomas thought to arise?	Arachnoid cap cells, though the true mechanism of pathogenesis is unclear
The majority of meningiomas harbor alterations in what gene, either by chromosomal loss or point mutation?	The *NF2* gene
Mutations in what two other genes are less commonly seen in meningiomas?	*AKT* and *SMO*
Describe four classic CT or MRI imaging characteristics of meningioma	Homogeneously enhancing Extra-axial "Dural tail" or "CSF cleft"
What are the two mainstays of treatment for meningiomas?	Surgery and/or Radiation therapy
What are three characteristics of a meningioma that might mean it is amenable to observation alone?	Incidentally found Small Asymptomatic

For which two categories of newly diagnosed meningioma patients is radiation typically recommended?	Subtotally resected WHO grade 2 meningiomas and all WHO grade 3 meningiomas
For which category of newly diagnosed meningioma patients is radiation felt controversial?	Gross totally resected WHO grade 2 meningiomas
What three chemotherapy options are included in the NCCN guidelines for treatment of meningiomas?	1. Bevacizumab 2. Sunitinib 3. SSTR-targeting approaches

QUESTIONS

1. Which of the following statements is true?
   a. Meningiomas represent the most common malignant brain tumors with an incidence of 500,000 per year.
   b. Meningiomas represent the most common intracranial tumors with an incidence of 20,000 per year.
   c. Meningiomas most commonly occur in children and are frequently associated with prior radiation exposure.
   d. The incidence of meningioma increases with age, and meningiomas tend to be more aggressive in older individuals.

2. Which of the following represents established risk factors for intracranial meningiomas?
   a. Prior radiation exposure and/or a diagnosis of NF2
   b. Breast cancer in hormone-receptor positive meningiomas
   c. Cellular phone use and head trauma.
   d. Hypertension, diabetes, hyperlipidemia

3. What is the origin of meningiomas?
   a. Meningiomas originate from arachnoid cap cells, and pathogenesis is incompletely understood.
   b. Meningiomas originate from the ependymal lining of the ventricles and disseminate via cerebrospinal fluid (CSF) spread.
   c. Meningiomas originate from glioma stem cells, and the exact pathogenesis is unclear.
   d. Meningiomas originate from arachnoid cap cells, and pathogenesis is driven by alterations in Merlin, which is encoded in the *NF2* gene.

4. Current potential medical treatment targets in meningiomas include all of the following, *except*
   a. *AKT* and *SMO*
   b. *SSTR2*
   c. *Merlin*
   d. *VEGF and VEGFR pathways*

5. Which statement is true about the WHO classification of meningiomas?
   a. WHO grade 2 tumors represent the majority of meningiomas (~80%).
   b. Secretory and papillary meningiomas are classified as WHO grade 1 meningiomas.
   c. Infiltration of underlying brain justifies diagnosis of a WHO grade 2 meningioma.
   d. WHO grade 3 tumors represent approximately 3% of all meningiomas.

6. A 26-year-old woman presents to the emergency room with a unrelenting headache. An MRI brain is obtained and reveals a 1.8×2.1 cm dural-based homogeneously enhancing mass at the base of the right middle temporal fossa. What would you suggest as the most appropriate next step in management?
   a. Neurosurgery consult for possible tumor resection
   b. Conservative and symptomatic headache management and short-term imaging surveillance. Surgical intervention if there is interval tumor growth and/or symptoms that clearly localize to the tumor
   c. Radiation Oncology consultation for consideration of stereotactic radiosurgery (SRS).
   d. Referral to palliative care for symptom management.

7. A 65-year-old man with hypertension, hyperlipidemia, and diabetes presents with a new-onset seizure. On exam, he has postictal right hemiparesis from which he recovers quickly. MRI brain reveals a 4.5×3.9 cm homogeneously enhancing extra-axial mass lesion overlying the left frontal motor cortex. You are consulted for recommendations in regards to next steps. What do you suggest?
   a. Seizure management per neurology recommendations and MRI brain and outpatient neuro-oncology follow-up in 1 month
   b. Systemic cancer workup including CT chest, abdomen, pelvis and oncology consultation.
   c. Radiation oncology consultation for consideration of SRS.
   d. Neurosurgery consult for tumor resection to establish diagnosis and tumor grade to inform further treatment recommendations
   e. Referral to palliative care for symptom management

8. A 45-year-old man presented with progressive headaches and cognitive changes. An MRI brain had revealed a 3.2×2.8 cm dural-based mass at the floor of the left frontal cranial fossa. He has undergone subtotal resection of the tumor, and pathology revealed a chordoid meningioma (WHO grade 2). The case is being discussed at brain tumor board. What is the most likely consensus recommendation in regards to further management?
   a. Observation, consider radiation at time of tumor progression
   b. Second-look surgery to achieve gross total tumor resection, then observe
   c. PET scan with SSTR-targeting tracer to evaluate for possible enrollment on a clinical trial
   d. Therapy with bevacizumab
   e. Given tumor-related symptoms and subtotal tumor resection, radiotherapy should be considered

9. A 52-year-old woman was diagnosed with and underwent resection of a right parietal WHO grade 2 meningioma 6 years ago. She received radiation at time of tumor recurrence 4 years ago and has now undergone repeat subtotal resection with the same pathology. What are the two most likely treatment options that could considered here?
   a. Repeat surgery with goal of gross total tumor resection

b. Re-irradiation, per radiation oncology discretion, either by involved field radiation or by STR
c. Participation in a clinical trial, if eligible
d. Immunotherapy
e. b and c

10. Which of the following recurrence rates for various meningioma scenarios are correct?
a. GTR WHO grade 1 tumors never recur.
b. GTR WHO grade 3 tumors recur in 50–60% of cases.
c. GTR WHO grade 2 tumors recur in about 50% of cases.
d. STR WHO grade 2 tumors always recur.

ANSWERS

1. b
2. a
3. a
4. c
5. d
6. b
7. d
8. e
9. e
10. c

REFERENCES

1. Louis DN, Ohgaki H, Wiestler OD, et al. The 2007 WHO classification of tumours of the central nervous system. *Acta Neuropathol.* 2007;114(2):97–109.
2. Ostrom QT, Cioffi G, Gittleman H, et al. CBTRUS statistical report: Primary brain and other central nervous system tumors diagnosed in the United States in 2012–2016. *Neuro Oncol.* 2019;21(Suppl 5):v1–v100.
3. Bondy M, Ligon BL. Epidemiology and etiology of intracranial meningiomas: A review. *J Neurooncol.* 1996;29(3):197–205.
4. Phillips LE, Frankenfeld CL, Drangsholt M, et al. Intracranial meningioma and ionizing radiation in medical and occupational settings. *Neurology.* 2005;64(2):350–352.
5. Ron E, Modan B, Boice JD Jr, et al. Tumors of the brain and nervous system after radiotherapy in childhood. *N Engl J Med.* 1988;319(16):1033–1039.
6. Sadetzki S, Flint-Richter P, Ben-Tal T, et al. Radiation-induced meningioma: A descriptive study of 253 cases. *J Neurosurg.* 2002;97(5):1078–1082.
7. Longstreth WT Jr, Phillips LE, Drangsholt M, et al. Dental X-rays and the risk of intracranial meningioma: A population-based case-control study. *Cancer.* 2004;100(5):1026–1034.
8. Phillips LE, Koepsell TD, van Belle G, et al. History of head trauma and risk of intracranial meningioma: Population-based case-control study. *Neurology.* 2002;58(12):1849–1852.
9. Custer B, Longstreth WT Jr, Phillips LE, et al. Hormonal exposures and the risk of intracranial meningioma in women: A population-based case-control study. *BMC Cancer.* 2006;6: 152.
10. Brastianos PK, Horowitz PM, Santagata S, et al. Genomic sequencing of meningiomas identifies oncogenic SMO and AKT1 mutations. *Nat Genet.* 2013;45(3):285–289.
11. Clark VE, Erson-Omay EZ, Serin A, et al. Genomic analysis of non-NF2 meningiomas reveals mutations in TRAF7, KLF4, AKT1, and SMO. *Science.* 2013;339(6123):1077–1080.
12. Norden AD, Ligon KL, Hammond SN, et al. Phase II study of monthly pasireotide LAR (SOM230C) for recurrent or progressive meningioma. *Neurology.* 2015;84(3):280–286.
13. Kaley T, Nabors LB. Management of central nervous system tumors. *J Natl Compr Canc Netw.* 2019;17(5.5):579–582.
14. Rogers L, Barani I, Chamberlain M, et al. Meningiomas: Knowledge base, treatment outcomes, and uncertainties. A RANO review. *J Neurosurg.* 2015;122(1):4–23.
15. Kaley T, Barani I, Chamberlain M, et al. Historical benchmarks for medical therapy trials in surgery- and radiation-refractory meningioma: A RANO review. *Neuro Oncol.* 2014;16(6):829–840.
16. Kaley TJ, Wen P, Schiff D, et al. Phase II trial of sunitinib for recurrent and progressive atypical and anaplastic meningioma. *Neuro Oncol.* 2015;17(1):116–121.
17. Nayak L, Iwamoto FM, Rudnick JD, et al. Atypical and anaplastic meningiomas treated with bevacizumab. *J Neurooncol.* 2012;109(1):187–193.

6 | EPENDYMOMA

IYAD ALNAHHAS, APPAJI RAYI, WAYNE SLONE, PETER KOBALKA, SHIRLEY ONG, PIERRE GIGLIO, AND VINAY K. PUDUVALLI

INTRODUCTION

Ependymomas are a subgroup of gliomas that arise from the ependymal lining of the cerebral ventricles and the central canal of the spinal cord. They are uncommon tumors that occur in both the pediatric and adult populations and remain to be fully characterized in their biological characteristics or clinical behavior. Conventional classification of these tumors has been based on histological features. However, recent studies have provided insights into the genetic makeup of these tumors and revealed several molecular subtypes that are associated with clinical behavior and outcome. Such an improved understanding of the biology of ependymomas has also yielded new directions for clinical treatments that are currently being explored. This chapter provides an overview of the diagnosis, classification, biology, and therapy of ependymal tumors.

EPIDEMIOLOGY, CLASSIFICATION, AND ANATOMIC DISTRIBUTION

Ependymomas are uncommon glial tumors designated by the US Food and Drug Administration (FDA) as an orphan disease due to their relatively low incidence. They are overall more common in males than females (incidence ratio male: female 1.32) and constitute 1.7% of all central nervous system (CNS) tumors. They also make up 5% of all pediatric/adolescent CNS tumors and 6.7% of all gliomas. Overall, 1-, 2-, 5-, and 10-year survival rates are 94.5%, 91.3%, 85.7%, and 80.6%, respectively, for all age groups as estimated by the Central Brain Tumor Registry of the United States (CBTRUS).[1]

> Ependymomas make up 5% of all pediatric CNS tumors and 6.7% of all gliomas.

They can occur along the entire neuroaxis, including the supratentorial, posterior fossa, and spinal compartments. Ependymal tumors were until recently classified based on microscopic features alone into four major subtypes according to the World Health Organization (WHO) classification: myxopapillary ependymoma (WHO grade 1),

subependymoma (WHO grade 1), classic ependymoma (WHO grade 2), and anaplastic ependymoma (WHO grade 3), but this has been revised recently to include molecular features. Characteristics and management of each subtype of ependymoma are outlined in the following sections.

SUBEPENDYMOMA

Subependymomas (WHO grade 1) typically occur in the fourth ventricle (75%) or less frequently in the lateral ventricles or spinal cord. They are often well-circumscribed, nodular, and small in size (≤2 cm; a feature that could distinguish them from infiltrative gliomas) and occur in any age group and in both sexes. While the majority of these tumors are often asymptomatic and incidentally identified, symptomatic presentation of tumors can occasionally occur especially in adults due to the development of obstructive hydrocephalus. Imaging characteristics are largely nonspecific. On magnetic resonance imaging (MRI) scans, these tumors appear as T1 hypointense and T2/fluid-attenuated inversion recovery (FLAIR) hyperintense non-enhancing well-demarcated, lobulated, and often asymmetric lesions arising from the ventricular wall and often clearly delineated from the surrounding normal brain (Figure 6.1A). Histologically, the tumors are hypocellular and show both ependymal and astrocytic characteristics.

> Subependymomas demonstrate ependymal and astrocytic histological characteristics.

They manifest as cellular clusters within a dense fibrillary matrix interspersed with microcalcifications and microcysts and could demonstrate blood products and hemosiderin deposits due to prior microhemorrhages (Figure 6.1B). They can also contain perivascular pseudorosettes typical of ependymal tumors and, less frequently, true ependymal rosettes but with only rare mitoses. Immunohistochemical analysis of these tumors shows positivity for vimentin, glial fibrillary acidic protein (GFAP), S-100 protein, and only rarely expression of epithelial membrane antigen (EMA).

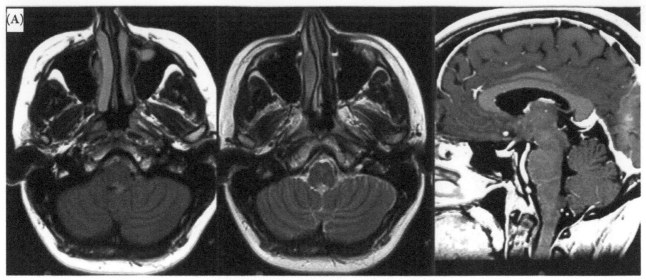

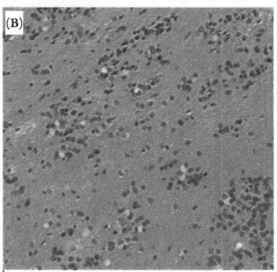

Figure 6.1 Subependymoma. (A) MRI characteristics of a subependymoma of the fourth ventricle: sharply demarcated, periventricular, non-enhancing nodular mass. (B) Histological characteristics of subependymoma: monomorphic cell clusters and microcysts within a dense fibrillary background with rare or no mitosis, necrosis, or vascular proliferation. H&E staining 20× magnification.

Management of these tumors depends on their mode of presentation; asymptomatic tumors found incidentally and without compression of the surrounding structures such as the brainstem or presence of hydrocephalus can be followed with MRI surveillance. For symptomatic tumors, surgical resection may be indicated as well as ventriculoperitoneal shunting. Patients who undergo a gross total resection (GTR) of the mass do not have tumor recurrence. A subset of these tumors can contain foci of classic ependymoma, which can portend a worse prognosis and may warrant a more aggressive management course.[2]

MYXOPAPILLARY EPENDYMOMA

Myxopapillary ependymomas (WHO grade 1) constitute about 20% of spinal cord tumors and predominantly occur in the conus medullaris, cauda equina, or filum terminale (~65%)

or thoracolumbar region (~32%) of the spinal cord. They are slow-growing, encapsulated tumors with a median age of presentation of ~35 years and are slightly more common in males. Low back pain is the most common symptom (~85%) followed by lower extremity weakness or numbness, urinary dysfunction, and impaired gait.[3]

Sixty-five percent of myxopapillary ependymomas occur in the conus medullaris, cauda equina, or filum terminale.

MRI scans typically show a solid elongated lobulated intradural lesion typically in the region of the filum terminale and cauda equina, which have a characteristic "sausage" shape with well-defined margins. The lesions are iso- to hypointense on T1-weighted sequences and hyperintense in T2/FLAIR sequences (Figure 6.2A). The mass can be associated with microhemorrhages, compression, and displacement of cauda

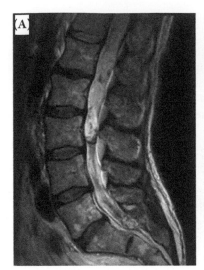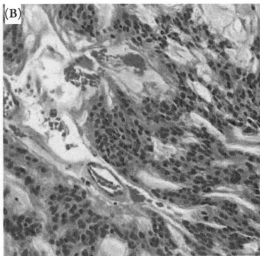

Figure 6.2 Myxopapillary ependymoma. (A) MRI lumbar spine (sagittal section) showing characteristic "sausage-shaped" mass filling the spinal canal with heterogeneous signal; enhancement is commonly noted, and scalloping of the posterior endplate of the vertebral body may also be seen. (B) Histology showing pseudorosettes and papillary structures lined by columnar or cuboidal cells admixed with myxoid elements. H&E staining 20× magnification.

equina nerve roots as well as scalloping of the posterior parts of the vertebral bodies and at times severe stenosis of the spinal canal. Post-contrast images show homogeneous or heterogeneous enhancement of the entire lesion.

These tumors are histologically characterized by papillary areas formed by well-differentiated cuboidal or columnar tumor cells and perivascular pseudorosettes with vessels enveloped by extracellular myxoid material comprised of mucin secreted by the tumor cells, which gives the tumors a gelatinous consistency and abundant collagenous fibrils (Figure 6.2B). Although occasionally pleomorphic, degenerative type nuclei may be seen, these tumors generally lack aggressive features or cellular atypia and only harbor rare mitoses.[4] Calcifications, vascular hyalinization, and endothelial proliferation can also be seen. Immunostaining is usually positive for GFAP, vimentin, for mucin by periodic acid-Schiff (PAS) or Alcian blue, and focally for S100, whereas cytokeratin staining is negative. Electron microscopy shows complex interdigitating tumor cell processes and microtubule aggregation within rough endoplasmic reticulum.

> Myxopapillary ependymomas have positive immunostaining for GFAP, vimentin, mucin, and S100.

The major goal of treatment of myxopapillary ependymomas is to achieve maximal safe resection. Given the importance of this step in the overall prognosis, it is critical that the treating surgeon recognizes this entity prior to surgery. Complete resection of the mass without capsular violation (marginal en bloc resection) can be curative; tumors at the conus are most amenable to such en bloc resection.[5] If this is not feasible, GTR of the mass, which can still confer an excellent prognosis, should be attempted whenever feasible, with meticulous microsurgical dissection and intraoperative monitoring of nerve function. This may require referral to centers with the necessary expertise and resources. Piece-meal resection can

result in neuroaxis dissemination, which can result in slow-growing tumor that extends through neural foramina into the surrounding structures, including the paraspinal and pelvic compartments and causes progressive symptoms. However, subtotal resection (STR) and biopsy alone may be necessary in complex multilobulated tumors that are intertwined with the surrounding spinal cord or nerve roots, in which case attempts at a more aggressive resection may result in irreversible neurological injury. Due to the high rate of recurrence in these instances, surgery should be followed by adjuvant radiation therapy given the benefit for this approach seen in several small series and retrospective studies.[5] While the optimal dose of radiation therapy has not been established, higher doses of 50.4–54 Gy have been recommended.

> Gross total (en bloc) resection can be curative in myxopapillary ependymomas.

Pediatric patients with myxopapillary ependymoma have been reported to present more frequently with disseminated spinal disease.[6] This has raised the possibility that myxopapillary ependymomas may behave similarly to spinal ependymomas in the younger age group, thus requiring closer monitoring and aggressive management in this patient population. The use of proton therapy and stereotactic fractionated radiotherapy to minimize radiation-induced side effects as well to reduce the risk of secondary cancers, especially in younger patients, has been considered.[3]

> Spinal cord dissemination of myxopapillary ependymomas occurs more frequently in pediatric patients, with an unclear influence on survival.

Additionally, extradural presentation of these tumors can also be associated with metastasis to extraneural structures such as the lymph nodes, liver, and lungs.[7] It has also been observed that disseminated disease or tumor recurrence does not necessarily influence overall survival (OS), which remains good for this tumor type.[5]

Medical therapies using various signal transduction agents, cytotoxic therapies, and antiangiogenic treatments have generally shown no efficacy in the setting of recurrent or disseminated myxopapillary ependymoma. However, treatment with temozolomide was reported to induce a complete and durable response in an anecdotal case of recurrent myxopapillary ependymoma with neuroaxis dissemination, which had failed radiotherapy suggesting that some tumors may exhibit chemosensitivity.[8] Single-agent sorafenib was reported to induce stability of disease in a patient with myxopapillary ependymoma with late pulmonary metastases.[9] Despite the adverse prognostic factors, which influence progression-free survival (PFS), OS from this disease remains excellent.

CLASSIC AND ANAPLASTIC EPENDYMOMA

OVERVIEW

Classic (WHO grade 2) and anaplastic (WHO grade 3) are the most common subtypes of ependymomas seen in adults and children. Supratentorial ependymomas arise from the walls of lateral or third ventricles, posterior fossa tumors typically arise in the region of the fourth ventricle, whereas spinal cord ependymomas can occur along the spinal canal or in the cauda equina or conus medullaris. Ependymomas occur more commonly in males, with an overall male-to-female ratio of 1.77:1.[10] Cerebrospinal fluid (CSF) dissemination can occur in up to 15% of cases and contributes to the morbidity of the disease.[11] In a retrospective review of the Surveillance, Epidemiology, and End Results (SEER) database, Rodriguez et al. noted that 88.5% of these tumors are classified as WHO grade 2 and the remainder as anaplastic (WHO grade 3).[12]

CLINICAL FEATURES AND DIAGNOSIS

In a large retrospective series of adults with ependymomas, pain was the most common presenting symptom for all tumor locations.[13] Since ependymomas arise from the ventricular system, common presentations include hydrocephalus and elevated intracranial pressure. Posterior fossa tumors may present with cranial nerve palsies or ataxia, whereas spinal ependymomas may present with back pain and focal motor and sensory deficits as well as urinary/bowel incontinence and gait disturbance.

> Ependymomas occur more commonly in males, with an overall male-to-female ratio of 1.77:1.

MRI is the imaging modality of choice for evaluating brain and spinal cord ependymal tumors. Ependymomas usually appear as well-circumscribed masses that are isointense on T1 imaging and hyperintense on T2 imaging with heterogeneous enhancement.[14] While imaging features can be strongly suggestive in posterior fossa and spinal ependymomas (Figure 6.3A), the differential diagnosis is usually wider for supratentorial ependymomas, which can share imaging characteristics with other gliomas (Figure 6.3B). All patients with higher risk grade 2 or 3 intracranial ependymomas should also have spine MRI and CSF studies to identify any drop metastases or leptomeningeal disease, as also endorsed by the NCCN guidelines.

> MR imaging is the ideal modality for ependymomas which are typically T1 isointense and T2 hyperintense.

Conversely, patients with spinal cord classic or anaplastic ependymomas should have MRI scans of the brain to determine if there is an intracranial primary lesion.

HISTOLOGICAL FEATURES

Initial approaches to ependymoma classification relied solely on microscopic histological features, several of which were noted to be characteristic for this tumor type. Classic ependymomas exhibit a monomorphic cell population that forms perivascular pseudorosettes as well as true ependymal rosettes, which are pathognomonic features of these tumors. Pseudorosettes are characterized by tumor cells that are radially arranged around blood vessels forming perivascular anucleate zones and are found practically in all ependymomas (Figure 6.3C), whereas true ependymal rosettes, found in 25% of cases, are composed of columnar tumor cells arranged around a central lumen.[10] Anaplastic ependymomas (grade 3) differ from their lower grade counterparts by the presence of hypercellularity and mitotic activity, with some tumors demonstrating pseudopalisading necrosis, and microvascular proliferation. Classic (WHO grade 2) ependymomas are further histologically classified into clear cell, papillary, and tanycytic (Figure 6.4).

> Classic ependymomas form perivascular pseudorosettes as well as true ependymal rosettes, which are pathognomonic features.

Most clear cell ependymomas show cells with rounded nuclei that have perinuclear clear halos and have focal perivascular pseudorosettes; these tumors present as supratentorial tumors and occur in younger patients. Papillary tumors demonstrate characteristic finger-like projections formed by single or multiple layers of cuboidal cells with a smooth contiguous surface and can hence mimic choroid plexus papillomas.[10] Tanycytic ependymomas, named for their resemblance to tanycytes and not their cell of origin, typically arise in the cervical or thoracic spinal cord; histologically, these tumors show slender cells are arranged in fascicles, separated by subtle perivascular pseudorosettes.

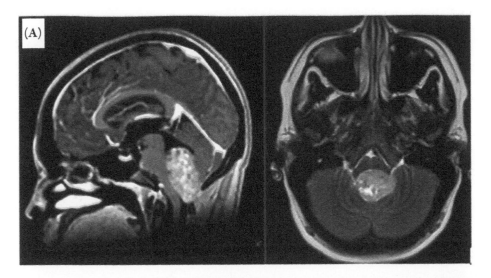

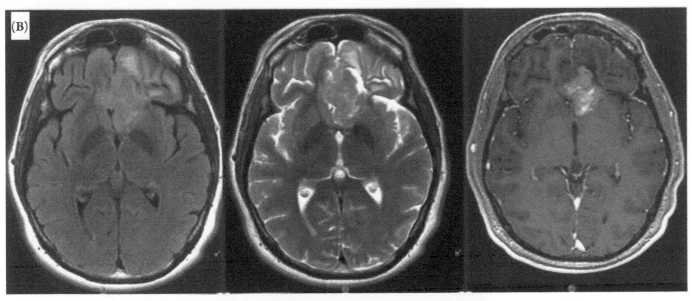

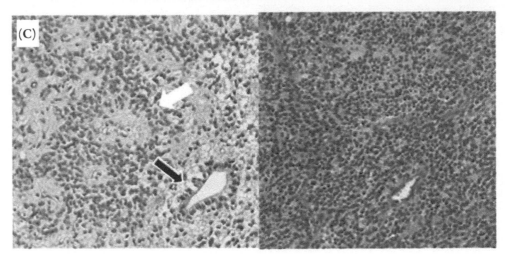

Figure 6.3 *Ependymoma. (A) MRI characteristics of posterior fossa classic ependymoma with sagittal T1 post-contrast and axial T2 images showing an asymmetrically placed predominantly rounded enhancing mass occupying the fourth ventricle and adjacent brain with local mass effect (right panel) and associated obstructive hydrocephalus (left panel). (B) MRI scan of a supratentorial anaplastic ependymoma: axial T2/fluid-attenuated inversion recovery (FLAIR) (left), T2 (middle), and post-contrast T1 images showing an infiltrative, partially enhancing left frontal mass with surrounding edema and mass effect. (C) Histological characteristics of a classic ependymoma (left) with perivascular pseudorosettes (white arrow) and true ependymal rosettes (black arrow), and an anaplastic ependymoma (right) which in addition also shows marked hypercellularity, nuclear atypia, and brisk mitotic activity often with microvascular proliferation (right). H&E staining 10× magnification.*

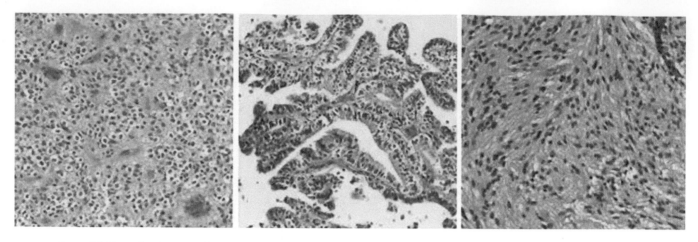

Figure 6.4 Clear cell (left), papillary (center) and tanycytic (right) subtypes of WHO grade 2 ependymoma. H&E staining 10× magnification.

> Tanycytic ependymomas typically arise in the cervical or thoracic spine and are named for their resemblance to tanycytes and not their cell of origin.

Despite the histological distinctions, including tumor grade, among these subtypes, their clinical implication remains debatable partly because of a high degree of interobserver variability in assigning such histological characteristics. Some studies reported no association between grade and clinical behavior,[15] while others suggested that hypercellularity, necrosis, microvascular proliferation, and elevated mitotic rate are associated with a worse PFS in posterior fossa ependymomas.[16] These issues raised the need for alternative methods of classifying these tumors in a manner that corresponds to clinical behavior or facilitates choice of treatment. Immunohistochemical analysis shows that GFAP and S-100 protein staining are seen in all ependymomas, especially in the perivascular pseudorosettes and true ependymal rosettes; in addition, keratin staining similar to the pattern of GFAP staining is noted in these tumors, whereas EMA reactivity occurs in the luminal portion of the true rosettes and tubules.

MANAGEMENT

GTR, whenever feasible, has been shown to be associated with longer PFS and improved survival rates in multiple retrospective studies.[17,18] Five-year PFS rates ranged from 50% to 70% after complete surgical resection compared with less than 30% after STR.[19] Data from the SEER database also support the importance of maximal safe resection; patients who had maximal surgical resection had a longer median survival (19.8 years vs. 18 years, p < 0.001) as well as improved 5-year survival rate (72.4% vs. 52.6%, P < 0.001).[12] Similar results have been seen in the pediatric population; Cage et al. noted in a retrospective review of 182 patients with pediatric ependymoma that GTR yielded better OS rates than STR in this population.[17]

Postsurgical management of ependymomas in both adults and pediatric patients includes consideration of radiation therapy and chemotherapy based on the grade and extent of the tumor. Analysis of the SEER database (following 2,408 patients with grade 2 or 3 ependymomas) indicated that in patients who had STR of their tumors, adjuvant radiation therapy provided a survival benefit; those who did not receive such treatment had a hazard ratio (HR) of 1.748 (p = 0.024).[12] This benefit of radiation therapy for subtotally resected or biopsied tumors has also been corroborated in several other studies.[20–22] For patients with anaplastic (WHO grade 3) ependymomas, there is broad consensus that postsurgical adjuvant conformal radiation therapy can provide benefit regardless of extent of resection.[23,24] On the other hand, the role of radiation postresection in the management of grade 2 ependymoma is more controversial. Some studies have reported that radiotherapy has no additional benefit in this tumor after GTR whereas improvement in PFS and OS was reported in patients who were of younger age, had an STR, and had infratentorial location.[25,26] A large prospective study of pediatric patients with supratentorial ependymomas showed benefit with postoperative radiotherapy for those with grade 2 and STR and in patients with grade 3 tumors.[23] Overall, these reports suggest that radiotherapy should be considered after surgical resection for all patients with anaplastic ependymomas but also in those with classic ependymoma after STR.

> Postsurgical adjuvant conformal radiation therapy can provide benefit in anaplastic ependymomas regardless of extent of resection.

The role of chemotherapy in treatment of ependymomas has been examined in both adult and pediatric patients; however, optimal regimens and selection of patients for such treatment remains under study. Both platinum- and nitrosourea-based regimens have been utilized when chemotherapy was felt appropriate in this setting. Combination therapies such as procarbazine, lomustine, and vincristine (PCV) as well as temozolomide have also been tried in smaller case series.[27] Pediatric Oncology Group study 9233, a large randomized controlled trial assessed the efficacy of dose-intensive combination chemotherapy compared to standard doses (cyclophosphamide, vincristine, cisplatin, and etoposide) in children younger than 3 years of age with newly diagnosed malignant brain tumors including ependymoma ($n = 82$). Patients with ependymoma, but not other tumors, showed improvement in event-free survival rate although this did not translate into an OS benefit. It was also noted that 40% of patients with ependymoma appeared to have long-term control with the dose-intensive regimen and without radiotherapy. It was, however, unclear whether this benefit was only derived from the chemotherapy regimen used or because patients with GTR had a better outcome than those with STR/biopsy given that their distribution in the ependymoma cohort was not provided.[28] While similar results have been reported by other groups as well,[29,30] use of dose-intensive regimens, including autologous stem cell rescue in children younger than 10 years, did not provide benefit over standard therapy and was associated with higher toxicity.[31]

> Chemotherapy regimens using a platinum- and nitrosourea-base have been utilized when appropriate in ependymomas.

Testing the efficacy of combining chemotherapy and radiation, ACNS0121, a Children's Oncology Group prospective phase II study in young patients (age 1–21 years) with intracranial ependymomas, included an arm in which patients with STR of either classic or anaplastic tumors received two cycles of induction chemotherapy (vincristine, carboplatin, and cyclophosphamide or etoposide) followed by further surgery when feasible and subsequent radiation therapy.[23] The 5-year EFS rates were 61.4%, 37.2%, and 68.5% for observation, STR, and near-total resection/GTR groups given immediate postoperative chemotherapy, respectively. The study has now led to the ongoing phase III similarly designed ACNS0831 study, which is expected to be completed by December 2020.[32] In contrast to the studies in the pediatric population, there are no prospective reports of use of chemotherapy in adults with newly diagnosed ependymomas. Hence, no recommendations can currently be made regarding the utility of chemotherapy in newly diagnosed grade 2 or 3 ependymomas in adults. Use of agents such as temozolomide alone in grade 3 or incompletely resected grade 2 tumors, or in combination with lapatinib in Her2+ ependymomas are potential approaches for study in such newly diagnosed patients after radiation therapy.

> There are no prospective reports of use of chemotherapy in adults with newly diagnosed ependymomas.

RECURRENT EPENDYMOMA

Recurrence occurs in the vast majority of patients with ependymomas, reaching up to 50% in some series.[19] A retrospective study of 182 pediatric patients identified extent of resection, infratentorial location, and use of radiotherapy to be positively associated with better PFS.[17] A Canadian population-based study of adults and children with ependymomas reported a median PFS of 55 months for all patients, but patients who were younger than 7 years had a significantly lower PFS of 20 months.[33] In a longitudinal study by the Collaborative Ependymoma Research Network (CERN) on 282 adult patients with ependymoma (spine [46%], infratentorial [35%], and supratentorial [19%]), a multivariate Cox proportional hazards model identified supratentorial location, grade 3, and STR as significantly increasing risk of early progression; influence of molecular subtypes was not reported, however.[34] Recurrence in this study occurred in 26% of patients, with a median time to progression of 14 years. In a retrospective literature review and meta-analysis incorporating 183 adult patients with ependymoma, Sayegh et al. reported that supratentorial ependymomas (despite having higher rates of GTR) and extraventricular location were associated with significantly poorer PFS and OS.[35] Thus, age, tumor location, extent of resection, and tumor grade have been identified across several studies as being prognostic for PFS, with additional benefit seen from radiotherapy in higher risk subsets of patients.

> A retrospective study of pediatric ependymomas positively associated extent of resection, infratentorial location, and use of radiotherapy with better PFS.

Treatment of recurrent ependymomas remains challenging, with no clear standards of care in both pediatric and adult patients. Most ependymomas exhibit ErbB2 overexpression and unmethylated MGMT promoter status; therefore, CERN 08-02 was a phase II study of dose-dense temozolomide 150 mg/m^2/day (7 days on and 7 days off) and lapatinib 1,250 mg/day in adult patients with recurrent classic or anaplastic ependymoma.[36] Forty-eight patients were evaluated: 25 had spinal cord ependymoma, 15 had supratentorial ependymoma, and 8 had infratentorial ependymoma. Median PFS was 0.65 years (95% confidence interval [CI] 0.46–1.02). One-year PFS was 38%. One patient had complete response and four patients had partial responses. Most patients experienced improvement in Karnofsky Performance Scale (KPS) and MD Anderson Symptom Inventory (MDASI) scores.

> CERN 08-02, a phase II study, used lapatinib and dose-dense temozolomide to treat adults with recurrent classic or anaplastic ependymomas.

ADVANCES IN MOLECULAR CLASSIFICATION OF EPENDYMOMAS

Recent advances in molecular studies of ependymomas have provided unique insights into the heterogeneity of these tumors and highlighted the limitations of current histological approaches to their classification and clinical course. Using an integrated genomic, cell of origin, and comparative oncology approach, Johnson et al. reported subtypes of ependymoma in preclinical genetic models to identify selective molecular pathways of relevance to the biology and classification of these tumors; they also identified *EPHB2* as a putative oncogene driving human supratentorial ependymomas.[37] Such subtypes have also been utilized in preclinical models to generate therapeutic leads against ependymomas.[38] Parker et al. first discovered C11orf95-RELA fusions driving oncogenic nuclear factor kappa-B (NFκB) signaling specifically in more than 70% of supratentorial ependymoma and associated with a poorer prognosis;[39] this was a result of clustered chromosomal rearrangements consistent with chromothripsis.[9] The study also identified a second oncogenic fusion event, YAP1-MAMLD1, in a subset of supratentorial ependymomas not having the RELA fusions.

> C11orf 95-RELA fusions are driver mutations in more than 70% of supratentorial ependymomas and are associated with a poorer prognosis.

In a similar study of posterior fossa ependymomas, Witt et al. described two distinct genetic subtypes with different clinical behaviors: group A (PFA), which occurs predominantly in infants, has a poor prognosis and is identifiable by expression of Laminin α-2; and group B (PFB), which occurs in older children and adults, has a better prognosis, and expresses neural epidermal growth factor like-2 (NELL-2) as a biomarker.[40] These two subtypes were found to have distinct methylomes, with PFA exhibiting aberrant methylation of tumor suppressor genes due to enhanced activity of PRC2 and presumed to be the reason for the poorer prognosis of this group.

A large-scale study using the DNA methylation profile analysis of a cohort of more than 500 patients with ependymomas further confirmed and expanded the identification of these subtypes of ependymoma within each CNS compartment (i.e., supratentorial [ST], posterior fossa [PF], and spine [SP]) with three subtypes within each group.[41] The study confirmed the genetic subtypes with the RELA (ST-EPN-RELA) and YAP1 (ST-EPN-YAP1) fusions respectively noted in both grade 2 and 3 tumors as well as the posterior fossa tumor subtypes Group A (PF-EPN-A) and Group B (PF-EPN-B). Both the supratentorial and posterior fossa additionally included subependymomas in the respective compartments (ST-SE and PF-SE). In addition,

General Consensus Statements

1. Outside of clinical trials, treatment decisions should not be based on grading (II vs III)
2. ST and PF ependymomas are different diseases although the impact on therapy is still evolving
3. Central radiological and histological review should be a principal component of future clinical trials
4. Molecular subgrouping should be part of all clinical trials henceforth
5. Submission of fresh-frozen tumor samples as well as of blood samples will mandatory in future clinical trials

Subgroup Consensus Statements

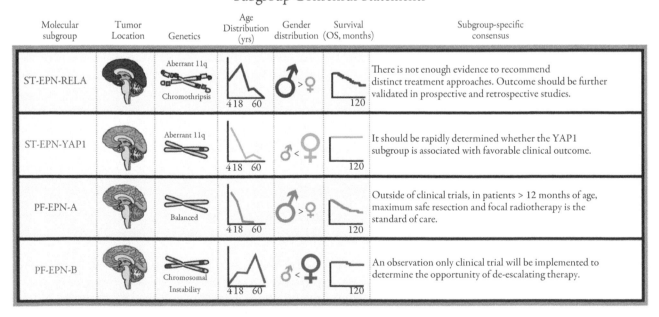

Molecular subgroup	Tumor Location	Genetics	Age Distribution (yrs)	Gender distribution	Survival (OS, months)	Subgroup-specific consensus
ST-EPN-RELA		Aberrant 11q / Chromothripsis	418 60	♂ > ♀	120	There is not enough evidence to recommend distinct treatment approaches. Outcome should be further validated in prospective and retrospective studies.
ST-EPN-YAP1		Aberrant 11q	418 60	♂ < ♀	120	It should be rapidly determined whether the YAP1 subgroup is associated with favorable clinical outcome.
PF-EPN-A		Balanced	418 60	♂ > ♀	120	Outside of clinical trials, in patients > 12 months of age, maximum safe resection and focal radiotherapy is the standard of care.
PF-EPN-B		Chromosomal Instability	418 60	♂ < ♀	120	An observation only clinical trial will be implemented to determine the opportunity of de-escalating therapy.

Figure 6.5 Consensus on clinical management of intracranial ependymoma by the Ependymoma Consensus conference.

From Pajtler et al. *Acta Neuropathologica.* 2017;133:5–12. Reproduced without modification under the Creative Commons license.

spinal ependymomas were classified as SP-EPN, SP-MPE, and SP-SE, corresponding to ependymomas, myxopapillary ependymoma, and subependymomas. The 2016 WHO classification of CNS tumors recognizes only the supratentorial RELA fusion subtype as a distinct molecular subtype of ependymoma given its distinctly poorer prognosis.

A more recent paper from the German Glioma Network correlated DNA methylation profiles with pathological characteristics in 122 adult patients with gliomas.[42] At a median follow-up of 86.7 months, only 22 patients experienced progression (18.0%) and 13 patients (10.7%) died. All histologic subependymomas corresponded to subependymoma (SE) DNA methylation subgroups. However, 19 histologic ependymomas (WHO grade 2) were allocated to molecular SE groups. Similarly, all histological myxopapillary ependymomas were assigned to the molecularly defined spinal myxopapillary ependymoma (SP-MPE) class, but also 15 WHO grade 2 ependymomas by histology fell under this methylation subgroup. The study highlighted the importance of methylation classification and its potential influence on treatment choices. Figure 6.5. illustrates the main molecular subtypes of ependymoma. For the most recent information on molecular groupings of ependymal tumors, see the 5th Edition of the WHO Classification of Central Nervous System Tumours. (WHO Classification of Tumours; 5th Edition. Cental Nervous System Tumours. Edited by the WHO Classification of Tumours Editorial Board. International Agency for Research for Researchg on Cancer 2021).

> The 2016 WHO recognizes only the supratentorial RELA fusion subtype as a distinct molecular ependymoma subtype, given its distinctly poorer prognosis.

Other biomarkers have been studied for their association with clinical outcome; CDKN2A loss in supratentorial ependymomas and gain of chromosome 1q in posterior fossa tumors have been associated with poor outcome.[43] Other studies showed that low levels of nucleolin expression (IHC) and TERT mRNA expression are independent favorable prognostic factors in pediatric intracranial ependymomas; nucleolin expression by immunohistochemistry (HR = 6.25; p = 0.008) and hTERT mRNA levels showed a strong association with PFS and OS upon multivariate analysis (HR = 9.9; p = 0.011).[44,45] These markers have also suggested potential therapeutic targets that are relevant to the specific subtype (Figure 6.5). For instance, targeting oncogenic NFκB pathway in ST-EPN-RELA tumors or the PRC2 complex driving aberrant methylation in the PF-EPN-A subgroups, which have poorer prognosis, are rational therapeutic targets.

CONCLUSION

Ependymomas are challenging tumors to manage in both the adult and pediatric populations. Although some of these tumors have excellent prognosis and can be cured with good surgical resection, the higher risk tumors have a poorer outcome. The relative rarity of these tumors, the poor understanding of the molecular underpinnings of ependymomas, and the limitations of histological classification have hampered development of effective therapies against ependymomas. However, the recent identification of distinct molecular subtypes of these tumors that better correlate with clinical outcome and the ongoing characterization of the pathways that drive their clinical behavior are being exploited to develop novel therapeutic approaches against these tumors.

FLASHCARDS

What is the glioma subgroup that arises from the ependymal lining of the ventricles and the central canal of the spinal cord from radial glia?	Ependymomas
Ependymomas can occur in which compartments?	Supratentorial, infratentorial, or spinal
Ependymoma: WHO grade 1 WHO grade 2 WHO grade 3	Subependymoma and myxopapillary ependymoma Classic ependymoma Anaplastic ependymoma*
This ependymoma variant predominantly affects the conus and cauda equina and should be resected en bloc without capsular violation whenever feasible	Myxopapillary variant
Classic ependymomas occur in children and adults, although posterior fossa tumors are more common in which group?	Children
In ependymoma, screening of the entire neuroaxis, including cerebrospinal fluid sampling when appropriate, is important for what reason?	Staging and prognostication
Signs and symptoms in ependymoma location: Hydrocephalus and increased ICP ataxia and cranial nerve palsies Back pain, focal limb, or urinary/bowel symptoms	Supratentorial Posterior fossa Spinal cord
Microscopic characteristics of ependymomas: Cells radially arranged around blood vessels Columnar cells arranged around a central lumen	Perivascular pseudorosettes True ependymal rosettes

*Please note that 2021 WHO classification for CNS Tumors has removed the term "anaplastic" and uses grading and molecular features for classification of ependymomas.

The three histologic types of grade 2 ependymomas are?	Papillary, clear cell, and tanycytic
Poor outcome in posterior fossa ependymomas is associated w/gain of	Chromosome 1q
In grade ___ ependymomas, gross total resection offers definitive treatment and extends survival	Grade 1
Radiation therapy is used mainly for which cases of ependymoma?	Anaplastic and subtotally resected classic ependymoma
The role of chemotherapy to treat ependymomas is less clear; when needed which class is commonly used?	Platinum-based regimens
Stratifying ependymomas into different risk groups to differentiate treatment modalities is being done based on these three characteristics:	Tumor location, tumor grade, and molecular patterns
Recurrence can occur in what percent of ependymomas?	50%
Using DNA methylation, these ependymomas were classified into the *supratentorial* subgroup:	Ependymomas with RELA fusions (worse prognosis) or YAP1 fusions and subependymomas
Using DNA methylation, these ependymomas were classified into the *posterior fossa* subgroup:	Group A (younger patients, worse prognosis), Group B (older patients) and subependymomas
Using DNA methylation, these ependymomas were classified into the *spinal cord* subgroup:	Myxopapillary ependymomas, classic ependymomas, and subependymomas

QUESTIONS

1. Classic ependymomas are classified as WHO grade:
   a. 1
   b. 2
   c. 3
   d. 4

2. Which of the following pathologic features is found in nearly all ependymomas?
   a. Pseudorosettes
   b. True ependymal rosettes
   c. Rosenthal fibers
   d. Homer Wright rosettes

3. The following characteristics in ependymomas carry worse prognosis *except*:
   a. Group A ependymoma
   b. RELA fusions
   c. YAP1 fusions
   d. Gain of chromosome 11

4. Dose-dense temozolomide has shown positive results in recurrent ependymoma in a phase II study when combined with which of the following agents?
   a. Bevacizumab
   b. Sunitinib
   c. Lapatinib
   d. Trastuzumab

5. RELA fusion is thought to activate which of the following signaling pathways?
   a. RTK pathway
   b. PI3K pathway
   c. Sonic hedgehog pathway
   d. NFKB pathway

6. An MRI scan shows a solid hyperintense elongated intradural lesion in the region of the cauda equina consistent with an ependymoma. The most likely pathology consistent with this lesion is:
   a. Subependymoma
   b. Myxopapillary ependymoma

   c. Classic ependymoma
   d. Anaplastic ependymoma

7. Tanycytic ependymoma is a histologic subtype of classic ependymoma that most commonly arises in which of the following compartments?
   a. Supratentorial
   b. Infratentorial
   c. Spinal cord
   d. Leptomeningeal

8. Radiation therapy is recommended in the management of ependymoma after which of the following scenarios?
   a. Gross total resection of a myxopapillary ependymoma
   b. Gross total resection of an anaplastic ependymoma
   c. Gross total resection of a posterior fossa Group B ependymoma
   d. Gross total resection of a classic ependymoma with YAP-1 fusion

9. Grade 2 versus 3 ependymoma has invariably shown consistent correlation with clinical outcome:
   a. True
   b. False

10. CSF dissemination is associated with worse overall survival in myxopapillary ependymoma:
    a. True
    b. False

ANSWERS

1. b
2. a
3. c
4. c
5. d
6. b
7. c
8. b
9. b
10. b

REFERENCES

1. Ostrom QT, Cioffi G, Gittleman H, et al. CBTRUS statistical report: Primary brain and other central nervous system tumors diagnosed in the United States in 2012–2016. *Neuro Oncol.* 2019;21(Suppl 5):v1–v100. doi:10.1093/neuonc/noz150

2. Bi Z, Ren X, Zhang J, Jia W. Clinical, radiological, and pathological features in 43 cases of intracranial subependymoma. *J Neurosurg.* 2015 Jan 1;122(1):49–60.

3. Weber DC, Wang Y, Miller R, et al. Long-term outcome of patients with spinal myxopapillary ependymoma: Treatment results from the MD Anderson Cancer Center and institutions from the Rare Cancer Network. *Neuro-Oncology.* 2015 Apr 1;17(4):588–595.

4. Kleinschmidt-DeMasters BK, Tihan T, Rodriguez F. *Diagnostic Pathology: Neuropathology.* Amsterdam: *Elsevier Health Sciences*; 2016 Feb 10;106–121.

5. Abdulaziz M, Mallory GW, Bydon M, et al. Outcomes following myxopapillary ependymoma resection: The importance of capsule integrity. *Neurosurg Focus.* 2015 Aug 1;39(2):E8.

6. Fassett DR, Pingree J, Kestle JR. The high incidence of tumor dissemination in myxopapillary ependymoma in pediatric patients: Report of five cases and review of the literature. *J Neurosurg Pediatr.* 2005 Jan 1;102(1):59–64.

7. Vagaiwala MR, Robinson JS, Galicich JH, et al. Metastasizing extradural ependymoma of the sacrococcygeal region: Case report and review of literature. *Cancer.* 1979 Jul;44(1):326–333.

8. Fujiwara Y, Manabe H, Izumi B, et al. Remarkable efficacy of temozolomide for relapsed spinal myxopapillary ependymoma with multiple recurrence and cerebrospinal dissemination: A case report and literature review. *Eur Spine J.* 2018 Jul 1;27(3):421–45.

9. Fegerl G, Marosi C. Stabilization of metastatic myxopapillary ependymoma with sorafenib. *Rare Tumors.* 2012 Sep 6;4(3):134–137.

10. Louis DN, Ohgaki H, Wiestler OD, Cavenee WK, eds. *WHO Classification of Tumours of the Central Nervous System.* 4th ed. rev. Lyon: IARC; 2016.

11. Gilbert MR, Ruda R, Soffietti R. Ependymomas in adults. *Curr Neurol Neurosci Rep.* 2010 May 1;10(3):240–247.

12. Rodríguez D, Cheung MC, Housri N, et al. Outcomes of malignant CNS ependymomas: An examination of 2408 cases through the Surveillance, Epidemiology, and End Results (SEER) database (1973–2005). *J Surg Res.* 2009 Oct 1;156(2):340–351.

13. Ellison DW, Kocak M, Figarella-Branger D, et al. Histopathological grading of pediatric ependymoma: Reproducibility and clinical relevance in European trial cohorts. *J Negative Results Biomed.* 2011 Dec 1;10(1):1–13.

14. Raghunathan A, Wani K, Armstrong TS, et al. Histological predictors of outcome in ependymoma are dependent on anatomic site within the central nervous system. *Brain Pathol.* 2013 Sep;23(5):584–594.

15. Armstrong TS, Vera-Bolanos E, Bekele BN, et al. Adult ependymal tumors: Prognosis and the M.D. Anderson Cancer Center experience. *Neuro Oncol.* 2010;12(8):862–870.

16. Cachia D, Johnson DR, Kaufmann TJ, et al. Case-based review: Ependymomas in adults. *Neuro-Oncology Pract.* 2018 Aug 3;5(3):142–153.

17. Cage TA, Clark AJ, Aranda D, et al. A systematic review of treatment outcomes in pediatric patients with intracranial ependymomas. *J Neurosurg Pediatr.* 2013;11(6):673Y681. doi:10.3171/ 2013.2. PEDS12345

18. Horn B, Heideman R, Geyer R, et al. A multi-institutional retrospective study of intracranial ependymoma in children: Identification of risk factors. *J Pediatr Hematol Oncol.* 1999;21(3):203Y211.

19. Dang M, Phillips PC. Pediatric brain tumors. *Continuum.* 2017 Dec 1;23(6):1727–1757.

20. Jung J, Choi W, Do Ahn S, et al. Postoperative radiotherapy for ependymoma. *Radiat Oncol J.* 2012 Dec;30(4):158.

21. Mansur DB, Perry A, Rajaram V, et al. Postoperative radiation therapy for grade II and III intracranial ependymoma. *Intl J Radiat Oncol Biol Physics.* 2005 Feb 1;61(2):387–391.

22. Oh MC, Ivan ME, Sun MZ, et al. Adjuvant radiotherapy delays recurrence following subtotal resection of spinal cord ependymomas. *Neuro-Oncology.* 2013 Feb 1;15(2):208–215.

23. Merchant TE, Bendel AE, Sabin ND, et al. Conformal radiation therapy for pediatric ependymoma, chemotherapy for incompletely resected ependymoma, and observation for completely resected, supratentorial ependymoma. *J Clin Oncol.* 2019;37(12):974–983. doi:10.1200/JCO.18.01765

24. Merchant TE, Li C, Xiong X, et al. Conformal radiotherapy after surgery for paediatric ependymoma: A prospective study. *Lancet Oncol.* 2009;10(3):258Y266. doi:10.1016/ S1470Y2045(08)70342Y5

25. Deng X, Lin D, Yu L, et al. The role of postoperative radiotherapy in pediatric patients with grade II intracranial ependymomas: A population-based, propensity score-matched study. *Cancer Manage Res.* 2018; 10:5515.

26. Metellus P, Guyotat J, Chinot O, et al. Adult intracranial WHO grade II ependymomas: Long-term outcome and prognostic factor analysis in a series of 114 patients. *Neuro-Oncology.* 2010 Sep 1;12(9):976–984.

27. Alnahhas I, Malkin MG. Chemotherapy of adult ependymoma. In Herbert Newton, ed. *Handbook of Brain Tumor Chemotherapy, Molecular Therapeutics, and Immunotherapy.* New York: Academic Press; 2018:483–485.

28. Strother DR, Lafay-Cousin L, Boyett JM, et al. Benefit from prolonged dose-intensive chemotherapy for infants with malignant brain tumors is restricted to patients with ependymoma: A report of the Pediatric Oncology Group randomized controlled trial 9233/34. *Neuro-Oncology.* 2014 Mar 1;16(3):457–465.

29. Geyer JR, Sposto R, Jennings M, et al. Multiagent chemotherapy and deferred radiotherapy in infants with malignant brain tumors: A report from the Children's Cancer Group. *J Clin Oncol.* 2005 Oct 20;23(30):7621–7631.

30. Grundy RG, Wilne SA, Weston CL, et al. Primary postoperative chemotherapy without radiotherapy for intracranial ependymoma in children: The UKCCSG/SIOP prospective study. *Lancet Oncol.* 2007 Aug 1;8(8):696–705.

31. Zacharoulis S, Ji L, Pollack IF, et al. Metastatic ependymoma: A multi-institutional retrospective analysis of prognostic factors. *Pediatr Blood Cancer.* 2008 Feb;50(2):231–235.

32. Children's Oncology Group. ACNS0831: Phase III randomized trial of post-radiation chemotherapy in patients with newly diagnosed ependymoma ages 1 to 21 years. (updated Jan 30, 2018). https://childrensoncologygroup.org/acns0831.

33. Urgoiti GB, Singh AD, Tsang RY, et al. Population based analysis ependymoma patients in Alberta from 1975 to 2007. *Can J Neurol Sci.* 2014 Nov;41(6):742–747.

34. Vera-Bolanos E, Aldape K, Yuan Y, et al. Clinical course and progression-free survival of adult intracranial and spinal ependymoma patients. *Neuro-Oncology.* 2015 Mar 1;17(3):440–447.

35. Sayegh ET, Aranda D, Kim JM, et al. Prognosis by tumor location in adults with intracranial ependymomas. *J Clin Neurosci.* 2014 Dec 1;21(12):2096–2101.

36. Armstrong T, Yuan Y, Wu J, et al. RARE-24. Objective response and clinical benefit in recurrent ependymoma in adults: Final report of CERN 08-02: A phase II study of dose-dense temozolomide and lapatinib. *Neuro-Oncology.* 2018;20(Suppl 6):vi241.

37. Johnson RA, Wright KD, Poppleton H, et al. Cross-species genomics matches driver mutations and cell compartments to model ependymoma. *Nature.* 2010 Jul;466(7306):632–636.

38. Atkinson JM, Shelat AA, Carcaboso AM, et al. An integrated in vitro and in vivo high-throughput screen identifies treatment leads for ependymoma. *Cancer Cell.* 2011 Sep 13;20(3):384–399.

39. Parker M, Mohankumar KM, Punchihewa C, et al. C11orf95-RELA fusions drive oncogenic NF-0B signalling in ependymoma. *Nature.* 2014;506(7489):451Y455. doi:10.1038/nature13109

40. Witt H, Mack SC, Ryzhova M, et al. Delineation of two clinically and molecularly distinct subgroups of posterior fossa ependymoma. *Cancer Cell.* 2011;20(2):143Y157. doi: 10.1016/j.ccr.2011.07.007

41. Pajtler KW, Witt H, Sill M, et al. Molecular classification of ependymal tumors across all CNS compartments, histopathological grades, and age groups. *Cancer Cell.* 2015 May 11;27(5):728–743.

42. Witt H, Gramatzki D, Hentschel B, et al. DNA methylation-based classification of ependymomas in adulthood: Implications for diagnosis and treatment. *Neuro-Oncology.* 2018 Nov 12;20(12):1616–1624.

43. Kilday JP, Mitra B, Domerg C, et al. Copy number gain of 1q25 predicts poor progression-free survival for pediatric intracranial ependymomas and enables patient risk stratification: A prospective European clinical trial cohort analysis on behalf of the Children's Cancer Leukaemia Group (CCLG), Societe Francaise d'Oncologie Pediatrique (SFOP), and International Society for Pediatric Oncology (SIOP). *Clin Cancer Res.* 2012 Apr;18(7):2001–2011.

44. Ridley L, Rahman R, Brundler MA, et al. Multifactorial analysis of predictors of outcome in pediatric intracranial ependymoma. *Neuro-Oncology.* 2008 Oct 1;10(5):675–689.

45. Modena P, Buttarelli FR, Miceli R, et al. Predictors of outcome in an AIEOP series of childhood ependymomas: A multifactorial analysis. *Neuro-Oncology.* 2012 Nov 1;14(11):1346–1356.

7 | TUMORS OF THE PITUITARY GLAND

REGINALD FONG AND ANDREW R. CONGER

INTRODUCTION

Tumors of the pituitary gland account for approximately 10–15% of intracranial neoplasms, with an incidence ranging from 1 to 20 cases per 100,000 per year.[1–4] Data from autopsy and radiographic studies suggest pituitary neoplasms in as many as 16% and 22% of the population, respectively.[2] The 2017 World Health Organization Classification of Tumors of Endocrine Organs lists 19 different pathologies originating from cell lines intrinsic to the pituitary gland.[3] The diverse variety of pathologies occurring in and around the sella turcica underscore the anatomic complexity of the pituitary gland and its environs. The anatomic complexity, long list of possible pathologies, and potential for pituitary gland dysfunction make diagnosis and management of these lesions complex, best managed with a multidisciplinary approach.[4]

PITUITARY GLAND ANATOMY AND PHYSIOLOGY

The pituitary gland sits in a bony depression of the cranial base called the *sella turcica*. The pituitary stalk connects the pituitary gland to the hypothalamus of the brain. The paired cavernous sinuses are lateral to the sella and contain the cavernous segment of the internal carotid arteries as well as cranial nerves III, IV, V_1, V_2, and VI. The optic chiasm lies a few millimeters above the sella, and the midline sphenoid sinus lies just below it.[5]

> Paired cavernous sinuses are lateral to the sella and contain the cavernous segment of the internal carotid arteries as well as cranial nerves III, IV, V_1, V_2, and VI.

The pituitary gland itself consists of an anterior lobe, or adenohypophysis, which forms from an upward evagination of embryologic pharyngeal ectoderm called Rathke's pouch and a posterior lobe or neurohypophysis, which forms from a downward evagination of the embryologic neuroectoderm. Rathke's pouch dissociates from the pharyngeal ectoderm and differentiates into neuroendocrine tissue of the adenohypophysis, accounting for 75% of the volume of the pituitary gland. The adenohypophysis attaches itself to the developing neurohypophysis, which remains connected to the central nervous system through the bundle of axons constituting the pituitary stalk. Both parts of the pituitary gland function under the direction of the hypothalamus: the adenohypophysis by hypothalamic releasing factors circulating through the associated venous portal circulation and the neurohypophysis via direct axonal transmission. The adenohypophysis produces and secretes the hormones growth hormone (GH), thyroid-stimulating hormone (TSH), adrenocorticotropic hormone (ACTH), luteinizing hormone (LH), follicle-stimulating hormone (FSH), and prolactin (PRL). Through their effects on end organs and other glands, these hormones direct broad systemic processes such as growth, metabolism, the stress response, and reproduction. The neurohypophysis releases antidiuretic hormone and oxytocin, which are produced in the hypothalamus and transported to neurosecretory vesicles in the neurohypophysis.[5]

CLINICAL PRESENTATION OF PITUITARY TUMORS

Pituitary tumors can present with various findings resulting from hormone hypersecretion, dysfunction of surrounding structures as a result of compression by the tumor, or a combination of both. Tumor hypersecretion of ACTH, GH, PRL, and TSH can cause Cushing's disease, acromegaly, hyperprolactinemia, and central hyperthyroidism, respectively. Mass effect caused by large tumors compressing surrounding structures can manifest itself in many ways including mild hyperprolactinemia (the so-called *stalk effect*) caused by distortion of the pituitary stalk and resultant loss of dopaminergic inhibition of PRL production. Tumor compression of the pituitary gland can cause pituitary hypofunction. Typically, production of gonadotropins (LH, FSH) is decreased first, followed in succession by TSH, GH, and finally ACTH. The respective clinical results of these pituitary hormone deficiencies are central hypogonadism, central hypothyroidism, growth hormone deficiency, and central adrenal insufficiency. Tumor-related dysfunction of the neurohypophysis is less common, but when present, ADH levels decline resulting in central diabetes insipidus with excessive urination and dehydration. Visual dysfunction can result from upward distortion of the optic chiasm causing homonymous hemianopsia or from extensive invasion in to one or both cavernous sinuses causing cranial neuropathies affecting the extraocular muscles with resultant double vision. Larger tumors can cause headaches which are usually retro-orbital in location and may radiate to the vertex or lateralize to the temporal region, suggesting involvement of the ipsilateral cavernous sinus. Acute-onset severe headache may represent pituitary apoplexy (hemorrhagic infarction of a pituitary tumor and/or the gland itself) and, if accompanied by acute visual loss, is considered a surgical emergency. Other rare presenting symptoms usually associated with extremely large tumors include cerebrospinal fluid (CSF) leak caused by a large tumor eroding through the base of the skull, seizures caused by compression of the medial temporal lobe, and personality changes caused by compression of the frontal lobes. Initial management of pituitary tumors should include evaluation for endocrinopathy and neuro-ophthalmologic exam, including visual field testing.[6] Surgery is the treatment of choice for most hypersecreting tumors (except for prolactin-secreting tumors) and all large tumors causing symptoms from mass effect. Radiation is a treatment option for tumors of the pituitary but risks hypopituitarism as well as radiation-induced optic neuropathy.

> Tumor hypersecretion of ACTH, GH, PRL, and TSH can cause Cushing's disease, acromegaly, hyperprolactinemia, and central hyperthyroidism, respectively.

TUMORS OF THE ADENOHYPOPHYSIS

PITUITARY ADENOMAS

The most common tumor of the pituitary gland is the pituitary adenoma.[2] These tumors originate from the neuroendocrine cells of the adenohypophysis and, as of the 2017 edition of the WHO classification scheme, are classified based on cell lineage differentiation as determined by the presence of specific transcription factors shown to play a role in regulation of hormone production and possibly tumorigenesis. Pituitary corticotroph cells secrete ACTH under the influence of the transcription factor Tpit. Lactotroph cells, thyrotroph cells, and somatotroph cells secrete PRL, TSH, and GH, respectively, all under the influence of the transcription factor Pit-1. The very rare Pit-1-positive plurihormonal adenoma secretes all three of these hormones under the influence of Pit-1, providing evidence that lactotrophs, thyrotrophs, and somatotrophs derive from a common cell precursor and perhaps that the transcription factors play a role in tumorigenesis. Gonadotroph cells secrete FSH and LH under the influence of the transcription factor SF-1. Subtypes within each cell lineage are delineated based on histological ultrastructural characteristics.[3,7] Magnetic resonance imaging (MRI) is the imaging modality of choice for suspected pituitary adenomas. These lesions are characteristically located within or just adjacent to the normal pituitary gland and enhance less brightly than the surrounding normal pituitary gland, characterized as hypoenhancement on T1 postgadolinium sequences. Pituitary microadenomas (tumors >1cm in diameter) can be difficult to discern on MRI, so dynamic pituitary imaging has been developed. Larger tumors, macroadenomas, are more readily identified (Figures 7.1 and 7.2). Dynamic pituitary imaging is performed at multiple time points after contrast administration. This technique takes advantage of differences in the rate of contrast absorption between the gland and the tumor, which absorbs the contrast more slowly.[8]

CORTICOTROPH ADENOMAS

Corticotroph adenomas can oversecrete ACTH (Figure 7.3) resulting in Cushing's disease, a rare disorder more common in women of child-bearing age and that in some cases may be related to loss of negative feedback of ACTH during pregnancy.[9] Clinically, these patients develop Cushing's syndrome of truncal obesity, supraclavicular and dorsocervical fat deposition ("buffalo hump"), proximal muscle wasting, abdominal striae, moon facies, hypertension, diabetes, hirsutism, and cognitive changes all as a result of excess exposure to cortisol.[10] Due to normal fluctuations in serum ACTH and cortisol levels, 24-hour urinary free cortisol testing and/or midnight salivary cortisol testing are required to verify hypercortisolemia. Once confirmed, dexamethasone

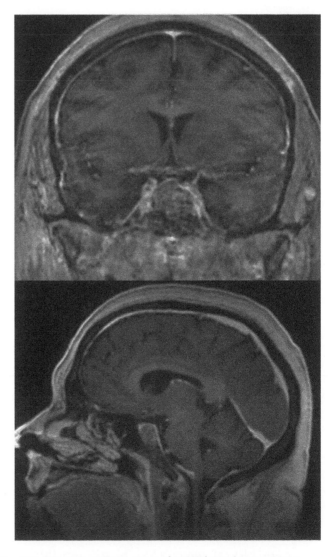

Figure 7.1 Post-contrast T1 sequences of an MRI brain demonstrating a pituitary macroadenoma. Coronal (top) and sagittal (bottom) views.

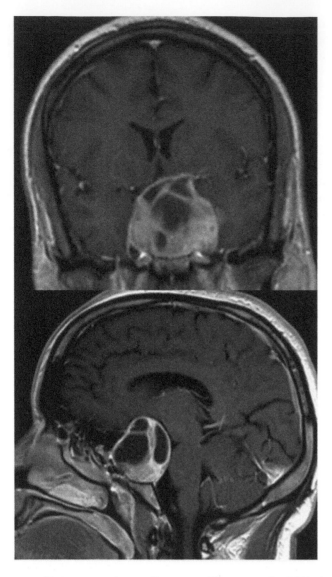

Figure 7.2 *Pituitary macroadenoma. Post-contrast T1 sequence of an MRI brain. Coronal (top) and sagittal (bottom) views.*

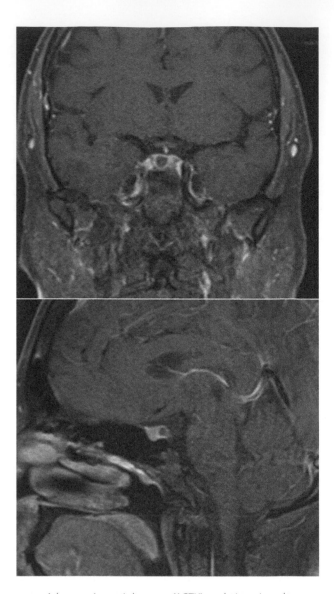

Figure 7.3 *Adrenocorticotropic hormone (ACTH)-producing microadenoma. Post-contrast T1 sequence of an MRI brain. Coronal (top) and sagittal (bottom) views.*

suppression testing can be performed to help distinguish between a pituitary adenoma and other sources of excess cortisol (ectopic ACTH source vs. cortisol-producing adrenal adenoma).[11] Suppression of ACTH release after administration of high-dose but not low-dose dexamethasone suggests a pituitary adenoma as the source. Pituitary MRI will usually reveal a pituitary adenoma which is the most likely cause. About 90% of ACTH-producing corticotroph adenomas are less than 1 cm, with about 20% being so small that the MRI appears negative. In cases of a negative pituitary MRI or ambiguous dexamethasone suppression testing, bilateral inferior petrosal sinus sampling (IPSS) of serum ACTH levels can suggest a pituitary versus peripheral source of ACTH production. If IPSS suggests a pituitary source, the patient is managed as such. If the IPSS suggests a peripheral source, additional imaging of the body should be performed to identify a potential source of ectopic ACTH production, usually by a bronchial, thymic, or pancreatic islet cell tumor which is more rare than pituitary Cushing's disease.[8] Surgical removal of the corticotroph

pituitary adenoma through a transsphenoidal approach is the treatment of choice for Cushing's disease with postoperative biochemical remission rates of 82–93% in corticotroph microadenomas and better success when an adenoma is visible on MRI. Even in MRI-negative cases, surgical exploration of the pituitary gland often reveals histologically proven corticotroph adenoma.[8] Postoperative remission is achieved in 40–86% of corticotroph macroadenomas, with lower rates seen when a portion of the tumor is not safely resectable. Cushing's disease has a high long-term recurrence risk, with recurrence in 5–27% of patients experiencing postoperative remission within the first 3–5 years of surgery.[12–17] Monitoring for recurrence of tumor and hypercortisolemia should be continued indefinitely. Reoperation is the ideal management at recurrence and might include hemi-hypophysectomy or complete hypophysectomy. In cases where surgery is contraindicated or repeat surgery has been unsuccessful, stereotactic radiosurgery (SRS) or fractionated stereotactic radiotherapy are treatment options with 63% remission at

12 months with 16% new hypopituitarism and 2% new visual deficit in patients treated with SRS after an initial resection.[18] Medical treatments for Cushing's disease exist, including the cortisol synthesis inhibitors metyrapone and ketoconazole. Both decrease cortisol levels but can have severe side effects.[19] Pasireotide is approved for the treatment of Cushing's disease but is effective in only about 20% of patients.[20] Bromocriptine has been used with varying degrees of success. Mifepristone antagonizes cortisol at the cellular receptor level and can decrease the symptoms of Cushing's disease, but it is difficult to monitor biochemically because it does not decrease cortisol levels and causes increases in ACTH levels.[21-23] In many cases, Cushing's disease can be refractory to all treatments, at which point bilateral adrenalectomy is considered to stop cortisol production altogether, with necessary supplementation of physiologic doses of glucocorticoids.

> Twenty-four-hour urinary free cortisol testing and/or midnight salivary cortisol testing are required to verify hypercortisolemia.

> Reoperation is the ideal management at recurrence and might include hemi-hypophysectomy or complete hypophysectomy.

LACTOTROPH ADENOMAS

Lactotroph adenomas typically oversecrete PRL. Hyperprolactinemia can cause galactorrhea, although this is uncommon in men. Elevated PRL also has an inhibitory effect on gonadotropin release resulting in hypogonadism with low libido and erectile dysfunction in men and amenorrhea and infertility in women. In a patient with hyperprolactinemia and a pituitary mass found on imaging, a lactotroph adenoma is often the correct diagnosis. However, as previously mentioned, distortion of the pituitary stalk by a tumor can decrease the normal dopaminergic inhibition of PRL release, resulting in "stalk effect" hyperprolactinemia. Because lactotroph adenomas can be treated medically with dopamine agonists, it is critically important to distinguish between them and other types of pituitary adenomas causing stalk effect hyperprolactinemia to avoid potentially unnecessary surgery on a lactotroph adenoma. To further complicate matters, there are numerous other causes of hyperprolactinemia including medications, systemic diseases, stress, or pregnancy. A systematic approach to hyperprolactinemia can assist with making this distinction. Usually stalk effect hyperprolactinemia does not exceed 150 μg/L. Hypersecretion of PRL by lactotroph macroadenomas (>1 cm) routinely causes hyperprolactinemia in excess of 200 μg/L, while lactotroph microadenomas (<1 cm) typically do not cause prolactin levels greater than 100 μg/L. Moderate-sized adenomas together with prolactin levels 100–200 μg/L can be difficult to diagnose as lactotroph adenomas or other pituitary adenomas with stalk effect hyperprolactinemia.[8] Once a lactotroph adenoma is presumed,

dopamine agonists can be initiated with either bromocriptine or cabergoline, with the latter being the treatment of choice due to higher efficacy and a lower side-effect profile. This is effective in 85–90% of lactotroph microadenomas and 65–70% of lactotroph macroadenomas.[24] Surgical removal is indicated after failed medical therapy due to intolerance of side effects, tumor resistance to treatment, persistent mass effect (common with cystic tumors), CSF leak as a result of shrinkage of a previously invasive tumor, or initial misdiagnosis as a lactotroph adenoma.[25-29] Prolactin levels are normalized by surgical removal in about 60–90% of microadenomas and 40–60% of macroadenomas.[30,31] If surgery is contraindicated for any reason, radiation including SRS or fractionated SRS are reasonable options resulting in normalized prolactin in about 63% of patients, but these treatments pose risk to pituitary and visual function, with 25% of patients developing new hypopituitarism and 3% developing a new visual complication.[32]

> Elevated PRL also has an inhibitory effect on gonadotropin release resulting in hypogonadism with low libido and erectile dysfunction in men and amenorrhea and infertility in women.

SOMATOTROPH ADENOMAS

Somatotroph adenomas produce excess levels of GH and result in acromegaly in adults or gigantism in children. In acromegaly, the increased GH causes enlarging hands and feet, arthritis, and nerve entrapment syndromes. Skin tags and colon polyps frequently occur. Enlargement of facial features occurs including frontal bossing, increased jaw size, and enlargement of the tongue, resulting in obstructive sleep apnea and, if left untreated, can progress to pulmonary hypertension and ultimately cardiomyopathy. Hypertension, diabetes mellitus, and insulin resistance are common. Untreated acromegaly has been shown to decrease life expectancy and should be treated once diagnosed.[33] Under normal circumstances, GH levels vary widely and may not test overtly abnormal. So, relevant laboratory data include elevations in insulin-like growth factor-1 (IGF-1), the systemic effector hormone stimulated by GH. Oral glucose tolerance testing confirms the diagnosis of acromegaly when GH levels greater than 5 μg/L fail to suppress below 1 μg/L after the administration of oral glucose. Sellar MRI to characterize the somatotroph adenoma should be obtained. Management of acromegaly is aimed at normalizing IGF-1. Medical treatment options with reasonable success rates exist for acromegaly, but the efficacy is improved following a cytoreductive surgery.[33,34] Surgical resection is the treatment of choice, with older studies showing normalization of IGF-1 levels in 85–91% of microadenomas and 70% of macroadenomas.[34-36] Newer studies following more stringent definitions of biochemical remission for acromegaly show 80–100% remission for microadenomas and 50–61% for macroadenomas, with larger tumor size, cavernous sinus invasion, and higher preop hormone levels predictive of unfavorable outcome.[37,38] Recurrence rates among those who achieve remission are relatively high around 8–10% at

10 years, and, as outlined earlier, many do not achieve remission at all. Reoperation is a reasonable option for recurrence if a resectable recurrent or residual mass is identified. In cases of persistent or recurrent acromegaly where reoperation is not recommended, medical options are available and effective.[39] Dopamine agonists, somatostatin analogs, and GH receptor antagonists have shown normalization of IGF-1 levels in 40%, 67%, and 89–97% of patients, respectively.[40-44] In refractory cases, stereotactic radiosurgery and fractionated stereotactic radiotherapy are treatment options, normalizing IGF-1 in 23% of patients with average time to normalization of 1.4 yrs.[45] Multimodality treatment is the emerging paradigm for recurrent acromegaly.[39]

> Recurrence rates among those who achieve remission are relatively high around 8–10% at 10 years, and, as outlined earlier, many do not achieve remission at all.

THYROTROPH ADENOMAS

Thyrotroph adenomas are a rare subtype, accounting for about 1% of all hypersecreting tumors. Clinical presentation reveals signs and symptoms of hyperthyroidism. Laboratory evaluation reveals elevated thyroid hormone with a concomitant elevation in TSH. Sellar MRI should reveal a pituitary adenoma, usually a small macroadenoma or larger microadenoma. Again, transsphenoidal surgery is the treatment of choice, with remission rates of 23–63%, better with smaller and non-invasive tumors. Surgery also establishes tissue diagnosis and verifies TSH secretion, both of which are necessary due to the overall rarity of thyrotroph adenomas.[46-49] Somatostatin analogues have shown success in normalizing TSH and thyroid hormones in refractory cases and as a primary treatment.[49,50] Stereotactic radiosurgery has also been used successfully, but there are limited data on biochemical remission specifically for thyrotroph adenomas.[51]

GONADOTROPH ADENOMAS

Gonadotroph adenomas are a common subtype of pituitary adenoma that often overproduce FSH and less commonly LH, but the elevations are modest and clinical evidence of this hypersecretion is exceedingly rare.[52] Case reports exist of both estrogen and testosterone hypersecretion syndromes caused by gonadotroph adenomas,[53-55] but the vast majority of this subtype are considered "non-functional" or "endocrine-inactive."

NULL CELL ADENOMAS

Null cell adenomas show no evidence of hypersecretion clinically or biochemically, and staining reveals no evidence of transcription factors or pituitary hormones. Null cells are found in the normal pituitary gland, and null cell adenomas are assumed to be neoplasms originating from these normal null cells. The roll of null cells in normal pituitary function is not well understood. Without the presence of a hypersecretion syndrome, both null cell and gonadotroph adenomas typically present as large tumors due to mass effect, most commonly visual deficit or pituitary hypofunction. Surgical removal is the recommended treatment to alleviate mass effect. Stereotactic radiosurgery has a high rate of tumor growth control but is typically not used as a primary treatment for larger tumors due to high risk of injury to the optic chiasm and normal pituitary gland.

"HIGH-RISK" PITUITARY ADENOMA SUBTYPES

The 2017 WHO classification of pituitary tumors no longer uses the classification atypical adenoma.[3] This diagnosis was based on several histopathological criteria which were ultimately shown to have little predictive value with respect to clinical course. Instead the scheme designates several subtypes of pituitary adenomas as "high-risk." These subtypes have been shown over time to behave more aggressively.[7] The *silent corticotroph adenoma* is a tumor that demonstrates the Tpit transcription factor and ACTH production consistent with other corticotroph adenomas in the absence of Cushing's disease. The silent corticotroph adenoma is usually more invasive into surrounding structures and has a higher recurrence rate than other corticotroph adenomas.[56,57] The *lactotroph adenoma* in male patients typically follows a more aggressive course.[58] The *sparsely granulated somatotroph adenoma* is less responsive to medical treatments, more invasive, and higher risk for recurrence.[59] The *pit-1-positive plurihormonal adenoma* demonstrates the Pit-1 transcription factor as well as evidence of production of GH, PRL, and TSH. There is typically no evidence of endocrinopathy. This subtype also follows a more aggressive clinical course, with high rates of invasion and recurrence and shorter interval to recurrence after primary treatment.[60]

PITUITARY CARCINOMA

According to the 2017 WHO classification scheme, the diagnosis of pituitary carcinoma is reserved for tumors that have spread beyond the sella, either by CSF dissemination or by hematogenous spread.[3,7] Management is multimodal, including surgery, radiation, and chemotherapy most commonly with temozolomide.[61]

PITUITARY BLASTOMA

Pituitary blastoma is a newly recognized diagnosis included for the first time in the 2017 WHO classification of pituitary tumors.[3] About 20 cases have been reported in the literature, mostly in infants less than 24 months of age who present with Cushing's disease and often ophthalmoplegia.[7] The prognosis is poor, with median overall survival of 8 months after diagnosis. The tumor consists of small, primitive-appearing cells, larger adenohypophyseal-appearing cells, and Rathke-type epithelial glands.[62,63]

NEURONAL AND PARANEURONAL TUMORS

Sellar gangliocytoma is a rare tumor with about 80 reported cases which is often a combined lesion with a pituitary adenoma.[64,65] Most of these lesions are hypersecreting, with GH the most common hormone produced.[64,65] Sellar neurocytoma has been reported nine times in the literature. All were treated surgically with varying degrees of success. Most patients present with visual loss and are initially misdiagnosed as having other pathologies based on imaging findings.[66] Sellar paraganglioma is another very rare diagnosis with 31 cases reported in the literature. In one study, attempts at surgical removal were aborted due to extreme vascularity of the tumor. After diagnosis was obtained, the tumors responded well to stereotactic radiosurgery.[67] Primary sellar neuroblastoma has been reported nine times in the literature. Clinical features include rapid tumor growth, hypopituitarism, visual loss, and oculomotor nerve palsy. Prognosis is likely poor but difficult to establish given the paucity of data.[68]

> Clinical features of primary sellar neuroblastoma include rapid tumor growth, hypopituitarism, visual loss, and oculomotor nerve palsy.

TUMORS OF THE NEUROHYPOPHYSIS AND INFUNDIBULUM

PITUICYTOMA

Pituicytomas represent a rare, low-grade glial neoplasm that originates in the neurohypophysis or infundibulum. To date, approximately 81 cases have been described in the literature. It has been referred to by other names such as *infundibuloma*, *granular cell tumor*, and *pilocytic astrocytoma* in the past but is a distinct entity. They are benign, slow-growing, and classified as WHO grade 1.

> Pituicytomas represent a rare, low-grade glial neoplasm that originates in the neurohypophysis or infundibulum.

Their cellular origin is from pituicytes, which are stromal support cells found in the neurohypophysis. Histologically, these tumors are characterized by dense, compact bipolar spindle cells. MRI shows T1 isointensity, contrast enhancing and heterogenous T2 signal intensity. A rich capillary network accounts for the contrast enhancement. Pituicytomas are slow-growing tumors that respond well to surgery when indicated. Subtotal resections (STRs) are associated with recurrence.

Genetic studies have found that thyroid transcription factor 1 (TTF-1) is strongly expressed in pituicytomas.[69] Further research discovered that TTF-1 is found in the pituicytes of the neurohypophysis and infundibulum.[6] TTF-1 expression was also found in other posterior pituitary tumors outlined in this chapter, which suggests suggest a possible common pituicyte origin.

GRANULAR CELL TUMORS

Granular cell tumors (GCTs) are rare, low-grade tumors that originate in the neurohypophysis or infundibulum. They are the most common primary tumor of the posterior pituitary.

Other names have been used for GCTs, such as *pituitary choristoma*, *Abrikossoff tumor*, and *pituicytoma*. It should be noted that pituicytomas are recognized as a separate entity, and this nomenclature is outdated.

Histologically, these tumors are characterized by abundant eosinophilic cytoplasm with periodic acid-Schiff (PAS)-positive granules, and focal spindled areas. They express TTF-1 like pituicytomas suggesting a common pituicyte origin. On MRI, they often appear heterogeneous with variable contrast enhancement. They appear to show a preference for the pituitary stalk and most commonly present as a suprasellar lesion. However, they also arise from the posterior pituitary and can present as an intrasellar mass.

> Granular cell tumors are the most common primary tumor of the posterior pituitary.

SPINDLE CELL ONCOCYTOMA

Spindle cell oncocytomas are rare, benign tumors of the neurohypophysis. They are classified as WHO grade 1. Only about 25 cases have been published in the literature. These tumors are defined histologically by their oncocytic cytoplasm, which means that it is abundant secondary to an accumulation of altered mitochondria. Like granular cell tumors and pituicytomas, spindle cell oncocytomas express TTF-1. This suggests that spindle cell oncocytomas might share a common origin arising from pituicytes. MRI shows a heterogenous enhancement pattern that may have calcifications. These have been managed surgically when symptomatic, but, due to their rarity and paucity of reported literature, long-term outcomes are unknown.

> Like granular cell tumors and pituicytomas, spindle cell oncocytomas express TTF-1.

CRANIOPHARYNGIOMAS

Craniopharyngiomas (CPs) are rare, histologically benign tumors classified as WHO grade 1 (Figure 7.4). They are thought to arise from remnants of Rathke's pouch and can appear anywhere along the craniopharyngeal duct. These commonly appear as midline tumors in the suprasellar region. They are near neurovascular structures such as the optic nerves and chiasm, perforating arteries, pituitary stalk, circle of Willis, third ventricle, hypothalamus, brainstem, and frontal/temporal lobes. Due to their proximity and aggressive nature, they are often found adherent to these neurovascular structures. As a result, CPs prove to be a challenging surgical entity despite their benign pathology.

CPs represent less than 1% of all primary CNS tumors but are the most common non-glial tumor in the pediatric population.[70] They account for 0.5–2.5 new cases per 1,000,000 population per year globally.[71]

There are two pathologic variants with distinct mutations and phenotypes. Adamantinomatous craniopharyngiomas

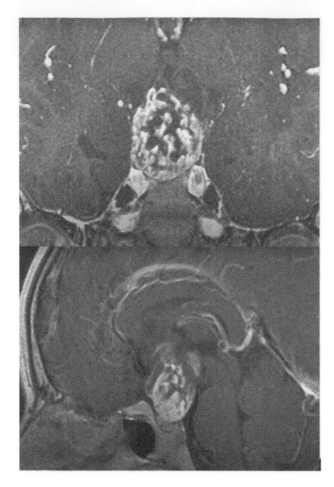

Figure 7.4 *Craniopharyngioma. Post-contrast T1 sequence of an MRI brain. Coronal (top) and sagittal (bottom) views.*

(ACPs) have a bimodal age distribution appearing in children ages 4–15 years and adults 45–60 years. They are thought to arise from neoplastic transformation of epithelial cell rests within the craniopharyngeal duct.[72] Genetic studies determined that 95% of ACPs show a *CTNNB1* mutation and aberrant nuclear expression of beta-catenin. This mutation has not yielded any targeted therapies to date. In contrast, papillary craniopharyngiomas (PCPs) occur exclusively in adults, at an average age of 45–55 years. PCPs are thought to arise from metaplasia of epithelial cells within the pituitary stalk.[73] Genetic

studies found that PCPs have a *BRAFV600E* mutation in 95% of cases. This has shown some promise in targeted therapies. Neither ACP nor PCP have shown any sex predilection. There may be an increased incidence in African Americans.[74]

Imaging shows that ACPs tend to have cystic components, and calcifications are frequent. PCPs tend to be more solid tumors on MRI. Despite their benign histology, they are quite aggressive. Indications for surgery are neurological deficits, pituitary dysfunction, obstructive hydrocephalus, and/or radiographic evidence of growth. Surgical goals are gross total resection or STR with adjuvant radiation therapy. In general, the guiding principle is a maximal safe resection while minimizing postoperative deficits, pituitary dysfunction, and hypothalamic dysfunction.

Surgical management has evolved considerably over the past 20 years. Traditionally, these were operated on by transcranial approaches. In more recent years, there has been a shift to endoscopic endonasal approaches. The advantages of the endoscopic endonasal approach are direct visualization and superior illumination of the pathology, a minimally invasive approach, and minimal retraction of brain and associated neurovascular structures that are often a significant source of morbidity. Surgical results are at least comparable if not superior to transcranial approaches.

There have been other proposed treatments, such as brachytherapy, but none has been shown to be effective. Currently, there are clinical trials investigating the roll of BRAF inhibitors for treating PCPs. Genetic analysis by Brastianos et al. was able to first identify a *BRAF V600E* mutation in 95% of histologically defined PCPs.[75] BRAF inhibitors have been used in the treatment of melanoma and colorectal cancer shown to have *BRAF* mutations.[72,76] Multiple case reports have been published detailing an arrest or regression in tumor volume with BRAF/MEK inhibitors. Brastianos et al. demonstrated an 85% reduction in tumor volume in a recurrence after 35 days of treatment with combined BRAF/MEK inhibitors.[77] Rostami et al. used combined BRAF/MEK inhibitors after a STR and saw a 91% reduction in tumor volume after 15 weeks of treatment.[78] Himes et al. had similar results in a patient treated with BRAF inhibitor alone for a recurrence of 4–5 mm that shrunk after 1 year of treatment.[79] This will require further investigation before any conclusions can be made; however, it does show promise.

Describe the anatomy of the cavernous sinus with respect to the sella turcica	Paired cavernous sinuses, lateral to the sella, and contain the cavernous segment of the internal carotid arteries as well as cranial nerves III, IV, V1, V2, and VI
What is the embryologic origin of the pituitary gland?	Neurohypophysis→posterior lobe→neuroectoderm Adenohypophysis→anterior lobe→pharyngeal ectoderm→Rathke's pouch
What is stalk effect?	Elevated prolactin levels (hyperprolactinemia) caused by mass effect/distortion of the pituitary stalk and resultant loss of dopaminergic inhibition of PRL production
What workup is required for Cushing's disease?	Twenty-four-hour urinary free cortisol testing and/or midnight salivary cortisol testing to verify hypercortisolemia, then Dexamethasone suppression testing to help distinguish between a pituitary adenoma and other sources of excess cortisol (ectopic ACTH source vs. cortisol-producing adrenal adenoma)
What is the incidence of pituitary tumors?	Incidence ranges from 1 to 20 cases per 100,000 per year
What is a silent corticotroph adenoma?	A tumor that demonstrates the Tpit transcription factor and ACTH production consistent with other corticotroph adenomas in the absence of Cushing's disease
Why is SRS not used for large pituitary tumors as primary treatment?	Stereotactic radiosurgery has a high rate of tumor growth control but is typically not used as a primary treatment for larger tumors due to high risk of injury to the optic chiasm and normal pituitary gland
What is the presentation for hyperprolactinemia?	Galactorrhea (uncommon for men), hypogonadism, low libido, erectile dysfunction in men, amenorrhea and infertility in women

How does oral glucose testing confirm acromegaly?

Oral glucose tolerance testing confirms the diagnosis of acromegaly when GH levels greater than 5 µg/L fail to suppress below 1 µg/L after the administration of oral glucose

When is inferior petrosal sinus sampling useful in the workup of Cushing's disease?

In cases of a negative pituitary MRI or ambiguous dexamethasone suppression testing, bilateral inferior petrosal sinus sampling (IPSS) of serum ACTH levels can suggest a pituitary vs. peripheral source of ACTH production

QUESTIONS

1. What mutation in craniopharyngiomas shows promise for a treatment target?
   a. PLD
   b. MEK
   c. BRAFV600E
   d. EGFR

2. Which subtype of craniopharyngioma shows the mutation that may prove to be a treatment target?
   a. Adamantinous
   b. Papillary
   c. None of the above
   d. Both a and b

3. Which of the following has become the gold standard approach for surgical intervention for pituitary pathologies?
   a. Transcranial
   b. Endonasal microscopic
   c. Transsphenoidal endonasal endoscopic
   d. Sublabial transsphenoidal

4. What is the embryologic origin of craniopharyngiomas?
   a. Mesoderm
   b. Neuroectoderm
   c. Neural crest cells
   d. Rathke's pouch remnant

5. In what tumors of the pituitary gland is TTF-1 expressed?
   a. Pituicytomas
   b. Spindle cell oncocytoma
   c. Granular cell tumor
   d. All of the above

6. What is the most common primary tumor of the posterior pituitary?
   a. Granular cell tumor
   b. Pituicytoma
   c. Spindle cell oncocytoma
   d. Pituitary blastoma

7. When is pituitary apoplexy a surgical emergency?
   a. Headache
   b. Visual loss
   c. Hormone dysfunction
   d. Imaging finding alone

8. What amount of prolactin is consistent with a secreting lactotroph pituitary adenoma?
   a. <100
   b. 100–150
   c. >200
   d. All of the above

9. What is the treatment for pituitary carcinoma?
   a. Surgery
   b. Chemotherapy
   c. Radiation
   d. All of the above

10. What imaging modality is useful for discerning microadenomas?
    a. CT with contrast
    b. Dynamic MRI
    c. Perfusion MRI
    d. Diffusor tensor imaging

ANSWERS

1. c
2. b
3. c
4. d
5. d
6. a
7. b
8. c
9. d
10. b

REFERENCES

1. Monson JP. The epidemiology of endocrine tumors. *Endocr Relat Cancer.* 2000;7:29–36.
2. Ezzat S, Asa SL, Couldwell WT, et al. The prevalence of pituitary adenomas: A systematic review. *Cancer.* 2004;101:613–661.
3. Lloyd RV, Osamura RY, Klöppel G, Rosai J, eds. *WHO Classification of Tumours of Endocrine Organs.* 4th ed. Lyon: IARC; 2017.
4. McLaughlin N, Laws ER, Oyesiku NM, et al. Pituitary centers of excellence. *Neurosurgery.* 2012;71(5):916–926.
5. Blumenfeld H. *Neuroanatomy Through Clinical Cases.* 2nd ed. Sunderland, MA: Sinauer; 2018:792–802.
6. Donangelo I, Melmed S. Pituitary adenomas. In Fink G, Pfaff D, Levine J, eds. *Handbook of Neuroendocrinology.* Waltham, MA: Elsevier Academic Press; 2012:746–756.
7. Mete O, Lopes MB. Overview of the 2017 WHO Classification of Pituitary Tumors *Endocr Pathol.* 2017:28:228–243.
8. Conger A, Barkhoudarian G, Kelly DF. Preoperative, intraoperative, and postoperative management following pituitary surgery. In Lavin N, ed. *Manual of Endocrinology and Metabolism.* 5th ed. Philadelphia, PA: Wolters Kluwer; 2019:117–118.
9. Palejwala SK, Conger AR, Eisenberg AA, et al. Pregnancy-associated Cushing's disease? An exploratory retrospective study. *Pituitary.* 2018;21(6):584–592.
10. Patil CG, Lad SP, Katznelson L, et al. Brain atrophy and cognitive deficits in Cushing's disease. *Neurosurg Focus.* 2007;23(3):E11.
11. Kunwar S. Pituitary tumors. In Bernstein M, Berger M, eds. *Neuro-Oncology: The Essentials.* 2nd ed. New York Thieme Medical; 2008:338–339.
12. Leinung MC, Kane LA, Scheithauer BW, et al. Long term follow up of transsphenoidal surgery for the treatment of Cushing's disease in childhood. *J Clin Endocrinol Metab.* 1995;80(8):2475–2479.
13. Estrada J, Boronat M, Mielgo M, et al. The long-term outcome of pituitary irradiation after unsuccessful transsphenoidal surgery in Cushing's disease. *N Engl J Med.* 1997;336(3):172–177.

14. Semple DM, Vance ML, Findling J, et al. Transsphenoidal surgery Cushing's disease: Outcome in patients with a normal magnetic resonance imaging scan. *Neurosurgery.* 2000. 46(3):553–558; discussion 558–559.
15. Prevedello DM, Pouration N, Sherman J, et al. Management of Cushing's disease: Outcome in patients with microadenoma detected on pituitary magnetic resonance imaging. *J Neurosurg.* 2008;109(4):751–759.
16. Hammer GD, Tyrrell JB, Lamborn KE, et al. Transsphenoidal microsurgery for Cushing's disease: Intitial outcome and long-term results. *J Clin Endocrinol Metab.* 2004;89(12):6348–6357.
17. Utz AL, Swearingen B, Biller BM. Pituitary surgery and postoperative management in Cushing's diease. *Endocrinol Metab Clin North Am.* 2005;34(2):459–478, xi.
18. Sheehan, JM, Vance ML, Sheehan JP, et al. Radiosurgery for Cushing's disease after failed transsphenoidal surgery. *J Neurosurg.* 2000. 93(5):738–742.
19. Lewis JH, Zimmerman HJ, Benson GD, et al. Hepatic injury associated with ketoconazole therapy. Analysis of 33 cases. *Gastroenterology.* 1984. 86(3):503–13.
20. Boscaro M, Ludlam WH, Atkinson B, et al. Treatment of pituitary-dependent Cushing's disease with the multireceptor ligand somatostatin analog pasireotide (SOM230): A multicenter, phase II trial. *J Clin Endocrinol Metab.* 2009;94(1):115–122.
21. Healy DL, Chrousos GP, Schulte HM, et al. Increased adrenocorticotropin, cortisol, and arginine vasopressin secretion in primates after the antiglucocorticoid steroid RU 486: Dose response relationships. *J Clin Endocrinol Metab.* 1985;60(1):1–4.
22. Nieman LK, Chrousos GP, Kellner C, et al. Successful treatment of Cushing's syndrome with the glucocorticoid antagonist RU 486. *J Clin Endocrinol Metab.* 1985;61(3):536–540.
23. Sartor O, Cutler GB, Mifepristone: Treatment of Cushing's syndrome. *Clin Obstet Gynecol.* 1996; 39(2):506–510.
24. Webster J, Piscitelli G, Polli A, et al. A comparison of cabergoline and bromocriptine in the treatment of hyperprolactinemic amenorrhea. Cabergoline Comparative Study Group. *N Engl J Med.* 1994;331(14):904–909.
25. Molitch ME, Pharmacologic resistance in prolactinoma patients. *Pituitary.* 2005;8(1):43–52.
26. Molitch ME. The cabergoline-resistant prolactinoma patient: New challenges. *J Clin Endocrinol Metab.* 2008;93(12):4643–4645.
27. Suliman SG, Gurlek A, Byrne JV, et al. Nonsurgical cerebrospinal fluid rhinorrhea in invasive macroprolactinoma: Incidence, radiological, and clinicopathological features. *J Clin Endocrinol Metab.* 2007;92(10):3829–3835.
28. Inder WJ, Macfarlane MR. Hyperprolactinaemia associated with a complex cystic pituitary mass: Medical versus surgical therapy. *Intern Med J.* 2004;34(9–10):573–576.
29. Bahuleyan B, Menon G, Nair S, et al. Non-surgical management of cystic prolactinomas. *J Clin Neurosci.* 2009;16(11):1421–1424.
30. Massoud F, Serri O, Hardy J, et al. Transsphenoidal adenomectomy for microprolactinomas: 10 to 20 years of follow-up. *Surg Neurol.* 1996;45(4):341–346.
31. Gokalp HZ, Deda H, Attar A, et al. The neurosurgical management of prolactinomas. *J Neurosurg Sci.* 2000;44(3):128–132.
32. Hung YC, Lee CC, Yang HC, et al. The benefit and risk of stereotactic radiosurgery for prolactinomas: An international multicenter cohort study [published online ahead of print, 2019 Aug 2]. *J Neurosurg.* 2019;1–10. doi:10.3171/2019.4.JNS183443
33. Clemmons DR, Chihara K, Freda PU, et al. Optimizing control of acromegaly: Integrating a growth hormone receptor antagonist into the treatment algorithm. *J Clin Endocrinol Metab.* 2003; 88(10):4759–4767.
34. Kreutzer J, Vance ML, Lopes MB, Laws ER Jr. Surgical management of GH-secreting pituitary adenomas: An outcome study using modern remission criteria. *J Clin Endocrinol Metab.* 2001;86(9):4072–4077.
35. Shimon I, Cohen ZR, Ram Z, Hadani M. Transsphenoidal surgery for acromegaly: Endocrinological follow-up of 98 patients. *Neurosurgery.* 2001;48(6):1239–1245.
36. Ahmed S, Elsheikh M, Stratton IM, et al. Outcome of transphenoidal surgery for acromegaly and its relationship to surgical experience. *Clin Endocrinol (Oxf).* 1999;50(5):561–567.
37. Minniti G, Jaffrain-Rea ML, Esposito V, Santoro A, Tamburrano G, Cantore G. Evolving criteria for post-operative biochemical remission of acromegaly: Can we achieve a definitive cure? An audit of surgical results on a large series and a review of the literature. *Endocr Relat Cancer.* 2003;10(4):611–619.
38. Jane JA Jr., Starke RM, Elzoghby MA, et al. Endoscopic transsphenoidal surgery for acromegaly: Remission using modern criteria, complications, and predictors of outcome. *J Clin Endocrinol Metab.* 2011;96(9):2732–2740.
39. Bollerslev J, Heck A, Olarescu NC. Management of endocrine disease: Individualised management of acromegaly. *Eur J Endocrinol.* 2019;181(2):R57–R71.
40. Freda PU. Somatostatin analogs in acromegaly. *J Clin Endocrinol Metab.* 2002;87(7):3013–3018.
41. Abs R, Verhelst J, Maiter D, et al. Cabergoline in the treatment of acromegaly: A study in 64 patients. *J Clin Endocrinol Metab.* 1998;83(2):374–378.
42. Trainer PJ, Drake WM, Katznelson L, et al. Treatment of acromegaly with the growth hormone–receptor antagonist pegvisomant. *N Engl J Med.* 2000;342:1171–1177.
43. Buchfelder M, van der Lely AJ, Biller BMK, et al. Long-term treatment with pegvisomant: Observations from 2090 patients in ACROSTUDY. *Eur J Endocrinol.* 2018 Dec 1;179(6):419–427.
44. van der Lely AJ, Hutson RK, Trainer PJ, et al. Long-term treatment of acromegaly with pegvisomant, a growth hormone receptor antagonist. *Lancet.* 2001;358(9295):1754–1759.
45. Attanasio R, Epaminonda P, Motti E, et al. Gamma-knife radiosurgery in acromegaly: A 4-year follow-up study. *J Clin Endocrinol Metab.* 2003;88(7):3105–3112.
46. Brucker-Davis F, Oldfield EH, Skarulis MC, et al. Thyrotropin-secreting pituitary tumors: Diagnostic criteria, thyroid hormone sensitivity, and treatment outcome in 25 patients followed at the National Institutes of Health. *J Clin Endocrinol Metab.* 1999;84(2):476–486.
47. Losa M, Giovanelli M, Persani L, et al. Criteria of cure and follow-up of central hyperthyroidism due to thyrotropin-secreting pituitary adenomas. *J Clin Endocrinol Metab.* 1996;81(8):3084–3090.
48. Laws ER, Vance ML, Jane JA Jr. TSH adenomas. *Pituitary.* 2006;9(4):313–315.
49. Socin HV, Chanson P, Delemer B, et al. The changing spectrum of TSH-secreting pituitary adenomas: Diagnosis and management in 43 patients. *Eur J Endocrinol.* 2003;148(4):433–442.
50. Rimareix F, Grunenwald S, Vezzosi D, et al. Primary medical treatment of thyrotropin-secreting pituitary adenomas by first-generation somatostatin analogs: A case study of seven patients. *Thyroid.* 2015;25(8):877–882.
51. Mouslech Z, Somali M, Sakali AK, et al. TSH-secreting pituitary adenomas treated by gamma knife radiosurgery: Our case experience and a review of the literature. *Hormones (Athens).* 2016;15(1):122–128.
52. Ho DM, Hsu CY, Ting LT, Chiang H. The clinicopathological characteristics of gonadotroph cell adenoma: A study of 118 cases. *Hum Pathol.* 1997;28(8):905–911.
53. Kihara M, Sugita T, Nagai Y, et al. Ovarian hyperstimulation caused by gonadotroph cell adenoma: A case report and review of the literature. *Gynecol Endocrinol.* 2006;22(2):110–113.
54. Cooper O, Geller JL, Melmed S. Ovarian hyperstimulation syndrome caused by an FSH-secreting pituitary adenoma. *Nat Clin Pract Endocrinol Metab.* 2008;4(4):234–238.
55. Dizon MN, Vesely DL. Gonadotropin-secreting pituitary tumor associated with hypersecretion of testosterone and hypogonadism after hypophysectomy. *Endocr Pract.* May-Jun 2002;8(3):225–231.
56. Cooper O, Ben-Shlomo A, Bonert V, et al. Silent corticogonadotroph adenomas: Clinical and cellular characteristics and long-term outcomes. *Horm Cancer.* 2010;1(2):80–92.
57. Ben-Shlomo A, Cooper O. Silent corticotroph adenomas. *Pituitary.* 2018;21(2):183–193.
58. Liu W, Zahr RS, McCartney S, et al. Clinical outcomes in male patients with lactotroph adenomas who required pituitary surgery: A retrospective single center study. *Pituitary.* 2018;21(5):454–462.
59. Trouillas J, Vasiljevic A, Lapoirie M, et al. Pathological markers of somatotroph pituitary neuroendocrine tumors predicting the response to medical treatment. *Minerva Endocrinol.* 2019;44(2):129–136.
60. García-Sáenz M, Uribe-Cortés D, González-Virla B, et al. Silent pituitary plurihormonal adenoma: Clinical relevance of immunohistochemical analysis. Adenoma hipofisario silente plurihormonal: Relevancia clínica de la inmunohistoquímica. *Rev Med Inst Mex Seguro Soc.* 2019;57(1):48–55.
61. Santos-Pinheiro F, Penas-Prado M, Kamiya-Matsuoka C, et al. Treatment and long-term outcomes in pituitary carcinoma: A cohort study. *Eur J Endocrinol.* 2019;181(4):397–407.
62. Scheithauer BW, Kovacs K, Horvath E, et al. Pituitary blastoma. *Acta Neuropathol.* 2008;116 (6):657–666.
63. Scheithauer BW, Horvath E, Abel TW, et al. Pituitary blastoma: A unique embryonal tumor. *Pituitary.* 2012;15(3):365–373.
64. Qiao N, Ye Z, Wang Y, et al. Gangliocytomas in the sellar region. *Clin Neurol Neurosurg.* 2014;126:156–161.
65. Yang B, Yang C, Sun Y, et al. Mixed gangliocytoma-pituitary adenoma in the sellar region: A large-scale single-center experience. *Acta Neurochir (Wien).* 2018;160(10):1989–1999.

66. Wang J, Song DL, Deng L, et al. Extraventricular neurocytoma of the sellar region: Case report and literature review. *Springerplus*. 2016;5(1):987.
67. Vasoya P, Aryan S, Thakar S, et al. Sellar-suprasellar paraganglioma: Report of 2 cases and review of literature [published online ahead of print, 2020 May 12]. *World Neurosurg*. 2020;S1878-8750(20):30864-0.
68. Yamamuro S, Fukushima T, Yoshino A, et al. Primary sellar neuroblastoma in an elderly patient: Case report. *NMC Case Rep J*. 2014;2(2):57–60.
69. Lee EB, Tihan T, Scheithauer BW, et al. Thyroid transcription factor 1 expression in sellar tumors: A histogenetic marker? *J Neuropathol Exp Neurol*. 2009;68:482–488.
70. Louis DN, Wiestler OD, Ohgaki H. *WHO Classification of Tumours of the Central Nervous System. Lyon: International Agency for Research on Cancer*; 2016.
71. Müller HL, Merchant TE, Warmuth-Metz M, et al. Craniopharyngioma. *Nat Rev Dis Primers*. 2019;5:75.
72. Cheng L, Lopez-Beltran A, Massari F, et al. Molecular testing for BRAF mutations to inform melanoma treatment decisions: A move toward precision medicine. *Mod Pathol*. 2018;31:24–38.
73. Prabhu VC, Brown HG. The pathogenesis of craniopharyngiomas. *Childs Nerv Syst*. 2005;21:622–627.
74. Zacharia BE, Bruce SS, Goldstein H, et al. Incidence, treatment and survival of patients with craniopharyngioma in the surveillance, epidemiology and end results program. *Neuro Oncol*. 2012;14:1070–1078.
75. Brastianos PK, Taylor-Weiner A, Manley PE, et al. Exome sequencing identifies BRAF mutations in papillary craniopharyngiomas. *Nat Genetics*. 2014;46:161–165.
76. Yeh JJ, Routh ED, Rubinas T, et al. KRAS/BRAF mutation status and ERK1/2 activation as biomarkers for MEK1/2 inhibitor therapy in colorectal cancer. *Mol Cancer Ther*. 2009;8:834–843.
77. Brastianos PK, Shankar GM, Gill CM, et al. Dramatic response of BRAF V600E mutant papillary craniopharyngioma to targeted therapy. *J Natl Cancer Inst*. 2016;108(2):djv310. https://academic.oup.com/jnci/article/108/2/djv310/2457803.
78. Rostami E, Witt Nyström P, Libard S, et al. Recurrent papillary craniopharyngioma with BRAFV600E mutation treated with neoadjuvant-targeted therapy. *Acta Neurochir*. 2017;159:2217–2221.
79. Himes BT, Ruff MW, Gompel JJV, et al. Recurrent papillary craniopharyngioma with BRAF V600E mutation treated with dabrafenib: Case report. *J Neurosurg*. 2018;1:1–5.

8 | GERM CELL TUMORS

HIROKAZU TAKAMI

INTRODUCTION

Central nervous system (CNS) germ cell tumors (GCTs) predominantly occur in pediatric and young adult males. Standard of care includes the diagnosis based on tumor markers and/or histopathological specimen and treatment composed of chemotherapy followed by radiation.[1] Clinical trials are ongoing in North America, Europe, and Japan, evaluating varying chemotherapy dosages and fields of radiation therapy to lessen the long-term sequelae of these treatments on the developing CNS. Molecular-targeted therapy for GCTs has yet to be developed as the molecular background of these tumors has not been fully unraveled. This chapter summarizes the updated knowledge of the clinical spectrum of CNS GCTs including clinical/radiological presentations, diagnostic methods, and treatments, as well as the biological backgrounds of its pathogenesis partially elucidated through next-generation sequencing.

GENERAL KNOWLEDGE

CLASSIFICATION

The World Health Organization (WHO) classification of CNS tumors defines five major histological subtypes for GCTs: germinoma, teratoma, choriocarcinoma, yolk sac tumor, and embryonal carcinoma.[2] Teratoma is further subdivided into mature teratoma, immature teratoma, and teratoma with malignant transformation. GCTs often consist of more than one of these components (mixed GCTs).[2] Germinoma accounts for approximately 40–60% of cases, followed by mixed GCT in approximately 30% of cases, and non-germinomatous GCTs (NGGCT) in approximately 10–20%.[3] From a clinical standpoint, GCTs are commonly divided into two major categories: germinoma and NGGCTs, with mixed GCT clinically categorized as a NGGCT. Except for mature teratoma and most germinomas, GCTs are invasive malignant tumors with poor prognoses, which can disseminate into the cerebrospinal fluid (CSF) space, including the ventricles and spinal canal. Germinoma is defined as WHO grade 4.

> Except for mature teratoma and most germinomas, GCTs are invasive malignant tumors with poor prognoses.

BIOLOGY

The biology of GCT reflects the normal development of embryos; teratoma consists of three embryonal germ-layer components, yolk sac tumor represents yolk sac epithelium, choriocarcinoma reflects tissues of a developing placenta, and embryonal carcinoma reflects embryonal stem cells, which have pluripotency. The cell of origin of GCT is hypothesized to be a primordial germ cell (PGC), which has totipotency but is or will be destined to become embryonal gonadal cells (sperm or ovarian cells). The development of germ cell tumor in the CNS is speculated to be caused by the mis-migration of PGCs.[4] GCTs in general occur in genital organs (testis and ovary) and the mediastinum, but the CNS is the most frequent site of extragonadal GCTs.[5]

> The CNS is the most frequent site of extragonadal GCTs.

EPIDEMIOLOGY AND CLINICAL FEATURES

GCTs occur in the pediatric and young adult population, with a peak incidence between 10 and 14 years.[1,6] There is a male preponderance (approximately 3:1).[7] GCTs account for 0.5% of primary brain tumors and 3.8% of pediatric brain tumors.[1] GCTs demonstrate characteristic geographic distributions, with gonadal GCTs predominating in Western countries,[8] whereas CNS GCTs arise more frequently in East Asia.[1,9–11] Tumors preferentially occur at the pineal region (38–54%) and neurohypophysis (13–37%), followed by basal ganglia.[3,6,12,13] Most (>90%) pineal region GCTs occur in men, but there is no gender difference for neurohypophysis GCT.[3,12]

IMAGING FEATURES

GCTs generally show contrast enhancement, except for teratomas. They usually show iso- to hypointensity on T1-weighted images and iso- to hyperintensity on T2-weighted images on magnetic resonance imaging (MRI) scans. Germinomas typically are well-demarcated, relatively homogeneously contrast-enhancing tumors. NGGCTs are generally more heterogeneously contrast-enhancing. Computed tomography (CT) scans may detect calcification (bone) or fat tissue in the tumor, which suggests the presence of a teratoma component. Intratumoral hemorrhage and necrosis

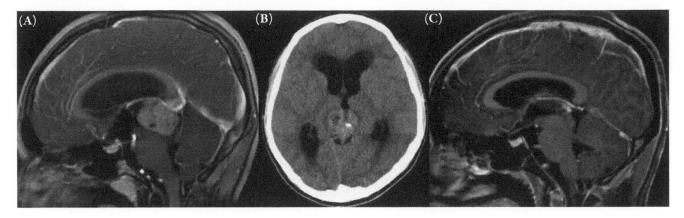

Figure 8.1 (A) MRI scan with gadolinium enhancement of a 16-year-old male patient with pineal germinoma. Germinomas are generally characterized as heterogeneously enhancing mass lesions, and pineal germ cell tumors often cause obstructive hydrocephalus, as in this case. (B) Plain CT image of the same case. Cysts and calcifications are present in the tumor. (C) Post-treatment MRI scan of the same case. Germinoma responds well to radiation and chemotherapy, and this image shows almost complete disappearance of the tumor.

suggests choriocarcinoma (Figure 8.1). However, radiograph-based examinations such as CT or angiography should be limited preoperatively, as these tumors are particularly radiation sensitive and exposure may shrink the tumor, particularly germinomas.[14] Presence of a bifocal tumor (also known as synchronous tumor) at the neurohypophysis and pineal gland is indicative of underlying germinoma but still requires histopathological confirmation because there are occasional exceptions, including NGGCT and primitive neuroectodermal tumor (PNET).[15,16]

SYMPTOMATOLOGY

Neurohypophyseal GCTs manifest prototypical symptoms due to their anatomic location, including pituitary insufficiency, visual deficits attributable to optic pathway compression or invasion, and hydrocephalus in large tumors compressing the third ventricle.[3] Diabetes insipidus is seen in most cases and is often the presenting symptom, but sometimes symptom onset is insidious and it takes some time before imaging reveals the tumor.[12]

Pineal region GCTs frequently involve the cerebral aqueduct or midbrain (tectal plate), with associated mass effect precipitating obstructive hydrocephalus or neuro-ophthalmologic abnormalities, respectively[13,17–20] The latter may present as dorsal midbrain or Parinaud's syndrome consisting of restrictions in upward gaze, convergence-retraction nystagmus, and pupillary hyporeflexia.[19,20]

Basal ganglia GCTs often represent germinomas that produce human chorionic gonadotropin (HCG), and, therefore, these tumors can present with hemiparesis, precocious puberty, or personality change.[21] Common clinical/pathological characteristics of these tumors are outlined in Table 8.1.

DIAGNOSIS

GCTs are diagnosed based on clinical presentation and tumor markers, along with imaging findings if a case presents with typical findings. Tumor marker examination for alpha-fetoprotein (AFP) and HCG is essential in blood serum, and, if possible, in CSF. CSF cytology is also recommended to screen for possible tumor dissemination into the CSF space. Imaging exams should include MRI with contrast of the entire CNS to screen for possible CNS dissemination.

> Tumor marker examination for alpha-fetoprotein (AFP) and HCG is essential in blood serum, and, if possible, in CSF.

TABLE 8.1 Clinical/pathological features and treatment of germ cell tumors according to tumor location

	PINEAL REGION	NEUROHYPOPHYSIS	BASAL GANGLIA
Sex	Dominantly male	Female : Male = 1 : 1	Mostly male
Histology	Mostly germinoma	Most commonly NGGCT	Variable
Typical symptom	Endocrine abnormalities (especially diabetes insipidus), visual disturbance	Hydrocephalus and ocular abnormalities (Parinaud's syndrome)	Hemiparesis, precocious puberty and personality change
Radiation coverage	Whole ventricle + focal radiation	Whole ventricle + focal radiation	Whole brain + focal radiation

NGGCT, non-germinomatous germ cell tumors.

Elevated HCG is typically associated with choriocarcinomas and elevated AFP with yolk sac tumors. Of note, mild to moderate elevation of HCG can be observed in germinomas, especially when syncytiotrophoblastic giant cells (STGCs) are present. Teratomas, especially immature teratomas, often show elevated HCG and AFP.[6] When tumor markers are negative, biopsy of the tumor is recommended for histopathological diagnosis. When at least one of the two tumor markers (AFP, HCG) is significantly elevated, histopathological diagnosis can be omitted, and the tumor is treated intensively as NGGCT. However, due to the possibility of mild to moderate HCG elevations in germinoma, elevations in HCG and AFP in teratomas, and marker-negative NGGCTs, there are many who recommend histopathological diagnosis in all cases.[6] In addition, there have been no standardized cutoff values for tumor markers, and there can be overlap in HCG values seen in germinoma and NGGCTs, for example.[22]

HISTOPATHOLOGY

GERMINOMA

Germinoma is characterized by densely packed large tumor cells with abundant glycogen-rich clear cytoplasm and round, prominent nucleoli. It is also characterized by abundant infiltration of small lymphocytes among tumor cells, and their histological appearance is often described as a "two-cell pattern" composed of large tumor cells and small lymphocytes. Germinomas occasionally harbor STGCs, which are gigantic cells with large cytoplasm and multiple nuclei. Germinoma cells are immunohistochemically positive for placental alkaline phosphatase (PLAP), c-Kit, OCT3/4, and NANOG. They occasionally show weak positivity for HCG, while STGCs are strongly positive for HCG.

NON-GERMINOMATOUS GERM CELL TUMORS

GCTs other than "pure" germinoma are clinically categorized as NGGCTs, including germinoma mixed with non-germinomatous components. Mature teratoma consists of well-differentiated somatic tissue derived from two or three germ layers (ectoderm, mesoderm, and endoderm). Tissues such as skin, respiratory epithelium, cartilage, bone, adipose tissue, and CNS are mixed in a disorderly fashion. Immature teratoma contains immature, embryonal, or fetal tissue. Teratoma with malignant transformation is known for the presence of malignant tumor in the teratoma tissue, such as squamous cell carcinoma, adenocarcinoma, and/or rhabdomyosarcoma.

In yolk sac tumors, epithelial tumor cells are arranged in sheets or cords and in papillary and ribbon-like patterns. The structure, similar to renal glomerulus, is known as a *Schiller-Duval body*. Tumor cells are arranged and connected with each other in a reticular pattern with a background of rich mucoid matrix. This recapitulates the yolk sac, allantois, and extra-embryonic mesenchyme. Tumor cells are positive for AFP, LIN28A, SALL4, and cytokeratin.

Choriocarcinomas often are characterized by intratumoral hemorrhage. Two types of cells that are similar to the syncytiotrophoblasts and the cytotrophoblasts in the placental villus are mixed together. Tumor cells are positive for HCG and cytokeratin.

Embryonal carcinoma consists of pluripotent stem cells that can differentiate into a large variety of cells, excluding germ cells. Large epithelioid cells are arranged in sheets and papillae. Tumor cells have abundant and clear cytoplasm with high nuclear atypia. They resemble the embryonic germ disc. Tumor cells are positive for cytokeratin, CD30, OCT4, NANOG, LIN28A, and PLAP. Tumor markers and typical histopathological appearances of germ cell tumors are demonstrated in Figure 8.2.

MOLECULAR BIOLOGY

The most frequent mutation in germ cell tumors is *KIT*, which is present in approximately 60% of germinoma cases but is less frequent in NGGCT (8.6%).[23] Other mutations are also found in the mitogen-activated protein kinase (MAPK) pathway (48.4%) and the PI3K pathway (12.9%), which include *RAS*, *CBL*, and *MTOR*.[24,25] GCT is also characterized by genomic instability and often harbors copy number alterations in many chromosomes.[23] In particular, gain of 1q, 12p, 21q, and X, and loss of 13q have been reported. Epigenetic analysis shows whole-genome demethylation in germinoma, which corroborates the hypothesis that germinoma resembles PGC tissues biologically, which is also globally hypomethylated.[26] To date, no targeted therapy has been developed and no clinical trials of targeted therapy have been initiated, presumably due to the rarity of the tumor and favorable response to available therapies.

TREATMENT

In general, up-front surgical resection of suspected tumor is not indicated for GCTs. Indications for surgical resection include histopathological diagnosis when the tumor markers are negative or non-diagnostic, mature teratoma pathology, and for removal of any remnant tissue after induction chemotherapy. Tissue for diagnostic purposes is obtained by stereotactic needle biopsy or endoscopic biopsy. If the histopathological diagnosis reveals a mature teratoma, gross total resection is indicated because this is a surgically curable disease.

> Indications for surgical resection include histopathological diagnosis when the tumor markers are negative or non-diagnostic, mature teratoma pathology, and for removal of any remnant tissue after induction chemotherapy.

Hydrocephalus associated with aqueduct stenosis or occlusion caused by pineal region tumors should be addressed by surgical intervention first. Acutely presenting

	Tumor marker	Hematoxylin-Eosin stain	Immunohistochemistry	Reflection at embryogenesis
Germinoma — Germinoma	HCG(±), PLAP	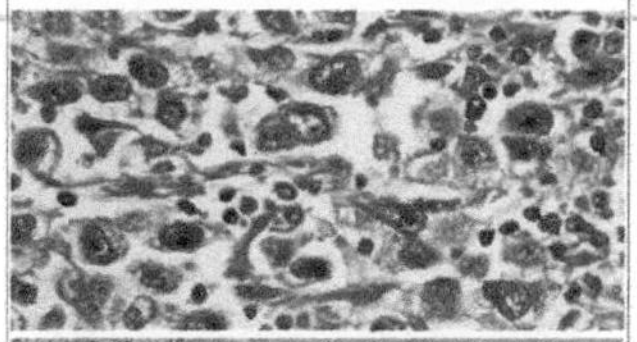	c-kit, PLAP, Oct4, NANOG	Developing to cells of gonads
Non-germinomatous germ cell tumor (NGGCT) — Mature teratoma	–	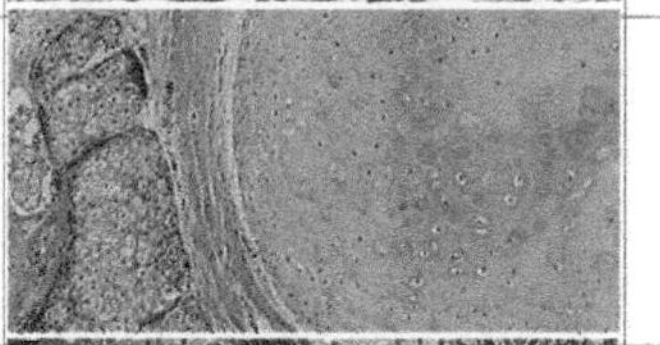	EMA, cytokeratin	Three germ layes, developing to systemic tissues /organs
Immature teratoma	AFP/HCG (±)	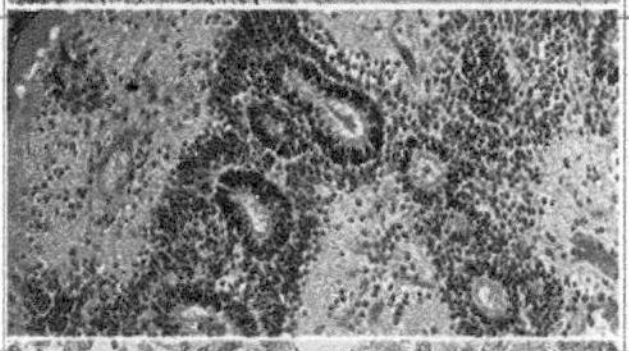	–	
Yolk sac tumor	AFP	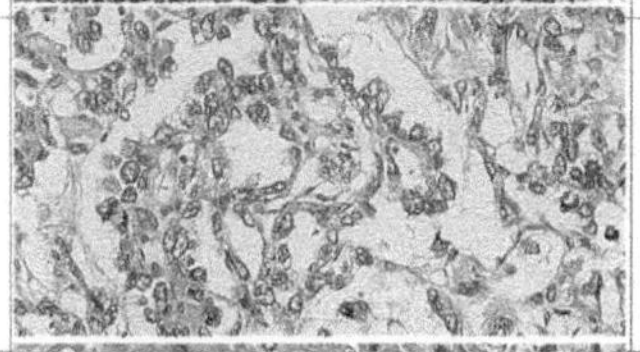	AFP, cytokeratin, LIN28A, SALL4	Yolk sac
Choriocarcinoma	HCG	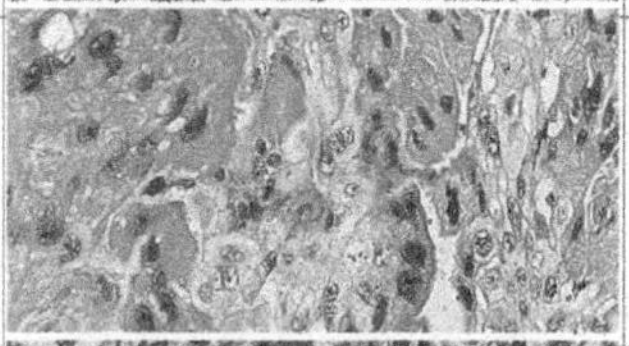	HCG, cytokeratin	Placenta
Embryonal carcinoma	–	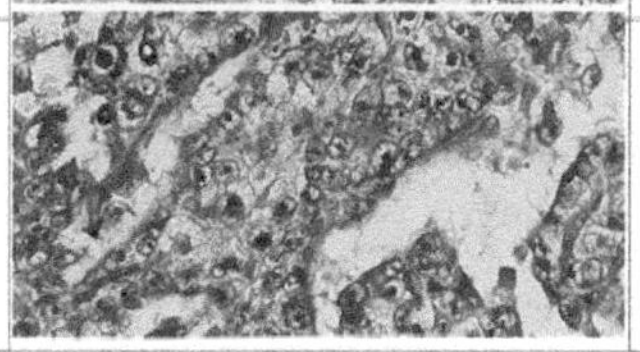	CD30, OCT4, NANOG, LIN28A, PLAP	Embryonal stem cell

Figure 8.2 Tumor markers, typical hematoxylin & eosin (HE) stain images, and immunohistochemistry patterns for each type of germ cell tumors

hydrocephalus can be treated by external ventricular drainage (EVD), but, otherwise, it is treated by endoscopic third ventriculostomy (ETV) and concurrent biopsy of the tumor, if possible. Ventriculo-peritoneal shunt (VPS) placement is not generally recommended as the tumor can resolve in response to chemotherapy and radiation therapy, and some argue that a shunt can disseminate tumor cells into the peritoneal cavity.[27]

> Hydrocephalus can be treated by external ventricular drainage (EVD), but, otherwise, it is treated by endoscopic third ventriculostomy (ETV) and concurrent biopsy of the tumor.

Standard-of-care treatment involves protocol-based chemotherapy and radiation, with the exception of mature teratomas, which do not respond to chemotherapy or radiation and therefore require surgical resection only. Per the Children's Oncology Group (COG) study protocol (ACNS1123), localized germinomas and NGGCTs are treated with platinum-based chemotherapy and whole ventricular irradiation/focal irradiation, which covers the tumor location and ventricles. Local (focal)-field radiation alone has been proved to be insufficient for tumor control[12,28,29] as recurrence most frequently occurs in the periventricular regions.[30] Therefore, whole ventricular irradiation is recommended above focal radiation or whole-brain radiation for non-disseminated disease because it provides the optimal balance between tumor control and reduction of long-term radiation sequela.[31] For disseminated CNS disease, radiation therapy covers the entire cerebrospinal axis in the form of craniospinal irradiation (CSI). Conventional external beam radiation therapy (EBRT) is commonly used, but other methods including intensity-modulated radiation therapy (IMRT) or three-dimensional conformal radiation therapy (3D-CRT) can be used depending on the treating institution. Sensitivity to chemotherapy and radiation therapy differs among the various GCTs. Germinomas are highly sensitive to radiation, while NGGCTs are more resistant. Thus, the dose of radiation is higher when treating NGGCTs compared to germinomas.

> Whole ventricular irradiation is recommended above focal radiation or whole-brain radiation for non-disseminated disease because it provides the optimal balance between tumor control and reduction of long-term radiation sequela.

Based on COG studies for germinoma (ACNS0232) and NGGCT (ACNS0122), the current recommended chemotherapy regimen consists of carboplatin and etoposide for germinoma and alternating carboplatin/etoposide and ifosfamide/etoposide for NGGCTs. Patients with germinomas and NGGCTs received four and six 21-day induction chemotherapy cycles, respectively. Based on the tumor response, this is followed by radiation therapy or second-look surgery.

> Standard-of-care treatment involves protocol-based chemotherapy and radiation, with the exception of mature teratomas, which do not respond to chemotherapy or radiation and therefore require surgical resection only.

Based on the ACNS1123 study, which represents the currently accepted standard-of-care protocol, the post-chemotherapy treatment paradigms has changed in recent years. For germinomas, it is now recommended that the radiation field be expanded to cover the whole ventricles in addition to the focal field in an effort to reduce relapse rates. For focal NGGCT, it is now recommended that the radiation field be reduced from CSI to cover the whole ventricles and the focal field. It has been proven that chemotherapy alone is insufficient for long-term tumor control, and radiation therapy is unavoidable for the treatment of GCTs.[28] For cases with poor response to induction chemotherapy and residual tumor on imaging, a "second-look" surgery is recommended. This allows for both further reduction of tumor mass and histopathological reassessment because diagnosis can change after initial treatment. The histopathology of the residual resected tissue is most often teratoma.[32]

> Chemotherapy alone is insufficient for long-term tumor control, and radiation therapy is an unavoidable treatment of GCTs.

Treatment of relapsed GCTs is often challenging, and no standard treatment has been established. Usually, craniospinal irradiation or high-dose chemotherapy with autologous stem cell transplant for relapsed germinomas and high-dose chemotherapy with autologous stem cell transplant for relapsed NGGCTs are utilized, but treatment response is often poor and the prognosis is dismal.[33]

PROGNOSIS

Progression-free survival (PFS) for germinoma is approximately 90% at 10 years.[3,30,34] Most germinomas respond well to chemotherapy and radiation therapy, while 10% of cases are challenging or more treatment-refractory. Five-year PFS and overall survival (OS) for NGGCTs range from 68% to 84% and 75% to 93%, respectively.[35-38] OS for relapsed germinoma is 55% at 5 years and 9% for relapsed NGGCT.[33]

LONG-TERM FOLLOW-UP

There is no consensus regarding how patients should be followed after treatment. Most often, recurrence occurs in the first 10 years following treatment. Annual imaging follow-up for 20 years is usually recommended for surveillance. There is no consensus if imaging of the entire neuroaxis (brain and spine) should be performed routinely, particularly for patients with focal/localized disease at the time of diagnosis. Tumor markers for all patients should be evaluated along with imaging for detection of recurrence.[39]

> Annual imaging follow-up for 20 years is usually recommended for surveillance.

Long-term sequelae secondary to chemotherapy and radiation therapy are problematic for survivors, particularly as the tumor occurs mainly in the pediatric population. Long-term complications for survivors include secondary neoplasms such as glioma, meningioma and cutaneous malignancy, vascular malformations such as Moyamoya disease and cavernous malformations, and cognitive decline.[40,41] A significant decline in working memory, processing speed, and visual memory in long-time survivors has been reported.[42] Endocrine disorders frequently persist after treatment, and long-term supplementation of hormones is often necessary.[12] Even in cases of long-term survival, life expectancy is shortened compared to age-matched peers, likely due to long-term complications of treatment.[34] For this reason, follow-up monitoring and management of sequelae of chemotherapy and radiation therapy are recommended for all survivors.[33]

> Long-term complications for survivors include secondary neoplasms such as glioma, meningioma and cutaneous malignancy, vascular malformations such as Moyamoya disease and cavernous malformations, and cognitive decline.

FUTURE PERSPECTIVE

Due to the radiation-induced sequelae experienced by long-term survivors, there is an effort to reduce the radiation dose. A recent report argues that lymphocyte-rich cases show better prognosis than tumor cell-rich cases in germinoma and suggests that the germinoma treatment regimen can be stratified based on lymphocyte density. The authors propose that perhaps the radiation dose could be reduced for lymphocyte-rich cases, but this is yet to be prospectively studied in patients.[6]

Additional potential future treatment strategies include therapies that target molecular alterations in GCTs and/or immunotherapy. Because GCTs harbor genomic abnormalities in the MAPK and PI3K pathway in more than half of the cases, targeted therapy with drugs that target these pathways could be an additional treatment option, particularly for relapsed or refractory disease. As PD-1/PD-L1 are often expressed in lymphocytes in the microenvironment and GCTs tumor cells, immune checkpoint inhibitors have additional future therapeutic potential.[43] Further molecular analyses are expected to unravel the genomic abnormalities to better clarify their role in the pathogenesis of GCTs and lead to novel treatments.

CONCLUSION

CNS GCTs are generally responsive to chemotherapy and radiation therapy with favorable OS. However, because this is a disease of adolescents and young adults, the long-term sequelae of these therapies can be detrimental in later life. Further efforts should be made to elaborate risk stratification of the cases and adjust the treatment intensities in future clinical trials. Better treatments for relapsed or refractory disease are also needed.

FLASHCARD

What is the most frequent site of germ cell tumors outside of the reproductive system?	Central nervous system
Geographically, germ tumors are most common in what part of the world?	East Asia
What are the two most common locations of CNS germ cell tumors?	Pineal gland and neurohypophysis
What are the histological subtypes of germ cell tumors?	Germinoma, non-germinomatous germ cell tumor (includes mature/immature teratoma), yolk sac tumor, choriocarcinoma, embryonal carcinoma
Human chorionic gonadotropin (HCG) and alpha fetoprotein (AFP) should be examined in which bodily fluids as part of work up for germ cell tumors?	Blood serum and cerebrospinal fluid
Markedly elevated HCG indicates	Choriocarcinoma
Markedly elevated AFP indicates	Yolk sac tumors and a subset of teratomas
What symptoms are associated with neurohypophyseal GCT?	Endocrine abnormalities, visual symptoms
What symptoms are associated with pineal GCT?	Visual symptoms, obstructive hydrocephalus
Which germ cell tumor is most sensitive to chemotherapy and radiation?	Germinoma
What is the 10-year survival for germinoma and non-germinoma germ cell tumors, respectively?	Germinoma: 95% NGGCTs: 75-90%
Long-term sequelae caused by radiation and chemotherapy include	Secondary malignancy, vascular abnormalities, cognitive/memory impairment

QUESTIONS

1. Which of the following statements is false with regards to germ cell tumors?
   a. Germinoma and non-germinomatous germ cell tumor are the major categories of germ cell tumors.
   b. The brain is the second most frequent site of occurrence of germ cell tumors after testis/ovary.
   c. Non-germinomatous germ cell tumors include teratoma (mature/immature), yolk sac tumor, choriocarcinoma, and embryonal carcinoma.
   d. Teratoma is the most common subtype, accounting for about 40% of cases.

2. Which of the following statements is false with regard to germ cell tumors?
   a. The cell of origin is considered to be primordial germ cells.
   b. There is a geographical difference in occurrence, and GTCs are more frequent in East Asia than in other areas.
   c. It comprises about 3.8% of pediatric brain tumors in the US population.
   d. The peak age is bimodal; occurring in teenagers and at 30–40 years of age.

3. Which of the following statements is false with regard to the histopathology of germ cell tumors?
   a. Germinoma is characterized by a "two-cell pattern."
   b. Embryonal carcinoma reflects embryonal stem cells at embryogenesis.
   c. Choriocarcinoma is characterized by large cells with glycogen-rich large cytoplasm and round nuclei.
   d. Teratoma contains constituents from three germ layers.

4. Which description is false with regard to tumor markers for germ cell tumors?
   a. AFP is elevated in embryonal carcinoma.
   b. AFP is elevated in immature teratoma.
   c. HCG is elevated in choriocarcinoma.
   d. HCG is elevated in germinoma with syncytiotrophoblastic giant cells.

5. Which of the following statements is true with regard to symptoms of germ cell tumors?
   a. Basal ganglia germ cell tumors cause diabetes insipidus.
   b. Neurohypophyseal germ cell tumors cause ophthalmic symptoms.
   c. Pineal germ cell tumors can cause endocrine dysfunction.
   d. Pineal germ cell tumors cause ophthalmic symptoms.

6. Which of the following statements is true with regards to the radiation treatment of germ cell tumors?
   a. Radiation to the focal field of tumors is recommended for localized germinoma.
   b. Craniospinal irradiation is recommended for all germinomas.
   c. Radiation after resection of mature teratoma is not recommended.
   d. Germinomas located in the basal ganglia only require focal radiation.

7. Which of the following statements is false with regard to chemotherapy for germ cell tumors?
   a. Chemotherapy is indicated for all histological subtypes of germ cell tumors.
   b. Chemotherapy without radiation therapy increases the chance of recurrence of germinoma
   c. Platinum-based chemotherapy is one of the standard chemotherapies used for germinomas.
   d. Chemotherapy regimens are different for germinomas and non-germinomatous germ cell tumors.

8. Which description is true with regards to treatment of germ cell tumors?
   a. Obstructive hydrocephalus is usually managed with ventriculo-peritoneal shunt placement.
   b. Endoscopic third ventriculostomy is useful as it allows for simultaneous tumor biopsy and resolution of hydrocephalus.
   c. Maximal surgical resection improves prognosis for patients with germinoma.
   d. Mature teratoma is sensitive to radiation therapy.

9. Which of the following statements is false with regard to the prognosis of germ cell tumors?
   a. The 10-year overall survival of germinoma is about 95%.
   b. The 10-year overall survival of non-germinomatous germ cell tumor is about 50%.
   c. Germinoma often disseminates along the ventricles.
   d. Histology can change at second-look surgery when compared with the initial diagnosis.

10. Which of the following statements is true with regard to the follow-up after treatment of germ cell tumors?
    a. Follow-up with tumor marker levels is not indicated.
    b. Follow-up after 10 years is not necessary.
    c. De novo neoplasms and cerebrovascular abnormalities can shorten survival 20 years after treatment.
    d. Chemotherapy rather than radiation therapy is considered to be the cause of long-term complications.

ANSWERS

1. d
2. d
3. c
4. a
5. c
6. c
7. a
8. b
9. b
10. c

REFERENCES

1. Ostrom QT, Gittleman H, Liao P, et al. CBTRUS Statistical Report: Primary brain and other central nervous system tumors diagnosed in the United States in 2010–2014. *Neuro Oncol.* 2017;19(suppl_5):v1–v88.
2. Louis D, Ohgaki H, Wiestler O, Cavenee W. *WHO Classification of Tumours of the Central Nervous System.* (4th ed. rev.). Lyon: International Agency for Research on Cancer (IARC); 2016.
3. Matsutani M, Sano K, Takakura K, et al. Primary intracranial germ cell tumors: A clinical analysis of 153 histologically verified cases. *J Neurosurg.* 1997;86(3):446–455.
4. Oosterhuis JW, Stoop H, Honecker F, Looijenga LH. Why human extragonadal germ cell tumours occur in the midline of the body: Old concepts, new perspectives. *Int J Androl.* 2007;30(4):256–263; discussion 263-254.
5. Oosterhuis JW, Looijenga LH. Testicular germ-cell tumours in a broader perspective. *Nat Rev Cancer.* 2005;5(3):210–222.
6. Takami H, Fukuoka K, Fukushima S, et al. Integrated clinical, histopathological, and molecular data analysis of 190 central nervous system germ cell tumors from the iGCT Consortium. *Neuro-Oncology.* 2019;21(12):1565–1577.
7. Shibui S. Report of brain tumor registry of Japan (2001–2004). *Neurol Med Chir (Tokyo).* 2014;54(suppl. 1):9–102.
8. Rosen A, Jayram G, Drazer M, Eggener SE. Global trends in testicular cancer incidence and mortality. *Eur Urol.* 2011;60(2):374–379.
9. Makino K, Nakamura H, Yano S, Kuratsu J. Incidence of primary central nervous system germ cell tumors in childhood: A regional survey in Kumamoto prefecture in southern Japan. *Pediatr Neurosurg.* 2013;49(3):155–158.
10. Kang J-M, Ha J, Hong EK, et al. A nationwide, population-based epidemiologic study of childhood brain tumors in Korea, 2005–2014: A comparison with United States data. *Cancer Epidemiol Biomarkers Prev.* 2019;28(2):409–416.
11. Takami H, Perry A, Graffeo CS, et al. Comparison on epidemiology, tumor location, histology, and prognosis of intracranial germ cell tumors between Mayo Clinic and Japanese consortium cohorts. *J Neurosurg.* 2020;1(aop):1–11.
12. Takami H, Graffeo CS, Perry A, et al. Epidemiology, natural history, and optimal management of neurohypophyseal germ cell tumors. *J Neurosurg.* 2020;1(aop):1-9.
13. Jennings MT, Gelman R, Hochberg F. Intracranial germ-cell tumors: Natural history and pathogenesis. *J Neurosurg.* 1985;63(2):155–167.
14. Ono H, Shin M, Takai K, et al. Spontaneous regression of germinoma in the pineal region before endoscopic surgery: A pitfall of modern strategy for pineal germ cell tumors. *J Neurooncol.* 2010;103(3):755–758.
15. Aizer AA, Sethi RV, Hedley-Whyte ET, et al. Bifocal intracranial tumors of nongerminomatous germ cell etiology: Diagnostic and therapeutic implications. *Neuro Oncol.* 2013;15(7):955–960.
16. Phuakpet K, Larouche V, Hawkins C, et al. Rare presentation of supratentorial primitive neuroectodermal tumors mimicking bifocal germ cell tumors: 2 case reports. *J Pediatr Hematol Oncol.* 2016;38(2):e67–e70.
17. Hoffman HJ, Otsubo H, Hendrick EB, et al. Intracranial germ-cell tumors in children. *J Neurosurg.* 1991;74(4):545–551.
18. Kyritsis AP. Management of primary intracranial germ cell tumors. *J Neurooncol.* 2010;96(2):143–149.
19. Hart MG, Sarkies NJ, Santarius T, Kirollos RW. Ophthalmological outcome after resection of tumors based on the pineal gland. *J Neurosurg.* 2013;119(2):420–426.
20. Hankinson EV, Lyons CJ, Hukin J, Cochrane DD. Ophthalmological outcomes of patients treated for pineal region tumors. *J Neurosurg Pediatr.* 2016;17(5):558–563.
21. Sonoda Y, Kumabe T, Sugiyama S-I, et al. Germ cell tumors in the basal ganglia: Problems of early diagnosis and treatment. *Journal of Neurosurgery: Pediatrics.* 2008;2(2):118–124.
22. Murray MJ, Bartels U, Nishikawa R, et al. Consensus on the management of intracranial germ-cell tumours. *Lancet Oncol.* 2015;16(9):e470–e477.
23. Fukushima S, Otsuka A, Suzuki T, et al. Mutually exclusive mutations of KIT and RAS are associated with KIT mRNA expression and chromosomal instability in primary intracranial pure germinomas. *Acta Neuropathol.* 2014;127(6):911–925.
24. Ichimura K, Fukushima S, Totoki Y, et al. Recurrent neomorphic mutations of MTOR in central nervous system and testicular germ cell tumors may be targeted for therapy. *Acta Neuropathol.* 2016;131(6):889–901.
25. Wang L, Yamaguchi S, Burstein MD, et al. Novel somatic and germline mutations in intracranial germ cell tumours. *Nature.* 2014;511(7508):241–245.
26. Fukushima S, Yamashita S, Kobayashi H, et al. Genome-wide methylation profiles in primary intracranial germ cell tumors indicate a primordial germ cell origin for germinomas. *Acta Neuropathol.* 2017;133(3):445–462.
27. Sawamura Y. Current diagnosis and treatment of central nervous system germ cell tumours. *Curr Opin Neurol.* 1996;9(6):419–423.
28. Balmaceda C, Heller G, Rosenblum M, et al. Chemotherapy without irradiation: A novel approach for newly diagnosed CNS germ cell tumors: Results of an international cooperative trial. The First International Central Nervous System Germ Cell Tumor Study. *J Clin Oncol.* 1996;14(11):2908–2915.
29. Uematsu Y, Tsuura Y, Miyamoto K, et al. The recurrence of primary intracranial germinomas: Special reference to germinoma with STGC (syncytiotrophoblastic giant cell). *J Neurooncol.* 1992;13(3):247–256.
30. Calaminus G, Kortmann R, Worch J, et al. SIOP CNS GCT 96: Final report of outcome of a prospective, multinational nonrandomized trial for children and adults with intracranial germinoma, comparing craniospinal irradiation alone with chemotherapy followed by focal primary site irradiation for patients with localized disease. *Neuro Oncol.* 2013;15(6):788–796.
31. Alapetite C, Brisse H, Patte C, et al. Pattern of relapse and outcome of non-metastatic germinoma patients treated with chemotherapy and limited field radiation: The SFOP experience. *Neuro Oncol.* 2010;12(12):1318–1325.
32. Ogiwara H, Kiyotani C, Terashima K, Morota N. Second-look surgery for intracranial germ cell tumors. *Neurosurgery.* 2015;76(6):658–661; discussion 661–652.
33. Murray MJ, Bailey S, Heinemann K, et al. Treatment and outcomes of UK and German patients with relapsed intracranial germ cell tumors following uniform first-line therapy. *Int J Cancer.* 2017;141(3):621–635.
34. Acharya S, DeWees T, Shinohara ET, Perkins SM. Long-term outcomes and late effects for childhood and young adulthood intracranial germinomas. *Neuro Oncol.* 2015;17(5):741–746.
35. Al-Hussaini M, Sultan I, Abuirmileh N, et al. Pineal gland tumors: Experience from the SEER database. *J Neurooncol.* 2009;94(3):351–358.
36. Breen WG, Blanchard MJ, Rao AN, et al. Optimal radiotherapy target volumes in intracranial nongerminomatous germ cell tumors: Long-term institutional experience with chemotherapy, surgery, and dose- and field-adapted radiotherapy. *Pediatr Blood Cancer.* 2017;64(11).
37. Calaminus G, Frappaz D, Kortmann RD, et al. Outcome of patients with intracranial non-germinomatous germ cell tumors: Lessons from the SIOP-CNS-GCT-96 trial. *Neuro Oncol.* 2017;19(12):1661–1672.
38. Goldman S, Bouffet E, Fisher PG, et al. Phase II trial assessing the ability of neoadjuvant chemotherapy with or without second-look surgery to eliminate measurable disease for nongerminomatous germ cell tumors: A Children's Oncology Group study. *J Clin Oncol.* 2015;33(22):2464–2471.
39. Fonseca A, Xia C, Lorenzo AJ, et al. Detection of relapse by tumor markers versus imaging in children and adolescents with nongerminomatous malignant germ cell tumors: A report from the Children's Oncology Group. *J Clin Oncol.* 2019;37(5):396.
40. Doyle DM, Einhorn LH. Delayed effects of whole brain radiotherapy in germ cell tumor patients with central nervous system metastases. *Int J Radiat Oncol Biol Phys.* 2008;70(5):1361–1364.
41. Sawamura Y, Ikeda J, Shirato H, et al. Germ cell tumours of the central nervous system: Treatment consideration based on 111 cases and their long-term clinical outcomes. *Eur J Cancer.* 1998;34(1):104–110.
42. Mabbott DJ, Monsalves E, Spiegler BJ, et al. Longitudinal evaluation of neurocognitive function after treatment for central nervous system germ cell tumors in childhood. *Cancer.* 2011;117(23):5402–5411.
43. Takami H, Fukushima S, Aoki K, et al. Intratumoural immune cell landscape in germinoma reveals multipotent lineages and exhibits prognostic significance. *Neuropathol Appl Neurobiol.* 2019.

9 | INTRAVENTRICULAR TUMORS

SAMANTHALEE C. S. OBIORAH, RICHARD S. DOWD, AND STEVEN A. TOMS

INTRODUCTION

Intraventricular tumors comprise a subset of lesions including developmental cysts, benign tumors, or malignant primary or secondary cancers that may be completely or partially within the ependyma of the lateral, third, and fourth ventricles. Lesions of adjacent structures including pituitary tumors and craniopharyngiomas near the sella, teratomas, germinomas, and primary pineal neoplasms in the pineal region, and primitive neuroectodermal tumors (PNETs), juvenile pilocytic astrocytomas (JPAs), and atypical teratoid rhabdoid (ATRT) tumors near the fourth ventricle are covered elsewhere. In this chapter, we review lesions which entirely (or primarily) arise within the ependymal lining of the lateral, third, and fourth ventricles. We discuss their origins, therapeutic options, and outcomes in order to better understand the complexity of these lesions.

COLLOID CYST

Colloid cysts are one of the most common primary intraventricular brain lesions.[1,2] They can be seen in patients ranging from neonates to the elderly, with most diagnoses occurring in men in the third and fourth decades of life.[3,4]

Colloid cysts are typically found in the anterior midline of the third ventricle (Figure 9.1) with the fornix surrounding the cyst.[4] They develop from embryonic foregut and are comprised of a fibrous external capsule surrounding a single layer of mucin-producing epithelium.[3] Therefore, rather than a neoplasm, these lesions are best thought of as developmental cysts.

Colloid cysts are most often found incidentally. When symptomatic, they present with progressively worsening positional paroxysmal headaches related to elevations in intracranial pressure (ICP).[2] Although uncommon, colloid cysts can result in sudden death from acute obstructive hydrocephalus[1] and be associated with physical examination findings related to an elevation in ICP such as nystagmus, papilledema, alterations in consciousness, and cerebellar signs.[4]

Radiographically, colloid cysts are simpler to view on computed tomography (CT) than on magnetic resonance imaging (MRI). Two-thirds of these cysts will display mild to moderate hyperdensity on CT.[3] The MRI appearance is variable (Table 9.1) and not always reliable for diagnosis.[1,3,4]

As the majority of colloid cysts are asymptomatic, the mainstay of treatment is expectant management. Yearly serial imaging can be performed safely with low risk of sudden death and should be continued with progressively longer (2–5 year) intervals for life.[5] Studies have shown a low progression rate of 8% of asymptomatic colloid cysts at 10 years.[5,6] Lesions less than 7 mm in size are amenable to observation while larger lesions are candidates for cyst resection or cerebrospinal fluid (CSF) shunting.[6] Surgical resection serves as the definitive treatment for symptomatic colloid cysts,[3] and recurrence is rare.[4,7]

> As the majority of colloid cysts are asymptomatic, the mainstay of treatment is expectant management.

CHOROID PLEXUS TUMORS

Choroid plexus tumors (CPTs) can be divided into three categories based on the World Health Organization's (WHO) 2016 classification: choroid plexus papilloma (CPP, WHO grade 1), atypical choroid plexus papilloma (ACPP, WHO grade 2), and choroid plexus carcinoma (CPC, WHO grade 3). CPPs are benign, with a histological architecture similar to normal choroid plexus with palm frond-like papillary structures and low mitotic activity. CPCs are invasive, with a minimum of four of the following characteristics: high mitotic activity, nuclear pleomorphism, necrosis, blurred papillary architecture, and increased cellularity. ACPPs are intermediary lesions with increased mitotic activity in comparison to CPPs; they are defined as having 2 or more mitoses per high powered field (HPF) while CPPs have fewer than 2 per HPF and CPCs have more than 5 per HPF.[8] ACPPs are the rarest of the three; the ratio of CPPs to CPCs is 5:1.[9] The median age at diagnosis for CPTs is 3 years.[10] In molecular profiling, CPCs may be distinguished from CPPs by frequent TP53 mutations and changes in DNA methylome.[11]

> CPCs may be distinguished from CPPs by the presence of frequent TP53 mutations and changes in DNA methylome.

Around 50% of CPTs develop in the lateral ventricles, particularly in the atrium, with another 40% occurring in the fourth ventricle. In pediatric patients, CPPs have a tendency to develop in the lateral ventricles, while in adults these tumors occur more commonly in the fourth ventricle.[12] Ninety-one

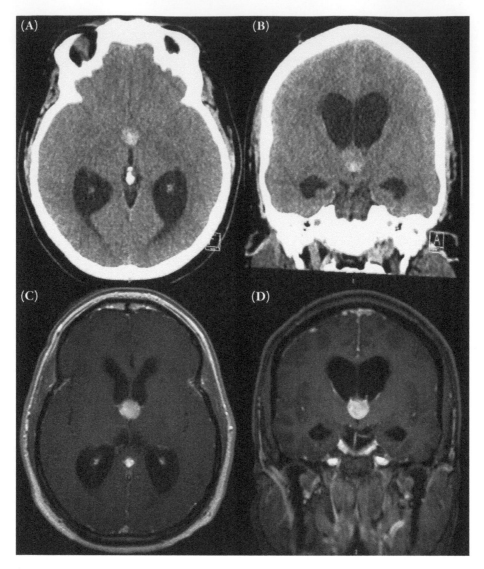

Figure 9.1 *CT and MRI imaging of a colloid cyst in the anterior third ventricle. (A) Axial CT showing dilated occipital horns and hyperdensity of the cyst in the third ventricle. (B) Coronal CT showing dilated lateral ventricles and hyperdense cyst in the third ventricle. (C) Axial T1 post-contrast MRI showing enhancement of the colloid cyst in the third ventricle; there is associated radiographic hydrocephalus as well. (D) Coronal T1 post-contrast MRI demonstrating dilation of the lateral ventricles and the temporal horns in relation to third ventricle obstruction by hyperintense cyst.*

percent of patients with a CPT will present with headaches and show symptoms of elevated ICP.[7]

> CPPs have a tendency to develop in the lateral ventricles in the pediatric population, while in adults these tumors occur more commonly in the fourth ventricle.

CPPs and CPCs can appear very similar or can have overlapping features on imaging, thus radiographic discrimination between CPP and CPC is considered unreliable. However, some imaging features are more likely to be associated with CPPs versus CPCs so are sometimes considered helpful indicators of tumor type. For example, papillomas typically have a lobulated contour while the contours of carcinomas are more irregular.[12] On CT most papillomas appear isodense to hyperdense with calcifications frequently seen.[1] CPPs are more commonly associated with hydrocephalus than are CPCs. Theoretically, this is

because aberrant CPP cells produce unregulated CSF, whereas CPC cells have become too undifferentiated to do so.

First-line treatment of symptomatic CPTs consists of surgical resection. Gross total resection (GTR) of CPP has a high probability of cure with a low probability of recurrence.[7,10] ACPPs have higher probabilities of recurrence.[10] Adjuvant radiotherapy can be useful for recurrent tumors unsuitable for re-resection.[10] The characteristic invasiveness of CPCs usually prevents GTR, leading to a poor prognosis with a median survival of 2.5–3 years.[12] Meta-analyses and retrospective studies have shown some benefit to the use of radiotherapy or chemotherapy following subtotal resection (STR).[10] In these studies, some patients have been treated in accordance with the CPT-SIOP 2009 protocol using cyclophosphamide carboplatin, vincristine, etoposide, and intrathecal cytarabine; others were treated using a different arm of this protocol and received high-dose methotrexate and intrathecal chemotherapy with an Ommaya reservoir.[10] Other patients have been treated

TABLE 9.1 Summary of the key imaging characteristics specific to intraventricular tumors

TUMOR TYPE	CT	MRI WITH CONTRAST	FLAIR	DWI
Colloid cyst	Ovoid/rounded masses in anterior third ventricle[3] 2/3 mild to moderate hyperdensity[3] Calcifications rare [1] Foramen of Monro[1]	T1WI 2/3 appear hyperintense[3] T2WI hypointense[3] Post-contrast mild enhancement of external capsule[3]		No diffusion restriction classically[80] Rare fluid-fluid levels[79]
Choroid plexus tumors	CPPs: Isodense to hyperdense; calcifications common[1] CPCs: Isodense to hyperdense; heterogeneous appearance, irregular borders[80]	CPPs: Isointense on both T1WI and T2WI[1] CPCs: Heterogenous; local invasion; surrounding edema[12,81]	CPCs: Heterogenous with encircling edema[82] CPPs: Hyperintense[80]	CPCs: No diffusion restriction[83] CPPs: Hyperintense[80]
Intraventricular meningioma	Hyperdense, well-defined[1]	Homogenous enhancement[12] Well-delineated[12] T1WI: Isointense to hypointense[12] T2WI: Isointense to hyperintense[12]		
Ependymoma	Cystic appearance[12]	Homogenous contrast enhancement[15] Cystic appearance[12] T1WI: Isointense to hypointense appearance[1,12] T2WI: Hyperintense[12]	Mid-high signal intensity[84]	Increased DWI signal[83]
Subependymoma	Well-demarcated Isodense to hyperdense[1]	Lobular appearance Little to no contrast enhancement[1,12] T1WI: Isointense or hypointense[1,12] T2WI: Isointense or hyperintense[1,12]	Hyperintense[84]	Mild increase in DWI signal[84]
Intraventricular lymphoma	Isodense to hyperdense[28]	T1WI: Isointense to hypointense[12,28] T2WI: Isointense to hyperintense[28] Immunocompromised: Irregular contrast enhancement with ring enhancement[28] Immunocompetent: Homogenous contrast enhancement, rare ring enhancement[28]	Hyperintense[29]	Increased DWI signal[85]
Central neurocytoma	Heterogenous appearance[35–37,40,41] Occasional calcifications[35–37,40,41]	Cystic and solid components[35–37,40,41] Heterogenous enhancement[35–37,40,41]	Hyperintense[87]	Increased DWI signal[86,87]
Subependymal giant cell tumor	Hyperdense[50] Calcified[50]	Homogeneously enhancing[50,51] T1WI: Isointense and hypointense[88] T2WI: Isointense and hyperintense[88]	Isointense and hyperintense[88]	
Astrocytoma	Isodense to hypodense lesion with surrounding edema[1]	Variable contrast enhancement depending on tumor grade[63] Low grade: T1WI hypointense; T2WI hyperintense; little to no contrast enhancement[1] Anaplastic: T1WI hypointense; T2WI hyperintensity; heterogeneous contrast enhancement[1]	FLAIR is variable[89]	High-grade tumors: Limited diffusion[90] Grade 2 tumors: Low signal[90] Grade 3: High signal[90]
Metastasis	Usually non-calcified[91] Solitary or multiple lesions[91]	Generally homogenous enhancement T1WI: Isointense or hypointense[91] T2WI: Hyperintense[91]	Hyperintensity[91]	

CPC, choroid plexus carcinoma; CPP, choroid plexus papilloma; DWI, diffusion weighted imaging; FLAIR, fluid-attenuated inversion recovery. T1WI, T1 weighted imaging; T2WI, T2 weighted imaging.

with either a combination of etoposide with vincristine or ifosfamide and cisplatin or carboplatin.[13]

> GTR of CPP has a high probability of cure with a low probability of recurrence.

INTRAVENTRICULAR MENINGIOMA

Intraventricular meningiomas (IVMs) account for only 0.5–5% of all intracranial meningiomas.[14] IVMs can be subdivided clinically into spontaneously arising meningiomas (SAM), neurofibromatosis-2-associated meningiomas (NF2-M), and radiation-induced meningiomas (RIM).[15] Eighty percent of IVMs develop from the lateral ventricle, with the majority of these found in the atrium.[16] They are twice as common in females, occurring most frequently between the ages of 30 and 60.[12] Meningiomas in patients with neurofibromatosis type 2 typically occur earlier in life, and RIMs are often more aggressive (WHO grade 2 and 3).[12]

> Eight percent of IVMs develop from the lateral ventricle, with the majority of these found in the atrium.

Typically, IVMs are slow-growing, reaching large volumes before symptoms appear (Figure 9.2).[17] Usually patients report headaches, nausea, vomiting, visual field deficits, speech difficulties, seizures, and sensorimotor deficits.[17] These tumors homogeneously enhance on post-contrast MRI.[12]

First-line treatment for IVMs is surgical resection.[16] However, due to the deep location of these tumors, resection is often a challenge.[17,18] Observation can also be employed in the case of asymptomatic IVMs, while radiosurgery can be employed for smaller IVMs.[18] Following total resection, patients have a good prognosis.[16] Further details on the management of meningiomas can be found in Chapter 5.

EPENDYMOMA

Ependymomas are rare tumors that develop from the ependymal cells lining the central canal of the spinal cord and the ventricular system.[12,19] They comprise approximately 5% of adult intracranial tumors and account for at most 10% of pediatric tumors of the central nervous system (CNS).[7,19] Pediatric patients account for roughly 30% of ependymoma patients. In children, the majority of these tumors lie infratentorially, while in adults the majority of tumors are spinal, followed by smaller numbers of infratentorial and supratentorial tumors.[12] The incidence of ependymomas peak at the ages of 5 and 35.[7] Of cranial tumors, they are most commonly grade 2; however, as many as 30% are grade 3, anaplastic.[20,21]

On histologic slides, ependymomas exhibit perivascular pseudorosettes and are moderately cellular.[19] Patients classically present with signs and symptoms of elevated ICP.[12,22] Ependymomas often exhibit cystic qualities that can be seen on both MRI and CT (Figure 9.3). Signs of hemorrhage can be seen in some cases.[12,15]

GTR with radiotherapy serves as the treatment of choice for ependymoma, with little data to support the use of chemotherapy.[7,19] Surgical resection is often difficult due to the locations of these tumors, leading to a high rate of STR as well as long-term neurological complications.[19] In cases of STR, radiation therapy can be helpful in long-term survival by decreasing the likelihood of recurrence.[7,19] Prognosis depends on multiple factors. These include age, extent of resection, and histologic grade. Children do worse than adults, and older children do worse than younger children.[22,23] Recurrence of tumor is local in 80% of cases, thus making extent of resection extremely important in these cases. The event-free survival rate in children is 68.8% at 10 years in the low-grade group and 49.8% for grade 3, anaplastic tumors.[23] Further details on evaluation and management of ependymomas can be found in Chapter 6.

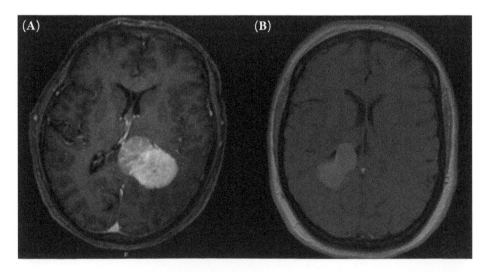

Figure 9.2 MRI imaging of interventricular meningiomas in two patients. (A) Axial T1 post-contrast imaging showing a homogenously enhancing mass arising the left atrium. (B) Axial fluid-attenuated inversion recovery (FLAIR) imaging showing a T2 hyperintense lesion arising in the right atrium.

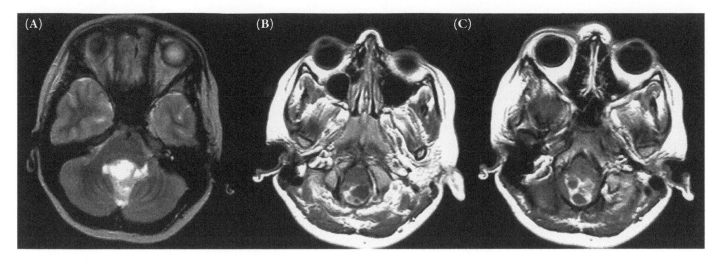

Figure 9.3 MRI of pediatric patient with ependymoma. (A) T2 weighted image showing hyperintensity to white matter. (B and C) Sequential axial images on T1 post-contrast showing heterogenous enhancement throughout the lesion.

SUBEPENDYMOMA

Subependymomas are exceedingly rare, benign tumors with a slow growth pattern that develop most often in middle-aged and older men.[24,25] They are most frequently found in the lateral ventricles (50–60%) and the fourth ventricle (30–40%) although they are occasionally found in the spinal cord and brain parenchyma itself.[12,25]

> Subependymomas are exceedingly rare, benign tumors with a slow growth pattern that develop most often in middle-aged and older men.

Subependymomas develop from subependymal glial precursor cells.[12,24] Subependymomas are clinically silent in up to 60% of cases and classically are less than 2 cm. Symptomatic patients will present with symptoms of obstructive hydrocephalus.[12] Other patients may present with symptoms related to tumor-induced compression of brain structures, such as sensorimotor deficits and seizures.[26]

On CT, subependymomas are well-demarcated lesions appearing isodense to hyperdense.[1] On MRI, these tumors show little to no enhancement due to their avascular nature.[1,12] In addition, they classically do not invade the local brain parenchyma or stimulate parenchymal edema.[12]

The rarity of subependymoma, accounting for only 0.51% of CNS tumors, has led to a lack of consensus on the best treatment guidelines.[24,25] GTR has been advocated as best for symptomatic tumors, but the location of these tumors can often make this difficult, leading to STRs.[25] Asymptomatic patients with imaging highly indicative of subependymoma can be managed with serial imaging.[25] Tumor recurrence following complete resection is a rarity.[12]

> The rarity of subependymoma, accounting for only 0.51% of CNS tumors, has led to a lack of consensus on the best treatment guidelines.

INTRAVENTRICULAR LYMPHOMA

Primary CNS lymphomas (PCNSLs) comprise 1–4% of all brain tumors and are a rare type of non-Hodgkin lymphoma.[27] Classically they are associated with immunodeficiency but are progressively being detected in immunocompetent patients without known risk factors.[27] In these patients, most PCNSL cases are diagnosed between the ages of 45 and 70, with an equal distribution between men and women.[28] Typically, PCNSL is found in the brain parenchyma, while secondary CNS lymphomas typically present as leptomeningeal metastases.[27] The singular intraventricular lymphoma lesion is exceedingly rare.[29] For most immunocompetent patients, the classic PCNSL presentation is a solitary, supratentorial tumor.[28]

Ninety-five percent of PCNSLs are histologically classified as diffuse large B-cell lymphomas.[28] Approximately 60% of patients present with symptoms of elevated ICP.[28] On MRI, PCNSLs classically have increased signal on diffusion weighted imaging (DWI).[28,29] Among immunocompromised patients, ring enhancement of the tumor is common with irregular overall contrast enhancement.[28] In contrast, immunocompetent patients rarely show ring enhancement and classically exhibit homogeneous contrast enhancement.[28] PCNSL is diagnosed based on the histopathological result of a brain biopsy and/or CSF analysis.[28] Further information, including management and prognosis is discussed in Chapter 11.

CENTRAL NEUROCYTOMA

Central neurocytoma (CN) is a rare tumor overall, making up only about 0.5% of all CNS tumors both benign and malignant.[30] However, it does account for about 50% of intraventricular tumors.[31] While infrequent variants can spread outside of the ventricular system, most CNs are found in the lateral ventricles.[31-33] Typical presenting symptoms are related to obstructive hydrocephalus, and the average age of presentation is around 34 years.[31,34,35]

CNs typically have a heterogenous appearance on CT scan, with occasional calcifications noted, but usually no hemorrhage. On MRI (Figure 9.4), they tend to have cystic and solid components and a heterogeneously enhancing pattern.[31,32,34–36] This can sometimes make them difficult to distinguish from high-grade glioma on imaging alone.[36]

Typically benign in nature, CNs arise from the cells of the septum pellucidum, which helps to explain their preference for the lateral ventricles. On pathology, they are composed of many well-differentiated small round cells with occasional pseudorosettes; on hemolysin and eosin (H&E) stains, they are difficult to distinguish from oligodendrogliomas.[30,31,35] Synaptophysin positivity is strongly correlated with CNs, however, which can help to distinguish this entity from other neoplasms. MIB-1 (Ki67) staining is important as a higher degree of mitoses is correlated with recurrence. A MIB-1 marker greater than 2% is considered an atypical CN. All CNs are WHO grade 2.[31,35,37,38]

> Central neurocytomas are composed of many well-differentiated small round cells with occasional pseudorosettes, and on H&E stains are difficult to distinguish from oligodendrogliomas.

Research has identified many genetic pathways that are overexpressed in CN including insulin-like growth factor 2 (IGF2) and WNT along with others that may be implicated in tumorigenesis, like neuregulin 2, N-Myc and platelet-derived growth factor (PDGF). Based on these findings there is evidence to suggest that therapies targeting these pathways could be effective.[39] Neuregulins bind to ErbB-3 and ErbB-4 receptors, part of the epidermal growth factor receptor (EGFR) family of tyrosine kinase receptors and there is at least one reported case of erlotinib, an EGFR inhibitor, being used in combination with temozolomide for neurocytoma, with stable disease reported over a year later.[40]

The mainstay of treatment is surgical resection. Most CNs are amenable to GTR which is associated with increased progression-free survival (PFS).[30,31,35,40,41] Adjuvant chemotherapy and radiation therapy have been studied but are not as effective as resection at increasing PFS.[42–44] Fractionated or stereotactic radiation is the treatment of choice for recurrence and STRs. Radiation therapy in this setting seems to significantly improve PFS at 10 years but does not change overall survival (OS).[45] The use of chemotherapy for CN does not have any standard guidelines, and studies show variation in the types and timing of its use. It has been used for both recurrent disease and as initial treatment. Temozolomide has been reported as being used for recurrent disease both as monotherapy and in combination with varied drugs; however, other chemotherapy combinations including vincristine, cisplatin, and etoposide, as well as procarbazine, lomustine, and vincristine, have been used as well. The results of these chemotherapy regimens are mixed without any true consensus on best practice.[40]

> Most CNs are amenable to GTR which is associated with increased progression-free survival (PFS).

Prognosis for CNs is generally good after GTR, with PFS of 54% at 5 years. However, this depends highly on the MIB-1 marker. PFS at 2 years is 90% and remains at 90% at 5 years for typical CNs with MIB-1 of less than 1%. For those with an MIB-1 of greater than 4%, PFS at 2 years is 48% and drops to 12% at 5 years. Luckily, even with recurrence, OS at 5 years is 96%.[37,41] Radiotherapy and re-resection have been used in cases of recurrence, and, as mentioned, temozolomide has been used in cases of recurrence with inconsistent results.[40]

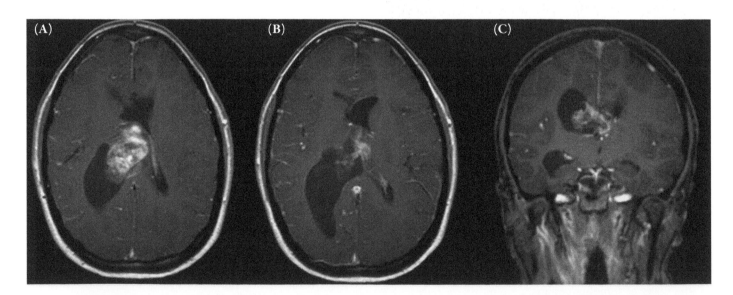

Figure 9.4 *MRI of patient with central neurocytoma. (A and B) axial representation through two consecutive areas of the ventricle on T1 post-contrast MRI demonstrates heterogenous enhancement and dilated ventricular system secondary to obstruction. (C) Coronal view of the same tumor on T1 post-contrast MRI, again demonstrating asymmetrically dilated ventricles and patchy enhancement.*

SUBEPENDYMAL GIANT CELL ASTROCYTOMA/TUMOR

A rare, benign tumor which is almost exclusively associated with tuberous sclerosis (TS) these tumors are referred to both as subependymal giant cell astrocytoma (SEGA) and subependymal giant cell tumors (SGCT).[46,47] They occur in 6–19% of patients with TS.[46–48] While isolated SGCT has been reported, it is limited to case reports.[49] Because they are associated with TS, they tend to become clinically apparent between the first and third decades of life.[47,48,50] Symptoms are related to increased ICP; however, they are often discovered incidentally in relation to imaging studies for the seizures common in TS patients.[48,51]

> Subependymal giant cell astrocytomas are rare, benign tumors that are almost exclusively associated with tuberous sclerosis.

SGCTs have a homogenously enhancing pattern on post contrast MRI (Figure 9.5).[50,51] They typically occur in the subependymal frontal horn of the lateral ventricle or at the foramen of Monro but can occur anywhere throughout the ventricular system.[50] SGCTs are thought to arise from subependymal nodules, common in TS patients. Part of the definition of a SGCT is a subependymal nodule which is bigger than 10 mm or is growing over serial scans.[50,52]

Under microscopic examination, these tumors have spindle cells and gemistocyte-like cells. They stain positively for both glial fibrillary acidic protein (GFAP) and neuronal markers.[48,51] They are classified as WHO grade 1. No known cases of malignant transformation have been described.[48,53] On the genetic level, SGCT, and TS in general, is caused by dysregulation of the mammalian target of rapamycin (mTOR) gene.[47,53,54]

Surgery remains a consideration for treatment of these tumors, but there is good evidence for the use of everolimus as a first-line treatment.[53,55–59] Everolimus is an mTOR inhibitor and therefore functions to inhibit the primary oncogenetic driving force of this disease. The EXIST-1 trial, a multicenter randomized controlled trial, showed 50% reduction in the volume of the tumor versus no reduction in the placebo group.[60,61] These patients were treated with a median dose intensity of 5.9 mg/m^2 per day with a range of 2.3 to 11.8 mg/m^2 to achieve trough blood concentrations of 5–15 ng/mL initially for 6 months as part of the EXIST-1 study.[60] The study continued with these same dosing parameters until all patients had received at least 60 months of everolimus treatment or discontinued the study.[61] Studies have shown no evidence contraindicating the use of stereotactic radiation for SGCTs and have shown a slow gradual response of the tumor to radiotherapy. However, there is a paucity of data on the use of radiotherapy alone or in combination with everolimus or surgery.[62]

> A multicenter randomized controlled trial showed that treatment of SGCTs with everolimus, an mTOR inhibitor, showed a 50% reduction in tumor volumes compared to no tumor volume reduction in the placebo group.

If surgery is necessary, following GTR, SGCTs tend not to recur and never metastasize. Patients are at higher risk of having a second SGCT after having had a first.[48] The overall prognosis related to SGCTs is strongly tied to the prognosis for the patient's underlying TS.

ASTROCYTOMA

Astrocytomas represent the most common primary brain tumors.[63,64] Intraventricular astrocytomas are very rare, but should be included on the differential for an intraventricular lesion.[63–65] These tumors appear the same as their extraventricular counterparts on imaging. Namely, they have variable contrast enhancement depending on the grade, with the highest grade showing ring enhancement and central necrosis.[63]

Astrocytomas are graded based on histochemical appearance and, as of 2016, genetic profiles.[66] They range from WHO grades 1 to 4 and carry significantly worse prognosis with higher grades.[63] Details on diagnosis, evaluation, treatment, and prognosis of astrocytomas are covered in other chapters of this book (Chapters 3, 4, 17, and 18).

METASTASIS

Metastases are the most common type of brain tumor, accounting for approximately 25–50% of intracranial lesions.[67] Purely intraventricular metastases are rare, accounting for

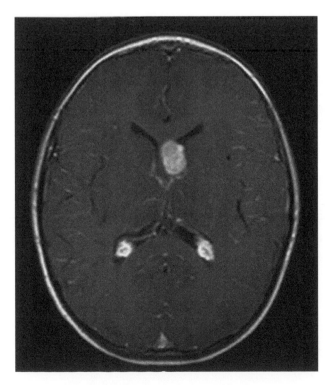

Figure 9.5 T1 post-contrast axial MRI image of a subependymal giant cell astrocytoma (SEGA) showing characteristic homogenous enhancement arising in the left frontal horn.

about 0.9–4.6% of all CNS metastases, but their occurrence has been documented throughout the literature in the form of case reports and series.[68-71] Metastases are thought to occur via hematogenous spread, and this seems to be supported by the fact that most intraventricular metastases are found in the choroid plexus, the area of highest blood flow in any organ.[72,73] Renal cell intraventricular metastasis are the most common and, on MRI, solidly enhance.[73-75] It must be noted that intraventricular metastases fall into two distinct groups: metastases to the choroid plexus, of which the predominant source is renal cell carcinoma, and subependymal metastases resulting from the spread of adjacent tumor along the ventricle.[75]

Treatment is either stereotactic radiosurgery or surgical resection followed by adjunctive radiation.[67,75] Chemotherapy is largely based on the primary tumor's chemosensitivity and the genetic profile thereof.[67,76]

Purely intraventricular metastases are rare, accounting for about 0.9–4.6% of all CNS metastases.

Leptomeningeal metastases can be seen as the result of intraventricular tumors presenting commonly with mental status changes and symptoms of hydrocephalus.[77] Treatment options include both intrathecal and systemic pharmacotherapy as well as radiotherapy.[78] Further details on the evaluation and management of patients with CNS metastases is covered in Chapter 12.

Intraventricular metastatic lesions with leptomeningeal spread commonly present with mental status changes and symptoms of hydrocephalus.

CONCLUSION

Lesions arising within the ventricles include benign and malignant neoplasms, infectious and inflammatory lesions, developmental cysts, and tumors arising from adjacent structures. Treatment is varied and includes surgical resection, stereotactic radiosurgery, and observation with serial imaging. Modern imaging techniques including MRI make preoperative differential diagnoses more reliable and have enabled more conservative management of many of these lesions than was possible historically.

What are common locations of intraventricular tumors?	Partially or completely within the lateral, third, or fourth ventricle Lesions bordering the ventricles such as pituitary tumors can mimic intraventricular tumors
Which developmental cysts are typically found incidentally within the third ventricle, most commonly asymptomatic but can cause sudden death due to sudden, significant increases in intracranial pressure?	Colloid cysts
Three categories of choroid plexus tumors:	1. Choroid plexus papilloma, WHO grade 1, most common and treated with surgical resection 2. Atypical choroid plexus papilloma, WHO grade 2, most rare subtype 3. Choroid plexus carcinoma, WHO grade 3, most aggressive with poorest prognosis; treatment usually includes surgical resection, radiation, and multiagent chemotherapy
Most commonly found in the lateral ventricles, these account for about 50% of intraventricular tumors. Mainstay of treatment is surgery with gross total resection; role of radiation and/or chemotherapy for recurrent disease is not yet well established	Central neurocytoma
Rare subtype of ependymoma that generally has a benign course, most commonly found in the lateral or fourth ventricles in adult men	Subependymoma
Intraventricular meningiomas	Rare, accounting for 0.5–5% of all meningiomas Eighty percent occur in the lateral ventricle
What is first-line treatment for subependymal giant cell tumors (SEGA) associated with tuberous sclerosis?	mTOR inhibitors
What are the most common intraventricular metastases?	Renal cell carcinoma, lung cancer, and colon cancer

QUESTIONS

1. Colloid cysts develop from
   a. Embryonic foregut
   b. Choroid plexus
   c. Neural tube
   d. Telencephalon

2. Colloid cysts can result in sudden death from
   a. Stroke
   b. Elevated intracranial pressure
   c. Acute obstructive hydrocephalus
   d. Acute hemorrhage

3. Among choroid plexus tumors, which of the following is true?
   a. Choroid plexus carcinomas appear more homogeneous on MRI than choroid plexus papillomas.
   b. Atypical choroid plexus papillomas have lower probabilities of recurrence than choroid plexus papillomas.
   c. The imaging characteristics of choroid plexus papillomas and choroid plexus carcinomas are vastly different.
   d. Gross total resection of choroid plexus papilloma has a high probability of cure with a low probability of recurrence.

4. The majority of intraventricular meningiomas develop from the
   a. Third ventricle
   b. Fourth ventricle
   c. Atrium of the lateral ventricles
   d. Anterior horn of the lateral ventricles

5. Adult ependymomas most commonly occur in the
   a. Spine
   b. Lateral ventricles
   c. Third ventricle
   d. Fourth ventricle

6. Among subependymomas, which of the following is true?
   a. Subependymomas are most commonly found in the third ventricle.
   b. The majority of subependymoma patients present with symptoms of elevated intracranial pressure.
   c. Subependymomas exhibit strong contrast enhancement on MRI.
   d. Subependymomas develop most often in middle-aged and older men.

7. Primary CNS lymphomas in immunocompromised patients classically exhibit
   a. No ring enhancement on MRI
   b. Overall irregular contrast enhancement on imaging
   c. Homogeneous contrast enhancement on imaging
   d. Decreased signal on diffusion-weighted imaging

8. Central neurocytomas arise from
   a. Septum pellucidum cells
   b. Glial precursor cells
   c. Ependymal cells
   d. B cells

9. Among subependymal giant cell tumors, which of the following is true?
   a. Malignant transformation is common.
   b. Even after gross total resection, these tumors tend to recur.
   c. These tumors most commonly occur in the sixth to seventh decades of life.
   d. The mammalian target of rapamycin (mTOR) inhibitor everolimus is a primary treatment.

10. Which of the following primary carcinomas does not commonly metastasize to the ventricles?
    a. Colon
    b. Renal cell
    c. Esophageal
    d. Lung

ANSWERS

1. a
2. c
3. d
4. c
5. a
6. d
7. b
8. a
9. d
10. c

REFERENCES

1. Hendricks B, Cohen-Gadol A. *Principles of Intraventricular Surgery. Neurosurgical Atlas.* Jan 2016. doi:10.18791/nsatlas.v4.ch05.1
2. Majmundar N, Ward M, Liu JK. Feasibility and challenges of microsurgical resection of colloid cysts in patients with preexisting ventriculoperitoneal shunts. *World Neurosurg.* 2020;133:e492–e497. doi:10.1016/j.wneu.2019.09.064
3. Aygun N, Shah G, Gandhi D. Colloid cyst. *Pearls and Pitfalls in Head and Neck and Neuroimaging.* Cambridge: Cambridge University Press; 2013:153–160. doi:10.1017/cbo9781139208420.056
4. Spears RC. Colloid cyst headache. *Curr Pain Headache Rep.* 2004;8(4):297–300. doi:10.1007/s11916-004-0011-2
5. Pollock BE, Huston J. Natural history of asymptomatic colloid cysts of the third ventricle. *J Neurosurg.* 1999;91(3): 364–369
6. Beaumont TL, Limbrick DD, Rich KM, Wippold FJ, Dacey Jr RG. Natural history of colloid cysts of the thrid ventricle. *J Neurosurg.* 2016;125:1420–1430. doi:10.3171/2015.11.JNS151396
7. Ahmed SI, Javed G, Laghari AA, et al. Third ventricular tumors: A comprehensive literature review. *Cureus.* October 2018. doi:10.7759/cureus.3417
8. Safaee M, Oh MC, Bloch O, et al. Choroid plexus papillomas: Advances in molecular biology and understanding of tumorigenesis. *Neuro-Oncology.* 2013;15(3):255–267. doi:10.1093/neuonc/nos289
9. Lehtinen MK, Bjornsson CS, Dymecki SM, et al. The choroid plexus and cerebrospinal fluid: Emerging roles in development, disease, and therapy. *J Neurosci.* 2013;33(45):17553–17559. doi:10.1523/JNEUROSCI.3258-13.2013

10. Bahar M, Hashem H, Tekautz T, et al. Choroid plexus tumors in adult and pediatric populations: The Cleveland Clinic and University Hospitals experience. *J Neurooncol.* 2017;132(3):427–432. doi:10.1007/s11060-017-2384-1

11. Merino DM, Shilien A, Villani A, et al. Molecular characterization of choroid plexus tumors reveals novel clinically relevant subgroups. *Clin Ca Res.* 2015;21(1):184–192. doi:10.1158/1078-0432

12. Muly S, Liu S, Lee R, et al. MRI of intracranial intraventricular lesions. *Clin Imaging.* 2018;52:226–239. doi:10.1016/j.clinimag.2018.07.021

13. Hosmann A, Hinker F, Dorfer C, et al. Management of choroid plexus tumors an institutional experience. *Acta Neurochirurgica.* 2019;161(4):745–754. doi:10.1007/s00701-019-03832-5

14. Jungwirth G, Warrta R, Beynon C, et al. Intraventricular meningiomas frequently harbor NF2 mutations but lack common genetic alterations in TTRAF7, AKTT1, SMO, KLF4, PIK3CA and TERT. *Acta Neuropathol Comm.* 2019;7. doi:10.1186/s40478-019-0793-4

15. Aygun N, Shah G, Gandhi D. Intraventricular masses. *Pearls and Pitfalls in Head and Neck and Neuroimaging.* Cambridge: Cambridge University Press; 2013:140–152. doi:10.1017/cbo9781139208420.056

16. Güngör A, Danyeli AE, Akbaş A, et al. Ventricular meningiomas: Surgical strategies and a new finding that suggest an origin from the choroid plexus epithelium. *World Neurosurg.* 2019;129:e177–e190. doi:10.1016/j.wneu.2019.05.092

17. Grujicic D, Cavallo LM, Somma T, et al. Intraventricular meningiomas: A series of 42 patients at a single institution and literature review. *World Neurosurg.* 2017;97:178–188. doi:10.1016/j.wneu.2016.09.068

18. Nanda A, Bir SC, Maiti T, Konar S. Intraventricular meningioma: Technical nuances in surgical management. *World Neurosurg.* 2016;88:526–537. doi:10.1016/j.wneu.2015.10.071

19. Figueiredo N, Santana SCBF. Intramedullary and myxopapillary ependymomas: An evidence-based approach. In Fowler R, ed. *Ependymomas: Prognostic Factors, Treatment Strategies and Clinical Outcomes.* New York: Nova Science Publishers; 2016:57–110.

20. Smyth M.D, Rubin J. Ependymoma. In Gupta N, Banerjee A, Haas-Kogan D, eds. *Pediatric CNS Tumors.* Berlin: Springer; 2010:67–87.

21. Massimino M, Miceli R, Giangaspero F, et al. Final results of the second prospective AIEOP protocol for pediatric intracranial ependymoma. *Neuro Oncol.* 2016;18(10):1451–1460. doi:10.1093/neuonc/now108

22. Chamberlain MC. Ependymomas. *Curr Neurol Neurosci Rep.* 2003;3:193–199.

23. Merchant TE, Bendel AE, Sabin ND, et al. Conformal radiation therapy for pediatric ependymoma, chemotherapy for incompletely resected ependymoma, and observation for completely resected, supratentorial ependymoma. *J Clin Oncol.* 2019;37(12):974–983. doi:10.1200/jco.18.01765

24. Bi Z, Ren X, Zhang J, Jia W. Clinical, radiological, and pathological features in 43 cases of intracranial subependymoma. *J Neurosurg.* 2015;122(1):49–60. doi:10.3171/2014.9.JNS14155

25. Nguyen HS, Doan N, Gelsomino M, Shabani S. Intracranial subependymoma: A SEER analysis 2004–2013. *World Neurosurg.* 2017;101:599–605. doi:10.1016/j.wneu.2017.02.019

26. Hou Z, Wu Z, Zhang J, et al. Clinical features and management of intracranial subependymomas in children. *J Clin Neurosci.* 2013;20(1):84–88. doi:10.1016/j.jocn.2012.05.026

27. Hsu HI, Lai PH, Tseng HH, Hsu SS. Primary solitary lymphoma of the fourth ventricle. *Int J Surg Case Rep.* 2015;14:23–25. doi:10.1016/j.ijscr.2015.07.006

28. Funaro K, Bailey KC, Aguila S, et al. A case of intraventricular primary central nervous system lymphoma. *J Radiol Case Rep.* 2014;8(3):1–8. doi:10.3941/jrcr.v8i3.1361

29. Suri V, Mittapalli V, Kulshrestha M, et al. Primary intraventricular central nervous system lymphoma in an immunocompetent patient. *J Pediatr Neurosci.* 2015;10(4):393–395. doi:10.4103/1817-1745.174433

30. Rades D, Fehlauer F, Lamszus K, et al. Well-differentiated neurocytoma: What is the best available treatment? *Neuro Oncol.* 2005;7(1):77–83. doi:10.1215/s1152851704000584

31. Sharma MC, Deb P, Sharma S, Sarkar C. Neurocytoma: A comprehensive review. *Neurosurg Rev.* 2006;29(4):270–285. doi:10.1007/s10143-006-0030-z

32. Ando K, Ishikura R, Morikawa T, et al. Central neurocytoma with craniospinal dissemination. *Magn Reson Med Sci.* 2002;1(3):179–182. doi:10.2463/mrms.1.179

33. Kane AJ, Sughrue ME, Rutkowski MJ, et al. Atypia predicting prognosis for intracranial extraventricular neurocytomas: Clinical article. *J Neurosurg.* 2012;116(2):349–354. doi:10.3171/2011.9.JNS10783

34. Byun J, Hong SH, Yoon MJ, et al. Prognosis and treatment outcomes of central neurocytomas: Clinical interrogation based on a single

center experience. *J Neurooncol.* 2018;140(3):669–677. doi:10.1007/s11060-018-2997-z

35. Bertalanffy A, Roessler K, Koperek O, et al. Recurrent central neurocytomas. *Cancer.* 2005;104(1):135–142. doi:10.1002/cncr.21109

36. Kocaoglu M, Ors F, Bulakbasi N, et al. Central neurocytoma: Proton MR spectroscopy and diffusion weighted MR imaging findings. *Magn Reson Imaging.* 2009;27(3):434–440. doi:10.1016/j.mri.2008.07.012

37. Vasiljevic A, François P, Loundou A, et al. Prognostic factors in central neurocytomas. *Am J Surg Pathol.* 2012;36(2):220–227. doi:10.1097/pas.0b013e31823b8232

38. Korshunov A, Sycheva R, Golanov A. Recurrent cytogenetic aberrations in central neurocytomas and their biological relevance. *Acta Neuropathol.* 2007;113(3):303–312. doi:10.1007/s00401-006-0168-3

39. Bonney PA, Boettcher LB, Krysiak III RS, et al. Histology and molecular aspects of central neurocytoma. *Neurosurg Clin N Am.* 2015;26(1):21–29. doi:10.1015/j.nec.2014.09.001

40. Johnson MO, Kirkpatrick JP, Patel MP, et al. The role of chemotherapy in the treatment of central neurocytoma. *CNS Oncol.* 2019;8(3):CNS41. doi:10.2217/cns-2019-0012

41. Imber BS, Braunstein SE, Wu FY, et al. Clinical outcome and prognostic factors for central neurocytoma: Twenty year institutional experience. *J Neurooncol.* 2016;126(1):193–200. doi:10.1007/s11060-015-1959-y

42. Paek SH, Han JH, Kim JW, et al. Long-term outcome of conventional radiation therapy for central neurocytoma. *J Neurooncol.* 2008;90(1):25–30. doi:10.1007/s11060-008-9622-5

43. Lee SJ, Bui TT, Chen CHJ, et al. Central neurocytoma: A review of clinical management and histopathologic features. *Brain Tumor Res Treat.* 2016;4(2):49. doi:10.14791/btrt.2016.4.2.49

44. Kim CY, Sun HP, Sang SJ, et al. Gamma knife radiosurgery for central neurocytoma: Primary and secondary treatment. *Cancer.* 2007;110(10):2276–2284. doi:10.1002/cncr.23036

45. Leenstra JL, Rodriguez FJ, Frechette CM, et al. Central neurocytoma: Management recommendations based on a 35-year experience. *Int J Radiat Oncol Biol Phys.* 2007;67(4):1145–1154. doi:10.1016/j.ijrobp.2006.10.018

46. Ess KC, Kamp CA, Tu BP, Gutmann DH. Developmental origin of subependymal giant cell astrocytoma in tuberous sclerosis complex. *Neurology.* 2005;64(8):1446–1449. doi:10.1212/01.wnl.0000158653.81008.49

47. Hallett L, Foster T, Liu Z, et al. Burden of disease and unmet needs in tuberous sclerosis complex with neurological manifestations: Systematic review. *Curr Med Res Opin.* 2011;27(8):1571–1583. doi:10.1185/03007995.2011.586687

48. Kim S-K, Wang K-C, Cho B-K, et al. Biological behavior and tumorigenesis of subependymal giant cell astrocytomas. *J Neuro-Oncol.* 2001;52:217–225.

49. Elousrouti LT, Lamchahab M, Bougtoub N, et al. Subependymal giant cell astrocytoma (SEGA): A case report and review of the literature. *J Med Case Rep.* 2016;10(1). doi:10.1186/s13256-016-0818-6

50. Torres OA, Roach E, Delgado MR, et al. Early diagnosis of subependymal giant cell astrocytoma in patients with tuberous sclerosis. *J Child Neurol.* 1998;13(4):173–177. doi:10.1177/088307389801300405

51. Nishio S, Morioka T, Suzuki S, et al. Subependymal giant cell astrocytoma: Clinical and neuroimaging features of four cases. *J Clin Neurosci.* 2001;8(1):31–34. doi:10.1054/jocn.2000.0767

52. O'Callaghan FJK, Martyn CN, Renowden S, et al. Subependymal nodules, giant cell astrocytomas and the tuberous sclerosis complex: A population-based study. *Arch Dis Child.* 2008;93(9):751–754. doi:10.1136/adc.2007.125880

53. Beaumont TL, Limbrick DD, Smyth MD. Advances in the management of subependymal giant cell astrocytoma. *Child's Nerv Syst.* 2012;28(7):963–968. doi:10.1007/s00381-012-1785-x

54. Crino PB, Henske EP. New developments in the neurobiology of the tuberous sclerosis complex. *Neurology.* 1999; 53(7):1384–1384. doi:10.1212/wnl.53.7.1384

55. Krueger DA, Northrup H, Krueger DA, et al. Tuberous sclerosis complex surveillance and management: Recommendations of the 2012 international tuberous sclerosis complex consensus conference. *Pediatr Neurol.* 2013;49(4):255–265. doi:10.1016/j.pediatrneurol.2013.08.002

56. Kotulska K, Borkowska J, Roszkowski M, et al. Surgical treatment of subependymal giant cell astrocytoma in tuberous sclerosis complex patients. *Pediatr Neurol.* 2014;50(4):307–312. doi:10.1016/j.pediatrneurol.2013.12.004

57. Goh S, Butler W, Thiele EA. Subependymal giant cell tumors in tuberous sclerosis complex. *Neurology.* 2004;63(8):1457–1461. doi:10.1212/01.wnl.0000142039.14522.1a

58. Jóźwiak S, Mandera M, Młynarski W. Natural history and current treatment options for subependymal giant cell astrocytoma in tuberous

sclerosis complex. *Semin Pediatr Neurol.* 2015;22(4):274–281. doi:10.1016/j.spen.2015.10.003

59. Berhouma M. Management of subependymal giant cell tumors in tuberous sclerosis complex: The neurosurgeon's perspective. *World J Pediatr.* 2010;6(2):103–110. doi:10.1007/s12519-010-0025-2

60. Franz DN, Belousova E, Sparagana S, et al. Efficacy and safety of everolimus for subependymal giant cell astrocytomas associated with tuberous sclerosis complex (EXIST-1): A multicentre, randomised, placebo-controlled phase 3 trial. *Lancet.* 2013;381(9861):125–132. doi:10.1016/S0140-6736(12)61134-9

61. Franz DN, Agricola K, Mays M, et al. Everolimus for subependymal giant cell astrocytoma: 5-year final analysis. *Ann Neurol.* 2015;78(6):929–938. doi:10.1002/ana.24523

62. Kamel R, Van den Berge D. Po04.03 Radiotherapy for subependymal giant cell astrocytoma: Time to challenge a historical ban? Case report and review of the literature. *Neuro-Oncology.* 2019;21(supplement):iii29. doi:10.1093/neuonc/noz126.098

63. Nsir AB, Gdoura Y, Thai QA, et al. Intraventricular glioblastomas. *World Neurosurg.* 2016;88:126–131. doi:10.1016/j.wneu.2015.12.079

64. Sattar S, Akhunzada N, Javed G, et al. Pilocytic astrocytoma: A rare presentation as intraventricular tumor. *Surg Neurol Int.* 2017;8(1). doi:10.4103/sni.sni_468_16

65. Ahn JS, Harrison W, Hughes E, McLendon RE. Intraventricular pilocytic astrocytoma with KIAA1549/BRAF fusion arising in a 44-year old. *J Neuropathol Exp Neurol.* 2019;78(2):187–190. doi:10.1093/jnen/nly116

66. Louis DN, Perry A, Reifenberger G, et al. The 2016 World Health Organization Classification of Tumors of the Central Nervous System: A summary. *Acta Neuropathol.* 2016;131(6):803–820. doi:10.1007/s00401-016-1545-1

67. Eichler AF, Loeffler JS. Multidisciplinary management of brain metastases. *Oncologist.* 2007;12(7):884–898. doi:10.1634/theoncologist.12-7-884

68. Sava I, Sava A, Şapte E, et al. Intraventricular metastatic clear cell renal carcinoma. *Rom J Morphol Embryol.* 2013;54(2):447–450. http://www.rjme.ro/

69. Vannier A, Gray F, Gherardi R, et al. Diffuse subependymal periventricular metastases: Report of three cases. *Cancer.* 1986;58(12):2720–2725. doi:10.1002/1097-0142(19861215)58:12<2720::aid-cncr2820581228>3.0.co;2-6

70. Chen H, Raza HK, Shi H, et al. A rare case of small cell carcinoma of lung with intraventricular metastasis. *Br J Neurosurg.* 2019;33(3):261–263. doi:10.1080/02688697.2017.1327020

71. Sharifi G, Bakhtevari MH, Alghasi M, et al. Bilateral choroid plexus metastasis from papillary thyroid carcinoma: Case report and review of the literature. *World Neurosurg.* 2015;84(4):1142–1146. doi:10.1016/j.wneu.2015.05.027

72. Quinones-Hinojosa A, Chang EF, Khan SA, et al. Renal cell carcinoma metastatic to the choroid mimicking intraventricular meningioma. *Can J Neurol Sci.* 2004;31(1):115–120. doi:10.1017/S0317167100002948

73. Singh S, Agarwal H, Singh P, Goel K. Intraventricular metastasis mimicking meningioma. *Surg Neurol Int.* 2018;9(1):149. doi:10.4103/sni.sni_68_18

74. Ji J, Gu C, Zhang M, et al. Pineal region metastasis with intraventricular seeding: A case report and literature review. *Medicine (Baltimore).* 2019;98(34):e16652. doi:10.1097/MD.0000000000016652

75. Siomin V, Lin JL, Marko NF, et al. Stereotactic radiosurgical treatment of brain metastases to the choroid plexus. *Int J Radiat Oncol Biol Phys.* 2011;80(4):1134–1142. doi:10.1016/j.ijrobp.2010.03.016

76. Shenoy S, Shenoy SN. Progeny in an inhospitable milieu: Solitary intraventricular metastasis from a triple-negative breast cancer mimicking central neurocytoma: Case report and review of diagnostic pitfalls and management strategies. *World Neurosurg.* 2019;135:309–315. doi:10.1016/j.wneu.2019.12.066

77. Bomgaars LR, Chamberlain MC, Poplack DG, Blaney SM. Leptomeningeal metastases. In Levin VA, ed. *Cancer in the Nervous System.* New York: Oxford University Press; 2002:375–394.

78. Le Rhun E, Preusser M, van den Bent M, et al. How we treat patients with leptomeningeal metastases. *ESMO Open.* 2019;4(Suppl 2):e000507. doi:10.1136/esmoopen-2019-000507

79. Algin O, Ozmen E, Arslan H. Radiologic manifestations of colloid cysts: A pictorial essay. *Can Assoc Radiol J.* 2013;64(1):56–60. doi:10.1016/j.carj.2011.12.011

80. Kim J, Moritani T, Kirby P. Restricted diffusion in benign CNS neoplasms: Imaging pitfalls and histopathological correlations. doi:10.1594/ecr2012/C-1968

81. Watts J, Yap KK, Ou D, et al. Intraventricular CNS lesions: A pictorial essay. *J Med Imaging Radiat Oncol.* 2015;59(4):453–460. doi:10.1111/1754-9485.12293

82. Salunke P, Sahoo SK, Madhivanan K, Radotra BD. A typical radiological presentation in a case of choroid plexus carcinoma. *Surg Neurol Int.* 2014;5(Suppl). doi:10.4103/2152-7806.132103

83. Yuh EL, Barkovich AJ, Gupta N. Imaging of ependymomas: MRI and CT. *Child's Nerv Syst.* 2009;25(10):1203–1213. doi:10.1007/s00381-009-0878-7

84. Abdel-Aal AK, Hamed MF, Al Naief NS, et al. Unusual appearance and presentation of supratentorial subependymoma in an adult patient. *J Radiol Case Rep.* 2012;6(8):8–16. doi:10.3941/jrcr.v6i8.999

85. Mansour A, Qandeel M, Abdel-Razeq H, Abu Ali HA. MR imaging features of intracranial primary CNS lymphoma in immune competent patients. *Cancer Imaging.* 2014;14(1). doi:10.1186/1470-7330-14-22

86. Zhang D, Wen L, Henning TD, et al. Central neurocytoma: Clinical, pathological and neuroradiological findings. *Clin Radiol.* 2006;61(4):348–357. doi:10.1016/j.crad.2006.01.002

87. Tlili-Graiess K, Mama N, Arifa N, et al. Diffusion weighted mr imaging and proton MR spectroscopy findings of central neurocytoma with pathological correlation. *J Neuroradiol.* 2014;41(4):243–250. doi:10.1016/j.neurad.2013.09.004

88. Stein JR, Reidman DA. Imaging manifestations of a subependymal giant cell astrocytoma in tuberous sclerosis. *Case Rep Radiol.* 2016:1–5. doi:10.1155/2016/3750450

89. Broen MPG, Smits M, Wijnenga MMJ, et al. The T2-FLAIR mismatch sign as an imaging marker for non-enhancing IDH-mutant, 1p/19q-intact lower-grade glioma: A validation study. *Neuro Oncol.* 2018;20(10):1393–1399. doi:10.1093/neuonc/noy048

90. Qin JB, Zhang H, Wang XC, et al. Combination value of diffusion-weighted imaging and dynamic susceptibility contrast-enhanced MRI in astrocytoma grading and correlation with GFAP, topoisomerase IIα and MGMT. *Oncol Lett.* 2019;18(3):2763–2770. doi:10.3892/ol.2019.10656

91. Fink K, Fink J. Imaging of brain metastases. *Surg Neurol Int.* 2013;4(Suppl 4). doi:10.4103/2152-7806.111298

10 | RARE TUMORS IN ADULTS, INCLUDING MEDULLOBLASTOMA

KEVIN SHIUE, LOGAN S. DEWITT, JOHN M. KINDLER, AND GORDON A. WATSON[†]

INTRODUCTION

In this chapter, we review a selection of rare adult central nervous system (CNS) tumors, including medulloblastoma in adults, cerebellar liponeurocytoma, diffuse leptomeningeal glioneuronal tumor (DLGNT), ganglioglioma (GG), pineal parenchymal tumors (PPTs), and pleomorphic xanthoastrocytoma (PXA). The focus is on epidemiology, important clinical characteristics, relevant histology and radiographic details, and general management and treatment paradigms. Discussion takes into account grade and molecular classification as noted in the 2016 World Health Organization (WHO) classification of brain tumors.

MEDULLOBLASTOMA IN ADULTS

Medulloblastoma is typically a disease of childhood but is also a rare cancer of adulthood, with an annual incidence in adults of approximately 0.5 per million. The median age of diagnosis in adults is around 30, with 80% of cases in patients under age 40 and only exceedingly rare reports of diagnoses above age 60.[1-4] Medulloblastoma is commonly a tumor of the posterior fossa, although there are rare reports of adults with supratentorial and/or multifocal involvement.[5,6]

> The median age of diagnosis in adults is around 30, with 80% of cases in patients under age 40 and only exceedingly rare reports of diagnoses above age 60.

Given its typical location, presenting symptoms most often include increased intracranial pressure and cerebellar dysfunction that progress in a subacute fashion over a period of weeks to months. Physical exam findings include truncal/gait ataxia, nystagmus, and dysmetria, among other usual signs of increased intracranial pressure. Work-up typically proceeds with computed tomography (CT), then follows with magnetic resonance imaging (MRI) of the brain pre- and (within 72 hours) postoperatively. MRI of the spine and cerebrospinal fluid (CSF) can be obtained preoperatively (i.e., when there is no concern for herniation) but typically is obtained more than 14 days postoperatively given risk of false positivity if obtained too soon after surgery.

Medulloblastoma is a WHO grade 4 tumor, with clinically relevant histological variants of classic, large cell/anaplastic, desmoplastic/nodular, and extensive nodularity. Historically, the classic and desmoplastic/nodular histologies have better prognosis, and this distinction is reflected in risk classification, with "standard-risk" disease including patients meeting all criteria of (a) M0 (meaning zero metastases), (b) gross total resection (GTR) or near GTR ($\leq$1.5 cm^2), and (c) classic or desmoplastic histology.

In the early 2010s, molecular analyses revealed that medulloblastoma could be divided into four distinct subgroups: WNT, SHH, Group 3, and Group 4. The WNT subgroup has the best prognosis, followed in order of worsening prognosis by SHH, Group 4, then Group 3.[7-10] In adults, most cases are histologically classic or desmoplastic/nodular. Molecularly, more than 50% are in the SHH subgroup (5-year overall survival [OS] 70%). Group 4 accounts for 25% (5-year OS 25%), and the WNT subgroup accounts for up to 15% (5-year OS 80%) of adult cases, but Group 3 is rare in adults.[3] The 2016 WHO classification has attempted to integrate the histology and molecular subgroups, which is well summarized in Louis et al.[11]

The imaging findings in adult medulloblastoma reflect the expected molecular subgroups and their distinct imaging phenotypes. On CT, adult medulloblastomas have similar appearance to pediatric medulloblastomas and are typically hyperintense, without calcification, and showing intense contrast uptake. On MRI, adult medulloblastomas (as compared to pediatric medulloblastomas) are less likely to localize to midline structures, more likely to have an atypical appearance (i.e., T1 isointense or hyperintense, T2 isointense or hypointense), less likely to have marked contrast enhancement, and more likely to have heterogeneous enhancement (Figure 10.1).[12]

Much—but not all—of the data informing our understanding of the management of adult medulloblastoma is derived from studies in children. Traditionally, adults are thought to tolerate radiotherapy (RT) better than children and chemotherapy worse than children. However, recent and primarily retrospective studies have demonstrated that (a) postoperative chemotherapy (at some point during initial therapy, most often adjuvant) may improve survival for adult patients, even

---

[†] Deceased

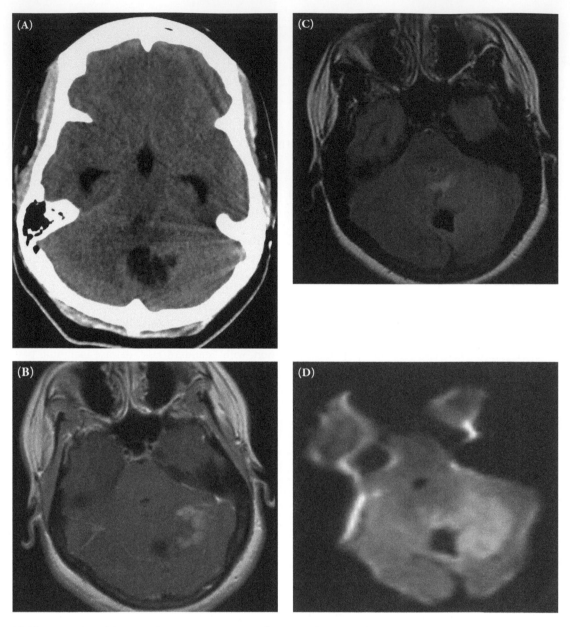

Figure 10.1 *Medulloblastoma. (A) Axial CT image demonstrating a posterior fossa mass that is partially cystic with mildly hyperdense margins reflective of the hypercellularity typical of medulloblastomas. (B and C) MRI T1 post-contrast (B) and T2/fluid-attenuated inversion recovery (FLAIR) (C) axial images with multifocal enhancement and mildly hyperintense to isointense FLAIR signal. This mass is primarily located within the left cerebellar hemisphere, an off-midline location suggestive of its histologic subtype of desmoplastic/nodular. (D) A diffusion weighted (DWI) MRI that shows strong diffusion restriction secondary to the hypercellularity typical of high-grade tumors.*

those who are M0,[13-15] and (b) adults who received lower-dose craniospinal irradiation (CSI) (i.e., as used in standard-risk children) with concurrent chemotherapy did not have worse survival as compared to those who received high-dose CSI (i.e., as is typically done when concurrent chemotherapy is not utilized).[16-18]

Adults who receive lower-dose CSI (i.e., as used in standard-risk children) with concurrent chemotherapy do not have worse survival as compared to those who receive high-dose CSI (i.e., as is typically done when concurrent chemotherapy is not utilized).

One prospective multicenter phase II study by Beier et al. (NOA-07) enrolled 15 adult patients (30% M+) and administered high-dose CSI concurrently with vincristine, followed by up to eight cycles of cisplatin, lomustine, and vincristine. This study demonstrated that four adjuvant cycles was feasible for 70% of patients (often with considerable dose reductions), and 3-year event-free survival (EFS), progression-free survival (PFS), and OS were 67%, 67%, and 70%, respectively. However, there was considerable toxicity as noted (a) during chemoradiation, with rates of 10–37% for grade 3 or 4 leukopenia, anemia, infection, and polyneuropathy; and (b) during adjuvant chemotherapy, with rates of 20–67% for grade 3 or 4 leukopenia, thrombocytopenia, anemia, polyneuropathy, and ototoxicity. Given such toxicity (notably in the setting of high-dose CSI with concurrent chemotherapy) this regimen is not routinely recommended.[19]

Another prospective phase II trial enrolled 11 adult high-risk patients after surgery to receive three cycles of pre-irradiation cisplatin, etoposide, cyclophosphamide, and vincristine followed by high-dose CSI with boost (without concurrent chemotherapy). Ultimately, this regimen was able to be delivered safely without compromising completion of CSI. However, there did not appear to be a benefit as compared to historical series in adults (5-year OS 55%), and this regimen is not recommended.[20]

In summary, for both standard- and high-risk adults, we would consider maximal safe resection followed by high-dose CSI with focal boost but without concurrent chemotherapy, then adjuvant combination chemotherapy.[21] Clinical trials or registry studies should be considered whenever possible, particularly when considering concurrent chemotherapy. CSI alone is a consideration in frail patients or patients with poor performance status.

CEREBELLAR LIPONEUROCYTOMAS

Cerebellar liponeurocytomas are a benign WHO grade 2 tumor primarily located in the posterior fossa of adults and typically seen between the third and fifth decades. There may be a slight female predilection, but this is not well established. Originally described in 1978,[22] it was first recognized in the WHO classification in 2000 as a grade 1 neuronal tumor.[23] In the 2016 WHO classification update, it was upgraded to a WHO grade glioneuronal 2 tumor (but still considered benign) due to its higher than expected rate of recurrence.[24] It has previously been described as "unusual medulloblastomas in adults," "lipomatous medulloblastomas," "neurolipocytomas," or "medullocytomas," with fewer than 100 total cases described in the literature.[25] Most patients present with some combination of headaches, nausea, vomiting, unsteadiness, ataxia, gait disturbance, or frequent falls. Given its typical location, obstruction of the cerebrospinal fluid is also a concern. The differential includes oligodendrogliomas, clear cell ependymomas, and medulloblastomas, among other posterior fossa tumors.

> In the 2016 WHO classification update, liponeurocytoma was upgraded to a WHO grade glioneuronal 2 tumor (but still considered benign) due to its higher than expected rate of recurrence.

Histopathologically, cerebellar liponeurocytomas are noted to have small cells and lipomatous cells (Figure 10.2). In one review, positive immunoreactivity was noted to synaptophysin (98.5% of 66 cases), neuron specific enolase (NSE) (100% of 27 cases), NeuN (100% of 16 cases), glial fibrillary acidic protein (GFAP) (85.5% of 62 cases), microtuble-associated protein (MAP-2) (100% of 20 cases), and S100-protein (82.1% of 28 cases). Less commonly, positive staining was also seen for chromogranin A (54.5% of 11 cases), neurofilament (32.3% of 31 cases), and tp53 (44.4% of 9 cases). Ki-67/MIB-I proliferation index was a mean of 3.7% (55 cases measured) at initial diagnosis and a mean of 9.2% at first recurrence.[25,26] Interestingly, there are rare reports of a possible familial predisposition, with one publication[27] describing cerebellar liponeurocytomas in a 37-year-old woman, her mother, her maternal grandfather, and her maternal uncle and a second publication[28] describing this tumor in two siblings. No clear genetic explanation has been identified to this date.

Radiologically, cerebellar liponeurocytomas are typically hypodense on CT with noted (but often irregular) contrast enhancement within the tumor. On MRI, the tumor is typically hypo- to isointense on T1-weighted images, although a minority of cases have been described as hyperintense. On T2-weighted images, the tumor is primarily hyperintense, with some described as isointense but only rarely as hypointense. On fluid-attenuated inversion recovery (FLAIR) and diffusion weighted imaging (DWI), the tumor typically appears hyperintense, but this is based on a very small number of reports. Contrast enhancement is observed in most cases.[25] On FDG positron emission tomography (PET), lower uptake was seen in tumor compared with normal cerebellar cortex.[29] Notably, there have been several reports of multifocality for this disease as well (Figure 10.3).[30–33]

Cerebellar liponeurocytomas are primarily treated with surgery, with a goal of GTR if safe. Overall, the lesion appears to be slow-growing, with one case report describing 1.2 × 0.5 cm growth in 4 years.[34] The extent of resection (complete vs. incomplete) and the use of postoperative RT (PORT) seems to have an impact on long term tumor control rates. The timing of PORT is also not well established, with some treating after first surgery and others treating only after multiple surgeries.[25] There is no apparent role for chemotherapy currently. Late and/or multiple recurrences are possible.[35]

In one review of 72 patients with known extent of resection, use of PORT was known for 57 patients. In patients with complete resection and adequate follow-up, 0% (0 of 6) of those who received PORT versus 26.1% (6 of 23) of those who

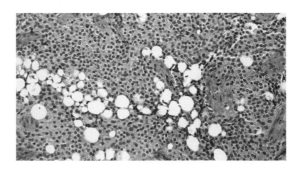

Figure 10.2 *The principle components of cerebellar liponeurocytoma include classic neurocytes (round, monomorphic cells with scant cytoplasm and stippled chromatin) and distinctive, variably lipidized cells resembling mature adipocytes. Mitotic figures are rare to absent.*

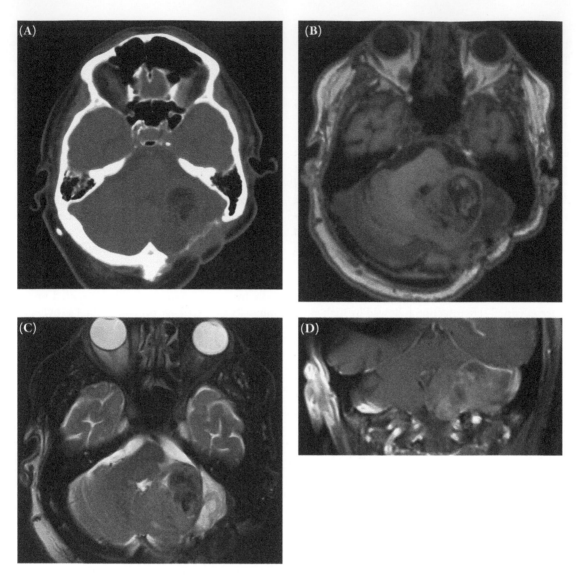

Figure 10.3 *Cerebellar liponeurocytoma. (A) Axial CT image demonstrating a recurrent cerebellar liponeurocytoma. (B and C) MRI T1 pre-contrast (B) and T2 fat saturation (C) axial images with intrinsic T1 hyperintensity that becomes null on fat saturation, consistent with macroscopic fat. (D) MRI T1 post-contrast fat saturation coronal image showing heterogeneous enhancement. With the fat signal nulled, the T1 hyperintensity is purely secondary enhancement and not intrinsic T1 hyperintensity.*

did not receive PORT had a recurrence. In patients with incomplete resection and adequate follow-up, 16.7% (1 of 6) of those who received PORT versus 77.8% (7 of 9) who did not receive PORT had a recurrence. When considering patients by use of PORT regardless of extent of resection (*n* = 59) who were followed, 8.3% (1 of 12) who received PORT versus 40.6% (13 of 32) who did not receive PORT had tumor recurrence. PORT dose was most often 54 Gy external beam RT, although there was wide variance in the literature.[25]

DIFFUSE LEPTOMENINGEAL GLIONEURONAL TUMOR

DLGNT was introduced as a distinct histopathologic entity in the 2016 WHO brain tumor classification within the group of neuronal and mixed neuronal-glial tumors.[36] It is most commonly seen in the pediatric/adolescent age group but has been

rarely reported in adults. The original description of these tumors had distinctive characteristics, including cystic lesions of the subarachnoid space with intense enhancement, diffuse leptomeningeal infiltration by glioneuronal cells with or without a primary mass, and an indolent clinical course.[37] The predominant cell type is a monomorphic clear glial cell often misidentified as oligodendroglial. Rarely, tumors will demonstrate elevated Ki-67 staining, high mitotic rate, and necrosis; clinically, such tumors will behave as aggressive, high-grade tumors with poor patient outcomes.[38,39]

Recently, DLGNTs were molecularly profiled via a genome-wide DNA methylation screening method.[40] All tumors displayed loss of chromosome 1p and were isocitrate dehydrogenase (IDH)-1-wildtype. DLGNTs harbored genetic alterations involving the mitogen-activated protein kinase (MAPK)/extracellular signal-regulated kinase (ERK) pathway in more than 80% of cases. This was most commonly a BRAF fusion mutation (65–77%). Many were also O[6]-methylguanine DNA methyltransferase (MGMT) promoter-methylated. Then, tumors could be divided into two subgroups with distinct clinical behaviors. DLGNT-1 tumors had co-deletion of 1p/19q (47%) while DLGNT-2 tumors display a gain of 1q and whole chromosome 8 (100%). DLGNT-1 tumors were seen only in pediatric patients and had an indolent clinical course (median age 5 years, 5-year OS 100%) compared to DLGNT-2 tumors (median age 14 years, 5-year OS 43%). All adults diagnosed with DLGNTs have been categorized as having subgroup 2 tumors. This clinical behavior would suggest DLGNT-1 tumors should be classified as WHO grade 1 and DLGNT-2 tumors as WHO grade 2-3.

MRI characteristics include diffuse leptomeningeal T1 post-contrast enhancement most often with associated cystic and/or nodular T2 hyperintense lesions.[41] Initial differential diagnosis for DLGNTs includes inflammatory diseases such as meningitis, IgG4 disease, neurosarcoid, and subdural abscess.[42] Thus, serologic and CSF examination for signs of inflammatory disease should be part of the initial workup. If results point more toward neoplastic processes, entities that can have leptomeningeal dissemination need to be considered. These include pilocytic astrocytoma, high-grade glioma, and metastatic disease. Biopsy is critical to making the diagnosis in DLGNT, but surgical resection is not usually possible except in the rare case when the patient presents with an intraparenchymal lesion. Once diagnosed, patients have been most often treated with combination RT and temozolomide (TMZ). RT has been either focal or craniospinal. A number of cases were treated with the addition of bevacizumab to RT/TMZ with reasonable outcomes.[43] Studies with MEK and RAF inhibitors suggest that they may have therapeutic potential for those tumors with BRAF fusion mutations.[44,45]

> Biopsy is critical to making the diagnosis in DLGNT, but surgical resection is not usually possible except in the rare case when the patient presents with an intraparenchymal lesion.

GANGLIOGLIOMAS

GGs are a group of tumors derived from dysplastic/atypical ganglion cells intermixed with neoplastic glial cells.[46,47] Most GGs are low grade (WHO grade 1) but can present as anaplastic GGs (grade 3).[36,48,49] These tumors are rare in adults, accounting for approximately 1.3% of primary brain tumors.[50] Typical location for GGs in adults is the frontal or temporal lobes. As such, the most common presentation is seizure, typically partial complex. GGs are the most common epilepsy-associated tumor in adults, with dysembryoplastic neuroepithelial tumors (DNETs) the second most common.[51,52] Together, GGs and DNETs make up the entity called "low-grade epilepsy-associated brain tumors (LEAT).

> GGs are the most common epilepsy-associated tumor in adults, with dysembryoplastic neuroepithelial tumors (DNETs) the second most common.

Gangliocytomas (GC) are WHO grade 1 tumors that are composed of dysplastic neuronal cells without admixed neoplastic glial cells.[53] This histologic variant has an incidence rate of only 2-4% of all GGs, depending on the published series.[54-56] The lack of neoplastic glial cells makes them difficult to diagnose, with significant discordance among experienced neuropathologists.[57] Dysplastic gangliocytomas of the cerebellum comprise the entity Lhermitte-Duclos disease (LDD), which is part of Cowden syndrome.[58] As almost all cases of LDD have associated PTEN gene mutations, they now are included in the PTEN hamartoma tumor syndrome (PHTS).[59-61]

Gangliogliomas are WHO grade 1 or 3 (if atypia is present) tumors of young adults that contain neoplastic astrocytic (90%) or oligodendroglial components (<10%). While most commonly occurring in the temporal lobes, they have been found in all supra- and infratentorial sites and the spinal cord. Most GGs harbor BRAF mutations (10-60%), the majority being the V600E mutation.[62-64] Those GGs without BRAF mutations harbor other genetic alterations associated with an activated MAPK signaling pathway. Of note, the presence of an IDH mutation implies a primary glial component and suggests at least a grade 2 diffusely infiltrative glioma.[65] Malignant transformation to anaplastic (WHO grade 3) or malignant (WHO grade 4) tumors (including anaplastic GG or primary glial tumors like glioblastoma) has been reported and related to prior RT.[48,66,67]

CT and MRI appearance for GGs can be quite variable, with the exception of the posterior fossa (PF) GCs. PF GCs are T1 hypointense and on T2 hyperintense with a classic "tiger-stripe" pattern.[58] GGs can have a variable appearance with cystic or solid patterns. MRI characteristics are perilesional/subcortical white matter signal change, T2-FLAIR hyperintensity, and focal cortical atrophy with prominent adjacent sulci. Approximately 50% of these tumors can have focal T1 post-contrast enhancement (Figure 10.4).[68]

Treatment for low-grade ganglioglioma is surgical resection, with recurrence rates after GTR between 1 and 12.5% in reported series.[48,69] Reported recurrence rates after subtotal resection (STR) vary between 8 and 50%.[68] Adjuvant RT has been used after STR. However, the low rates of progression and the risk of malignant transformation have been used to argue against its use. Currently RT, either fractionated or stereotactic radiosurgery, is used only for salvage therapy after surgical options have been exhausted. Adjuvant radiation is recommended for WHO grade 3 tumors after maximal surgical resection, but outcomes have been poor.[48,70]

> RT for treatment of ganglioglioma, either as fractionated or stereotactic radiosurgery, is used only for salvage therapy after surgical options have been exhausted.

PINEAL PARENCHYMAL TUMORS

Pineal region tumors include many different potentially benign and malignant processes. Most common neoplasms in this location include germ cell tumors, PPTs, and gliomas

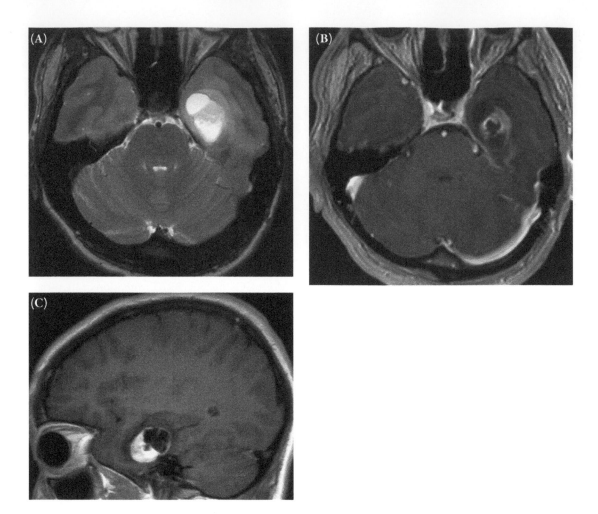

Figure 10.4 *Ganglioglioma. (A) MRI T2 axial image with a well-defined, partially cystic, and cortically based temporal lobe mass, consistent with the most common location and morphology for gangliogliomas. (B and C) MRI axial T1 (B) and sagittal T1 (C) post-contrast images demonstrating an enhancing nodule associated with the cystic mass.*

(59%, 30%, and 5%, respectively). This section focuses on PPTs, which account for fewer than 1% of adult CNS tumors.[71] Other reported but much rarer histologies include ependymomas, choroid plexus papillomas, meningiomas, epidermoid tumors, and metastases, among many others (not an exhaustive list).[72-77]

Tumors of the pineal region, including PPTs, often present with headaches, visual abnormalities, nausea, vomiting, and/or ataxia or other gait abnormalities. These symptoms are often due to hydrocephalus and increased intracranial pressure due to the location of the pineal gland. On exam, clinicians should pay attention to papilledema, loss of upward gaze and pupillary dysfunction (known as Parinaud syndrome), ataxia, and tremor. Cranial neuropathies and hypothalamic dysfunction are seen as well. Higher grade tumors may lead to leptomeningeal dissemination. Work-up often starts with a CT of the head, followed by MRI (ideally of the entire neuraxis). Serum and CSF levels of alpha-fetoprotein (AFP) and beta-human chorionic gonadotropin (HCG) should be obtained given the differential includes germ cell tumors. Of note, CSF can be obtained preoperatively if safe but is often obtained postoperatively. No serum CSF markers exist specifically for PPTs, although serum melatonin profile is of investigative interest[78] and melatonin synthesis-related mRNAs are partially preserved in PPTs.[79]

> On exam, clinicians should pay attention to papilledema, loss of upward gaze and pupillary dysfunction (known as Parinaud syndrome), ataxia, and tremor.

The pineal gland is composed of specialized neuronal endocrine cells called pinealocytes, which are phylogenetically related to photoreceptor cells in the retina (clinically evidenced by the entity of trilateral retinoblastoma). Pinealocytes secrete melatonin, which regulates circadian rhythm. Immunohistochemically, pinealocytes stain positive for synaptophysin, NSE, and neurofilament. Cone-rod homeobox (CRX) protein is found in both normal pineal glands and PPTs, but GFAP is found in interstitial cells only (in contrast to gliomas).[80-82] As discussed, this staining is maintained for lower grade, well-differentiated tumors but less so for higher grade, more advanced tumors.

The WHO classification system divides PPTs into four groups: pineocytomas (WHO grade 1, 20% of PPTs), PPTs of intermediate differentiation (PPTID, WHO grade 2 or 3, 45%), papillary tumors of the pineal region (PTPR, WHO grade 2 or 3, <1%), and pineoblastomas (WHO grade 4, 35%).[24]

> The WHO classification system divides PPTs into four groups: pineocytomas (WHO grade 1, 20% of PPTs), PPTs of intermediate differentiation (PPTID, WHO grade 2 or 3, 45%), papillary tumors of the pineal region (PTPR, WHO grade 2 or 3, <1%), and pineoblastomas (WHO grade 4, 35%).

- Pineocytomas contain aggregates of round, uniform cells with a well-circumscribed border, no (or rare) necrosis, no (or rare) mitotic activity (mean Ki-67 0%).[83] Pineocytomatous rosettes are present in pineocytomas but not in normal pineal gland tissue; however, absence in pineocytomas (i.e., representing lack of neuronal differentiation) portends worse prognosis. It retains the staining profile of normal pinealocytes (positive synaptophysin, NSE, neurofilament) and has no (or rare) chromosomal abnormalities. Pleomorphism does not upgrade the tumor.[84-86]

- Pineoblastomas contain irregular and patternless aggregates of small cells with high nucleus-to-cytoplasm ratios, infiltration, and high mitotic activity (mean Ki-67 36.4%).[83] Necrosis, hypercellularity, and hemorrhage are frequently seen. No pineocytomatous rosettes are seen, but rosettes associated with medulloblastoma/neuroblastoma (Homer-Wright) and retinoblastoma (Flexner-Wintersteiner) are seen in some cases. Pineoblastomas continue to stain for synaptophysin and NSE but in a more diffuse and less intense manner; however, neurofilament is negative or rare.[84-86] Two studies describe molecular subgroups related to Rb1 and DICER1/DROSHA, FOXR2, and MYC alterations.[87,88] More work needs to be done to refine these findings and incorporate them into clinical care, as is being done in medulloblastoma.

- PPTIDs are morphologically divided into three subtypes: (1) an endocrine-like lobulated pattern with high vascularity, (2) a diffuse growth pattern similar to oligodendroglioma or neurocytoma, and (3) a transitional type that is a combination of the previous two subtypes intermixed with pineocytomatous rosettes.[85,89] Mitotic activity is typically intermediate (mean Ki-67 5.2% in grade 2, 11.2% grade 3).[83] PPTIDs retain staining for synaptophysin and NSE, but neurofilament staining is variable and is incorporated into grading. Grade 3 tumors include any subtype with strong neurofilament staining and 0–5 mitoses per 10 high-power field (HPF). Grade 3 tumors include lobulated and diffuse subtypes with (a) 0–5 mitoses per 10 HPF and no neurofilament staining, or (b) 6+ mitoses per 10 HPF. Like pineocytomas, pleomorphism does not appear to upgrade the tumor.[85]

- PTPR, as a neuroepithelial tumor, is a distinct entity with its eponymous papillary architecture and some solid areas (sheets of epitheliod tumor cells with variable perivascular pseudorosettes but without pineocytomatous rosettes). Mitotic activity is variable. PTPRs sometimes stain for synaptophysin and commonly stain for NSE; however, they typically do not stain for neurofilament.[90] The distinction between grade 2 and 3 is not well established, but grade 2 tumors typically have 0–5 mitoses per 10 HPF and Ki-67 of 10% or less, whereas grade 3 tumors typically have higher mitotic counts and Ki-67 or the presence of necrosis, microvascular proliferation, and nuclear atypia.[91,92] One study has shown that lack of BRAF V600E may help differentiate PTPRs from other non-PPT pineal region tumors.[93] Another study demonstrated that staining for CRX and not FOXJ1 is suggestive of pineal parenchymal differentiation, whereas weak or absent CRX staining and positive staining for FOXJ1 (in additional to other features of ependymal differentiation) is suggestive of PTPR, which resembles tissue from the ependymal circumventricular subcommissural organ (SCO) of the posterior third ventricle.

On CT, pineocytomas are most often isodense and contrast-enhance homogeneously, with associated peripheral calcifications and sometimes cystic areas (making them hard to distinguish from pineal cysts). In contrast, pineoblastomas are hyperdense and typically do not have associated calcifications. They are not well demarcated, with heterogeneous contrast enhancement. On MRI, lower grade PPTs typically have a more expansive growth pattern resulting in compression, rather than direct invasion, of adjacent structures, although invasion is certainly possible (especially for higher grade tumors). Pineocytomas are typically 3 cm or smaller, well-circumscribed, and more homogeneous, with hypointensity on T1 but hyperintensity on T2 (see Figure 10.5A–D). Pineoblastomas are typically larger than 3 cm, poorly circumscribed, and hypo- to isointense on T1 and iso- to mildly hyperintense on T2 with heterogeneous contrast enhancement (see Figure 10.6A–D). PPTIDs in general have variable features reflecting their intermediate status, with features of both pineocytomas and pineoblastomas depending on each individual tumor[86,90,94] (see Figure 10.7A–D). PTPRs are moderate in size (2.5–4 cm) and well-circumscribed, with T1 hyperintensity and increased T2 signal as well as heterogeneous contrast enhancement on MRI.[95]

Given the rarity of PPTs, there are no randomized trials to inform their management. The first step is maximal safe resection for (a) diagnosis; (b) relief of hydrocephalus, if present; and (c) cytoreduction.

- Pineocytomas require maximal safe resection, but those with GTR may not require additional therapy. Adjuvant fractionated RT is considered in the setting of STR or biopsy only, especially for tumors that lack neuronal differentiation or otherwise behave more like higher grade tumors.[96] Pineocytomas may be relatively radioresistant, and there are some data for radiosurgery as definitive or adjuvant treatment (20-year PFS and OS 81% and 76%).[97] Chemotherapy is not utilized.

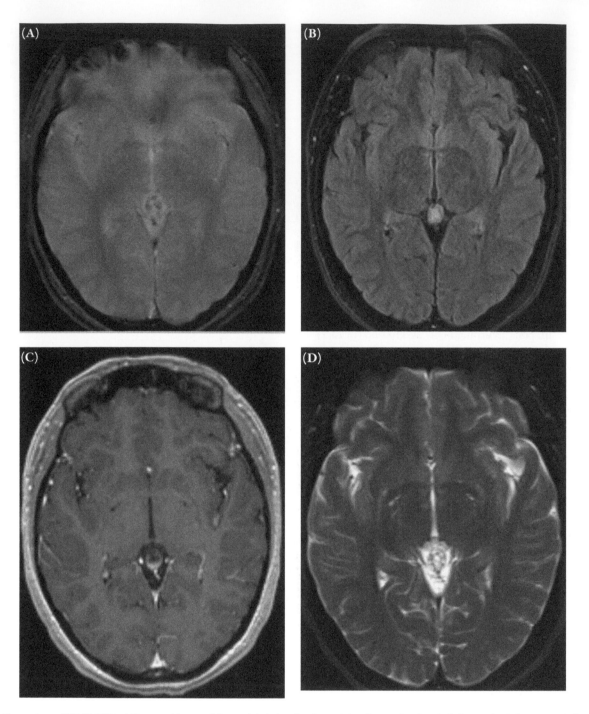

Figure 10.5 Pineocytoma. (A) MRI GRE axial image with a small focus of dark signal at the peripheral secondary "exploded" pineal calcification typically seen in pineocytomas. (B) MRI fluid-attenuated inversion recovery (FLAIR) axial image with hyperintensity in the pineal mass. (C and D) MRI T1 post-contrast (C) and T2 fat saturation (D) axial images of a partially cystic mass with strong peripheral enhancement.

- Pineoblastomas are treated similarly to medulloblastomas, with maximal safe resection followed by CSI and focal boost. Interestingly, there is some limited evidence that adult pineoblastomas patients do better than pediatric patients. GTR plays a significant role in pediatric pineoblastomas, but some adult patients may demonstrate long-term survival even with STR.[98] However, we feel GTR should be a goal if safe, given very limited experience in adults. Adjuvant chemotherapy should be considered, and the role of concurrent chemotherapy is not well established.[99,100] Radiosurgery has no role in the definitive setting, with poor 5-year PFS and OS of 27% and 48%, respectively.[97]

- PPTIDs comprise a heterogeneous group of tumors, and it is difficult to determine a specific set of recommendations. Adjuvant radiation is typically recommended, especially if less than GTR, grade 3, recurrent, or with other features suggesting aggressive behavior (e.g., more pineoblastomas-like features). Although leptomeningeal dissemination is possible, its

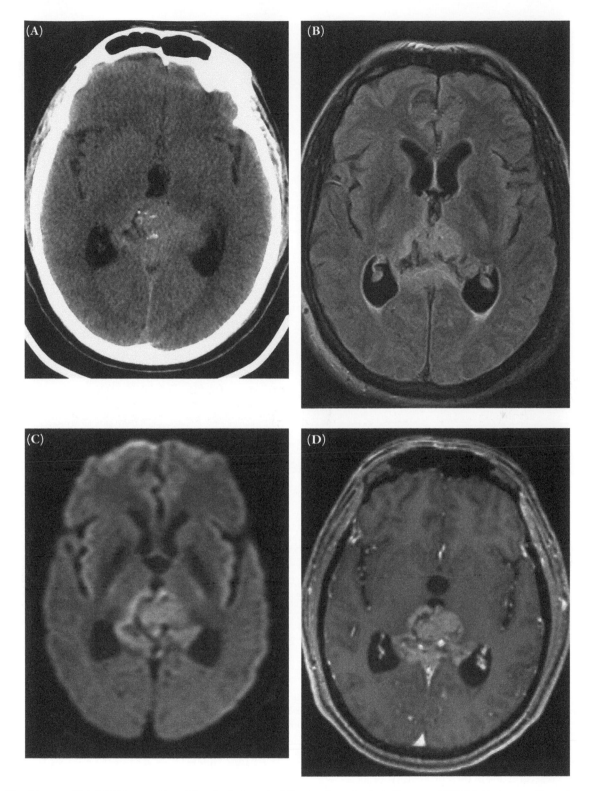

Figure 10.6 Pineoblastoma. (A) Axial CT image with peripherally distributed calcifications in an "exploded" pattern. (B) MRI fluid-attenuated inversion recovery (FLAIR) axial image of a large mass infiltrating the adjacent corpus callosum and thalami with obstructive hydrocephalus. (C) MRI diffusion-weighted imaging (DWI) axial image with diffusion restriction reflective of the expected hypercellularity. (D) MRI T1 post-contrast image with marked heterogeneous enhancement.

relatively low frequency (11.8% in one series) suggests that CSI should be reserved for those with evidence of leptomeningeal spread, and focal RT should be used in most cases.[101] The role of chemotherapy is even more controversial and does not appear to benefit patients with PPTIDs.[101,102] We would consider chemotherapy in cases with recurrent disease or leptomeningeal spread. Radiosurgery has no role in the definitive setting (except possibly in select grade 2 cases), with poor 5-year PFS and OS (50% and 56%, respectively).[97]

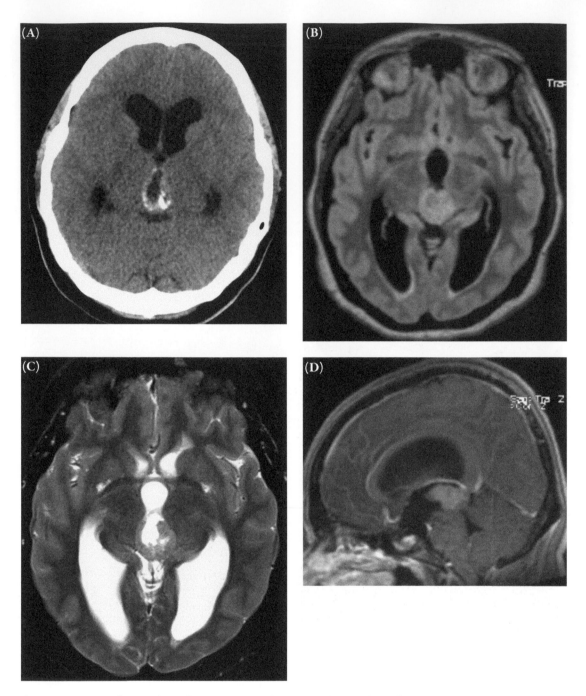

Figure 10.7 Pineal parenchymal tumor of intermediate differentiation. (A) Axial CT image with a partially calcified and cystic mass with indistinct margins. (B) MRI fluid-attenuated inversion recovery (FLAIR) axial image of the same with obstructive hydrocephalus, possibly with invasion into the thalami. (C) MRI T2 axial image with a hyperintense cystic component and an isointense solid component. (D) MRI T1 post-contrast sagittal image with marked enhancement in the solid component.

- PTPRs are typically considered for adjuvant radiation after maximal safe resection due to their propensity for local recurrence, particularly for recurrent or grade 3 tumors. However, the data about adjuvant radiation are conflicting, with some series demonstrating good control after adjuvant RT and others showing no benefit. Radiosurgery has been used as well in a small number of cases with reasonable outcome.[103–106]

Pineoblastomas are treated similarly to medulloblastomas, with maximal safe resection followed by CSI and focal boost.

PLEOMORPHIC XANTHOASTROCYTOMAS

Pleomorphic xanthoastrocytoma (PXA) is a glial tumor seen in young adults with a median age of 19 years.[107] However, the age range is quite broad, with cases reported from younger than 1 year to 84 years.[108] These tumors are mostly WHO grade 2 (77–80%) but can be WHO grade 3 if they have anaplastic features and behavior (20–23%). Presenting symptoms are, most commonly, signs of increased intracranial pressure (25–47%) and seizure (33–75%). The most common location is the temporal lobes (36–40%), followed by multifocal or spanning lobes (16–22%) and frontal lobes (7.5–10%). Rarely, patients can present with disease in the spinal cord or with diffuse leptomeningeal disease.[109]

Classically, PXAs appear as a cystic supratentorial mass with a solid mural nodule adjacent to the leptomeninges. However, these tumors can have a predominantly solid component with or without associated cyst or fluid-containing components.[110] MRI characteristics typically are bright/high T2-weighted signal but isointense by T1-weighted imaging. The solid component of PXAs enhance with gadolinium on T1-weighted imaging.[111] The cystic components do not typically show contrast enhancement but can in 25–33% of cases. The fluid in the cysts usually has an attenuation signal that is slightly higher than that of CSF (Figure 10.8).

Histologically, PXAs have a densely cellular glial component with large, multinucleated xanthomatous cells with foamy cytoplasm. WHO grade 3 PXAs will have anaplastic features with more atypical mitotic figures, a mitotic index of 5 or more per 10 HPF, necrosis, and/or endothelial proliferation.[112] The BRAF V600E mutation is found in 60–78% of PXAs, most notably in younger patients, suggesting that activation of the RAS/RAF/MEK/ERK pathway plays a role in tumorogenesis.[113–115]

> With the BRAF V600E mutation being common, BRAF inhibitors are being used with increasing frequency and have been shown to have efficacy in patients with PXA.

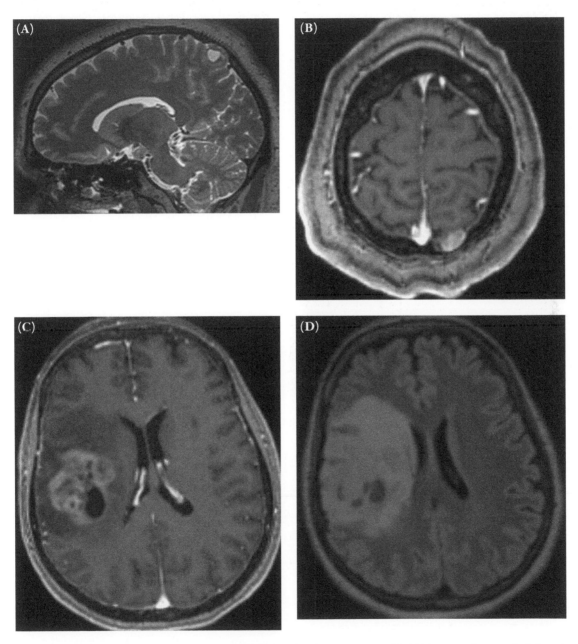

Figure 10.8 Pleomorphic xanthoastrocytoma. (A and B) sagittal T2 weighted (A) and axial T1 post contrast (B) MRI demonstrating a cortically based cystic lesion with enhancing mural nodule contacting the leptomeninges, with resulting calvarial remodeling. (C and D) MRI T1 post-contrast (C) and fluid-attenuated inversion recovery (FLAIR) (D) axial images of the anaplastic variant of pleomorphic xanthoastrocytomas with relatively larger size and robust surrounding vasogenic edema resembling that of high-grade gliomas.

Treatment of PXAs is surgical with a goal of GTR. SEER dataset analysis documented both an OS and PFS advantage for GTR versus STR or biopsy only with a hazard ratio of 2.8.[116] The median survival for patients WHO grade 2 tumors is 209 months, compared to 49 months for those with grade 3 tumors.[108] Adjuvant radiation after GTR has not been shown to provide either an OS or PFS benefit.[108,117,118] After STR, adjuvant radiation or chemotherapy is controversial, with conflicting data. A risk-adapted approach to adjuvant treatment is recommended, with more aggressive therapy appropriate for WHO grade 3 tumors. At recurrence, repeat surgery followed by salvage radiation and chemotherapy is typically recommended. With the BRAF V600E mutation being common, BRAF inhibitors such as vemurafenib and dabrafenib are being used with increasing frequency.[119-121] In a large non-randomized trial, more than 40% of PXA patients treated with BRAF-inhibiting monotherapy exhibited both radiographic and clinical response.[122]

SEER dataset analysis documented both an OS and PFS advantage for GTR versus STR or biopsy only with a hazard ratio of 2.8.

CONCLUSION

Rare CNS tumors in adults comprise a wide variety, most with limited evidence regarding management. Here, we reviewed the available literature pertinent to general management paradigms for a select number of rare tumors. Importantly, current knowledge on molecular advancements within the study of each of these tumors is reviewed and is a key theme as new molecular discoveries are incorporated into evolving treatment approaches. Multidisciplinary management, often at centers with specialized neuro-oncology providers, is recommended for these rare tumors.

What are the epidemiology and characteristics of medulloblastomas in adult?	0.5 per 1 million adults Average age at diagnosis is 30 years old Posterior fossa is the most common location
After maximal safe resection, treatment for medulloblastoma in adults often includes	Craniospinal radiation, plus concurrent/adjuvant chemotherapy
What is the WHO grade of cerebellar liponeurocytomas?	Always WHO grade 2
What are the epidemiology and tumor location of liponeurocytomas?	Average age at diagnosis is 49, most commonly located in the posterior fossa
Radiation therapy is used in liponeurocytomas in these situations:	At time of recurrence and occasionally after subtotal resection (if gross total resection is not possible)
What is the WHO grade of diffuse leptomeningeal glioneural tumor (DLGNT)?	WHO grade 2 or 3
What are the epidemiology and characteristics of DLGNT?	Rarely seen in adults Clinically and radiographically can mimic sarcoidosis, other malignant leptomeningeal process (i.e., leptomeningeal metastases), IgG4 disease, etc.
What is the treatment of DLGNT?	CSI or focal radiation with or without adjuvant chemotherapy; MEK or RAF inhibitors may be useful for BRAF fusion mutant tumors
Most common epilepsy-associated tumor is:	Ganglioglioma
Treatment of ganglioglioma involves:	Gross total resection; adjuvant XRT for grades 3–4 tumors; targeted therapies may be useful in BRAF V600E mutant tumors

Categories of pineal parenchymal tumors include:	Pineocytomas (WHO grade 1), pineal parenchymal tumors of intermediate differentiation (WHO grade 2 or 3), papillary tumors of the pineal region (WHO grade 2 or 3), and pineoblastomas (WHO grade 4)
What type of pineal tumor always requires CSI postoperatively?	Pineoblastomas
What are the WHO grades of pleomorphic xanthoastrocytoma (PXA)?	WHO grade 2 or 3
Common appearance of PXA on imaging includes:	Temporal lobe location, cystic mass with solid enhancing mural nodule
What is the most common potentially targetable mutation in PXA?	BRAF V600E mutations

QUESTIONS

1. Patients with gangliogliomas most commonly present with the following symptom:
   a. Headache
   b. Seizure
   c. Stroke
   d. Hearing loss

2. Gangliocytomas are tumors that typically are found in the
   a. Temporal lobe
   b. Brainstem
   c. Spinal cord
   d. Cerebellum

3. The most common genetic abnormality found in gangliogliomas is
   a. IDH-mutation
   b. MGMT promoter methylation
   c. BRAF V600E mutation
   d. BRAF fusion mutation

4. Diffuse leptomeningeal glioneuronal tumors (DLGNT) harbor alterations in this molecular pathway in 80% of cases:
   a. VEG-F
   b. PTEN
   c. EGFR
   d. MAPK/ERK

5. Gross total resection is the recommended therapy for DLGNT.
   a. True
   b. False

6. Pleomorphic xanthoastrocytomas (PXAs) are tumors that can arise in
   a. Frontal lobe
   b. Temporal lobe
   c. Spinal cord
   d. All of the above

7. Recommended therapy for PXA is gross total resection.
   a. True
   b. False

8. Following subtotal resection of a grade 2 PXA, adjuvant radiation therapy provides improved
   a. Overall survival
   b. Progression-free survival
   c. Both
   d. Neither

9. Patients with "standard-risk" medulloblastoma include those with
   a. M0 disease, STR (>1.5 cm^2 residual), anaplastic histology
   b. M$^+$ disease, GTR, classic histology
   c. M0 disease, NTR (≤1.5 cm^2 residual), desmoplastic histology
   d. M0 disease, GTR, extensive nodularity histology

10. This molecular subgroup of medulloblastoma is rarely seen in adults.
    a. WNT
    b. SHH
    c. Group 3
    d. Group 4

11. Medulloblastomas are more common in adults than children.
    a. True
    b. False

12. Cerebellar liponeurocytomas are typically treated with radiation therapy alone.
    a. True
    b. False

13. PPTs are the most common tumor of the pineal region.
    a. True
    b. False

14. All of the following are correct, *except*
    a. PPTIDs can be grade 2 or 3.
    b. Pineocytomas often do not require adjuvant RT after GTR.
    c. PTPRs are neuroepithelial tumors that resemble tissue of ependymal origin (SCO).
    d. Pineoblastomas exhibit pineocytomatous rosettes.

15. Pineoblastoma molecular subgroups include all of the following, *except*
    a. FOR2
    b. MYC
    c. MAPK
    d. DICER1/DROSHA

ANSWERS

1. b
2. d
3. c
4. d
5. b
6. d
7. a
8. d
9. c
10. c
11. b
12. b
13. b
14. d
15. c

REFERENCES

1. Shonka N, Brandes A, De Groot JF. Adult medulloblastoma, from spongioblastoma cerebelli to the present day: A review of treatment and the integration of molecular markers. *Oncology (Williston Park)*. Nov 2012;26(11):1083–1091.

2. Murase M, Saito K, Abiko T, et al. Medulloblastoma in older adults: A case report and literature review. *World Neurosurg*. Sep 2018;117:25–31. doi:10.1016/j.wneu.2018.05.216

3. Spreafico F, Ferrari A, Mascarin M, et al. Wilms tumor, medulloblastoma, and rhabdomyosarcoma in adult patients: Lessons learned from the pediatric experience. *Cancer Metastasis Rev*. Dec 2019;38(4):683–694. doi:10.1007/s10555-019-09831-3

4. Yong RL, Kavanagh EC, Fenton D, et al. Midline cerebellar medulloblastoma in a seventy-one-year-old patient. *Can J Neurol Sci*. Feb 2006;33(1):101–4. doi:10.1017/s0317167100004789

5. Saad AG, Balik V, Parvez A, El Jamal SM. Multifocal supra and infratentorial medulloblastoma in an adult: Histologic, immunohistochemical, and molecular evaluation of a rare case and review of the literature. *Appl Immunohistochem Mol Morphol*. Nov/Dec 2017;25(10):e89–e94. doi:10.1097/pai.0000000000000447

6. Ciccarino P, Rotilio A, Rossetto M, et al. Multifocal presentation of medulloblastoma in adulthood. *J Neurooncol*. Apr 2012;107(2):233–7. doi:10.1007/s11060-011-0746-7

7. Northcott PA, Korshunov A, Pfister SM, Taylor MD. The clinical implications of medulloblastoma subgroups. *Nat Rev Neurol*. May 8 2012;8(6):340–51. doi:10.1038/nrneurol.2012.78

8. Taylor MD, Northcott PA, Korshunov A, et al. Molecular subgroups of medulloblastoma: The current consensus. *Acta Neuropathol*. Apr 2012;123(4):465–72. doi:10.1007/s00401-011-0922-z

9. Ramaswamy V, Taylor MD. Medulloblastoma: From myth to molecular. *J Clin Oncol*. Jul 20 2017;35(21):2355–2363. doi:10.1200/jco.2017.72.7842

10. Juraschka K, Taylor MD. Medulloblastoma in the age of molecular subgroups: A review. *J Neurosurg Pediatr*. Oct 1 2019;24(4):353–363. doi:10.3171/2019.5.Peds18381

11. Louis DN, Perry A, Reifenberger G, et al. The 2016 World Health Organization Classification of Tumors of the Central Nervous System: A summary. *Acta Neuropathol*. Jun 2016;131(6):803–820. doi:10.1007/s00401-016-1545-1

12. Beier D, Kocakaya S, Hau P, Beier CP. The neuroradiological spectra of adult and pediatric medulloblastoma differ: Results from a literature-based meta-analysis. *Clin Neuroradiol*. Mar 2018;28(1):99–107. doi:10.1007/s00062-016-0517-0

13. Atalar B, Ozsahin M, Call J, et al. Treatment outcome and prognostic factors for adult patients with medulloblastoma: The Rare Cancer Network (RCN) experience. *Radiother Oncol*. Apr 2018;127(1):96–102. doi:10.1016/j.radonc.2017.12.028

14. Kann BH, Lester-Coll NH, Park HS, et al. Adjuvant chemotherapy and overall survival in adult medulloblastoma. *Neuro Oncol*. Feb 1 2017;19(2):259–269. doi:10.1093/neuonc/now150

15. Kocakaya S, Beier CP, Beier D. Chemotherapy increases long-term survival in patients with adult medulloblastoma: A literature-based meta-analysis. *Neuro Oncol*. Mar 2016;18(3):408–416. doi:10.1093/neuonc/nov185

16. Padovani L, Sunyach MP, Perol D, et al. Common strategy for adult and pediatric medulloblastoma: A multicenter series of 253 adults. *Int J Radiat Oncol Biol Phys*. Jun 1 2007;68(2):433–440. doi:10.1016/j.ijrobp.2006.12.030

17. De B, Beal K, De Braganca KC, et al. Long-term outcomes of adult medulloblastoma patients treated with radiotherapy. *J Neurooncol*. Jan 2018;136(1):95–104. doi:10.1007/s11060-017-2627-1

18. Friedrich C, von Bueren AO, von Hoff K, et al. Treatment of adult nonmetastatic medulloblastoma patients according to the paediatric HIT 2000 protocol: A prospective observational multicentre study. *Eur J Cancer*. Mar 2013;49(4):893–903. doi:10.1016/j.ejca.2012.10.006

19. Beier D, Proescholdt M, Reinert C, et al. Multicenter pilot study of radiochemotherapy as first-line treatment for adults with medulloblastoma (NOA-07). *Neuro Oncol*. Feb 19 2018;20(3):400–410. doi:10.1093/neuonc/nox155

20. Moots PL, O'Neill A, Londer H, et al. Preradiation chemotherapy for adult high-risk medulloblastoma: A trial of the ECOG-ACRIN Cancer Research Group (E4397). *Am J Clin Oncol*. Jun 2018;41(6):588–594. doi:10.1097/coc.0000000000000326

21. Majd N, Penas-Prado M. Updates on management of adult medulloblastoma. *Curr Treat Options Oncol*. Jun 24 2019;20(8):64. doi:10.1007/s11864-019-0663-0

22. Bechtel JT, Patton JM, Takei Y. Mixed mesenchymal and neuroectodermal tumor of the cerebellum. *Acta Neuropathol*. Mar 15 1978;41(3):261–3. doi:10.1007/bf00690447

23. Kleihues P, Cavanee WK, IARC. *Pathology and Genetics of Tumours of the Nervous System*. Lyon: International Agency for Research on Cancer; 2000.

24. Louis DN, Cancer IAfRo, Wiestler OD, Ohgaki H. *WHO Classification of Tumours of the Central Nervous System*. Lyon: International Agency for Research on Cancer; 2016.

25. Gembruch O, Junker A, Monninghoff C, et al. Liponeurocytoma: Systematic review of a rare entity. *World Neurosurg*. Dec 2018;120:214–233. doi:10.1016/j.wneu.2018.09.001

26. Xu L, Du J, Wang J, et al. The clinicopathological features of liponeurocytoma. *Brain Tumor Pathol*. Jan 2017;34(1):28–35. doi:10.1007/s10014-017-0279-7

27. Wolf A, Alghefari H, Krivosheya D, et al. Cerebellar liponeurocytoma: A rare intracranial tumor with possible familial predisposition. Case report. *J Neurosurg*. Jul 2016;125(1):57–61. doi:10.3171/2015.6.Jns142965

28. Pikis S, Fellig Y, Margolin E. Cerebellar liponeurocytoma in two siblings suggests a possible familial predisposition. *J Clin Neurosci*. Oct 2016;32:154–6. doi:10.1016/j.jocn.2016.04.004

29. Takami H, Mukasa A, Ikemura M, et al. Findings from positron emission tomography and genetic analyses for cerebellar liponeurocytoma. *Brain Tumor Pathol*. Jul 2015;32(3):210–5. doi:10.1007/s10014-014-0210-4

30. Khatri D, Bhaisora KS, Das KK, et al. Cerebellar liponeurocytoma: The dilemma of multifocality. *World Neurosurg*. Dec 2018;120:131–137. doi:10.1016/j.wneu.2018.08.156

31. Pelz D, Khezri N, Mainprize T, et al. Multifocal cerebellar liponeurocytoma. *Can J Neurol Sci*. Nov 2013;40(6):870–872. doi:10.1017/s0317167100016048

32. Scoppetta TL, Brito MC, Prado JL, Scoppetta LC. Multifocal cerebellar liponeurocytoma. *Neurology*. Nov 24 2015;85(21):1912. doi:10.1212/wnl.0000000000002156

33. Sivaraju L, Aryan S, Ghosal N, Hegde AS. Cerebellar liponeurocytoma presenting as multifocal bilateral cerebellar hemispheric mass lesions. *Neurol India*. Mar-Apr 2017;65(2):422–424. doi:10.4103/neuroindia.NI_1379_15

34. Hamzaoglu V, Ozalp H, Karatas D, et al. Clinical course of the untreated calcified big cerebellar liponeurocytoma. *J Surg Case Rep*. Nov 2018;2018(11):rjy316. doi:10.1093/jscr/rjy316

35. Limaiem F, Bellil S, Chelly I, et al. Recurrent cerebellar liponeurocytoma with supratentorial extension. *Can J Neurol Sci*. Sep 2009;36(5):662–665. doi:10.1017/s0317167100008222

36. Becker AJ, Wiestler OD, Figarella-Branger D, et al. Ganglioglioma. In Louis DN, Cancer IAfRo, Wiestler OD, Ohgaki H, eds. *WHO Classification of Tumours of the Central Nervous System*. Lyon: International Agency for Research on Cancer; 2016:138–141 (vol. v.1).

37. Gardiman MP, Fassan M, Orvieto E, et al. Diffuse leptomeningeal glioneuronal tumors: A new entity? *Brain Pathol*. Mar 2010;20(2):361–366. doi:10.1111/j.1750-3639.2009.00285.x

38. Rodriguez FJ, Perry A, Rosenblum MK, et al. Disseminated oligodendroglial-like leptomeningeal tumor of childhood: A distinctive clinicopathologic entity. *Acta Neuropathol*. Nov 2012;124(5):627–641. doi:10.1007/s00401-012-1037-x

39. Cho HJ, Myung JK, Kim H, et al. Primary diffuse leptomeningeal glioneuronal tumors. *Brain Tumor Pathol*. Jan 2015;32(1):49–55. doi:10.1007/s10014-014-0187-z

40. Deng MY, Sill M, Chiang J, et al. Molecularly defined diffuse leptomeningeal glioneuronal tumor (DLGNT) comprises two subgroups with distinct clinical and genetic features. *Acta Neuropathol*. Aug 2018;136(2):239–253. doi:10.1007/s00401-018-1865-4

41. Demir MK, Yapicier O, Yilmaz B, Kilic T. Magnetic resonance imaging findings of mixed neuronal-glial tumors with pathologic correlation: A review. *Acta Neurol Belg*. Sep 2018;118(3):379–386. doi:10.1007/s13760-018-0981-1

42. Fiaschi P, Badaloni F, Cagetti B, et al. Disseminated oligodendroglial-like leptomeningeal tumor in the adult: Case report and review of the literature. *World Neurosurg*. Jun 2018;114:53–57. doi:10.1016/j.wneu.2018.02.160

43. Xu H, Chen F, Zhu H, et al. Diffuse leptomeningeal glioneuronal tumor in a Chinese adult: A novel case report and review of literature. *Acta Neurol Belg*. Apr 2020;120(2):247–256. doi:10.1007/s13760-019-01262-9

44. Sievert AJ, Lang SS, Boucher KL, et al. Paradoxical activation and RAF inhibitor resistance of BRAF protein kinase fusions characterizing pediatric astrocytomas. *Proc Natl Acad Sci U S A*. Apr 9 2013;110(15):5957–5962. doi:10.1073/pnas.1219232110

45. Maraka S, Janku F. BRAF alterations in primary brain tumors. *Discov Med*. Aug 2018;26(141):51–60.

46. Zentner J, Wolf HK, Ostertun B, et al. Gangliogliomas: Clinical, radiological, and histopathological findings in 51 patients. *J Neurol Neurosurg Psychiatry*. Dec 1994;57(12):1497–1502. doi:10.1136/jnnp.57.12.1497

47. Blumcke I, Wiestler OD. Gangliogliomas: An intriguing tumor entity associated with focal epilepsies. *J Neuropathol Exp Neurol*. Jul 2002;61(7):575–584. doi:10.1093/jnen/61.7.575

48. Rumana CS, Valadka AB. Radiation therapy and malignant degeneration of benign supratentorial gangliogliomas. *Neurosurgery*. May 1998;42(5):1038–1043. doi:10.1097/00006123-199805000-00049

49. Schittenhelm J, Reifenberger G, Ritz R, et al. Primary anaplastic ganglioglioma with a small-cell glioblastoma component. *Clin Neuropathol*. Mar-Apr 2008;27(2):91–95. doi:10.5414/npp27091

50. Zhang D, Henning TD, Zou LG, et al. Intracranial ganglioglioma: Clinicopathological and MRI findings in 16 patients. *Clin Radiol*. Jan 2008;63(1):80–91. doi:10.1016/j.crad.2007.06.010

51. Thom M, Blumcke I, Aronica E. Long-term epilepsy-associated tumors. *Brain Pathol*. May 2012;22(3):350–79. doi:10.1111/j.1750-3639.2012.00582.x

52. Blumcke I, Aronica E, Becker A, et al. Low-grade epilepsy-associated neuroepithelial tumours: The 2016 WHO classification. *Nat Rev Neurol*. Dec 2016;12(12):732–740. doi:10.1038/nrneurol.2016.173

53. Giorgianni A, Pellegrino C, De Benedictis A, et al. Lhermitte-Duclos disease. A case report. *Neuroradiol J*. Dec 2013;26(6):655–660. doi:10.1177/197140091302600608

54. Zülch KJ. *Atlas of Gross Neurosurgical Pathology*. New York: Springer-Verlag; 1975.

55. Brain tumor registry of Japan. *Neurol Med Chir (Tokyo)*. 1992;32(7 Spec No):381–547.

56. Suh YL, Koo H, Kim TS, et al. Tumors of the central nervous system in Korea: A multicenter study of 3221 cases. *J Neurooncol*. Feb 2002;56(3):251–259. doi:10.1023/a:1015092501279

57. McLendon RE, Provenzale J. Glioneuronal tumors of the central nervous system. *Brain Tumor Pathol*. 2002;19(2):51–58. doi:10.1007/bf02478927

58. Jiang T, Wang J, Du J, et al. Lhermitte-Duclos disease (dysplastic gangliocytoma of the cerebellum) and Cowden syndrome: Clinical experience from a single institution with long-term follow-up. *World Neurosurg*. Aug 2017;104:398–406. doi:10.1016/j.wneu.2017.04.147

59. Ngeow J, Eng C. Germline PTEN mutation analysis for PTEN hamartoma tumor syndrome. *Methods Mol Biol*. 2016;1388:63–73. doi:10.1007/978-1-4939-3299-3_6

60. Yakubov E, Ghoochani A, Buslei R, et al. Hidden association of Cowden syndrome, PTEN mutation and meningioma frequency. *Oncoscience*. 2016;3(5-6):149–155. doi:10.18632/oncoscience.305

61. Leslie NR, Longy M. Inherited PTEN mutations and the prediction of phenotype. *Semin Cell Dev Biol*. Apr 2016;52:30–38. doi:10.1016/j.semcdb.2016.01.030

62. Chappe C, Padovani L, Scavarda D, et al. Dysembryoplastic neuroepithelial tumors share with pleomorphic xanthoastrocytomas and gangliogliomas BRAF(V600E) mutation and expression. *Brain Pathol*. Sep 2013;23(5):574–583. doi:10.1111/bpa.12048

63. Chen X, Pan C, Zhang P, et al. BRAF V600E mutation is a significant prognosticator of the tumour regrowth rate in brainstem gangliogliomas. *J Clin Neurosci*. Dec 2017;46:50–57. doi:10.1016/j.jocn.2017.09.014

64. Koelsche C, Wohrer A, Jeibmann A, et al. Mutant BRAF V600E protein in ganglioglioma is predominantly expressed by neuronal tumor cells. *Acta Neuropathol*. Jun 2013;125(6):891–900. doi:10.1007/s00401-013-1100-2

65. Horbinski C. What do we know about IDH1/2 mutations so far, and how do we use it? *Acta Neuropathol*. May 2013;125(5):621–636. doi:10.1007/s00401-013-1106-9

66. Ulutin HC, Onguru O, Pak Y. Postoperative radiotherapy for ganglioglioma: Report of three cases and review of the literature. *Minim Invasive Neurosurg*. Dec 2002;45(4):224–227. doi:10.1055/s-2002-36202

67. Tarnaris A, O'Brien C, Redfern RM. Ganglioglioma with anaplastic recurrence of the neuronal element following radiotherapy. *Clin Neurol Neurosurg*. Dec 2006;108(8):761–767. doi:10.1016/j.clineuro.2005.09.005

68. Song JY, Kim JH, Cho YH, et al. Treatment and outcomes for gangliogliomas: A single-center review of 16 patients. *Brain Tumor Res Treat*. Oct 2014;2(2):49–55. doi:10.14791/btrt.2014.2.2.49

69. Liauw SL, Byer JE, Yachnis AT, et al. Radiotherapy after subtotally resected or recurrent ganglioglioma. *Int J Radiat Oncol Biol Phys*. Jan 1 2007;67(1):244–247. doi:10.1016/j.ijrobp.2006.08.029

70. Luyken C, Blumcke I, Fimmers R, et al. Supratentorial gangliogliomas: Histopathologic grading and tumor recurrence in 184 patients with a median follow-up of 8 years. *Cancer*. Jul 1 2004;101(1):146–155. doi:10.1002/cncr.20332

71. Al-Hussaini M, Sultan I, Abuirmileh N, et al. Pineal gland tumors: Experience from the SEER database. *J Neurooncol*. Sep 2009;94(3):351–358. doi:10.1007/s11060-009-9881-9

72. Choque-Velasquez J, Hernesniemi J. Unedited microneurosurgery of a pineal region ependymoma. *Surg Neurol Int*. 2018;9:260. doi:10.4103/sni.sni_355_18

73. Dinc C, Iplikcioglu AC, Ozek E. Pineal epidermoid tumors: Report of five cases. *Turk Neurosurg*. 2013;23(4):446–450. doi:10.5137/1019-5149.Jtn.6219-12.0

74. Hogan R, Almira-Suarez I, Li S, et al. Clinical management of prostate cancer metastasis to pineal gland: Case report and review of literature. *World Neurosurg*. Feb 2019;122:464–468. doi:10.1016/j.wneu.2018.11.111

75. Ji J, Gu C, Zhang M, et al. Pineal region metastasis with intraventricular seeding: A case report and literature review. *Medicine (Baltimore)*. Aug 2019;98(34):e16652. doi:10.1097/md.0000000000016652

76. Lee KH, Lall RR, Chandler JP, et al. Pineal chordoid meningioma complicated by repetitive hemorrhage during pregnancy: Case report and literature review. *Neuropathology*. Apr 2013;33(2):192–198. doi:10.1111/j.1440-1789.2012.01337.x

77. Sasani M, Solmaz B, Oktenoglu T, Ozer AF. An unusual location for a choroid plexus papilloma: The pineal region. *Childs Nerv Syst*. Jul 2014;30(7):1307–1311. doi:10.1007/s00381-014-2361-3

78. Leston J, Mottolese C, Champier J, et al. Contribution of the daily melatonin profile to diagnosis of tumors of the pineal region. *J Neurooncol*. Jul 2009;93(3):387–394. doi:10.1007/s11060-008-9792-1

79. Fevre-Montange M, Champier J, Szathmari A, et al. Histological features and expression of enzymes implicated in melatonin synthesis in pineal parenchymal tumours and in cultured tumoural pineal cells. *Neuropathol Appl Neurobiol*. Jun 2008;34(3):296–305. doi:10.1111/j.1365-2990.2007.00891.x

80. Jimenez-Heffernan JA, Barcena C, et al. Cytologic features of the normal pineal gland of adults. *Diagn Cytopathol*. Aug 2015;43(8):642–645. doi:10.1002/dc.23282

81. Coy S, Dubuc AM, Dahiya S, et al. Nuclear CRX and FOXJ1 expression differentiates non-germ cell pineal region tumors and supports the ependymal differentiation of papillary tumor of the pineal region. *Am J Surg Pathol*. Oct 2017;41(10):1410–1421. doi:10.1097/pas.0000000000000903

82. Manila A, Mariangela N, Libero L, et al. Is CRX protein a useful marker in differential diagnosis of tumors of the pineal region? *Pediatr Dev Pathol*. Mar-Apr 2014;17(2):85–8. doi:10.2350/13-06-1346-oa.1

83. Fevre-Montange M, Vasiljevic A, Frappaz D, et al. Utility of Ki67 immunostaining in the grading of pineal parenchymal tumours: A multicentre study. *Neuropathol Appl Neurobiol*. Feb 2012;38(1):87–94. doi:10.1111/j.1365-2990.2011.01202.x

84. Borit A, Blackwood W, Mair WG. The separation of pineocytoma from pineoblastoma. *Cancer*. Mar 15 1980;45(6):1408–1418. doi:10.1002/1097-0142(19800315)45:6<1408::aid-cncr2820450619>3.0.co;2-0

85. Jouvet A, Saint-Pierre G, Fauchon F, et al. Pineal parenchymal tumors: A correlation of histological features with prognosis in 66 cases. *Brain Pathol*. Jan 2000;10(1):49–60. doi:10.1111/j.1750-3639.2000.tb00242.x

86. Amato-Watkins AC, Lammie A, Hayhurst C, Leach P. Pineal parenchymal tumours of intermediate differentiation: An evidence-based review of a new pathological entity. *Br J Neurosurg*. 2016;30(1):11–15. doi:10.3109/02688697.2015.1096912

87. Pfaff E, Aichmuller C, Sill M, et al. Molecular subgrouping of primary pineal parenchymal tumors reveals distinct subtypes correlated with clinical parameters and genetic alterations. *Acta Neuropathol*. Feb 2020;139(2):243–257. doi:10.1007/s00401-019-02101-0

88. Liu APY, Gudenas B, Lin T, et al. Risk-adapted therapy and biological heterogeneity in pineoblastoma: Integrated clinico-pathological analysis from the prospective, multi-center SJMB03 and SJYC07 trials. *Acta Neuropathol*. Feb 2020;139(2):259–271. doi:10.1007/s00401-019-02106-9

89. Han SJ, Clark AJ, Ivan ME, et al. Pathology of pineal parenchymal tumors. *Neurosurg Clin N Am*. Jul 2011;22(3):335–340, vii. doi:10.1016/j.nec.2011.05.006

90. Dahiya S, Perry A. Pineal tumors. *Adv Anat Pathol*. Nov 2010;17(6):419–427. doi:10.1097/PAP.0b013e3181f895a4

91. Heim S, Beschorner R, Mittelbronn M, et al. Increased mitotic and proliferative activity are associated with worse prognosis in papillary tumors of the pineal region. *Am J Surg Pathol*. Jan 2014;38(1):106–110. doi:10.1097/PAS.0b013e31829e492d

92. Verma A, Epari S, Bakiratharajan D, et al. Primary pineal tumors: Unraveling histological challenges and certain clinical myths. *Neurol India*. Mar-Apr 2019;67(2):491–502. doi:10.4103/0028-3886.258045

93. Cimino PJ, Gonzalez-Cuyar LF, Perry A, Dahiya S. Lack of BRAF-V600E mutation in papillary tumor of the pineal region. *Neurosurgery*. Oct 2015;77(4):621–628. doi:10.1227/neu.0000000000000877

94. Nakamura M, Saeki N, Iwadate Y, et al. Neuroradiological characteristics of pineocytoma and pineoblastoma. *Neuroradiology*. Jul 2000;42(7):509–514. doi:10.1007/s002349900243

95. Vaghela V, Radhakrishnan N, Radhakrishnan VV, et al. Advanced magnetic resonance imaging with histopathological correlation in papillary tumor of pineal region: Report of a case and review of literature. *Neurol India*. Nov-Dec 2010;58(6):928–932. doi:10.4103/0028-3886.73750

96. Clark AJ, Ivan ME, Sughrue ME, et al. Tumor control after surgery and radiotherapy for pineocytoma. *J Neurosurg*. Aug 2010;113(2):319–324. doi:10.3171/2009.12.Jns091683

97. Iorio-Morin C, Kano H, Huang M, et al. Histology-stratified tumor control and patient survival after stereotactic radiosurgery for pineal region tumors: A report from the International Gamma Knife Research Foundation. *World Neurosurg*. Nov 2017;107:974–982. doi:10.1016/j.wneu.2017.07.097

98. Gener MA, Conger AR, Van Gompel J, et al. Clinical, pathological, and surgical outcomes for adult pineoblastomas. *World Neurosurg*. Dec 2015;84(6):1816–1824. doi:10.1016/j.wneu.2015.08.005

99. Mynarek M, Pizer B, Dufour C, et al. Evaluation of age-dependent treatment strategies for children and young adults with pineoblastoma: Analysis of pooled European Society for Paediatric Oncology (SIOP-E) and US Head Start data. *Neuro Oncol*. Apr 1 2017;19(4):576–585. doi:10.1093/neuonc/now234

100. Gaito S, Malagoli M, Depenni R, et al. Pineoblastoma in adults: A rare case successfully treated with multimodal approach including craniospinal irradiation using helical tomotherapy. *Cureus*. Oct 7 2019;11(10):e5852. doi:10.7759/cureus.5852

101. Mallick S, Benson R, Rath GK. Patterns of care and survival outcomes in patients with pineal parenchymal tumor of intermediate differentiation: An individual patient data analysis. *Radiother Oncol*. Nov 2016;121(2):204–208. doi:10.1016/j.radonc.2016.10.025

102. Choque-Velasquez J, Resendiz-Nieves JC, Jahromi BR, et al. Pineal parenchymal tumors of intermediate differentiation: A long-term follow-up study in Helsinki neurosurgery. *World Neurosurg*. Feb 2019;122:e729–e739. doi:10.1016/j.wneu.2018.10.128

103. Lancia A, Becherini C, Detti B, et al. Radiotherapy for papillary tumor of the pineal region: A systematic review of the literature. *Clin Neurol Neurosurg*. Mar 2020;190:105646. doi:10.1016/j.clineuro.2019.105646

104. Fauchon F, Hasselblatt M, Jouvet A, et al. Role of surgery, radiotherapy and chemotherapy in papillary tumors of the pineal region: A multicenter study. *J Neurooncol*. Apr 2013;112(2):223–231. doi:10.1007/s11060-013-1050-5

105. Fernandez-Mateos C, Martinez R, Vaquero J. Long-term follow-up after radiosurgery of papillary tumor of pineal region: 2 case reports and review of literature. *World Neurosurg*. Aug 2018;116:190–193. doi:10.1016/j.wneu.2018.05.080

106. Choque-Velasquez J, Colasanti R, Resendiz-Nieves J, et al. Papillary tumor of the pineal region in children: Presentation of a case and comprehensive literature review. *World Neurosurg*. Sep 2018;117:144–152. doi:10.1016/j.wneu.2018.06.020

107. Lipper MH, Eberhard DA, Phillips CD, et al Pleomorphic xanthoastrocytoma, a distinctive astroglial tumor: Neuroradiologic and pathologic features. *AJNR Am J Neuroradiol*. Nov-Dec 1993;14(6):1397–1404.

108. Mallick S, Giridhar P, Benson R, et al. Demography, pattern of care, and survival in patients with xanthoastrocytoma: A systematic review and individual patient data analysis of 325 cases. *J Neurosci Rural Pract*. Jul 2019;10(3):430–437. doi:10.1055/s-0039-1697873

109. Benjamin C, Faustin A, Snuderl M, Pacione D. Anaplastic pleomorphic xanthoastrocytoma with spinal leptomeningeal spread at the time of diagnosis in an adult. *J Clin Neurosci*. Aug 2015;22(8):1370–1373. doi:10.1016/j.jocn.2015.02.026

110. Crespo-Rodriguez AM, Smirniotopoulos JG, Rushing EJ. MR and CT imaging of 24 pleomorphic xanthoastrocytomas (PXA) and a review of the literature. *Neuroradiology*. Apr 2007;49(4):307–315. doi:10.1007/s00234-006-0191-z

111. Tien RD, Cardenas CA, Rajagopalan S. Pleomorphic xanthoastrocytoma of the brain: MR findings in six patients. *AJR Am J Roentgenol*. Dec 1992;159(6):1287–1290. doi:10.2214/ajr.159.6.1442403

112. Rutkowski MJ, Oh T, Niflioglu GG, et al. Pleomorphic xanthoastrocytoma with anaplastic features: Retrospective case series. *World Neurosurg*. Nov 2016;95:368–374. doi:10.1016/j.wneu.2016.07.068

113. Dias-Santagata D, Lam Q, Vernovsky K, et al. BRAF V600E mutations are common in pleomorphic xanthoastrocytoma: Diagnostic and therapeutic implications. *PLoS One*. Mar 29 2011;6(3):e17948. doi:10.1371/journal.pone.0017948

114. Schindler G, Capper D, Meyer J, et al. Analysis of BRAF V600E mutation in 1,320 nervous system tumors reveals high mutation frequencies in pleomorphic xanthoastrocytoma, ganglioglioma and extra-cerebellar pilocytic astrocytoma. *Acta Neuropathol*. Mar 2011;121(3):397–405. doi:10.1007/s00401-011-0802-6

115. Ida CM, Rodriguez FJ, Burger PC, et al. Pleomorphic xanthoastrocytoma: Natural history and long-term follow-up. *Brain Pathol*. Sep 2015;25(5):575–586. doi:10.1111/bpa.12217

116. Perkins SM, Mitra N, Fei W, Shinohara ET. Patterns of care and outcomes of patients with pleomorphic xanthoastrocytoma: A SEER analysis. *J Neurooncol*. Oct 2012;110(1):99–104. doi:10.1007/s11060-012-0939-8

117. Lim S, Kim JH, Kim SA, et al. Prognostic factors and therapeutic outcomes in 22 patients with pleomorphic xanthoastrocytoma. *J Korean Neurosurg Soc*. May 2013;53(5):281–287. doi:10.3340/jkns.2013.53.5.281

118. Oh T, Kaur G, Madden M, et al. Pleomorphic xanthoastrocytomas: Institutional experience of 18 patients. *J Clin Neurosci*. Oct 2014;21(10):1767–1772. doi:10.1016/j.jocn.2014.04.002

119. Hussain F, Horbinski CM, Chmura SJ, et al Response to BRAF/MEK inhibition after progression with BRAF inhibition in a patient with anaplastic pleomorphic xanthoastrocytoma. *Neurologist*. Sep 2018;23(5):163–166. doi:10.1097/nrl.0000000000000194

120. Brown NF, Carter T, Mulholland P. Dabrafenib in BRAFV600-mutated anaplastic pleomorphic xanthoastrocytoma. *CNS Oncol*. Jan 2017;6(1):5–9. doi:10.2217/cns-2016-0031

121. Migliorini D, Aguiar D, Vargas MI, et al. BRAF/MEK double blockade in refractory anaplastic pleomorphic xanthoastrocytoma. *Neurology*. Mar 28 2017;88(13):1291–1293. doi:10.1212/wnl.0000000000003767

122. Kaley T, Touat M, Subbiah V, et al. BRAF inhibition in BRAF(V600)-mutant gliomas: Results from the VE-BASKET Study. *J Clin Oncol*. Oct 23 2018:Jco2018789990. doi:10.1200/jco.2018.78.9990

11 | PRIMARY CENTRAL NERVOUS SYSTEM LYMPHOMA AND HEMATOPOIETIC NEOPLASMS AFFECTING THE NERVOUS SYSTEM

MARY JANE LIM-FAT AND LAKSHMI NAYAK

INTRODUCTION

Primary central nervous system lymphoma (PCNSL) is a rare and aggressive variant of extranodal non-Hodgkin lymphoma (NHL), which, by definition, involves compartments of the central nervous system (CNS) (brain, leptomeninges, eyes, or spinal cord) in the absence of systemic disease. Ninety percent of PCNSL cases consist of diffuse large cell lymphomas (DLBCL), and the remaining 10% include T-cell lymphomas, Burkitt lymphomas, or low-grade lymphomas.[1] Compared to other subtypes of extranodal lymphoma, PCNSL has a worse prognosis, with only about 50% of patients achieving remission and with high risk of recurrence. PCNSL remains unique in its diagnosis, management, and surveillance compared to other CNS tumors. Advances in molecular profiling and ongoing clinical trials promise to shape the oncologist's approach to PCNSL disease. The first part of this chapter covers primary and secondary lymphomas affecting the CNS; in the second part other hematopoietic neoplasms affecting the nervous system are discussed.

> Primary CNS lymphoma is a variant of non-Hodgkin lymphoma that can involve the brain, leptomeninges, eyes, and spinal cord in the absence of systemic disease.

PRIMARY CENTRAL NERVOUS SYSTEM LYMPHOMAS

EPIDEMIOLOGY

There are around 1,500 new cases of PCNSL diagnosed in the United States every year. PCNSL makes up about 4% of all newly diagnosed primary tumors of the CNS. The previous trend in the 1980s–1990s of higher incidence in males age 20–64 years was attributed to the human immunodeficiency virus (HIV) and acquired immune deficiency syndrome (AIDS) epidemic. This is no longer observed due to effective antiretroviral therapy. The highest incidence is now observed in immunocompetent patients older than 65 years and is predicted to increase with the growing aging population. Immunodeficiency syndromes are strong risk factors that predispose patients to PCNSL and most are those

infected with Epstein-Barr virus (EBV). These also include HIV, iatrogenic immune suppression (patients with autoimmune conditions or organ transplant), and congenital immune disorders (ataxia-telangiectasia, Wiskott-Aldrich syndrome, severe combined immunodeficiencies, or X-linked lymphoproliferative disease). The association between PCNSL and autoimmune diseases such as rheumatoid arthritis, Sjögren syndrome, systemic lupus erythematosus, sarcoidosis, vasculitis, and myasthenia gravis is in part due to disease-modifying therapies but might also be secondary to the autoimmune disease itself.[3]

> The highest incidence of PCNSL is now observed in immunocompetent patients older than 65.

PATHOGENESIS

The exact mechanisms and events leading to the development of PCNSL have not been clearly elucidated. Studies were previously limited by, among several factors, the rarity of the disease and lack of molecular characterization due to often limited tissue at the time of diagnosis.

The histopathological appearance of PCNSL comprises malignant B cells with a high proliferative index, organized in an angiocentric pattern and intermixed with other reactive cells (i.e., small lymphocytes, macrophages, and activated microglial cells). A large proportion of these malignant cells express pan B-cell markers such as CD19, CD20, CD22, and CD79a. In the 2000s, a seminal paper subclassified non-CNSL DLBCLs into three molecular groups based on gene expression profiling: germinal center B-cell like (GCB), activated B-cell like (ABC)/non-germinal center (non-GCB), and a smaller subset of type 3 large B-cell lymphoma.[4] Immunohistochemistry (IHC) markers CD10, CD138, MUM1, and BCL-6 are useful to distinguish these DLBCL subtypes.[5] Applying these markers on PCNSL tissue samples, the majority of PCNSL (>85%) have been classified as non-GCB subtype.[6]

The invasion of the CNS by malignant large B cells could be due to intrathecal proliferation of transformed B cells or, alternatively, via systemic invasion of malignant cells through the blood–brain barrier aided by chemokines and mutations in cell-adhesion molecules such as *MUM1*, *CXCL13*, and

TABLE 11.1 Genetic alterations associated with the pathogenesis of primary central nervous system lymphoma

TYPE OF MUTATION	GENE	FUNCTION
Point mutation (non-somatic hypermutation/ aberrant somatic hypermutation)	ATM, TP53, PTEN, PIK3CA, JAK3, CTNNB1, PTPN11, KRAS, PIM1, BTG2, MYD88, CD79B, MALT1, CARD11	
Somatic hypermutation/aberrant somatic hypermutation	BCL6 PIM1, PX5, RhoH/TTF, MYC IGH	Promoter substitution Proto-oncogene activation IGH translocation
Gain of genetic material	12q (STAT6, MDM2, CDK4, GLI1), 1q, 7q, 18q 9p24.1 (CD274 (PD-L1)/PDCD1LG2(PD-L2)	NF-κB activation Tumor-immune evasion
Loss of genetic material	6p21 (HLA) 9P21 (CKDN2A) 6q21-23 (PTPRK, PRDM1, A20 (TNFAIP3)	Immune escape Proliferation Decreased cell adhesion, increased tumor activation, NF-κB activation
DNA hypermethylation	CKDN2A, DPAK, p14^{ARF} p16^{INK4}α, RFC, MGMT	Decreased expression

From Cai Q, Fang Y, Young KH.[84]

CHI3L1.[7] These genes are differentially expressed in PCNSL compared to systemic DLBCL.

Next-generation sequencing has also identified high prevalence of *MYD88, CD79B* mutations, and less frequently *CARD11* and *TNFAIP3* mutations associated with activation of the B-cell receptor (BCR), toll-like receptor (TLR), and nuclear factor-kappa beta (NF-κβ) pathways.[8] Another genomic alteration noted in PCNSL is frequent inactivation of *CDKN2A.* In addition, analysis of the immunoglobulin variable heavy gene (IgHV) demonstrates that most PCNSL cells have somatic hypermutation and intraclonal heterogeneity, which supports the derivation of mutated germinal center B cells.[9] Recently, *9p24.1/PD-L1(CD274)/PD-L2 (PDCD1LG2)* copy-number alterations and associated increased expression of the programmed cell death protein 1 (PD-1) ligands PD-L1 and PD-L2 have been shown in PCNSL and, less commonly, chromosomal rearrangements involving *PD-L1* or *PD-L2* and selective overexpression of the respective ligand, suggesting a potential mechanism for immune evasion.[10] The genetic alterations involved in the pathogenesis of PCNSL are summarized in Table 11.1.

Last, a causal EBV relationship to PCNSL remains controversial. While genomic material has been detected in PCNSL cells in both immunocompromised and immunocompetent patients, most immunocompetent patients do not have EBV genomic DNA within their tumors, and presence of EBV within spinal fluid is not always associated with PCNSL.[11,12]

CLINICAL PRESENTATION
The clinical presentation of PCNSL can vary greatly depending on the CNS compartment involved. Up to 70% of patients present with focal neurological deficits if eloquent brain parenchyma or leptomeninges are involved.[13] Up to 45% of patients can also present with non-specific cognitive or neuro-psychiatric disturbances, which could lead to delayed diagnosis in the absence of a high level of suspicion. Up to 35% of patients experience increased signs and symptoms of intracranial pressure (headache, nausea, vomiting, and confusion). Cortical lesions can cause seizures, although this is less

frequent compared to other brain tumors (<15%). Visual or ocular symptoms occur in 15–20% of patients (mostly blurry vision, decreased acuity, floaters, and more rarely diplopia) and ocular involvement can be present in up to 25% of newly diagnosed PCNSL cases.[14] While leptomeningeal involvement is not uncommon, less than a third of patients with leptomeningeal dissemination exhibit focal neurological symptoms. Leptomeningeal involvement or spinal cord lesions are typically associated with an intraparenchymal brain lesion and are very rarely observed in isolation. Spinal cord involvement from CNS lymphoma tends to be intramedullary and can present with sensory deficits, long-tract signs, and bowel/bladder dysfunction.

> Up to 45% of patients with PCNSL can present with nonspecific cognitive or neuro-psychiatric disturbances, which could lead to delayed diagnosis in the absence of a high level of suspicion.

DIAGNOSIS

The diagnostic evaluation of suspected PCNSL entails (1) identification of any CNS lesion and (2) extent of disease evaluation to assess for involvement of other CNS compartments and to rule out systemic disease.

IMAGING FEATURES

Imaging of the neuro-axis with gadolinium-enhanced magnetic resonance imaging (MRI) is the preferred imaging modality in cases of suspected PCNSL. Contrast-enhanced computed tomography (CT) can be obtained in patients with contraindications to MRI, although this is not as sensitive nor specific. Classically, the lesions associated with PCNSL are well-circumscribed with homogeneous enhancement after gadolinium contrast and modest surrounding edema. These lesions are less likely associated with necrosis, calcification,

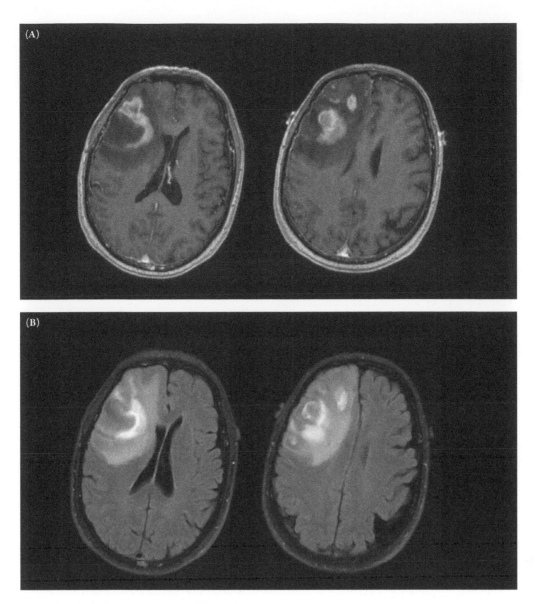

Figure 11.1 (A) MRI brain (T1 post-gadolinium sequence) showing large contrast-enhancing lesion in right frontal lobe. Biopsy was later consistent with diffuse large B-cell lymphoma; extent of disease evaluation confirmed primary CNS lymphoma. (B) T2/fluid-attenuated inversion recovery (FLAIR) sequence showing surrounding vasogenic edema.

or hemorrhage. PCNSL lesions are highly cellular and show restricted diffusion on diffusion weighted images. Multiple ring-enhancing lesions can be present in immunocompromised patients, but immunocompetent patients tend to present with a solitary lesion, without a ring-enhancing pattern (Figure 11.1). While the majority of PCNSL patients develop solitary brain lesions, 25% can have multifocal disease. Up to 60% of intracranial lesions tend to be periventricular, particularly in the thalamus, basal ganglia, or corpus callosum. Other locations include the frontal (20%), parietal (18%), temporal (15%), and occipital (4%) lobes.[15] MRI of the spine can detect spinal cord and leptomeningeal involvement.

PATHOLOGY

Pathologic confirmation with brain biopsy of an accessible lesion remains the gold standard in the diagnosis of PCNSL.

Diagnostic yield of biopsies can be significantly compromised by the use of corticosteroids, in particular dexamethasone, which is often used to decrease the burden of neurological symptoms. Even a single dose (or a short course) of corticosteroids can cause the disappearance of PCNSL lesions due to their lymphocytotoxic activity and lead to false-negative biopsies. In the absence of acute neurological emergencies, holding off on corticosteroids until biopsy is obtained is a reasonable recommendation. Steroid use preoperatively in PCNSL cases has been associated with diagnostic delay and a higher risk of additional biopsies.[16] Intraoperative rapid diagnosis of PCNSL includes intraoperative cytological preparations and frozen section slides with a reported rate of agreement of 83–96% with postoperative definitive diagnosis.[17] PCNSL can be histologically indistinguishable from malignant gliomas or demyelination on frozen section because the edge of the lesions can contain a combination of gliosis, demyelinating features, macrophages, and non-neoplastic perivascular lymphocytes. Flow cytometry on tissue specimen is often helpful in these cases. Postoperative confirmation with examination of permanent sections is preferred. Immunohistochemical, pathological, and molecular features of primary CNS lymphoma were described earlier.

CEREBROSPINAL FLUID ANALYSIS

Malignant cells are present in the cerebospinal fluid (CSF) of about 40% of patients with PCNSL, and CSF analysis for extent of disease of evaluation is therefore recommended when deemed safe (no significant mass effect or clinical signs of high intracranial pressure). CSF evaluation should include cell count, protein, glucose, cytology, flow cytometry, and IgH gene rearrangement studies (by polymerase chain reaction [PCR]).

The typical CSF profile in PCNSL includes lymphocytic pleocytosis, elevated protein concentration, and normal or occasionally lowered glucose. Malignant cells confirming lymphoma can be found in 10–30% of patients. Immunophenotypic analysis by flow cytometry can be helpful to identify antibodies against lymphocytic antigens and identify both the lymphoid lineage (B- vs. T-cell subtype) and clonality of the abnormal cells. Combination of both PCR for IgH genes and CSF cytologic examination is preferred because the information can be complementary, rather than concordant, and help with establishing a diagnosis of meningeal involvement.[18] Detection of $MYD88^{L265P}$ PCR in CSF can increase the yield of diagnostic testing.

While identification of lymphoma cells or IgH gene rearrangement patterns yields a diagnosis of lymphoma involving the leptomeninges, "bland" CSF does not exclude the diagnosis of PCNSL, and imaging of the neuraxis, combined with the extent of disease evaluation needs to be completed.

OPHTHALMOLOGIC EVALUATION AND VITREOUS ANALYSIS

Involvement of the retina, vitreous humor, or optic nerves should be excluded with a comprehensive evaluation by an ophthalmologist that includes a slit-lamp examination. A vitreous biopsy is recommended in case of isolated eye involvement or inability to obtain brain biopsy. Interleukin (IL)-10 levels, IL10/IL6 ratio, and $MYD88^{L265P}$ PCR can aid diagnosis.

EXTENT OF DISEASE EVALUATION

A thorough history with identification of possible risks of immunosuppression should be obtained and a detailed physical and neurological examination should be performed. In addition to evaluation of the neuroaxis, it is important to rule out systemic involvement with at least a CT scan of the chest, abdomen, and pelvis, and preferably fluorodeoxyglucose (FDG) body positron emission tomography (PET). The International PCNSL Collaborative Group (IPCG) has developed guidelines for extent of disease evaluation, summarized in Table 11.2.

TABLE 11.2 Recommended extent of disease evaluation based on guidelines of the International Primary Central Nervous System Lymphoma Collaborative Group (IPCG)

Physical examination	Lymph node evaluation Testicular evaluation Comprehensive neurological evaluation
Laboratory studies	Complete blood count with differential Comprehensive metabolic panel Lactate dehydrogenase level Serologic testing for HIV
CSF studies	Cell count, protein, glucose Cytology Flow cytometry IgH gene rearrangement
Full ophthalmological testing	Slit lamp testing
Imaging	MR imaging: brain and spine CT/PET: chest, abdomen and pelvis
Cognitive/functional assessment	Karnofsky performance status or Eastern Cooperative Oncology Group Mini-Mental State Examination.
Additional tests	Testicular ultrasound (can be considered in older men) Bone marrow aspirate and biopsy (can be considered) Vitreous biopsy (if necessary)

It is critical to follow International PCNLS Collaborative Group guidelines for extent of disease evaluation in every patient with newly diagnosed PCNSL and at the time of relapse.

PROGNOSTIC FACTORS

Age and performance status have consistently emerged as the two most important prognostic factors for PCNSL. The two scoring systems developed for PCNSL include the International Extranodal Lymphoma Study Group (IELSG) scoring system and the Memorial Sloan Kettering Cancer Center (MSKCC) prognostic model.[19,20] The scoring systems and attributed outcome measures are shown in Table 11.3A and B.

TREATMENT FOR NEWLY DIAGNOSED PCNSL

Prompt initiation of therapy can avoid neurological sequelae and improve survival and functional status.[21] Therapy for PCNSL includes two phases: induction and consolidation. Response assessment during these stages has been defined by the IPCG by evaluation of imaging, eye, CSF, and corticosteroid dosing (Table 11.4).[22] Outside of the standard regimens, patients should also be encouraged to participate in clinical trials where and when available.

TABLE 11.3 A. International Extranodal Lymphoma Study Group prognostic scoring system and 2-year survival rate

Total score	2-year overall survival rate	Prognostic factors scored 1 point each if present:
0–1	80%	Age >60 years Eastern Cooperative Oncology Group Performance Status >2
2–3	48%	Elevated serum lactate dehydrogenase Elevated CSF protein concentration
4–5	15%	Involvement of deep structures of the brain

B. The Memorial Sloan Kettering Cancer Center prognostic model for primary central nervous system lymphoma (PCNSL) patients

		AGE ≤ 50	AGE > 50
Class 1 (irrespective of KPS)		Class 2: KPS ≥ 70	Class 3: < 70
Median overall survival (years)	8.5	3.2	1.1
Median progression-free survival (years)	2.0	1.8	0.6

From Ferreri et al.[19]
From Abrey et al.[20]

TABLE 11.4 International PCNSL Collaborative Group (IPCG) response criteria for primary central nervous system lymphoma (PCNSL)

RESPONSE	BRAIN IMAGING	CORTICOSTEROID DOSE	EYE EXAMINATION	CEREBROSPINAL FLUID CYTOLOGY
Complete response (CR)	No contrast enhancement	None	Normal	Negative
Unconfirmed complete response (CRu)	No contrast enhancement	Any	Normal	Negative
	Minimal abnormality	Any	Minor retinal pigment epithelium (RPE) abnormality	Negative
Partial response (PR)	50% decrease in enhancing tumor	Irrelevant	Minor RPE abnormality or normal	Negative
	No contrast enhancement	Irrelevant	Decrease in vitreous cells or retinal infiltrate	Persistent or suspicious
Progressive disease (PD)	25% increase in lesion	Irrelevant	Recurrent or new ocular disease	Recurrent or positive
	Any new site of disease (CNS or systemic)			

From Abrey et al.[22]

There is no clear survival benefit of surgical resection in PCNSL, particularly because of the widespread, infiltrative nature of the disease. A retrospective analysis of the German PCNSL Study Group-1 phase III trial demonstrated increase in progression-free survival (PFS) and overall survival (OS) in patients with a subtotal/gross total resection compared to patients with a biopsy only, but this benefit was not significant for OS when corrected for the number of lesions.[23] Rae et al. also showed benefit of craniotomy over biopsy in a subset of patients with favorable prognostic features.[24] As PCNSL lesions can be deep and multifocal, the role of surgery is primarily for obtaining a diagnosis, and stereotactic biopsy is the preferred approach to prevent morbidity and mortality.

INDUCTION

While there is no uniform gold standard regimen for induction, a high-dose methotrexate (HD-MTX)- based intravenous (IV) polychemotherapy regimen is the recommended first-line treatment and has been shown to confer survival benefit.[25,19] The primary goal of the induction phase of treatment is to induce a complete response (CR).

Clinical trials with various doses of HD-MTX from 3.5 to 8 g/m² IV have been studied. No randomized trial has compared different doses of HD-MTX. Any dose of 3 g/m² IV or higher achieves adequate CSF concentrations and is recommended. There is no clear role for intrathecal methotrexate in treating PCNSL.

The New Approaches to Brain Tumor Therapy (NABTT) prospective phase II trial studied single-agent HD-MTX in newly diagnosed PCNSL.[26] In this trial, 52% achieved a CR, and 22% achieved PR for an response rate of 74%. Median PFS was 12.8 months and median OS was more than 23 months. Combination therapy with HD-MTX was found to further increase response rates and duration of response. A randomized study enrolling 79 patients

(International Extranodal Lymphoma Study Group [IELSG] 20) investigated the addition of (high-dose cytarabine) HD-ARA-C to HD-MTX compared to HD-MTX alone for induction, which demonstrated a significant improvement in CR and PFS with the combination.[27] Subsequently, a large phase II trial (IELSG32) enrolled 227 PCNSL patients who were randomly assigned (1:1:1) to three groups for induction[28] (Group A: HD-MTX and HD-ARA-C, Group B: HD-MTX, HD-ARA-C, and rituximab; and Group C: HD-MTX, HD-ARA-C, rituximab, and thiotepa). At a median follow-up of 30 months, the MATRix regimen (Group C) was associated with a CR rate of 49% compared with 23% for Group A, and 30% with Group B. Overall response was also higher in Group C (87%) compared to 40% in Group A and 51% in Group B. Other effective HD-MTX-based combination regimens include HD-MTX, temozolomide, and rituximab (MTR regimen)[21]; HD-MTX, rituximab, procarbazine, and vincristine (R-MPV)[29]; and HD-MTX, carmustine, teniposide, and prednisolone (MBVP).[30] Based on some of these studied regimens, 6–8 doses of HD-MTX are required to achieve CR.[31,28,29] However, most of these different combination regimens have not been compared, except one study comparing HD-MTX and temozolomide with MPV in patients older than 60 years of age that demonstrated no difference in median OS although the results favored the MPV arm.[32] In general, there is currently no proven standard-of-care combination regimen as reflected in the heterogeneity of chemotherapy induction treatments used across institutions.

> While there is no uniform gold standard regimen for induction, a high-dose methotrexate (HD-MTX)- based intravenous (IV) polychemotherapy regimen is the recommended first-line treatment for PCNSL and has been shown to confer survival benefit.

RITUXIMAB IN INDUCTION THERAPY

Rituximab is an anti-CD20 chimeric monoclonal antibody that has been showed to have clear efficacy in systemic NHL and is routinely part of the systemic regimen. However, its role in the treatment of PCNSL remains uncertain. As a large molecule, its ability to cross the blood–brain barrier is unclear. Rituximab monotherapy was associated with radiographic responses in 36% in a multicenter cohort of 12 patients with recurrent PCNSL.[33] Several trials have included rituximab as part of a combination regimen for induction, as just described. In the IELSG32 trial, the addition of rituximab was associated with better response rates.[28] Conversely, a multicenter phase III study that assigned patients with newly diagnosed PCNSL to MBVP or R-MVBP found no clear benefit from the addition of rituximab as measured by event-free survival at 1 year of 49% versus 52%, although younger patients seemed to benefit. Of note, in this trial, "event" was defined as absence of CR/CRu or progression/death at the end of protocol treatment.[34] A large retrospective study of 1,002 patients indicated survival benefit from the addition of rituximab in newly diagnosed PCNSL, although this treatment group had better baseline prognostic scores (younger with higher performance status) and the difference was only observed in a univariate analysis.[35]

CONSOLIDATION

After completion of induction therapy, consolidation is considered in eligible patients. The role of consolidation therapy is to prevent disease recurrence and improve PFS and OS. Various consolidation approaches include whole-brain radiation therapy (WBRT), high-dose chemotherapy followed by autologous stem cell transplantation (HDT-ASCT), and chemotherapy alone.

PCNSL was historically effectively treated with whole-brain irradiation,[36] although responses were not sustained. In addition, concerns for delayed neurotoxicity have led experts to favor high-dose chemotherapy while avoiding WBRT for the consolidation phases in PCNSL.[37,38] Moreover, the addition of WBRT (45 Gy) after treatment with an HD-MTX–based regimen (HD-MTX or HD-MTX and ifosfamide) was not found to improve OS in a large multicenter randomized phase III study of 551 patients[39] and was associated with more neurotoxicity and worse quality of life.[40] Reduced-dose WBRT for consolidation has demonstrated reduction in neurotoxicity. A multicenter phase II randomized study of rituximab, methotrexate, vincristine, procarbazine, and cytarabine (R-MPV-A) with or without low-dose (LD) WBRT (23.4 Gy) met its primary endpoint and demonstrated improved 2-year PFS on the LD WBRT arm (NCT1399372).[41] The data for long-term neurotoxicity and OS are yet to mature.

The phase II study CALGB 50202, which introduced non-myeloablative high-dose chemotherapy consolidative therapy, included 44 patients first treated with MT-R followed by high-dose infusional etoposide and cytarabine (EA).[21] This study reported outcomes superior to chemotherapy-alone regimens and comparable to consolidative regimens incorporating WBRT, with a 2-year PFS rate of 57%.

> Concerns regarding delayed neurotoxicity have led experts to favor high-dose chemotherapy rather than WBRT for consolidation in treatment of PCNSL.

A multicenter phase II study of 79 patients with newly diagnosed PCNSL treated with induction treatment with MATRix followed by high-dose carmustine/thiotepa and auto-HCT reported an overall response rate of 91% and a 2-year OS rate of 87%, with three deaths related to toxicity (9%).[42]

Two multicenter phase II clinical trials have compared WBRT to HDT/ASCT for consolidation. The IELSG32 study included patients older than 70 years and showed no significant difference in the 2-year PFS (80% in the WBRT arm and 69% in the HDT/ASCT arm).[43] The Intergroup ANOCEF-GOELAMS phase II PRECIS study enrolled patients younger than 60 years and showed slightly better efficacy in the ASCT arm (2-year PFS 87% vs. 63%), although transplant-related mortality was high at 11% in this study.[44] Both studies monitored long-term cognitive outcomes and found the WBRT to be associated with a higher rate of cognitive decline at 2–3 years of follow-up, thus highlighting the need to consider patient factors and risk of severe adverse events when contemplating WBRT versus HDT/ASCT for consolidation.

> Despite response to initial therapy, most patients will eventually relapse within 5 years of completing treatment. Additionally, approximately 10–25% of patients have disease refractory to initial induction therapy.

MANAGEMENT OF RELAPSED/RECURRENT PCNSL

Despite completion and response to induction and consolidation, most patients will eventually relapse within 5 years of completing treatment. Additionally, approximately 10–25% of patients have disease refractory to initial induction therapy. Patients who relapse within a year of completing therapy have a prognosis similar to that of chemotherapy-refractory patients. Other prognostic factors at first relapse/progression include Karnofsky Performance Scale (KPS) of greater than 70 versus KPS of less than 70, sensitivity to first-line therapy (relapsed vs. refractory disease), duration of first remission (PFS 1 year vs. <1 year), and management at relapse/progression (palliative vs. salvage therapy).[45]

Extent of disease evaluation at the time of relapse/recurrence is recommended (including all of the CNS compartments, as well as systemically). Treatment can include HD-MTX rechallenge in patients who previously had durable response. A study of 22 patients with relapsed PCNSL retreated with HD-MTX showed overall response rates of 91% to first rechallenge and median survival of 61.9 months after first relapse.[46] HDT/ASCT, if not initially part of the patient's prior therapy, has shown some efficacy in recurrent PCNSL patients,[47] and, in rare cases, a second ASCT has been successful in carefully selected patients.[48] In addition, other chemotherapies such as cytarabine and pemetrexed can also be considered. Salvage WBRT has been associated with radiographic response of up to 74–79% when used in the recurrent/refractory setting in radiation-naïve patients.[49,50]

> WBRT has been associated with high radiographic response rates of up to 79% in recurrent/refractory, radiation-naïve PCNSL patients.

Novel targeted agents including Bruton's tyrosine kinase (BTK) inhibitors, phosphoinositide 3-kinase (pI3K) inhibitors, mTOR inhibitors, and other immunomodulatory strategies such as immunomodulatory imide drugs (IMiDs) (including lenalidomide and pomalidomide), immune checkpoint inhibitors, and CD19-directed chimeric antigen receptor (CAR). T cells are being investigated in relapsed and refractory PCNSL.[51-55] Single-agent ibrutinib, a BTK inhibitor, demonstrated an overall response rate of 52–77% in patients with relapsed/refractory PCNSL in two separate studies,[51] with a median PFS of approximately 5 months.[52] Ibrutinib-based combination regimens with HD-MTX and rituximab,[56] or with temozolomide, etoposide, liposomal doxorubicin, dexamethasone, and rituximab (TEDDI-R) in phase I studies have demonstrated promising results.[54] Lenalidomide alone and in combination with rituximab has been studied in phase I and II trials of relapsed/refractory PCNSL[55] and was associated with an overall response rate of 64–67%. Both ibrutinib and lenalidomide are now included in the National Comprehensive Cancer Network (NCCN) guidelines as options for salvage therapy in recurrent PCNSL.

MONITORING AND FOLLOW-UP

Following CR with initial therapy, the NCCN guidelines recommend clinical and imaging follow-up at 3 months for the first 2 years, every 6 months for the following 3 years, then annually for at least 5 years, based on the IPCG consensus guidelines.[22] During these follow-up evaluations, history, physical examination, cognitive evaluation (e.g., with Mini Mental State Examination), and gadolinium-enhanced MRI of the brain are needed at minimum. In addition, CSF analysis and ophthalmologic examination should be considered based on symptoms and initial site of disease.

OTHER SUBTYPES OF PRIMARY NERVOUS SYSTEM LYMPHOMA

Other rare types of primary CNS lymphoma exist, and their diagnosis relies on a thorough extent of disease evaluation to rule out synchronous lesion. Primary vitreoretinal lymphoma (PVRL) is a high-grade and rare subtype of PCNSL that presents solely in the eye, without parenchymal brain disease. Presenting symptoms can include floaters, blurry vision, and decreased acuity, and ophthalmologic testing may include vitreous and subretinal tumor infiltration. Diagnosis is made by identification of malignant cells with aspiration, vitrectomy, or retinal biopsy. Treatment can include local therapy (intravitreal therapy, ocular radiation) or systemic therapy with HD-MTX.

Primary leptomeningeal lymphoma (PLL) occurs in fewer than 10% of PCNSL patients and is defined as isolated leptomeningeal disease involvement without any intraparenchymal, ophthalmic, or spinal cord lesions.

> Primary leptomeningeal lymphoma (PLL) occurs in less than 10% of PCNSL patients.

Fewer than 10% of PCNSL patients present with isolated leptomeningeal disease, and they can have symptoms such as headaches, cranial nerve palsies, meningismus, and radiculopathies. CSF profile may show malignant lymphocytes and IgH gene rearrangement, while MRI spine occasionally reveals nodular enhancement especially around the lumbar nerve roots. The treatment of PLL does not differ significantly from classic PCNSL; HD-MTX, in combination with other agents, is typically used to treat PLL.

Primary intramedullary spinal cord lymphoma is a rare but recognized entity characterized by intramedullary spinal lesions in the absence of other areas of CNS or systemic involvement. It can present with myelopathy, cauda equina, or conus medullaris syndrome. In addition to the standard approach to PCNSL, focal RT may help in alleviating symptoms if severe myelopathic symptoms do not respond to high-dose steroids.

PCNSL IN THE IMMUNOCOMPROMISED: ACQUIRED IMMUNODEFICIENCY SYNDROME AND POST-TRANSPLANT LYMPHOPROLIFERATIVE DISEASE

HIV-related PCNSL is now a rarely seen AIDS-defining malignancy which typically occurs in patients with low CD4+ counts and typically high viral load, and it is strongly related to EBV infection. Clinically, HIV-related PCNSL can present in a fashion similar to PCNSL in an immunocompetent host, however MRI lesions tend to be solitary or multifocal with ring enhancement. Given the other possible CNS lesions that may present in patient with AIDS (toxoplasmosis, progressive multifocal leukoencephalopathy, and other opportunistic bacterial and fungal infections), a stereotactic biopsy or CSF studies are encouraged to reach a pathological diagnosis. Antiretroviral therapy to enhance the immune system is a key therapeutic goal, and tumor-targeted therapy in the form of HD-MTX can be used concurrently (recommended dose of 3 g/m²),[57] with an effort to avoid WBRT.

Chronic immunosuppression in solid organ and hematopoietic cell transplant (HCT) recipients can also lead to emergence of post-transplant lymphoproliferative disorders (PTLD). This is typically rare, with an incidence of about 1%, and is typically more frequent in solid transplant patients (highest in intestinal and multiorgan transplant, followed by heart and lung transplant, then less frequently in renal transplant and HCT). The pathogenesis is also related to proliferation of EBV-positive B cells in the setting of chronic T-cell immunosuppression, although EBV-negative and T-cell tumors can also occur. Risk factors include overall degree of immunosuppression, EBV serostatus of the transplant recipient, and time post-transplant.[58]

Post-transplant lymphoproliferative disorders (PTLD) are more frequent in solid organ transplant patients. The highest incidence is seen in intestinal and multiorgan transplants, followed by heart and lung transplants, with a lower incidence in renal and HCTs.

Although CNS involvement can present with focal neurological deficits or more subtle cognitive changes, nonspecific constitutional symptoms (weight loss, fever, and fatigue) can be more common than in immunocompetent PCNSL patients. The diagnosis of PTLD is usually based on clinical features, and a history of transplant accompanied by pertinent symptoms or imaging findings (such as radiological evidence of a mass) should prompt further investigations. Evaluation for systemic involvement with PET scanning is recommended, and tissue biopsy with review from a hematopathologist is an essential step in reaching an accurate diagnosis. Prevention of PTLD involves limiting exposure to aggressive immunosuppressive regimens along with antiviral prophylaxis and occasionally EBV monitoring in high-risk patients. Patients diagnosed with PTLD are first and foremost managed by reducing immunosuppression if clinically possible. In addition, anti-CD20 therapy with rituximab has been found to improve outcomes in patients with tumors expressing CD20.[59] Chemotherapy or radiation therapy can also be used concurrently or sequentially.[60]

PRIMARY T-CELL LYMPHOMA

Primary CNS T-cell lymphoma is a rare subtype of PCNSL and makes up less than 5% of all PCNSL cases, although it may be more prevalent in Japan compared to Western countries. Based on very small cohort studies, patients tend to have presentations similar to DLBCL PCNSL. Extent of disease workup is required similar to DLBCL. Treatment of these cases was heterogeneous in the literature, with most patients receiving HD-MTX, although chemotherapy and irradiation have also been described. In a cohort of 45 patients, use of HD-MTX and performance status were associated with disease-specific survival. Median PFS and OS were 22 months and 25 months, respectively.[61]

Primary CNS T-cell lymphoma is a rare subtype of PCNSL and makes up less than 5% of all PCNSL cases, although it may be more prevalent in Japan compared to Western countries.

CENTRAL NERVOUS SYSTEM INVOLVEMENT BY OTHER SYSTEMIC HEMATOLOGICAL MALIGNANCIES

SYSTEMIC NON-HODGKIN LYMPHOMA (SECONDARY CNS LYMPHOMA)

Systemic NHL may involve any area of the nervous system either by direct invasion, compression, or paraneoplastic effects. Secondary involvement of the CNS (SCNSL) occurs in a minority of patients and is usually in the setting of relapsed disease within the first year after completion of therapy. The majority of cases are histologically high-grade

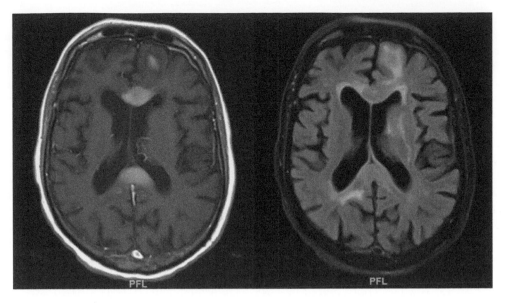

Figure 11.2 *MRI brain showing T1 contrast-enhanced image (left) and T2/fluid-attenuated inversion recovery (FLAIR) image (right) in a case of secondary CNS lymphoma.*

lymphomas such as DLBCL or Burkitt lymphoma. An international prognostic index (IPI) has identified risk factors contributing to CNS relapse that include older age, poor performance status, elevated lactate dehydrogenase (LDH), involvement of extranodal sites, stage III/IV disease, and kidney or adrenal involvement. Presentation can include symptoms due to leptomeningeal disease (most common), parenchymal brain involvement, and, rarely, intramedullary spinal dissemination. MRI with gadolinium is the most sensitive imaging (Figure 11.2). All patients with suspected SCNSL should undergo imaging of the entire neuraxis (brain and spine with gadolinium) as well as CSF studies including cell count, protein, glucose, cytology, flow cytometry, and IgH gene rearrangement studies. The radiological differential diagnosis includes infections, inflammatory processes, and late effects of therapy. While management focuses on preventing neurologic morbidity and improving quality of life, survival in these patients depends on control of both CNS and systemic disease.[62]

> Secondary involvement of the CNS by systemic non-Hodgkins lymphoma (SCNSL) occurs in a minority of patients and is usually in the setting of relapsed disease within the first year after completion of therapy.

Treatment can consist of high-dose chemotherapy, and, in some carefully selected patients with prior response to chemotherapy, HDT/ASCT. Intrathecal therapy for leptomeningeal disease, either through an Ommaya reservoir or serial lumbar punctures, is slowly falling out of favor. Ibrutinib as a single agent and in combination with rituximab and HD-MTX has shown promising clinical response in patients with SCNSL.

Lenalidomide has also showed activity in refractory SCNSL from DLBCL and mantle cell lymphoma.[63,64] A case series of CD19-directed CAR T-cells demonstrated encouraging results in patients with SCNSL.[65]

Radiation therapy (WBRT or SRS) can be used as a salvage option in the appropriate patient. CNS prophylaxis with systemic HD-MTX or intrathecal MTX remains part of the routine care of patients with highly aggressive subtypes of NHL such as lymphoblastic lymphoma/acute lymphoblastic leukemia, Burkitt lymphoma, and NHL with high CNS IPI, but not in more indolent forms of NHL such as follicular lymphoma.

Additional nervous system complications from systemic lymphoma include neurolymphomatosis and intravascular lymphoma, which can involve the brain, spinal cord, or peripheral nerves. Primary neurolymphomatosis (invasion of the cranial or spinal nerves without involvement of the CNS) is exceedingly rare, and direct nerve root infiltration is more typical in systemic B-cell NHL, underscoring the need for systemic screening with whole-body PET imaging in addition to screening the entire neuraxis. Neurolymphomatosis can present with nerve root or cranial nerve involvement (including cauda dysfunction, asymmetric weakness, radicular pain, and cranial nerve findings). The treatment of neurolymphomatosis often consists of rituximab in combination with chemotherapy (often rituximab, cyclophosphamide, hydroxydaunorubicin hydrochloride [doxorubicin hydrochloride], vincristine [Oncovin], and prednisone [R-CHOP]), but prognosis remains poor with lack of durability of response.[66]

Intravascular large B-cell lymphoma is rare and has a highest prevalence in elderly patients. Forty percent of cases typically have CNS involvement, and the skin is frequently involved. The characteristic pathological findings include pleomorphic large lymphoid cells confined within small arteries, veins, and capillaries. Patients may present with constitutional symptoms such as fever and rash, and neurological symptoms can be caused by cerebral ischemia, although subacute encephalopathy is also common. Diagnosis is achieved with biopsy, and early recognition and treatment is key in improving an otherwise poor prognosis. Skin biopsies prior to brain biopsies can also increase the yield of diagnosis, with a reported sensitivity of about 75%, although steroid use may yield false-negative results.[67] Regimens including HD-MTX interlaced with R-CHOP are typically used in patients with intravascular large B-cell lymphoma who have both CNS and systemic involvement.

BING-NEEL SYNDROME

Bing-Neel syndrome (BNS) is a rare entity caused by CNS invasion from malignant lymphoplasmacytic cells, with or without systemic progression of systemic Waldenstrom's macroglobulinemia (WM).[68] The neurological presentation can be diverse (headache, seizures, cognitive decline, ataxia), and imaging of the brain and spinal cord can reveal diffuse parenchymal or leptomeningeal enhancement or T2/fluid-attenuated inversion recovery (FLAIR) changes, as well as a tumoral appearance. CSF studies can be helpful in demonstrating a lymphoplasmacytic lymphoma and monoclonal B cells. Ig rearrangement analysis or $MYD88^{L265P}$ mutation detection can be present. Because WM is often indolent, treatment is often only initiated with symptomatic disease. Similarly, treatment of BNS would aim only to slow or reverse clinical symptoms and increase PFS, not necessarily aim for CR. A 3-year OS rate of 60% has been described in BNS, with age older than 65 years, low platelet counts, and prior treatment for WM associated with worse outcome.[69] Treatment regimens, such as those used in PCNSL including HD-MTX and HD-ARA-C, have been used for BNS,[70] and other regimens such as fludrabine, cladribine, and bendamustine have also been used as first-line with some response.[69,71,72] Last, ibrutinib is approved by the US Food and Drug Administration (FDA) for systemic WM and has been shown to be effective in BNS.[73]

CNS INVOLVEMENT FROM ACUTE LEUKEMIAS

Neurological complications from acute leukemias can be a consequence of direct infiltration of leukemic cells (hyperleukocytosis causing disseminated intravascular coagulation or tumor lysis syndrome, leukemic meningitis, or leptomeningeal involvement); direct CNS involvement from acute myeloid leukemia (AML) is rare (<5%), and has been associated with higher LDH levels and WBC counts at diagnosis, as well as chromosome 16 inversion and chromosome 11 abnormalities.[74] Acute lymphoblastic leukemia (ALL), in contrast, has a higher incidence in the pediatric compared to the adult population, and about 10% of adult cases are associated with CNS involvement, which is a marker of poor prognosis.[75,76] Specific to the pediatric population, rates of CNS

involvement of 3–5% have been reported at initial diagnosis and significantly higher rates of 30–40% at relapse[77] despite newer chemotherapy-based protocols yielding 80–90% cure rates.[78] All current chemotherapy regimens, which involve intensive chemotherapy and potential hematopoietic bone marrow transplant, also include CNS prophylaxis, typically with intrathecal methotrexate and cytarabine.[77] Synchronous CNS occurrence is associated with younger age, mature B- or T-cell phenotype, and Philadelphia chromosome positivity.[77] Suspected CNS involvement based on neurological symptoms should include a thorough workup including CSF cytology and flow cytometry as well as MRI of the neuraxis with contrast. CSF presence of leukemic cells can provide confirmation of CNS involvement; however, these results need to be interpreted with caution as CNS hemorrhage or traumatic LPs may introduce false-positive results.[67] If confirmed, treatment of CNS-ALL can include cranial irradiation, intrathecal chemotherapy, and HD-MTX-based systemic therapy.[79] CNS relapse carries a dismal prognosis, and no clear regimen has been proved superior in this scenario.

CNS INVOLVEMENT FROM CHRONIC LEUKEMIAS (CLL)

In a large cohort study of 4,174 patients, 172 patients were investigated for neurological symptoms and 18 were identified as having CNS involvement from CLL.[80] The majority of patients with CLL are more likely to have neurological symptoms from other etiologies, including infections and autoimmune/inflammatory conditions. Imaging of the neuraxis and CSF analysis or tissue biopsy is recommended in all patients with CLL presenting with neurological symptoms to assess for these other etiologies and to rule out malignant transformation to a more aggressive lymphoma. Richter syndrome has been described as occurring in 2–10% of CLL patients during their disease course. There is no standard regimen for CNS CLL or Richter syndrome, and treatment of advanced disease in such patients should be individualized and can depend on prior therapy, disease location, and extent. However, some case reports have demonstrated activity of systemic fludrarabine-based therapy for CLL patients with CNS disease. Lenolidomide and ibrutinib have also shown promise in CLL, although further studies are warranted for CNS CLL. Despite these possible treatments, the prognosis remains dismal for patients with CNS CLL with a median OS of 12 months.[80]

> The majority of patients with CLL are more likely to have neurological symptoms from other etiologies, including infections and autoimmune/inflammatory conditions.

HISTIOCYTIC TUMORS OF THE CNS

Histiocytic tumors of the CNS are a diverse but rare group of proliferative disorders involving dendritic cells and macrophages. These include, broadly, Langerhans cell histiocytosis (LCH) and the non-LCH disorders such as Erdheim-Chester disease,

Rosai-Dorfman disease, juvenile xanthogranuloma, and histiocytic sarcoma.

LCH is defined by the presence of pathological Langerhans cells that are positive for CD1a, CD207, and S100. Patients can present clinically with diverse clinical symptoms. Although involvement of the CNS tends to be in the form of diabetes insipidus, a parenchymal brain lesion can occasionally be present as well. Treatment consists of chemotherapy (such as cladribine or cytarabine) and focal radiation, alone or in combination. More recently, mutations in *BRAF* V600E has been detected in about 50–60% of cases, identifying a potential for targeted therapy with dabrafenib or vemurafenib.[81] CNS neurodegenerative disease (CNS-ND) from LCH is also a well-recognized entity and is a devastating irreversible complication that occurs up to 10 years after resolution of the CNS lesions. CNS-ND consists of a cerebellar syndrome, and cognitive difficulties and dysarthria, ataxia, dysmetria, and behavioral changes may be present. Neuro-imaging may reveal bilateral symmetric lesions in the dentate nucleus of the cerebellum or basal ganglia. Treatment of CNS-ND with IV gamma-globulin or retinoic acid has been associated with stabilization of progression in pediatric patients.[82,83] Cytarabine with or without vincristine has also been reported in a small cohort to help stabilize symptoms and radiological findings of CNS-ND.[83]

CONCLUSION

CNS lymphomas, while generally rare conditions, are relatively common in neuro-oncologic practice. Knowing most commonly encountered lymphomas (diffuse large B-cell), their presentation, diagnostic workup, and treatment is critically important for a practicing neuro-oncologist. Familiarity with treatment options and mastery of methotrexate-based regimens is vital. It has to be emphasized that there is no consensus on the optimal management of patients with PCNSL, although methotrexate-based regimens are uniformly utilized as the backbone of induction therapy. Multiple clinical trials are ongoing. Novel agents are emerging and are already entering the clinical arena, particularly in the recurrent setting. Systemic lymphomas and leukemias can also affect CNS. ALLs have a high incidence of CNS involvement and most of the current chemotherapy regimens, which involve intensive chemotherapy and potential hematopoietic bone marrow transplant, also include CNS prophylaxis.

What is the definition of primary CNS lymphoma?	It is a rare and aggressive variant of extranodal non-Hodgkin lymphoma which involves compartments of the central nervous system (brain, leptomeninges, eyes, or spinal cord) without evidence of systemic disease
What lymphoma subtype makes up 90% of PCNSL cases?	Diffuse large cell lymphoma
What three lymphoma subtypes make up the other 10%?	1. T-cell lymphoma (<5% of all cases) 2. Burkitt lymphoma 3. Poorly characterized low-grade lymphoma
Describe three classic histological characteristics of PCNSL	1. High proliferative index 2. Organized in an angiocentric pattern 3. Malignant cells expressing B-cell markers such as CD19, CD20, CD22, and CD79a
How does the prognosis of PCNSCL compare with that of other subtypes of extranodal lymphoma?	The prognosis is worse, with only about 50% achieving remission
What percentage of PCNSL patients present with focal neurological deficits, and how many have nonspecific cognitive or neuro-psychiatric disturbances?	Up to 70%, and 45%, respectively
What components should be included in evaluation for suspected PCNSL?	1. Imaging of the neuro-axis with contrast-enhanced MRI 2. CSF analysis 3. Testicular ultrasound 4. PET-CT 5. Slit lamp examination 6. Pathologic evaluation via biopsy (brain, vitreous)

What are the two stages of therapy for PCNSL?	Induction and consolidation
What criteria are used for response assessment in PCNSL?	The IPCG response criteria
What is the optimal induction regimen for PCNSL?	There is little consensus beyond inclusion of high-dose methotrexate-based chemotherapy
What options can be included in consolidation regimens?	High-dose chemotherapy with autologous hematopoietic stem cell transplantation or whole-brain radiation therapy
What patient population has higher risk of radiation-induced symptomatic neurotoxicity?	Patients older than 60 years
What are salvage options at relapse?	1. Rechallenge with HD-MTX 2. Alternative chemo, such as cytarabine and etoposide with auto-SCT 3. WBRT
What factor is strongly related to HIV-related PCNSL?	EBV infection
Which two lymphoma types are most common with CNS involvement from systemic lymphoma?	DLBCL Burkitt lymphoma
What is Bing-Neel syndrome?	It is a rare entity caused by CNS invasion from malignant lymphoplasmacytic cells, with or without systemic progression of systemic Waldenstrom's macroglobulinemia
Is CNS involvement more common from acute lymphoblastic leukemias or acute myeloid leukemias?	More common from ALL than AML (10% vs. 5%)

Name five histiocytic tumors of the CNS

1. Langerhans cell histiocytosis
2. Erdheim-Chester disease
3. Rosai-Dorfman disease
4. Juvenile xanthogranuloma
5. Histiocytic sarcoma

What are possible causes of neurological symptoms in patients with CLL?

1. Infection
2. Autoimmune/inflammatory conditions
3. Richter syndrome (transformation to aggressive lymphoma, occurs in 2–10% of cases)

1. Which of the following is the *least* helpful CSF test to pursue in the workup of possible PCNSL?
   a. CSF cytology
   b. MYD88 testing
   c. IgH rearrangement studies
   d. CSF lactate dehydrogenase

2. Evaluation of suspected PCNSL should always include all of the following *except*
   a. PET-CT (skull to mid-thighs)
   b. Slit lamp examination
   c. Biopsy (brain, vitreous)
   d. Bone marrow biopsy

3. Reasonable induction regimens in PCNSL include all of the following *except*
   a. HD-MTX alone
   b. HD-MTX with rituximab and temozolomide
   c. HD-MTX with WBRT
   d. HD-MTX, rituximab, procarbazine, and vincristine

4. According to the IELSG prognostic score, which of the following patients with PCNSL has a relatively better prognosis compared to the others?
   a. A 61-year-old man with an Eastern Cooperative Oncology Group (ECOG) score of 1, ocular involvement alone, elevated CSF protein, normal LDH
   b. A 61-year-old man with thalamic involvement, elevated CSF protein, normal LDH, and ECOG of 3
   c. A 49-year-old man with ECOG of 2, basal ganglia involvement, normal LDH, and normal CSF protein
   d. A 59-year-old man with ECOG of 2, frontal lobe involvement, normal LDH and normal CSF protein

5. According to the MSKCC prognostic scale for PCNSL, a 45-year-old patient with a KPS of 70 would have a median overall survival of
   a. 1.1 years
   b. 5.4 years
   c. 8.5 years
   d. 14.6 years

6. Which of the following markers on malignant cells would not be in keeping with a diagnosis of diffuse large B-cell PCNSL?
   a. CD4
   b. CD19
   c. CD20
   d. CD79a

7. The complete response rate with a HD-MTX-based regimen based on past clinical trials is
   a. 0–30%
   b. 30–60%

   c. 60–90%
   d. Greater than 90%

8. A 45-year-old patient has achieved complete response after HD-MTX-based induction and consolidative high-dose chemotherapy with autologous stem cell transplant. He is now 3 years post-treatment completion and has no evidence of disease recurrence. What is the ideal follow-up interval for this patient according to the IPCG consensus guidelines?
   a. Every 3 months
   b. Every 6 months
   c. Every year
   d. No follow-up needed as he is now 3 years post-treatment

9. The following are all risk factors for the development of post-transplant lymphoproliferative disorder *except*
   a. Long duration of immunosuppressive treatment
   b. Positive EBV status
   c. Solid organ transplant
   d. Age older than 50

10. Which of the following about Bing-Neel syndrome is false?
    a. It can be associated with $MYD88^{L265P}$ mutation.
    b. It can present with leptomeningeal enhancement on MRI.
    c. Chemotherapy is always indicated.
    d. Therapy using ibrutinib has been showed to be of some benefit.

11. Intrathecal prophylaxis remains part of the routine care of patients with which of the following?
    a. Follicular lymphoma
    b. Chronic lymphocytic leukemia
    c. Waldenstrom's macroglobulinemia
    d. Lymphoblastic lymphoma

12. A 70-year-old patient with a history of CLL presents with a 2-week history of altered mental status. Which of the following would you consider for a workup of this patient?
    a. MRI brain with and without contrast
    b. MRI whole spine with and without contrast
    c. CSF studies with flow cytometry and cytology
    d. All of the above

13. A 30-year-old patient with history of Langerhans cell histiocytosis presents with new learning difficulties, abnormal eye movements, and gait instability. Imaging reveals T2/FLAIR changes in the dentate region of the cerebellum. Which of the following is not a suitable treatment option?
    a. Cytarabine
    b. Intravenous gamma-globulin (IVIg)
    c. Retinoic acid
    d. Focal RT to cerebellum

ANSWERS

1. d
2. d
3. c
4. d
5. c
6. a
7. b
8. b
9. d
10. c
11. d
12. d
13. d

REFERENCES

1. Swerdlow SH, Campo E, Pileri SA, et al. The 2016 revision of the World Health Organization classification of lymphoid neoplasms. *Blood.* 2016;127(20):2375–2390. doi:10.1182/blood-2016-01-643569

2. Ostrom QT, Gittleman H, Truitt G, et al. CBTRUS Statistical Report: Primary Brain and Other Central Nervous System Tumors Diagnosed in the United States in 2011-2015 Introduction. *Neuro Oncol.* 2018;20(S4):1–86. doi:10.1093/neuonc/noy131

3. Bhagavathi S, Wilson JD. Primary central nervous system lymphoma. *Arch Pathol Lab Med.* 2008;132(11):1830–1834. doi:10.1043%2F1543-2165-132.11.1830

4. Alizadeh AA, Elsen MB, Davis RE, et al. Distinct types of diffuse large B-cell lymphoma identified by gene expression profiling. *Nature.* 2000;403(6769):503–511. doi:10.1038/35000501

5. Hans CP, Weisenburger DD, Greiner TC, et al. Confirmation of the molecular classification of diffuse large B-cell lymphoma by immunohistochemistry using a tissue microarray. *Blood.* 2004;103(1):275–282. doi:10.1182/blood-2003-05-1545

6. Camilleri-Broët S, Criniè E, Broët P, et al. A uniform activated B-cell-like immunophenotype might explain the poor prognosis of primary central nervous system lymphomas: Analysis of 83 cases. *Blood.* 2006;107(1):190–196. doi:10.1182/blood-2005-03-1024

7. Smith JR, Braziel RM, Paoletti S, et al. Expression of B-cell-attracting chemokine 1 (CXCL13) by malignant lymphocytes and vascular endothelium in primary central nervous system lymphoma. *Blood.* 2003;101(3):815–821. doi:10.1182/blood-2002-05-1576

8. Fukumura K, Kawazu M, Kojima S, et al. Genomic characterization of primary central nervous system lymphoma. *Acta Neuropathol.* 2016;131:865–875. doi:10.1007/s00401-016-1536-2

9. Montesinos-Rongen M, Kü R, Schlüter D, et al. Primary central nervous system lymphomas are derived from germinal-center b cells and show a preferential usage of the v4-34 gene segment.

10. Chapuy B, Roemer MGM, Stewart C, et al. Targetable genetic features of primary testicular and primary central nervous system lymphomas. *Blood.* 2016;127(7):869–881. doi:10.1182/blood-2015-10-673236

11. Miller DC, Hochberg FH, Harris NL, et al. Pathology with clinical correlations of primary central nervous system non-Hodgkin's lymphoma. The Massachusetts General Hospital experience 1958-1989. *Cancer.* 1994;74(4):1383–1397. doi:10.1002/1097-0142(19940815)74:4<1383::AID-CNCR2820740432>3.0.CO;2-1

12. Martelius T, Lappalainen M, Palomäki M, Anttila VJ. Clinical characteristics of patients with Epstein Barr virus in cerebrospinal fluid. *BMC Infect Dis.* 2011;11:281. doi:10.1186/1471-2334-11-281

13. Bataille B, Delwail V, Menet E, et al. Primary intracerebral malignant lymphoma: Report of 248 cases. *J Neurosurg.* 2000;92(2):261–266. doi:10.3171/jns.2000.92.2.0261

14. Hong JT, Chae JB, Lee JY, et al. Ocular involvement in patients with primary CNS lymphoma. *J Neurooncol.* 2011;102(1):139–145. doi:10.1007/s11060-010-0303-9

15. Bataille B, Delwail V, Menet E, et al. Primary intracerebral malignant lymphoma: Report of 248 cases. *J Neurosurg.* 2000;92(2):261–266. doi:10.3171/jns.2000.92.2.0261

16. Velasco R, Mercadal S, Vidal N, et al. Diagnostic delay and outcome in immunocompetent patients with primary central nervous system lymphoma in Spain: A multicentric study. *J Neurooncol.* 2020;148(3):545–554. doi:10.1007/s11060-020-03547-z

17. Sugita Y, Terasaki M, Nakashima S, et al. Intraoperative rapid diagnosis of primary central nervous system lymphomas: Advantages and pitfalls. *Neuropathology.* 2014;34(5):438–445. doi:10.1111/neup.12126

18. Fischer L, Martus P, Weller M, et al. Meningeal dissemination in primary CNS lymphoma: Prospective evaluation of 282 patients. *Neurology.* 2008;71(14):1102–1108. doi:10.1212/01.wnl.0000326958.52546.f5

19. Ferreri AJM, Blay JY, Reni M, et al. Prognostic scoring system for primary CNS lymphomas: The International Extranodal Lymphoma Study Group experience. *J Clin Oncol.* 2003;21(2):266–272. doi:10.1200/JCO.2003.09.139

20. Abrey LE, Ben-Porat L, Panageas KS, et al. Primary central nervous system lymphoma: The Memorial Sloan-Kettering Cancer Center prognostic model. *J Clin Oncol.* 2006;24(36):5711–5715. doi:10.1200/JCO.2006.08.2941

21. Rubenstein JL, Hsi ED, Johnson JL, et al. Intensive chemotherapy and immunotherapy in patients with newly diagnosed primary CNS lymphoma: CALGB 50202 (Alliance 50202). *J Clin Oncol.* 2013;31:3061–3068. doi:10.1200/JCO.2012.46.9957

22. Abrey LE, Batchelor TT, Ferreri AJM, et al. Report of an international workshop to standardize baseline evaluation and response criteria for primary CNS lymphoma. *J Clin Oncol.* 2005;23(22):5034–5043. doi:10.1200/JCO.2005.13.524

23. Weller M, Martus P, Roth P, et al., German PCNSL Study Group. Surgery for primary CNS lymphoma? Challenging a paradigm. *Neuro Oncol.* 2012;14(12):1481–1484. doi:10.1093/neuonc/nos159

24. Rae AI, Mehta A, Cloney M, et al. Craniotomy and survival for primary central nervous system lymphoma. *Neurosurgery.* 2019;84(4):935–944. doi:10.1093/neuros/nyy096

25. Schultz C, Scott C, Sherman W, et al. Preirradiation chemotherapy with cyclophosphamide, doxorubicin, vincristine, and dexamethasone for primary CNS lymphomas: Initial report of radiation therapy oncology group protocol 88-06. *J Clin Oncol.* 1996;14(2):556–564. doi:10.1200/JCO.1996.14.2.556

26. Batchelor T, Carson K, O'Neill A, et al. Treatment of primary CNS lymphoma with methotrexate and deferred radiotherapy: A report of NABTT 96-07. *J Clin Oncol.* 2003;21(6):1044–1049. doi:10.1200/JCO.2003.03.036

27. Ferreri AJ, Reni M, Foppoli M, et al. High-dose cytarabine plus high-dose methotrexate versus high-dose methotrexate alone in patients with primary CNS lymphoma: A randomised phase 2 trial. *Lancet.* 2009;374(9700):1512–1520. doi:10.1016/S0140-6736(09)61416-1

28. Ferreri AJ, Cwynarski K, Pulczynski E, et al. Chemoimmunotherapy with methotrexate, cytarabine, thiotepa, and rituximab (MATRix regimen) in patients with primary CNS lymphoma: Results of the first randomisation of the International Extranodal Lymphoma Study Group-32 (IELSG32) phase 2 trial. *Lancet Haematol.* 2016;3(5):e217–e227. doi:10.1016/S2352-3026(16)00036-3

29. Morris PG, Correa DD, Yahalom J, et al. Rituximab, methotrexate, procarbazine, and vincristine followed by consolidation reduced-dose whole-brain radiotherapy and cytarabine in newly diagnosed primary CNS lymphoma: Final results and long-term outcome. *J Clin Oncol.* 2013;31(31):3971–3979. doi:10.1200/JCO.2013.50.4910

30. Poortmans PMP, Kluin-Nelemans HC, Haaxma-Reiche H, et al. High-dose methotrexate-based chemotherapy followed by consolidating radiotherapy in non-AIDS-related primary central nervous system lymphoma: European Organization for Research and Treatment of Cancer Lymphoma Group Phase II Trial 20962. *J Clin Oncol.* 2003;21(24):4483–4488. doi:10.1200/JCO.2003.03.108

31. Batchelor T, Carson K, O'Neill A, et al. Treatment of primary CNS lymphoma with methotrexate and deferred radiotherapy: A report of NABTT 96-07. *J Clin Oncol.* 2003;21(6):1044–1049. doi:10.1200/JCO.2003.03.036

32. Omuro A, Chinot O, Taillandier L, et al. Methotrexate and temozolomide versus methotrexate, procarbazine, vincristine, and cytarabine for primary CNS lymphoma in an elderly population: An intergroup ANOCEF-GOELAMS randomised phase 2 trial. *Lancet Haematol.* 2015;2(6):e251–e259. doi:10.1016/S2352-3026(15)00074-5

33. Batchelor TT, Grossman SA, Mikkelsen T, et al. Rituximab monotherapy for patients with recurrent primary CNS lymphoma. *Neurology.* 2011;76(10):929–930. doi:10.1212/WNL.0b013e31820f2d94

34. Bromberg JEC, Issa S, Bakunina K, et al. Rituximab in patients with primary CNS lymphoma (HOVON 105/ALLG NHL 24): A randomised, open-label, phase 3 intergroup study. *Lancet Oncol.* 2019;20(2):216–228. doi:10.1016/S1470-2045(18)30747-2

35. Houillier C, Soussain C, Ghesquì H, et al. Management and outcome of primary CNS lymphoma in the modern era: An LOC network study. 2020. doi:10.1212/WNL.0000000000008900

36. Nelson DF, Martz KL, Bonner H, et al. Non-Hodgkin's lymphoma of the brain: Can high dose, large volume radiation therapy improve survival? Report on a prospective trial by the Radiation therapy Oncology Group (RTOG): RTOG 8315. *Int J Radiat Oncol Biol Phys*. 1992;23(1):9–17. doi:10.1016/0360-3016(92)90538-S

37. Doolittle ND, Korfel A, Lubow MA, et al. Long-term cognitive function, neuroimaging, and quality of life in primary CNS lymphoma. *Neurology*. 2013;81(1):84–92. doi:10.1212/WNL.0b013e318297eeba

38. Juergens A, Pels H, Rogowski S, et al. Long-term survival with favorable cognitive outcome after chemotherapy in primary central nervous system lymphoma. *Ann Neurol*. 2010;67(2):182–189. doi:10.1002/ana.21824

39. Thiel E, Korfel A, Martus P, et al. High-dose methotrexate with or without whole brain radiotherapy for primary CNS lymphoma (G-PCNSL-SG-1): A phase 3, randomised, non-inferiority trial. *Lancet Oncol*. 2010;11(11):1036–1047. doi:10.1016/S1470-2045(10)70229-1

40. Herrlinger U, Schäfer N, Fimmers R, et al. Early whole brain radiotherapy in primary CNS lymphoma: Negative impact on quality of life in the randomized G-PCNSL-SG1 trial. *J Cancer Res Clin Oncol*. 2017;143(9):1815–1821. doi:10.1007/s00432-017-2423-5

41. Omuro A, DeAngelis L, Karrison T et al. Randomized phase II study of rituximab, methotrexate (MTX), procarbazine, vincristine, and cytarabine (R-MPV-A) with and without low-dose whole-brain radiotherapy (LD-WBRT) for newly diagnosed primary CNS lymphoma (PCNSL). *J Clin Oncol*. 2020;38. https://meetinglibrary.asco.org/record/185073/abstract

42. Omuro A, Correa DD, DeAngelis LM, et al. R-MPV followed by high-dose chemotherapy with TBC and autologous stem-cell transplant for newly diagnosed primary CNS lymphoma. *Blood*. 2015;125(9):1403–1410. doi:10.1182/blood-2014-10-604561

43. Ferreri AJM, Cwynarski K, Pulczynski E, et al. Whole-brain radiotherapy or autologous stem-cell transplantation as consolidation strategies after high-dose methotrexate-based chemoimmunotherapy in patients with primary CNS lymphoma: Results of the second randomisation of the International Extranodal Lymphoma Study Group-32 phase 2 trial. *Lancet Haematol*. 2017;4(11):e510–e523. doi:10.1016/S2352-3026(17)30174-6

44. Houillier C, Taillandier L, Dureau S, et al. Radiotherapy or autologous stem-cell transplantation for primary CNS lymphoma in patients 60 years of age and younger: Results of the Intergroup ANOCEF-GOELAMS Randomized Phase II PRECIS Study. *J Clin Oncol*. 2019;37:823–833. doi:10.1200/JCO.18

45. Langner-Lemercier S, Houillier C, Soussain C, et al. Primary CNS lymphoma at first relapse/progression: Characteristics, management, and outcome of 256 patients from the French LOC network. *Neuro-Oncology*. doi:10.1093/neuonc/now033

46. Plotkin SR, Betensky RA, Hochberg FH, et al. Treatment of relapsed central nervous system lymphoma with high-dose methotrexate. *Clin Cancer Res*. 2004;10(17):5643–5646. doi:10.1158/1078-0432.CCR-04-0159

47. Soussain C, Hoang-Xuan K, Taillandier L, et al. Intensive chemotherapy followed by hematopoietic stem-cell rescue for refractory and recurrent PCNSL and IOL. *J Clin Oncol*. 2008;26(15):2512–2518. doi:10.1200/JCO.2007.13.5533

48. Kasenda B, Schorb E, Fritsch K, et al. Primary CNS lymphoma-radiation-free salvage therapy by second autologous stem cell transplantation. *Biol Blood Marrow Transplant*. 2011;17(2):281–283. doi:10.1016/j.bbmt.2010.11.011

49. Hottinger AF, Deangelis LM, Yahalom J, Abrey LE. Salvage whole brain radiotherapy for recurrent or refractory primary CNS lymphoma. *Neurology*. 2007;69(11):1178–1182. doi:10.1212/01.wnl.0000276986.19602.c1

50. Nguyen PL, Chakravarti A, Finkelstein DM, et al. Results of whole-brain radiation as salvage of methotrexate failure for immunocompetent patients with primary CNS lymphoma. *J Clin Oncol*. 2005;23(7):1507–1513. doi:10.1200/JCO.2005.01.161

51. Grommes C, Pastore A, Palaskas N, et al. Ibrutinib unmasks critical role of bruton tyrosine kinase in primary CNS lymphoma. *Cancer Discov*. 2017;7(9):1018–1029. doi:10.1158/2159-8290.CD-17-0613

52. Soussain C, Choquet S, Blonski M, et al. Ibrutinib monotherapy for relapse or refractory primary CNS lymphoma and primary vitreoretinal lymphoma: Final analysis of the phase II 'proof-of-concept' iLOC study by the Lymphoma study association (LYSA) and the French oculo-cerebral lymphoma (LOC) network. *Eur J Cancer*. 2019;117:121–130. doi:10.1016/j.ejca.2019.05.024

53. Grommes C, Nayak L, Tun HW, Batchelor TT. Introduction of novel agents in the treatment of primary CNS lymphoma. *Neuro-Oncology*. doi:10.1093/neuonc/noy193

54. Lionakis MS, Dunleavy K, Roschewski M, et al. Inhibition of B cell receptor signaling by ibrutinib in primary CNS lymphoma. *Cancer Cell*. 2017;31(6):833–843.e5. doi:10.1016/j.ccell.2017.04.012

55. Rubenstein JL, Geng H, Fraser EJ, et al. Phase 1 investigation of lenalidomide/rituximab plus outcomes of lenalidomide maintenance in relapsed CNS lymphoma. *Blood Adv*. 2018;2(13):1595–1607. doi:10.1182/bloodadvances.2017014845

56. Grommes C, Tang SS, Wolfe J, et al. Phase 1b trial of an ibrutinib-based combination therapy in recurrent/refractory CNS lymphoma. *Blood*. 2019;133(5):436–445. doi:10.1182/blood-2018-09-875732

57. Moulignier A, Lamirel C, Picard H, et al. Long-term AIDS-related PCNSL outcomes with HD-MTX and combined antiretroviral therapy. *Neurology*. 2017;89(8):796–804. doi:10.1212/WNL.0000000000004265

58. Dierickx D, Habermann TM. Post-transplantation lymphoproliferative disorders in adults. Longo DL, ed. *N Engl J Med*. 2018;378(6):549–562. doi:10.1056/NEJMra1702693

59. Trappe RU, Dierickx D, Zimmermann H, et al. Response to rituximab induction is a predictive marker in B-cell post-transplant lymphoproliferative disorder and allows successful stratification into rituximab or r-chop consolidation in an international, prospective, multicenter Phase II trial. *J Clin Oncol*. 2017;35:536–543. doi:10.1200/JCO.2016.69.3564

60. Cavaliere R, Petroni G, Lopes MB, et al. Primary central nervous system post-transplantation lymphoproliferative disorder: An international primary central nervous system lymphoma collaborative group report. *Cancer*. 2010;116(4):863–870. doi:10.1002/cncr.24834

61. Shenkier TN, Blay JY, O'Neill BP, et al. Primary CNS lymphoma of T-cell origin: A descriptive analysis from the international primary CNS Lymphoma Collaborative Group. *J Clin Oncol*. 2005;23(10):2233–2239. doi:10.1200/JCO.2005.07.109

62. Wasserstrom WR, Glass JP, Posner JB. Diagnosis and treatment of leptomeningeal metastases from solid tumors: Experience with 90 patients. *Cancer*. 1982;49(4):759–772. doi:10.1002/1097-0142(19820215)49:4<759::AID-CNCR2820490427>3.0.CO;2-7

63. Rubenstein JL, Treseler PA, Stewart PJ. Regression of refractory intraocular large B-cell lymphoma with lenalidomide monotherapy. *J Clin Oncol*. 2011;29(20). doi:10.1200/JCO.2011.34.7252

64. Cox MC, Mannino G, Lionetto L, et al. Lenalidomide for aggressive B-cell lymphoma involving the central nervous system? *Am J Hematol*. 2011;86(11):957–957. doi:10.1002/ajh.22148

65. Frigault MJ, Maus MV, Dietrich J, et al. Tisagenlecleucel CAR T-cell therapy in secondary CNS lymphoma. *Blood*. 2019;134(11):860–866. doi:10.1182/blood.2019001694

66. Gan HK, Azad A, Cher L, Mitchell PLR. Neurolymphomatosis: Diagnosis, management, and outcomes in patients treated with rituximab. doi:10.1093/neuonc/nop021

67. Yamada E, Ishikawa E, Watanabe R, et al. Random skin biopsies before brain biopsy for Intravascular large B-cell lymphoma. *World Neurosurg*. 2019;121:e364–e369. doi:10.1016/j.wneu.2018.09.110

68. Kulkarni T, Treon S, Manning R, Xu L, Rinne M. Clinical characteristics and treatment outcome of CNS involvement (Bing-Neel syndrome) in Waldenstrom's macroglobulinemia. 2013. https://ashpublications.org/blood/article-abstract/122/21/5090/11241

69. Castillo JJ, D'Sa S, Lunn MP, et al. Central nervous system involvement by Waldenström macroglobulinaemia (Bing-Neel syndrome): A multi-institutional retrospective study. *Br J Haematol*. 2016;172(5):709–715. doi:10.1111/bjh.13883

70. Hoang-Xuan K, Bessell E, Bromberg J, et al. Diagnosis and treatment of primary CNS lymphoma in immunocompetent patients: Guidelines from the European Association for Neuro-Oncology. *Lancet Oncol*. 2015;16(7):e322–e332. doi:10.1016/S1470-2045(15)00076-5

71. Simon L, Fitsiori A, Lemal R, et al. Bing-Neel syndrome, a rare complication of waldenström macroglobulinemia: Analysis of 44 cases and review of the literature. A study on behalf of the French Innovative Leukemia Organization (FILO). *Haematologica*. 2015;100(12):1587–1594. doi:10.3324/haematol.2015.133744

72. Varettoni M, Marchioni E, Bonfichi M, et al. Successful treatment with rituximab and bendamustine in a patient with newly diagnosed Waldenström's macroglobulinemia complicated by Bing-Neel syndrome. *Am J Hematol*. 2015;90(8):E152–E153. doi:10.1002/ajh.24059

73. Mason C, Savona S, Rini JN, et al. Ibrutinib penetrates the blood brain barrier and shows efficacy in the therapy of Bing Neel syndrome. *Br J Haematol*. 2017;179(2):339–341. doi:10.1111/bjh.14218

74. Shihadeh F, Reed V, Faderl S, et al. Cytogenetic profile of patients with acute myeloid leukemia and central nervous system disease. *Cancer*. 2012;118(1):112–117. doi:10.1002/cncr.26253

75. Lazarus HM, Richards SM, Chopra R, et al. Central nervous system involvement in adult acute lymphoblastic leukemia at diagnosis: Results from the international ALL trial MRC UKALL XII/ECOG E2993. *Blood.* 2006;108(2):465–472. doi:10.1182/blood-2005-11-4666

76. Thomas X, Le QH. Central nervous system involvement in adult acute lymphoblastic leukemia. *Hematology.* 2008;13(5):293–302. doi:10.1179/102453308X343374

77. Thomas X, Boiron JM, Huguet F, et al. Outcome of treatment in adults with acute lymphoblastic leukemia: Analysis of the LALA-94 Trial. *J Clin Oncol.* 2004;22(20):4075–4086. doi:10.1200/JCO.2004.10.050

78. Pui C-H, Evans WE. Treatment of acute lymphoblastic leukemia. *N Engl J Med.* 2006;354(2):166–178. doi:10.1056/NEJMra052603

79. Pui CH. Central nervous system disease in acute lymphoblastic leukemia: Prophylaxis and treatment. *Hematology Am Soc Hematol Educ Program.* 2006;2006(1):142–146. doi:10.1182/asheducation-2006.1.142

80. Strati P, Uhm JH, Kaufmann TJ, et al. Prevalence and characteristics of central nervous system involvement by chronic lymphocytic leukemia. *Haematologica.* 2016;101(4):458–465. doi:10.3324/haematol.2015.136556

81. Berres ML, Lim KPH, Peters T, et al. BRAF-V600E expression in precursor versus differentiated dendritic cells defines clinically distinct LCH risk groups. *J Exp Med.* 2014;211(4):669–683. doi:10.1084/jem.20130977

82. Idbaih A, Donadieu J, Barthez MA, et al. Retinoic acid therapy in "degenerative-like" neuro-langerhans cell histiocytosis: A prospective pilot study. *Pediatr Blood Cancer.* 2004;43(1):55–58. doi:10.1002/pbc.20040

83. Imashuku S, Fujita N, Shioda Y, et al. Follow-up of pediatric patients treated by IVIG for Langerhans cell histiocytosis (LCH)-related neurodegenerative CNS disease. *Int J Hematol.* 2015;101(2):191–197. doi:10.1007/s12185-014-1717-5

84. Cai Q, Fang Y, Young KH. Primary central nervous system lymphoma: Molecular pathogenesis and advances in treatment. *Transl Oncol.* 2019;12(3):523–538. doi:10.1016/j.tranon.2018.11.011

12 | METASTATIC DISEASE IN THE CENTRAL NERVOUS SYSTEM

JESSICA A. WILCOX AND ADRIENNE A. BOIRE

INTRODUCTION

As many as one-third of all patients with cancer will develop metastases of the central nervous system (CNS), a clinical scenario that carries a high degree of morbidity and mortality. As improvements in available therapies and diagnostic techniques lead to an increase in survival among patients with cancer, more patients are living long enough to develop this unfortunate complication. Consequently, oncologists must be competent to diagnose CNS dissemination and choose appropriate treatments. Whereas solely palliative treatments were utilized in the past, the therapeutic arsenal against brain and leptomeningeal metastases has rapidly evolved to afford improvements in survival outcomes and quality of life. A collaborative effort between neurosurgeons, radiation oncologists, medical oncologists, and neuro-oncologists is critical in devising a targeted approach for each individual encounter.

EPIDEMIOLOGY

Brain metastases are a common occurrence in patients with systemic malignancies. An estimate of up to 200,000 new cases of brain metastases are diagnosed each year in the United States, as compared to only 17,000 new cases of primary brain tumors.[1] The frequency with which brain metastases arise varies based on the primary cancer, stage of disease, and study methodology. Current epidemiologic studies rely heavily on hospital- and population-based analyses, which predict that up to 10% of all adults with cancer will develop parenchymal brain metastases.[2-4] Older, autopsy series suggests that brain metastasis frequency may be even higher, with as many as 30% of cancer patients harboring symptomatic or asymptomatic brain metastases at the time of death.[5,6] While autopsy series are thought to offer a more reliable reflection of disease burden, the decline in autopsy rates combined with the change in oncologic trends in the past 30 years suggests that autopsy data may not accurately depict our current cancer era. That being said, the increase in overall survival (OS), advent of more sensitive imaging techniques, and development of immune-based and targeted therapies for brain metastases has led to an overall rise in the frequency of brain metastases in recent years.

In modern practice, the most common cancers to spread to the brain are from lung, breast, melanoma, renal, and colorectal primary neoplasms. While typically associated with advanced disease, brain metastases can be diagnosed at any time in the clinical course and may be independent of extracranial progression. The estimated incidences of brain metastases are 19.9% for lung, 6.9% for melanoma, 5.1% for breast, 6.5% for renal, and 1.8% for colorectal cancers.[2] Certain cancers, however, have a higher predilection to spread to the central nervous system (CNS) earlier in their disease course. For example, up to 28% of patients with de novo metastatic melanoma will harbor brain metastases, as compared to 27% of lung adenocarcinoma, 24% of small cell lung cancer (SCLC), 11% of renal cell carcinoma (RCC), and 8% of breast cancer patients.[7]

> The most common cancers to spread to the CNS include lung, breast, melanoma, renal, and colorectal.

Leptomeningeal metastases are nearly universally associated with advanced cancer, present in 3–8% of patients with solid tumor malignancies[5,6] and are highest among breast, melanoma, and lung primaries. Many patients with leptomeningeal metastases will also have synchronous growth of parenchymal metastases, indicating a common driver in metastatic progression within the two compartments.

PROGNOSIS

Despite advances in oncologic care affording increased OS in patients with metastatic cancer, those with brain metastases continue to face high morbidity and mortality. Median OS from the diagnosis of parenchymal brain metastases is on the order of 4–6 months.[8-10] Conversely, patients with leptomeningeal metastases have a historical life expectancy of only 2–4 months, with slightly better outcomes among breast cancer as opposed to melanoma and lung cancer patients.[11-15]

Certain prognostic variables confer a longer survival, such as young age (<65 years), female gender, higher performance status (Karnofsky Performance Status [KPS] ≥70), solitary parenchymal brain metastasis, and lack of extracranial disease.[8-10] The presence of certain molecular phenotypes, particularly those that open the avenues of targeted therapy and/or immunotherapy, tend to improve intracranial response rates and extend OS by several months.[16-20] Similarly for patients with leptomeningeal disease, additional factors such as response to radiation therapy, availability of systemic therapy, lower symptomatology, and lower serum lactate dehydrogenase (serum LDH <500 U/L) leads to prolonged survival.[21] A number of prognostication calculators, such as the recursive partitioning analysis (RPA)[8,22] and diagnosis-specific graded prognostic assessment (DS-GPA),[23,24] have been designed to predict survival and potential benefit to interventional therapies for patients with brain metastases.

PATHOPHYSIOLOGY

Stephen Paget's original "seed and soil" hypothesis of 1889 proposed that the metastatic colonization of specific organs is not due to chance but instead is a complex process requiring a favorable interaction between the tumor cell ("the seed") and the end-organ microenvironment ("the soil").[25] An overwhelming body of literature has come to support this theory in the past century. However, a central tenet of metastatic progression, termed the "metastatic cascade," is preserved across primary tumor types: selection of tumor cells with metastatic potential, invasion through stromal tissue, capillary intravasation, hematogenous dissemination, arrest within end-organ capillaries, extravasation into the surrounding tissue, and proliferation within a new foreign microenvironment.[26] In the setting of brain metastases, tumor cell arrest tends to occur at areas of narrowed cerebral microvasculature, hence the predilection for seeding watershed vascular territories and the highly vascularized gray–white junction.[27] An alternative pattern for lymphatic and retrograde venous spread along Batson's plexus into the CNS also exists.[28] It is essential to underline that tumor cell entry into the CNS alone is insufficient to enable metastatic growth. Tumor cells must overcome multiple selective pressures within the unfamiliar niche. To acquire these traits, metastatic cancer cells leverage genetic, epigenetic, and transcriptional heterogeneity. A reflection of this, cancer cells disseminated to the CNS are often genetically divergent from the primary tumor,[29] an important principle when considering treatment options.

Anatomic barriers of the CNS, protecting the "immuno-privileged" brain and spinal cord from systemic pathogens and toxic insults, provide an added layer of complexity to CNS metastasis development. The CNS comprises of three distinct compartments: the parenchyma, leptomeninges, and pachymeninges. Variability exists in terms of vascular access, distinct microenvironment, and metastatic potential for each site, and so will be discussed separately.

PARENCHYMAL METASTASES

To gain access to the brain parenchyma, tumor cells must first penetrate the blood–brain barrier (BBB). This vascular gateway is a selective semi-permeable border at the level of cerebral capillaries, comprised of endothelial cells, pericytes, and astrocytic end-feet.[30] Tumor cell arrest and extravasation through the endothelial cell layer requires a combination of CNS-tropic and inflammatory arrest signals, mediated by tumor and endothelial cell interactions.[31-33] Once safely secured on the extraluminal side of the capillary network, cancer cells compete with adjacent pericytes for space and nestle near the basal lamina, a microenvironment typically inhabited by neural stem cells. Micrometastases within this perivascular niche then acquire blood supply through two major mechanisms. This first, *vessel co-option*, involves cohesive interactions with preexisting capillaries for signals that induce plasticity, nutrients such as glucose and oxygen, and endothelial-produced angiocrine factors to support proliferation.[34,35] The second, *sprouting angiogenesis*, involves the formation of new blood vessels from preexisting capillaries.[36] The newly formed neurovascular–tumor unit marks an inherently leaky blood-tumor barrier (BTB), lacking the tight junctions and astrocytic end-feet that regulate the BBB.[36] Additional considerations, such as upregulation of drug efflux pumps at the BTB and hijacking of growth factors and cytokines released by astrocytes and microglia, contribute to the complexity and resistance mechanisms of metastatic brain tumors.[30]

LEPTOMENINGEAL METASTASES

The leptomeninges are composed of two meningeal layers, the pia mater and arachnoid mater, separated by the subarachnoid space. Cerebrospinal fluid (CSF) courses through the subarachnoid space and intraventricular system and, through unclear mechanisms, provides a suitable microenvironment for metastatic dissemination. In some ways analogous to the BBB, a multifunctional blood-CSF barrier (BCSFB) exists within the choroid plexus. While the BCSFB does function in part to impede transit of blood-borne products into CSF and facilitates exchange of nutrients and waste, the main responsibility of the BCSFB lies in production of CSF by the choroid plexus epithelium. The main pathway of CSF egress occurs by diffusion through arachnoid granulations into the dural venous sinuses, and the pressure gradient between these two systems maintains intracranial pressure (ICP) homeostasis.

The pathway of metastatic tumor infiltration into the CSF space to cause leptomeningeal carcinomatosis is not fully understood. A number of routes have been proposed based mainly on mouse model observations: hematogenous seeding from the fenestrated capillaries of the choroid plexus,[37] venous dissemination following bridging veins or Batson's plexus,[38,39] perineural invasion,[40] and direct seeding from parenchymal, dural, or osseous tumors near the CSF spaces.[41] Surgical resection of brain metastases, particularly superficial lesions and those within the posterior fossa, confers a risk of subsequent leptomeningeal cancer development hypothetically due to intraoperative tumor spillage.[42,43] Once within the meninges, leptomeningeal cancer cells disseminate widely through the subarachnoid space and ependymal lining but have a predilection for depositing along low-flow and gravity-dependent areas such as the posterior fossa, basal cisterns, and lumbar cistern.

How cancer cells survive within the hypoxic, nutrient-sparse CSF represents another gray area. Levels of glucose, protein, oxygen, and other metabolic resources, otherwise essential in tumor growth, are devoid within the CSF compartment.[44] In addition, the development of leptomeningeal metastases induces a vast inflammatory infiltrate of neutrophils, macrophages, and lymphocytes that share the subarachnoid space—hence the term "carcinomatous meningitis"—further policing this microenvironment and competing for nutrients. Mouse model experiments illuminate one potential mechanism by which leptomeningeal metastases overcome this challenge: tumor cell expression of complement C3.[45] Subsequent activation of the complement cascade at the level of the choroid plexus disrupts epithelial border tight junctions, leading to loss of BCSFB integrity and spillage of nutrient-rich plasma into the CSF to support leptomeningeal cell proliferation.

PACHYMENINGEAL METASTASES

The pachymeninges consist of dura mater, the outermost protective covering of the CNS. Dural metastases, in stark contrast to parenchymal and leptomeningeal metastases, do not reside behind a BBB or BCSFB and therefore are amenable to systemic treatments regardless of CNS penetrance. Cancer cells metastasize to the dura either through hematogenous spread or by direct extension of skull metastases.[46] As one might expect, the most common cancers to metastasize to the dura are also those with highest propensity for osseous spread: breast and prostate.[47]

> There are three main types of CNS metastatic disease: parenchymal metastases, leptomeningeal metastases, and pachymeningeal metastases.

PRESENTATION AND DIAGNOSIS

PARENCHYMAL METASTASES

Patients with new or worsening parenchymal metastases present with a wide variety of symptoms, and so all treating clinicians must maintain a high level of suspicion when faced with subtle neurologic complaints. The most common presenting symptoms of parenchymal brain metastases are headache, hemiparesis, aphasia, dysarthria, gait instability, visual disturbances, confusion, and seizures. Headaches often intensify when supine or bending forward. However, the "classic" brain tumor headache triad—worse in the morning, severe intensity, associated nausea or vomiting—is only present in approximately 17% of patients, and is indicative of increased ICP.[48]

A comprehensive neurologic examination can often localize the symptomatic lesion(s). Gadolinium-enhanced magnetic resonance imaging (MRI) is the preferred imaging modality for brain metastasis diagnosis, particularly since small metastases might be missed with computed topography (CT) scans. If gadolinium is contraindicated, then CT scans with iodine-based contrast is an alternative. Parenchymal metastases appear as contrast-enhancing lesions at the gray–white junction, often with a disproportionate amount of vasogenic edema and/or central necrosis, reflecting rapid tumor growth (Figure 12.1). Traditional teaching dictates that brain metastases with the highest rates of intratumoral hemorrhage include melanoma, RCC, choriocarcinoma, and papillary thyroid cancer. However, due to preponderance of lung and breast cancer metastases in the population, hemorrhage within these lesions is more frequently encountered in clinical practice.

Screening for CNS metastases in the form of MRI or CT scans, in the absence of neurologic symptoms, is not standard of care for all cancer types. The exception to this rule lies in

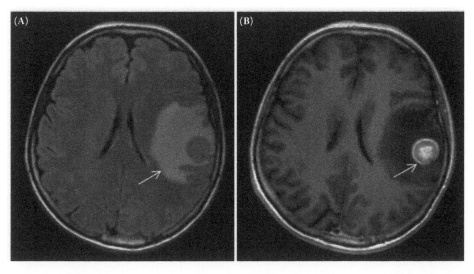

Figure 12.1 Solitary brain metastasis with associated vasogenic edema. (A) MRI brain, fluid-attenuated inversion recovery (FLAIR). Vasogenic edema surrounding the tumor (arrow). (B) T1 pre-contrast showing solitary brain metastasis with hemorrhage.

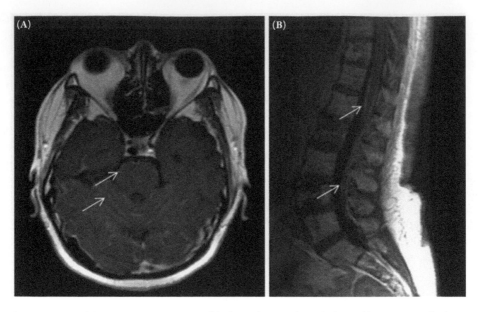

Figure 12.2 Leptomeningeal carcinomatosis. (A) T1 post-contrast images of the brain showing classic findings of leptomeningeal enhancement in cerebellar folia and pre-pontine area. (B) T1 post-contrast images of the lumbar spine showing linear enhancement of the conus medullaris and cauda equina.

malignancies with a high propensity for CNS invasion, for which early diagnosis and treatment would provide a survival benefit. For this reason, expert consensus guidelines from the National Comprehensive Cancer Network (NCCN) recommend screening MRIs for all patients with grade 3C and 4 melanoma, stage 2 to 4 non-small cell lung cancer (NSCLC), and SCLC of any stage.[49] Asymptomatic patients with breast and renal cell cancer do not require baseline CNS screening per NCCN guidelines.

LEPTOMENINGEAL METASTASES

Leptomeningeal metastases cause a wide array of symptoms and signs depending on the site of deposition, leading to a medley of cranial neuropathies, radiculopathies, and pressure-mediated symptoms. These can include diplopia (cranial nerve III, IV, or VI), lower motor neuron facial weakness (cranial nerve VII), facial numbness or paresthesias (cranial nerve V), dysphagia (cranial nerve IX, X, and XII), vocal cord paralysis (cranial nerve X), ataxia (cerebellar folia), radiculopathies (cervical and lumbar roots), or bowel/bladder dysfunction with saddle anesthesia (conus medullaris, cauda equina). Elevated ICP due to impaired CSF reabsorption manifests as headaches, nausea, confusion, and even obtundation in severe or acute cases.

The diagnosis of leptomeningeal cancer can at times be elusive, and clinical symptoms are often out of proportion to imaging findings. Radiographic findings include ependymal and leptomeningeal enhancement in any region of the neuro-axis, with particular attention to the cerebellar folia, cranial nerves, and cauda equina (Figure 12.2). Skull base metastases causing compressive cranial neuropathies are a common mimic for leptomeningeal metastases, and so calvarial lesions should be excluded. Communicating hydrocephalus with increased trans-ependymal flow may be seen

in some, but not all, cases of elevated ICP. Lumbar puncture is a critical component in the workup of leptomeningeal metastases as this procedure offers both diagnostic and therapeutic benefit. Detection of malignant cells on cytologic examination of the CSF is the gold standard for diagnosis, a test that has high specificity (>95%) but unfortunately low sensitivity (50%). Cytologic samples should contain 5–10 cc of fluid and be processed immediately to maximize yield. If the initial cytologic specimen is negative for malignant cells, lumbar puncture can be repeated, with sensitivity approaching 90% after the third spinal tap.[50] In the setting of elevated opening pressure of greater than 20 cm CSF, large volume fluid removal (30–40 cc) can provide prompt relief of symptoms, albeit only temporarily. CSF is produced at a rate of 20 cc per hour, therefore symptoms attributed to increased ICP are likely to return within 1 day without a more permanent solution, such as ventriculoperitoneal shunting (Figure 12.5).

In only the past decade, circulating tumor cell (CTC) enumeration has begun to complement traditional CSF cytology within specialized medical centers. CTC enumeration provides a quantitative measure of malignant cells of epithelial origin (breast, lung, colorectal, prostate, ovarian) in the CSF with approximately 95% sensitivity, notably higher than that of standard cytologic testing.[51–53] This technique was adapted from the Veridex CellSearch assay, a technique approved by the US Food and Drug Administration (FDA) which detects cancer cells expressing epithelial cell adhesion molecule (EpCAM) in the peripheral blood. Additional available assays include the Biocept TargetSelector assay. Peripheral blood CTC burden serves as a useful biomarker of systemic disease status and response to treatment for many epithelial solid tumor malignancies,[54–57] and recent studies suggest that CSF CTCs operate similarly in breast and NSCLC cohorts.[58,59]

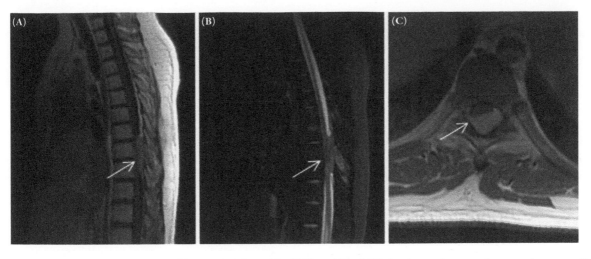

Figure 12.3 *Malignant spinal cord compression. MRI of the spine. (A) Sagittal T1, (B) T2, and (C) axial T1 showing cord compression secondary to a malignancy. Note cord impingement and loss of cerebrospinal fluid (CSF) signal.*

EPIDURAL SPINE METASTASES

Epidural metastases carry a high risk of causing significant neurologic morbidity. Spinal metastases will occur in up to 20% of cancer patients, with prostate and breast cancers responsible for the highest proportion of cases.[60] Patients with epidural spinal metastases may report gnawing back pain which awakens them from sleep, termed "biological pain" due to the relative reduction in endogenous cortisol production in the late evening. Epidural metastases may also be asymptomatic, particularly if they have not yet encroached on neighboring osseous or spinal cord structures. However, when epidural metastases grow to the extent of spinal cord compression, pain at the symptomatic lesion is nearly universally reported.[61] Additional common complaints of cord compression include motor or sensory deficits below the level of the lesion, urinary retention, fecal incontinence, and saddle anesthesia. The neurologic examination may also uncover myelopathic signs, reduced rectal tone, and a sensory level. The absence of hyperreflexia, however, does not reliably rule out clinical cord compression because acute spinal cord ischemia initially results in hyporeflexia. A concurrent cauda equina syndrome with lower motor neuron findings will also mask brisk reflexes.

A definitive diagnosis for malignant spinal cord compression relies on emergent MRI (Figure 12.3). Complete spine imaging should be pursued to also evaluate the extent of disease, particularly as sensory levels can falsely localize to several levels below the site of compression. Epidural metastases localize to the thoracic spine in approximately 70% of affected patients but are also present in the lumbar spine in 20% and cervical spine in 10% of cases.[61] Additional information on diagnosis and management of epidural metastases can be found in Chapter 25.

DURAL METASTASES

Dural metastases are typically asymptomatic, but if large enough to compress adjacent brain parenchyma might induce headaches, seizures, and/or focal neurologic deficits. The vast majority of dural metastases will appear as diffuse or nodular contrast-enhancing plaques on a gadolinium-enhanced brain MRI. The leading alternative diagnosis in the differential for dural-enhancing lesion is a meningioma; factors such as rapid tumor growth, the lack of calcification, synchronous increase of multiple lesions, and active systemic disease would be supportive of metastatic disease.[62] Some cases remain elusive, however, and require biopsy for definitive diagnosis. Treatment of symptomatic lesions involves radiation to the symptomatic lesion. As discussed before, dural metastases do not lie within the confines of the BBB and thus are amenable to systemic cancer therapies.

MANAGEMENT

The general approach to managing CNS metastases involves first identifying the symptomatic lesion(s), offering stabilizing treatments for immediate symptom management, and involving a team of neurosurgeons, radiation oncologists, medical oncologists, and neuro-oncologists to develop an appropriate treatment plan based on anatomic constraints, functional status, and goals of care. Psychosocial factors also require close attention, as the development of CNS metastases often precipitates anxiety, depression, and reduction in quality of life for patients.

Corticosteroids, generally in the form of dexamethasone, are commonly employed in the immediate setting to quickly reduce peri-tumoral edema and improve neurologic symptoms. Seizures may be suspected based on the site of metastases and symptoms. Electroencephalography may guide the clinician if the diagnosis is unclear, but empiric treatment with anti-epileptics is often necessary, preferably with non-enzyme inducing agents (levetiracetam, lacosamide, zonisamide) to minimize risk of potential drug interactions with systemic cancer treatments. Potential systemic aberrations, such as hyponatremia and infection, should be investigated as these may worsen neurologic symptoms and lower the seizure threshold. Hyponatremia is particularly common in brain tumor patients due to volume depletion states and the syndrome of inappropriate secretion of antidiuretic hormone

(SIADH). Opiates, antiemetics, anxiolytics, laxatives, and urine catheterization are all additional palliative considerations.

In the case of hemorrhagic metastases, management often becomes complex. Patients with metastatic disease are at increased risk for thrombotic events and are therefore likely to require anticoagulation (typically with low-molecular-weight heparin). Because the vascular supply generated by brain metastases is imperfect, patients on anticoagulation with brain metastases are at slight but elevated risk for intracranial hemorrhage.[63] Such patients therefore represent a therapeutic dilemma. Current clinical practice therefore generally entails a discussion among the medical oncologist, neuro-oncologist, and the patient, followed by serial non-contrast CTs to determine the stability of metastasis after initiation of anticoagulation. Importantly, hemorrhagic brain metastases are more epileptogenic than their non-hemorrhagic counterparts. In the case of a cortically based hemorrhagic metastasis, seizure prophylaxis with a non–enzyme-inducing antiepileptic such as levetiracetam or lacosamide is recommended.[64]

Once the tumor-directed treatment is initiated, NCCN guidelines advise that patients with CNS metastases follow with their oncologist every 8–12 weeks for clinical evaluations, including neurologic exam and review of neuro-axial imaging.[49] After 1–2 years of stability, the surveillance window may be extended on a case-by-case basis. In the setting of leptomeningeal metastases, serial CSF sampling may also be considered, as needed, to monitor response to treatment.

PARENCHYMAL METASTASES

When approaching a patient with parenchymal metastases, a combination of surgical resection, focal radiation therapy, and/or whole-brain radiation therapy (WBRT) is employed to achieve prompt local control. Small, minimally symptomatic or asymptomatic metastases of certain cancer types may be addressed with a trial of CNS-penetrant systemic treatments alone; however, this is the exception, not the rule.

> Small, asymptomatic or minimally symptomatic parenchymal CNS metastases caused by certain cancer types can be treated with a trial of systemic CNS-penetrant therapy prior to focal or particularly whole-brain irradiation.

The specific choice of therapy is predicted by a number of factors: cancer type, number and size of metastases, lesion location, degree of symptoms, mass effect, prognosis, and functional status (Figure 12.4).

Brain Metastasis Management Algorithm

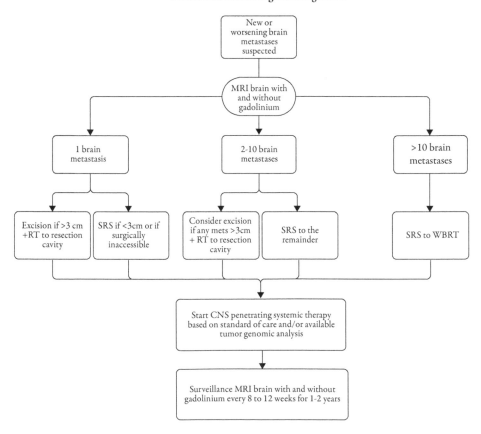

Figure 12.4 *Schema for management of brain metastases for patients with Karnofsky Performance Score (KPS) >70. In the setting of KPS <70 or uncontrolled systemic disease, foregoing surgical excision in favor of radiation or palliative measures is reasonable. Of note, select patients with small asymptomatic brain metastases and a highly efficacious CNS-penetrant systemic therapy option (i.e., immunotherapy for melanoma, targeted therapy for EGFR or ALK mutated non-small cell lung cancer [NSCLC]) may first trial systemic treatments without local control on a case-by-case basis.*
Abbreviations: RT, radiation therapy; SRS, stereotactic radiosurgery; WBRT, whole-brain radiation therapy.

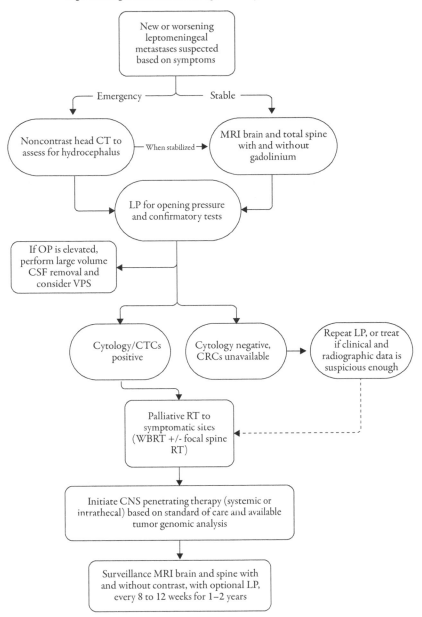

Leptomeningeal Metastases Management Algorithm

New or worsening leptomeningeal metastases suspected based on symptoms

— Emergency — Stable —

Noncontrast head CT to assess for hydrocephalus — When stabilized → MRI brain and total spine with and without gadolinium

LP for opening pressure and confirmatory tests

If OP is elevated, perform large volume CSF removal and consider VPS

Cytology/CTCs positive

Cytology negative, CRCs unavailable

Repeat LP, or treat if clinical and radiographic data is suspicious enough

Palliative RT to symptomatic sites (WBRT +/- focal spine RT)

Initiate CNS penetrating therapy (systemic or intrathecal) based on standard of care and available tumor genomic analysis

Surveillance MRI brain and spine with and without contrast, with optional LP, every 8 to 12 weeks for 1–2 years

Figure 12.5 Diagnosis and management of leptomeningeal metastases. Symptoms such as severe headache, nausea, emesis, and obtundation warrant emergent head CT and LP. Candidacy for palliative ventriculoperitoneal shunt (VPS), if indicated, should take into consideration Karnofsky Performance Score (KPS), overall prognosis, and remaining available treatments. Confirmatory cerebrospinal fluid (CSF) testing includes cell count with differential, protein, glucose, cytology, circulating tumor cells (CTCs) (where available), and tumor-derived cell free DNA (where available) as this might influence treatment decisions. Abbreviations: LP, lumbar puncture; OP, opening pressure; WBRT, whole-brain radiation therapy; RT, radiation therapy.

Surgery is typically indicated for patients with good prognoses who harbor large (>3 cm), symptomatic, surgically accessible brain metastases.[65] Deep-seated lesions, or those located within eloquent areas, pose more of a surgical dilemma. The most compelling argument for surgical resection is for a patient with a solitary, accessible brain mass from oligometastatic disease to the CNS. Nevertheless, in the setting of multiple brain metastases, removal of up to three dominant lesions can afford palliative benefit.[66] The benefit of surgical resection is twofold; not only has this been shown to provide a survival benefit,[67,68] but genomic analysis of this tissue also may reveal valuable targetable mutations inherent to CNS metastases.[29]

The risk of local recurrence with surgery alone approaches 50%, a percentage which can be mitigated with the use of adjuvant radiotherapy. Historically, surgery had been followed by WBRT to prevent recurrence at the surgical bed and impede growth of distant metastases.[69–71] However, WBRT has not been proved to improve OS[70] and leads to functional decline and cognitive dysfunction.[72] Therefore, postoperative focal radiation, such as stereotactic radiosurgery (SRS) or intensity modulated radiation therapy (IMRT), to the surgical cavity is preferred over WBRT with similar survival rates and less toxicity.[73–75] SRS may also be employed to treat distant, small metastases

(<3 cm) that are not amenable to surgical resection, with similar local control rates.[76,77]

For surgically inaccessible tumors, or for patients with high burden of intracranial disease for which surgical resection may not be beneficial, SRS for up to 10 metastases is generally acceptable. Similar to the surgical data, the addition of WBRT to SRS in such patients improves distant failure rates but does not translate into a survival benefit.[78] One small, randomized study also found the probability of significant memory and learning impairment at 4 months to be twice as likely in the WBRT plus SRS patients (52%) as compared to the SRS only group (24%).[79] Literature supports the efficacy of SRS or gamma knife radiosurgery alone for patients with more than 10 metastases,[80-83] however, at this stage, WBRT may be more appropriate based on the clinical scenario. Owing to the high burden of disease among brain metastasis patients receiving WBRT, the OS for these patients is on the order of 5–6 months.[84,85]

Both short- and long-term survivors following WBRT are at risk for radiation-induced CNS toxicity. The neurocognitive domains most affected include verbal and non-verbal memory, sustained attention, processing speed, and executive function, owing to the impact of radiation on the hippocampus and prefrontal cortex.[86] The risk of radiation-induced toxicity is heightened by several factors: advanced age, aggressive malignancy, chemotherapies administered (particularly methotrexate), higher total radiation doses and fractionation schemes, and larger treatment fields. Three phases of WBRT-induced cognitive toxicity have been observed with differing mechanisms.[87,88] The acute (days to weeks) and early delayed (1–6 months) side effects involve cerebral edema and transient demyelination, respectively, and tend to cause symptoms of headaches, somnolence, and worsening of preexisting neurologic deficits. These early symptoms are typically reversible and may be shortened with a course of steroids. Patients who develop late delayed toxicity (>6 months after radiation), conversely, suffer more permanent and progressive symptoms including seizures, hypertonicity, ataxia, dementia, and, in severe cases, death. Histologic samples of those with late delayed toxicity reveal vascular insult, demyelination, and gliosis. Delayed radiation toxicity is primarily a clinical diagnosis; radiographic findings of periventricular leukoencephalopathy and diffuse cerebral atrophy, however, are supportive. Strategies to minimize the cognitive toxicity associated with WBRT, such as memantine prophylaxis[89] and hippocampal-sparing techniques,[90] are currently being investigated with modest meaningful benefit.

> There are three distinct phases of WBRT-induced neurotoxicity: acute (days to weeks), early delayed (1–6 months), and late delayed (>6 months post treatment).

LEPTOMENINGEAL METASTASES

Treatment of leptomeningeal metastases is notoriously challenging. The leptomeningeal cavity is not easily accessible with systemic treatments, intrathecal (IT) treatments are met with only a small increase in survival, and radiation to one site does not eradicate disease in another. As such, treatment of leptomeningeal metastases is focused on palliation.

Patients with signs and symptoms of increased ICP should undergo prompt lumbar puncture as this affords near-immediate relief of symptoms. Ventriculoperitoneal shunt offers a more permanent solution, with a survival gain of 2–6 months from the time of CSF diversion[91-94]; this benefit is longer in patients who are amenable to further targeted therapies.[95]

Symptomatic sites of cancer deposition can be targeted with radiation, with neurologic stabilization in approximately 75%.[21] WBRT may be indicated for those with cranial involvement, particularly those with elevated ICP, albeit without an appreciable survival benefit.[96] Full craniospinal irradiation (CSI) with photons is not feasible due to the severe myelosuppressive effect.[97] The use of proton CSI as a means of treating the entire neuro-axis while limiting toxicity to the bone marrow is currently under investigation.

IT chemotherapy does not penetrate beyond a few cell layers and depends on unimpeded CSF flow. Therefore, the use of such treatments requires normal CSF fluid dynamics and a lack of bulky, nodular leptomeningeal deposits. Available IT treatments for eligible patients include methotrexate, cytarabine, thiotepa, topotecan, etoposide, and rituximab, to name the most common.[98] No randomized control trial has been conducted to formally compare each treatment, but efficacy is estimated to be similar.[98-101] A few small retrospective studies suggest that IT trastuzumab for eligible HER2-positive breast cancer patients can be efficacious and result in long-term survival.[102,103] Clinical trial results of this approach are pending. Administration through an Ommaya reservoir is preferred over lumbar puncture. Beyond patient comfort, this approach overcomes risk of infiltration of chemotherapy into the skin and surrounding tissues, improving drug delivery.[98] Aseptic meningitis and treatment-related leukoencephalopathy are common side effects of IT treatments, particularly when combined with WBRT in the latter.

> Intraventricular administration of chemotherapy via Ommaya reservoir is preferred as it is associated with improved drug delivery and improved patient comfort as compared to conventional approach via lumbar puncture.

EPIDURAL METASTASES

Cord compression from an epidural metastasis is a neurologic emergency and must be treated promptly to reduce the risk of permanent disability (see also Chapter 25). High-dose dexamethasone should be administered immediately upon clinical suspicion for cord compression while awaiting confirmatory imaging. Historically, physicians recommended a 100 mg intravenous bolus of dexamethasone up-front, followed by 96 mg/day in divided doses; however, a randomized trial found that a 10 mg bolus followed by 16 mg/day is not inferior in terms of pain scores and outcomes.[104]

The severity of neurologic compromise relies on both clinical and radiographic factors, for which validated scoring systems have been designed to stratify patients into different treatment algorithms. For example, the epidural spinal cord compression (ESCC) radiographic score, developed by the Spine Oncology Study Group, delineates compressive tumors on T2-weighted axial images from low grade (scores 0–1) to high grade (scores 2–3).[105] Similarly, the spinal instability neoplastic score (SINS) classifies the degree of mechanical instability, with higher number (scores 7–18 on an 18-point scale) warranting surgical consultation.[106] These results are then integrated with factors such as radiation sensitivity of the tumor, extent of systemic disease, and functional status in determining therapeutic approach. This algorithm, known as the NOMS (neurologic, oncologic, mechanical, systemic) framework, helps to guide physicians in determining whether a complex patient should be offered radiation, surgery, or a combination of both.[60] Most patients with a low SINS and radiosensitive malignancies (breast, prostate, lymphoma, multiple myeloma, small cell lung cancer, germ cell tumors) may be treated with conventional external beam radiation therapy (cEBRT) regardless of ESCC score, although solid tumor malignancies may require initial surgical decompression based on the severity of neurologic deficits. Any patient with spinal instability or a radioresistant malignancy (melanoma, RCC, NSCLC, gastrointestinal tumors, sarcoma) with high-grade ESCC score should undergo surgical decompression prior to radiation therapy. Stereotactic body radiation therapy (SBRT), which delivers a high dose of radiation with greater precision than cEBRT, may be considered as an alternative for radioresistant tumors with low-grade ESCC scores, when available.

> Any patient with spinal instability or a radioresistant malignancy (melanoma, RCC, NSCLC, gastrointestinal tumors, sarcoma) with high-grade ESCC score should undergo surgical decompression prior to radiation therapy.

Despite these interventions, patients with metastatic epidural cord compression suffer a high rate of neurologic sequelae. Low-quality evidence suggests that the duration and severity of neurologic deficits are most predictive of postoperative outcomes,[107] and so every effort should be made to achieve clinical stabilization as soon as safely feasible.

SYSTEMIC THERAPIES FOR CNS METASTASES

IMMUNOTHERAPY

The immune checkpoint inhibitors (ICI), a class of monoclonal antibodies against cytotoxic T-lymphocyte–associated antigen-4 (CTLA-4) and programmed death-1 (PD-1) or ligand-1 (PD-L1), have gained tremendous traction in the treatment of a variety of extracranial solid tumor malignancies. These agents interfere with malignant evasion of the immune system by blocking the inhibitory signals on T cells at both the nodal (CTLA-4) and tumor (PD-1 and PD-L1) microenvironments,

thereby unleashing cytotoxic T cells to attack malignant cells. Healthy non-neoplastic tissues may also be endangered by such a mechanism, and, as such, autoimmune reactions are commonly observed with these treatments. Available agents include ipilimumab (CTLA-4), nivolumab (PD-1), pembrolizumab (PD-1), and atezolizumab (PD-L1). Perhaps owing to the immunoprivileged misconception regarding brain tumors, patients with intracranial metastases were commonly excluded from clinical trials for systemic malignancies. Nevertheless, mounting data support the use of ICIs for brain metastases from melanoma, NSCLC, and, to a lesser extent, RCC.[108]

Among patients with small, asymptomatic melanoma brain metastases, the combination of ipilimumab and nivolumab achieves an intracranial control rate as high as 57% with improvement in OS, a regimen which is now first-line therapy in this target population.[109,110] Tumors with high PD-L1 expression (PD-L1 >5%) tend to achieve better response rates. Select patients may opt for a trial of immunotherapy without up-front cranial irradiation on a case-by-case basis, thus saving radiation for a later time point should systemic treatments fail. Similarly, multiple checkpoint inhibitors have demonstrated intracranial response rates ranging from 27% to 39% in NSCLC[111–113]; the combination of pembrolizumab, pemetrexed, and a platinum-based agent has become first-line therapy for epidermal growth factor receptor (EGFR) negative and anaplastic lymphoma kinase (ALK)-negative NSCLC.[114] The intense inflammatory infiltrate into metastatic lesions being treated with immunotherapy leads to a transient increase in tumor enhancement and surrounding edema, a phenomenon known as *pseudoprogression*.[115] This radiographic finding may falsely mimic tumor progression and lead to the inappropriate discontinuation of an effective treatment. The immunotherapy response assessment in neuro-oncology (iRANO) criteria was therefore devised to help clinicians differentiate pseudoprogression from true progression.

While select patients with minimal CNS disease can forego up-front SRS upon initiation of ICI, it is worth noting that a synergistic effect has been observed with the combination of radiation with immunotherapy.[116] *Abscopal effects*, where non-irradiated metastases regress at sites distant from the primary site of irradiation, have also been reported both intracranially and extracranially following CNS irradiation.[116,117] It is hypothesized that these findings occur due to the radiation-induced breakdown of the BBB and release of tumor antigens into the circulation, thus making tumors more amenable to immunotherapy.

TARGETED THERAPY

Molecular targeted therapy has revolutionized the current landscape of oncologic care. These drugs exploit oncogenic driver mutations inherent to cancer development, disrupting neoplastic growth and survival at the source. Whereas traditional chemotherapy agents tend to poorly penetrate the BBB, most targeted agents are small-molecule tyrosine kinase inhibitors (TKIs) with reasonable CNS distribution and therefore brain and leptomeningeal metastasis activity. Because brain metastases often harbor mutations genetically divergent from those of the primary tumor,[29] confirmation of such oncogenes via genomic sequencing of a resected brain metastasis or tumor-derived cell-free DNA within the CSF is preferred whenever feasible.[118] Targeted therapies are generally used as adjunctive treatments for brain metastases following local control with surgery and/ or radiation therapy, aiming to minimize recurrence and prevent development of future metastases. A summary of CNS-penetrant targeted agents is available in Table 12.1, with a few notable mentions detailed here.

Activating mutations within the *EGFR* gene, predominantly exon 19 deletions and exon 21 L858R mutations,

TABLE 12.1 Targeted therapies with central nervous system (CNS) efficacy

NAME	TARGET AGENT DOSE	ROUTE	CNS RESPONSE RATES	SIDE EFFECTS	PROSPECTIVE TRIALS
NSCLC					
EGFR–mutant					
Erlotinib[a]	1,200 mg QD (day 1–2), 50 mg QD (day 2–7)	PO	75%	Rash	Arbour 2018
Gefitinib	250 mg QD	PO	27–88%	Rash, diarrhea	Ceresoli 2004, Iuchi 2013
Afatinib	40 mg QD	PO	54–75%	Diarrhea, rash, paronychia	Schuler 2016, Park 2016
Osimertinib	80 mg–160 mg QD	PO	40–91%, 41–62% for LM	Diarrhea, rash, paronychia	Mok 2017, Goss 2018, Wu 2018, Reungwetwattana 2018, Yang 2020
ALK–alteration					
Crizotinib	250 mg BID	PO	18–33%	Nausea, vomiting, diarrhea, transaminitis, edema	Costa 2015, Peters 2017, Nishio 2018
Ceritinib	750 mg QD	PO	23–47%	Nausea, vomiting, diarrhea, transaminitis	Crino 2016, Kim 2016, Shaw 2017, Soria 2017
Alectinib	300 mg–600 mg BID	PO	34–59%	Anemia, myalgias, nausea, vomiting, diarrhea, transaminitis	Gadgeel 2014, Gadgeel 2016, Peters 2017, Nishio 2018
Brigatinib[b]	90 mg–180 mg QD	PO	41–57%	Nausea, diarrhea, headache	Gettinger 2016, Kim 2017
Lorlatinib	100 mg QD	PO	40–88%	Hypercholesteroleima, hypertriglyceridemia, edema, neuropathy	Solomon 2018, Shaw 2019, Bauer 2020
Melanoma					
BRAF–mutant					
Vemurafenib	960 mg BID	PO	18–42%	Rash, photosensitivity, arthralgia, headache	McArthur 2017, Dummer 2014
Dabrafenib	150 mg BID	PO	31–50%	Fatigue, hyperkeratosis, cutaneous SCC	Long 2012, Falchook 2012
BRAF + MEK Combinations					
Dabrafenib + Trametinib	150 mg BID/2 mg QD	PO	44–59%	Pyrexa, headache, asthenia, nausea, diarrhea	Davies 2017
Vemurafenib + Cobimetinib	960 mg BID/60 mg QD	PO	n/a	Rash, diarrhea, nausea, fatigue, pyrexia, CPK elevation	Ascierto 2016
Encorafenib + Binimetinib	450 mg QD/45 mg BID	PO	n/a	Nausea, diarrhea, fatigue, CPK elevaton	Dummer 2018
Breast					
HER2/ERBB2–amplified					

TABLE 12.1 Continued

NAME	TARGET AGENT DOSE	ROUTE	CNS RESPONSE RATES	SIDE EFFECTS	PROSPECTIVE TRIALS
Lapatinib[c]	750 mg BID	PO	6%	Diarrhea, rash, nausea, vomiting	Lin 2009
Lapatinib + Capecitabine	1,250 mg QD	PO	20–66%	Hand–foot syndrome, diarrhea, nausea	Lin 2009, Bachelot 2013
Neratinib	240 mg QD	PO	8%	Diarrhea, fatigue	Freedman 2016
Neratinib + Capecitabine	240 mg QD	PO	33–49%	Diarrhea, nausea, vomiting, fatigue	Freedman 2019
Tucatinib + Trastuzumab + Capecitabine	300 mg BID	PO	47%	Diarrhea, hand–foot syndrome, nausea, vomiting, fatigue	Lin 2020

NSCLC, non-small cell lung cancer; EGFR, epidermal growth factor receptor; ALK, anaplastic lymphoma kinase; HER2, human epidermal growth factor receptor 2; LM, leptomeningeal metastases.

[a]Pulse/continuous dosing.

[b]ALK and EGFR inhibitor.

[c]HER2 and EGFR inhibitor.

are present in 20–40% of NSCLC patients.[119] Furthermore, brain metastases arise in approximately 70% of *EGFR*-mutant NSCLC, as opposed to only 30% in the *EGFR*-wildtype cohort. Erlotinib, a first-generation TKI targeting EGFR, heralded tremendous benefit in the treatment *EGFR*-mutant NSCLC patients, but with poor intracranial activity. Pulse-dosing regimens help to improve the delivery of erlotinib into the CNS,[120,121] and multiple EGFR-TKIs have since been developed with superior CNS penetration.[119,122–125] Nevertheless, nearly one-third of *EGFR*-mutant NSCLC patients will develop intracranial progression while receiving first-generation TKIs.[126] Metastatic progression following first- and second-generation EGFR-inhibitor therapy typically occurs through the acquisition of a T790M resistance mutation. Osimertinib, a third-generation TKI, maintains efficacy despite this escape mutation and demonstrates impressive CNS activity, with an objective response rate (ORR) of 54–91% for brain metastases[127–130] and 41–62% for leptomeningeal disease.[131] *EML4-ALK* translocations are present in approximately 5% on NSCLC; however, up to 20% of this population will harbor brain metastases at initial diagnosis.[132] Crizotinib, a first-generation ALK and ROS1 inhibitor, achieved only modest intracranial response rates of short duration.[133–135] Second- and third-generation ALK-inhibitors (ceritinib, alectinib, brigatinib, and lorlatinib) offer greater control of both brain and leptomeningeal metastases and are also able to overcome resistance to early-generation TKIs.[17,134–148]

Approximately one-half of advanced melanoma patients harbor mutations in the *BRAF* gene, with V600E representing more than 90% of these mutations.[149] *BRAF*-mutant melanomas are more biologically aggressive than their *BRAF*-wildtype counterparts and also more likely to metastasize to the brain. The duration of intracranial responses with BRAF-inhibitors, such as with dabrafenib[150,151] and vemurafenib,[152,153] is limited due to acquired resistance mutation involving the mitogen-activated protein kinase pathway.[154] Supplementing dabrafenib therapy with the MEK inhibitor, trametinib, raises the intracranial

ORR to 44–59% with an improvement in OS.[149,155] Additional clinical trials evaluating other BRAF/MEK inhibitor combination regimens (vemurafenib/cobimetinib,[156] encorafenib/binimetinib[157]) are ongoing. Retrospective studies suggest that the combination of BRAF inhibition with radiation may provide a synergistic effect, but prospective trials are lacking.[158]

Among patients with breast cancer, the use of HER2/ERBB2-targeting monoclonal antibody trastuzumab has long been associated with development of brain metastases, perhaps secondary to poor BBB penetration and also a genetic predilection for CNS disease in this patient population. Lapatinib, an oral TKI targeting both the ERBB2 and EGFR pathways, has emerged as an efficacious option in combination with capecitabine in patients with HER2-positive brain metastases that have progressed on trastuzumab, though intracranial response rates approach only 30% in a pooled analysis.[18,159,160] When used as monotherapy, lapatinib achieves only a 6% CNS ORR following trastuzumab failure and prior CNS radiation.[160] Neratinib, an irreversible HER2-TKI, carries similar single- and dual-agent response rates to lapatinib.[161,162] Tucatinib, a third-generation and highly selective HER2 inhibitor, in combination with trastuzumab and capecitabine, demonstrated significant intracranial efficacy as well as a survival benefit in the HER2CLIMB study, with a CNS ORR of 47.3% versus 20.0% in the placebo plus combination arm.[163] Patients harboring germline *BRCA1/2* mutations are amenable to treatment with poly (adenosine diphosphate-ribose) polymerase (PARP) inhibitors, and case reports suggest that olaparib confers CNS activity in select patients with breast[164] and ovarian[165] cancers. Similarly, the cyclin-dependent kinases 4/6 (CDK4/6) inhibitors abemaciclib[166] and palbociclib[167] have shown early success in the treatment of breast and other solid tumor CNS metastases; however, more large-scale studies are pending.

> Both immunotherapy and targeted therapy show promise in treatment of CNS metastases, and their use in neuro-oncology is likely to increase in the coming years.

Finally, the vascular endothelial growth factor (VEGF)-inhibitor, bevacizumab, has gained FDA approval for a number of extracranial malignancies. This anti-angiogenic monoclonal antibody prevents VEGF from binding to its receptor on endothelial cells, thereby regulating vascular permeability, shrinking peri-tumoral edema, and reducing radiographic enhancement. While not FDA-approved specifically for brain metastases, this agent is highly effective in the treatment of cerebral radiation necrosis after an initial trial of corticosteroids, which can have deleterious effects when used long term.[168] Consequently, the administration of bevacizumab provides a steroid-sparing palliative benefit in the treatment of cerebral radiation necrosis across cancer types. Known adverse effects of bevacizumab therapy include increased arterial and venous thromboembolic events, impaired wound healing, hypertension, and renal injury. Increased risk of hemorrhagic events can also be seen with bevacizumab use, and so clinicians should proceed with caution when administering to patients with hemorrhagic brain metastases.

NON-TARGETED THERAPY

Since the advent of targeted therapies, the use of traditional non-targeted chemotherapies has been generally reserved for the recurrent setting. The BBB serves as a sanctuary for brain metastases against large water-soluble chemotherapies and monoclonal antibodies, therefore the list of chemotherapies able to penetrate the BBB is small. Standard chemotherapies carry a high rate of toxic side effects, and the radiographic response rates for such agents tend to fall below 40%. Agents such as high-dose methotrexate, temozolomide, capecitabine, pemetrexed, cisplatin, carboplatin, etoposide, and vinorelbine fall into this category. Some regimens supplement non-targeted chemotherapies with either a targeted agent or immunotherapy to boost the efficacy of either agent alone, as is seen with lapatinib plus capecitabine[169] and pembrolizumab plus pemetrexed and carboplatin.[114]

CONCLUSION

The diagnosis and management of CNS metastases has evolved tremendously in the twenty-first century, and commonly harmful therapies of the past are being replaced with better-tolerated and targeted strategies. Advances in our understanding of the molecular drivers and microenvironments of tumor formation have been indispensable to the current landscape of oncologic care. The direct consequences of these discoveries include wider access to genomic testing, targeted treatments to exploit cell signaling aberrations, and immune-based approaches with efficacy both systemically and in the CNS. Large-scale studies have also displaced WBRT in favor of focal radiation strategies, thus mitigating long-term neurotoxic effects in brain tumor survivors. As modern therapies lead to improvements in progression-free survival and OS for patients with cancer, continued advances in basic, translational, and clinical CNS metastasis research remain critical.

FLASHCARD

What is the incidence of brain metastases (BM) per year in the US?	20,000
The most common primary malignancies to metastasize to the brain include	Lung (19.9%), breast (5.1%), melanoma (6.9%), renal (6.5%), and colorectal (1.8%)
What is the percentage of patients with metastatic melanoma or non-small cell lung cancer (NSCLC) with BM at time of cancer diagnosis?	25%
What is the prevalence of leptomeningeal metastases among patients with solid tumor malignancies?	3–8%
Median overall survival for patients with BM and for leptomeningeal metastases (LM) is	Less than 6 months for patients with BM, less than 4 months for patients with (LM)
Good prognostic indicators for patients with CNS metastases include	Age <65, KPS ≥70, female gender, solitary brain metastasis, controlled extracranial disease, and targetable mutations
What is the sensitivity of CSF cytology on initial and third lumbar puncture (LP)?	~50% on first LP, close to 90% on third LP. CSF circulating tumor cells is a more sensitive confirmatory test for LM of epithelial origin
What is typical initial management of large metastases (>3 cm), particularly if single BM?	Surgery followed by postop radiation to the surgical bed
What is typical initial management of smaller BM, particularly if multiple?	Stereotactic radiosurgery (SRS)
Whole-brain radiation is generally reserved for which clinical situations?	Patients with high intracranial BM burden (>10 BMs) and LM
Intrathecal treatments should be avoided in which patients with LM?	Patients with abnormal CSF flow dynamic, and/or large, bulky, nodular LM

Molecular sequencing is recommended for CNS metastases for what reason?	CNS metastases are often genetically divergent from the primary tumor, and results could lead to new therapeutic options for the patient
CNS EGFR-mutant NSCLC may be treated with	Pulse-dose erlotinib, or osimertinib
CNS ALK-rearranged NSCLC may be treated with	Crizotinib, alectinib, or lorlatinib
CNS $BRAF^{V600E}$- mutant melanoma may be treated with	Dabrafenib combined with MEK inhibitor trametinib
CNS HER2-amplified breast cancer may be treated with	Lapatinib
Synergistic effect may be seen when combining SRS with which therapies?	Immunotherapies and tyrosine kinase inhibitors
Up-front radiation for BM may be held in which cases?	Small, asymptomatic CMs from melanoma or EGFR/ALK-mutant NSCLC in favor of CNS-penetrant targeted treatments

CASE 1

A 32-year old right-handed woman with metastatic breast cancer (ER⁺, PR⁻, HER2⁺) with osseous and lung metastases is currently receiving anastrozole, trastuzumab, and pertuzumab with stable systemic disease and a KPS of 90. She presents to the hospital with 2 weeks of intermittent confusion, language disturbances, and severe headaches. Her family states that at times "her speech is gibberish" for minutes at a time, and, after a period of fatigue, she returns to near baseline but with more mild word-finding difficulties. On exam, she appears uncomfortable and has paraphasic errors, right arm pronator drift, and subtle dysmetria in her left arm. MRI brain with and without gadolinium demonstrates four ring-enhancing lesions with vasogenic edema, the largest of which is 3.5 cm in the left temporal lobe. She has additional smaller (2–3 cm) metastases in the right frontal lobe, left occipital lobe, and left cerebellum.

1. What is the next *immediate* step in management?
   a. Lumbar puncture to assess for leptomeningeal metastases
   b. Start dexamethasone 4 mg BID and levetiracetam 500 mg BID
   c. Send her home with outpatient follow-up with her medical oncologist
   d. Consult radiation oncology for whole-brain radiation therapy

She is admitted to the hospital, started on symptomatic treatment and feels much better. Her paraphasic errors and headaches have resolved. However, in the evening she has an abrupt episode of confusion, described as not answering staff correctly, perseverating on the same word, and not following commands. The neurology team sees her and diagnoses her with a receptive aphasia, which has been ongoing for now 20 minutes.

2. How should her aphasia be investigated and managed?
   a. STAT non-contrast head CT to rule out increasing edema or new hemorrhage
   b. Give lorazepam 2 mg IV and increase levetiracetam to 1,000 mg BID
   c. Consult radiation oncology for emergent radiation of her left temporal metastasis
   d. Start video EEG monitoring
   e. a, b, and d

3. Once she is stabilized, what is the next best step for managing her brain metastases?
   a. Neurosurgical consultation to resect her four brain metastases
   b. Neurosurgical consultation to resect her dominant, left temporal brain metastasis
   c. Radiation oncology consultation for whole-brain radiation therapy
   d. Radiation oncology consultation for stereotactic radiosurgery
   e. b and d

Following local control with resection of her left temporal metastasis and SRS to the surgical bed and remaining metastases, she is recovering well at home. MRI brain 1 month after treatment shows mild expected postoperative enhancement around the resection cavity, and her remaining three metastases are smaller. Left temporal pathology confirms metastatic breast cancer (ER⁻, PR⁻, HER2⁺).

4. What is true about the pathophysiology of her brain metastases?
   a. Patients with HER2⁺ breast cancer treated with trastuzumab have a high incidence of brain metastases, partially due to its poor blood–brain barrier (BBB) penetration.
   b. The development of brain metastases in this woman is highly unusual given her stable systemic disease.
   c. Trastuzumab has dose-dependent penetration through the BBB, so increasing her dose is appropriate as her brain tumor is still positive for HER2.
   d. Anastrozole has dose-dependent penetration through the BBB, so increasing her dose is appropriate as her brain tumor is still positive for HER2.

5. What is a reasonable next line of therapy which will also target her brain metastases?
   a. Capecitabine
   b. Intrathecal methotrexate
   c. Lapatinib
   d. a and c

CASE 2

A 64-year old right-handed man, previous smoker, is diagnosed with EGFR mutant non-small cell lung cancer (T2N1M1a). He is started on initial therapy with erlotinib, and his cancer remains stable for 6 months. On his next series of staging, however, he is found to have new metastases in his contralateral lung, liver, and abdominal lymph nodes. At his oncologist's office to discuss these results, he endorses also new posterior headaches waking him from sleep, associated with nausea and frequent vomiting. He's also been experiencing increasing gait difficulty. He is sent to the hospital for emergent non-contrast head CT, which demonstrates a space-occupying hypodensity in the left cerebellum with surrounding edema, effacement of the fourth ventricle, and early mild hydrocephalus.

6. What is the next best *immediate* step in his management?
   a. Arrange for outpatient neurosurgical consultation
   b. Perform lumbar puncture to measure opening pressure and lower elevated pressure
   c. Bolus with dexamethasone 10 mg IV followed by standing 6 mg BID
   d. b and c

7. MRI brain confirms a 3.8 cm left cerebellar metastasis with surrounding vasogenic edema. He has no additional enhancing lesions. How should this metastasis be treated?
   a. Cerebellar metastasis resection alone
   b. Cerebellar metastasis resection followed by postoperative radiation to the surgical bed
   c. Whole-brain radiation therapy
   d. SRS to the cerebellum
   e. Pulse-dose erlotinib

The patient is started on dexamethasone and undergoes suboccipital craniotomy for resection of his cerebellar metastasis. Postoperative imaging confirms a gross total resection, and the surgical bed is subsequently treated with hypofractionated radiation to lessen the risk of recurrence. The cerebellar tumor pathology returns positive for lung adenocarcinoma with an EGFR T790M mutation.

8. What targeted treatment should be started next to treat both his CNS and systemic disease?
   a. Crizotinib
   b. Afatinib
   c. Ceritinib
   d. Osimertinib

Eight months later, the patient returns to his oncologist's office with recurrent headaches and nausea. He is now also experiencing double vision, which improves if he covers one eye; difficulty swallowing; left facial droop; and pain shooting into his right leg. On examination, he has a right abducens nerve palsy, left lower motor neuron facial palsy, left hypoglossal weakness, and 3/5 strength of dorsiflexion in his right leg with an absent right ankle jerk.

9. What is true about the development and workup of leptomeningeal metastases?
   a. CSF cytology is highly sensitive and specific, and so a negative result reliably rules out this diagnosis.
   b. His history of cerebellar metastasis resection places him at a higher risk of developing leptomeningeal metastases.
   c. Osimertinib has no proved efficacy for treating leptomeningeal disease.
   d. All of the above.

MRI brain and total spine demonstrate leptomeningeal enhancement involving his cerebellar folia, multiple cranial nerves, patchy involvement of his cerebral sulci, and cauda equina. His ventricle size is mildly increased. His lumbar puncture demonstrates an opening pressure of 18 cm CSF, nucleated cells 55 per microliter (neutrophils 12%, lymphocytes 70%, monocytes 10%, extrinsic cells 8%), red blood cells <1 per microliter, protein 120 mg/dL, glucose 45 mg/dL. Cytology is positive for adenocarcinoma, and CSF circulating tumor cell count is 150 cells/3.0 mL. CSF bacterial cultures are negative.

10. What is the next best step in his management?
    a. Consult neurosurgery for ventriculoperitoneal shunt placement.
    b. Consult radiation oncology for palliative radiation to the symptomatic areas.
    c. Consult radiation oncology for cranio-spinal photon radiation.
    d. Consult infectious disease and begin empiric acyclovir for herpes meningitis.

STAND-ALONE QUESTIONS

11. Which combination therapy has been proved to have high intracranial activity in BRAF-wildtype metastatic melanoma to the brain?
    a. Ipilimumab and nivolumab
    b. Pembrolizumab, pemetrexed, and carboplatin
    c. Dabrafenib and trametinib
    d. Lapatinib and capecitabine

12. What are the five most common solid-tumor malignancies to metastasize to the brain?
    a. Lung, breast, thyroid, urothelial, melanoma
    b. Breast, melanoma, hepatocellular, renal, colorectal
    c. Lung, breast, melanoma, renal, colorectal
    d. Melanoma, lung, breast, prostate, colorectal

13. Which of the following tyrosine kinase inhibitors is correctly matched to its target mutation?
    a. Erlotinib—anaplastic lymphoma kinase (ALK)
    b. Dabrafenib—B-raf (BRAF)
    c. Olaparib—epidermal growth factor receptor (EGFR)
    d. Lorlatinib—human epidermal growth factor receptor 2 (HER2)

14. What is the most common class of adverse events that should be monitored for when administering immune checkpoint inhibitor therapy?
    a. Autoimmune reactions
    b. Bone marrow suppression
    c. Stevens-Johnson syndrome
    d. Venous thromboembolism

15. Which of the following is not true regarding metastatic tumor infiltration into the CNS?
    a. Circulating tumor cells must extravasate through the capillary cells of the BBB to establish micrometastases.
    b. Tumor cells inhabiting the CNS acquire blood supply from both vessel co-option and neo-angiogenesis.
    c. The mechanism of tumor cell invasion into the leptomeningeal space is not confirmed but hypothesized to be partially mediated by interactions with the blood–CSF barrier in the choroid plexus.
    d. Brain metastases most commonly seed the deep white matter because this is where capillary size is most narrow to facilitate tumor cell arrest and entry.

ANSWERS

1. b
2. e
3. e
4. a
5. d
6. c
7. b
8. d
9. b
10. b
11. a
12. c
13. b
14. a
15. d

REFERENCES

1. Kohler BA, et al. Annual report to the nation on the status of cancer, 1975–2007, featuring tumors of the brain and other nervous system. *J Natl Cancer Inst.* 2011;103:714–736. doi:10.1093/jnci/djr077

2. Barnholtz-Sloan JS, et al. Incidence proportions of brain metastases in patients diagnosed (1973 to 2001) in the Metropolitan Detroit Cancer Surveillance System. *J Clin Oncol.* 2004;22:2865–2872.

3. Schouten LJ, Rutten J, Huveneers HAM, Twijnstra A. Incidence of brain metastases in a cohort of patients with carcinoma of the breast, colon, kidney, and lung and melanoma. *Cancer.* 2002;94:2698–2705.

4. Goncalves PH, et al. Risk of brain metastases in patients with non-metastatic lung cancer: Analysis of the Metropolitan Detroit Surveillance, Epidemiology, and End Results (SEER) data. *Cancer.* 2016;122:1921–1927.

5. Posner JB, Chernik NL. Intracranial metastases from systemic cancer. *Adv Neurol.* 1978;19:579–592.

6. Takakura K, Sano K, Hojo S, Hirano A. *Metastatic Tumors of the Central Nervous System.* Tokyo: Igaku-Shoin; 1982.

7. Cagney DN, et al. Incidence and prognosis of patients with brain metastases at diagnosis of systemic malignancy: A population-based study. *Neuro Oncol.* 2017;19:1511–1521. doi:10.1093/neuonc/nox077

8. Gaspar L, et al. Recursive partitioning analysis (RPA) of prognostic factors in three Radiation Therapy Oncology Group (RTOG) brain metastases trials. *Int J Radiat Oncol Biol Phys.* 1997;37:745–751. doi:10.1016/s0360-3016(96)00619-0

9. Suteu P, Fekete Z, Todor N, Nagy V. Survival and quality of life after whole brain radiotherapy with 3D conformal boost in the treatment of brain metastases. *Med Pharm Rep.* 2019;92:43–51. doi:10.15386/cjmed-1040

10. Rastogi K, et al. Palliation of brain metastases: Analysis of prognostic factors affecting overall survival. *Indian J Palliat Care.* 2018;24:308–312. doi:10.4103/ijpc.Ijpc_1_18

11. Harstad L, Hess KR, Groves MD. Prognostic factors and outcomes in patients with leptomeningeal melanomatosis. *Neuro Oncol.* 2008;10:1010–1018. doi:10.1215/15228517-2008-062

12. Park JH, et al. Clinical outcomes of leptomeningeal metastasis in patients with non-small cell lung cancer in the modern chemotherapy era. *Lung Cancer.* 2012;76:387–392. doi:10.1016/j.lungcan.2011.11.022

13. Stelzer KJ. Epidemiology and prognosis of brain metastases. *Surg Neurol Int.* 2013;4:S192–202. doi:10.4103/2152-7806.111296

14. Kingston B, et al. Treatment and prognosis of leptomeningeal disease secondary to metastatic breast cancer: A single-centre experience. *Breast.* 2017;36:54–59. doi:10.1016/j.breast.2017.07.015

15. Morikawa A, et al. Characteristics and outcomes of patients with breast cancer with leptomeningeal metastasis. *Clin Breast. Cancer.* 2017;17:23–28. doi:10.1016/j.clbc.2016.07.002

16. Tawbi HA, et al. Combined nivolumab and ipilimumab in melanoma metastatic to the brain. *N Engl J Med.* 2018;379:722–730. doi:10.1056/NEJMoa1805453

17. Solomon BJ, et al. Lorlatinib in patients with ALK-positive non-small-cell lung cancer: Results from a global phase 2 study. *Lancet Oncol.* 2018;19:1654–1667. doi:10.1016/s1470-2045(18)30649-1

18. Petrelli F, et al. The efficacy of lapatinib and capecitabine in HER-2 positive breast cancer with brain metastases: A systematic review and pooled analysis. *Eur J Cancer.* 2017;84:141–148. doi:10.1016/j.ejca.2017.07.024

19. Petrelli F, et al. Efficacy of ALK inhibitors on NSCLC brain metastases: A systematic review and pooled analysis of 21 studies. *PLoS One.* 2018;13, e0201425. doi:10.1371/journal.pone.0201425

20. Reungwetwattana T, et al. CNS response to osimertinib versus standard epidermal growth factor receptor tyrosine kinase inhibitors in patients with untreated EGFR-mutated advanced non-small-cell lung cancer. *J Clin Oncol.* 2018;Jco2018783118. doi:10.1200/jco.2018.78.3118

21. El Shafie RA, et al. Palliative radiotherapy for leptomeningeal carcinomatosis: Analysis of outcome, prognostic factors, and symptom response. *Front Oncol.* 2019;8. doi:10.3389/fonc.2018.00641

22. Gaspar LE, Scott C, Murray K, Curran W. Validation of the RTOG recursive partitioning analysis (RPA) classification for brain metastases. *Int J Radiat Oncol Biol Phys.* 2000;47:1001–1006. doi:10.1016/s0360-3016(00)00547-2

23. Sperduto PW, et al. Diagnosis-specific prognostic factors, indexes, and treatment outcomes for patients with newly diagnosed brain metastases: A multi-institutional analysis of 4,259 patients. *Int J Radiat Oncol Biol Phys.* 2010;77:655–661. doi:10.1016/j.ijrobp.2009.08.025

24. Sperduto PW, et al. Summary report on the graded prognostic assessment: An accurate and facile diagnosis-specific tool to estimate survival for patients with brain metastases. *J Clin Oncol.* 2012;30:419–425. doi:10.1200/jco.2011.38.0527

25. Paget S. The distribution of secondary growths in cancer of the breast. 1889. *Cancer Metastasis Rev.* 1989;8:98–101

26. Preusser M, et al. Brain metastases: Pathobiology and emerging targeted therapies. *Acta Neuropathol.* 2012;123:205–222. doi:10.1007/s00401-011-0933-9

27. Hwang TL, Close TP, Grego JM, Brannon WL, Gonzales F. Predilection of brain metastasis in gray and white matter junction and vascular border zones. *Cancer.* 1996;77:1551–1555. doi:10.1002/(sici)1097-0142(19960415)77:8<1551::Aid-cncr19>3.0.Co;2-z

28. Carr I. Lymphatic metastasis. *Cancer Metastasis Rev.* 1983;2:307–317. doi:10.1007/bf00048483

29. Brastianos PK, et al. Genomic characterization of brain metastases reveals branched evolution and potential therapeutic targets. *Cancer Discov.* 2015;5:1164–1177. doi:10.1158/2159-8290.CD-15-0369

30. Sprowls SA, et al. Improving CNS delivery to brain metastases by blood–tumor barrier disruption. *Trends Cancer.* 2019;5:495–505. doi:https://doi.org/10.1016/j.trecan.2019.06.003

31. Bos PD, et al. Genes that mediate breast cancer metastasis to the brain. *Nature.* 2009;459:1005–1009. doi:10.1038/nature08021

32. Liu W, et al. AKR1B10 (Aldo-keto reductase family 1 B10) promotes brain metastasis of lung cancer cells in a multi-organ microfluidic chip model. *Acta Biomater.* 2019;doi:10.1016/j.actbio.2019.04.053

33. Guo Q, et al. LRP1–upregulated nanoparticles for efficiently conquering the blood-brain barrier and targetedly suppressing multifocal and infiltrative brain metastases. *J Control Release.* 2019;303:117–129. doi:10.1016/j.jconrel.2019.04.031

34. Rafii S, Butler JM, Ding BS. Angiocrine functions of organ-specific endothelial cells. *Nature.* 2016;529:316–325. doi:10.1038/nature17040

35. Holash J, et al. Vessel cooption, regression, and growth in tumors mediated by angiopoietins and VEGF. *Science.* 1999;284:1994–1998

36. Arvanitis CD, Ferraro GB, Jain RK. The blood–brain barrier and blood–tumour barrier in brain tumours and metastases. *Nature Rev Cancer.* 2020;20:26–41. doi:10.1038/s41568-019-0205-x

37. Garzia L, et al. A hematogenous route for medulloblastoma leptomeningeal metastases. *Cell.* 2018;173:1549. doi:10.1016/j.cell.2018.05.033

38. Yao H, et al. Leukaemia hijacks a neural mechanism to invade the central nervous system. *Nature.* 2018;560:55–60. doi:10.1038/s41586-018-0342-5

39. Bubendorf L, et al. Metastatic patterns of prostate cancer: An autopsy study of 1,589 patients. *Hum Pathol.* 2000;31:578–583. doi:10.1053/hp.2000.6698

40. Kokkoris CP. Leptomeningeal carcinomatosis. How does cancer reach the pia-arachnoid? *Cancer.* 1983;51:154–160.

41. Boyle R, Thomas M, Adams JH. Diffuse involvement of the leptomeninges by tumour--a clinical and pathological study of 63 cases. *Postgrad Med J.* 1980;56:149–158. doi:10.1136/pgmj.56.653.149

42. van der Ree TC, et al. Leptomeningeal metastasis after surgical resection of brain metastases. *J Neurol Neurosurg Psychiatry.* 1999;66:225–227. doi:10.1136/jnnp.66.2.225

43. Ahn JH, et al. Risk for leptomeningeal seeding after resection for brain metastases: Implication of tumor location with mode of resection. *J Neurosurg.* 2012;116:984–993. doi:10.3171/2012.1.Jns111560

44. Spector R, Robert Snodgrass S, Johanson CE. A balanced view of the cerebrospinal fluid composition and functions: Focus on adult humans. *Exp Neurol.* 2015;273:57–68. doi:10.1016/j.expneurol.2015.07.027

45. Boire A, et al. Complement component 3 adapts the cerebrospinal fluid for leptomeningeal metastasis. *Cell.* 2017;168:1101–1113 e1113. doi:10.1016/j.cell.2017.02.025

46. Heo MH, Cho YJ, Kim HK, Kim JY, Park YH. Isolated pachymeningeal metastasis from breast cancer: Clinical features and prognostic factors. *Breast.* 2017;35:109–114. doi:10.1016/j.breast.2017.07.006

47. Nayak L, Abrey LE, Iwamoto FM. Intracranial dural metastases. *Cancer.* 2009;115:1947–1953. doi:10.1002/cncr.24203

48. Forsyth PA, Posner JB. Headaches in patients with brain tumors: A study of 111 patients. *Neurology.* 1993;43:1678–1683. doi:10.1212/wnl.43.9.1678

49. NCCN Clinical Practice Guidelines in Oncology. *National Comprehensive Cancer. Network*

50. Wasserstrom WR, Glass JP, Posner JB. Diagnosis and treatment of leptomeningeal metastases from solid tumors: Experience with 90 patients. *Cancer.* 1982;49:759–772

51. Li X, et al. Clinical significance of detecting CSF-derived tumor cells in breast cancer patients with leptomeningeal metastasis. *Oncotarget.* 2017;9:2705–2714. doi:10.18632/oncotarget.23597

52. Nayak L, et al. Rare cell capture technology for the diagnosis of leptomeningeal metastasis in solid tumors. *Neurology.* 2013;80:1598–1605;discussion 1603. doi:10.1212/WNL.0b013e31828f183f

53. Lee JS, et al. Detection of cerebrospinal fluid tumor cells and its clinical relevance in leptomeningeal metastasis of breast cancer. *Breast Cancer Res Treat.* 2015;154:339–349. doi:10.1007/s10549-015-3610-1

54. Krebs MG, Hou, J.-M, Ward TH, Blackhall FH, Dive C. Circulating tumour cells: Their utility in cancer management and predicting outcomes. *Thera Adv Med Oncol.* 2010;2:351–365. doi:10.1177/1758834010378414

55. Yan WT, et al. Circulating tumor cell status monitors the treatment responses in breast cancer patients: A meta-analysis. *Sci Rep.* 2017;7:43464. doi:10.1038/srep43464

56. Cohen SJ, et al. Relationship of circulating tumor cells to tumor response, progression-free survival, and overall survival in patients with metastatic colorectal cancer. *J Clin Oncol.* 2008;26:3212–3221. doi:10.1200/JCO.2007.15.8923

57. de Bono JS, et al. Circulating tumor cells predict survival benefit from treatment in metastatic castration-resistant prostate cancer. *Clin Cancer Res.* 2008;14:6302–6309

58. Malani R, et al. CMET-04. Cerebrospinal fluid circulating tumor cells (CSF CTCs) for patient monitoring and response to treatment. *Neuro-Oncology.* 2017;19:vi39–vi39. doi:10.1093/neuonc/nox168.153

59. Nevel KS, et al. A retrospective, quantitative assessment of disease burden in patients with leptomeningeal metastases from non-small-cell lung cancer. *Neuro-Oncology.* 2020 May 15;22(5):675–683. doi:10.1093/neuonc/noz208

60. Laufer I, et al. The NOMS framework: Approach to the treatment of spinal metastatic tumors. *Oncologist.* 2013;18:744–751. doi:10.1634/theoncologist.2012-0293

61. Gilbert RW, Kim JH, Posner JB. Epidural spinal cord compression from metastatic tumor: Diagnosis and treatment. *Ann Neurol.* 1978;3:40–51. doi:10.1002/ana.410030107

62. Scherer K, Johnston J, Panda M. Dural based mass: Malignant or benign. *J Radiol Case Rep.* 2009;3:1–12. doi:10.3941/jrcr.v3i11.189

63. Chai-Adisaksopha C, et al. Outcomes of low-molecular-weight heparin treatment for venous thromboembolism in patients with primary and metastatic brain tumours. *Thromb Haemost.* 2017;117:589–594. doi:10.1160/th16-09-0680

64. Rudà, R Mo F, Pellerino A. Epilepsy in brain metastasis: An emerging entity. *Curr Treat Options Neurol.* 2020;22:6. doi:10.1007/s11940-020-0613-y

65. Marenco-Hillembrand L, Alvarado-Estrada K, Chaichana KL. Contemporary surgical management of deep-seated metastatic brain tumors using minimally invasive approaches. *Front Oncol.* 2018; Article 558. Pages 1–5. doi:10.3389/fonc.2018.00558

66. Pollock BE, Brown PD, Foote RL, Stafford SL, Schomberg PJ. Properly selected patients with multiple brain metastases may benefit from aggressive treatment of their intracranial disease. *J Neurooncol.* 2003;61:73–80

67. Patchell RA, et al. A randomized trial of surgery in the treatment of single metastases to the brain. *N Engl J Med.* 1990;322:494–500. doi:10.1056/NEJM199002223220802

68. Vecht CJ, et al. Treatment of single brain metastasis: Radiotherapy alone or combined with neurosurgery? *Ann Neurol.* 1993;33:583–590. doi:10.1002/ana.410330605

69. McPherson CM, et al. Adjuvant whole-brain radiation therapy after surgical resection of single brain metastases. *Neuro Oncol.* 2010;12:711–719. doi:10.1093/neuonc/noq005

70. Patchell RA, et al. Postoperative radiotherapy in the treatment of single metastases to the brain: A randomized trial. *JAMA.* 1998;280:1485–1489. doi:10.1001/jama.280.17.1485

71. Kocher M, et al. Adjuvant whole-brain radiotherapy versus observation after radiosurgery or surgical resection of one to three cerebral metastases: Results of the EORTC 22952–26001 study. *J Clin Oncol.* 2011;29:134–141. doi:10.1200/jco.2010.30.1655

72. Soffietti R, et al. A European Organisation for Research and Treatment of Cancer phase III trial of adjuvant whole-brain radiotherapy versus observation in patients with one to three brain metastases from solid tumors after surgical resection or radiosurgery: Quality-of-life results. *J Clin Oncol.* 2013;31:65–72. doi:10.1200/jco.2011.41.0639

73. Mahajan A, et al. Post-operative stereotactic radiosurgery versus observation for completely resected brain metastases: A single-centre, randomised, controlled, phase 3 trial. *Lancet Oncol.* 2017;18:1040–1048. doi:10.1016/s1470-2045(17)30414-x

74. Brown PD, et al. Postoperative stereotactic radiosurgery compared with whole brain radiotherapy for resected metastatic brain disease (NCCTG N107C/CEC.3): A multicentre, randomised, controlled, phase 3 trial. *Lancet Oncol.* 2017;18:1049–1060. doi:10.1016/S1470-2045(17)30441-2

75. Kayama T, et al. Effects of surgery with salvage stereotactic radiosurgery versus surgery with whole-brain radiation therapy in patients with one to four brain metastases (JCOG0504): A phase III, noninferiority, randomized controlled trial. 2018;*J Clin Oncol.*, JCO2018786186. doi:10.1200/JCO.2018.78.6186

76. Muacevic A, et al. Microsurgery plus whole brain irradiation versus gamma knife surgery alone for treatment of single metastases to the brain: A randomized controlled multicentre phase III trial. *J Neurooncol.* 2008;87:299–307. doi:10.1007/s11060-007-9510-4

77. Churilla TM, et al. Comparison of local control of brain metastases with stereotactic radiosurgery vs surgical resection: A secondary analysis of a randomized clinical trial. *JAMA Oncol.* 2019;5:243–247. doi:10.1001/jamaoncol.2018.4610

78. Aoyama H, et al. Stereotactic radiosurgery plus whole-brain radiation therapy vs stereotactic radiosurgery alone for treatment of brain metastases: A randomized controlled trial. *JAMA.* 2006;295:2483–2491. doi:10.1001/jama.295.21.2483

79. Chang EL, et al. Neurocognition in patients with brain metastases treated with radiosurgery or radiosurgery plus whole-brain irradiation: A randomised controlled trial. *Lancet Oncol.* 2009;10:1037–1044. doi:10.1016/s1470-2045(09)70263-3

80. Kim CH, et al. Gamma knife radiosurgery for ten or more brain metastases. *J Korean Neurosurg Soc.* 2008;44:358–363. doi:10.3340/jkns.2008.44.6.358

81. Grandhi R, et al. Stereotactic radiosurgery using the Leksell Gamma Knife Perfexion unit in the management of patients with 10 or more brain metastases. *J Neurosurg.* 2012;117:237–245. doi:10.3171/2012.4.JNS11870

82. Rava P, et al. Survival among patients with 10 or more brain metastases treated with stereotactic radiosurgery. *J Neurosurg.* 2013;119:457–462. doi:10.3171/2013.4.JNS121751

83. Yamamoto M, et al. Stereotactic radiosurgery for patients with multiple brain metastases (JLGK0901): A multi-institutional prospective observational study. *Lancet Oncol.* 2014;15:387–395. doi:10.1016/S1470-2045(14)70061-0

84. Mehta MP, et al. Survival and neurologic outcomes in a randomized trial of motexafin gadolinium and whole-brain radiation therapy in brain metastases. *J Clin Oncol.* 2003;21:2529–2536. doi:10.1200/JCO.2003.12.122

85. Hyun MK, et al. Survival outcomes after whole brain radiation therapy and/or stereotactic radiosurgery for cancer patients with metastatic brain tumors in Korea: A systematic review. *Asian Pac J Cancer Prev.* 2013;14:7401–7407. doi:10.7314/apjcp.2013.14.12.7401

86. McDuff SG, et al. Neurocognitive assessment following whole brain radiation therapy and radiosurgery for patients with cerebral metastases. *J Neurol Neurosurg Psychiatry.* 2013;84:1384–1391. doi:10.1136/jnnp-2013-305166

87. Laack NN, Brown PD. Cognitive sequelae of brain radiation in adults. *Semin Oncol.* 2004;31:702–713. doi:https://doi.org/10.1053/j.seminoncol.2004.07.013

88. Makale MT, McDonald CR, Hattangadi-Gluth JA, Kesari S. Mechanisms of radiotherapy-associated cognitive disability in patients with brain tumours. *Nat Rev Neurol.* 2017;13:52–64. doi:10.1038/nrneurol.2016.185

89. Brown PD, et al. Memantine for the prevention of cognitive dysfunction in patients receiving whole-brain radiotherapy: A randomized, double-blind, placebo-controlled trial. *Neuro Oncol.* 2013;15:1429–1437. doi:10.1093/neuonc/not114

90. Gondi V, et al. Preservation of memory with conformal avoidance of the hippocampal neural stem-cell compartment during whole-brain radiotherapy

for brain metastases (RTOG 0933): A phase II multi-institutional trial. *J Clin Oncol.* 2014;32:3810–3816. doi:10.1200/JCO.2014.57.2909

91. Omuro AM, Lallana EC, Bilsky MH, DeAngelis LM. Ventriculoperitoneal shunt in patients with leptomeningeal metastasis. *Neurology.* 2005;64:1625–1627. doi:10.1212/01.WNL.0000160396.69050.DC

92. Jung TY, Chung WK, Oh IJ. The prognostic significance of surgically treated hydrocephalus in leptomeningeal metastases. *Clin Neurol Neurosurg.* 2014;119:80–83. doi:10.1016/j.clineuro.2014.01.023

93. Nigim F, Critchlow JF, Kasper EM. Role of ventriculoperitoneal shunting in patients with neoplasms of the central nervous system: An analysis of 59 cases. *Mol Clin Oncol.* 2015;3:1381–1386. doi:10.3892/mco.2015.627

94. Kim HS, et al. Clinical outcome of cerebrospinal fluid shunts in patients with leptomeningeal carcinomatosis. *World J Surg Oncol.* 2019;17:59–59. doi:10.1186/s12957-019-1595-7

95. Mitsuya K, et al. Palliative cerebrospinal fluid shunting for leptomeningeal metastasis-related hydrocephalus in patients with lung adenocarcinoma: A single-center retrospective study. *PloS One.* 2019;14, e0210074–e0210074. doi:10.1371/journal.pone.0210074

96. Morris PG, et al. Leptomeningeal metastasis from non-small cell lung cancer: Survival and the impact of whole brain radiotherapy. *J Thorac Oncol.* 2012;7:382–385. doi:10.1097/JTO.0b013e3182398e4f

97. Mehta M, Bradley K. Radiation therapy for leptomeningeal cancer. *Cancer Treat Res.* 2005;125:147–158. doi:10.1007/0-387-24199-x_9

98. Beauchesne P. Intrathecal chemotherapy for treatment of leptomeningeal dissemination of metastatic tumours. *Lancet Oncol.* 2010;11:871–879. doi:10.1016/S1470-2045(10)70034-6

99. Siegal T, Lossos A, Pfeffer MR. Leptomeningeal metastases: Analysis of 31 patients with sustained off-therapy response following combined-modality therapy. *Neurology.* 1994;44:1463–1469. doi:10.1212/wnl.44.8.1463

100. Hitchins RN, Bell DR, Woods RL, Levi JA. A prospective randomized trial of single-agent versus combination chemotherapy in meningeal carcinomatosis. *J Clin Oncol.* 1987;5:1655–1662. doi:10.1200/JCO.1987.5.10.1655

101. Grossman SA, et al. Randomized prospective comparison of intraventricular methotrexate and thiotepa in patients with previously untreated neoplastic meningitis. Eastern Cooperative Oncology Group. *J Clin Oncol.* 1993;11:561–569. doi:10.1200/JCO.1993.11.3.561

102. Figura NB, et al. Intrathecal trastuzumab in the management of HER2+ breast leptomeningeal disease: A single institution experience. *Breast Cancer Res Treat.* 2018;169:391–396. doi:10.1007/s10549-018-4684-3

103. Dumitrescu C, Lossignol D. Intrathecal trastuzumab treatment of the neoplastic meningitis due to breast cancer: A case report and review of the literature. *Case Rep Oncol Med.* 2013;2013:154674–154674. doi:10.1155/2013/154674

104. Vecht CJ, et al. Initial bolus of conventional versus high-dose dexamethasone in metastatic spinal cord compression. *Neurology.* 1989;39:1255–1257. doi:10.1212/wnl.39.9.1255

105. Bilsky MH, et al. Reliability analysis of the epidural spinal cord compression scale. *J Neurosurg Spine.* 2010;13:324–328. doi:10.3171/2010.3.Spine09459

106. Fisher CG, et al. Reliability of the Spinal Instability Neoplastic Score (SINS) among radiation oncologists: An assessment of instability secondary to spinal metastases. *Radiat Oncol.* 2014;9:69. doi:10.1186/1748-717x-9-69

107. Laufer I, et al. Predicting neurologic recovery after surgery in patients with deficits secondary to MESCC: Systematic review. *Spine (Phila Pa 1976).* 2016;41 Suppl 20, S224–S230. doi:10.1097/BRS.0000000000001827

108. Di Giacomo AM, et al. Immunotherapy of brain metastases: Breaking a "dogma." *J Exp Clin Cancer Res.* 2019;38:419. doi:10.1186/s13046-019-1426-2

109. Tawbi HA, et al. Combined nivolumab and ipilimumab in melanoma metastatic to the brain. *N Engl J Med.* 2018;379:722–730

110. Long GV, et al. Combination nivolumab and ipilimumab or nivolumab alone in melanoma brain metastases: A multicentre randomised phase 2 study. *Lancet Oncol.* 2018;19:672–681. doi:10.1016/S1470-2045(18)30139-6

111. Goldberg SB, et al. Pembrolizumab for patients with melanoma or non-small-cell lung cancer and untreated brain metastases: Early analysis of a non-randomised, open-label, phase 2 trial. *Lancet Oncol.* 2016;17:976–983. doi:10.1016/S1470-2045(16)30053-5

112. Crino L, et al. Nivolumab and brain metastases in patients with advanced non-squamous non-small cell lung cancer. *Lung Cancer.* 2019;129:35–40. doi:10.1016/j.lungcan.2018.12.025

113. Hendriks LEL, et al. Outcome of patients with non-small cell lung cancer and brain metastases treated with checkpoint inhibitors. *J Thorac Oncol.* 2019;14:1244–1254. doi:10.1016/j.jtho.2019.02.009

114. Gandhi L, et al. Pembrolizumab plus chemotherapy in metastatic non-small-cell lung cancer. *N Engl J Med.* 2018;378:2078–2092. doi:10.1056/NEJMoa1801005

115. Okada H, et al. Immunotherapy response assessment in neuro-oncology: A report of the RANO working group. *Lancet Oncol.* 2015;16, e534–e542. doi:10.1016/S1470-2045(15)00088-1

116. Lehrer EJ, et al. Stereotactic radiosurgery and immune checkpoint inhibitors in the management of brain metastases. *Intl J Mol Sci.* 2018;19:3054. doi:10.3390/ijms19103054

117. Lin X, et al. Extracranial abscopal effect induced by combining immunotherapy with brain radiotherapy in a patient with lung adenocarcinoma: A case report and literature review. *Thorac Cancer.* 2019;10:1272–1275. doi:10.1111/1759-7714.13048

118. Boire A, et al. Liquid biopsy in central nervous system metastases: A RANO review and proposals for clinical applications. *Neuro Oncol.* 2019;21:571–584. doi:10.1093/neuonc/noz012

119. Kelly WJ, Shah NJ, Subramaniam DS. Management of brain metastases in epidermal growth factor receptor mutant non-small-cell lung cancer. *Front Oncol.* 2018;8:Article 208. Pages 1–9. https://www.ncbi.nlm.nih.gov/pmc/articles/PMC6037690/pdf/fonc-08-00208.pdf

120. Grommes C, et al. "Pulsatile" high-dose weekly erlotinib for CNS metastases from EGFR mutant non-small cell lung cancer. *Neuro Oncol.* 2011;13:1364–1369. doi:10.1093/neuonc/nor121

121. Arbour KC, et al. Twice weekly pulse and daily continuous-dose erlotinib as initial treatment for patients with epidermal growth factor receptor-mutant lung cancers and brain metastases. *Cancer.* 2018;124:105–109. doi:10.1002/cncr.30990

122. Ceresoli GL, et al. Gefitinib in patients with brain metastases from non-small-cell lung cancer: A prospective trial. *Ann Oncol.* 2004;15:1042–1047. doi:10.1093/annonc/mdh276

123. Iuchi T, et al. Phase II trial of gefitinib alone without radiation therapy for Japanese patients with brain metastases from EGFR-mutant lung adenocarcinoma. *Lung Cancer.* 2013;82:282–287. doi:10.1016/j.lungcan.2013.08.016

124. Schuler M, et al. First-line afatinib versus chemotherapy in patients with non-small cell lung cancer and common epidermal growth factor receptor gene mutations and brain metastases. *J Thorac Oncol.* 2016;11:380–390. doi:10.1016/j.jtho.2015.11.014

125. Park K, et al. Afatinib versus gefitinib as first-line treatment of patients with EGFR mutation-positive non-small-cell lung cancer (LUX-Lung 7): A phase 2B, open-label, randomised controlled trial. *Lancet Oncol.* 2016;17:577–589. doi:10.1016/s1470-2045(16)30033-x

126. Heon S, et al. The impact of initial gefitinib or erlotinib versus chemotherapy on central nervous system progression in advanced non-small cell lung cancer with EGFR mutations. *Clin Cancer Res.* 2012;18:4406–4414

127. Reungwetwattana T, et al. CNS response to osimertinib versus standard epidermal growth factor receptor tyrosine kinase inhibitors in patients with untreated EGFR-mutated advanced non–small-cell lung cancer. *J Clin Oncol.* 2018;36:3290–3297. doi:10.1200/jco.2018.78.3118

128. Mok TS, et al. Osimertinib or platinum-pemetrexed in EGFR T790M-positive lung cancer. *N Engl J Med.* 2017;376:629–640. doi:10.1056/NEJMoa1612674

129. Wu YL, et al. CNS efficacy of osimertinib in patients with T790M-positive advanced non-small-cell lung cancer: Data from a randomized phase III Trial (AURA3). *J Clin Oncol.* 2018;36:2702–2709. doi:10.1200/JCO.2018.77.9363

130. Goss G, et al. CNS response to osimertinib in patients with T790M-positive advanced NSCLC: Pooled data from two phase II trials. *Ann Oncol.* 2018;29:687–693. doi:10.1093/annonc/mdx820

131. Yang, JCH, et al. Osimertinib in patients with epidermal growth factor receptor mutation-positive non-small-cell lung cancer and leptomeningeal metastases: The BLOOM Study. *J Clin Oncol.* 2020;38:538–547. doi:10.1200/jco.19.00457

132. Rangachari D, et al. Brain metastases in patients with EGFR-mutated or ALK-rearranged non-small-cell lung cancers. *Lung Cancer.* 2015;88:108–111

133. Costa DB, et al. Clinical experience with crizotinib in patients with advanced ALK-rearranged non-small-cell lung cancer and brain metastases. *J Clin Oncol.* 2015;33:1881–1888. doi:10.1200/JCO.2014.59.0539

134. Peters S, et al. Alectinib versus crizotinib in untreated ALK-positive non-small-cell lung cancer. *N Engl J Med.* 2017;377:829–838. doi:10.1056/NEJMoa1704795

135. Nishio M, et al. Analysis of central nervous system efficacy in the J-ALEX study of alectinib versus crizotinib in ALK-positive non-small-cell lung cancer. *Lung Cancer.* 2018;121:37–40. doi:10.1016/j.lungcan.2018.04.015

136. Petrelli F, et al. Efficacy of ALK inhibitors on NSCLC brain metastases: A systematic review and pooled analysis of 21 studies. *PloS One.* 2018;13, e0201425–e0201425. doi:10.1371/journal.pone.0201425

137. Shaw AT, et al. Lorlatinib in non-small-cell lung cancer with ALK or ROS1 rearrangement: An international, multicentre, open-label, single-arm first-in-man phase 1 trial. *Lancet Oncol.* 2017;18:1590–1599. doi:10.1016/s1470-2045(17)30680-0

138. Gafer H, de Waard Q, Compter A, van den Heuvel M. Rapid regression of neurological symptoms in patients with metastasised ALK+ lung cancer who are treated with lorlatinib: A report of two cases. *BMJ Case Rep.* 2019;12. doi:10.1136/bcr-2018-227299

139. Crino L, et al. Multicenter phase II study of whole-body and intracranial activity with ceritinib in patients with ALK-rearranged non-small-cell lung cancer previously treated with chemotherapy and crizotinib: Results from ASCEND-2. *J Clin Oncol.* 2016;34:2866–2873. doi:10.1200/jco.2015.65.5936

140. Kim DW, et al. Activity and safety of ceritinib in patients with ALK-rearranged non-small-cell lung cancer (ASCEND-1): Updated results from the multicentre, open-label, phase 1 trial. *Lancet Oncol.* 2016;17:452–463. doi:10.1016/s1470-2045(15)00614-2

141. Shaw AT, et al. Ceritinib versus chemotherapy in patients with ALK-rearranged non-small-cell lung cancer previously given chemotherapy and crizotinib (ASCEND-5): A randomised, controlled, open-label, phase 3 trial. *Lancet Oncol.* 2017;18:874–886. doi:10.1016/s1470-2045(17)30339-x

142. Soria JC, et al. First-line ceritinib versus platinum-based chemotherapy in advanced ALK-rearranged non-small-cell lung cancer (ASCEND-4): A randomised, open-label, phase 3 study. *Lancet.* 2017;389:917–929. doi:10.1016/s0140-6736(17)30123-x

143. Gadgeel SM, et al. Safety and activity of alectinib against systemic disease and brain metastases in patients with crizotinib-resistant ALK-rearranged non-small-cell lung cancer (AF-002JG): Results from the dose-finding portion of a phase 1/2 study. *Lancet Oncol.* 2014;15:1119–1128. doi:10.1016/S1470-2045(14)70362-6

144. Gadgeel SM, et al. Pooled analysis of CNS response to alectinib in two studies of pretreated patients with ALK-positive non-small-cell lung cancer. *J Clin Oncol.* 2016;34:4079–4085. doi:10.1200/jco.2016.68.4639

145. Gettinger SN, et al. Activity and safety of brigatinib in ALK-rearranged non-small-cell lung cancer and other malignancies: A single-arm, open-label, phase 1/2 trial. *Lancet Oncol.* 2016;17:1683–1696. doi:10.1016/s1470-2045(16)30392-8

146. Kim DW, et al. Brigatinib in patients with crizotinib-refractory anaplastic lymphoma kinase-positive non-small-cell lung cancer: A randomized, multicenter phase II Trial. *J Clin Oncol.* 2017;35:2490–2498. doi:10.1200/jco.2016.71.5904

147. Bauer TM, et al. Brain penetration of lorlatinib: Cumulative incidences of CNS and non-CNS progression with lorlatinib in patients with previously treated ALK-positive non-small-cell lung cancer. *Targeted Oncol.* 2020;15:55–65. doi:10.1007/s11523-020-00702-4

148. Shaw AT, et al. Lorlatinib in advanced ROS1–positive non-small-cell lung cancer: A multicentre, open-label, single-arm, phase 1–2 trial. *Lancet Oncol.* 2019;20:1691–1701. doi:10.1016/S1470-2045(19)30655-2

149. Cheng L, Lopez-Beltran A, Massari F, MacLennan GT, Montironi R. Molecular testing for BRAF mutations to inform melanoma treatment decisions: A move toward precision medicine. *Mod Pathol.* 2018;31:24–38. doi:10.1038/modpathol.2017.104

150. Long GV, et al. Dabrafenib in patients with Val600Glu or Val600Lys BRAF-mutant melanoma metastatic to the brain (BREAK-MB): A multicentre, open-label, phase 2 trial. *Lancet Oncol.* 2012;13:1087–1095. doi:10.1016/s1470-2045(12)70431-x

151. Falchook GS, et al. Dabrafenib in patients with melanoma, untreated brain metastases, and other solid tumours: A phase 1 dose-escalation trial. *Lancet.* 2012;379:1893–1901. doi:10.1016/s0140-6736(12)60398-5

152. McArthur GA, et al. Vemurafenib in metastatic melanoma patients with brain metastases: An open-label, single-arm, phase 2, multicentre study. *Ann Oncol.* 2017;28:634–641. doi:10.1093/annonc/mdw641

153. Dummer R, et al. Vemurafenib in patients with BRAF(V600) mutation-positive melanoma with symptomatic brain metastases: Final results of an open-label pilot study. *Eur J Cancer.* 2014;50:611–621. doi:10.1016/j.ejca.2013.11.002

154. Kim KB, et al. Phase II study of the MEK1/MEK2 inhibitor Trametinib in patients with metastatic BRAF-mutant cutaneous melanoma previously treated with or without a BRAF inhibitor. *J Clin Oncol.* 2013;31:482–489. doi:10.1200/jco.2012.43.5966

155. Davies MA, et al. Dabrafenib plus trametinib in patients with BRAF(V600)-mutant melanoma brain metastases (COMBI-MB): A multicentre, multicohort, open-label, phase 2 trial. *Lancet Oncol.* 2017;18:863–873. doi:10.1016/S1470-2045(17)30429-1

156. Ascierto PA, et al. Cobimetinib combined with vemurafenib in advanced BRAF(V600)-mutant melanoma (coBRIM): Updated efficacy results from a randomised, double-blind, phase 3 trial. *Lancet Oncol.* 2016;17:1248–1260. doi:10.1016/s1470-2045(16)30122-x

157. Dummer R, et al. Overall survival in patients with BRAF-mutant melanoma receiving encorafenib plus binimetinib versus vemurafenib or encorafenib (COLUMBUS): A multicentre, open-label, randomised, phase 3 trial. *Lancet Oncol.* 2018;19:1315–1327. doi:10.1016/s1470-2045(18)30497-2

158. Chowdhary M, Patel KR, Danish HH, Lawson DH, Khan MK. BRAF inhibitors and radiotherapy for melanoma brain metastases: Potential advantages and disadvantages of combination therapy. *OncoTargets Ther.* 2016;9:7149–7159. doi:10.2147/OTT.S119428

159. Bachelot T, et al. Lapatinib plus capecitabine in patients with previously untreated brain metastases from HER2–positive metastatic breast cancer (LANDSCAPE): A single-group phase 2 study. *Lancet Oncol.* 2013;14:64–71. doi:10.1016/S1470-2045(12)70432-1

160. Lin NU, et al. Multicenter phase II study of lapatinib in patients with brain metastases from HER2–positive breast cancer. *Clin Cancer Res.* 2009;15:1452–1459. doi:10.1158/1078-0432.CCR-08-1080

161. Freedman RA, et al. Translational Breast Cancer Research Consortium (TBCRC) 022: A phase II trial of neratinib for patients with human epidermal growth factor receptor 2–positive breast cancer and brain metastases. *J Clin Oncol.* 2016;34:945–952. doi:10.1200/jco.2015.63.0343

162. Freedman RA, et al. TBCRC 022: A phase II trial of neratinib and capecitabine for patients with human epidermal growth factor receptor 2–positive breast cancer and brain metastases. *J Clin Oncol.* 2019;37:1081–1089. doi:10.1200/jco.18.01511

163. Lin NU, et al. Intracranial efficacy and survival with tucatinib plus trastuzumab and capecitabine for previously treated HER2–positive breast cancer with brain metastases in the HER2CLIMB Trial. *J Clin Oncol.* 2020;38:2610–2619. doi:10.1200/JCO.20.00775

164. Pascual T, et al. Significant clinical activity of olaparib in a somatic BRCA1–mutated triple-negative breast cancer with brain metastasis. *JCO Precision Oncol.* 2019;1–6. doi:10.1200/PO.19.00012

165. Sakamoto I, et al. Durable response by olaparib for a Japanese patient with primary peritoneal cancer with multiple brain metastases: A case report. *J Obstet Gynaecol Res.* 2019;45:743–747. doi:10.1111/jog.13851

166. Anders CK, et al. A phase II study of abemaciclib in patients (pts) with brain metastases (BM) secondary to HR+, HER2– metastatic breast cancer (MBC). *J Clin Oncol.* 2019;37:1017–1017. doi:10.1200/JCO.2019.37.15_suppl.1017

167. Brastianos P, et al. CMET-33: Phase II study of palbociclib in brain metastases harboring cdk pathway alterations. *Neuro-Oncology.* 2019;21, vi58–vi59. doi:10.1093/neuonc/noz175.234

168. Zhuang H, Shi S, Yuan Z, Chang JY. Bevacizumab treatment for radiation brain necrosis: Mechanism, efficacy and issues. *Mol Cancer.* 2019;18:21–21. doi:10.1186/s12943-019-0950-1

169. Cameron D, et al. A phase III randomized comparison of lapatinib plus capecitabine versus capecitabine alone in women with advanced breast cancer that has progressed on trastuzumab: Updated efficacy and biomarker analyses. *Breast Cancer Res.*

13 | TUMORS AFFECTING THE SPINAL CORD

TERRENCE VERLA, KARA L. CURLEY, MATTHEW T. NEAL, AND ALEXANDER ROPPER

INTRODUCTION

Spinal tumors are uncommon neoplasms that can cause significant neurologic morbidity and mortality if left undiagnosed and untreated. Spinal tumors are characterized into three different groups based on their relationship with the spinal cord and dura mater: intradural intramedullary, intradural extramedullary, and extradural.[1] Intradural intramedullary account for 20–30% of intradural tumors and are most commonly ependymomas, astrocytomas, or hemangioblastomas. The remaining 70–80% of intradural lesions are extramedullary tumors, such as meningioma, schwannoma, and neurofibroma. Extradural tumors are most commonly metastatic in nature, with common primary malignancies being lung cancer, breast cancer, prostate cancer, renal cell carcinoma, or colorectal cancer.[2] Primary bone tumors have diverse pathologies and make up less than 10% of extradural tumors.[3]

INTRAMEDULLARY SPINAL CORD TUMORS

EPIDEMIOLOGY

Intradural intramedullary spinal cord tumors (IMSCTs) comprise 20–30% of all intradural tumors.[4] IMSCTs are most commonly gliomas, accounting for approximately 80–90%. Gliomas can be further divided into ependymomas and astrocytomas. Ependymomas comprise 60% of IMSCTs and have a higher incidence in the adult population. Astrocytomas represent 30% of IMSCTs and are more common in pediatric patients.[1]

> Intramedullary spinal cord tumors (IMSCTs) are most commonly gliomas, accounting for approximately 80–90%.

After gliomas, the next most common IMSCTs are hemangioblastomas, accounting for approximately 2–8% of IMSCTs. The remaining pathologies include metastatic lesions which, may include up to 2% of IMSCTs. Lipomas represent 1–2% of IMSCTs, and other rare tumors include various neuroepithelial lesions, neurofibromas, dermoid tumors, and germ cell tumors.[1,4]

IMSCTs have been found to be associated with certain genetic factors and clinical syndromes, including neurofibromatosis type 1 (NF1) and type 2 (NF2), and Von Hippel-Lindau disease (VHL). Patients with NF1 may develop IMSCTs, with astrocytomas being the most common.[4] In NF2, ependymomas are the more common IMSCT. Additionally, meningiomas may be seen in NF2, which are extramedullary. A variety of tumor types are associated with VHL, most commonly hemangioblastomas. With VHL, approximately 20% of hemangioblastomas are found in the spinal cord.[1]

Given the rarity of occurrence, poor prognosis, and often poor tissue sampling, high-grade gliomas of the spinal cord have historically been incompletely characterized. However, molecular aberrations have been identified more recently, allowing improved classification of central nervous system (CNS) tumors.

> Historically, high-grade gliomas of the spinal cord have been incompletely characterized because of the rarity of occurrence, poor prognosis, and often poor tissue sampling. However, molecular tumor biomarkers are increasingly identified that will contribute to the better characterization of these tumors.

Molecular analysis of high-grade gliomas has revealed recurrent lysine to methionine substitution at codon 27 (K27M) in histone H3 variants encoded predominantly by H3.3 gene H3F3A and in H3.1 gene HIST1H3B, less commonly.[5] The H3 K27M mutation now defines a group of gliomas referred to as diffuse midline gliomas (DMG), which includes tumors that were previously described as diffuse intrinsic pontine glioma (DIPG) but also includes tumors along the midline structures of the CNS, such as the thalamus, midbrain, pons, medulla, and spinal cord.[6] These K27M-mutant gliomas have been associated with more aggressive qualities compared to wildtype equivalents in pediatric patients, but the frequency and behavior is less defined in the adult population.[5,7]

Ependymomas have differing biology and molecular features based on where they arise in the CNS. Supratentorial ependymomas include a RELA fusion-positive subtype which accounts for the majority of supratentorial tumors in pediatric populations.[6] RELA fusion-negative subtypes alternatively have YAP1-MAMLD1 fusions; however, both fusion types are oncogenic in nature.[8] Spinal ependymomas are commonly associated with NF2 and typically have a more indolent disease course than non-NF2 spinal ependymomas. Spinal ependymomas have increased expression of homeobox (HOX) family genes which encode transcription factors. The subtype myxopapillary ependymoma (WHO grade 1) is only found in the spinal cord.[8]

> Spinal ependymomas are commonly associated with NF2 and typically have a more indolent disease course than non-NF2 spinal ependymomas.

CLINICAL MANIFESTATIONS

IMSCTs can present with a multitude of nonspecific symptoms. The most common presenting symptom is back pain, which is often related to dural distention. This results in constant pain that may be exacerbated in a supine position. An eccentric lesion may cause unilateral radiculopathy, while a centrally located lesion may cause myelopathy. Compromise of spinal tracts will lead to tract-specific deficits. Autonomic pathways can also be disrupted, causing parasympathetic and sympathetic system dysfunction. Furthermore, if a lesion extends cranially, cranial nerve dysfunction is also possible; most commonly the hypoglossal nerve (CN XII) from foramen magnum lesions and accessory nerve (CN XI) from high cervical lesions are affected.[4]

DIAGNOSTICS AND IMAGING

Currently, magnetic resonance imaging (MRI) is the preferred diagnostic imaging modality for IMSCT as the anatomical detail allows for characterization of lesions.[9] Each tumor type has characteristics that may be revealed with high-quality MRI. However, radiographic differentiation between ependymomas, astrocytomas, hemangioblastomas, and other IMSCTs remains inherently challenging, and therefore imaging appearance alone is not sufficient for treatment recommendations. MRI is critical for surgical planning as cord–tumor interface, as well as associated cysts and syringes, can be assessed.[4]

Gliomas, including ependymomas (Figure 13.1A–C) and astrocytomas (Figure 13.2A–C), may cover multiple vertebral levels and variably enhance with contrast. Both ependymomas and astrocytomas are hypo- or isointense on T1 weighted imaging (T1WI) and hyperintense on T2 weighted imaging (T2WI).[4,9] Ependymomas typically have enhancing margins, whereas astrocytomas will enhance heterogeneously or not at all. Ependymomas are more centrally located within the spinal cord, and astrocytomas are more eccentric and sometimes have an exophytic component. Astrocytomas may present with nodular features and do not have well-defined borders. Satellite cysts may also be present.[9,10] Both gliomas can be associated with intraparenchymal hemorrhage, although hemorrhage is more commonly seen with ependymomas.[4]

Hemangioblastomas (Figure 13.3A–C) appear as highly vascularized lesions with often extensive associated edema and may be associated with syringomyelia, which can be appreciated on MRI. They are isointense on T1WI and hyperintense on T2WI and enhance with contrast in a homogeneous fashion.[4,10] Given their complex vascular nature, hemangioblastomas may be further evaluated via spinal angiography to detect feeding vessels and draining veins.[9]

IMSCTs of metastatic origin are typically well-encapsulated, singular, and eccentrically located lesions. They appear isointense on T1WI and hyperintense on T2WI with significant surrounding edema that may be out of proportion given the size of the metastatic lesion.[4,9] A "rim sign" describes a rim of enhancement, and a "flame sign" describes a flame-like enhancement at the superior or inferior margin of the tumor which may help distinguish lesions as metastatic.[11]

Rare IMSCTs may be more difficult to distinguish. Lipomas appear as other fatty tissue and are hyperintense T1WI appearance. Oligodendrogliomas are mildly hyperintense on T1WI and have poorly defined borders. Intramedullary lymphoma lesions are typically associated with supratentorial disease.[9]

TUMOR-SPECIFIC CONSIDERATIONS

EPENDYMOMAS

Ependymomas, typically considered benign and slow-growing lesions, represent 60% of IMSCTs and are more common in adult populations. Approximately half of all CNS ependymomas are found in the spine, with a slight predilection for cord lesions over cauda equina lesions.[12] Spinal ependymomas are most commonly located in the cervical or thoracic regions and arise from the ependymal lining of the central canal; therefore, they tend to expand centrally and vertically across 3–4 vertebral bodies. Syrinx formation is common with ependymomas and occurs in approximately 65%. Ependymomas are less likely to invade adjacent tissue as they are typically encapsulated creating a clear margin.[12] Subtypes of ependymomas include typical lesions (WHO grade 2), tanycytic (WHO grade 2), myxopapillary (WHO grade 1), anaplastic (WHO grade 3), and subependymomas (WHO grade 1).[4,11] Leptomeningeal metastasis of intramedullary tumors is uncommon; however, ependymomas are more likely to metastasize than astrocytomas.[13]

> Syrinx formation is common with ependymomas and occurs in approximately 65%.

ASTROCYTOMAS

Astrocytomas are the second most common IMSCT, representing 30%, but they have a higher incidence in pediatric patients and make up 90% of IMSCTs in the pediatric population.[1] Only 3% of astrocytomas occur in the spinal cord, and they are more common in the cervical spine. They are typically expansile, extending across 5–6 vertebral levels, and are infiltrative in nature.[4] They have ill-defined borders between tumor and normal cord tissue.[9] Syrinx formation is associated with approximately 20% of astrocytomas. Malignant transformation may occur in a quarter of adult tumors.[4]

> Only 3% of astrocytomas occur in the spinal cord, and they are more common in the cervical spine.

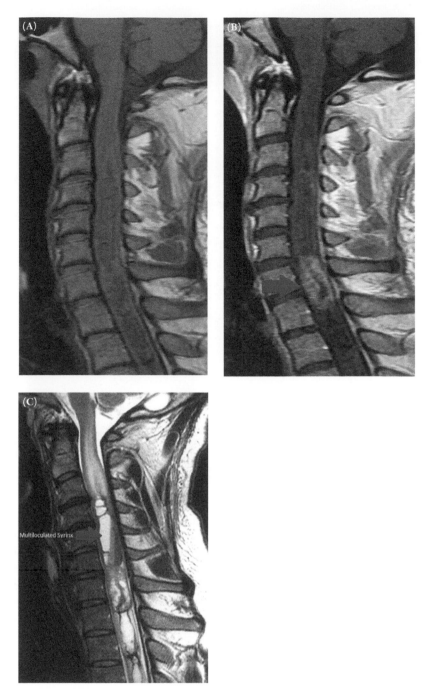

Figure 13.1 *MRI, sagittal views of a cervical intradural intramedullary ependymoma. (A) The tumor appears isointense to normal spinal cord on T1 non–contrast-enhanced imaging. (B) demonstrates inhomogeneous enhancement on T1 contrast-enhanced imaging. (C) T2 sequences illustrate multiloculated syrinx formation.*

HEMANGIOBLASTOMAS

Hemangioblastomas are the third most common IMSCT and are solitary, small, vascularized lesions with well-defined margins and a capsule. The lesions consist of a dense web of capillary channels with endothelial cells, pericytes, and lipid-containing stromal cells with larger feeding vessels and draining veins.[4] It is hypothesized that the cells of origin are vascular endothelial growth factor (VEGF)-secreting in nature.[12] They are most commonly found in the cervical and thoracic regions, subpial in location and along the posterior aspect of the cord.[1,9]

Syrinx formation is common and occurs in up to 60–70% of lesions. Additionally, enhancing nodules and formation of cysts are also characteristic of hemangioblastomas and tend to outgrow the lesion itself, causing mass effect.[12] The incidence of leptomeningeal dissemination of hemangioblastoma in the CNS is rare; however, it is higher in patients with sporadic hemangioblastoma than with VHL-related hemangioblastoma. The mechanism of dissemination is unknown but in cases without a genetic predisposition dissemination may be iatrogenic in nature and related to intraoperative tumor cell disruption.[14]

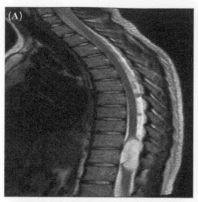
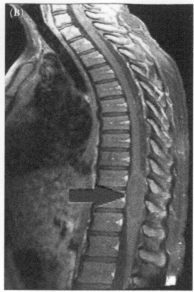
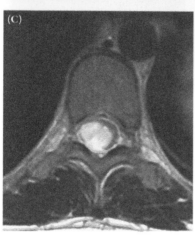

Figure 13.2 *MRI of a low-grade spinal cord astrocytoma. (A) The tumor appears hyperintense compared to spinal cord on sagittal T2 and (B) isointense compared to spinal cord on sagittal T1 non-contrast sequences. (C) Axial T1 contrast-enhanced imaging demonstrate homogeneous enhancement with ill-defined borders.*

METASTATIC LESIONS

IMSCTs are rarely metastatic in origin and are diagnosed in less than 1% of patients with cancer. When present, lung and breast cancers are the most common source, and it is hypothesized that cord infiltration occurs through hematogenous spread. Theories include retrograde infiltration and tumor cell seeding via the venous system and parenchyma penetrating vessels or through perforating osseous veins, cerebrospinal fluid (CSF) dissemination through perineural sheaths, and antidromic cellular migration.[4,12]

> IMSCTs are rarely metastatic in origin and are diagnosed in less than 1% of patients with cancer.

LIPOMAS

Lipomas are rare and benign IMSCTs that are slow-growing in nature and become symptomatic due to mass effect. They may be solitary lesions or occurs as multiples.[4,12] There is a mixing of the neural and lipomal tissue creating a lack of a clear marginal plane, and there is firm attachment to the dura.[6]

RARE INTRAMEDULLARY LESIONS

Primary intramedullary lymphomas can occur with other CNS lymphomatous lesions or may be solitary intramedullary

tumors; they are highly aggressive and have a poor prognosis. Gangliogliomas are benign glial lesions and are more common in pediatric patients, where they are found in the upper cervical region.[1,4,12] Vascular malformations, such as cavernomas, may hemorrhage recurrently and may have associated syrinxes, although less commonly than hemangioblastomas. Oligodendrogliomas are exceptionally rare and may have associated calcifications and hemorrhages like their cranial counterparts. Other rare lesions include melanoma, paraganglioma, melanocytoma, fibrosarcomas, neuroectodermal tumors, and amyloid angiopathies.[4,12]

TREATMENT

Surgical intervention has become the standard for many symptomatic IMSCTs as it allows for tissue diagnosis, decompression/debulking to stabilize or improve neurologic function, and potential cure with gross total resection (GTR) for some subtypes.[15]

The most important factor in determining neurologic outcomes following surgical resection is the patient's preoperative neurologic status.[15] The tumor's histopathology and WHO grade are critical for prognostic assessment but are confirmed only after surgical intervention or biopsy. Presence of defined margins, which can be predicted preoperatively on imaging, lends to a GTR. Ependymomas and hemangioblastomas typically have a defined tumor–cord interface and consequently are

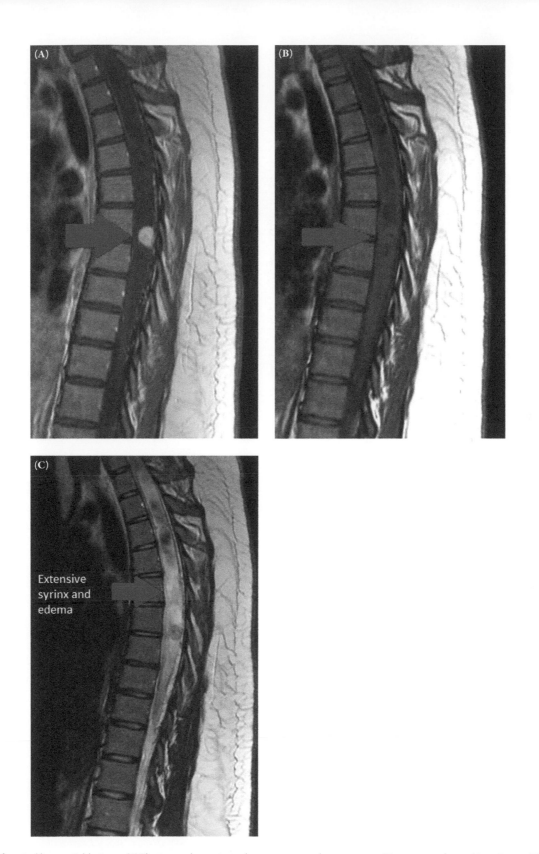

Figure 13.3 *MRI of a spinal hemangioblastoma. (A) The tumor demonstrates homogeneous enhancement on T1 contrast-enhanced imaging and (B) is isointense compared to spinal cord on T1 non–contrast-enhanced sequences. (C) T2 sequence demonstrates extensive amount of vasogenic spinal cord edema and extensive syringomyelia.*

well-resected, leading to lower rates of recurrence. Therefore, surgical resection for these lesions is considered the treatment of choice. Preoperative embolization of hemangioblastomas can further facilitate surgical resection.[6,15] In contrast, astrocytomas are infiltrative in nature and are more challenging to resect: subtotal resections (STR) are common to preserve neurologic function. Lesion residuals are followed serially with MRI to monitor for progression.[12]

Adjuvants to surgical resection, such as chemotherapy and radiation therapy, are typically reserved for recurrent or residual high-grade IMSCTs.[12] Given the infiltrative and malignant nature of high-grade astrocytomas, radiation is common after STR. Typical doses of radiation range from 40 to 54 Gy in 25 to 30 fractions over a course of 5 weeks.[1,15] Postoperative radiation has been shown to improve progression-free survival (PFS) for high-grade astrocytoma; unfortunately, long-term survival remains poor despite adjuvant therapy.[1,15] Given the more benign nature of spinal ependymomas, radiation is more commonly used in the setting of recurrence or for anaplastic subtypes.

Chemotherapy is preferred to radiation therapy in pediatric IMSCTs because it is better tolerated in the pediatric population.[12] In metastatic IMSCTs, a combination of surgical resection, chemotherapy, and radiation is considered and tailored based on the primary source.[15] For astrocytomas, temozolomide is an option for adjuvant therapy with radiation. Oral etoposide, a topoisomerase 2 inhibitor, has been used for recurrent ependymoma after failure of surgical resection and radiation.[1,15] Antiangiogenic agents, specifically bevacizumab, have been used as adjuvant therapy for hemangioblastoma.[1] Other targeted agents are also being evaluated in clinical trials.

For asymptomatic patients with incidental radiographic evidence of IMSCT, prophylactic resection is not recommended secondary to the intrinsic risks of surgical resection.[15] After surgery, new symptoms may suggest postoperative complications requiring further treatment. Development of arachnoiditis, syringomyelia, tumor recurrence, or CSF leakage can cause neurologic compromise. Wound dehiscence or infection may occur following any surgical intervention and can delay recovery. Destabilization of the spine and progressive mechanical pain may develop up to years postoperatively following laminectomy during IMSCT resection.[6] Fortunately, advancing operative techniques, use of surgical adjuncts including intraoperative neuromonitoring, the operative microscope, and ultrasonography have decreased the risks and complications associated with IMSCT resection.

INTRADURAL EXTRAMEDULLARY SPINAL TUMORS

MENINGIOMA

Meningiomas are the most common intradural extramedullary spinal tumors.[16] They are thought to arise from the arachnoid cap cells in the dura and are typically slow growing. They are more common in women, and the most frequent location is the thoracic spine. Most spinal meningiomas are solitary lesions. However, when associated with NF2, they can present at multiple locations within the spinal column. Radiographically, they are similar in appearance to their intracranial counterparts and are characterized as circumscribed dural-based lesions on MRI associated with homogenous contrast enhancement. A characteristic CSF cleft or dural tail is frequently described. Calcifications may be present and better appreciated on computed tomography (CT). Due to the slow-growing nature of meningiomas and their location within the spinal canal, patients often present with gradual progressive neurologic deficits consistent with myelopathy; these range from gait disturbances and motor and sensory changes, to bowel and bladder dysfunction. Histologically, most spinal cord meningiomas are WHO grade 1 lesions. These benign lesions have a number of tumor subtypes such as meningothelial, psammomatous, and transitional, being the most common. Figure 13.4 shows an example of a thoracic meningioma.

SCHWANNOMA

These are the second most common intradural extramedullary spinal tumors and are the most common nerve sheath tumors. They most frequently arise from the Schwann cells in the nerve roots and are slow growing.[16] They are sporadic but can also be associated with NF2. Patients typically present first with

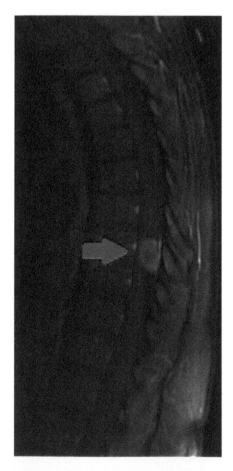

Figure 13.4 *Sagittal T1 contrast-enhanced imaging demonstrates a thoracic meningioma characterized by homogeneous contrast enhancement and a dural tail.*

radicular pain. Based on the size of the lesion and proportion within the canal, more neurologic deficits can develop. Schwannomas are well-defined lesions on MRI, with homogenous contrast enhancement. Often, there is remodeling of adjacent bony elements, with the typical widening of the spinal foramen. They protrude out into the extraforaminal compartment and form the characteristic dumbbell shape. Grossly, they are separate from the nerve roots and are encapsulated. Histologically, they are benign lesions, WHO grade 1, with a network of dense hypercellular Antoni type A cells with palisading Verocay bodies and loosely arranged stellate cells, Antoni type B.[17-19] They stain positive for S100, epithelial membrane antigen (EMA), and vimentin. Figure 13.5 shows a cervical schwannoma originating from the left C3 nerve root.

> Schwannoma are the second most common intradural extramedullary spinal tumors and are the most common nerve sheath tumors.

NEUROFIBROMA

Neurofibromas are radiographically similar to schwannomas, and patients present with the same clinical signs and symptoms. They also originate from Schwann cells but grow within the neuronal tissue with proliferation of all elements of the nerve. They consist of abundant fibrous tissue with a stroma of dense nerve fibers, resulting in a fusiform enlargement of the nerve.[19] They are mostly sporadic in nature but can be syndromic-associated, as in NF1. Like schwannoma, they are positive for S100. However, they are negative for EMA. Histologically, they consist of loosely arranged spindle cells without the typical Antoni A/B cells or Verocay bodies seen in schwannomas. They are mostly benign, WHO grade 1 lesions. Though rare,

they can transform into more aggressive malignant peripheral nerve sheath tumors.

> Neurofibromas also originate from Schwann cells but grow within the neuronal tissue with proliferation of all elements of the nerve.

MALIGNANT PERIPHERAL NERVE SHEATH TUMORS

Malignant peripheral nerve sheath tumors (MPNST) are believed to represent a malignant transformation of both schwannomas and neurofibromas. In some cases, however, they may arise de novo. Risk factors for malignant transformation include prior radiation treatment, plexiform neurofibromas, and NF1 germline mutations.[20-22]

> Malignant peripheral nerve sheath tumors (MPNST) are believed to represent a malignant transformation of both schwannomas and neurofibromas.

MPNSTs are often large, palpable, and tender when they occur outside the spinal foramen. Within the spinal canal, the large tumor can cause compression of neural elements, resulting in pain and neurologic deficits. Histologically, they are hypercellular, with high vascularity, areas of necrosis, and frequent mitotic figures.[23] Radiographically, they are large with irregular borders.[24] They have a high rate of recurrence after resection. The NF1 gene, which codes for neurofibromin, plays a critical role in the pathogenesis of MPNST because disruption in NF1 can affect the RAS signaling pathway, resulting in the development of tumor oncogens.[25] Once the RAS pathway is hyperactive, there is secondary downstream activation of other signaling pathways, including PI3K/AKT/mTOR, with the subsequent effect being proliferation and survival of tumor cells.[26] As such, research efforts are targeting the inhibition of these activated downstream signaling pathways.

> Risk factors for malignant transformation include prior radiation treatment, plexiform neurofibromas, and NF1 germline mutations.

SOLITARY FIBROUS TUMOR

These are rare soft tissue lesions that could be intradural or extradural. Their imaging appearance often mimics other pathologies such as meningioma or schwannoma when intradural, and fibrosarcoma, disc herniation, or osteosarcoma when extradural. They usually enhance on post-contrast MRI (Figure 13.6) and patients present with radicular symptoms depending on the location of the lesion. Histologically, they are benign, WHO grade 1 lesions with low mitotic activity. They show reactivity for CD43 and STAT-6 and are S100-negative.[27]

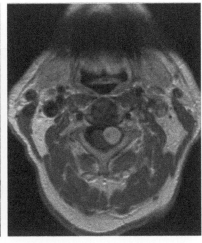

Figure 13.5 Sagittal (left) and axial (right) T1 contrast-enhanced MRI demonstrates a schwannoma arising from the left C3 nerve root with avid contrast enhancement and local expansion of the neural foramina.

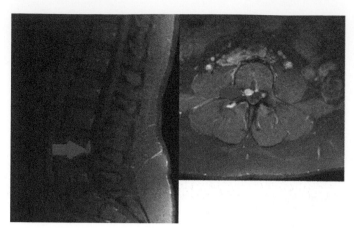

Figure 13.6 Sagittal (left) and axial (right) T1 contrast-enhanced MR imaging shows a solitary fibrous tumor with homogenous contrast enhancement at the level of the L4 pedicle, effacing the thecal sac and nerve root.

TREATMENT OF INTRADURAL EXTRAMEDULLARY SPINE TUMOR

Surgical resection is the primary and optimal treatment option for patients with symptomatic intradural extramedullary spinal tumors. For more benign lesions, local recurrence is rare after *en bloc* resection, and, in many cases, there is a plane between the tumor and the neural elements, making *en bloc* resection possible.

> Surgical resection is the primary and optimal treatment option for patients with symptomatic intradural extramedullary spinal tumors.

In patients with asymptomatic spinal meningiomas, observation with serial imaging is often recommended. However, in symptomatic patients or whenever treatment is needed, surgical resection is the primary modality with very low recurrence rates. For recurrent tumors, surgically unresectable tumors, or incomplete resection, there is benefit in conventional external beam fractionated radiotherapy or stereotactic radiosurgery in halting tumor progression.[28-30] The true efficacy, however, remains controversial. The role of systemic or targeted therapy remains very limited, mainly due to the good outcomes from surgery and also the slow-growing nature of spinal meningiomas. Studies have investigated targeted therapies such as tyrosine kinase inhibitors, mammalian target of rapamycin (mTOR) inhibitors, and platelet-derived growth factor receptor (PDGFR) inhibitors but there is no consensus on their therapeutic advantage in the management of spinal meningiomas.[31,32]

Similarly, asymptomatic spinal schwannomas and neurofibromas can be observed with serial imaging. Surgical resection is recommended as the main treatment modality, with complete resection being the goal. For unresectable

nerve sheath tumors or in poor surgical candidates, studies have shown a beneficial role in stereotactic radiosurgery with minimal neurotoxicity.[33-36] However, patients with NF1 should be cautioned appropriately because radiation can result in malignant degeneration and tumor transformation.[37] Targeted therapies for benign nerve sheath tumor are mostly investigational and not standard of care. Similar to meningioma, tyrosine kinase inhibitors and mTOR inhibitors are molecular targets with promising results. Chemotherapy is mainly reserved for malignant peripheral nerve sheath tumors whereby there is dysregulation of the RAS signaling pathway resulting in activation of PI3K/AKT/mTOR. Targeted therapy such as e.g., a farnesyltransferase inhibitor, which inhibits the hyperactivated RAS pathway, can potentially block cellular proliferation in the tumor.[38]

Regardless, surgical resection with negative margins in appropriate cases has been shown to be most effective in tumor control. In unresectable or metastatic MPNST, doxorubicin-based therapy such as Adriamycin, has been shown to reduce progression.[26,39] Investigational efforts are being directed at downstream RAS signaling pathways involving PI3K/AKT/mTOR and combinational therapy including epidermal growth factor receptor (EGFR), angiogenesis, mTOR, tyrosine kinase and MEK inhibitors with potential benefits in treatment response.[26,40]

EXTRADURAL SPINAL TUMORS

METASTATIC BONE TUMORS OF THE SPINE

Metastasis to the spinal column represents the most common extradural tumor. These metastatic lesions result from a variety of primary cancers, the most common of which are lung cancer, breast cancer, prostate cancer, renal cell carcinoma, and colorectal cancer. Surgical management for these patients is not curative but is a palliative option.

Patients with refractory pain, progressive neurologic deficit, or segmental instability from tumor invasion/bony destruction are generally considered for surgery.[2] The Neurologic, Oncologic, Mechanical and Systemic (NOMS) framework is a widely utilized decision-making tool to guide surgical intervention since radiation therapy is a viable option for some oncologic pathologies.[2,41] The NOMS framework assesses neurologic status from the extent of epidural compression and myelopathy, oncologic status based on radiation responsiveness, mechanical stability of the spinal column, and systemic burden of disease with respect to ability to tolerate surgical intervention. Thus, tumor histology and sensitivity to radiation are the major branch points for most patients in this treatment algorithm.

> Metastasis to the spinal column represents the most common extradural tumor.

Examples of radiation- and/or chemotherapy-sensitive metastatic lesions include lymphoma, myeloma, seminoma, breast cancer, prostate cancer, and neuro-endocrine tumors. For these, conventional external beam radiation (cEBRT) is the preferred treatment in the absence of spinal instability.[2] For radioresistant tumors such as renal cell carcinoma, lung cancer, colon cancer, and sarcoma, stereotactic spinal radiosurgery (SSRS) can provide good outcomes with respect to tumor control.[2]

> The Neurologic, Oncologic, Mechanical and Systemic (NOMS) framework is a widely utilized decision-making tool to guide surgical intervention since radiation therapy is a viable option for some oncologic pathologies.

For patients undergoing surgery, the primary goal is decompression of neural elements (spinal cord and nerve roots) and stabilization of the spinal column in order to safely deliver SSRS. This is the main concept of "separation surgery," whereby adequate decompression is performed to create a satisfactory margin around the dura for delivery of a tumoricidal dose of radiation. In the category of patients with high-grade epidural compression and radioresistant tumors, direct decompression plus SSRS has been shown to provide superior outcomes compared to SSRS only.[42]

PRIMARY BONE TUMORS OF THE SPINE

Among all neoplasms of the spinal column, primary bone tumors account for fewer than 5%.[43] They often occur in a single location, unlike metastases. Benign tumors include osteoblastoma, osteoid osteoma, hemangioma, eosinophilic granuloma, aneurysmal bone cyst (ABC), osteochondroma, and giant cell tumor (GCT). While the pathology is generally classified as benign, their behavior can be locally aggressive. Malignant tumors include chordoma, osteosarcoma, Ewing's sarcoma, chondrosarcoma, lymphoma, plasmacytoma, and multiple myeloma. Inappropriate treatment of primary bone tumors, which can be a potentially curable pathology, may cause transformation into a deadly disease.[44] Hemangioma is the most common benign primary bone tumor in adults, representing about 20–30% of benign tumor of the spine.[45] Plasmacytoma is the most common malignant primary bone tumor of the spine in adults, accounting for about 30%.[46]

It is recommended by the Spine Oncology Study Group that surgery be the primary treatment for most primary bone tumors of the spine with respect to local disease control and PFS.[2] For large benign tumors such as osteochondroma, ABC, and GCT, *en bloc* resection is the primary treatment modality. Figures 13.7 and 13.8 show a representative management of a patient with thoracic GCT. For large, inoperable GCT, the use of denosumab (a RANKL inhibitor) has been shown to reduce

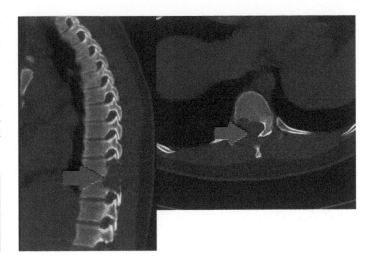

Figure 13.7 *Sagittal (left) and axial (right) CT shows a giant cell tumor of the thoracic spine with extensive bony destruction and soft tissue invasion.*

the size of these tumors and facilitate surgical resection.[47] The management of patients with malignant primary bone tumor of the spine requires a multidisciplinary approach since there is significant morbidity associated with surgery and the majority of patients require pre-/postoperative chemotherapy and radiation.

Plasmacytoma, multiple myeloma, and lymphoma are very sensitive to chemotherapy and radiation therapy, and these modalities should be the primary treatment for patients. Surgery is reserved for spinal instability, deformity correction, or rapidly progressive neurologic deficits.

> For large benign tumors such as osteochondroma, ABC, and GCT, *en bloc* resection is the primary treatment modality.

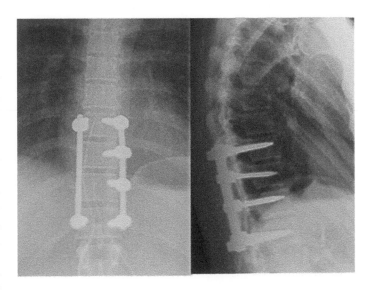

Figure 13.8 *X-ray with coronal (left) and sagittal (right) views after gross total surgical resection of a thoracic giant cell tumor with instrumentation for stability.*

TABLE 13.1 Classification of intramedullary spinal cord tumors

TUMOR ORIGIN	TUMOR TYPE	SUBTYPE	INCIDENCE	WHO GRADE
Neuroepithelial tumors			90%	
	Ependymal cell tumors		60%	
		Ependymoma		2
		Anaplastic ependymoma*		3
		Subependymoma		1
		Myxopapillary ependymoma		1
	Astrocytic tumors		30%	
		Pilocytic astrocytoma		1
		Fibrillary astrocytoma		2
		Anaplastic astrocytoma*		3
		Glioblastoma multiforme		4
	Oligodendroglioma tumors		<1%	
		Oligodendroglioma		2
		Anaplastic oligodendroglioma*		3
Mixed neuronal/glial tumors			<1%	
		Ganglioma		1
		Gangliocytoma		1
Mesenchymal tumors			<8%	
		Hemangioblastoma	2–8%	1
		Lipoma	2%	
		Melanocytoma		
Metastatic tumors			2%	
Hematopoietic tumors		Primary CNS lymphoma		
		Leukemia		

* Please note 2021 WHO classification of tumors removed the term "anaplastic" in lieu of grading.

Data from Mechtler, Nandigam K[1] and Louis et al.[6]

Classification of intramedullary spinal cord tumors

CONCLUSION

While spinal tumors are rare, significant neurologic morbidity and mortality can occur without proper diagnosis and treatment. Intradural intramedullary tumors are most commonly gliomas, such as ependymoma or astrocytoma, and hemangioblastomas. Symptomatic lesions are typically treated with surgery followed by chemotherapy/radiation therapy in cases with recurrent or residual tumor. Intradural extramedullary tumors include meningioma, schwannoma, and neurofibroma. These are preferably managed with *en bloc* resection and possibly radiation in the setting of residual or infiltrative lesions. Extradural tumors are most commonly metastatic in nature and may be treated with a combination of palliative surgical resection and adjuvant therapies. Primary bone tumors are a minority of extradural tumors and have diverse pathologies and are commonly resected surgically.

What are the most common types of intramedullary spinal cord tumors?	Ependymomas, astrocytomas, and hemangioblastomas
Spinal cord ependymomas are characterized as	Slow-growing lesions that arise from the ependymal lining of the central canal. They tend to expand centrally and are commonly associated with syrinxes and cysts. They are typically encapsulated with a clear margin separating them from the spinal cord tissue
Spinal cord astrocytomas typically appear as	Expansile and infiltrative intramedullary tumors with ill-defined borders between tumor and normal spinal cord tissue
Hemangioblastomas are characterized as	Highly vascularized lesions with associated cord edema. They are frequently associated with syrinxes
The finding of an intramedullary spinal cord tumor should always raise suspicion of and investigation for what?	Presence of certain genetic factors and clinical syndromes, including Neurofibromatosis type 1 and type 2 and von Hippel-Lindau syndrome
Clinical manifestations of intramedullary spinal cord tumors are characterized as	Diverse and based on location. They may include symptoms and findings of radiculopathy, myelopathy, cranial nerve dysfunction, neuropathic pain syndromes, and symptoms of hydrocephalus
If safe and feasible, what is the treatment of choice for a intramedullary spinal cord tumor?	Surgical resection because it allows for tissue diagnosis and decompression/debulking, which may result in stabilization or improvement of neurologic function. There is the potential for cure, depending on pathology and if gross total resection can be achieved
What is the most common intradural extramedullary spinal tumor?	Meningiomas. They are more prevalent in women and most often occur in the thoracic region. On MRI, they appear as contrast-enhancing tumors, frequently associated with a dural tail

What is the characteristic appearance of spinal schwannomas?

Schwannomas are the second most common intradural extramedullary spinal tumors. They arise from Schwann cells at the nerve roots. On MRI, they appear as homogeneously enhancing tumors with a typical dumbbell appearance when extraforaminal. The neural foramen is typically expanded. Histologically, they show densely packed Antoni Type A cells, loosely arranged Antoni Type B cells, and palisading Verocay bodies

How can neurofibromas be differentiated from schwannomas?

Imaging appearance of neurofibromas is similar to schwannomas. Histologically, they consist of loosely arranged spindle cells that differentiate them from schwannomas

Which of the intradural extramedullary spinal tumors are at risk for malignant transformation?

Although rare, both schwannoma and neurofibroma can undergo malignant transformation into malignant peripheral nerve sheet tumors (MPNSTs)

What is the primary treatment for intradural extramedullary spinal tumors?

Surgical resection remains the primary treatment for intradural extramedullary tumors. For benign lesions, *en bloc* resection could be curative. For malignant tumors, adjuvant radiation may reduce the risk for local recurrence

What are the most frequently observed spinal tumor in extradural location?

Extradural spinal tumors mainly consist of metastatic lesions and primary bony tumors of the spinal column. Metastases remain the most common tumors and originate from a variety of underlying oncological diseases

What is the preferred treatment for extradural spinal tumors?

Surgical management is only palliative in these patients and is reserved for patients with refractory pain, progressive neurologic deficit, or segmental instability

For radiosensitive tumors and in the absence of spinal instability, external beam radiation may be preferred

For radioresistant tumors, stereotactic radiosurgery may provide tumor control

What are the most common primary bone tumors of the spine?

Hemangiomas and plasmacytomas

Most patients with primary bone tumors present with what symptom?	Non-specific back pain
What is the preferred treatment for hematologic malignancies of the spine?	Plasmacytoma, multiple myeloma, and lymphoma are very sensitive to chemotherapy and radiation. Surgery is reserved for spinal instability, deformity correction, or rapidly progressive neurologic deficits

QUESTIONS

1. In adults, the most common type of intramedullary spinal cord tumor (IMSCT) is
   a. Ependymoma
   b. Astrocytoma
   c. Hemangioblastoma
   d. Metastatic lesion

2. In patients with von Hippel-Lindau (VHL) disease, the most common IMSCT is
   a. Ependymoma
   b. Astrocytoma
   c. Hemangioblastoma
   d. Neurofibroma

3. Prior to surgical resection, preoperative embolization may be most helpful for the following type of lesion.
   a. Ependymoma
   b. Astrocytoma
   c. Hemangioblastoma
   d. Oligodendroglioma

4. MRI features including heterogeneous enhancement, eccentric location, and ill-defined borders are most consistent with which IMSCT?
   a. Ependymoma
   b. Astrocytoma
   c. Hemangioblastoma
   d. Lipoma

5. The most important factor in determining neurologic outcomes following surgical resection is
   a. Patient's preoperative neurologic status
   b. Tumor histopathology
   c. Well-circumscribed tumor
   d. Tumor location

6. The best course of treatment for the ependymoma patient is
   a. *En bloc* resection
   b. Chemotherapy
   c. Neo-adjuvant radiation therapy
   d. Stereotactic radiosurgery

7. Spinal cord ependymomas are associated with which syndrome?
   a. NF1
   b. NF2
   c. Down syndrome
   d. Von Hippel-Lindau

8. A ring of enhancement or "flame sign" on T1 gadolinium-weighted MRI at the periphery of a intramedullary spinal cord tumor is suggestive of what pathology?
   a. Astrocytoma
   b. Ependymoma
   c. Hemangioblastoma
   d. Metastasis

9. All of the following are histologic characteristics of schwannoma, *except*
   a. Antoni A fibers
   b. Verocay bodies
   c. Spindle cells
   d. Antoni B fibers

10. Malignant peripheral nerve sheath tumors (MPNSTs) may develop from all *except*
    a. Degeneration of schwannomas
    b. Degeneration of meningiomas
    c. Degeneration of neurofibromas
    d. They may arise *de novo*

11. The following metastases to the spine are radiosensitive to conventional external beam radiotherapy (cEBRT), *except*
    a. Prostate
    b. Breast
    c. Lymphoma
    d. Renal cell

12. The most common intradural extramedullary tumor is
    a. Schwannoma
    b. Meningioma
    c. Metastasis
    d. Neurofibroma

13. Presentation with multiple spinal meningiomas would be most likely with which condition?
    a. Charcot-Marie-Tooth disease
    b. Von Hippel-Lindau syndrome
    c. Tay-Sachs disease
    d. Neurofibromatosis type 2 (NF2)

14. Risk factors for malignant transformation of peripheral nerve sheath tumors include the following *except*
    a. Prior radiation treatment
    b. Presence of plexiform neurofibromas
    c. Smoking
    d. NF1 germline mutations

15. Syringomyelia is common with which intradural intramedullary lesion?
   a. Astrocytoma
   b. Ependymoma
   c. Hemangioblastoma
   d. All of the above

ANSWERS

1. a
2. c
3. c
4. b
5. a
6. a
7. b
8. d
9. c
10. b
11. d
12. b
13. d
14. c
15. d

REFERENCES

1. Mechtler LL, Nandigam K. Spinal cord tumors: New views and future directions. *Neurol Clin.* 2013;31(1):241–268. doi:10.1016/j.ncl.2012.09.011
2. Liu JKC, Laufer I, Bilsky MH. Update on management of vertebral column tumors. *CNS Oncol.* 2014;3(2):137–147. doi:10.2217/cns.14.3
3. Chi JH, Bydon A, Hsieh P, Witham T, Wolinsky JP, Gokaslan ZL. Epidemiology and demographics for primary vertebral tumors. *Neurosurg Clin N Am.* 2008;19(1):1–4. doi:10.1016/j.nec.2007.10.005
4. Samartzis D, Gillis CC, Shih P, O'Toole JE, Fessler RG. Intramedullary spinal cord tumors: Part I-epidemiology, pathophysiology, and diagnosis. *Glob Spine J.* 2015;5(5):425–435. doi:10.1055/s-0035-1549029
5. Alvi MA, Ida CM, Paolini MA, et al. Spinal cord high-grade infiltrating gliomas in adults: Clinico-pathological and molecular evaluation. *Mod Pathol.* 2019;32:1236–1243. doi:10.1038/s41379-019-0271-3
6. Louis DN, Perry A, Reifenberger G, et al. The 2016 World Health Organization Classification of Tumors of the Central Nervous System: A summary. *Acta Neuropathol.* 2016;131(6):803–820. doi:10.1007/s00401-016-1545-1
7. Solomon DA, Wood MD, Tihan T, et al. Diffuse midline gliomas with histone H3-K27M mutation: A series of 47 cases assessing the spectrum of morphologic variation and associated genetic alterations. doi:10.1111/bpa.12336
8. Wu J, Armstrong T, Gilbert M. Biology and management of ependymomas. *Neuro- Oncol.* 2016;18(7):902–913. https://www.ncbi.nlm.nih.gov/pmc/articles/PMC4896548/
9. Abul-Kasim K, Thurnher MM, McKeever P, Sundgren PC. Intradural spinal tumors: Current classification and MRI features. *Neuroradiology.* 2008;50(4):301–314. doi:10.1007/s00234-007-0345-7
10. Arima H, Hasegawa T, Togawa D, et al. Feasibility of a novel diagnostic chart of intramedullary spinal cord tumors in magnetic resonance imaging. *Spinal Cord.* 2014;52(10):769–773. doi:10.1038/sc.2014.127
11. Rykken JB, Diehn FE, Hunt CH, et al. Rim and flame signs: Postgadolinium MRI findings specific for Non-CNS intramedullary spinal cord metastases. *Am J Neuroradiol.* 2013;34(4):908–915. doi:10.3174/ajnr.A3292
12. Harrop JS, Ganju A, Groff M, Bilsky M. Primary intramedullary tumors of the spinal cord. *Spine (Phila Pa 1976).* 2009;34(22 Suppl). doi:10.1097/BRS.0b013e3181b95c6f
13. De Amoreira Gepp R, Mauro J, Couto C, Dorvalina Da Silva M, Rolando M, Quiroga S. Mortality is higher in patients with leptomeningeal metastasis in spinal cord tumors. *Arq Neuropsiquiatr.* 2013 Jan;71(1):40–45. doi:10.1590/s0004-282x2012005000019. Epub 2013 Jan 8.
14. Koo H-W, Park JE, Cha J, et al. Hemangioblastomas with leptomeningeal dissemination: Case series and review of the literature. doi:10.1007/s00701-016-2798-0
15. Samartzis D, Gillis CC, Shih P, O'Toole JE, Fessler RG. Intramedullary spinal cord tumors: Part II: Management options and outcomes. *Glob Spine J.* 2015;6(2):176–185. doi:10.1055/s-0035-1550086
16. Ottenhausen M, Ntoulias G, Bodhinayake I, et al. Intradural spinal tumors in adults: Update on management and outcome. *Neurosurg Rev.* 2019;42(2):371–388. doi:10.1007/s10143-018-0957-x
17. Wippold FJ, Lubner M, Perrin RJ, Lämmle M, Perry A. Neuropathology for the neuroradiologist: Antoni A and Antoni B tissue patterns. *Am J Neuroradiol.* 2007;28(9):1633–1638. doi:10.3174/ajnr.A0682
18. Zhang E, Zhang J, Lang N, Yuan H. Spinal cellular schwannoma: An analysis of imaging manifestation and clinicopathological findings. *Eur J Radiol.* 2018;105:81–86. doi:10.1016/j.ejrad.2018.05.025
19. Meyer A, Billings SD. What's new in nerve sheath tumors. *Virchows Arch.* 2020;476(1):65–80. doi:10.1007/s00428-019-02671-0
20. Tucker T, Wolkenstein P, Revuz J, Zeller J, Friedman JM. Association between benign and malignant peripheral nerve sheath tumors in NF1. *Neurology.* 2005;65(2):205–211. doi:10.1212/01.wnl.0000168830.79997.13
21. Yamanaka R, Hayano A. Radiation-induced malignant peripheral nerve sheath tumors: A systematic review. *World Neurosurg.* 2017;105:961–970. e8. doi:10.1016/j.wneu.2017.06.010
22. De Raedt T, Brems H, Wolkenstein P, et al. Elevated risk for MPNST in NF1 microdeletion patients. *Am J Hum Genet.* 2003;72(5):1288–1292. doi:10.1086/374821
23. Pekmezci M, Reuss DE, Hirbe AC, et al. Morphologic and immunohistochemical features of malignant peripheral nerve sheath tumors and cellular schwannomas. *Mod Pathol.* 2015;28(2):187–200. doi:10.1038/modpathol.2014.109
24. Lang N, Liu XG, Yuan HS. Malignant peripheral nerve sheath tumor in spine: Imaging manifestations. *Clin Imaging.* 2012;36(3):209–215. doi:10.1016/j.clinimag.2011.08.015
25. DeClue JE, Papageorge AG, Fletcher JA, et al. Abnormal regulation of mammalian p21ras contributes to malignant tumor growth in von Recklinghausen (type 1) neurofibromatosis. *Cell.* 1992;69(2):265–273. doi:10.1016/0092-8674(92)90407-4
26. Prudner BC, Ball T, Rathore R, Hirbe AC. Diagnosis and management of malignant peripheral nerve sheath tumors: Current practice and future perspectives. *Neuro-oncology Adv.* 2019;2(Suppl 1):i40–i49. doi:10.1093/NOAJNL/VDZ047
27. Wushou A, Jiang YZ, Liu YR, Shao ZM. The demographic features, clinicopathologic characteristics, treatment outcome and disease-specific prognostic factors of solitary fibrous tumor: A population-based analysis. *Oncotarget.* 2015;6(39):41875–41883. doi:10.18632/oncotarget.6174
28. Setzer M, Vatter H, Marquardt G, Seifert V, Vrionis FD. Management of spinal meningiomas: Surgical results and a review of the literature. *Neurosurg Focus.* 2007;23(4):E14. doi:10.3171/FOC-07/10/E14
29. Sandalcioglu IE, Hunold A, Müller O, Bassiouni H, Stolke D, Asgari S. Spinal meningiomas: Critical review of 131 surgically treated patients. *Eur Spine J.* 2008;17(8):1035–1041. doi:10.1007/s00586-008-0685-y
30. Ryu SI, Chang SD, Kim DH, et al. Image-guided hypo-fractionated stereotactic radiosurgery to spinal lesions. *Neurosurgery.* 2001;49(4):838–846. doi:10.1097/00006123-200110000-00011
31. Kaley T, Barani I, Chamberlain M, et al. Historical benchmarks for medical therapy trials in surgery-and radiation-refractory meningioma: A RANO review. doi:10.1093/neuonc/not330
32. Blakeley J. Development of drug treatments for neurofibromatosis type 2-associated vestibular schwannoma. *Curr Opin Otolaryngol Head Neck Surg.* 2012;20(5):372–379. doi:10.1097/MOO.0b013e328357d2ee
33. Shin DW, Sohn MJ, Kim HS, et al. Clinical analysis of spinal stereotactic radiosurgery in the treatment of neurogenic tumors. *J Neurosurg Spine.* 2015;23(4):429–437. doi:10.3171/2015.1.SPINE14910
34. Gersztenne PC, Quader M, Novotny J, Flickinger JC. Radiosurgery for benign tumors of the spine: Clinical experience and current trends. *Technol Cancer Res Treat.* 2012;11(2):133–139. doi:10.7785/tcrt.2012.500242
35. Marchetti M, De Martin E, Milanesi I, Fariselli L. Intradural extramedullary benign spinal lesions radiosurgery. Medium- to long-term results from a single institution experience. *Acta Neurochir (Wien).* 2013;155(7):1215–1222. doi:10.1007/s00701-013-1756-3
36. Gersztenne PC, Burton SA, Ozhasoglu C, McCue KJ, Quinn AE. Radiosurgery for benign intradural spinal tumors. *Neurosurgery.* 2008;62(4):887–895. doi:10.1227/01.neu.0000318174.28461.fc
37. Evans DGR, Birch JM, Ramsden RT, Sharif S, Baser ME. Malignant transformation and new primary tumours after therapeutic radiation for

benign disease: Substantial risks in certain tumour prone syndromes. *J Med Genet.* 2006;43(4):289–294. doi:10.1136/jmg.2005.036319

38. Khalaf WF, Yang F-C, Chen S, et al. K-ras is critical for modulating multiple c-kit-mediated cellular functions in wild-type and Nf1 +/– mast cells. *J Immunol.* 2007;178(4):2527–2534. doi:10.4049/jimmunol.178.4.2527

39. Chamberlain MC, Tredway TL. Adult primary intradural spinal cord tumors: A review. *Curr Neurol Neurosci Rep.* 2011;11(3):320–328. doi:10.1007/s11910-011-0190-2

40. Abd-El-Barr M, Huang K, Moses Z, Iorgulescu J, Chi J. Recent advances in intradural spinal tumors. *Neuro Oncol.* 2017;20(6):729–742. https://www.ncbi.nlm.nih.gov/pmc/articles/PMC5961256/pdf/nox230.pdf. Accessed July 22, 2020.

41. Laufer I, Rubin DG, Lis E, et al. The NOMS Framework: Approach to the treatment of spinal metastatic tumors. *Oncologist.* 2013;18(6):744–751. doi:10.1634/theoncologist.2012-0293

42. Patchell RA, Tibbs PA, Regine WF, et al. Direct decompressive surgical resection in the treatment of spinal cord compression caused by metastatic cancer: A randomised trial. *Lancet.* 2005;366(9486):643–648. doi:10.1016/S0140-6736(05)66954-1

43. Boriani S, Biagini R, De Iure F, et al. Primary bone tumors of the spine: A survey of the evaluation and treatment at the Istituto Ortopedico Rizzoli: PubMed. *Orthopedics.* 1995;18(10):993–1000.

44. Charest-Morin R, Fisher CG, Sahgal A, et al. Primary bone tumor of the spine: An evolving field: What a general spine surgeon should know. *Glob Spine J.* 2019;9(1_suppl):108S–116S. doi:10.1177/2192568219828727

45. Fox MW, Onofrio BM. The natural history and management of symptomatic and asymptomatic vertebral hemangiomas. *J Neurosurg.* 1993;78(1):36–45. doi:10.3171/jns.1993.78.1.0036

46. Kelley S, Ashford R, Rao A, Dickson R. Primary bone tumours of the spine: A 42-year survey from the Leeds Regional Bone Tumour Registry. *Eur Spine J.* 2007;16(3):405–409. Accessed June 25, 2020.

47. Charest-Morin R, Boriani S, Fisher CG, et al. Benign tumors of the spine: Has new chemotherapy and interventional radiology changed the treatment paradigm? *Spine (Phila Pa 1976).* 2016;41:S178–S185. doi:10.1097/BRS.0000000000001818

PART III. | PEDIATRIC NEURO-ONCOLOGY

14 | EPIDEMIOLOGY AND GENERAL OVERVIEW OF PEDIATRIC CENTRAL NERVOUS SYSTEM TUMORS

SCOTT L. COVEN

INTRODUCTION

Central nervous system (CNS) tumors are the most common solid tumor in children between 1 and 19 years of age. Additionally, CNS tumors are the leading disease-related cause of death in children under 19 years of age in the United States.[1-2] Despite advances in diagnostic modalities, surgical interventions, and treatment methods, children with CNS tumors continue to experience significant morbidity and mortality. Children with brain tumors require a multidisciplinary team, with expertise in nursing, pediatric neurosurgery, pediatric neuro-oncology, pediatric radiology, pediatric neuropathology, pediatric radiation oncology, pediatric rehab, palliative care, and other subspecialties.

BACKGROUND

The Central Brain Tumor Registry of the United States (CBTRUS) is a not-for-profit corporation established by a grant from the Pediatric Brain Tumor Foundation in 1992. The CBTRUS has grown into the largest, centralized aggregation of population-based data on the incidence of CNS tumors in the United States. The CBTRUS acquires data from state cancer registries and publishes yearly statistical reports.[3]

> The CBTRUS has grown into the largest, centralized aggregation of population-based data on the incidence of CNS tumors in the United States.

The CBTRUS published the most recent pediatric update in 2019, reflecting CNS tumors diagnosed in the United States from 2012 to 2016. Between 0 and 14 years of age, CNS tumors were the most common location for cancer. The average incidence for children in this age group was 5.74 per 100,000 population, ahead of leukemia (4.99 per 100,000 population). The incidence rate for all CNS tumors increased slightly to 6.06 per 100,000 population (0–19 years) when including adolescents.[4,5]

The incidence rates for CNS tumors for the age group 15–19 years (6.98 per 100,000 population) exceeded the incidence rates of those observed in the age groups 0–4 years (6.22 per 100,000 population), 5–9 years (5.38 per 100,000 population), and 10–14 years (5.65 per 100,000 population). Males and females have a similar overall incidence rate in children 0–19 years. With respect to race, white children have the highest incidence rate of 6.29 per 100,000 population. The next highest incidence rates were among Asian/Pacific Islander (5.17 per 100,000 population) and Hispanic (5.14 per 100,000 population); black children had an incidence rate of 4.71 per 100,000 population.[4]

According to the CBTRUS, there are estimated to be 4,750 new cases of primary CNS tumors among children age 0–19 years in 2019 and 2020. The overall survival (OS) for children age 0–19 years, including all histologic subtypes, is 88.5% at 1 year and 75.5% at 5 years.[4]

DISTRIBUTION BY HISTOLOGIC TUMOR TYPE

There are more than 100 histologically distinct types of primary CNS tumors. Unlike other types of cancer, CNS tumors are not staged.[6] They are classified by grade (1 through 4) according to the World Health Organization (WHO) 2000 Classification of Tumours of the Central Nervous System.[7] This grading system aims to characterize the histological subtype by its predicted clinical behavior. The updated classification from 2016 includes the implementation of molecular biomarkers in addition to the histologic diagnosis.[8] Despite the challenges in the collection of these markers, state cancer registries began reporting these data in early 2018.[4,6-9]

GLIOMA

Gliomas are tumors that arise from glial cells and include a heterogenous group of histologic diagnoses. Despite the differences in histology among gliomas, many divide them further into malignant and non-malignant.[6-9] Gliomas account for around 45% of all CNS tumors in children age 0–19 years.[4-5,10] Gliomas are graded according to the WHO classification as grades 1 to 4, with low-grade gliomas (LGGs) representing grades 1 and 2 and high-grade gliomas (HGGs) representing grades 3 and 4.[4-10] Additionally, gliomas tend to occur in any anatomical region throughout the CNS. Pilocytic astrocytomas and other gliomas are known to occur in children with neurofibromatosis type 1.[4,5]

"Pediatric low-grade glioma" is a basket term used to include pilocytic astrocytoma (WHO grade 1), diffuse astrocytoma (WHO grade 2), oligodendroglioma, ganglioglioma, pilomyxoid astrocytoma, and pleomorphic astrocytoma. Together, this group represents more than 40% of all primary brain tumors in children.[4,10,11] Pilocytic astrocytoma of the cerebellum represents the most common pediatric low-grade glioma. While the age of low-grade glioma varies throughout childhood, cerebellar pilocytic astrocytoma has a peak age at diagnosis of 5–15 years.[12] White children have a significantly higher incidence of pilocytic astrocytoma at a rate of 0.97 per 100,000, with no sex predominance.[4] Children with low-grade gliomas most commonly experience alterations and dysregulation of the mitogen-activated protein kinase (MAPK) pathway, which has become the focus of recent drug development and up-front clinical trial design.[11-14]

> Children with low-grade gliomas most commonly experience alterations and dysregulation of the mitogen-activated protein kinase (MAPK) pathway, which has become the focus of recent drug development and up-front clinical trial design.

Pediatric high-grade glioma includes diagnoses such as anaplastic astrocytoma (WHO grade 3) and glioblastoma (WHO grade 4). High-grade gliomas represent around 8–12% of all primary brain tumors in children.[10] Additionally, brainstem gliomas account for another 10–20% of CNS tumors in children, with the majority of these representing diffuse intrinsic pontine gliomas (DIPG).[11,15] This group of tumors often peaks between 5 and 15 years of age, occurring more in white children, with no specific sex predominance.[4] As with pediatric low-grade glioma, children with high-grade glioma and DIPG may possess alterations in the MAPK pathway. Other significant molecular drivers, such as platelet-derived growth factor receptor (PDGFRA), epidermal growth factor receptor (EGFR), and DNA-repair enzyme (MGMT) likely contribute to the more aggressive biologic features of high-grade gliomas.[10,14,15] More recently, tumors in the midline (thalamus, brainstem, spinal cord) have been characterized by discovery of K27M mutations in the histone H3 gene H3F3A. The 2016 WHO classification defined this as a new entity, diffuse midline glioma, H3 K27M-mutant and it includes DIPG.[8,10,11-17] Drug development and prospective clinical trial design have incorporated biopsy techniques to evaluate molecular characteristics and targeted therapies.[11,12]

The standard treatment for children with gliomas varies widely and is often dependent on a multitude of factors including neurologic symptoms, radiographic progression, tumor location, and diagnosis. For example, children with biologically indolent lesions may be observed with surveillance imaging until symptoms necessitate further intervention. Surgery is often curative for low-grade gliomas when a complete resection is achievable. However, many lesions are located in deep and essential structures and are inaccessible to aggressive surgical intervention.[13] Therefore, surgical biopsy with adequate tissue sampling for diagnosis and molecular characterization is imperative. Long-term OS for children with high-grade gliomas has been linked to the degree of surgical resection. Radiation therapy is often avoided or considered a last option for children with low-grade gliomas due to the long-term risks to the developing brain.[10,11] However, radiation therapy for high-grade gliomas and DIPG is the standard treatment modality.[12-15] Chemotherapy is the standard treatment for children with low-grade gliomas not amenable to surgical resection. Recently, new clinical trials are attempting to demonstrate efficacy of molecular targeted agents to replace the front-line standard of carboplatin and vincristine.[13] Unfortunately, chemotherapy has not greatly improved OS for children with high-grade gliomas. The 5-year OS for children with low-grade glioma remains greater than 90%; however, in children with tumors not amenable to surgical resection, low-grade gliomas often resemble a chronic disease.[4,5,10-13] In sharp contrast, the OS for children with high-grade glioma remains poor, with a 5-year OS of 20–30%.[4] Despite the significant advancements in the biologic understanding of DIPG, the median survival remains around 12 months from initial diagnosis.[13-15]

> Surgery is often curative for low-grade gliomas when a complete resection is achievable. However, many lesions are located in deep and essential structures and are inaccessible to aggressive surgical intervention.

MEDULLOBLASTOMA

Embryonal tumors are a heterogenous group of tumors that may disseminate throughout the CNS.[18,19] Prior to 2016, medulloblastoma and other embryonal tumors were grouped together and referred to as primitive neuroectodermal tumor (PNET), but this term has been removed and replaced with "embryonal tumors" in the updated WHO classification.[8] Embryonal tumors account for 11.5% of all CNS tumors for children age 0–19 years, and medulloblastoma is the most common histology accounting for 64.9% in this age group.[4,5] Medulloblastomas by definition occur in the posterior fossa and account for 40% of all posterior fossa tumors.[18] Additionally, children with Gorlin syndrome are at an increased risk for developing medulloblastoma.[5] Children with Gorlin syndrome with germline patched-1 gene (PTCH1) mutations have been associated with a risk of medulloblastoma of less than 2%; however, limited studies describe a substantially higher risk of up to one-third in those Gorlin syndrome patients with germline suppressor of fused gene (SUFU) mutations.[19]

> Medulloblastomas by definition occur in the posterior fossa and account for 40% of all posterior fossa tumors.

Medulloblastoma is a highly aggressive childhood brain tumor (WHO grade 4) that represents a heterogenous group of complex histological and molecular variants. While previously considered a singular entity, molecular profiling and genomics have transformed our understanding of medulloblastoma.[18-22] The updated 2016 WHO classification married histologic and molecular findings, definitively characterizing medulloblastoma into four groups: wingless (WNT)-activated, sonic hedgehog (SHH)-activated, "group 3" and "group 4."[8,20,22] Within these four established groups, additional subtypes and genetic drivers exist. The WNT-activated and SHH-activated subgroups are considered low-risk medulloblastoma due to their improved OS, while "group 3" and "group 4" subgroups are often considered high-risk medulloblastoma due to their propensity for CNS dissemination and treatment challenges.[18-22]

These tumors occur throughout childhood, with peak incidence at 3–4 years and 7–10 years.[12] Additionally, around 20% occur in infants. There is variation with age and sex with respect to molecular subtypes. WNT-activated tumors occur in older children with no sex predominance. SHH-activated tumors occur in infants and adults with no sex predominance. Group 3-activated tumors occur in infants and children with a male predominance. Group 4-activated tumors occur at all ages with a male predominance.[12] Last, white children have the highest age-adjusted incidence rate at 0.42 per 100,000.[4]

The standard treatment for children with medulloblastoma begins with maximal safe surgical resection and confirmatory diagnosis. Since medulloblastoma can seed the neuro-axis, cerebrospinal fluid (CSF) sampling needs to occur 14 days after surgical resection. Radiotherapy (including craniospinal) and chemotherapy play significant roles in the treatment of medulloblastoma depending on age.[18-20] Risk-adapted treatment strategies with intensive chemotherapy to avoid irradiation for children less than 3 years and even up to 10 years of age (for low-risk subtypes) are currently under investigation. Additional radiotherapy strategies, such as proton therapy and tailored volumes and doses to reduce long-term treatment effects, are also under consideration.[18] The 5-year OS for all children with medulloblastoma regardless of histologic and molecular classification is 72.3%.[4,5,18] However, children with WNT-activated pathway medulloblastoma have a 5-year OS that approaches 100%.[20-22] Treatment failures for children with medulloblastoma are likely dependent on molecular subtype, extent of dissemination, and extent of surgical resection (or presence of residual disease).[18]

EPENDYMOMA

Ependymomas arise from neuroepithelial cells and occur throughout the CNS. Among children, ependymomas account for around 10% of all CNS tumors in children and have a predilection for males over females.[4,5,23] Ependymomas can vary by WHO classification and are graded 1, 2, and 3. Grade 2 is the most common histology across all age groups. The major peak for children with this tumor occurs at 0–4 years. Again, ependymal tumors have a predilection for white children more so than other races.[4] Pediatric ependymoma occurs predominantly intracranially, with two-thirds occurring in the posterior fossa.[23-28] Additionally, spinal ependymomas occur primarily in familial cancer syndromes, such as neurofibromatosis type 2.[5] The average age at diagnosis for supratentorial ependymoma is 7.8 years, for infratentorial ependymoma is 5 years, and for spinal ependymoma is 12 years.[29]

> The average age at diagnosis for supratentorial ependymoma is 7.8 years, for infratentorial ependymoma is 5 years, and for spinal ependymoma is 12 years.

Myxopapillary ependymomas (WHO grade 1) are predominantly found in adults. Grade 2 ependymomas, often referred to as "classic" ependymomas, and grade 3, anaplastic ependymomas, commonly occur in children. Along with the histological features that characterize grades 2 and 3 tumors, pediatric ependymoma has evolved with the addition of molecular profiling.[23,26-28] The average age at diagnosis for patients with myxopapillary ependymoma is 36 years, although it has been described in pediatric patients as young as 6 years.[29] An international collaborative study established a molecular classification approach that further divides ependymoma into nine distinct subtypes, with three in each anatomical compartment (spinal, posterior fossa, and supratentorial) of the CNS. An example is the *RELA* fusion-positive (ST-EPN-RELA) and *YAP1* (ST-EPN-YAP1) ependymomas, which define the two distinct molecular subtypes in the supratentorial region. Additionally, the posterior fossa (PF) has been divided into PF-EPN-A and PF-EPN-B. These two subtypes vary in molecular findings, age at diagnosis, and clinical outcomes.[23,27,28] PF-EPN-A occurs primarily in infants and young children, whereas PF-EPN-B occurs more often in adolescents and young adults. The molecular subgroup of supratentorial ependymomas with the *YAP1* fusion are primarily seen in children.[13]

The standard treatment for children with intracranial ependymoma includes maximal safe neurosurgical intervention followed by focal radiotherapy.[30-32] Ependymoma is known to seed the CSF so sampling at an appropriate time after surgical resection is required. Chemotherapy has failed to show improvements in OS among children, although this remains controversial when discussing radiation deferral for infants.[5,25,30-32] Based on the CBTRUS data, the 5-year OS for children 0–19 years with ependymoma is 78.9%.[4] However, if gross total resection is not achieved, the OS drops to 32.5%.[30-32] Furthermore, ST-EPN-RELA, which primarily occurs in children, and PF-EPN-A, which primarily occurs in infants and children, have a worse 10-year OS of 50% and 56%, respectively.[23-32] Last, children with ependymoma may experience very late recurrences or relapses, up to 10 years after initial diagnosis.

RARER TUMORS

Several other tumors are worth mentioning that primarily exist in children, but they often occur in much rarer frequency. Examples include CNS germ cell tumors, craniopharyngioma, and atypical teratoid/rhabdoid tumors (AT/RT). Germ cell tumors account for approximately 4% of all childhood CNS tumors in the United States but account for up to 11% in Asian countries such as Japan.[4,13] CNS germ cell tumors are often subdivided into pure germinoma and non-germinomatous germ cell tumors, and the tumors may secrete specific proteins (e.g., AFP and bHCG) in either the blood or CSF. Germinoma accounts for more than 50% of all intracranial germ cell tumors.[13] There is a slightly higher incidence in males than females.[4] Chemotherapy and radiotherapy are the primary treatment modalities for children with germ cell tumors, with a 5-year OS near 96%.[4,33]

Craniopharyngioma is an epithelial tumor arising from Rathke's pouch in the sellar and suprasellar regions, accounting for around 3.5% of all childhood CNS tumors.[4,34] Craniopharyngioma has the highest rate of incidence from 5 to 9 years, has no sex predominance, and is one of the few pediatric brain tumors with a higher rate of incidence among black children than white children.[4] The location of these tumors provides a challenge when determining optimal treatment strategy. Surgery is often the primary treatment modality. Chemotherapy has not been shown to be an effective treatment for craniopharyngioma. Radiotherapy significantly improves local control while increasing the risk of long-term effects. Despite the high 5-year OS (95%), many children with craniopharyngioma experience treatment-related complications such as endocrinopathies, visual deficits, or obesity.[4,34]

AT/RT is a rare embryonal tumor that accounts for approximately 1.5–2% of all primary CNS tumors in children 0–19 years.[35] However, AT/RT tends to occur in the youngest children, often affecting those younger than 3 years. There is no predominance among sex or race.[4] The 5-year OS based on historical CBTRUS data is around 35%, but many cohorts have demonstrated an improved OS for children older than 3 years.[4,35] Additionally, improved OS correlates with multimodality treatment including maximal safe surgical resection, intensive chemotherapy, and radiotherapy.

Despite the high 5-year OS (95%), many children with craniopharyngioma experience treatment-related complications such as endocrinopathies, visual deficits, or obesity.

SPINAL CORD TUMORS

Primary spinal cord tumors account for around 4–6% of all CNS, with an annual incidence of near 1 per 100,000 children.[12,13] Ependymal tumors are the most common histological subtype (20.6%) followed by nerve sheath tumors (17.8%).[4] Spinal cord tumors are challenging to diagnose given their presenting symptoms and gradual onset.[13] The incident rate among children is highest for adolescents age 15–19 years. There is no significant sex predominance, but a higher incidence in whites over blacks.[4]

DISTRIBUTION BY TUMOR LOCATION

The tumor location often influences the presenting signs and symptoms for children with primary CNS tumors. The predominant tumor location for children and adolescents is in the pituitary and craniopharyngeal duct (16.5%). The cerebellum (12.9%), other brain areas (12.8%), and brainstem (10.9%) are the next most common tumor locations.[4] Additional sites throughout the CNS are represented in much lesser frequency (Figure 14.1).[2–4] Histologic diagnosis

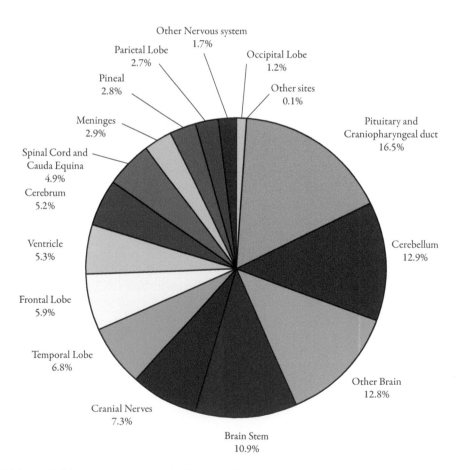

Figure 14.1 Distribution in children and adolescents (age 0-19 year s) of location of primary CNS tumors (5-year total = 24,931; annual average).

often varies with tumor location, impacting treatment strategies, quality of life, and OS.

> Histologic diagnosis often varies with tumor location, impacting treatment strategies, quality of life, and OS.

Intracranial CNS tumors are often divided by their compartment location within the brain: supratentorial or infratentorial. There is a nearly equivalent distribution between tumor types that arise supratentorial versus infratentorial.[12] Supratentorial tumors have a bimodal peak, occurring in infants and children younger than 3 years and after age 10 years. Infratentorial tumors are more common in children between 4 and 10 years.[13] Younger children have a higher incidence of embryonal tumors, whereas older children have a higher incidence of gliomas.[13]

RISK FACTORS FOR CNS TUMORS

Although the cause of most childhood CNS tumors is relatively unknown, there are two well-known risk factors for the development of a CNS tumor: exposure to ionizing radiation and genetic predisposition. Given that many CNS tumors require high-dose irradiation as a primary treatment strategy, this significantly increases the risk for second malignancies within the radiation field.[5] Parental age has been debated as a risk factor for childhood brain tumors, although with limited reports.[1] Maternal genetic effects are currently understudied with their potential connection to pediatric CNS tumors.[1] Allergic conditions such as asthma and eczema have been studied and may show a potential protective factor for the development of pediatric brain tumors, although more research is needed.[1] Exposure to infection has been studied through cancer registries, but no definitive associations have been demonstrated.[1] Several studies have documented an increased risk of brain tumor development in children with congenital anomalies.[1] Numerous other risk factors for childhood brain tumors are currently under investigation (Box 14.1).[36]

> Two well-known risk factors for the development of a CNS tumor include exposure to ionizing radiation and genetic predisposition.

There is some debate on the frequency, often quoted at around 10%, of genetic predisposition of childhood cancer.[5] However, several syndromes have been identified that increase the risk of developing a CNS tumor. Neurofibromatosis (NF) is an autosomal dominant neurocutaneous disorder associated with an array of clinical features and associated with CNS tumors such as optic pathway gliomas, extraoptic pathway tumors, vestibular schwannomas, meningiomas, and spinal cord tumors (ependymomas). NF1 occurs in one in 2,500 to 5,000 live births and is the most common familial syndrome associated with CNS tumors.[37] Around 15–20% of patients with NF will develop a low-grade glioma, which includes optic pathway gliomas.[12,37] Neurofibromas are another stigmata that

must be watched closely because approximately 15% undergo malignant transformation.[37] NF2 is less common, with the classic characteristic of vestibular schwannomas occurring in roughly 95% of patients.[37] Additionally, up to 50% of NF2 patients develop multiple meningiomas and approximately 2–5% of patients develop ependymomas.[36]

Tuberous sclerosis (TS) is an autosomal dominant neurocutaneous disorder, affecting 1 in 6,000 to 1 in 30,000 people, associated with brain lesions such as hamartomas and subependymal giant cell astrocytomas (SEGAs).[37] SEGAs develop in 5–15% of TS patients.[37] Von Hippel-Lindau (VHL) syndrome is an autosomal dominant disorder associated with CNS lesions such as hemangioblastomas, occurring in 60–80% of patients.[37] Gorlin syndrome is caused by a germline mutation in the patched gene (tumor suppressor gene) and confers an increased risk of medulloblastoma, specifically the SHH subtype. Gorlin syndrome is characterized by multiple basal cell cancers, affecting 1 in 60,000 live births, with medulloblastoma occurring in 3–5% of patients.[37] Rhabdoid tumor predisposition syndrome is predominantly caused by a germline mutation in the *SMARCB1* gene. This syndrome is associated with atypical teratoid/rhabdoid tumors (AT/RTs). Li-Fraumeni syndrome (LFS) is an autosomal dominant disorder characterized by a germline mutation in the *TP53* gene and increases the risk of many malignancies including CNS tumors. Overall, about 10% of LFS patients will develop a glioma before the age of 45, and another 5% will develop a medulloblastoma or choroid plexus carcinoma.[37] Turcot syndrome (brain tumor-polyposis syndrome) describes the association of familial colon cancer with brain tumors (medulloblastomas and gliomas).[5]

> Gorlin syndrome is characterized by multiple basal cell cancers, affecting 1 in 60,000 live births, with medulloblastoma occurring in 3–5% of patients.

CONCLUSION

CNS tumors in children represent the most common childhood cancer, now surpassing leukemia. The Central Brain Tumor Registry in the United States relies on state cancer registries and accounts for the largest, most comprehensive database for indexing CNS tumors for children age 0–19 years. The CBTRUS allows for monitoring of incidence trends and changes in outcomes since its inception in 1992. The 2016 CNS WHO classification system incorporated molecular biomarkers to enhance brain tumor diagnoses. The collection of this new information within state registries will allow for improved understanding of pediatric CNS tumors.[3,8] Despite advances in treatment and knowledge, pediatric CNS tumors represent the largest cause of years of potential life lost, with an estimate of an individual's life shortened by premature death to cancer of nearly 80 years.[4]

What is the most common solid tumor of children 1–19 years of age?	CNS tumors
What is the overall survival for children with CNS tumors?	Approximately 75% at 5 years
Most common location of CNS tumors include	Intracranial; spinal cord tumors account for only about 6% of all childhood CNS tumors
Annual incidence of CNS tumors in: All children 0–19 years Children 0–14 years Adolescents 15–19 years	6.06 per 100,000 people 5.74 per 100,000 people 6.98 per 100,000 people
Annual incidence of CNS tumors in: Females Males	6.13 per 100,000 people 5.98 per 100,000 people
What is the most common tumor of the brain and spinal cord in children?	Low grade glioma, accounting for approximately 40% of tumors
Distribution of CNS tumors in children by overall percentage: Embryonal tumors Gliomas (including high-grade) Ependymoma Germ cell tumors Craniopharyngioma	11.5% of all children 45% of all children 10% all children, males > females 4% in US, 11% in East Asia 3.5% of all children
Two known, definitive risk factors for CNS tumors in childhood are:	Prior exposure to ionizing radiation and genetic predisposition

QUESTIONS

1. What is the most common histology of childhood CNS tumors?
   a. Glioma
   b. Medulloblastoma
   c. Craniopharyngioma
   d. Ependymoma

2. What is the 5 year median overall survival for children with CNS tumors?
   a. 20%
   b. 45%
   c. 95%
   d. 75%

3. What is the median survival for children with DIPG?
   a. 6 months
   b. 24 months
   c. 12 months
   d. 18 months

4. What subtype of medulloblastoma has the best overall survival?
   a. SHH-activated
   b. WNT-activated
   c. "Group 4"
   d. "Group 3"

5. What inherited syndrome has a risk of gliomas and ependymomas?
   a. Neurofibromatosis
   b. Li-Fraumeni syndrome
   c. Tuberous sclerosis
   d. Gorlin syndrome

6. Males have a higher incidence of CNS tumors.
   a. True
   b. False

7. What year did the CBTRUS begin collecting vital information from state cancer registries?
   a. 1995
   b. 1988
   c. 1999
   d. 1992

8. Primary spinal cord tumors in children make up what percentage of all CNS tumors?
   a. 6%
   b. 15%
   c. 10%
   d. 25%

9. What is the predominant tumor location for childhood CNS tumors?
   a. Pituitary
   b. Brainstem
   c. Spine
   d. Cerebellum

10. What tumor is associated with tuberous sclerosis?
    a. Ependymoma
    b. SEGAs
    c. Medulloblastoma
    d. AT/RT

11. Pediatric low-grade glioma accounts for approximately what percentage of all childhood brain and spinal cord tumors?
    a. 25%
    b. 55%
    c. 40%
    d. 75%

12. What tumor histology was removed from the 2016 WHO classification?
    a. *PNET*
    b. Embryonal
    c. Diffuse midline glioma
    d. Ependymoma

13. Children younger than what age tend to do worse with AT/RT?
    a. 5 years
    b. 12 months
    c. 3 years
    d. 10 years

ANSWERS

1. a
2. d
3. c
4. b
5. a
6. b
7. d
8. a
9. a
10. b
11. c
12. a
13. c

REFERENCES

1. Johnson KJ, Cullen J, Barnholtz-Sloan JS, et al. Childhood brain tumor epidemiology: A brain tumor epidemiology consortium review. *Cancer Epidemiol Biomarkers Prev.* 2014;23(12):2716–2736.
2. Ostrom QT, de Blank PM, Kruchko C, et al. Alex's Lemonade Stand Foundation infant and childhood primary brain and central nervous system tumors diagnosed in the United States in 2007-2011. *Neuro Oncol.* 2015;16 Suppl 10:x1–x36.

3. Central Brain Tumor Registry of the United States. http://www.cbtrus.org/ www.cbtrus.org/aboutus/aboutus.html

4. Ostrom QT, Cioffi G, Gittleman H, et al, CBTRUS statistical report: Primary brain and other central nervous system tumors diagnosed in the United States in 2012–2016. *Neuro Oncol.* 2019;21(5):v1–v100. https://doi.org/10.1093/neuonc/noz150

5. Epidemiology of central nervous system tumors in children. https://www-uptodate-com/contents/epidemiology-of-central-nervous-system-tumors-in-children

6. McCarthy BJ, Surawicz T, Bruner JM, Kruchko C, Davis F. Consensus conference on brain tumor definition for registration. *Neuro Oncol.* 2002;4(2):134–145.

7. Kleihues P, Cavenee W, eds. Tumours of the nervous system. *World Health Organization Classification of Tumours.* Lyon: IARC Press; 2000.

8. Louis DN, Perry A, Reifenberger G, et al. The 2016 World Health Organization classification of tumors of the central nervous system: A summary. *Acta Neuropathol.* 2016;131(6):803–820.

9. Louis DN, Ohgaki H, Wiestler OD, et al. The 2007 WHO classification of tumours of the central nervous system. *Acta Neuropathol.* 2007;114:97–109.

10. Mintum JE, Fisher MJ. Gliomas in children. *Curr Treat Options Neurol.* 2013;15(3):316–327.

11. Packer RJ, Pfister S, Bouffet E, et al. Pediatric low-grade gliomas: Implications of the biologic era. *Neuro Onc.* 2017;19(6):750–761.

12. Wells EM, Packer RJ. Pediatric brain tumors. *Continuum.* 2015;21(2):373–396.

13. Udaka YT, Packer RJ. Pediatric brain tumors. *Neurol Clin.* 2018;36:533–556.

14. Sturm D, Pfister SM, Jones DTW. Pediatric gliomas: Current concepts on diagnosis, biology and clinical management. *J Clin Oncol.* 2017;35:2370–2377.

15. Hennika T, Becher OJ. Diffuse intrinsic pontine glioma: Time for cautious optimism. *J Child Neurol.* 2016;31(12):1377–1385.

16. Paugh BS, Qu C, Jones C, et al. Integrated molecular genetic profiling of pediatric high-grade gliomas reveals key differences with the adult disease. *J Clin Oncol.* 2010;28:3061–3068.

17. Schroeder KM, Hoeman CM, Becher OJ. Children are not just little adults: Recent advances in understanding of diffuse intrinsic pontine glioma biology. *Pediatr Res.* 2014;75:205–209.

18. PDQ Pediatric Treatment Editorial Board. Childhood medulloblastoma and other central nervous system embryonal tumors treatment (PDQ®): Health Professional Version. 2020 Mar 23. PDQ Cancer Information Summaries. Bethesda, MD: National Cancer Institute (US); 2002. https://www-ncbi-nlm-nih-gov/NBK65981/

19. Millard NE, De Braganca KC. Medulloblastoma. *J Child Neurol.* 2016;31(12):1341–1353.

20. Gajjar A, Packer RJ, Foreman NK, et al. Children's Oncology Group's 2013 blueprint for research: Central nervous system tumors. *Pediatr Blood Cancer.* 2013;60:1022–1026.

21. Cavalli FMG, Remke M, Rampasek L, et al. Intertumoral heterogeneity within medulloblastoma subgroups. *Cancer Cell.* 2017;31:737–754.

22. Northcott PA, Buchhalter I, Morrissy AS, et al. The whole genome landscape of medulloblastoma subtypes. *Nature.* 2017;547:311–317.

23. Hübner JM, Kool M, Pfister SM, Pajtler KW. Epidemiology, molecular classification and WHO grading of ependymoma. *J Neurosurg Sci.* 2018;62:46–50. doi:10.23736/S0390-5616.17.04152-2.

24. Villano JL, Parker CK, Dolecek TA. Descriptive epidemiology of ependymal tumours in the united states. *Br J Cancer.* 2013;108:2367–2371.

25. Purdy E, Johnston DL, Bartels U, et al. Ependymoma in children under the age of 3 years: A report from the Canadian pediatric brain tumour consortium. *J Neurooncol.* 2014;117:359–364.

26. Kilday JP, Rahman R, Dyer S, Ridley L, Lowe J, Coyle B, et al. Pediatric ependymoma: Biological perspectives. *Mol Cancer Res.* 2009;7:765–786.

27. Pajtler KW, Witt H, Sill M, et al. Molecular classification of ependymal tumors across all CNS compartments, histopathological grades, and age groups. *Cancer Cell.* 2015;27:728–743.

28. Khatua S, Ramaswamy V, Bouffet E. Current therapy and the evolving molecular landscape of paediatric ependymoma. *Eur J Cancer.* 2017;70:34–41.

29. Vitanza NA, Partap S. *J Child Neurol.* 2016;31(12):1354–1366.

30. Cage TA, Clark AJ, Aranda D, et al. A systematic review of treatment outcomes in pediatric patients with intracranial ependymomas. *J Neurosurg Pediatr.* 2013;11:673–681.

31. Merchant TE, Li C, Xiong X, Kun LE, Boop FA, Sanford RA. Conformal radiotherapy after surgery for paediatric ependymoma: A prospective study. *Lancet Oncol.* 2009;10:258–266.

32. Merchant TE. Current clinical challenges in childhood ependymoma: A focused review. *J Clin Oncol.* 2017;35(21):2364–2369.

33. Allen J, Chacko J, Donahue B, et al. Diagnostic sensitivity of serum and lumbar CSF bHCG in newly diagnosed CNS germinoma. *Pediatr Blood Cancer.* 2012;59:1180–1182.

34. Winkfield KM, Tsai HK, Yao X, et al. Long-term clinical outcomes following treatment of childhood craniopharyngioma. *Pediatr Blood Cancer.* 2011;56:1120–1126.

35. Ostrom QT, Chen Y, de Blank PM, et al. The descriptive epidemiology of atypical teratoid/rhabdoid tumors in the United States, 2001–2010. *Neuro Onc.* 2014;16(10):1392–1399.

36. McNeill KA. Epidemiology of brain tumors. *Neurol Clin.* 2016;34:981–998.

37. Ranger AM, Patel YK, Chaudhary N, Ram V. Familial syndromes associated with intracranial tumours: A review. *Childs Nerv Syst.* 2014;30:47–64.

15 | NEUROSURGICAL MANAGEMENT OF PEDIATRIC CENTRAL NERVOUS SYSTEM TUMORS

NIR SHIMONY, MOHAMMAD HASSAN A. NOURELDINE, CAMERON BRIMLEY, AND GEORGE I. JALLO

CONSIDERATIONS FOR DECISION-MAKING PROCESSES IN THE CHILD WITH BRAIN TUMOR

DIAGNOSTIC ROLE OF ADVANCED IMAGING AND BIOPSY

Most pediatric brain and spinal cord tumors have specific imaging characteristics that provide for relatively accurate tumor identification; however, tissue diagnosis and molecular profiling are often beneficial when a safe surgery is possible. The various imaging modalities (computed tomography [CT], magnetic resonance imaging [MRI], nuclear studies, x-ray, ultrasound, etc.) and sequence types typically present patterns that provide sufficient variation to successfully differentiate tumor types in most of the cases (see Table 15.1). Many pediatric brain tumor types have a distinct presentation based on location of the tumor and the age of the patient that, combined with the different imaging characteristics, provides for a high rate of accurate diagnosis without the necessity of obtaining tissue. For example, a patient between 5 and 9 years old with a pontine mass with poorly defined border that is T2/fluid-attenuated inversion recovery (FLAIR) hyperintense and T1 hypointense, with infrequent contrast enhancement, has a high probability of being diffuse intrinsic pontine glioma with few alternative diagnoses.[1,2] Another example is a posterior fossa mass that fills the fourth ventricle, is contrast-enhancing and diffusion-restricting, in a 3-year-old child; this has a very high probability of being a medulloblastoma.

Conventional MR imaging sequences help detail the anatomical structure of the tumor and brain tissue while advanced techniques provide physiologic and functional information. Advanced MR sequences include magnetic resonance spectroscopy (MRS), perfusion weighted, diffusion weighted (DWI), susceptibility-weighted (SWI), diffusion tensor (DTI), and functional imaging. DWI for example, will show high intensity (diffusion restriction) when water is unable to move as freely, thus indicating a higher level of cellularity (e.g., medulloblastoma). This helps to determine cellular metabolism, regional hemodynamics, tumor cellularity, circuitry pathways and tracts, and physiological functionality. In addition, techniques such as proton MRS have

been designed to allow for molecular profiling, including identifying DNA methylation[3]; however, these have not yet been commonly incorporated in many clinical practices. In recent years, there is a growing interest in the utility of advanced MRI sequences in order to differentiate not only subtypes of tumors (e.g., ependymoma vs. medulloblastoma), but also to be able to delineate the specific subgroup and molecular subtype of the tumor just from analyzing the MRI. *Radiomics*, which is the term used for analyzing tumor specific parameters from radiographic studies, applies advanced computational methods to convert medical images into a large number of quantitative descriptors of oncologic tissues.[4,5] The use of these techniques is gaining more attention as their diagnostic accuracy improves. Presently, tools to best estimate the tumor molecular subtype prior to surgery is of primary academic importance; however, we can imagine that future advances in cancer diagnostics might allow for limiting or removal of the need for surgery in specific cases. Several groups have used radiomics to give a more precise prognostic evaluation for glioblastoma.[6-13] Similar work has been conducted for some types of pediatric brain tumors, most notably medulloblastomas, focusing on the qualitative characterization of these tumors and trying to delineate between the different subgroups of medulloblastomas according to the tumor location and the enhancement pattern.[14-20] For example, group 3 and group 4 medulloblastomas often arise in the midline and tend to have less enhancement, sonic hedgehog (SHH)-activated tumors occur most frequently in the cerebellar hemispheres, while Wingless (WNT)-activated tumors occur both midline and laterally around the cerebellopontine angle cistern. Different imaging methodologies and sequences are continually under investigation and are becoming even more productive with the recent addition of applied machine learning.[21]

> Techniques such as proton MRS have been designed to allow for molecular profiling, including identifying DNA methylation.

Although radiomics provides a high probability of accurate diagnosis, in today's environment of extensive tumor

IMAGING MODALITY	METHOD	FINDING	USE IN PEDIATRIC BRAIN TUMORS
Diffusion-weighted imaging (DWI)	Qualitative and quantitative assessments of water diffusion reflecting tumor cellularity	High intensity (diffusion restriction) when water is unable to move as freely indicating a higher level of cellularity. Correlate with a low signal on the apparent diffusion coefficient (ADC)	Medulloblastoma, PNET, occasionally glioblastoma are tumors with high cellularity and typically exhibit diffusion restriction
Diffusion tensor imaging (DTI)	Uses at least 6 diffusion-sensitizing gradient directions and identifies anisotropic water diffusion in the brain, primarily along white matter tracts.	Helps identify directional water flow and labels the directionality with color mapping	Used to identify fiber tracts, particularly useful for surgical planning
Functional MRI	Uses blood oxygen level differentials based on tasks being performed	Allows for identification of portions of cortex that is used for speech, motor, and vision function	Used to identify key functional cortex for surgical planning
Perfusion imaging Dynamic susceptibility contrast Arterial spin labeling	Dynamic T2-weighted gradient-echo echo-planar image derived from T2 susceptibility effect post gadolinium. Uses endogenous arterial water as a diffusible tracer to identify cerebral blood flow	Provides the degree of neovascularity or tumor angiogenesis, helps with tumor grading and prognostication. Cerebral blood volume (rCBV), relative cerebral blood flow (rCBF), and mean transit time	Most useful in its negative predictive value in helping to exclude high-grade tumors from the differential. May help differentiate ATRT from medulloblastoma, hemangioblastoma from pilocytic astrocytoma, as well as differentiate between viable tumor and radiation necrosis or tumor progression from pseudoprogression.
Proton MR spectroscopy	Uses single voxel, with either long or short echo times (T2 relaxation) to detect cerebral metabolites, typically in ratios	Measures metabolites: taurine, glutamine/glutamate, myoinositol, glycine, alanine, N-acetyl aspartate (NAA), choline (Cho), and creatine (Cr)	Brain tumors have elevated Cho and decreased NAA. High grade tumors have a higher Cho:Cr ratio and lower NAA:Cr ratio. Medulloblastomas exhibit higher taurine levels. Grade 2 astrocytomas, ependymomas, and choroid plexus papillomas have elevated myoinositol levels
Susceptibility-weighted imaging	Identifies microvasculature and substances with magnetic susceptibilities	Shows blood products and calcium	Useful for identifying low grade tumors

genetic and molecular testing, relying solely on imaging is likely subpar. Knowing the genetics, gene mutations, molecular profile, and other cellular variations allows physicians to mold and customize multiple available treatment options and help determine prognosis and potential response to therapies. With the exception of a few tumor pathologies with limited treatment options, there remains multiple advantages to accurate tissue characterization and diagnosis through safe biopsy or resection.

"Radiomics," which is the term used for analyzing tumor specific parameters from radiographic studies, applies advanced computational methods to convert medical images into a large number of quantitative descriptors of oncologic tissues.

TREATMENT DECISION-MAKING: WATCHFUL WAITING VERSUS SURGICAL RESECTION

Over the past four decades, the management of pediatric central nervous system (CNS) tumors has fluctuated between gross total resection (GTR),[22] maximal safe resection,[23] obtaining a biopsy for tissue diagnosis with debulking if possible,[24] and watchful waiting.[25] Many variables factor into the decision-making process, which explains this wide management spectrum. Arguably, knowledge of the natural history of different pediatric CNS tumors is among the most important factors. For example, watchful waiting with serial clinical and radiographic assessments may be the best strategy for asymptomatic, incidental, and radiographically benign brain lesions.[26] However, any signs of radiographic or symptomatic progression, suspicion of malignancy, and parental preference may prompt a discussion about pursuit of surgical resection.[27] Approaching newly diagnosed pediatric brain tumors with biopsy only is typically reserved for infiltrative tumors residing in highly eloquent anatomical locations such as the thalamus and brainstem. There is also a need to obtain tissue to further characterize tumors to tailor medical and radiation treatment. The treatment dilemma is more significant with incidentally found tumors that appear to be low grade.

Adults with presumed primary low-grade glial tumors have in the past been managed with watchful waiting; however, there has been a paradigm shift based on evidence that early surgical intervention in primary brain tumors is associated with improved survival, decreased tumor recurrence, and delay of malignant transformation.[28–30] The idea of early resection of asymptomatic tumors is being raised in the pediatric realm as well. Recent data have shown that 3% of pediatric low-grade gliomas undergo malignant transformation.[31–33] Some publications have shown that tumors exhibiting certain molecular markers, such as BRAF V600E mutations and CDKN2A deletion, are at even greater risk for malignant transformation. This means that, in order to anticipate this behavior, having tissue diagnosis from pathology is vital because imaging modalities are not yet able to assess for these alterations. In recent years, there is a growing trend favoring resection of incidental brain tumors in the pediatric population.[32,34] If watchful waiting is elected, the surgeon should ensure that the patient does not harbor a genetic predisposition that increases the likelihood for tumor malignant transformation (e.g., Li-Fraumeni syndrome, Turcot syndrome, etc.).

> About 3% of pediatric low-grade gliomas undergo malignant transformation.

ANATOMICAL LOCATION OF THE TUMOR AS CONSIDERATION FOR TREATMENT

Tumor location is a significant prognostic variable and is a key determinant in the management strategy for pediatric CNS tumors. Many of these tumors are frequently and consistently identified in and associated with specific anatomical locations, and, when taken into account with other parameters such as age of the patient and advanced imaging characteristics, the diagnostic differential diagnostic can be significantly narrowed. Additionally, the tumor location has significant implications for the development of future neurological injury and deficits. One example is a midbrain/tectal tumor that compresses the cerebral aqueduct and leads to the development of obstructive hydrocephalus. Additionally, small tumors in the spinal cord and other midline CNS structures would be expected to eventually disrupt white matter tracts as they continue to grow. Prognosis for pediatric CNS tumors is related to tumor type and genetic and molecular profile, but also to location based on its accessibility, resectability, and the potential resultant neurological sequelae of the tumor. All these factors combine to help determine if surgery is appropriate for a patient. Fortunately, the majority of pediatric CNS tumors originate in the cerebral and cerebellar hemispheres. Many tumors in these locations are amenable to gross surgical resection or near total surgical resection, whereas the rest may extend into eloquent areas such as the internal capsule or primary motor and speech cortices, rendering subtotal resection (STR) a viable option to decompress critical neurovascular structures and modify the natural history of the disease.[35]

> Tumor location is a significant prognostic variable and is a key determinant in the management strategy for pediatric CNS tumors.

> Prognosis for pediatric CNS tumors is related to tumor type and genetic and molecular profile, but also to location based on its accessibility, resectability, and the potential resultant neurological sequelae of the tumor.

NON-DIAGNOSTIC NEUROSURGICAL INTERVENTIONS

Hydrocephalus develops typically in pediatric patients with CNS tumors in the posterior fossa, including the cerebellum, fourth ventricle, and brainstem (midbrain/tectum/pons/medulla). This occurs as the tumor grows to the point of blocking cerebrospinal fluid (CSF) pathways. Hydrocephalus may develop over a long period of time preoperatively, which is typically less morbid and frequently resolves after surgical resection and removal of the obstruction. This entity is in contrast to the acute symptomatic hydrocephalus that may develop in the immediate postoperative period. This could result from a surgical cavity hematoma or cerebellar swelling, warranting a emergent CSF diversion such as insertion of an external ventricular drain (EVD).[36] Additionally, although good restoration of the CSF pathways may be achieved, some patients with posterior fossa tumors may still require permanent CSF diversion, sometimes in a delayed fashion. All pediatric patients with brain or spinal cord tumors should be closely monitored in the subacute postoperative period for the development of symptomatic hydrocephalus. Asymptomatic ventricular enlargement may occur but typically does not require any intervention. In patients with posterior fossa tumors, perioperative shunting was performed in as many as 42% of subjects.[36] In certain patients with continued obstructive hydrocephalus secondary to a lesion, endoscopic third ventriculostomy (ETV) can be an attractive alternative to shunting as it may obviate the need for permanent placement of a ventriculoperitoneal shunt in many patients.[37]

> In patients with posterior fossa tumors, perioperative shunting was performed in as many as 42% of subjects.

SPECIAL CONSIDERATIONS IN NEUROFIBROMATOSIS (CHAPTER 27)

For patients with neurofibromatosis type 1 (NF1), annual physical examination, including visual field and funduscopic testing is used for early detection of lesions growing in locations that may compromise critical neurovascular structures. NF1 patients typically have a large number of lesions in many locations, making aggressive surgical reection impractical. Typically, only symptomatic or expectedly deleterious lesions that can be safely pursued should be treated surgically.[38–41] Radiation therapy is typically avoided due to the neuropsychological and endocrine adverse effects and the potential increased risk of malignant transformation of existing lesions, as well as the risk of developing secondary malignancies.[42–47] For NF1 patients with optic pathway gliomas, surgical intervention is not recommended as the initial treatment of choice.[48] Systemic chemotherapy seems to be associated with favorable visual outcomes as well as better survival outcomes compared to non-NF1 patients with similar lesions.[49-52] Surgical resection is reserved for painful and disfiguring plexiform neurofibromas as well as large compressive lesions. A growing number of targeted therapy studies are producing better medical treatment options that may replace surgery for these lesions in the future.[53,54]

> Radiation therapy is typically avoided due to the neuropsychological and endocrine adverse effects and the potential increased risk of malignant transformation of existing lesions, as well as the risk of developing secondary malignancies.

In NF2 patients, vestibular schwannomas (VSs) are the most concerning lesions due to eventual hearing loss with progression to bilateral symptoms in many patients. Unfortunately, NF2-associated VSs seem to be less responsive to radiosurgery compared to their sporadic counterparts.[55] Radiosurgery also leads to malignant transformation and radiation-induced cancer induction more frequently compared to sporadic vestibular schwannomas, though the overall incidence is very low.[56] Surgery is indicated for large lesions, especially those compressing the brainstem.[57] Iatrogenic facial nerve injury is a potential complication during resection of large VSs even in the most skilled hands.[58] Targeted biologic therapies may have a role in managing these NF2-associated VSs in the future,[59-62] but watchful waiting remains a mainstay until the risks of conservative management outweigh the benefits of radiosurgery or surgical resection. Multidisciplinary follow-up with audiology and medical neuro-oncology is beneficial in these cases.

> NF2-associated VSs seem to be less responsive to radiosurgery compared to their sporadic counterparts.

SIGNIFICANCE OF EXTENT OF RESECTION IN PEDIATRIC BRAIN TUMORS

Many pediatric brain and spinal cord tumors demonstrate a limited response to conventional chemotherapies and biologic therapies. In these cases, the utilization of radiation therapy is avoided because of the morbidity from radiation at a young age. However, HhHexceptions to this rule exist, such as the standard radiation of high-grade gliomas. Maximal safe resection reduces the tumor burden and allows for genetic and molecular analysis for tailoring adjuvant therapy.

MEDULLOBLASTOMA (CHAPTER 16)

Partial surgical resection of medulloblastomas is commonly considered high-risk for disease progression and overall disease status.[63] This notion is somewhat controversial,

but drives aggressive surgical resections, "second-look" surgeries, and/or intensified adjuvant therapy.[64] The previous grading system for risk stratification depended partially on the postoperative assessment of any tumor remnant, categorized by GTR, with no tumor remnant left on the postoperative imaging; near total resection (NTR, <1.5 cm^2), or STR (≥1.5 cm^2). The 1.5 cm^2 residual tumor cutoff was largely based on the CCG921 protocol which enrolled patients in the 1980s and early 1990s. It is mainly based on postoperative CT[65,66] rather than the high-resolution MRI now in use. This protocol also was not utilizing modern cisplatin-based chemotherapy or any molecular subtyping technology. Recent publications led to the new classification for the medulloblastoma subtypes (WNT, SHH, Group 3, Group 4),[67,68] which have led to significant evolution in our understanding of the genetics and molecular aspects of this tumor type. In recent years, several publications have shown that the benefit of extent of resection is attenuated when accounting for the molecular subgroup of medulloblastoma, meaning that, aside from achieving maximal safe resection, there is no significant prognostic difference between NTRs and GTRs.[64] When considering the different subtypes, with the exception of subtotally resected Group 4 patients, there is no correlation between extent of resection and overall survival (OS). These Group 4 cases have a significantly worse OS compared to NTR or GTR. Hence, the notion that GTR is best for the patient's OS or that prognosis is better if less than 1.5 cm^2 of tumor remains after surgery is being reevaluated in the setting of our understanding of the medulloblastoma molecular subtypes. In recent literature, some groups found a correlation between GTR and better progression-free survival (PFS)[64,69] while others have not.[70] The aim of surgery should still be maximal safe resection rather than pursuing GTR at any cost. The idea of second-look surgeries might also be considered for these tumors.

> When considering the different subtypes, with the exception of subtotally resected Group 4 medulloblastoma, there is no correlation between extent of resection and OS.

EPENDYMOMA (CHAPTER 6)

Significant progress has been made in recent years toward our understanding of ependymal tumors. In 2016, the WHO classification included changes in supratentorial ependymomas, adding the new molecular subtyping of RELA and Yap1,[71] an advancement beyond the histopathology classification. The literature has been showing that ependymomas that harbor the C11orf95-RELA gene fusion have less favorable outcome than those that have the YAP1 gene fusions, also on chromosome 11.[72,73] For posterior fossa ependymomas, present literature discusses ependymoma subtypes Group A (PF-EPN-A) and B (PF-EPN-B), although these have yet to be incorporated into the official WHO classification. Unlike adults, in whom ependymomas most frequently occur in the spinal cord, the pediatric patient population experiences almost all ependymomas intracranially (>90% of patients), with the vast majority of these in the posterior fossa.[74] There is an age correlation to the subtypes, with Group A most commonly associated with patients younger than 3 years and Group B with patients older than 5 years.[75,76] Group A has been described to carry a much worse prognosis.[77] Most of the studies still do not incorporate this subtyping, leaving prognostic correlation to be done by age group. Extent of resection is a dominant parameter for posterior fossa ependymomas, with GTR shown to be the most significant factor in OS. Some suggest that for the cases where STR rather than GTR was achieved initially, a second-look surgery should be considered, especially for patients in Group A, where the response to radiation therapy is questionable.[78] The treatment paradigm is a combination of surgical resection, adjuvant radiation therapy, and enrollment in clinical trials. For a newly diagnosed tumor, the first step is usually maximal safe resection. If GTR was achieved and there are no anaplastic features on histopathology, some argue for no further immediate treatment with clinical and imaging follow-up.[79] In most cases, the classic treatment after maximal safe resection includes focal radiation and, in some cases, chemotherapy (Children's Oncology Group study ACNS0831). This same paradigm continues whenever there is tumor relapse. Histopathology including anaplastic features has failed to demonstrate any prognostic significance.[80] Some studies suggest that, regardless of the molecular subtyping, achieving GTR or NTR is an independent parameter that can overcome the deleterious effects of C11orf95-RELA fusion on survival in these patients.[81] A recently published prospective study by St. Jude (Young Children 07/SJYC07) included children 3 years and younger with supratentorial or infratentorial ependymoma who were treated with a combination of surgery, chemotherapy, and radiation therapy.[82] This study found no difference in PFS for any type of ependymoma when surgery achieved GTR or NTR and that histologic subtype did not impact outcomes.[82] The study reported that all subtypes demonstrated a worse prognosis when only a STR was achieved, regardless of adjuvant treatment modality.[82] This was especially true in the PF-EPN-A with 1q gain.[82] This study further supported the finding that the ST-EPN-RELA group had a favorable outcome with combined therapy, which could also have been attributed to the high rate of GTR/NTR achieved (89%).[82] The St. Jude study advocated for the use of chemotherapy with the addition of second-look surgery with a goal to achieve GTR/NTR prior to initiating radiation therapy when possible.[82]

In 2016, the WHO classification included changes in supratentorial ependymomas, adding the new molecular subtyping of RELA and Yap1.

Unlike adults, in whom ependymomas most frequently occur in the spinal cord, the pediatric patient population experiences almost all ependymomas intracranially (>90% of patients), with the vast majority of these in the posterior fossa.

PEDIATRIC LOW-GRADE GLIOMA (CHAPTER 17)

As with many pediatric brain tumors, the goal to achieve a maximal safe surgical resection followed by adjuvant therapy to treat the remnant of the tumor is paramount to decreasing the risks for tumor recurrence and improving patient outcomes.[83-85] This approach is advocated by many, including the authors of this chapter, but remains unproved.[86] The LGG subgroup of tumors is quite diverse and treatment must to be tailored accordingly. For example, optic pathway glioma might not require any surgical intervention while hypothalamic tumors might only need a biopsy. Other considerations need to be taken with regard to the anatomical location and the need to surgically alleviate the consequences of mass effect (e.g., hydrocephalus secondary to tectal low-grade glioma that is resolved by performing ETV). For pilocytic astrocytomas, achieving a GTR is curative and recommended, even at the expense of a second-look surgery. For ganglioglioma tumors, the extent of resection regardless the WHO grade, has been demonstrated to be the strongest predictive parameter for recurrence-free survival. As such, GTR should be aimed to be achieved in every case of ganglioglioma. Some authors found that a resection percentage of 94% was the cutoff for surgery to offer progression-free advantage and any beneficial results.[87] Surgical resection of midline gliomas (with histone mutations) is complicated by high risk for neurologic injury. The discovery of the BRAF V600E mutation and the possibility of targeted treatment options will likely allow patients to receive treatment without incurring the risk of significant neurological injury by an attempted extensive resection.[88] Oligodendrogliomas are relatively rare tumors among the pediatric population. In a recent study, it was found that STR, initial presentation of headache, mixed pathologies, and location of the tumor in the parietal lobe are all significant predictors of tumor progression or recurrence, as well as OS.[89] To summarize, unless a pediatric low-grade tumor resides in an eloquent anatomical location (e.g., hypothalamus, brainstem), the first step in treatment should be achieving maximal safe resection. Targeted therapy should be considered when there is an active residual or recurrence in most situations, although with pilocytic astrocytoma and gangliogliomas a second-look surgery could be considered before the conventional chemotherapy and radiation therapy.

In ganglioglioma tumors the extent of resection regardless the WHO grade has been demonstrated to be the strongest predictive parameter for recurrence-free survival.

PEDIATRIC HIGH-GRADE GLIOMA, ATRT (CHAPTER 18)

This group of tumors is fairly rare in the pediatric population. The management paradigm is derived primarily from the adult literature, although pediatric studies and research are growing rapidly. These tumors tend to be infiltrative in nature, and surgery cannot be a standalone treatment. Maximal safe resection is the first treatment step whenever feasible, as described in the results of the CCG 945 study.[90] This study showed that the

5-year PFS among the children who underwent GTR was twice as long as those who had only STR, irrespective of histology. The same group published their analysis for midline high-grade gliomas and found that they have much worse prognosis when compared to other subtypes and concluded that the midline location makes it hard to achieve meaningful resection.[90] From this and other studies, the treatment concept supports the surgeon aiming for GTR or NTR as much as possible in order to leave the smallest tumor burden possible for adjuvant therapy.

Other types of pediatric malignant brain tumor are treated in similar fashion. Atypical teratoid rhabdoid tumors (ATRT), were found in different studies to have a dismal prognosis in general, but achieving GTR has the most significant impact on survival. When comparing the results of NTR to STR or biopsy, results also showed significantly better survival for NTR.[91]

> The CCG 945 study showed that the 5-year PFS after GTR was twice as long as those who had only STR, irrespective of histology.

WHEN THE GOAL OF SURGERY IS NOT MEANINGFUL RESECTION

Tumors in this category are becoming fewer due to emerging surgical technologies that allow for more meaningful and safer surgery in anatomical locations previously considered inaccessible. On the other hand, better understanding of the molecular subtypes and their biological behavior allows us to use adjuvant therapy in more effective ways, potentially limiting the need for repeated resections. One of the more promising treatment modalities is the use of BRAF and MEK inhibitors (e.g., Dabrafenib) for those tumors harboring the BRAF V600E mutation, regardless if they are LGG or HGG.[92-94] While the use of these therapies demonstrate promise, there is a high rate of adverse events which might limit the feasibility of chronic treatment in some cases.[93,94] However, there is potential benefit to delay further surgery or other more complex treatment modalities.[92] In pathologies such as diffuse intrinsic pontine glioma (DIPG) or in most cases of optic pathway glioma (OPG), open surgical resection is not a meaningful approach and is typically aimed at diagnostic biopsy or tumor molecular characterization.[95] A detailed discussion of these types of tumors is beyond the scope of this chapter.

CONCLUSION

Pediatric brain and spinal cord tumors cause significant morbidity in the life of a growing child. Fortunately, pediatric spinal cord tumors are quite rare. However, pediatric brain tumors are the most common solid tumors among children and vary widely from adult brain tumors when it comes to neurosurgical decision-making. While up-front maximal safe surgical resection remains the standard for most pediatric brain tumors, adjunctive treatment strategies utilizing targeted or conventional chemotherapy and radiotherapy have been helpful to inform the need for more surgery. Our knowledge in the field is expanding rapidly with the use of better imaging modalities and with informative tumor molecular markers that guide our therapeutic decision-making. There is a growing motivation in the field to utilize advanced brain tumor imaging techniques to guide treatment next steps. Furthermore, genetic and molecular subtyping, such as identification of BRAF alterations or tumors harboring variable histone mutations, are significant today for the diagnosis and clinical prognostication of these tumors. There is yet a long way to go in the field, and it remains a priority to continue enrolling patients into collaborative clinical trials in order to develop evidence-based approaches in pediatric brain tumors. Table 15.1 provides a list of variable MRI modalities useful to evaluate pediatric brain tumors.

FLASHCARD

Advanced imaging modalities help to determine:	Cellular metabolism, regional hemodynamics, tumor cellularity, circuitry pathways and tracts, physiological functionality, and can support molecular profiling (i.e., identifying DNA methylation)
Biopsy of newly diagnosed pediatric brain tumors is utilized in:	Infiltrative tumors in eloquent anatomical locations (thalamus and brainstem) that require a tissue diagnosis to tailor nonsurgical treatment to the tumor's genetic and molecular profile
Prognosis for pediatric CNS tumors is driven by:	Tumor type, genetic/molecular profile, tumor location (accessibility, resectability, and risk for deficit)
Perioperative shunting was performed in up to 42% of patients with which tumor location?	Posterior fossa
Radiation therapy for neurofibromas in patients with NF1 is typically avoided due to what?	Potential for adverse neuropsychological and endocrine effects, increased risk for malignant transformation, or the development of secondary malignancies
When considering extent of resection and survival in the different medulloblastoma subtypes:	There seems to be no correlation between extent of resection and overall survival, with the exception of Group 4 subtype
In adults, ependymomas most frequently occur in the _____ versus in the _____ in pediatrics	Spinal cord, posterior fossa (In pediatric patients, >90% of ependymomas occur intracranially)
For gangliogliomas, the extent of resection has been demonstrated to be the strongest predictive parameter for recurrence free survival irrespective of what?	The WHO grade

In high-grade gliomas, the CCG 945 study demonstrated that the 5-year progression free survival was what?

Doubled in children who underwent gross total resection as compared to those with subtotal resection, irrespective of histology

Better understanding of the tumor molecular subtype informs on tumor biological behavior as well as on what else?

The selection of adjuvant therapy, and it could limit the need for repeated surgical resections

QUESTIONS

1. Name the different molecular subtypes of medulloblastoma?
   a. Atypical, anaplastic, and malignant
   b. WNT-activated, RELA, and Group 3A
   c. WNT-activated, SHH-activated (TP53 mutant or wildtype), and non-WNT/non-SHH Group 3 and 4
   d. Posterior fossa group A/B and YAP1

2. What are the different molecular subtypes of ependymoma affecting the brain?
   a. H327KM, BRAF V600E, RELA
   b. YAP1, RELA, Group A and B
   c. Papillary, clear cell, and tanycytic
   d. IDH (mutant and wildtype), 1p/19q co-deleted

3. Pediatric ependymomas are more likely to be located ___ _____ as compared to adults where these tumors tend to present more frequently in the _____.
   a. Intracranially, spinal cord
   b. Extracranially, posterior fossa
   c. Extra-axial, cerebrum
   d. Extracranially, spinal vertebrae

4. The best course of treatment for newly diagnosed suspected medulloblastoma is
   a. Observation and follow-up
   b. Maximal surgical resection and adjuvant chemotherapy +/− radiotherapy
   c. Maximal safe resection, then observation and repeat resection at recurrence
   d. Diagnostic biopsy followed by radiation therapy

5. BRAF inhibitors can be considered for use as a targeted therapy when
   a. Tumor is positive for BRAF V600E mutation
   b. Tumor is positive for BRAF KIAA1549 fusion
   c. Radiomic tumor imaging demonstrates BRAF mutation
   d. All of the above

6. The best course of treatment for newly diagnosed suspected ATRT includes maximal safe resection, adjuvant chemotherapy, and +/− radiotherapy.
   a. True
   b. False

7. In a newly diagnosed pilocytic astrocytoma with postoperative residual tumor, the next treatment steps include
   a. Second-look surgery with active or large remnant for feasibility of further resection
   b. Watchful follow-up in the case of inactive or small remnant
   c. Chemotherapy and +/− radiotherapy with residual tumor without feasible safe resection
   d. All of the above

8. What is true in regard to the BRAF V600E mutation?
   a. Most commonly found in ganglioglioma
   b. Most commonly found in pilocytic astrocytomas
   c. Is found in combination with H3K27M in LGG
   d. Has no clinical importance

9. For patients with NF2 and vestibular schwannomas (VS), it is best to
   a. Use stereotactic radiosurgery since response is good and hearing can be preserved
   b. Operate immediately to preserve hearing
   c. Avoid all interventions in patients with NF2 and VS despite symptoms and tumor size
   d. None of the above

10. Which of the below item(s) best apoly to patients with NF1?
    a. they tend to have multiple T2 signal abnormalities which are nonurgent
    b. their most common brain tumor is ganglioglioma of the brainstem
    c. in a newly diagnosed patient, optic pathway glioma treatment should start immediately
    d. none of the above

11. Which advanced imaging technique can detect biochemical aspects of lesions?
    a. Contrasted CT
    b. MR perfusion
    c. Diffusion tensor imaging
    d. MR spectroscopy
    e. Susceptibility weighted imaging

12. Diffusion-weighted imaging (DWI). MRI is used to identify
    a. Cerebral blood flow in a tumor relative to the water content of parenchymal tissue
    b. High tissue cellularity that may limit the movement of water
    c. Cerebral blood volume compared to net water content
    d. The amount of CSF diffusion through the arachnoid villi

13. The use of radiomics is an advanced imaging modality that extracts a large number of quantitative features from tumor images.
    a. True
    b. False

14. A patient with newly diagnosed posterior fossa tumor presents with signs of acute hydrocephalus. What are the treatment options?
    a. Resection of the tumor to free the mass effect from the CSF pathways
    b. Installation of ventriculo-peritoneal shunt
    c. Endoscopic third ventriculostomy
    d. All of the above

15. Pediatric brain tumors are commonly found in which anatomic location?
   a. Cerebral or cerebellar hemispheres
   b. Extra-axially, attached to the dura with an arachnoid cap cell origin
   c. Thoracic spinal cord
   d. Conus medullaris

ANSWERS

1. c
2. b
3. a
4. b
5. a
6. a
7. d
8. a
9. d
10. a
11. d
12. b
13. a
14. d
15. a

REFERENCES

1. Bartels U, Hawkins C, Vézina G, et al. Proceedings of the diffuse intrinsic pontine glioma (DIPG) Toronto Think Tank: advancing basic and translational research and cooperation in DIPG. *J Neurooncol.* 2011;105:119–125.
2. Dellaretti M, Touzet G, Reyns N, et al. Correlation among magnetic resonance imaging findings, prognostic factors for survival, and histological diagnosis of intrinsic brainstem lesions in children. *J Neurosurg Pediatr.* 2011;8:539–543.
3. Lequin M, Hendrikse J. Advanced MR imaging in pediatric brain tumors, clinical applications. *Neuroimaging Clin N Am.* 2017;27:167–190.
4. Gillies RJ, Kinahan PE, Hricak H. Radiomics: images are more than pictures, they are data. *Radiology.* 2016;278:563–577.
5. Lambin P, Rios-Velazquez E, Leijenaar R, et al. Radiomics: extracting more information from medical images using advanced feature analysis. *Eur J Cancer.* 2012;48:441–446.
6. Cui Y, Tha KK, Terasaka S, et al. Prognostic imaging biomarkers in glioblastoma: development and independent validation on the basis of multiregion and quantitative analysis of MR images. *Radiology.* 2016;278:546–553.
7. Gevaert O, Mitchell LA, Achrol AS, et al. Glioblastoma multiforme: exploratory radiogenomic analysis by using quantitative image features. *Radiology.* 2014;273:168–174.
8. Grossmann P, Narayan V, Chang K, et al. Quantitative imaging biomarkers for risk stratification of patients with recurrent glioblastoma treated with bevacizumab. *Neuro Oncol.* 2017;19:1688–1697.
9. Itakura H, Achrol AS, Mitchell LA, et al. Magnetic resonance image features identify glioblastoma phenotypic subtypes with distinct molecular pathway activities. *Sci Transl Med.* 2015;7:303ra138.
10. Kickingereder P, Burth S, Wick A, et al. Radiomic profiling of glioblastoma: identifying an imaging predictor of patient survival with improved performance over established clinical and radiologic risk models. *Radiology.* 2016;280:880–889.
11. Kickingereder P, Götz M, Muschelli J, et al. Large-scale radiomic profiling of recurrent glioblastoma identifies an imaging predictor for stratifying anti-angiogenic treatment response. *Clin Cancer Res.* 2016;22:5765–5771.
12. Kickingereder P, Neuberger U, Bonekamp D, et al. Radiomic subtyping improves disease stratification beyond key molecular, clinical, and standard imaging characteristics in patients with glioblastoma. *Neuro Oncol.* 2018;20:848–857.
13. Yang D, Rao G, Martinez J, et al. Evaluation of tumor-derived MRI-texture features for discrimination of molecular subtypes and prediction of 12-month survival status in glioblastoma. *Med Phys.* 2015;42:6725–6735.
14. Gibson P, Tong Y, Robinson G, et al. Subtypes of medulloblastoma have distinct developmental origins. *Nature.* 2010;468:1095–1099.
15. Patay Z, DeSain LA, Hwang SN, et al. MR imaging characteristics of wingless-type-subgroup pediatric medulloblastoma. *AJNR Am J Neuroradiol.* 2015;36:2386–2393.
16. Perreault S, Ramaswamy V, Achrol AS, et al. MRI surrogates for molecular subgroups of medulloblastoma. *AJNR Am J Neuroradiol.* 2014;35:1263–1269.
17. Teo WY, Shen J, Su JM, et al. Implications of tumor location on subtypes of medulloblastoma. *Pediatr Blood Cancer.* 2013;60:1408–1410.
18. Yeom KW, Mobley BC, Lober RM, et al. Distinctive MRI features of pediatric medulloblastoma subtypes. *AJR Am J Roentgenol.* 2013;200:895–903.
19. Zhao F, Li C, Zhou Q, et al. Distinctive localization and MRI features correlate of molecular subgroups in adult medulloblastoma. *J Neuro-Oncol.* 2017;135:353–360.
20. Łastowska M, Jurkiewicz E, Trubicka J, et al. Contrast enhancement pattern predicts poor survival for patients with non-WNT/SHH medulloblastoma tumours. *J Neuro-Oncol.* 2015;123:65–73.
21. Iv M, Zhou M, Shpanskaya K, et al. MR Imaging-based radiomic signatures of distinct molecular subgroups of medulloblastoma. *AJNR Am J Neuroradiol.* 2019;40:154–161.
22. Pollack IF. The role of surgery in pediatric gliomas. *J Neuro-Oncology.* 1999;42:271–288.
23. Shimony N, Hartnett S, Osburn B, et al. Malignant intramedullary spinal cord tumors. In Arnautović KI, Gokaslan ZL, eds., *Spinal Cord Tumors.* Cham: Springer; 2019:337–364
24. Puget S, Beccaria K, Blauwblomme T, et al. Biopsy in a series of 130 pediatric diffuse intrinsic Pontine gliomas. *Child Nerv Syst.* 2015;31:1773–1780.
25. Ali ZS, Lang S-S, Sutton LN. Conservative management of presumed low-grade gliomas in the asymptomatic pediatric population. *World Neurosurg.* 2014;81:368–373.
26. Bredlau A-L, Constine LS, Silberstein HJ, et al. Incidental brain lesions in children: to treat or not to treat? *J Neuro-Oncology.* 2012;106:589–594.
27. Jumah F, Rallo MS, Quinoa T, et al. Incidental brain tumors in the pediatric population: a systematic review and reappraisal of literature. *World Neurosurg.* 2020;139:121–131.
28. Cochereau J, Herbet G, Rigau V, Duffau H. Acute progression of untreated incidental WHO Grade II glioma to glioblastoma in an asymptomatic patient. *J Neurosurg.* 2016;124:141–145.
29. Lima GLO, Dezamis E, Corns R, et al. Surgical resection of incidental diffuse gliomas involving eloquent brain areas. Rationale, functional, epileptological and oncological outcomes. *Neurochirurgie.* 2017;63:250–258.
30. Potts MB, Smith JS, Molinaro AM, Berger MS. Natural history and surgical management of incidentally discovered low-grade gliomas. *J Neurosurg.* 2012;116:365–372.
31. Mistry M, Zhukova N, Merico D, et al. BRAF mutation and CDKN2A deletion define a clinically distinct subgroup of childhood secondary high-grade glioma. *J Clin Oncol.* 2015;33:1015–1022.
32. Roth J, Soleman J, Paraskevopoulos D, et al. Incidental brain tumors in children: an international neurosurgical, oncological survey. *Child Nerv Syst.* 2018;34:1325–1333.
33. Soleman J, Roth J, Ram Z, et al. Malignant transformation of a conservatively managed incidental childhood cerebral mass lesion: controversy regarding management paradigm. *Child Nerv Syst.* 2017;33:2169–2175.
34. Broniscer A. Malignant transformation of low-grade gliomas in children: lessons learned from rare medical events. *J Clin Oncol.* 2015;33:978–979.
35. Keles GE, Lamborn KR, Berger MS. Low-grade hemispheric gliomas in adults: a critical review of extent of resection as a factor influencing outcome. *J Neurosurg.* 2001;95:735–745.
36. Gjerris F, Agerlin N, Børgesen S, et al. Epidemiology and prognosis in children treated for intracranial tumours in Denmark 1960–1984. *Child Nerv Sys.* 1998;14:302–311.
37. Tamburrini G, Pettorini B, Massimi L, et al. Endoscopic third ventriculostomy: the best option in the treatment of persistent hydrocephalus after posterior cranial fossa tumour removal? *Child Nerv Syst.* 2008;24:1405.
38. Astrup J. Natural history and clinical management of optic pathway glioma. *Br J Neurosurg.*1 2003;7:327–335.
39. Medlock MD, Scott M. Optic chiasm astrocytomas of childhood. *Pediatr Neurosurg.* 1997;27:129–136.
40. Pollack IF, Shultz B, Mulvihill JJ. The management of brainstem gliomas in patients with neurofibromatosis 1. *Neurology.* 1996;46:1652–1660.

41. Turgut M, Özcan E, Sağlam S. Central neurofibromatosis. *Eur Neurol.* 1991;31:188–192.
42. Grill J, Couanet D, Cappelli C, et al. Radiation-induced cerebral vasculopathy in children with neurofibromatosis and optic pathway glioma. *Ann Neurol.* 1999;45:393–396.
43. Madden J, Rush S, Stence N, et al. Radiation-induced gliomas in 2 pediatric patients with neurofibromatosis type 1: case study and summary of the literature. *J Pediatr Hematol Oncol.* 2014;36:e105–108.
44. Merchant T, Conklin H, Wu S, et al. Late effects of conformal radiation therapy for pediatric patients with low-grade glioma: prospective evaluation of cognitive, endocrine, and hearing deficits. *J Clin Oncol.* 2009;27:3691–3697.
45. Sharif S, Ferner R, Birch JM, et al. Second primary tumors in neurofibromatosis 1 patients treated for optic glioma: substantial risks after radiotherapy. *J Clin Oncol.* 2006;24:2570–2575.
46. Singhal S, Birch J, Kerr B, et al. Neurofibromatosis type 1 and sporadic optic gliomas. *Arch Dis Child.* 2002;87:65–70.
47. Wentworth S, Pinn M, Bourland J, et al. Clinical experience with radiation therapy in the management of neurofibromatosis-associated central nervous system tumors. *Int J Radiation Oncol Biol Physics.* 2009;73:208–213.
48. Walker DA, Liu J, Kieran M, et al. A multi-disciplinary consensus statement concerning surgical approaches to low-grade, high-grade astrocytomas and diffuse intrinsic pontine gliomas in childhood (CPN Paris 2011) using the Delphi method. *Neuro-Oncology.* 2013;15:462–468.
49. Fisher MJ, Loguidice M, Gutmann DH, et al. Visual outcomes in children with neurofibromatosis type 1–associated optic pathway glioma following chemotherapy: a multicenter retrospective analysis. *Neuro-Oncology.* 2012;14:790–797.
50. Gnekow AK, Falkenstein F, von Hornstein S, et al. Long-term follow-up of the multicenter, multidisciplinary treatment study HIT-LGG-1996 for low-grade glioma in children and adolescents of the German Speaking Society of Pediatric Oncology and Hematology. *Neuro-Oncology.* 2012;14:1265–1284.
51. Gururangan S, Cavazos C, Ashley D, et al. Phase II study of carboplatin in children with progressive low-grade gliomas. *J Clin Oncol.* 2002;20:2951–2958.
52. Kalamarides M, Acosta M, Babovic-Vuksanovic D, et al. Neurofibromatosis 2011: a report of the Children's Tumor Foundation annual meeting. *Acta Neuropathol.* 2012;123:369–380.
53. Robertson KA, Nalepa G, Yang F-C, et al. Imatinib mesylate for plexiform neurofibromas in patients with neurofibromatosis type 1: a phase 2 trial. *Lancet Oncol.* 2012;13:1218–1224.
54. Widemann BC, Dombi E, Gillespie A, et al. Phase 2 randomized, flexible crossover, double-blinded, placebo-controlled trial of the farnesyltransferase inhibitor tipifarnib in children and young adults with neurofibromatosis type 1 and progressive plexiform neurofibromas. *Neuro-Oncology.* 2014;16:707–718.
55. Rowe J, Radatz M, Kemeny A. Radiosurgery for type II neurofibromatosis. *Prog Neurol Surg.* 2008;21:176–182.
56. Balasubramaniam A, Shannon P, Hodaie M, et al. Glioblastoma multiforme after stereotactic radiotherapy for acoustic neuroma: case report and review of the literature. *Neuro-Oncol.* 2007;9:447–453.
57. Blakeley JO, Evans DG, Adler J, et al. Consensus recommendations for current treatments and accelerating clinical trials for patients with neurofibromatosis type 2. *Am J Med Gen Part A* 158:24–41.
58. Grey P, Moffat D, Palmer C, et al. Factors which influence the facial nerve outcome in vestibular schwannoma surgery. *Clin Otolaryngol Allied Sci.* 1996;21:409–413.
59. Karajannis M, Ferner R. Neurofibromatosis-related tumors: emerging biology and therapies. *Curr Opin Pediatr.* 2015;27:26–33.
60. Karajannis MA, Legault G, Hagiwara M, et al. Phase II trial of lapatinib in adult and pediatric patients with neurofibromatosis type 2 and progressive vestibular schwannomas. *Neuro-Oncology.* 2012;14:1163–1170.
61. Plotkin S, Stemmer-Rachamimov A, Halpin C, et al. Hearing improvement after bevacizumab in patients with neurofibromatosis type 2. *N Engl J Med.* 2009;361:358–367.
62. Plotkin SR, Merker VL, Halpin C, et al. Bevacizumab for progressive vestibular schwannoma in neurofibromatosis type 2: a retrospective review of 31 patients. *Otol Neurotol.* 2012;33:1046–1052.
63. Thompson EM, Bramall A, Herndon JE, et al. The clinical importance of medulloblastoma extent of resection: a systematic review. *J Neurooncol.* 2018;139:523–539.
64. Thompson EM, Hielscher T, Bouffet E, et al. Prognostic value of medulloblastoma extent of resection after accounting for molecular subgroup: a retrospective integrated clinical and molecular analysis. *Lancet Oncol.* 2016;17:484–495.
65. Albright AL, Wisoff JH, Zeltzer PM, et al. Effects of medulloblastoma resections on outcome in children: a report from the Children's Cancer Group. *Neurosurgery.* 1996;38:265–271.
66. Zeltzer PM, Boyett JM, Finlay JL, et al. Metastasis stage, adjuvant treatment, and residual tumor are prognostic factors for medulloblastoma in children: conclusions from the Children's Cancer Group 921 randomized phase III study. *J Clin Oncol.* 1999;17:832–845.
67. Taylor MD, Northcott PA, Korshunov A, et al. Molecular subgroups of medulloblastoma: the current consensus. *Acta Neuropathol.* 2012;123:465–472.
68. Wen PY, Huse JT. 2016 World Health Organization Classification of Central Nervous System Tumors. *Continuum (Minneap Minn).* 2017;23:1531–1547.
69. Schwalbe EC, Lindsey JC, Nakjang S, et al. Novel molecular subgroups for clinical classification and outcome prediction in childhood medulloblastoma: a cohort study. *Lancet Oncol.* 2017;18:958–971.
70. Pietsch T, Schmidt R, Remke M, et al. Prognostic significance of clinical, histopathological, and molecular characteristics of medulloblastomas in the prospective HIT2000 multicenter clinical trial cohort. *Acta Neuropathol.* 2014;128:137–149.
71. Louis DN, Perry A, Reifenberger G, et al. The 2016 World Health Organization Classification of Tumors of the Central Nervous System: a summary. *Acta Neuropathol.* 2016;131:803–820.
72. Khatua S, Ramaswamy V, Bouffet E. Current therapy and the evolving molecular landscape of paediatric ependymoma. *Eur J Cancer.* 2017;70:34–41.
73. Pajtler KW, Mack SC, Ramaswamy V, et al. The current consensus on the clinical management of intracranial ependymoma and its distinct molecular variants. *Acta Neuropathol.* 2017;133:5–12.
74. Kilday JP, Rahman R, Dyer S, et al. Pediatric ependymoma: biological perspectives. *Mol Cancer Res.* 2009;7:765–786.
75. Pajtler KW, Witt H, Sill M, et al. Molecular classification of ependymal tumors across all CNS compartments, histopathological grades, and age groups. *Cancer Cell.* 2015;27:728–743.
76. Ramaswamy V, Hielscher T, Mack SC, et al. Therapeutic impact of cytoreductive surgery and irradiation of posterior fossa ependymoma in the molecular era: a retrospective multicohort analysis. *J Clin Oncol.* 2016;34:2468–2477.
77. Snider CA, Yang K, Mack SC, et al. Impact of radiation therapy and extent of resection for ependymoma in young children: A population-based study. *Pediatr Blood Cancer.* 2018;65.
78. Godfraind C, Kaczmarska JM, Kocak M, et al. Distinct disease-risk groups in pediatric supratentorial and posterior fossa ependymomas. *Acta Neuropathol.* 2012;124:247–257.
79. Aizer AA, Ancukiewicz M, Nguyen PL, et al. Natural history and role of radiation in patients with supratentorial and infratentorial WHO grade II ependymomas: results from a population-based study. *J Neurooncol.* 2013;115:411–419.
80. Raghunathan A, Wani K, Armstrong TS, et al. Histological predictors of outcome in ependymoma are dependent on anatomic site within the central nervous system. *Brain Pathol.* 2013;23:584–594.
81. Lillard JC, Venable GT, Khan NR, et al. Pediatric supratentorial ependymoma: surgical, clinical, and molecular analysis. *Neurosurgery.* 2019;85:41–49.
82. Upadhyaya SA, Robinson GW, Onar-Thomas A, et al. Molecular grouping and outcomes of young children with newly diagnosed ependymoma treated on the multi-institutional SJYC07 trial. *Neuro Oncol.* 2019;21:1319–1330.
83. Dirven CM, Mooij JJ, Molenaar WM. Cerebellar pilocytic astrocytoma: a treatment protocol based upon analysis of 73 cases and a review of the literature. *Childs Nerv Syst.* 1997;13:17–23.
84. Hirsch JF, Sainte Rose C, Pierre-Kahn A, et al. Benign astrocytic and oligodendrocytic tumors of the cerebral hemispheres in children. *J Neurosurg.* 1989;70:568–572.
85. Wisoff JH, Sanford RA, Heier LA, et al. Primary neurosurgery for pediatric low-grade gliomas: a prospective multi-institutional study from the Children's Oncology Group. *Neurosurgery.* 2011;68:1548–1554; discussion 1554–1545.
86. Whittle IR. What is the place of conservative management for adult supratentorial low-grade glioma? *Adv Tech Stand Neurosurg.* 2010;35:65–79.

87. Haydon DH, Dahiya S, Smyth MD, et al. Greater extent of resection improves ganglioglioma recurrence-free survival in children: a volumetric analysis. *Neurosurgery.* 2014;5:37–42.

88. Lassaletta A, Zapotocky M, Mistry M, et al. Therapeutic and prognostic implications of BRAF V600E in pediatric low-grade gliomas. *J Clin Oncol.* 2017;35:2934–2941.

89. Wang KY, Vankov ER, Lin DDM. Predictors of clinical outcome in pediatric oligodendroglioma: meta-analysis of individual patient data and multiple imputation. *J Neurosurg Pediatr.* 2018;21:153–163.

90. Eisenstat DD, Pollack IF, Demers A, et al. Impact of tumor location and pathological discordance on survival of children with midline high-grade gliomas treated on Children's Cancer Group high-grade glioma study CCG-945. *J Neurooncol.* 2015;121:573–581.

91. Richards A, Ved R, Murphy C, et al. Outcomes with respect to extent of surgical resection for pediatric atypical teratoid rhabdoid tumors. *Child Nerv Syst.* 2020;36:713–719.

92. Hargrave DR, Bouffet E, Tabori U, et al. efficacy and safety of dabrafenib in pediatric patients with cancer. *Clin Cancer Res.* 2019;25:7303–7311.

93. Nakano Y, Yamasaki K, Sakamoto H, et al. A long-term survivor of pediatric midline glioma with H3F3A K27M and BRAF V600E double mutations. *Brain Tumor Pathol.* 2019;36:162–168.

94. Toll SA, Tran HN, Cotter J, et al. Sustained response of three pediatric BRAF. *Oncotarget.* 2019;10:551–557.

95. Pfaff E, El Damaty A, Balasubramanian GP, et al. Brainstem biopsy in pediatric diffuse intrinsic pontine glioma in the era of precision medicine: the INFORM study experience. *Eur J Cancer.* 2019;114:27–35.

16 | PEDIATRIC EMBRYONAL TUMORS

AARON MOCHIZUKI AND SONIA PARTAP

INTRODUCTION

Embryonal tumors are malignant central nervous system (CNS) tumors that account for 11.5% of all CNS cancers in children and adolescents age 0–19 years and 13% in children age 0–14 years with an age-adjusted incidence rate of 0.6 per 100,000 population.[1] In the World Health Organization (WHO)'s 2016 classification system, embryonal tumors are divided into medulloblastoma, atypical teratoid/rhabdoid tumor (ATRT), pineoblastoma, embryonal tumor with multilayered rosettes (ETMR), and other embryonal tumors. Histopathologically, these entities are described as small, round, blue cell tumors and are all designated WHO grade 4. Please, refer to Chapter 1, for additional information on the classification of the embryonal tumors and 2021 WHO classification.

MEDULLOBLASTOMA

EPIDEMIOLOGY AND CLINICAL PRESENTATION

Medulloblastoma accounts for approximately two-thirds of CNS embryonal tumors diagnosed in children age 0–19, peaking between 5 and 9 years and occurring 1.5–2 times as frequently in boys compared to girls.[1] By definition, medulloblastomas occur in the posterior fossa, although they can spread throughout the neuroaxis. With increasing age, tumors can occur in the cerebellar hemispheres.[2,3] Previously, medulloblastoma had commonly been recognized in certain genetic syndromes such as Turcot and Gorlin, which are known to be associated with specific mutations in *WNT* and *SHH*, respectively. However, recent studies have shown a multitude of germline mutations as outlined in Table 16.1 (e.g., *APC*, *BRCA2*, *PALB2*, *PTCH1*, *SUFU*, *TP53*,[4] and *GPR161*).[5] Patients with medulloblastoma commonly present with symptoms of increased intracranial pressure and hydrocephalus, which include nocturnal and morning headaches, vomiting, and nausea. Owing to cerebellar and brainstem involvement, patients may present with truncal ataxia, head bobbing/titubation, dysmetria, double vision, or dizziness.[6] Classically, medulloblastomas appear as a round mass of the cerebellar vermis that is T1 iso- to hypointense on magnetic resonance imaging (MRI) (Figure 16.1A–B) compared to white matter, with heterogeneous enhancement.[7] Small, focal cysts are frequently present; cysts larger than 1 cm are less common.[6,8] There can be significant heterogeneity in MRI findings with varying enhancement pattern, although distinct subtypes may be discernible by machine-learning approaches.[6,9,10] Peritumoral edema

TABLE 16.1 Age of incidence and molecular characteristics of embryonal tumors

TUMOR TYPE	AGE	SOMATIC TUMOR MUTATIONS	GERMLINE MUTATIONS
Medulloblastoma			
WNT	All ages	Beta-Catenin	APC
SHH – TP53 wildtype	Infants and adults	GL1, GL2, MYCN*, PTCH1, SMO, SUFU, TP53	PTCH1, SUFU PALB2, BRCA2, TP53
SHH – TP53 mutant	7–17 years		
Group 3 – non-WNT/non-SHH	4–15 years	MYCC*, MYCN^	PALB2, BRCA2
Group 4 – non-WNT/non-SHH	Predominantly 4–15 years, adults	CDK6*, MYCN*	
ATRT	0–3 years	SMARCB1 (INI1), SMARCA4 (BRG1)	SMARCB1, SMARCA4
EMTR	0.5–6 years	C19MC*	
Pineoblastoma	Younger than 9 years		DICER1

WNT, wingless; SHH, sonic hedgehog; APC, adenomatous polypolis coli; ATRT, atypical teratoid/rhabdoid tumor; ETMR, embryonal tumor with multilayered rosettes.

*Indicates amplification.

^Indicates amplification or gain.

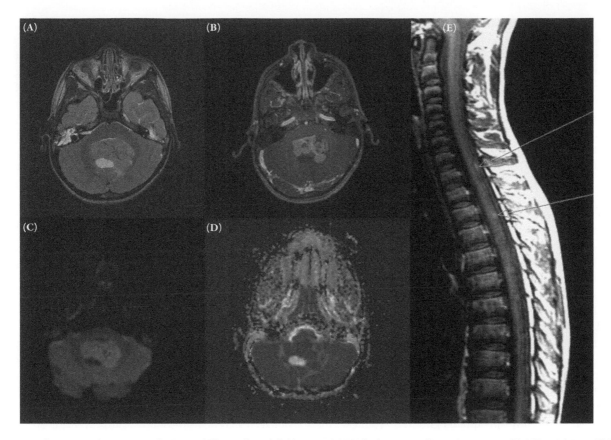

Figure 16.1 MRI with contrast administration of a 7-year-old boy with medulloblastoma. (A) T2/ fluid-attenuated inversion recovery (FLAIR), axial view. (B) T1 weighted with gadolinium. (C) Diffusion weighted imaging (DWI), axial view. (D) Apparent diffusion coefficient (ADC) sequence, axial view. (E) T1 weighted sagittal view with gadolinium of the cervical and thoracic spine. Open arrows denote areas of metastatic disease.

and T2 hyperintensity are often seen. Restricted diffusion, as a feature of the tumor's hypercellularity, is visible on diffusion-weighted imaging (DWI) and apparent diffusion coefficient (ADC) (Figure 16.1C–D).[11] Supratentorial and spinal cord metastasis as well as leptomeningeal dissemination are seen in 30% of new diagnoses (Figure 16.1E).[4] Recurrent disease can be seen in the cerebellum or cerebrum, or isolated in the brain or spinal cord. This is reliably associated with restricted diffusion on MRI, which is the recommended sequence for early detection of relapse.[12]

> Classically, medulloblastomas appear as a round mass of the cerebellar vermis that is T1 iso- to hypointense compared to white matter with heterogeneous enhancement.

PATHOLOGY

Medulloblastomas are considered grade 4 tumors in the WHO classification. Prior to the advent of integrated molecular diagnosis, these medulloblastomas were grouped morphologically into classic, desmoplastic/nodular, large cell/anaplastic medulloblastoma, and medulloblastoma with extensive nodularity. Classic medulloblastoma is described as a small, round, blue cell tumor; it is made up of a syncytial arrangement of densely packed undifferentiated embryonal cells with mitoses and apoptotic bodies. Homer-Wright

(neuroblastic) rosettes are found in some classic and large cell/anaplastic medulloblastomas (Figure 16.2). Desmoplastic/nodular medulloblastoma typically demonstrates nodular, reticulin-free "pale islands" surrounded by undifferentiated, densely packed, highly proliferative cells. Large cell/anaplastic medulloblastoma contains large, monomorphic cells with

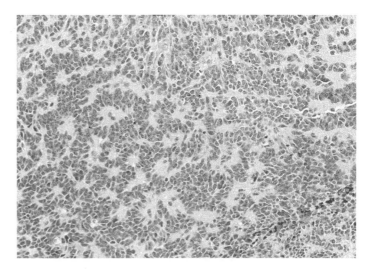

Figure 16.2 Histopathological section from a classical medulloblastoma. Hematoxylin & eosin (H&E) stain demonstrates a typical syncytial arrangement of undifferentiated tumor cells with Homer Wright (neuroblastic) rosettes. 400× magnification.

Courtesy of H. Vogel, MD.

intervening areas of anaplasia; high mitotic rates and apoptotic bodies are present throughout.[13] Medulloblastoma with extensive nodularity is described as having larger reticulin-free zones compared to desmoplastic/nodular medulloblastomas that are enriched in neuropil-like tissue.[13]

In 2012, international consensus divided medulloblastomas into four distinct molecular subgroups (Figure 16.3): wingless (WNT)-activated, sonic hedgehog (SHH)-activated, Group 3, and Group 4.[14–17] WNT-activated tumors account for approximately 10% of medulloblastoma cases and are characterized by WNT pathway activation, commonly with chromosome 6 loss and *CTNNB1* mutation but few other aberrations. Most WNT-activated medulloblastomas demonstrate classic histology and nuclear accumulation of beta-catenin. They can occur in almost any age group, but are uncommon in infancy.[16] When treated with maximal resection and craniospinal irradiation, this molecular subtype has been associated with a very good prognosis, with 5- and 10-year overall survival (OS) and progression-free survival (PFS) of approximately 95%.[15,18–20]

SHH-activated medulloblastoma comprises approximately 30% of medulloblastoma cases and is further divided into *TP53*-wildtype and *TP53*-mutant in the 2016 WHO classification. The most commonly mutated genes are *TP53*, *PTCH1*, *SMO* (enriched in adults), and *SUFU* (almost exclusively in children 3 years of age or younger).[21] SHH-activated medulloblastomas occur most frequently in infants/children younger than

3 years and in children/adults older than 16 years. They are the most common subtype in both age groups, affecting males and females in a roughly equal distribution.[16] Histologically, almost all nodular/desmoplastic medulloblastomas are SHH-activated; however, only about 50% of SHH-activated medulloblastomas are nodular/desmoplastic.[16] These tumors can readily be identified with a panel of antibodies, including Gab1, YAP1, P75-NGFR, and others.[22] *TP53* mutation is associated with complex, catastrophic chromosome breakage, termed *chromothripsis*,[23] and decreased OS in patients with SHH medulloblastomas.

> SHH-activated medulloblastomas occur most frequently in infants/children younger than 3 years and in children/adults older than 16 years

In one retrospective, multi-institution study, *TP53* mutation was the only factor associated with a poorer 5-year OS of 41% ± 9% in patients with SHH medulloblastoma compared to 81% ± 5% for those without the mutation in multivariate analysis.[24] In infants with SHH-activated medulloblastoma, two distinct groups have been delineated on methylation profiling, designated iSHH-I/SHHβ and iSHH-II/SHHγ. Patients in the iSHH-I/SHHβ group often demonstrate *SUFU* mutations and chromosome 2 gains, whereas *SMO* mutations

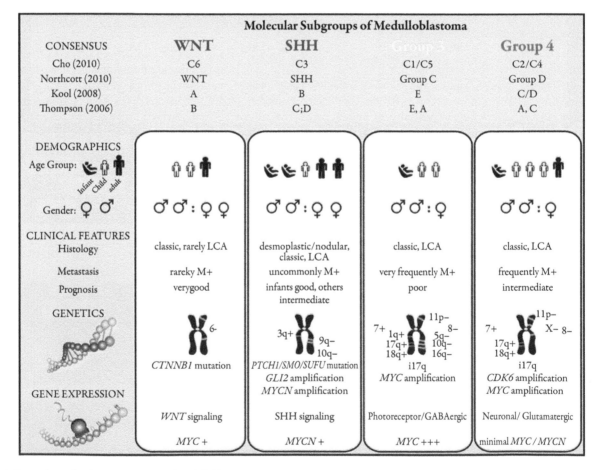

Figure 16.3 Comparison of molecular subgroups of medulloblastoma.

and chromosome 9q deletions are enriched in iSHH-II/SHHγ group.[25,26] In St. Jude Children's Research Hospital's (SJCRH) multi-institution study of young children less than 3 years of age, SJYC07, both groups demonstrated a median age of 2 years and male:female ratio of 1.3:1, although iSHH-II occurred across a wider age distribution. Patients in the iSHH-I/SHHβ exhibited poorer 5-year PFS compared to iSHH-II/SHHγ (27.8% vs. 75.4%).[27]

Group 3 (approximately 20% of medulloblastoma cases) and Group 4 (approximately 40% of medulloblastoma cases) have historically been considered provisional variants as they do not separate as distinctly as WNT- and SHH-activated medulloblastomas in clustering analyses. They are associated with established high-risk disease features, such as *MYC* or *MYCN* amplification, large cell/anaplastic or classic histopathology, and metastatic disease,[28] though they demonstrate marked heterogeneity in clinical course. They are not readily distinguishable on immunohistochemistry and thus are often designated as non-WNT/non-SHH medulloblastoma. Assignment to Group 3 or Group 4 requires DNA methylation or mRNA expression profiling; however, this terminology continues to evolve: higher resolution subtyping approaches (e.g., methylation assays, proteomics, etc.) have further partitioned Group 3/4 tumors into multiple subtypes.[25,29]

> Group 3 medulloblastoma (20% of cases) and Group 4 medulloblastoma (40% of cases) have historically been considered provisional variants as they do not separate as distinctly as WNT- and SHH-activated medulloblastomas in clustering analyses.

DIAGNOSIS AND STAGING

Risk-adapted therapy has become standard of care as the delineation of risk factors and staging criteria continue to evolve. Patients have historically been risk-stratified by modified Chang M staging (Table 16.2),[30] age, and extent of resection: children years of age or older with near-total or gross total resection were assigned to the average risk stratum, whereas those with greater than 1.5 cm² residual disease (measured by postoperative gadolinium-enhanced MRI) were considered

TABLE 16.2 Chang M staging

STAGE	DEFINITION
M_0	No evidence of gross subarachnoid or hematogenous metastasis
M_1	Microscopic tumor cells found in the cerebrospinal fluid
M_2	Gross nodular seedings demonstrated in the cerebellar, cerebral subarachnoid space or in the third or lateral ventricles
M_3	Gross nodular seeding in spinal subarachnoid space
M_4	Extraneuroaxial metastasis

Adapted from Chang et al.[30]

high-risk. Following imaging, maximal safe resection remains a crucial step in management as this has been associated with improved relapse free survival, taking molecular subtype into account.[31,32] Generally, there is no role for biopsy alone unless there is diffuse tumor that precludes any feasible resection.

> Maximal safe resection remains a critical step in management of medulloblastoma as this has been associated with improved relapse free survival, taking molecular subtype into account.

Following surgery, patients should be staged with spinal imaging if not obtained beforehand. As postsurgical changes such as leptomeningeal enhancement can occur after surgery, staging MRI is recommended 7–10 days postoperatively. CSF cytology should be obtained by lumbar puncture, which is superior to ventricular sampling,[33] to evaluate for microscopic metastasis by microfiltration or cytospin techniques 14 or more days postsurgery to reduce the risk of false positivity from surgical debris. Tissue should be sent to an accredited laboratory for molecular testing as current recommendations incorporate molecular data into risk stratification (Table 16.3).[17]

TREATMENT

In the 1970s, standard treatment consisted of maximal surgery followed by craniospinal irradiation, with 10-year OS rates of 44%.[34] However, debilitating neuroendocrine and neurocognitive adverse effects, correlated with craniospinal radiation dose and inversely associated with age, were subsequently noted in long-term survivors.[35,36] Recognizing these detrimental effects, the International Society of Pediatric Oncology (SIOP), Pediatric Oncology Group (POG), and Children's Cancer Group (CCG) sought to improve outcomes through randomized trials of craniospinal irradiation alone versus the addition of adjuvant chemotherapy (lomustine or procarbazine plus vincristine) and reduction or elimination of radiation.[37-39] Although an improvement in OS was not noted for all patients, patients with bulky residual or metastatic disease appeared to derive benefit from chemotherapy. Drawing on these and subsequent experiences, alkylators, vinca alkaloids, and platinum agents became the backbone of chemotherapy regimens for medulloblastoma.

In children older than 3 years, conventional treatment has evolved to include surgical resection, craniospinal radiation with radiation boosts to the tumor bed and any visible metastases, plus adjuvant chemotherapy. In the late 1990s, the Children's Oncology Group (COG) trial A9961 enrolled 379 children with average risk medulloblastoma, treating them with 23.4 Gy of craniospinal irradiation with a boost to 55.8 Gy to the posterior fossa. Patients were then randomized to receive cisplatin and vincristine plus either lomustine or cyclophosphamide. The 5-year event-free survival (EFS) and OS rates were 81 ± 2% and 87 ± 2%; the 10-year EFS and OS were 76 ± 2% and 81 ± 2%, respectively.[40] The St. Jude Medulloblastoma-96 trial, conducted from 1996 to 2003, enrolled 86 children with average-risk medulloblastoma, treating them with 23.4 Gy

TABLE 16.3 Molecularly based risk stratification for non-infant childhood medulloblastoma

	WNT	SHH	GROUP 3	GROUP 4	OTHER
Low risk	Younger than 16 y			Non-metastatic and chromosome 11 loss	
Standard risk		TP53 wildtype, no MYCN amplification, non-metastatic	No MYC amplification and non-metastatic	Non-metastatic and no chromosome 11 loss	
High risk		Metastatic and/or MYCN amplification		Metastatic	
Very high risk		TP53-mutated	Metastatic		
Unknown	Metastatic		Non-metastatic with MYC amplification Anaplasia Isochromosome 17q	Anaplasia	Metastatic medulloblastoma Medullomyoblastoma Boundary between Groups 3 and 4 Definition of MYC and MYCN amplification

Adapted from Ramaswany et al.[17]

craniospinal radiotherapy, 36 Gy to the posterior fossa and 55.8 Gy to the tumor bed. Patients subsequently received 4 cycles of high-dose chemotherapy (cisplatin, vincristine, and cyclophosphamide) followed by autologous stem cell rescue. The 5-year EFS was 83% (95% confidence interval [CI] 73–93).[41]

> In children older than 3 years, conventional treatment includes surgical resection, craniospinal radiation with radiation boosts to the tumor bed and any visible metastases, plus adjuvant chemotherapy.

In children older than 3 years with high-risk disease (subtotal resection and/or metastatic disease on imaging or CSF analysis), optimal treatment is less well established. In a phase I/II COG study of 161 children age 3–21 years, patients received 36 Gy craniospinal irradiation with boosts to sites of disease as well as concurrent carboplatin and vincristine. Maintenance chemotherapy consisted of vincristine and cyclophosphamide with or without cisplatin. The 5-year EFS and OS was 66 ± 6% and 80 ± 5%, respectively.[42] St. Jude Medulloblastoma-96 enrolled 48 patients with high-risk medulloblastoma. Following surgery, patients received 6 weeks of topotecan and/ or went on to receive 36 to 39.6 Gy craniospinal radiation depending on Chang M stage, with boosts to 50.4 Gy to sites of metastasis and 55.8 Gy to the tumor bed. Adjuvant chemotherapy consisted of the same regimen as given to patients with average-risk medulloblastoma, as detailed earlier. In this cohort, the 5-year EFS was 70% (95% CI 55–85).[41]

> Treatment of infants and children (<3 years) with medulloblastoma has not met the same successes as in older pediatric patients.

The treatment of infants and children younger than 3 years with medulloblastoma has not met the same successes as in older pediatric patients. In this age group, radiation is delayed or avoided to spare patients the associated high risk of severe neurologic deficits. Chemotherapy-only regimens can avoid the attendant complications of craniospinal radiation; however, approximately 50% of patients require salvage therapy, often including craniospinal radiation.[43] In the German HIT-SKK '92 study conducted from 1992 to 1997, 43 children younger than 3 years received three cycles of intravenous cyclophosphamide, vincristine, methotrexate, carboplatin, and etoposide and intraventricular methotrexate in lieu of radiation. The 5-year PFS and OS rates were 58 ± 9% and 66 ± 7%, respectively; 16 patients in total received further treatment at progression or relapse.[44] SJCRH's SJYC07 utilized an up-front induction chemotherapy regimen of methotrexate, vincristine, cisplatin, and cyclophosphamide with additional vinblastine for high-risk patients. Following induction, risk-adapted consolidation chemotherapy was administered: low-risk patients received cyclophosphamide, etoposide, and carboplatin; intermediate-risk patients received focal radiation (54 Gy) to the tumor bed; high-risk patients received topotecan and cyclophosphamide. Maintenance chemotherapy consisted of cyclophosphamide, topotecan, and erlotinib. The 5-year EFS was 31.3% (95% CI 19.3–43.3) for all patients; 55.3% (95% CI 33.3–77.3) for the low-risk group; 24.6% (95% CI 3.6–45.6) for the intermediate-risk cohort, and 16.7% (95% CI 3.4–30.0) in the high-risk cohort. This study also included methylation subgrouping in its statistical analyses. Stratified in this way, the 5-year PFS was 51.1% (95% CI 34.6–67.6) in the SHH subgroup, 8.3% (95% CI 0.0–24.0) in the Group 3 subgroup, and 13.3% (95% CI 0.0–37.6) in the Group 4 subgroup.[27]

The incidence of medulloblastoma declines exponentially after 9 years of age, reaching a rate of approximately 0.05 case per 100,000 annually.[3,45] Adults, however, comprise approximately 12% of cases of medulloblastoma overall.[15] OS and EFS rates are similar between adults and children; however, prognostic factors are dissimilar.[45] Medulloblastomas in adults harbor biologically distinct features compared to tumors in pediatric patients and are comprised of three molecular subgroups: WNT, SHH, and the non-WNT/non-SHH Group 4 (or D).[46] WNT-driven tumors are typically associated with the most favorable prognosis, whereas Group 4 tumors are associated with the least.[46,47] Whereas the extent and dose of radiation have been positively correlated with disease-free survival,[48,49] consensus on the role of chemotherapy in the treatment of adult patients with medulloblastoma has not been achieved.[50,51] A German study of 33 adults with medulloblastoma prospectively analyzed the combination of radiation and adjuvant cisplatin, lomustine, and vincristine, demonstrating a 3-year EFS of 67% and 3-year OS of 70%. The investigators found that although four cycles of multiagent maintenance chemotherapy is feasible in most patients, older adults experience increased rates of toxicity.[52] The long-term effects of radiation therapy in patients treated for medulloblastoma as adults include executive dysfunction, weakness/ataxia, and depression/anxiety, suggesting that select patients may benefit from reduced doses of radiation.[53]

In both pediatric and adult patients with medulloblastoma, consensus on subgrouping has led to the development of multiple molecularly based, risk-adapted trials.[27,54,55] In SHH-activated medulloblastoma, targeted therapy with smoothened (SMO) receptor inhibitors (e.g., vismodegib, sonidegib) has demonstrated anti-tumor activity in both adults and children[56-59]; additional clinical trials are under way (e.g., NCT01878617).

OUTCOMES

Relapse, which occurs in 20–30% of patients, generally takes place within 2 years of original diagnosis and is unlikely beyond 8 years.[60] Salvage therapy often includes a combination of second surgery, reirradiation, platinum-based chemotherapy, or high-dose chemotherapy with autologous stem cell rescue. Outcomes are poor, with median OS ranging from 1 to 1.8 years.[60-62]

> Relapses occur in 20–30% of patients with medulloblastoma, generally within the first 2 years after original diagnosis. Relapses are uncommon beyond 8 years after the diagnosis.

Posterior fossa syndrome, also known as cerebellar mutism or cerebellar cognitive affective syndrome, is a known postoperative complication caused by injury to the inferior cerebellar outflow pathway and inferior vermis.[63] It occurs in approximately 25% of patients 1–2 days after surgery. Patients demonstrate decrement in expressive language progressing to mutism, impairment in executive function, ataxia, and emotional lability; symptoms can last for weeks to months.[64] Some neurocognitive effects may be long term: in the multi-institutional trial SJMB03 for patients with newly diagnosed medulloblastoma, 77 (24%) patients experienced posterior fossa syndrome. These patients exhibited impaired processing speed and below-average intellectual disability at 1 year post diagnosis and poorer cognitive developmental trajectories over the course of 5 years post diagnosis compared to a matched cohort of patients who did not experience posterior fossa syndrome.[65]

As previously mentioned, the long-term effects of chemotherapy and radiation are well described in patients with a history of medulloblastoma. Endocrinologic effects can include hypothyroidism, growth hormone deficiency, delayed puberty onset, and hypogonadism. Patients have a higher risk of grade 3 to 4 hearing loss, particularly in cases of cisplatin-containing chemotherapy regimens; ophthalmologic complications are frequent. Cardiovascular conditions, such as cerebrovascular disease (including stroke, stroke-like migraine variants, and vascular malformations), coronary heart disease, and other blood clots have also been noted.[66] In patients who receive cranial radiation therapy, stroke risk increases in a dose-dependent manner.[67] Additionally, longitudinal studies in patients with malignant posterior fossa tumors have demonstrated persistent declination in neurocognitive function over time following cranial radiation.[35,68] Children treated for medulloblastoma are at increased risk of academic remediation, unemployment, difficulties with psychosocial functioning, and decreased quality of life.[69]

> Children who were treated for medulloblastoma are at increased risk of academic remediation, unemployment, difficulties with psychosocial functioning, and decreased quality of life.

In a follow-up of the COG trial A9961 wherein patients with non-metastatic, completely resected medulloblastoma were treated with 23.4 Gy CSI and adjuvant chemotherapy, researchers evaluated the long-term data on 379 patients and found that 15 (4.2%) had developed subsequent neoplasms at 10 years, including malignant gliomas, osteosarcoma, and myelodysplastic syndrome.[40] In a study of 1,311 patients with medulloblastoma in the Childhood Cancer Survivor Study, those who received standard-risk multimodal therapy had a 9.5% incidence of subsequent neoplasms at 15 years from diagnosis.[70]

ATYPICAL TERATOID/RHABDOID TUMOR

EPIDEMIOLOGY AND CLINICAL PRESENTATION

ATRT is defined by alterations in *SMARCB1* (*INI1*) or, rarely, *SMARCA4* (*BRG1*),[13] comprising 15.9% of all embryonal tumors diagnosed in children age 0–19 years with an incidence of 0.09 per 100,000 population.[1] It most commonly occurs between ages 0 and 3 years and accounts for 40–50% of all embryonal CNS tumors in children younger than 1 year.[71] There is a slight male predominance. Tumors occur infratentorially more often in younger children, whereas in older patients, supratentorial disease is more common. ATRT in the nonbrain CNS, including the pituitary gland and spine, occurs at a relatively stable frequency (~8%) across all age groups.[72]

Patients with ATRT often present with a relatively short prodrome of symptoms owing to the tumor's rapid growth; CSF flow is frequently obstructed, leading to acute hydrocephalus that commonly requires operative intervention. Supratentorial

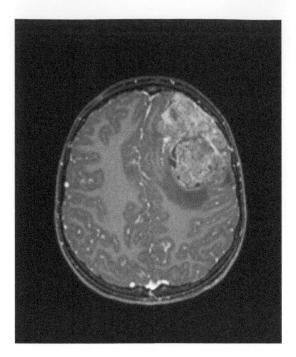

Figure 16.4 *T1 weighted axial view of MRI with gadolinium contrast administration of a 4-year-old boy with left frontal lobe atypical teratoid/ rhabdoid tumor (ATRT).*

PATHOLOGY

ATRTs often contain populations of cells exhibiting classic rhabdoid features and nuclear atypia as well as primitive neuroectodermal, mesenchymal, and, least commonly, epithelial components (Figure 16.5A). In general, ATRTs are heterogeneous and difficult to recognize on histopathology alone, and they were often misdiagnosed as primitive neuroectodermal tumors/medulloblastoma before loss of SMARCB1 (INI1) was identified as a characteristic finding on immunohistochemistry (Figure 16.5B).[81] DNA methylation analysis of 325 ATRT cases identified three main subgroups: ATRT-SHH, ATRT-TYR, and ATRT-MYC. These subgroups were confirmed in a separate analysis of the gene expression profiles in an additional 172 cases.[82] ATRT-TYR tumors overexpress tyrosinase and are diagnosed at a median age of 12 months, most commonly presenting in an infratentorial location. ATRT-SHH tumors overexpress sonic hedgehog (SHH) and Notch pathway proteins and can be further subgrouped into ATRT-SHH-1, which present primarily in a supratentorial location and ATRT-SHH-2, which more frequently occur infratentorially. Tumors in the ATRT-MYC subgroup overexpress several HOXC cluster genes, often arising in the supratentorial region or in the spinal column.

disease may present with seizures due to mass effect on cortical structures or direct involvement.[73] Metastatic disease is present in approximately 12–24% at diagnosis.[74-76] Radiographically, ATRT demonstrates significant heterogeneity, with some tumors demonstrating intratumoral hemorrhage, calcification, cysts, and necrosis. Similar to other embryonal tumors, restricted diffusion is often evident on DWI and ADC, owing to the tumors' hypercellularity.[11] T1 hypointensity, T2 hyperintensity, and a "wavy" band-like enhancement pattern are often seen[77-79] (Figure 16.4). The prognosis of this tumor has historically been poor, with a reported median OS of approximately 17 months.[80] This tumor occurs very rarely in adults.

Patients with ATRT often present with a relatively short prodrome of symptoms owing to the very rapid tumor growth.

TREATMENT

There is no international consensus on a standardized treatment for ATRT. One study reported a 2-year EFS and OS of 78% ± 14% and 89% ± 11%, respectively, in 31 children age 3 years or older treated with high-dose alkylator-based therapy. For younger patients who did not receive radiotherapy, the EFS and OS were 11% ± 6% and 17% ± 8%, respectively.[83] In another study from the Canadian ATRT registry, of 26 age 12 months or younger at diagnosis of ATRT, 22 patients (84.6%) experienced recurrent or progressive disease at a median time of 1.6 months (range 0.0–8.3 months).[84] The median survival time for patients of 6 months or younger was 3.0 months (range 0.03–14.3 months) compared to 9.7 months (range 1.3–87.0 months) for older children (P = 0.02). Twenty-two patients died of disease. When omitting patients treated

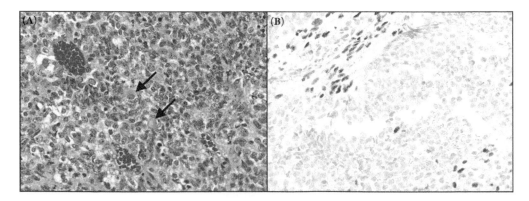

Figure 16.5 *Histopathological sections from an atypical teratoid/rhabdoid tumor (ATRT). (A) Hematoxylin & eosin (H&E) stain demonstrating a highly cellular tumor with primitive cells and scant cytoplasm. Two cells demonstrate rhabdoid morphology, with prominent eosinophilic cytoplasm and nuclear displacement (closed arrows). (B) SMARCB1 (INI1) stain demonstrating loss of nuclear expression in tumor cells but retention in non-neoplastic endothelial nuclei. Both images at 400× magnification.*
Courtesy of H. Vogel, MD.

with surgery alone, the 5-year PFS and 5-year OS were 18.9 ± 11.7 and 14.3 ± 9.4%, respectively.

In the only formal clinical trial specific for ATRT currently published (NCT00084838), 20 patients received an intensive anthracycline-based chemotherapy including intrathecal therapy, early radiotherapy, and chemotherapy. The 2-year OS and EFS were 70% ± 10% and 53% ± 13%, respectively, but with significant toxicities, including one toxic death and severe adverse events, including one episode of transverse myelitis and two of radiation recall.[85]

In the European registry for rhabdoid tumors (EU-RHAB), 143 uniformly treated patients with ATRT were analyzed, demonstrating a 5-year OS and EFS of 34.7 ± 4.5% and 30.5 ± 4.2%, respectively.[86] The authors performed DNA methylation subtyping on all tumors, classifying tumors based on the established molecular subgroups ATRT-SHH, ATRT-TYR, and ATRT-MYC described earlier.[26,82] In an adjusted multivariable model, the authors found that age younger than 1 year and non-TYR DNA methylation signature were negatively associated with OS. There was no statistically significant association between high-dose chemotherapy with stem cell rescue and EFS or OS. Based on evolving understanding of this tumor's biology, clinical trials with the aurora kinase inhibitor alisertib[87] (NCT02114229) and the EZH2 inhibitor tazemetostat[88] (NCT03213665) are currently under way. There are no well-established treatment recommendations for adult patients with ATRT.

EMBRYONAL TUMOR WITH MULTILAYERED ROSETTES

ETMR is a rare, malignant brain tumor that occurs almost exclusively in children age 0.5–6 years,[89] with a male:female ratio of 1:2.[90,91] ETMR is most commonly located supratentorially; approximately 20–25% of patients have metastatic disease at diagnosis.[89–91] Patients manifest symptoms depending on the brain structures affected; in one study, these often included unilateral weakness, increased intracranial pressure, confusion, seizures, and cerebellar syndrome.[90] The term "ETMR" encompasses three previously designated histological variants of the embryonal rosette-forming neuroepithelial brain tumor family: embryonal tumor with abundant neuropil and true rosettes (ETANTR), ependymoblastoma, and medulloepithelioma.[92] These three variants were found to exhibit uniform molecular signatures by DNA methylation and copy number profiling as well as highly similar clinicopathological features. As a single entity, ETMR is characterized morphologically by the presence of multilayered true ependymoblastic rosettes and genetically by C19MC (19q13.42) amplification,[93] most frequently, followed by DICER1 mutation and amplification of the miR-17-92 miRNA cluster on chromosome 13.[94] However, in the WHO 2016 classification system, ETMR without C19MC amplification is referred to as "embryonal tumor with multilayered rosettes, not otherwise specified (NOS)," and medulloepithelioma, if it possesses the hallmark histological features (e.g., sheets of embryonal cells with neural tube-like structures of pseudostratified neuroepithelium).[13]

Radiographically, ETMRs demonstrate minimal heterogeneous enhancement without surrounding T2/ fluid-attenuated inversion recovery (FLAIR) abnormality. The tumors tend to be solid without cystic components and demonstrate restricted diffusion.[95] In general, ETMRs are often chemoradiotherapy-resistant and are associated with a poor prognosis.[96] Treatment is typically multimodal but nonstandardized, based largely on small series and case reports given the rarity of this diagnosis.[96,97] However, retrospective reviews suggest that irradiation and adjuvant chemotherapy confer a survival benefit in patients with ETMR.[98,99] As an instance, one retrospective review of 38 children treated at multiple French centers utilized a protocol combining surgery and conventional chemotherapy with carboplatin and etoposide, followed by high-dose chemotherapy with melphalan, cisplatin, and thiotepa and peripheral stem cell transplantation with reduced dose radiation. The 1-year EFS and OS were 36% (95% CI 23–55) and 45% (95% CI 31–64), respectively.[90]

> Embryonal tumors with multilayered rosettes are often chemoradiotherapy-resistant and are associated with a poor prognosis.

PINEOBLASTOMA

Pineoblastoma is a rare embryonal neoplasm that arises from the pineal gland, more commonly occurring in children younger than 9 years of age with a median of 7 years, though it can occur through young adulthood. The male:female ratio is approximately 0.7:1.[13] Patients frequently present with hydrocephalus (93% in a case series of 41 patients from SJCRH)[100] necessitating surgical intervention, headache, ocular disturbances (including Parinaud syndrome), and ataxia[101]; metastases are found in 20–35% of patients at diagnosis.[101,102] Radiographically, pineoblastomas can demonstrate calcification, restricted diffusion, homogeneous enhancement, and internal cystic changes (Figure 16.6).[103,104] Histologically, they are highly cellular, typically demonstrating sheets of small, immature neuroepithelial cells with a high proliferative index and evidence of necrosis.[13,105] Pineoblastoma has been associated with germline mutations in DICER1[106] as well as in the RB1 gene in cases of the rare trilateral retinoblastoma.[107] Historically, pineoblastoma is associated with a poor prognosis,[108] with a median survival of 24–35 months.[100,109] In addition to metastatic disease at presentation and recurrent tumor, age younger than 5 years was found to portend a significantly worse prognosis.[100] This may be due to the avoidance of craniospinal radiation therapy in infants.[100,101] In older patients, typical radiation doses are approximately 25–38 Gy to the craniospinal axis with boost to 44–55 Gy to the tumor bed.[110,111] Given the infrequent incidence of these tumors, the optimal management of pineoblastoma beyond maximal safe resection[111] and radiation remains unclear. Adjuvant chemotherapy agents often include vincristine, a platinum agent, cyclophosphamide, etoposide, or lomustine.[110] Some groups have also attempted the use of high-dose chemotherapy with

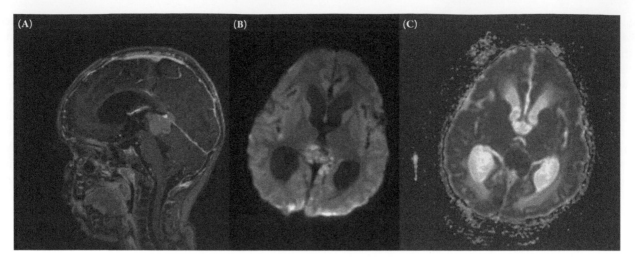

Figure 16.6 *MRI of a 4-year-old girl with pineoblastoma. (A) T1 weighted gadolinium contrast-enhanced sagittal view. (B) Diffusion weighted imaging (DWI), axial view, with positivity in the pineal region. (C) Apparent diffusion coefficient (ADC) sequence, axial view.*

stem cell rescue to reduce or eliminate radiation[112]; however, most evidence suggests that radiation is a crucial component of treatment.[111,113,114]

> Radiographically, pineoblastomas can demonstrate calcifications, restricted diffusion, homogeneous enhancement, and internal cystic changes.

OTHER EMBRYONAL TUMORS

In the WHO 2016 classification scheme, a group of tumors lacking the specific histopathological features described in the entities so far was also delineated as a category. The group is comprised of CNS embryonal tumors that at the time lacked a characteristic genetic alteration: medulloepithelioma, CNS neuroblastoma, CNS ganglioneuroblastoma, and CNS embryonal tumor, NOS. However, expression and epigenetic analyses have elucidated some of these previously unclassifiable entities (and reclassified some to known diagnoses, e.g., high-grade glioma, ependymoma, and ATRT). Of the remaining tumors, four new CNS tumor entities have been proposed: CNS neuroblastoma with *FOXR2* activation (CNS NB-FOXR2), CNS Ewing sarcoma family tumor with *CIC* alteration (CNS EFT-CIC), CNS high-grade neuroepithelial tumor with *MN1* alteration (CNS HGNET-MN1), and CNS high-grade neuroepithelial tumor with *BCOR* alteration (CNS HGNET-BCOR).[115] The subgrouping of embryonal tumors with *FOXR2* activation or *BCOR* alteration has been

recapitulated in other studies.[116] Due to the rarity of these novel diagnoses, the clinical characteristics, prognostic factors, and optimal treatment strategy remain to be ascertained. Highlighting the importance of molecular characterization, 85 patients institutionally diagnosed with CNS primitive neuroectodermal (embryonal) tumors/pineoblastoma were enrolled as part of the COG study ACNS0332 and were randomized to receive carboplatin during radiation and/or adjuvant isotretinoin after standard intensive therapy. Although no benefit was initially demonstrated, 77 patients underwent retrospective DNA methylation profiling, which identified 18 high-grade gliomas, 3 CNS NB-FOXR2, and other distinct entities. Patients with high-grade gliomas had significantly poorer outcomes than those with supratentorial embryonal tumors or pineoblastomas, thus underlining the utility of molecularly based profiling.[117]

CONCLUSION

Since the publication of the WHO's 2016 classification of CNS tumors, our understanding of pediatric tumors has continued to evolve at a rapid rate. Although medulloblastoma is one of the most common malignant pediatric brain tumors, other CNS embryonal tumors, such as CNS high-grade neuroepithelial tumor with *BCOR* alteration are exceptionally uncommon. Pediatric brain tumors are rare; thus it is imperative that patients be enrolled in multicenter clinical trials. Doing so will enable researchers to define more efficacious and less toxic treatments to mitigate, and hopefully cure, these aggressive tumors.

FLASHCARD

Medulloblastoma is the most common brain tumor in children between which ages?	Five and nine
List the molecular subgroups of medulloblastoma:	1. Wingless (WNT)-activated 2. Sonic hedgehog (SHH)-activated 3. Group 3 4. Group 4
Which medulloblastoma is associated with the best prognosis?	WNT-activated
Which type of medulloblastoma is typically metastatic at diagnosis?	Group 3
What is the age distribution for SHH-activated medulloblastoma?	SHH-activated medulloblastomas occur most frequently in infants/children younger than 3 years of age and children/adults older than 16 years
In children older than 3 years conventional treatment for medulloblastoma includes	Surgical resection, craniospinal radiation with radiation boosts to the tumor bed and any visible metastases, plus adjuvant chemotherapy
List genetic alterations seen in ATRT: **Molecular subtypes of ATRT:** 1. SHH 2. TYR 3. MYC	*SMARCB1* (*INI1*) *SMARCA4* (*BRG1*)—rare -SHH; -TYR; -MYC
ATRT is:	1. One of the most common CNS embryonal tumors in infants 2. Typically, infratentorial in younger children 3. Age younger than 1 and non-TYR subtype is associated with poor prognosis

Embryonal tumor with multilayered rosettes (ETMR) is:

1. Characterized by *C19MC* amplification
2. Almost exclusively occurs in children younger than 6 years of age
3. Female:male ratio of 2:1
4. Most commonly arises in a supratentorial location
5. Prognosis is poor
6. Multimodal treatment is recommended; few published data exist

Pineoblastoma:

1. Arises from the pineal gland
2. Has slight female predominance
3. Median age of onset is 7 years
4. Associated with germline *DICER1* mutations and *RB1* mutations in cases of trilateral retinoblastoma

QUESTIONS

1. A 3-year-old boy presents with vomiting and ataxia and is noted to have a fourth ventricular mass. Histopathologically, the tumor is composed of small, round blue cells, consistent with medulloblastoma. Of the four molecular subtypes of medulloblastoma, the one associated with the worst prognosis is
   a. WNT
   b. SHH
   c. Group 3
   d. Group 4

2. A 7-year-old boy is found to have medulloblastoma and undergoes a gross total resection with no evidence of metastasis. You recommend adjuvant radiation therapy. Clinical trials are currently under way to reduce radiation doses in which medulloblastoma subgroup?
   a. WNT
   b. SHH
   c. Group 3
   d. Group 4

3. A patient with history of medulloblastoma status post resection, radiation, and chemotherapy undergoes their routine surveillance imaging. Given the highly cellular nature of medulloblastoma, which MRI finding is most suggestive of recurrent disease?
   a. Contrast enhancement
   b. T2/FLAIR hyperintensity
   c. T1 hyperintensity
   d. Positivity on diffusion weighted imaging

4. A 31-month-old girl presents with vomiting and hydrocephalus. She is found to have a fronto-parietal supratentorial mass and is ultimately diagnosed with embryonal tumor with multilayered rosettes (ETMR). This tumor is characterized by amplification of
   a. PTCH1
   b. MYCN
   c. C19MC
   d. SHH

5. A patient presents with a left frontal mass. Histologically, it demonstrates rhabdoid components and a characteristic genetic alteration that confirms the diagnosis of ATRT. This alteration is in
   a. SMARCD2 or SMARCB1
   b. SMARCB1 or SMARCA4
   c. SMARCA4 or SUFU
   d. MYC or TYR

6. Medulloblastoma most commonly occurs in which age group in children?
   a. 0–4 years
   b. 5–9 years
   c. 10–14 years
   d. 15–19 years

7. What is the most common molecular subtype of medulloblastoma in adults?
   a. WNT
   b. SHH
   c. Group 3
   d. Group 4

8. A 3-year-old girl presents with a calcified metastatic pineal mass. Small, round blue cells are noted on histopathology with a high proliferative index and evidence of necrosis. You find that the patient has a significant family history of cancer. Based on this, you recommend genetic testing for germline mutations specifically in
   a. PTCH2
   b. BRCA2
   c. DICER1
   d. FOXR2

9. A 4-year-old patient is found to have a calcified pineal mass with areas of restricted diffusion. Preliminary pathology suggests a small, round blue cell tumor. Alpha-fetoprotein (AFP) and beta-human chorionic gonadotropin (BhCG) are within normal limits. Based on these findings, you suspect
   a. Pineal cyst
   b. Germ cell tumor
   c. Pineoblastoma
   d. Medulloblastoma

10. Which of the following CNS embryonal tumors has the highest incidence in children?
    a. Medulloblastoma
    b. ETMR
    c. ATRT
    d. Pineoblastoma

11. A 9-month-old patient is diagnosed with ATRT. For which of the following reasons would you recommend avoiding or delaying radiation therapy?
    a. Radiation therapy is ineffective in patients with ATRT.
    b. Patients with ATRT only need observation after surgical resection.
    c. Patients of this age are at high risk of severe neurocognitive deficits with radiation.
    d. Chemotherapy is sufficient for a complete response in patients with ATRT.

12. A 5-year-old boy presents with a posterior fossa mass. The mass is completely resected; pathology is consistent with medulloblastoma. As part of the staging workup, you recommend
    a. MRI of the spine with and without gadolinium to evaluate for metastases
    b. Lumbar puncture to evaluate the CSF for malignant cells
    c. Serum AFP and BhCG
    d. a and b

13. A 3-year-old girl presents with new-onset vomiting, convergence-retraction nystagmus, and upward gaze paralysis. You astutely recommend brain imaging. Which of the following embryonal tumors are you most concerned about?
    a. Medulloblastoma
    b. ETMR of the frontal lobe
    c. Pineoblastoma
    d. ATRT of the posterior fossa

14. A 9-year-old boy presents with a posterior fossa mass and is found to have medulloblastoma. Family history is significant for multiple relatives with innumerable colonic polyps. You suspect a germline mutation in
    a. RB1
    b. APC
    c. TP53
    d. DICER1

15. A pediatric patient is found to have a brain tumor. The histopathological diagnosis is CNS embryonal tumor, NOS; however, the lab is unable to give you more information. You suggest
    a. Send out for molecular profiling to better characterize the tumor
    b. Watchful waiting with serial imaging
    c. 36 Gy craniospinal irradiation with boost to 54 Gy to the tumor bed
    d. High-dose chemotherapy with stem cell rescue

ANSWERS

1. c
2. a
3. d
4. c
5. b
6. b
7. b
8. c
9. c
10. a
11. c
12. d
13. c
14. b
15. a

REFERENCES

1. Ostrom QT, Cioffi G, Gittleman H, et al. CBTRUS statistical report: Primary brain and other central nervous system tumors diagnosed in the United States in 2012-2016. *Neuro Oncol.* 2019;21(Suppl_5):v1–v100.
2. Riffaud L, Saikali S, Leray E, et al. Survival and prognostic factors in a series of adults with medulloblastomas. *J Neurosurg.* 2009;111(3):478–487.
3. Giordana MT, Schiffer P, Lanotte M, et al. Epidemiology of adult medulloblastoma. *Int J Cancer.* 1999;80(5):689–692.
4. Waszak SM, Northcott PA, Buchhalter I, et al. Spectrum and prevalence of genetic predisposition in medulloblastoma: A retrospective genetic study and prospective validation in a clinical trial cohort. *The Lancet Oncology.* 2018;19(6):785–798.
5. Begemann M, Waszak SM, Robinson GW, et al. Germline GPR161 mutations predispose to pediatric medulloblastoma. *J Clin Oncol.* 2020;38(1):43–50.
6. Yeom KW, Mobley BC, Lober RM, et al. Distinctive MRI features of pediatric medulloblastoma subtypes. *AJR Am J Roentgenol.* 2013;200(4):895–903.
7. Koeller KK, Rushing EJ. From the archives of the AFIP: Medulloblastoma: A comprehensive review with radiologic-pathologic correlation. *Radiographics.* 2003;23(6):1613–1637.
8. Poretti A, Meoded A, Huisman TA. Neuroimaging of pediatric posterior fossa tumors including review of the literature. *J Magn Reson Imaging.* 2012;35(1):32–47.
9. Perreault S, Ramaswamy V, Achrol AS, et al. MRI surrogates for molecular subgroups of medulloblastoma. *AJNR Am J Neuroradiol.* 2014;35(7):1263–1269.
10. Iv M, Zhou M, Shpanskaya K, et al. MR imaging-based radiomic signatures of distinct molecular subgroups of medulloblastoma. *AJNR Am J Neuroradiol.* 2019;40(1):154–161.
11. Shih RY, Koeller KK. Embryonal tumors of the central nervous system: From the radiologic pathology archives. *Radiographics.* 2018;38(2):525–541.
12. Aboian MS, Kline CN, Li Y, et al. Early detection of recurrent medulloblastoma: The critical role of diffusion-weighted imaging. *Neurooncol Pract.* 2018;5(4):234–240.
13. Louis DN, Perry A, Reifenberger G, et al. The 2016 World Health Organization Classification of Tumors of the Central Nervous System: A summary. *Acta Neuropathol.* 2016;131(6):803–820.
14. Northcott PA, Korshunov A, Witt H, et al. Medulloblastoma comprises four distinct molecular variants. *J Clin Oncol.* 2011;29(11):1408–1414.
15. Kool M, Korshunov A, Remke M, et al. Molecular subgroups of medulloblastoma: An international meta-analysis of transcriptome, genetic aberrations, and clinical data of WNT, SHH, Group 3, and Group 4 medulloblastomas. *Acta Neuropathol.* 2012;123(4):473–484.
16. Taylor MD, Northcott PA, Korshunov A, et al. Molecular subgroups of medulloblastoma: The current consensus. *Acta Neuropathol.* 2012;123(4):465–472.
17. Ramaswamy V, Remke M, Bouffet E, et al. Risk stratification of childhood medulloblastoma in the molecular era: The current consensus. *Acta Neuropathol.* 2016;131(6):821–831.
18. Clifford SC, Lusher ME, Lindsey JC, et al. Wnt/Wingless pathway activation and chromosome 6 loss characterize a distinct molecular sub-group of medulloblastomas associated with a favorable prognosis. *Cell Cycle.* 2006;5(22):2666–2670.
19. Ellison DW, Onilude OE, Lindsey JC, et al. beta-Catenin status predicts a favorable outcome in childhood medulloblastoma: The United Kingdom Children's Cancer Study Group Brain Tumour Committee. *J Clin Oncol.* 2005;23(31):7951–7957.
20. Ellison DW, Kocak M, Dalton J, et al. Definition of disease-risk stratification groups in childhood medulloblastoma using combined clinical, pathologic, and molecular variables. *J Clin Oncol.* 2011;29(11):1400–1407.
21. Kool M, Jones DT, Jager N, et al. Genome sequencing of SHH medulloblastoma predicts genotype-related response to smoothened inhibition. *Cancer Cell.* 2014;25(3):393–405.
22. Pietsch T, Haberler C. Update on the integrated histopathological and genetic classification of medulloblastoma: A practical diagnostic guideline. *Clin Neuropathol.* 2016;35(6):344–352.
23. Rausch T, Jones DT, Zapatka M, et al. Genome sequencing of pediatric medulloblastoma links catastrophic DNA rearrangements with TP53 mutations. *Cell.* 2012;148(1-2):59–71.
24. Zhukova N, Ramaswamy V, Remke M, et al. Subgroup-specific prognostic implications of TP53 mutation in medulloblastoma. *J Clin Oncol.* 2013;31(23):2927–2935.
25. Cavalli FMG, Remke M, Rampasek L, et al. Intertumoral heterogeneity within medulloblastoma subgroups. *Cancer Cell.* 2017;31(6):737–754 e736.
26. Capper D, Jones DTW, Sill M, et al. DNA methylation-based classification of central nervous system tumours. *Nature.* 2018;555(7697):469–474.
27. Robinson GW, Rudneva VA, Buchhalter I, et al. Risk-adapted therapy for young children with medulloblastoma (SJYC07): Therapeutic and molecular outcomes from a multicentre, phase 2 trial. *Lancet Oncology.* 2018;19(6):768–784.

28. Pizer BL, Clifford SC. The potential impact of tumour biology on improved clinical practice for medulloblastoma: Progress towards biologically driven clinical trials. *Br J Neurosurg.* 2009;23(4):364–375.

29. Sharma T, Schwalbe EC, Williamson D, et al. Second-generation molecular subgrouping of medulloblastoma: An international meta-analysis of Group 3 and Group 4 subtypes. *Acta Neuropathol.* 2019;138(2):309–326.

30. Chang CH, Housepian EM, Herbert C, Jr. An operative staging system and a megavoltage radiotherapeutic technic for cerebellar medulloblastomas. *Radiology.* 1969;93(6):1351–1359.

31. Zeltzer PM, Boyett JM, Finlay JL, et al. Metastasis stage, adjuvant treatment, and residual tumor are prognostic factors for medulloblastoma in children: Conclusions from the Children's Cancer Group 921 randomized phase III study. *J Clin Oncol.* 1999;17(3):832–845.

32. Thompson EM, Bramall A, Herndon JE, 2nd, et al. The clinical importance of medulloblastoma extent of resection: A systematic review. *J Neurooncol.* 2018;139(3):523–539.

33. Gajjar A, Fouladi M, Walter AW, et al. Comparison of lumbar and shunt cerebrospinal fluid specimens for cytologic detection of leptomeningeal disease in pediatric patients with brain tumors. *J Clin Oncol.* 1999;17(6):1825–1828.

34. Hughes EN, Shillito J, Sallan SE, et al. Medulloblastoma at the joint center for radiation therapy between 1968 and 1984.The influence of radiation dose on the patterns of failure and survival. *Cancer.* 1988;61(10):1992–1998.

35. Moxon-Emre I, Bouffet E, Taylor MD, et al. Impact of craniospinal dose, boost volume, and neurologic complications on intellectual outcome in patients with medulloblastoma. *J Clin Oncol.* 2014;32(17):1760–1768.

36. Gudrunardottir T, Lannering B, Remke M, et al. Treatment developments and the unfolding of the quality of life discussion in childhood medulloblastoma: A review. *Childs Nerv Syst.* 2014;30(6):979–990.

37. Tait DM, Thornton-Jones H, Bloom HJ, et al. Adjuvant chemotherapy for medulloblastoma: The first multi-centre control trial of the International Society of Paediatric Oncology (SIOP I). *Eur J Cancer.* 1990;26(4):464–469.

38. Evans AE, Jenkin RD, Sposto R, et al. The treatment of medulloblastoma. Results of a prospective randomized trial of radiation therapy with and without CCNU, vincristine, and prednisone. *J Neurosurg.* 1990;72(4):572–582.

39. Krischer JP, Ragab AH, Kun L, et al. Nitrogen mustard, vincristine, procarbazine, and prednisone as adjuvant chemotherapy in the treatment of medulloblastoma. A Pediatric Oncology Group study. *J Neurosurg.* 1991;74(6):905–909.

40. Packer RJ, Zhou T, Holmes E, et al. Survival and secondary tumors in children with medulloblastoma receiving radiotherapy and adjuvant chemotherapy: Results of Children's Oncology Group trial A9961. *Neuro Oncol.* 2013;15(1):97–103.

41. Gajjar A, Chintagumpala M, Ashley D, et al. Risk-adapted craniospinal radiotherapy followed by high-dose chemotherapy and stem-cell rescue in children with newly diagnosed medulloblastoma (St Jude Medulloblastoma-96): Long-term results from a prospective, multicentre trial. *Lancet Oncology.* 2006;7(10):813–820.

42. Jakacki RI, Burger PC, Zhou T, et al. Outcome of children with metastatic medulloblastoma treated with carboplatin during craniospinal radiotherapy: A Children's Oncology Group Phase I/II study. *J Clin Oncol.* 2012;30(21):2648–2653.

43. Dhall G, Grodman H, Ji L, et al. Outcome of children less than three years old at diagnosis with non-metastatic medulloblastoma treated with chemotherapy on the "Head Start" I and II protocols. *Pediatr Blood Cancer.* 2008;50(6):1169–1175.

44. Rutkowski S, Bode U, Deinlein F, et al. Treatment of early childhood medulloblastoma by postoperative chemotherapy alone. *N Engl J Med.* 2005;352(10):978–986.

45. Li Q, Dai Z, Cao Y, Wang L. Comparing children and adults with medulloblastoma: A SEER based analysis. *Oncotarget.* 2018;9(53):30189–30198.

46. Remke M, Hielscher T, Northcott PA, et al. Adult medulloblastoma comprises three major molecular variants. *J Clin Oncol.* 2011;29(19):2717–2723.

47. Zhao F, Ohgaki H, Xu L, et al. Molecular subgroups of adult medulloblastoma: A long-term single-institution study. *Neuro Oncol.* 2016;18(7):982–990.

48. Hubbard JL, Scheithauer BW, Kispert DB, et al. Adult cerebellar medulloblastomas: The pathological, radiographic, and clinical disease spectrum. *J Neurosurg.* 1989;70(4):536–544.

49. Berry MP, Jenkin RD, Keen CW, Nair BD, Simpson WJ. Radiation treatment for medulloblastoma. A 21-year review. *J Neurosurg.* 1981;55(1):43–51.

50. Moots PL, O'Neill A, Londer H, et al. Preradiation chemotherapy for adult high-risk medulloblastoma: A trial of the ECOG-ACRIN Cancer Research Group (E4397). *Am J Clin Oncol.* 2018;41(6):588–594.

51. Franceschi E, Bartolotti M, Paccapelo A, et al. Adjuvant chemotherapy in adult medulloblastoma: Is it an option for average-risk patients? *J Neurooncol.* 2016;128(2):235–240.

52. Beier D, Proescholdt M, Reinert C, et al. Multicenter pilot study of radiochemotherapy as first-line treatment for adults with medulloblastoma (NOA-07). *Neuro Oncol.* 2018;20(3):400–410.

53. De B, Beal K, De Braganca KC, et al. Long-term outcomes of adult medulloblastoma patients treated with radiotherapy. *J Neurooncol.* 2018;136(1):95–104.

54. Khatua S, Song A, Citla Sridhar D, Mack SC. Childhood medulloblastoma: Current therapies, emerging molecular landscape and newer therapeutic insights. *Curr Neuropharmacol.* 2018;16(7):1045–1058.

55. Brandes AA, Bartolotti M, Marucci G, et al. New perspectives in the treatment of adult medulloblastoma in the era of molecular oncology. *Crit Rev Oncol Hematol.* 2015;94(3):348–359.

56. Robinson GW, Orr BA, Wu G, et al. Vismodegib exerts targeted efficacy against recurrent sonic hedgehog-subgroup medulloblastoma: Results from phase II Pediatric Brain Tumor Consortium studies PBTC-025B and PBTC-032. *J Clin Oncol.* 2015;33(24):2646–2654.

57. Kieran MW, Chisholm J, Casanova M, et al. Phase I study of oral sonidegib (LDE225) in pediatric brain and solid tumors and a phase II study in children and adults with relapsed medulloblastoma. *Neuro Oncol.* 2017;19(11):1542–1552.

58. Li Y, Song Q, Day BW. Phase I and phase II sonidegib and vismodegib clinical trials for the treatment of paediatric and adult MB patients: A systemic review and meta-analysis. *Acta Neuropathol Commun.* 2019;7(1):123.

59. Robinson GW, Kaste SC, Chemaitilly W, et al. Irreversible growth plate fusions in children with medulloblastoma treated with a targeted hedgehog pathway inhibitor. *Oncotarget.* 2017;8(41):69295–69302.

60. Tsang DS, Sarhan N, Ramaswamy V, et al. Re-irradiation for children with recurrent medulloblastoma in Toronto, Canada: A 20-year experience. *J Neurooncol.* 2019;145(1):107–114.

61. Bowers DC, Gargan L, Weprin BE, et al. Impact of site of tumor recurrence upon survival for children with recurrent or progressive medulloblastoma. *J Neurosurg.* 2007;107(1 Suppl):5-10.

62. Gupta T, Maitre M, Sastri GJ, et al. Outcomes of salvage re-irradiation in recurrent medulloblastoma correlate with age at initial diagnosis, primary risk-stratification, and molecular subgrouping. *J Neurooncol.* 2019;144(2):283–291.

63. Albazron FM, Bruss J, Jones RM, et al. Pediatric postoperative cerebellar cognitive affective syndrome follows outflow pathway lesions. *Neurology.* 2019;93(16):e1561–e1571.

64. Levisohn L, Cronin-Golomb A, Schmahmann JD. Neuropsychological consequences of cerebellar tumour resection in children: Cerebellar cognitive affective syndrome in a paediatric population. *Brain.* 2000;123(Pt 5):1041–1050.

65. Schreiber JE, Palmer SL, Conklin HM, et al. Posterior fossa syndrome and long-term neuropsychological outcomes among children treated for medulloblastoma on a multi-institutional, prospective study. *Neuro Oncol.* 2017;19(12):1673–1682.

66. Morris B, Partap S, Yeom K, Gibbs IC, Fisher PG, King AA. Cerebrovascular disease in childhood cancer survivors: A Children's Oncology Group Report. *Neurology.* 2009;73(22):1906–1913.

67. Mueller S, Fullerton HJ, Stratton K, et al. Radiation, atherosclerotic risk factors, and stroke risk in survivors of pediatric cancer: A report from the Childhood Cancer Survivor Study. *Int J Radiat Oncol Biol Phys.* 2013;86(4):649–655.

68. Spiegler BJ, Bouffet E, Greenberg ML, Rutka JT, Mabbott DJ. Change in neurocognitive functioning after treatment with cranial radiation in childhood. *J Clin Oncol.* 2004;22(4):706–713.

69. Chevignard M, Camara-Costa H, Doz F, Dellatolas G. Core deficits and quality of survival after childhood medulloblastoma: A review. *Neurooncol Pract.* 2017;4(2):82–97.

70. Salloum R, Chen Y, Yasui Y, et al. Late morbidity and mortality among medulloblastoma survivors diagnosed across three decades: A report from the Childhood Cancer Survivor Study. *J Clin Oncol.* 2019;37(9):731–740.

71. Ostrom QT, de Blank PM, Kruchko C, et al. Alex's Lemonade Stand Foundation infant and childhood primary brain and central nervous system tumors diagnosed in the United States in 2007-2011. *Neuro Oncol.* 2015;16 Suppl 10:x1-x36.

72. Ostrom QT, Chen Y, P MdB, et al. The descriptive epidemiology of atypical teratoid/rhabdoid tumors in the United States, 2001-2010. *Neuro Oncol.* 2014;16(10):1392–1399.

73. Nesvick CL, Nageswara Rao AA, Raghunathan A, Biegel JA, Daniels DJ. Case-based review: Atypical teratoid/rhabdoid tumor. *Neurooncol Pract.* 2019;6(3):163–178.

74. Lau CS, Mahendraraj K, Chamberlain RS. Atypical teratoid rhabdoid tumors: A population-based clinical outcomes study involving 174 patients from the Surveillance, Epidemiology, and End Results database (1973–2010). *Cancer Manag Res.* 2015;7:301–309.

75. Buscariollo DL, Park HS, Roberts KB, Yu JB. Survival outcomes in atypical teratoid rhabdoid tumor for patients undergoing radiotherapy in a Surveillance, Epidemiology, and End Results analysis. *Cancer.* 2012;118(17):4212–4219.

76. Meyers SP, Khademian ZP, Biegel JA, Chuang SH, Korones DN, Zimmerman RA. Primary intracranial atypical teratoid/rhabdoid tumors of infancy and childhood: MRI features and patient outcomes. *AJNR Am J Neuroradiol.* 2006;27(5):962–971.

77. Warmuth-Metz M, Bison B, Dannemann-Stern E, et al. CT and MR imaging in atypical teratoid/rhabdoid tumors of the central nervous system. *Neuroradiology.* 2008;50(5):447–452.

78. Nowak J, Nemes K, Hohm A, et al. Magnetic resonance imaging surrogates of molecular subgroups in atypical teratoid/rhabdoid tumor. *Neuro Oncol.* 2018;20(12):1672–1679.

79. Arslanoglu A, Aygun N, Tekhtani D, et al. Imaging findings of CNS atypical teratoid/rhabdoid tumors. *AJNR Am J Neuroradiol.* 2004;25(3):476–480.

80. Athale UH, Duckworth J, Odame I, Barr R. Childhood atypical teratoid rhabdoid tumor of the central nervous system: A meta-analysis of observational studies. *J Pediatr Hematol Oncol.* 2009;31(9):651–663.

81. Judkins AR, Mauger J, Ht A, et al. Immunohistochemical analysis of hSNF5/INI1 in pediatric CNS neoplasms. *Am J Surg Pathol.* 2004;28(5):644–650.

82. Ho B, Johann PD, Grabovska Y, et al. Molecular subgrouping of atypical teratoid/rhabdoid tumors (ATRT): A reinvestigation and current consensus. *Neuro Oncol.* 2019.

83. Tekautz TM, Fuller CE, Blaney S, et al. Atypical teratoid/rhabdoid tumors (ATRT): Improved survival in children 3 years of age and older with radiation therapy and high-dose alkylator-based chemotherapy. *J Clin Oncol.* 2005;23(7):1491–1499.

84. Fossey M, Li H, Afzal S, et al. Atypical teratoid rhabdoid tumor in the first year of life: The Canadian ATRT registry experience and review of the literature. *J Neurooncol.* 2017;132(1):155–162.

85. Chi SN, Zimmerman MA, Yao X, et al. Intensive multimodality treatment for children with newly diagnosed CNS atypical teratoid rhabdoid tumor. *J Clin Oncol.* 2009;27(3):385–389.

86. Fruhwald MC, Hasselblatt M, Nemes K, et al. Age and DNA-methylation subgroup as potential independent risk factors for treatment stratification in children with Atypical Teratoid/Rhabdoid Tumors (ATRT). *Neuro Oncol.* 2019.

87. Wetmore C, Boyett J, Li S, et al. Alisertib is active as single agent in recurrent atypical teratoid rhabdoid tumors in 4 children. *Neuro Oncol.* 2015;17(6):882–888.

88. Kurmasheva RT, Sammons M, Favours E, et al. Initial testing (stage 1) of tazemetostat (EPZ-6438), a novel EZH2 inhibitor, by the Pediatric Preclinical Testing Program. *Pediatr Blood Cancer.* 2017;64(3).

89. Korshunov A, Sturm D, Ryzhova M, et al. Embryonal tumor with abundant neuropil and true rosettes (ETANTR), ependymoblastoma, and medulloepithelioma share molecular similarity and comprise a single clinicopathological entity. *Acta Neuropathol.* 2014;128(2):279–289.

90. Horwitz M, Dufour C, Leblond P, et al. Embryonal tumors with multilayered rosettes in children: The SFCE experience. *Childs Nerv Syst.* 2016;32(2):299–305.

91. Picard D, Miller S, Hawkins CE, et al. Markers of survival and metastatic potential in childhood CNS primitive neuro-ectodermal brain tumours: An integrative genomic analysis. *Lancet Oncol.* 2012;13(8):838–848.

92. Buccoliero AM, Castiglione F, Rossi Degl'Innocenti D, et al. Embryonal tumor with abundant neuropil and true rosettes: Morphological, immunohistochemical, ultrastructural and molecular study of a case showing features of medulloepithelioma and areas of mesenchymal and epithelial differentiation. *Neuropathology.* 2010;30(1):84–91.

93. Korshunov A, Remke M, Gessi M, et al. Focal genomic amplification at 19q13.42 comprises a powerful diagnostic marker for embryonal tumors with ependymoblastic rosettes. *Acta Neuropathol.* 2010;120(2):253–260.

94. Lambo S, Grobner SN, Rausch T, et al. The molecular landscape of ETMR at diagnosis and relapse. *Nature.* 2019;576(7786):274–280.

95. Wang B, Gogia B, Fuller GN, Ketonen LM. Embryonal tumor with multilayered rosettes, C19MC-altered: Clinical, pathological, and neuroimaging findings. *J Neuroimaging.* 2018;28(5):483–489.

96. Choi SH, Kim SH, Shim KW, et al. Treatment outcome and prognostic molecular markers of supratentorial primitive neuroectodermal tumors. *PLoS One.* 2016;11(4):e0153443.

97. Hartman LLR, Oaxaca DM, Carcamo B, et al. Integration of a personalized molecular targeted therapy into the multimodal treatment of refractory childhood embryonal tumor with multilayered rosettes (ETMR). *Case Rep Oncol.* 2019;12(1):211–217.

98. Alexiou GA, Stefanaki K, Vartholomatos G, et al. Embryonal tumor with abundant neuropil and true rosettes: A systematic literature review and report of 2 new cases. *J Child Neurol.* 2013;28(12):1709–1715.

99. Shah AH, Khatib Z, Niazi T. Extracranial extra-CNS spread of embryonal tumor with multilayered rosettes (ETMR): Case series and systematic review. *Childs Nerv Syst.* 2018;34(4):649–654.

100. Parikh KA, Venable GT, Orr BA, et al. Pineoblastoma—the experience at St. Jude Children's Research Hospital. *Neurosurgery.* 2017;81(1):120–128.

101. Tate M, Sughrue ME, Rutkowski MJ, et al. The long-term postsurgical prognosis of patients with pineoblastoma. *Cancer.* 2012;118(1):173–179.

102. Villa S, Miller RC, Krengli M, et al. Primary pineal tumors: Outcome and prognostic factors--a study from the Rare Cancer Network (RCN). *Clin Transl Oncol.* 2012;14(11):827–834.

103. Choudhri AF, Whitehead MT, Siddiqui A, et al. Diffusion characteristics of pediatric pineal tumors. *Neuroradiol J.* 2015;28(2):209–216.

104. Jaju A, Hwang EI, Kool M, et al. MRI features of histologically diagnosed supratentorial primitive neuroectodermal tumors and pineoblastomas in correlation with molecular diagnoses and outcomes: A report from the Children's Oncology Group ACNS0332 trial. *AJNR Am J Neuroradiol.* 2019;40(11):1796–1803.

105. Jouvet A, Saint-Pierre G, Fauchon F, et al. Pineal parenchymal tumors: A correlation of histological features with prognosis in 66 cases. *Brain Pathol.* 2000;10(1):49–60.

106. de Kock L, Sabbaghian N, Druker H, et al. Germ-line and somatic DICER1 mutations in pineoblastoma. *Acta Neuropathol.* 2014;128(4):583–595.

107. de Jong MC, Kors WA, de Graaf P, et al. Trilateral retinoblastoma: A systematic review and meta-analysis. *The Lancet Oncology.* 2014;15(10):1157–1167.

108. Deng X, Yang Z, Zhang X, et al. Prognosis of pediatric patients with pineoblastoma: A SEER analysis 1990-2013. *World Neurosurg.* 2018;118:e871–e879.

109. Mena H, Rushing EJ, Ribas JL, et al. Tumors of pineal parenchymal cells: A correlation of histological features, including nucleolar organizer regions, with survival in 35 cases. *Human Pathology.* 1995;26(1):20–30.

110. Tate MC, Rutkowski MJ, Parsa AT. Contemporary management of pineoblastoma. *Neurosurg Clin N Am.* 2011;22(3):409–412, ix.

111. Gilheeney SW, Saad A, Chi S, et al. Outcome of pediatric pineoblastoma after surgery, radiation and chemotherapy. *J Neurooncol.* 2008;89(1):89–95.

112. Mynarek M, Pizer B, Dufour C, et al. Evaluation of age-dependent treatment strategies for children and young adults with pineoblastoma: Analysis of pooled European Society for Paediatric Oncology (SIOP-E) and US Head Start data. *Neuro Oncol.* 2017;19(4):576–585.

113. Timmermann B, Kortmann RD, Kuhl J, et al. Role of radiotherapy in supratentorial primitive neuroectodermal tumor in young children: Results of the German HIT-SKK87 and HIT-SKK92 trials. *J Clin Oncol.* 2006;24(10):1554–1560.

114. Jakacki RI, Zeltzer PM, Boyett JM, et al. Survival and prognostic factors following radiation and/or chemotherapy for primitive neuroectodermal tumors of the pineal region in infants and children: A report of the Childrens Cancer Group. *J Clin Oncol.* 1995;13(6):1377–1383.

115. Sturm D, Orr BA, Toprak UH, et al. New brain tumor entities emerge from molecular classification of CNS-PNETs. *Cell.* 2016;164(5):1060–1072.

116. Li BK, Al-Karmi S, Huang A, Bouffet E. Pediatric embryonal brain tumors in the molecular era. *Expert Rev Mol Diagn.* 2020:1–11.

117. Hwang EI, Kool M, Burger PC, et al. Extensive molecular and clinical heterogeneity in patients with histologically diagnosed CNS-PNET treated as a single entity: A report from the Children's Oncology Group randomized ACNS0332 trial. *J Clin Oncol.* 2018:JCO2017764720.

17 | PEDIATRIC LOW-GRADE GLIOMA

SHEETAL PHADNIS AND THEODORE NICOLAIDES

INTRODUCTION

Tumors of the central nervous system (CNS) are the most common solid tumors in children and the second most common childhood malignancy. The most frequently diagnosed pediatric CNS tumors are gliomas, with pediatric low-grade gliomas (PLGGs) being the most common subgroup. Historically, low-grade gliomas included WHO grade 1 and 2 tumors. Modern classification of gliomas is based on the World Health Organization (WHO) Classification of Central Nervous System Tumors, first published in 1979 and revised several times since then, most recently in 2021.[1] Low-grade gliomas are brain tumors that originate from glial cells, which have a role in support and nourishment of neurons. Pediatric low-grade gliomas are a diverse set of tumors encompassing tumors of astrocytic, oligodendroglial, and mixed glial-neuronal histology. The most common pediatric tumors are described here because other astrocytic tumors or oligodendrogliomas are less common. The majority of PLGGs are pilocytic astrocytomas while diffuse astrocytomas, pleomorphic xanthoastrocytoma (PXA), subependymal giant cell astrocytoma (SEGA), and pilomyxoid astrocytoma are less common variants. Pilocytic astrocytoma and SEGA are considered WHO grade 1 tumors while PXA and diffuse astrocytoma are considered grade 2 tumors. Several other and rarer PLGGs are also described here, including oligodendroglioma, astroblastoma, mixed glioneuronal tumors, and angiocentric glioma.

Management of PLGG depends on the location of tumor and age of the patient. Complete surgical removal of PLGG is usually curative but can be challenging in deep-seated tumors. In those cases, limited surgery for diagnostic purposes followed by chemotherapy or radiation is undertaken. Non-surgical treatment options confer short- and long-term toxicities and sequelae, but overall prognosis of PLGG is very good. More recently, characteristic molecular signatures of PLGG have been identified that allow for use of targeted therapies as a suitable treatment option.

EPIDEMIOLOGY

The CNS is the most common cancer site among patients age 0–14 years, with an annual age-adjusted incidence rate for CNS tumors of 5.74 per 100,000 persons in the United States in 2012–2016.[2] PLGGs are the most common pediatric CNS tumors with an annual age-adjusted incidence rate of 2.1 cases per 100,000 persons. As estimated by the Central Brain Tumor Registry of the United States (CBTRUS), 1,200 new diagnoses were anticipated in 2020.[2]

> PLGGs are the most common pediatric CNS tumors with an annual age-adjusted incidence rate of 2.1 cases per 100,000 persons.

While PLGG are idiopathic in most patients, they are associated with an underlying tumor predisposition syndrome in 2–5% of cases.[3] Table 17.1 lists the most common tumor predisposition syndromes that are known to have associations with PLGG.[4] In some patients, prior radiation exposure can be a contributing factor in the development of CNS tumors. As such, moderate- to high-dose ionizing radiation (IR) is the only established environmental risk factor for brain and CNS tumors, as confirmed by studies of atomic bomb survivors and children irradiated for benign medical conditions and first primary tumors.[5] In a recent meta-analysis of radiation-induced gliomas, 9.6% of the 296 cases reviewed had low-grade gliomas after radiation therapy.[6] In contrast, other potential risk factors, including exposure to cell phones, parental exposure to pesticides, dietary elements, prenatal exposure to certain medications, and heat have all been queried but were not found to be associated with the development of brain tumors, including PLGGs.[7]

> While PLGG are idiopathic in most patients, they are associated with an underlying tumor predisposition syndrome in 2–5% of cases.

NEUROCUTANEOUS AND TUMOR PREDISPOSITION SYNDROMES

NEUROFIBROMATOSIS TYPE 1

Neurofibromatosis type 1 (NF1) is an autosomal dominant genetic disorder with an annual incidence rate of approximately 1 in 2,600–3,000 individuals. Compared to the general population, patients with NF1 are more likely to develop an intracranial neoplasm before they reach adulthood. Pilocytic astrocytomas and, to a lesser extent, diffuse astrocytomas are the most common tumors seen in NF1 patients. NF1 related

TABLE 17.1 Tumor predisposition syndromes associated with pediatric low-grade gliomas

SYNDROME	GENE MUTATION
Ataxia telangiectasia (Louis-Bar)	ATM
Beckwith Wiedemann (EMG) syndrome	CDKN1C, NSD1, H19, KCNQ1OT1
Cowden syndrome	PTEN
Dysplastic nevus syndrome	CDKN2A
Familial adenomatous polyposis	APC
Li-Fraumeni syndrome	TP53
Melanoma-astrocytoma syndrome	CDKN2A
Neurofibromatosis type1	NF1
Neurofibromatosis type 2	NF2
Noonan syndrome	PTPN11, KRAS, SOS1, BRAF
Tuberous sclerosis	TSC1, TSC2

PLGGs most often occur in the optic pathway, are estimated to occur in 15% of patients with NF1,[8] are less aggressive, and tend to have a better clinical outcome than sporadic PLGG, with several reports of spontaneous regression.[9]

Gliomagenesis in NF1 patients is frequently driven by activation of the RAS/MAPK pathway through loss of NF1 gene function. Histologically, gliomas in NF1 patients can demonstrate morphologic features similar to SEGAs in patients with tuberous sclerosis complex (TSC; discussed later), and these tumors have therefore been coined "SEGA-like astrocytomas." Recently, NF1-associated high-grade astrocytomas with co-existing alterations such as ATRX mutations and an alternative lengthening of telomeres (ALT) phenotype have been identified.[10]

TUBEROUS SCLEROSIS

TSC is an autosomal dominant genetic disorder with an incidence rate of approximately 1 in 5,000–10,000 live births. TS is associated with a germline mutation in one of two tumor suppressor genes, TSC1 (hamartin on Chr 9q34) and TSC2 (tuberin on 16p13.3). TSC1 and TSC2 are part of the TSC within the mammalian target of rapamycin (mTOR) signaling pathway.[11] SEGAs are the most common intracranial gliomas associated with TS and are seen to develop in approximately 15% of patients.[12]

The lack of tuberin (or lack of a functional tuberin-hamartin complex) results in loss of GTPase activity, which in turn causes inappropriate activation of these proteins and releases the inhibitory effect on the cell cycle. Hamartin and tuberin function together to inhibit mTOR-mediated signaling of two distinct proteins: eukaryotic initiation factor 4E-binding protein 1 (4E-BP1) and ribosomal protein S6 kinase 1 (S6K1), making TS tumors exquisitely sensitive to mTOR inhibitors.[13]

CLINICAL PRESENTATION

PLGG has similar presenting features for early adolescents, young adults, and children, with characteristic symptoms depend on location of the lesion and tumor biology.

In infants, unfused cranial sutures can accommodate rising intracranial pressure (ICP) without acutely compromising the child's neurological status but resulting in increased head circumference; hence, macrocephaly is the most common presenting symptom in this age group.[14] After fusion of cranial sutures is complete, young children often present with failure to thrive or to achieve developmental milestones. School-age children may present with developmental delay, personality changes, irritability, altered psychomotor function, apathy, and declining school performance.[15]

More than 50% of children with supratentorial tumors present with seizures, and often these are generalized tonic-clonic seizures. Children with posterior fossa tumors frequently show signs of raised intracranial pressure due to obstruction of the fourth ventricle, such as headache, papilledema, nausea, and vomiting.[7]

Furthermore, focal neurologic signs and cranial nerve deficits can be useful to localize an intracranial tumor (e.g., optic pathway lesions cause visual symptoms such as decreased visual acuity, double vision, eye deviation, proptosis, strabismus, visual field loss, or even cortical blindness). Cerebellar tumors usually cause cerebellar signs such as ataxia, dysmetria, and speech changes.[16] Suprasellar and pineal lesions affect the hypothalamus and pituitary gland causing endocrine disturbances leading to precocious puberty, growth disturbances, diabetes insipidus, and visual field changes due to compression of optic chiasm.

Of note, the neurologic findings seen in these patients can be subtle and difficult to elucidate, in particular in younger pediatric patients. Therefore, a thorough neurological exam is vital to making an early diagnosis.

RADIOLOGY

MAGNETIC RESONANCE IMAGING

Magnetic resonance imaging (MRI) is the most important imaging tool for identification and localization of any brain tumor, including PLGG. In addition, MRI characteristics can help narrow the differential diagnosis. Axial and coronal T1 sequences, both pre- and post-gadolinium contrast administration, as well as T2, fluid-attenuated inversion recovery (FLAIR), and diffusion-weighted imaging (DWI) sequences should be part of any MRI scan. In addition, advanced imaging technologies, including MR spectroscopy, perfusion weighted imaging (PWI), and functional MRI may provide some insight into the functional and biochemical properties of a tumor and may help guide management and predict prognosis.

Classic MRI appearance of a PLGG is that of a T1 iso- to hypointense and T2/FLAIR hyperintense mass as lesion that most often is not associated with enhancement after gadolinium contrast administration (see Figure 17.1). However, the

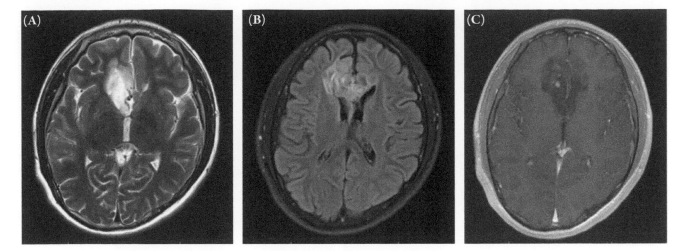

Figure 17.1 14-year-old with bifrontal low-grade glioma seen as a T2 and fluid-attenuated inversion recovery (FLAIR) hyperintense expansile intra-axial mass centered in the corpus callosum genu/rostrum extending to both sides of midline (A and B) with no gadolinium enhancement seen on T1 sequence (C).

presence or absence of enhancement is not a reliable indicator of tumor grade (e.g., many pilocytic astrocytomas can present as contrast-enhancing lesions due to the commonly found microvascular proliferation; see Figure 17.2). In the absence of contrast enhancement, FLAIR signal is useful to determine extent of tumor infiltration.[17]

MRI of spine is usually not absolutely indicated in intracranial PLGG. Solitary posterior fossa tumors are rarely associated with leptomeningeal disease although often spine imaging is undertaken at diagnosis for staging.[18]

Optic pathway gliomas tend to have a fusiform appearance and enlargement of optic nerve and chiasm. Detailed imaging of the sella in optic pathway glioma patients is necessary due to likelihood of suprasellar pituitary involvement and the potential profound impact on growth and development in these cases. FLAIR sequence in optic pathway glioma reveals an infiltrative component along the optic tracts. Children without NF1 may sporadically develop optic pathway gliomas which

tend to be more aggressive. This is reflected radiographically by more prominent evidence of infiltration on FLAIR imaging, enhancement with gadolinium contrast, and commonly associated cysts. Often, NF1 patients without evidence of optic nerve glioma are found to have extensive streaking along the optic pathway or optic nerve involvement with non-specific T2 white matter changes on surveillance imaging which do not warrant oncologic treatment (Figure 17.3). NF1 patients diagnosed with optic pathway glioma often have bilateral lesions.

Oligodendrogliomas are usually superficial cortical lesions which typically do not enhance on post-contrast MRI. Intrinsic calcifications are present in 60–90% of cases.[15] Pilocytic astrocytomas tend to be well-circumscribed lesions with associated cystic changes. Diffuse astrocytomas (WHO grade 2) are less circumscribed, infiltrative, and non-enhancing unless there is a higher-grade component to the tumor.[16]

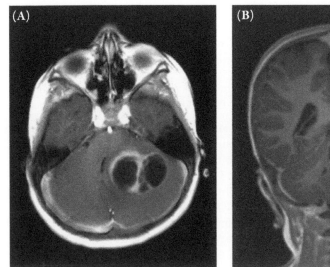
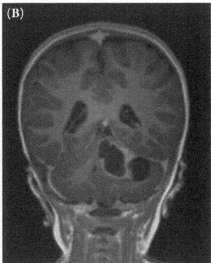
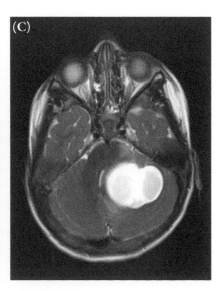

Figure 17.2 A 2-year-old with a well-circumscribed left cerebellar multiseptated cystic pilocytic astrocytoma with preoperative MRI showing gadolinium contrast enhancement on axial T1 (A) and coronal (B) sequences; T2 hyperintensity is well-visualized on axial T2 sequence (C).

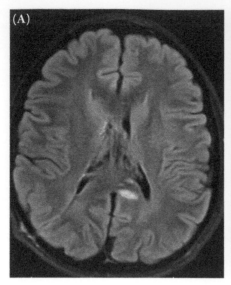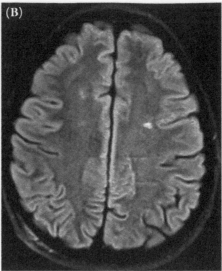

Figure 17.3 *Non-specific T2 white matter changes seen within cortex of a patient with neurofibromatosis type 1 (NF1) on routine surveillance MRI with no clinical symptoms (A and B).*

COMPUTER TOMOGRAPHY

Computerized tomography (CT), although not preferred, can identify intracranial PLGG as iso- or hypodense, non-enhancing masses. Contrast enhancement and calcifications may be seen in some PLGGs with CT imaging.

SURVEILLANCE IMAGING

According to the current standard of practice followed by most clinicians, a post-operative MRI scan is obtained within 48 hours of the surgical procedure in order to determine extent of resection. Thereafter, surveillance imaging is obtained again at 2–3 months from surgery followed by periodic imaging every 3 months to determine extent of disease, response to treatment/disease progression, and need for further treatment. In addition, MRI surveillance is useful to delineate radiation- or treatment-related changes and to differentiate these changes from tumor progression.

PATHOLOGY OF PEDIATRIC LOW-GRADE GLIOMAS

As of the 2016 edition of the WHO classification, gliomas are classified based not only on histopathologic appearance but also on well-established molecular parameters. The incorporation of molecular features has most notably impacted the classification of astrocytic and oligodendroglial tumors, which are now grouped together as diffuse gliomas on the basis of growth pattern, behavior, and shared isocitrate dehydrogenase (IDH) genetic status. The 2016 CNS WHO classification did not include any major revisions addressing PLGGs. Genetic characteristics of PLGG such as BRAF V600E status or BRAF fusion status have important diagnostic, prognostic, and therapeutic implications. Methylation profiling is a powerful tool to evaluate the epigenetic landscape of brain tumors and may be

added to histologic and genetic classification of brain tumors in the future.[1]

> Genetic characteristics of PLGG, such as BRAF V600E status or BRAF fusion status, have important diagnostic, prognostic, and therapeutic implications.

HISTOLOGY

Pilocytic astrocytomas microscopically exhibit elongated cells with long processes that form a densely fibrillary background, alternating with regions of loose and microcystic appearance. Rosenthal fibers are frequently encountered and are a useful pathologic hallmark in differentiating these tumors from other astrocytic gliomas. Additionally, microvascular proliferation is a common finding on routine hemolysin and eosin (H&E) staining of pilocytic astrocytomas. Currently, PLGG undergo robust molecular workup in addition to conventional histologic evaluation to identify potential therapeutically useful molecular characteristics.

MOLECULAR PATHOLOGY

Pilocytic astrocytomas are associated with a molecular profile that may be helpful in distinguishing these tumors from other gliomas and that may eventually provide an opportunity for targeted therapy. Pilocytic astrocytomas often have a tandem duplication of chromosome 7q34, which is associated with a KIAA1549-BRAF fusion gene (Figure 17.4).

Alterations in BRAF component of the Ras-Raf-MEK pathway characterize specific subsets of gliomas.

KIAA1549-BRAF fusion: Tandem duplication of chromosome 7q34 with subsequent fusion of the BRAF and KIAA1549 genes is observed in 60–80% of sporadic pilocytic astrocytomas.[19] A FISH probe can demonstrate duplication at 7q34, and this technique is most often used to confirm evidence of KIAA1549-BRAF fusion. Reverse-transcription polymerase chain reaction (RT-PCR) can detect 96% of BRAF fusions; the most common fusion is between exon 16 of *KIAA1549* and exon 9 of *BRAF* (63%), with less common fusion variants including exon 15-exon 9 (23%) and exon 16-exon 11 (10%).[20] However, polymerase chain reaction (PCR) can still miss a large number of different combinations of KIAA1549 and BRAF exons involved in the duplication.

BRAF V600E mutation: V600E point mutations in the BRAF gene are present in numerous PLGGs, including 10% of pilocytic astrocytomas.[21] BRAF V600E mutation is easily identified by immunohistochemistry using a specific antibody. BRAF V600E can also be detected by sequencing. In PLGG, presence of BRAF V600E poses an increased risk of recurrence after standard therapy, particularly when seen in combination with CDKN2A deletion.[22]

RAS-RAF-MAP KINASE PATHWAY

The Ras-Raf-MEK pathway is a chain of proteins in the cell that communicates a signal from a receptor on the surface of the cell to the DNA in the nucleus of the cell. When a signaling molecule binds to the receptor on the cell surface, there is a downstream effect that causes the DNA in the nucleus to express a protein and produce some change in the cell, namely cell division. The Ras-Raf-MEK pathway includes proteins including mitogen-activated protein kinases (MAPK) which play a role in protein phosphorylation, which in turn has a promoting or hindering effect on cell division. A mutation in the pathway proteins can present an imbalance between cell proliferation and apoptosis,

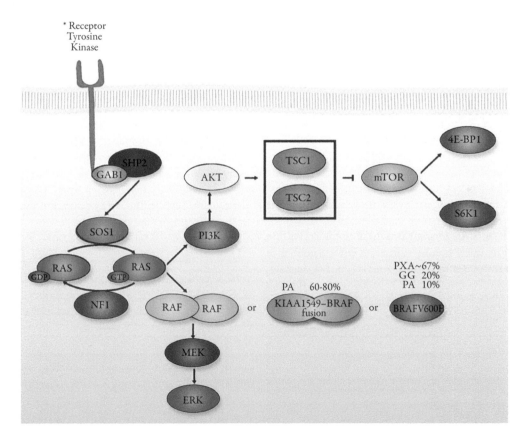

Figure 17.4 *Schematic diagram of the intracellular RAS/RAF/MAPK and the PI3K pathways in pediatric low-grade glioma (PLGG). Growth factor stimulated receptor tyrosine kinases (RTKs) phosphorylation results in RAS activation. This leads to phosphorylation of RAF and PI3K. Phosphorylated RAF activates MAPK kinases/extracellular signal-regulated kinases (MEK), which in turn phosphorylates and activates ERK. Activation of ERK regulates both cytosolic proteins and transcription factors involved in cell cycle progression and tumor survival. BRAFV600E point mutation and BRAF-KIAA1549 are the most common RAF mutations in PLGG, and their incidence is shown here. On the other hand, PI3K phosphorylation activates AKT, which controls transcriptional activity and cellular growth and survival. The signal proceeds through the tuberous sclerosis complex (TSC) and mammalian target of rapamycin (mTOR), primarily affecting protein synthesis. Mutations in several RTKs including fibroblast growth factor receptor 1/2 (FGFR1/2), neurotrophic tyrosine receptor kinase (NTRK), platelet derived growth factor receptor A (PDGFRA), anaplastic lymphoma kinase (ALK), orphan tyrosine kinase receptor (ROS 1), and MET fusions are being documented but with limited clinical significance.*

Abbreviations: 4E-BP1, eukaryotic initiation factor 4E binding protein 1; AKT, serine-threonine protein kinase; ERK, extracellular signal-regulated kinase; GAB1, GRB2-associated binding protein 1; GAP, GTPase activating protein; GG, ganglioglioma; MEK, MAPK kinases/extracellular-signal-regulated kinases; mTOR, mammalian target of Rapamycin; NF1, neurofibromatosis type 1; PA, pilocytic astrocytoma; PI3K, phosphatidylinositol-3-kinase; PXA, pleomorphic xanthoastrocytoma; RAF, rapidly accelerated fibrosarcoma; S6K1, ribosomal protein S6 kinase 70 kDa polypeptide 1; SHP2, SH2-domain-containing protein tyrosine phosphatase-2; SOS1, son of sevenless; TSC1, tuberous sclerosis complex 1; TSC2, tuberous sclerosis complex 2.

Figure courtesy of Daniel Muldoon.

which is the hallmark of all cancer cells. Increasing insights into molecular biology has revealed that a majority of PLGGs are driven by a single genetic event resulting in up-regulation of the Ras-Raf-MEK pathway. It is now well known that 10–15% of patients with NF1 develop PLGG, and a majority of these tumors harbor alterations in the Ras-Raf-MEK pathway.[23] In fact, recent molecular profiling efforts have uncovered that PLGGs are almost exclusively associated with a single abnormality of the MAPK pathway leading to the terminology one-pathway disease.[24] Recent recommendations have suggested analyzing biopsy specimens of presumed gliomas in individuals with NF1 for immunohistochemical assessment of ATRX and CDKN2A/B.[25] The LANDING (genomic LANDscape in NF1-mutant Glioma) Consortium throws light on the loss-of-function genetic alterations of ATRX, CDKN2A, and TP53 and their implications in different age groups within the NF1 population.[26]

> Ten to fifteen percent of patient with NF 1 develop PLGGs, and a majority of these tumors harbor alterations in the Ras-Raf-MEK pathway.

PI3-KINASE-AKT-MTOR PATHWAY

The PI3K/AKT/mTOR pathway is another intracellular signaling pathway important in regulating the cell cycle and often implicated in PLGG. It is directly related to maintenance of cellular quiescence and replication, in turn related to cancer and cell longevity. PI3K activation leads to phosphorylation and activation of the AKT molecule within the plasma membrane, which in turn has a number of downstream effects, the most important of which is the activation of mTOR. There are many factors that are known to enhance the PI3K/AKT pathway including EGF, SHH, IGF-1, insulin, and CAM. The pathway is antagonized by various factors including PTEN, GSK3B, and HB9. This pathway is necessary to promote maintenance of neural stem cells. In many PLGGs, this pathway is overactive, thus reducing apoptosis and allowing proliferation.[27]

> In many PLGGs, the PI3K/AKT/mTOR pathway is overactive, thus reducing apoptosis and allowing proliferation.

Activation of mTOR protein kinase in turn regulates protein synthesis, cell growth, and proliferation. There are two distinct mTOR complexes, mTORC1 and mTORC2. mTORC1 plays a role in relaying signals following PI3K-AKT activation, while the mTORC2 complex leads to the phosphorylation of AKT on serine 473. AKT phosphorylation in known to play an important role in the aggressiveness of many cancers, especially PLGG. The PI3K-AKT-mTOR pathway has important prognostic and treatment implications.[28] It is now well known that mTORC1 is strongly inhibited by rapamycin while mTORC2 is less affected by this drug.

TREATMENT OF PEDIATRIC LOW-GRADE GLIOMAS

SURGICAL OPTIONS

Surgery is curative therapy for PLGGs in areas of the brain amenable to complete resection. However, when LGGs are located in areas where complete resection is not possible, they can impact life expectancy and quality of life. These tumors can often be thought of as a chronic disease, and treatment after biopsy or subtotal resection is recommended.

CHEMOTHERAPY

The currently best available data with regards to a chemotherapy approach for patients with PLGGs are derived from a randomized study conducted by the Children's Oncology Group (COG) This study compared two chemotherapy regimens in 274 children younger than 10 years for whom tumor resection was contraindicated and radiotherapy (RT) was considered high-risk for neurodevelopmental injury. Patients were randomly assigned to receive carboplatin and vincristine (CV) or thioguanine, procarbazine, lomustine, and vincristine (TPCV). The overall survival (OS) at 5 years was comparable in both groups (86% in CV and 87% in TPCV). While the 5-year event-free survival (EFS) rate appeared lower in the CV (39 ± 4%) compared to the TPCV group (52 ± 5%), this difference did not reach statistical significance. Toxicity was slightly worse with TPCV.[29] Because of the increased toxicity seen with TPCV and because of the risk for infertility and secondary malignancies associated with alkylating chemotherapy agents, most oncologists favor CV over TPCV as first-line chemotherapy.[30] Of note, the risk of secondary malignancies from use of alkylating agent is particularly high in the NF1 population due to a germline loss of the NF1 tumor suppressor gene.

> Because of the increased toxicity seen with TPCV and because of the risk for infertility and secondary malignancies associated with alkylating chemotherapy agents, most oncologists favor CV over TPCV as first-line chemotherapy.

More recently, a retrospective analysis of monthly single-agent carboplatin showed comparable efficacy to historical multiagent chemotherapy for the treatment of patients with unresectable PLGG. Equivalent outcomes were achieved with less chemotherapy, reduced side effects, and fewer hospital visits.[31]

Furthermore, monotherapy with temozolomide, vinblastine, or cyclophosphamide has been evaluated in phase II studies, although with mixed results.[30] Phase II studies examining the efficacy of these single-agent therapies are hampered by slow accrual. Therefore, the generalized use of these agents as first-line therapy cannot be recommended.

RADIOTHERAPY

Historically, RT was considered the treatment of choice for unresectable, progressive PLGG with an expected 10-year progression-free survival (PFS) and OS rates of approximately 70% and 80%, respectively.[32] However, RT has been associated with toxicities including second malignancy, cerebral vasculopathy, neurocognitive deficits, and endocrine dysfunction.[33] Several studies have reported particularly worse outcomes in children who received RT prior to age 10. A large retrospective evaluation of adult patients who received up-front RT for PLGG as children revealed a worse OS and greater risk of disease-associated death compared to those who were not treated with radiation therapy.[34]

Yet these toxicities are overshadowed by the need for treatment options in deep-seated tumors not amenable to resection and not responsive to systemic therapy, including chemotherapy or targeted therapy. Additionally, advances in three-dimensional radiation planning and proton beam RT may allow for highly conformal delivery of radiation with relative sparing of normal adjacent brain tissue. Two important studies have therefore demonstrated the efficacy of highly conformal RT for PLGGs either as up-front therapy or salvage therapy with comparable outcomes. A prospective study conducted at Dana-Farber Cancer Institute evaluated conformal RT for newly diagnosed, biopsy-confirmed PLGG and demonstrated 5-year PFS of 82.5% and OS of 97.5%.[35] A phase II study of conformal RT at St. Jude Children's Research Hospital conducted in children with progressive PLGG showed 5-year PFS of 87% and OS of 96%.[36] However, Merchant et al. reported cognitive effects to be inversely correlated with age by observing a steeper decline in IQ in younger children. Therefore, there is an overall shift toward avoiding radiation therapy in younger patients, especially in those younger than 15 years. In general, PLGGs most often do not progress rapidly after surgery, and, therefore, radiation can be reserved and is typically used as salvage for aggressive cases. Usually, a dose of 50–54 Gy with a margin of 1 cm margin or less is typically considered the upper limit of the radiation dose used in PLGG.

> PLGGs most often do not progress rapidly after surgery, and, therefore, radiation can be reserved, particularly in those younger than 15 years of age and is typically used as salvage for aggressive cases.

TARGETED THERAPIES

BRAF INHIBITORS

First-generation BRAFV600E inhibitors such as dabrafenib and vemurafenib have been proven to show excellent results in melanoma patients harboring the BRAF V600E mutation. These agents have been investigated in PLGG by way of a phase I multicenter trial which noted an initial impressive response rate of 41%.[37] A follow-up trial optimizing the dosing safety and tolerability is currently under way (NCT01677741). It is now well known that despite their efficacy in BRAF V600E tumors, first-generation BRAF inhibitors are associated with a paradoxical activation of RAS/MAPK signaling when used as monotherapy

in KIAA1549-BRAF or BRAF wildtype tumors.[38] This was in fact demonstrated clinically when a clinical trial using the BRAF inhibitor sorafenib in unselected PLGGs showed rapid increased growth in patients harboring KIAA1549-BRAF fusions.[39] A current phase II multicenter open-label trial is investigating the role of concomitant use of the BRAF inhibitor dabrafenib and MEK inhibitor trametinib to limit this paradoxical RAS/MAPK activation.[40] There is a need for careful molecular characterization of PLGGs to assist therapeutic decision-making.[23]

> First-generation BRAF inhibitors are associated with a paradoxical activation of RAS/MAPK signaling when used as monotherapy in KIAA1549-BRAF or BRAF wildtype tumors, leading to rapid increased tumor growth.

MEK INHIBITORS

MEK inhibitors are emerging as a promising therapeutic strategy for PLGGs especially those that are resistant to treatment with cytotoxic chemotherapy and also as a first-line approach in those that are known to have a KIAA1549-BRAF fusion. Currently, the clinical utility of four MEK inhibitors—selumetinib, trametinib, cobimetinib, and binimetinib—has been or is being assessed in both NF1-associated and non–NF1-associated tumors. Selumetinib has demonstrated an impressive response in phase I and II trials. The phase I study focused on NF1-associated as well as sporadic and treatment-refractory PLGG and showed tumor stability or reduction in 32 out of 38 patients (84%).[41] A phase II study investigating selumetinib in recurrent NF1-associated PLGG exhibited similar results, with 40% of patients achieving a partial response to treatment and only one patient progressing while on treatment.[42] Similar trials using other MEK inhibitors are currently under way. Rash is the most common side effect from MEK inhibitors, with rare reports of serious ocular or cardiac toxicities. Due to encouraging results in phase II trials with selumetinib for recurrent PLGG, a randomized, up-front trial comparing carboplatin/vincristine with selumetinib is currently under way, both in those patients with NF1 (NCT03871257) and in patients with sporadic PLGG (NCT04166409).

> Currently, the clinical utility of four MEK inhibitors—selumetinib, trametinib, cobimetinib, and binimetinib—has been or is being assessed in both NF1-associated and non–NF1-associated tumors.

OTHER AGENTS

Alterations in FGFR1, ALK, ROS1, and NTRK are relatively rare in PLGG. Agents targeting these pathways have been used in smaller cohorts of glioma patients. There are ongoing trials investigating the utility of FGFR1 inhibitors (e.g., AZD4547 [NCT02824133]) as well as TRK inhibitors (NCT02637687, NCT02576431). There is an ongoing phase I/Ib study being conducted in pediatrics to evaluate NTRK inhibitor entrectinib in primary CNS tumors.[43]

TOXICITIES AND FOLLOW-UP

While PLGGs in general are associated with excellent survival outcomes and studies have reported on 5-year survival outcomes close to 90% at 5 years. Nevertheless, there are many short- and long-term treatment-related implications that patients, families, and oncologists need to bear in mind when deciding on treatment strategies.[44] Cognitive and social disabilities are important long-term consequences seen in nearly half of the patients treated for PLGG.[45]

SURGICAL TOXICITY

Surgery-related toxicity for cerebellar and cerebral lesions include intellectual disability and difficulties with adaptive behavior.[46] Left hemispheric lesions can cause more postoperative difficulties likely due to associated problems with language function.[47]

TOXICITY DUE TO CHEMOTHERAPY AND OTHER MEDICAL THERAPY

Multiple chemotherapeutic treatment regimens are associated with various short- and long-term morbidities. Peripheral neuropathy is a well-known toxicity of vincristine, while platinum compounds like carboplatin and cisplatin are notorious for causing significant ototoxicity. As previously discussed, cytotoxic agents like procarbazine and lomustine pose a significant risk of secondary hematologic cancers especially in the NF1 patient population.[48] Cisplatin and etoposide are well-known to be associated with secondary malignancies.

RADIATION-ASSOCIATED TOXICITY

Due to the well-recognized long-term neurotoxicities associated with RT, cranial irradiation is avoided as much as possible. Radiation-associated toxicity includes impairment of executive functioning, behavioral problems, difficulties with visuospatial skills and expressive language, and verbal memory deficits. Long-term neurocognitive deficits are clearly associated with higher radiation dose and volume.[49] Neurovascular disease due to vascular injury, endothelial proliferation, and loss of structural integrity of the neural vascular ecosystem are other important toxicities associated with radiation. However, it is worth mentioning that tumor location and associated tumor-related symptoms are important confounding factors for the development and magnitude of radiation associated long-term disability.[50] Additionally, treatment with radiation at a younger age is more likely to be associated with a higher drop in IQ than radiation at an older age. One study suggested that up to 34% of long-term survivors of PLGG have an IQ below average. This was associated with younger age of diagnosis, epilepsy, and shunt placement. Long-term toxicity continues to become more apparent after the 5-year survival time point.[51]

OTHER TOXICITIES

Endocrine abnormalities and hypothalamic dysfunction are common for midline PLGGs and those that are located in the diencephalic region. These have been described repeatedly in the literature, and it is unclear whether they are related to location of tumor, surgery-related anatomic disruption, or adverse effects of chemotherapy and radiation.[52] A unique and rare entity called *diencephalic syndrome* is potentially fatal and characterized by extreme cachexia and failure to thrive despite adequate calorie intake. Other well-known long-term sequelae related to PLGGs and their therapies are visual impairment, pituitary dysfunction, obesity, motor deficits, cerebellar signs, and seizures, as well as psychologic and psychiatric disorders.[53]

Thorough neuropsychological testing prior to and following treatment is essential in all pediatric patients with CNS tumors to identify areas of need. Multidisciplinary follow-up through adulthood, psychosocial support, and access to adequate resources may be needed to improve quality of life in the setting of multiple of intellectual, physical, and emotional challenges commonly encountered in PLGG survivors.

CONCLUSION

In conclusion, PLGGs are a heterogenous group of pediatric tumors with overall favorable prognosis. Although complete resection is the best curative option, tumor location may not always be amenable to surgery. Increasing knowledge of molecular characteristics of PLGGs is allowing for application of targeted treatment in lieu of cytotoxic chemotherapy. Radiation therapy remains an important treatment option although reserved for recurrent or progressive PLGGs due to the long-term neurocognitive consequences for the pediatric population. The general approach for treatment of PLGG remains very targeted therapy, be it surgical or medical, with a shift toward avoiding radiation therapy to mitigate long-term toxicity.

FLASHCARD

What are the most common CNS tumors in children 0–19 years old?	Pilocytic astrocytoma, WHO grade 1
What is the annual incidence of PLGGs?	2.1 per 100,000 in the United States
Underlying tumor predisposition syndrome is seen in this percentage of cases of pediatric LGGs	2–5%
What is the most common intracranial neoplasm in patients with NF1?	Optic glioma
Subependymal giant cell astrocytomas, harboring mTOR signal pathway aberrations, occur in what percentage of patients with tuberous sclerosis?	15%
Most PLGG are non-enhancing, with exception of this tumor which can enhance when microvascular proliferation is present	Pilocytic astrocytoma
This is a common distinguishing histopathologic feature of pilocytic astrocytomas	Rosenthal fibers
These molecular aberrations are commonly observed in pilocytic astrocytomas (60–80%)	Tandem duplication of chromosome 7q34 with subsequent fusion of the BRAF and KIAA1549 genes
Presence of BRAFV600E point mutation is associated with what prognostically?	Increased risk of recurrence after standard therapy
Majority of PLGGs are driven by a single genetic event resulting in up-regulation of this pathway.	Ras-Raf-MEK pathway; though the PI3K/AKT/mTOR pathway is another important intracellular signaling pathway in PLGG
What is the most common chemotherapies given for PLGG, when needed?	Carboplatin plus vincristine, due to significant risk of secondary malignancies with alkylating agents
What treatment is usually reserved as salvage for aggressive cases of PLGG?	Radiation

1. A 12-year-old boy with a history of ataxia and nystagmus was found to have a well-circumscribed, non-enhancing, posterior fossa tumor with cystic component. Patient underwent a complete resection of the tumor and pathology confirmed a WHO grade 1 pilocytic astrocytoma of the cerebellum. What is the appropriate management for this patient?
   a. Spine MRI and lumbar puncture for CSF cytopathology
   b. Conformational radiation therapy to posterior fossa
   c. Observation with interval exam and MRI brain every 3–6 months.
   d. Craniospinal radiation with adjuvant chemotherapy

2. An 8-year-old girl is followed by her pediatrician for findings of several café-au-lait macules and learning disability with a diagnosis of sporadic NF1. She recently started to complain of decreased vision in both eyes for the past 2 months. She was referred to you for further management. What is the next best step?
   a. Refer to neurosurgery
   b. Refer to ophthalmology and obtain MRI brain and orbits
   c. Refer to dermatology for skin biopsy
   d. Refer to developmental pediatrics

3. A 6-year-old boy is noted to have right-sided sixth and seventh nerve palsies on a routine annual exam. Family further reports some ataxia, dysphagia, and clumsiness due to left-sided weakness over the last 3–4 months. An MRI reveals an exophytic, contrast-enhancing mass approximating the brainstem, not involving the basilar artery and pushing the pons to the side. What is the likely diagnosis?
   a. High-grade astrocytoma
   b. High-grade midline glioma
   c. Pilocytic astrocytoma
   d. Ependymoma

4. A 12-year-old girl with a diagnosis of tuberous sclerosis recently started complaining of headaches associated with nausea and early morning vomiting. An MRI brain reveals a mass at the level of foramen of Monroe with evidence of obstructive hydrocephalus. What is the most likely diagnosis?
   a. Dysembryoplastic neuroepithelial tumor (DNET)
   b. Primitive neuroepithelial tumor (PNET)
   c. Subependymal giant cell astrocytoma (SEGA)
   d. Benign hamartoma

5. An 11-year-old boy with familial NF1 recently had a disease surveillance MRI showing optic pathway enhancement without thickening of optic nerves. Ophthalmology evaluation does not identify any visual deficits, and the patient is visually asymptomatic. What is the best management approach?
   a. Biopsy of tumor to obtain a pathological diagnosis
   b. Close ophthalmology follow-up with interval imaging
   c. Full-body MRI to identify other tumors
   d. Referral for initiation of radiation therapy

6. Identify the incorrect pair:
   a. Gorlin's syndrome—Ependymoma
   b. NF1—Optic pathway glioma
   c. Tuberous sclerosis—Subependymal giant cell astrocytoma
   d. Li Fraumeni syndrome—Choroid plexus carcinoma

7. A 14-year-old girl with tuberous sclerosis with known fourth ventricular subependymal giant cell astrocytoma presents with increased seizure frequency. MRI reveals three additional ventricular nodules with heterogenous appearance. She underwent partial resection of the fourth ventricular tumor with ventriculoperitoneal shunt placement 2 years ago. Family is inquiring about treatment options. What will be your recommendation?
   a. Surgical resection of residual SEGA
   b. Targeted therapy with mTOR inhibitor
   c. Optimize antiseizure medication doses
   d. Close observation with periodic MRI scans

8. An 11-year-old boy with slowly worsening ataxia noted over the past 6 months is found to have a cerebellar tumor that is non-enhancing on MRI with a cystic component. The tumor is resected and pathology confirms a low-grade glioma. What is the most likely molecular event?
   a. KIAA1549-BRAF
   b. C-Myc overexpression
   c. Bcl-2 deletion or loss of heterozygosity (LOH)
   d. Trk-C overexpression

9. With respect to PLGGs, IHC can be reliably utilized in the detection of which clinically relevant molecular finding?
   a. FGFR1
   b. CDKN2A deletion
   c. BRAF p.V600E
   d. KIAA1549: BRAF fusion

10. An 8-year-old boy with a history of cervico-medullary exophytic mass that was partially resected 6 months ago presents with significant tumor progression over the past 3 months. Pathology confirmed a pilocytic astrocytoma with IHC positive for BRAF p.V600E. Based on existing data, what would you recommend as front-line adjuvant therapy at this time?
    a. Conventional chemotherapy with carboplatin, vincristine
    b. Targeted therapy with MEK inhibitor
    c. Targeted therapy with FGFR1 inhibitor
    d. Targeted therapy with BRAF inhibitor

11. A 2-year-old boy presents with nystagmus ongoing for 6 months. An MRI reveals a large optic pathway glioma which was partially resected. Diagnosis of pilocytic astrocytoma is made; the tumor is positive for KIAA1549-BRAF fusion. Patient had tumor progression after 3 months of adjuvant treatment with carboplatin/vincristine. What is the next best treatment option?
    a. MEK inhibitor
    b. FGFR1 inhibitor
    c. mTOR inhibitor
    d. NTRK inhibitor

12. Which of the following have been linked with development of low-grade glioma in children?
    a. Exposure to HSV infection in utero
    b. Maternal folate intake during pregnancy
    c. Prior cranial irradiation
    d. Head trauma

13. Tuberous sclerosis complex is associated with activation of which of the following intracellular signaling molecules?
    a. MAPK
    b. mTOR
    c. BRAF
    d. EGFR

14. Neurofibromatosis type 1 is associated with activation of which intracellular signaling pathway?
    a. NF-kB
    b. RAS/MEK/MAPK
    c. Notch
    d. WNT

15. A 3-year-old child presents to your clinic with proptosis and poor vision in the left eye. An MRI reveals an enhancing, expansile mass of the intraorbital left optic nerve. Skin exam reveals multiple café-au-lait lesions. What is the most likely clinical syndrome?
    a. Li-Fraumeni syndrome
    b. Tuberous sclerosis complex
    c. Neurofibromatosis type 1
    d. Cowden syndrome

ANSWERS

1. c
2. b
3. c
4. c
5. b
6. a
7. b
8. a
9. c
10. a
11. a
12. c
13. b
14. b
15. c

REFERENCES

1. Louis DN, Perry A, Wesseling P, et al. The 2021 WHO Classification of Tumors of the Central Nervous System: a summary. *Neuro Oncol.* 2021 Aug 2;23(8):1231–1251. doi: 10.1093/neuonc/noab106. PMID: 34185076; PMCID: PMC8328013.
2. Ostrom QT, Cioffi G, Gittleman H, et al. CBTRUS Statistical Report: Primary brain and other central nervous system tumors diagnosed in the United States in 2012–2016. *Neuro-Oncology.* October 2019. https://doi-org.ezproxy.med.nyu.edu/10.1093/neuonc/noz150
3. Halperin EC, Wazer DE, Perez CA. *Perez and Brady's Principles and Practice of Radiation Oncology.* 6th ed. Philadelphia: Lippincott Williams & Wilkins; 2013.
4. Bleeker FE, Hopman SM, Merks JH, et al. Brain tumors and syndromes in children. *Neuropediatrics.* 2014 Jun;45(3):137–161. doi:10.1055/s-0034-1368116
5. Braganza MZ, Kitahara CM, Berrington de González A, et al. Ionizing radiation and the risk of brain and central nervous system tumors: A systematic review. *Neuro Oncol.* 2012;14(11):1316–1324. doi:10.1093/neuonc/nos208
6. Yamanaka R, Hayano A, Kanayama T. Radiation-induced gliomas: A comprehensive review and meta-analysis. *Neurosurg Rev.* 2018;41(3):719–731. doi:10.1007/s10143-016-0786-8. Epub 2016 Oct 5.
7. Dulac O, Lassonde M, Sarnat H, eds. Pediatric neurology, part II. In *Handbook of Clinical Neurology* (vol. 112). Amsterdam: Elsevier; 2013.
8. Levin MH, Armstrong GT, Broad JH, et al. Risk of optic pathway glioma in children with neurofibromatosis type 1 and optic nerve tortuosity or nerve sheath thickening *Br J Ophthalmol.* 2016;100:510–514.
9. Rodriguez FJ, Perry A, Gutmann DH, et al. Gliomas in neurofibromatosis type 1: A clinicopathologic study of 100 patients. *J Neuropathol Exp Neurol.* 2008;67(3):240–249. doi:10.1097/NEN.0b013e318165eb75
10. Nix JS, Blakeley J, Rodriguez FJ. An update on the central nervous system manifestations of neurofibromatosis type 1. *Acta Neuropathol.* 2020;139:625–641. https://doi.org/10.1007/s00401-019-02002-2
11. Randle SC. Tuberous sclerosis complex: A review. *Pediatr Ann.* 2017 Apr 1;46(4):e166–e171. doi:10.3928/19382359-20170320-01
12. Hargrave D. Pediatric high and low grade glioma: The impact of tumor biology on current and future therapy. *Br J Neurosurg.* 2009, 23(4):351–363.
13. Tee AR, Fingar DC, Manning BD, et al. Tuberous sclerosis complex-1 and -2 gene products function together to inhibit mammalian target of rapamycin (mTOR)-mediated downstream signaling. *Proc Natl Acad Sci U S A.* 2002;99(21):13571–13576. doi:10.1073/pnas.202476899
14. Wilne S, Collier J, Kennedy C, et al. Presentation of childhood CNS tumours: A systematic review and meta-analysis. *Lancet Oncol.* 2007 Aug;8(8):685–695.
15. Gupta N, Banerjee A, Haas-Kogen D. *Pediatric CNS Tumors.* New York: Springer; 2004.
16. Sievert AJ, Fisher MJ. Pediatric low-grade gliomas. *J Child Neurol.* 2009;24(11):1397–1408. doi:10.1177/0883073809342005
17. Alkonyi B, Nowak J, Gnekow AK, et al. Differential imaging characteristics and dissemination potential of pilomyxoid astrocytomas versus pilocytic astrocytomas. *Euroradiology.* 2015 Jun;57(6):625–638. doi:10.1007/s00234-015-1498-4
18. Roth J, Fischer N, Limbrick DD, et al. The role of screening spinal MRI in children with solitary posterior fossa low-grade glial tumors. *J Neurosurg Pediatr.* 2019 Nov 15:1–5. doi:10.3171/2019.9.PEDS19358
19. Jones DT, Kocialkowski S, Liu L, et al. Tandem duplication producing a novel oncogenic BRAF fusion gene defines the majority of pilocytic astrocytomas. *Cancer Res.* 2008;68(21):8673–8677. doi:10.1158/0008-5472.CAN-08-2097
20. Faulkner C, Ellis HP, Shaw A, et al. BRAF fusion analysis in pilocytic astrocytomas: KIAA1549-BRAF 15-9 fusions are more frequent in the midline than within the cerebellum. *J Neuropathol Exp Neurol.* 2015;74(9):867–872. doi:10.1097/NEN.0000000000000226
21. Dougherty MJ, Santi M, Brose MS, et al. Activating mutations in BRAF characterize a spectrum of pediatric low-grade gliomas. *Neuro Oncol.* 2010;12(7):621–630. doi:10.1093/neuonc/noq007
22. Lassaletta A, Zapotocky M, Mistry M, et al. Therapeutic and prognostic implications of BRAF V600E in pediatric low-grade gliomas. *J Clin Oncol.* 2017;35(25):2934–2941. doi:10.1200/JCO.2016.71.8726

23. Ryall S, Tabori U, Hawkins C. Pediatric low-grade glioma in the era of molecular diagnostics. *Acta Neuropathol Commun.* 2020;8(1):30. doi:10.1186/s40478-020-00902-z

24. Collins VP, Jones DT, Giannini C. Pilocytic astrocytoma: Pathology, molecular mechanisms and markers. *Acta Neuropathol.* 2015 Jun;129(6):775–788. doi:10.1007/s00401-015-1410-7. Epub 2015 Mar 20.

25. Packer RJ, Iavarone A, Jones DTW, et al. Implications of new understandings of gliomas in children and adults with NF1: Report of a Consensus Conference, Neuro-Oncology, 2020. https://doi.org/10.1093/neuonc/noaa036

26. D'Angelo F, Ceccarelli M, Tala, et al. The molecular landscape of glioma in patients with neurofibromatosis 1. *Nat Med.* 2019;25(1):176–187. doi:10.1038/s41591-018-0263-8

27. Santarpia L, Lippman SM, El-Naggar AK. Targeting the MAPK-RAS-RAF signaling pathway in cancer therapy. *Expert Opin Ther Targets.* 2012;16(1):103–119. doi:10.1517/14728222.2011.645805

28. Rodriguez EF, Scheithauer BW, Giannini C, et al. PI3K/AKT pathway alterations are associated with clinically aggressive and histologically anaplastic subsets of pilocytic astrocytoma. *Acta Neuropathol.* 2011;121(3):407–420. doi:10.1007/s00401-010-0784-9

29. Ater JL, Zhou T, Holmes E, et al. Randomized study of two chemotherapy regimens for treatment of low-grade glioma in young children: A report from the Children's Oncology Group. *J Clin Oncol.* 2012 Jul 20;30(21):2641–2647. doi:10.1200/JCO.2011.36.6054

30. Bergthold G, Bandopadhayay P, Bi WL, et al. Pediatric low-grade gliomas: How modern biology reshapes the clinical field. *Biochim Biophys Acta.* 2014;1845(2):294–307. doi:10.1016/j.bbcan.2014.02.004

31. Dodgshun A, Hansford J, Sullivan M. LG-15: Risk assessment in paediatric glioma: Time to move on from the binary classification. *Neuro Oncol.* 2016;18(Suppl 3):iii81. doi:10.1093/neuonc/now075.15

32. Jahraus CD, Tarbell N. Optic pathway gliomas. *Ped Blood Cancer.* 2006;46(5):586–596. https://doi.org/10.1002/pbc.20655

33. Packer RJ, Sutton LN, Atkins TE, et al. A prospective study of cognitive function in children receiving whole-brain radiotherapy and chemotherapy: 2-year results. *J Neurosurg.* 1989 May;70(5):707–713.

34. Bandopadhayay P, Bergthold G, London WB, et al. Long-term outcome of 4,040 children diagnosed with pediatric low-grade gliomas: An analysis of the Surveillance Epidemiology and End Results (SEER) database. *Pediatr Blood Cancer.* 2014 Jul;61(7):1173–1179. doi:10.1002/pbc.24958

35. Marcus KJ, Goumnerova L, Billett AL, et al. Stereotactic radiotherapy for localized low-grade gliomas in children: Final results of a prospective trial. *Int J Radiat Oncol Biol Phy.* 2005;61(2):374–379. https://doi.org/10.1016/j.ijrobp.2004.06.012

36. Merchant TE, Conklin HM, Wu S, et al. Late effects of conformal radiation therapy for pediatric patients with low-grade glioma: Prospective evaluation of cognitive, endocrine, and hearing deficits. *J Clin Oncol.* 2009;27(22):3691–3697. doi:10.1200/JCO.2008.21.2738

37. Kieran MW, Sun Y, Pilarz C, et al. LG-47: Type II RAF inhibitors inhibit BRAF mutations and truncated fusions in pediatric low-grade gliomas. *Neuro Oncol.* 2016;18(Suppl 3):iii89. doi:10.1093/neuonc/now075.47

38. Sievert AJ, Lang SS, Boucher KL, et al. Paradoxical activation and RAF inhibitor resistance of BRAF protein kinase fusions characterizing pediatric astrocytomas [published correction appears in *Proc Natl Acad Sci U S A.* 2013 May 21;110(21):8750. *Proc Natl Acad Sci U S A.* 2013;110(15):5957–5962. doi:10.1073/pnas.1219232110

39. Karajannis MA, Legault G, Fisher MJ, et al. Phase II study of sorafenib in children with recurrent or progressive low-grade astrocytomas. *Neuro Oncol.* 2014;16(10):1408–1416. doi:10.1093/neuonc/nou059

40. Ryall S, Zapotocky M, Fukuoka K, et al. Integrated molecular and clinical analysis of 1,000 pediatric low-grade gliomas. *Cancer Cell.* 2020 Apr 13;37(4):569–583.e5. doi:10.1016/j.ccell.2020.03.011

41. Banerjee A, Jakacki RI, Onar-Thomas A, et al. A phase I trial of the MEK inhibitor selumetinib (AZD6244) in pediatric patients with recurrent or refractory low-grade glioma: A Pediatric Brain Tumor Consortium (PBTC) study. *Neuro Oncol.* 2017;19(8):1135–1144. doi:10.1093/neuonc/now282

42. Fangusaro JR, Onar-Thomas A, Poussaint TY, et al. LTBK-01: Updates on the phase II and re-treatment study of AZD6244 (selumetinib) for children with recurrent or refractory pediatric low grade glioma: A Pediatric Brain Tumor Consortium (PBTC) study. *Neuro Oncol.* 2018;20(Suppl 2):i214. doi:10.1093/neuonc/noy109

43. Drilon A, Siena S, Ou SI, et al. Safety and antitumor activity of the multitargeted pan-TRK, ROS1, and ALK inhibitor entrectinib: Combined results from two phase I Trials (ALKA-372-001 and STARTRK-1). *Cancer Discov.* 2017;7(4):400–409. doi:10.1158/2159-8290.CD-16-1237

44. Wisoff JH, Sanford RA, Heier LA, et al. Primary neurosurgery for pediatric low-grade gliomas: A prospective multi-institutional study from the Children's Oncology Group. *Neurosurgery.* 2011;68(6):1548–1555. https://doi.org/10.1227/NEU.0b013e318214a66e

45. Aarsen FK, Paquier PF, Reddingius RE, et al. Functional outcome after low-grade astrocytoma treatment in childhood. *Cancer.* 2006 Jan 15;106(2):396–402.

46. Pollack IF. Multidisciplinary management of childhood brain tumors: A review of outcomes, recent advances, and challenges. *J Neurosurg Pediatr.* 2011 Aug;8(2):135–418. doi:10.3171/2011.5.PEDS1178

47. Roncadin, C, Dennis, M, Greenberg, ML, et al. Adverse medical events associated with childhood cerebellar astrocytomas and medulloblastomas: Natural history and relation to very long-term neurobehavioral outcome. *Childs Nerv Syst.* 2008;24:995. https://doi.org/10.1007/s00381-008-0658-9

48. Leone G, Mele L, Pulsoni A, et al. The incidence of secondary leukemias. *Haematologica.* 1999 Oct;84(10):937–945.

49. Fuss M, Poljanc K, Hug EB, et al. Full scale IQ changes in children treated with whole brain and partial brain irradiation. A review and analysis. *Strahlenther Onkol.* 2000;176(12):573–581.

50. Fouladi M, Wallace D, Langston JW, et al. Survival and functional outcome of children with hypothalamic/chiasmatic tumors. *Cancer.* 2003;97(4):1084–1092.

51. Armstrong GT, Liu W, Leisenring W, et al. Occurrence of multiple subsequent neoplasms in long-term survivors of childhood cancer: A report from the childhood cancer survivor study. *Neuro Onc 2011 J Clin Oncol.* 2011 Aug 1;29(22):3056–3064. doi:10.1200/JCO.2011.34.6585

52. Siffert J, Allen JC. Late effects of therapy of thalamic and hypothalamic tumors in childhood: Vascular, neurobehavioral and neoplastic. *Pediatr Neurosurg.* 2000;33(2):105–111.

53. Kilday JP, Bartels U, Huang A, et al. Favorable survival and metabolic outcome for children with diencephalic syndrome using a radiation-sparing approach. *J Neurooncol.* 2014;116(1):195–204.

18 | PEDIATRIC HIGH-GRADE GLIOMA

SAMEER FAROUK SAIT, MORGAN FRERET, AND MATTHIAS KARAJANNIS

INTRODUCTION

Pediatric high-grade gliomas (pHGGs) represent 8–12% of all pediatric central nervous system (CNS) tumors and comprise a spectrum of histologies that includes anaplastic astrocytoma (World Health Organization [WHO] grade 3), glioblastoma (WHO grade 4), and diffuse midline glioma (DMG), H3K27M mutant (WHO grade 4).[1] The incidence in children up to 19 years of age is approximately 0.85 per 100,000 person-years.[2] pHGGs seem to affect boys and girls equally, with a peak in children age 5–9 years.[2] Diffuse intrinsic pontine gliomas (DIPGs) are pHGGs of the brainstem that can be diagnosed based on clinical and imaging findings alone. However, biopsy is now increasingly performed, and pathology reveals DMG, H3K27M mutant, with rare exceptions.[3,4] Median age at diagnosis is 6–7 years, with median survival of 9 months.[4,5]

At present, the only known environmental risk factor for developing pHGG is prior radiation therapy.[6] Other rare risk factors include genetic syndromes including neurofibromatosis type 1 (NF1), constitutional mismatch repair deficiency (CMMRD), and Li-Fraumeni syndrome (LFS).[7] Transformation from a low-grade glioma (LGG) into HGG in children is very rare (<10%) as opposed to in adults.[8]

CLINICAL PRESENTATION

The clinical manifestations of pHGGs depend on the anatomic location and the age of the patient. The clinical prodrome is usually short and rapidly evolving, with signs and symptoms of elevated intracranial pressure (ICP), focal neurologic deficits, and/or seizures.

Approximately half of patients with DIPG initially present with the classic triad of cranial neuropathies (e.g., abducens palsy, facial weakness), long tract signs (e.g., extremity weakness, hyperreflexia), and cerebellar signs (e.g., ataxia).[9,10] Hydrocephalus resulting from dorsal tumor extension and CSF obstruction occurs in fewer than 10% of cases at presentation.[9,10]

It is important to obtain a detailed family history, perform a comprehensive physical exam, and consider referral to genetics in all patients with pHGG at diagnosis. Current recommendation is to screen for germline *TP53* mutations (i.e., LFS) in all individuals presenting either with a HGG or a family history of LFS tumors.[11] NF1 is an autosomal dominant

tumor predisposition syndrome with affected individuals developing a combination of dermatologic, skeletal, ophthalmic, and neurologic findings and is diagnosed based on National Institutes of Health (NIH) criteria.[12] CMMRD is inherited in an autosomal recessive fashion and should be considered for young children who present with hematologic malignant disease, brain tumors, and/or Lynch syndrome (LS)-related cancers, in conjunction with (1) café-au-lait macules and/or other signs of NF1 and/or hypopigmented skin lesions, (2) consanguineous parents, (3) a family history of LS-related cancers, (4) a second malignant tumor, and/or (5) siblings with childhood cancer. Because CMMRD shares clinical features with NF1, familial adenomatous polyposis (FAP), and LFS, and it is important to keep this diagnosis in mind when evaluating children who present with one or more of these features.[13,14]

> Current recommendation is to screen for germline *TP53* mutations (i.e., LFS) in all individuals presenting either with a HGG or a family history of LFS tumors.

CNS dissemination at presentation, including distant sites, is present in approximately 3% of pHGG patients,[15] and secondary dissemination can be observed in more than 20%.[16] In patients with DIPG, leptomeningeal dissemination is present in up to 20% of patients at diagnosis.[17] Complete neuroimaging of the entire neuraxis (brain and total spine) in all patients with pHGG, including DIPG, is recommended. Lumbar puncture is not considered a standard part of initial staging.[15]

NEUROIMAGING

Magnetic resonance imaging (MRI) of the brain and spine should be performed at diagnosis. MR imaging should include T1-weighted sequences (pre- and post-contrast), T2-weighted and fluid attenuated inversion recovery (FLAIR) sequences, and diffusion-weighted imaging (DWI).

> Complete neuroimaging of the entire neuraxis (brain and total spine) in all patients with pHGG, including DIPG, is recommended.

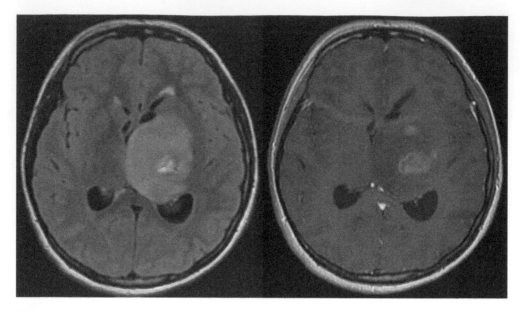

Figure 18.1 A 15-year-old female presented with right hemiparesis and facial weakness. MRI brain demonstrated an expansile, T2/FLAIR hyperintense, infiltrating, expansile mass measuring 6.0 x 4.1 cm which is centered within the left thalamus with effacement of the third and lateral ventricles, post-obstructive dilatation of the atrium and temporal horn of the left lateral ventricle (left panel), with heterogeneous contrast enhancement on T1-weighted post-contrast imaging (right panel). Biopsy was performed and pathology demonstrated a WHO grade 4 diffuse midline glioma H3K27 mutant. MSK-IMPACT testing demonstrated the following alterations - H3F3A Missense Mutation K28M (c.83A>T) exon 2, TERT Non-coding g.1295228C>T Promoter, PDGFRA Missense Mutation D576G (c.1727A>G) exon 12.

There is no pathognomonic appearance to differentiate pHGGs from other tumors on MRI. Pediatric HGGs are hypointense on T1-weighted images and hyperintense on T2-weighted sequences with heterogeneous contrast enhancement post gadolinium administration. The differential diagnosis based on imaging appearance includes ependymomas, embryonal tumors, germ cell tumors, and pleomorphic xanthoastrocytoma (PXAs).

The diagnosis of DIPG is based on the clinical history and examination combined with imaging findings. Typical imaging findings include a diffusely infiltrative tumor with ill-defined margins centered in the pons. The tumor is non-gadolinium contrast enhancing and frequently encases the basilar artery.[9,18] The differential diagnosis of brainstem lesions also includes embryonal tumors,[9,10,12] germ cell tumors, neurodegenerative (Alexander disease, acute demyelinating encephalomyelitis), and infectious conditions.[14]

> The diagnosis of DIPG is based on the clinical history and examination combined with imaging findings. Typical imaging findings include a diffusely infiltrative tumor with ill-defined margins centered in the pons. The tumor is non-gadolinium contrast enhancing and frequently encases the basilar artery.

Several additional MR sequences may be used as adjuncts to assist with diagnosis and assessing response to therapy. MR perfusion-weighted imaging (PWI) detects abnormal hemodynamic changes related to increased angiogenesis and vascular permeability, or "leakiness" that occur with aggressive tumor histology. These are reflected by changes in cerebral blood volume (CBV) and permeability.[19] Malignant brain tumors, including pHGG, typically have elevated rCBV values (ratio of tumoral CBV to normal appearing white matter CBV) compared to normal brain. Pooled data from a meta-analysis indicate that the utility of PWI in differentiating LGG from pHGG is limited due to the frequently elevated perfusion values seen in LGGs.[19] PWI metrics can help differentiate between viable/recurrent tumor and posttreatment changes with good accuracy. However, significant variability exists in optimal reported thresholds, and standardization is needed before implementing a universal approach.[20] MR spectroscopy (MRS) allows for the measurement of the relative composition of metabolites, including N-acetyl aspartate (NAA), choline, creatinine, lipid, and lactate. Choline is a component of cell membranes, while NAA is found primarily in normal functioning neurons. HGG is often associated with lower levels of NAA and creatine and higher levels of choline and lactate. In select cases, MRS may serve as an adjunct to standard MRI to help differentiate tumor from normal tissue and recurrent disease from treatment-related changes.[21] Metabolic imaging using 18F-fluorodeoxyglucose positron emission tomography (FDG-PET) is of limited utility in the management of pHGG and therefore rarely performed.[22] While PET-directed radiation planning is not done routinely, this remains an area of future investigation, and alternative radiotracers may be of greater utility relative to FDG-PET.[23]

NEUROPATHOLOGY

Diffusely infiltrative gliomas represent a heterogeneous group of neoplasms wherein the predominant tumor cell population shares morphological features with astrocytes (anaplastic astrocytoma and glioblastoma) and, less commonly, with oligodendrocytes (anaplastic oligodendroglioma) or a mixture of both astrocytes and oligodendrocytes (anaplastic oligoastrocytoma).[24] Grade 3 gliomas maybe distinguished from low-grade tumors based on demonstration of nuclear atypia, increased cellularity, multiple mitoses, and a high degree of cellular pleomorphism.[25] Grade 4 diffuse glioma, also referred to as *glioblastoma* (GBM) is defined by the presence of additional features of necrosis and/or endothelial proliferation.[25]

Additional rarer subtypes of pHGG are anaplastic variants of PXA, ganglioglioma, and pilocytic astrocytoma,[1] which can pose diagnostic challenges. While prior studies demonstrated a strong correlation between proliferation index and outcome of pHGGs,[26] more recent data demonstrate that molecular classification provides better prognostication, independent of proliferation index.[27] Isocitrate dehydrogenase (*IDH*)-wildtype grade 3 astrocytomas have a dismal prognosis, similar to GBM.[28] Samples obtained at autopsy from DIPG patients universally show grade 3 or 4 histology, whereas DIPG biopsy samples at initial diagnosis may occasionally appear as lower grade (grade 2), likely due to sampling bias.[29,30]

The application of high-throughput genome and epigenome-wide molecular profiling techniques revolutionized our understanding of the origin and biological features of pHGGs.[31] The WHO 2016 classification incorporates both microscopic and molecular parameters when classifying CNS tumors and provides a major restructuring to pHGGs with meaningful clinical correlation, particularly related to age at presentation, anatomical location, and prognosis.[1] Therefore, it is important to highlight specific disease terminologies that are no longer considered relevant while simultaneously clarifying the new designations that now represent them. For instance, *gliomatosis cerebri* is a clinico-radiologic pattern of exceptionally widespread tumor growth which represents a phenotypic extreme and not a separate disease entity.[32] pHGGs arising in midline locations (thalamus or spinal cord) demonstrate overlapping molecular features and share the dismal survival encountered in DIPG patients. As such, these tumors are viewed as a spectrum along a single molecular and clinicopathological entity,[31,33] termed *DMGs with K27M histone mutations* and designated WHO grade 4, regardless of histology.[1] The prognostic/biologic relevance of the grade 3 and grade 4 distinction in children is not clear and experts propose the designation of molecular glioblastoma for *IDH*-wildtype astrocytomas regardless of the WHO grade determined at histologic analysis.[25,34]

O6-METHYLGUANINE-DNA-METHYLTRANSFERASE METHYLATION

O6-Methylguanine-DNA-Methyltransferase (MGMT) is a DNA repair gene which functions to eliminate methylated adducts (DNA damage) from the O6-guanine position. Methylation of the MGMT promoter and subsequent gene silencing leads to reduced proficiency of DNA damage repair induced by alkylating agent chemotherapy. Hypomethylation of the MGMT promoter is associated with alkylator chemotherapy/temozolomide (TMZ) resistance. There are no randomized controlled HGG trials in pediatrics comparing radiotherapy and TMZ to radiotherapy alone; hence, the value of MGMT promoter methylation as a predictive biomarker for benefit from TMZ is unproven in the pediatric population. It has been noted that the MGMT promoter is hypomethylated in the vast majority of *H3K27M*-mutant midline gliomas and hypermethylated in most *G34R/V*-mutant

HGG. However, in pHGG patients treated with TMZ, there is no association between MGMT promoter methylation status and progression-free survival (PFS) or overall survival (OS) in multivariate analysis.[35,36] This finding is in striking contrast to adult glioblastoma patients, where MGMT promoter methylation status has been validated as a highly reproducible prognostic and predictive biomarker across prospective, randomized clinical trials using radiotherapy and radiotherapy and TMZ.[37] Therefore, the utility of MGMT promoter methylation status as an independent prognostic biomarker in pHGG is not supported by the current data, and its role as a predictive biomarker for benefit from TMZ in this population is unproven as well.

> In pHGG patients treated with TMZ, there is no association between MGMT promoter methylation status and PFS or OS in multivariate analyses.

MOLECULAR GENETICS

Multiple genome-wide studies have demonstrated that pHGGs arising in children are biologically distinct from those occurring in adults.[38–43] Subsequently, the identification of novel histone mutations connecting tumorigenesis, chromatin modification, and neural developmental pathways dramatically altered the molecular landscape of pHGG.[44,45] The resulting data have led to a fundamental reclassification of pHGGs, moving from a solely histology-based classification to molecular-based categorization into groups with meaningful clinical correlation, particularly in terms of age predilection, anatomical locations, and survival.[33,46,47] Furthermore, these studies have transformed our understanding of the cellular origins and evolution of HGGs in children. Distinct cell-of-origin populations of neural stem cells, susceptible to unique selective pressures in the developing brain, give rise to biologically distinct groups of tumors harboring unique oncogenic driver mutations, DNA methylation profiles, and gene expression.[31,34] The most important molecular groups are (1) the histone mutations related pHGG, that is, *H3.K27*-mutated midline, which includes DIPGs and *H3.G34*-mutated hemispheric pHGG; (2) the rare IDH-1/2-mutated pHGG occurring mainly in young adults; (3) the BRAFV600-mutant tumors, which transform from low-grade precursors to malignant astrocytomas; and (4) H3-/IDH-/BRAF-wildtype tumors.

The majority of pHGGs have complex genomic signatures, with significant copy number alterations (CNAs), single nucleotide variants (SNVs), and structural variants (SVs) resulting from chromothripsis.[48] In general, pHGGs have a greater mutational burden (with a median of 15 non-synonymous coding mutations per tumor) than other pediatric cancers but lower than that detected in adult GBM.[49–52] However, the genomic complexity of pHGG spans a wide range, with infant non-brainstem high-grade glioma (NBS-HGG; median mutational burden of 2) and pHGGs from patients with inherited mutations in mismatch repair genes (with a median of >6,000 non-synonymous coding mutations per tumor) at either end of the spectrum.[31]

PHGGs demonstrate molecular alterations in canonical cancer pathways, including the TP53 pathway, the PI3-kinase/Akt/mTOR pathway, and the retinoblastoma (RB) pathway, similar to adult HGGs. However, the specific effectors that are altered by mutation vary between childhood and adult tumors.[47,53–58] Genes encoding receptor tyrosine kinases (RTKs) are commonly mutated/amplified in pHGG; however, the frequency of affected genes varies between particular age groups.[53] PDGFRA is one of the most frequently altered genes encoding a RTK in pHGG, including DIPGs (30%). By contrast, mutations in EGFR, which are frequently found in adult GBM, are uncommon in pHGG.[31,40,41,56] FGFR1 hotspot mutations (thalamic midline gliomas) and amplifications of MET and IGF1R have also been reported in pHGGs. Mosaic heterogeneity (i.e., the stable coexistence of different clones within the same tumor harboring amplification of different RTK genes in a mutually exclusive fashion) has been described, which carries important clinical implications for tumor resistance to targeted therapies.[59] Alterations involving the RB pathway include chromosome 13q loss in one-third of pHGGs,[41,52] homozygous deletions of CDKN2A/B in 25% of supratentorial pHGG,[40,52,60] and amplification of the components of the cyclin–CDK complex (CDK4, CDK6) demonstrated across all pHGG subgroups.[61]

HISTONE-MUTANT GLIOMAS

Histones play an integral role in chromatin remodeling and transcriptional regulation/gene expression via post-translational modification (PTMs) (i.e., acetylation and methylation of lysine residues localized in histone H3 tail regions).[31] PTMs are regulated by specific enzymes that promote their addition ("writers") or removal ("erasers"). Specific recurrent mutations in the genes encoding the H3.3 (H3F3A) and H3.1 (HIST1H3B, HIST1H3C) histone variants result in amino acid substitutions at two key residues in the histone tail: lysine-to-methionine at position 27 (K27M) and glycine-to-arginine or -valine at position 34 (G34R/V). These mutations are mutually exclusive and delineate distinct subgroups of histone-mutant pHGG as defined by numerous molecular and clinical parameters and will be discussed later.

> Presence of the H3 K27M or the H3 G34R/V mutation is mutually exclusive.

DIFFUSE MIDLINE GLIOMAS, H3 K27M-MUTANT

H3 K27M-mutant DMGs are defined by the WHO 2016 as "infiltrative midline high-grade glioma with predominantly astrocytic differentiation and a K27M mutation in either H3F3A or HIST1H3B/C."[1,62] DMGs are associated with aggressive clinical behavior and poor prognosis,[33,63] regardless of histological grade,[49] and are therefore always designated as WHO grade 4. Demonstration of the H3 K27M mutation, either by direct sequencing or via immunohistochemistry (IHC), is a prerequisite for diagnosis (see Figure 18.1 and Figure 18.2). The H3 K27M antibody detects both the H3.3 and H3.1 K27M mutation and will demonstrate diffuse nuclear positivity (non-neoplastic cells serve as negative control), whereas the H3 K27me3 antibody will show loss of nuclear staining.[64,65]

Trimethylation at the K27 position is associated with repression of gene expression that modulates stem cell differentiation and development.[31] The enhancer of zeste homologue 2 (EZH2) catalytic site of the polycomb repressive complex 2 (PRC2) is responsible for this methylation. The K27M mutation is always heterozygous and interferes with EZH2/PRC2 methyltransferase activity, resulting in globally diminished H3K27me3 levels (hypomethylated state) and derepression of PRC2 target genes.[31,66]

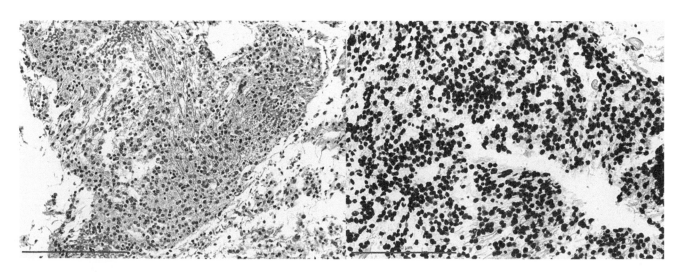

Figure 18.2 A 9-year-old girl with diffuse midline glioma (DIPG) (Hematoxylin & Eosin [H&E], left), IHC using a K27M mutant-specific antibody demonstrates brown nuclear staining while non neoplastic cells serve as negative control (right). IMPACT (next-generation sequencing) demonstrated the following alterations: H3F3A exon2 p.K27M mutation, PDGFRA exon12 p.Y555C (c.1664A>G), PDGFRA exon4 p.V129_F178del (c.385_534del), and TERT promoter variant (g.1295228C>T).

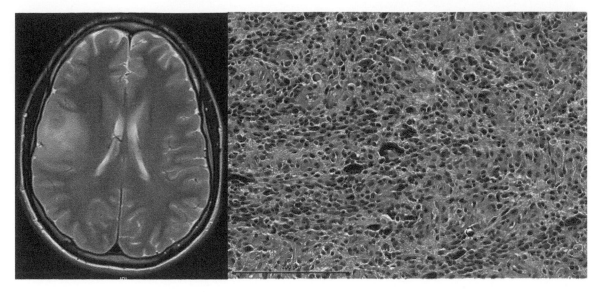

Figure 18.3 *A 17-year-old male presented with left sided focal seizures and headaches. MRI brain demonstrates a T2 hyperintense right parieto-temporal lesion (left panel). H&E stain shows hypercellular infiltrative astrocytoma - cells are markedly atypical with hyperchromatic nuclei. Mitotically active with Ki-67 and MIB-1 index of 30%.*

Differences exist between the H3 histone variants in which the mutations occur. The K27M mutation results in a lysine-to-methionine substitution at position K27 in *H3F3A* (encoding histone H3.3) or *HIST1H3B/HIST1H3C* (encoding histone H3.1). *H3.3* and *H3.1 K27M* mutations are mutually exclusive, associate with distinct genetic alterations,[5,67] and also segregate by clinical features, highlighting that these represent specific molecular subgroups.[5]

H3 G34-MUTANT TUMORS

H3.3 G34R/V-mutant tumors are restricted to the cerebral hemispheres[31] and typically manifest during adolescence or young adulthood (10–25 years).[47,68] Up to a third of all hemispheric HGGs are defined by G34R and G34V mutations of histone H3.

Histologically, *H3 G34*-mutant tumors seem to have a heterogeneous appearance with microscopic characteristics typical of either GBM or CNS primitive neuroectodermal tumors (CNS-PNET)[46] (see Figure 18.3). However, both histological variants demonstrate similar clinical, demographic, and DNA methylation profiles. Some studies suggest that *H3 G34*-mutant HGG patients have a more favorable outcome (median OS is 22 months) than *H3 K27M*-mutant glioma patients,[33,69] which may be related to the cortical location and surgical resectability, as well as relatively higher frequency of MGMT promoter methylation and better response to TMZ chemotherapy.[46] *H3.3 G34R/V* mutant HGG also demonstrate *TP53* mutations as well as alterations in other chromatin regulators including *ATRX/DAXX* (see Figure 18.4).

The anatomical distribution of cortical pHGGs arising during late adolescence through young adulthood suggests a potential difference in tumor susceptibility associated with

developmental context.[31] For instance, *IDH1/2*-mutant gliomas more frequently occur within the frontal lobe, while the mutually exclusive population of histone *H3 G34*-mutant tumors are more commonly found in the temporal and parietal lobes of the cerebral cortex.[33,44,53]

> The anatomical distribution of cortical pHGGs arising during late adolescence through young adulthood suggests a potential difference in tumor susceptibility associated with developmental context.

IDH1/2-MUTANT GLIOMAS

IDH1/2 gene hotspot mutations associated with a global hypermethylation (G-CIMP)[33,53,70] represent a small subgroup of pHGG. They likely represent the younger tail of an age distribution for these primarily adult-onset tumors with whom they share similar molecular characteristics and a more favorable prognosis,[25,70] as reviewed elsewhere.

BRAFV600-MUTANT GLIOMAS

The *BRAFV600E* mutation is detected in a group (5–10%) of predominantly cortical tumors, most commonly in the context of secondary pHGG arising from tumors that were originally low-grade, such as gangliogliomas[71,72] or PXA.

H3/IDH/BRAF-WILDTYPE

Recent further refinements in the molecular subclassification demonstrate additional diversity within *H3-/IDH-/BRAF* wildtype tumors that are associated with recurrent amplifications of the *MYCN*, *EGFR*, and *PDGFRA* oncogenes.[46,47]

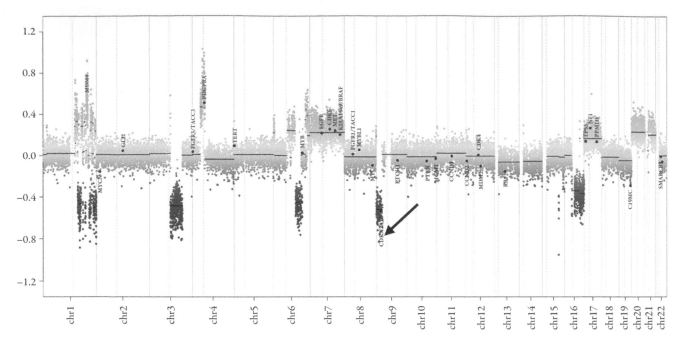

Figure 18.4 *A 17-year-old male presented with left sided focal seizures and headaches and was diagnosed with WHO grade 3 (anaplastic astrocytoma). Depicted here is a Copy number alteration plot using genome-wide methylation profiling. Arrow points to CDKN2A/B loss. Next generation sequencing (Foundation One) demonstrated the following alterations - Histone3 G34/35 (p.G35R H3F3A), TP53 Frameshift Deletion H214Qfs*7 (c.642_643del) exon 6, ATRX Nonsense Mutation K183* (c.547A>T) exon 7, and CDKN2A loss. Diagnosis was later changed to molecular glioblastoma, hemispheric H3.G34 variant.*

INFANT HGGS

The genomic and clinical features NBS-HGGs arising in children younger than 3 years are distinct,[52] with lower mutational burdens and a significantly better survival, respectively, compared to NBS-HGGs in older children.[73] Oncogenic gene fusions including *NTRK1/2/3* (neurotrophic tropomyosin-related kinase), *ROS* (protein tyrosine kinase encoded by the ROS1 gene), or *ALK* (anaplastic lymphoma kinase)[74] are commonly observed.[75–77]

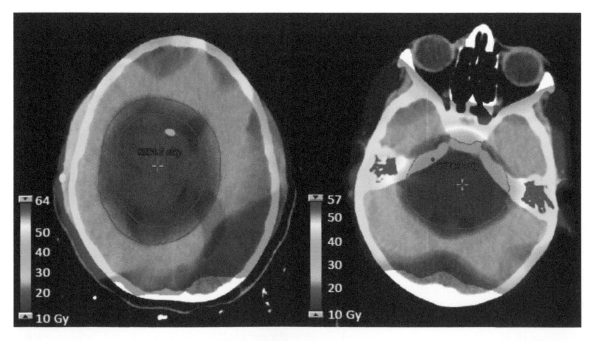

Figure 18.5 *Intensity-modulated radiation therapy (IMRT) plans showing standard treatment approaches in non-brainstem pHGG and DIPG. (A) In non-brainstem pHGG, there are typically two radiation planning target volumes (PTVs), a larger PTV1 (pink outline) treated with 54 Gy designed to encompass any residual microscopic disease after GTR and a smaller "boost" volume treated with 59.4 Gy (red outline). (B) DIPGs typically have a single PTV (blue outline) treated with 54 Gy.*

PEDIATRIC HGGS IN THE CONTEXT OF CANCER PREDISPOSITION SYNDROMES

The Pediatric Cancer Genome Project (PCGP) reported that the prevalence of germline mutations that were pathogenic or probably pathogenic among patients with HGG is 9.1%.[78] LFS, NF1, and CMMRD are three prominent cancer predisposition syndromes (CPS) associated with an increased incidence of pHGG.[52,79] The molecular landscape in HGGs associated with *NF1* and *P53* germline mutations is similar to those seen in sporadic cases.[7,52,79] Identifying a tumor predisposition syndrome is important for diagnostics, therapeutics, screening, risk reduction, and family planning.[80–83] For example, irradiation may promote the development of new tumors in some syndromes such as LFS and NF1,[84] where irradiation-sparing therapeutic approaches are strongly preferable. More recently, molecular targeted therapies have begun to emerge for some conditions, a prominent example being the molecular targeted treatment of recurrent/refractory LGGs with MEK inhibitors in patients with NF1.[85] Clinical implications with a focus on underlying biology, diagnosis, and treatment are discussed here.

> Identifying a tumor predisposition syndrome is important for diagnostics, therapeutics, screening, risk reduction, and family planning.

CONSTITUTIONAL MISMATCH REPAIR DEFICIENCY

CMMRD is an autosomal recessive disorder which results from germline biallelic (homozygous or compound heterozygous) mutations in one of the MMR genes (*MSH2*, *MSH6*, *MLH1*, and *PMS2*).[86] This disorder is distinct from patients who develop hereditary non-polyposis colorectal carcinoma HNPCC, also known as Lynch syndrome, characterized by monoallelic mutations in DNA mismatch repair (MMR) genes and associated with a 3% lifetime risk of developing a brain tumor, notably glioblastoma.[87] MMR genes play essential roles in maintaining genome integrity by correcting errors that arise during DNA replication, and mutations in MMR genes lead to "hypermutant" cancer,[7] characterized by point mutations (SNVs) and microsatellite instability (MSI) in which mutation repetitive sequences (microsatellites) are not adequately repaired.[7,86] Establishing a molecular diagnosis of CMMRD can be accomplished in a stepwise manner beginning with testing for MSI and/or loss of expression of an MMR protein, followed by mutational analysis of the appropriate MMR genes.[88]

Astrocytomas, primarily GBMs, are the most prevalent brain tumors in patients with biallelic MMR mutations and usually present in the second decade of life (3% lifetime risk).[87,89] Some patients are initially diagnosed with LGGs, but these tend to transform to high-grade tumors. Some of these patients with HGGs have been reported as long-term survivors, possibly suggesting a somewhat more favorable prognosis compared to other pHGGs.[90–92]

> GBMs and other tumors associated with CMMRD have a high mutational load compared with sporadic tumors, predicting that they may be responsive to immune checkpoint inhibition.

There are limited data regarding the optimal treatment of cancers in patients with CMMRD. However, increased toxicity and reduced efficacy of chemotherapy, as well as increased risk of second primary malignant tumors should be kept in mind.[93,94] GBMs and other tumors associated with CMMRD have a high mutational load compared with sporadic tumors, predicting that they may be responsive to immune checkpoint inhibition, and at least one case report describes an impressive response to nivolumab in two children with recurrent GBM related to CMMRD.[95]

LI-FRAUMENI SYNDROME

LFS is an autosomal dominant condition with an estimated incidence of 1 in 5,000–10,000 person-years. Germline mutations in the tumor suppressor gene *TP53* located at chromosome 17p13.1 were linked to LFS in the early 1990s.[96] Referred to as the "gatekeeper of the genome," TP53 represents one of the key proteins that maintain genome integrity after DNA damage, hypoxia, and other stressors. The CHK2 checkpoint homolog gene, *CHEK2*, which is located on the long (q) arm of chromosome 22, also has been implicated in some families with classic LFS.[97] Brain tumors are found in about 14% of the patients with *TP53* germline mutations; the frequency is particularly high (21%) in patients with mutations in the L2 and L3 loop of *TP53* that mediates the binding to the minor groove of DNA.[98]

Malignant gliomas can occur throughout childhood, but more commonly in young adults (average age of onset is 16 years). No data currently exist regarding the prognostic significance of germline *TP53* mutations in pHGGs. Although no molecular targeted therapy for *TP53* mutated tumors is currently available, detection of a germline *TP53* mutation has significant prognostic and therapeutic implications for the patient. Both children and adults with LFS have been considered to be at an increased risk for developing radiation therapy–induced secondary malignant tumors,[99,100] as well as secondary myelodysplastic syndrome following specific chemotherapies.[101] Furthermore, surveillance protocols have identified several LGGs, perhaps suggesting that some of LFS-associated GBMs arise as secondary glioblastomas and may benefit from early intervention. These observations imply that genetic counseling followed by an aggressive surveillance protocol may change our management and the need for toxic therapies for tumors, which may have a significant beneficial effect on survival and quality of life of individuals with LFS.[102]

NEUROFIBROMATOSIS TYPE 1

NF1 results from germline loss-of-function mutations in the *NF1* gene located on chromosome *17q11.2*. The *NF1*-encoded protein (neurofibromin) inhibits the oncoprotein RAS, which promotes cell growth and survival via downstream effector pathways including the RAS-MEK-ERK and the PI3K-AKT-mTOR pathways. Loss of neurofibromin due to biallelic inactivation of the *NF1* gene leads to deregulated RAS activity, thereby permitting oncogenesis.[103–105] NF1-associated pHGG (NF1-pHGG) may arise secondary to transformation of low-grade lesions or can be primary pHGG.[106]

NF1-pHGGs share many of the same molecular alterations as sporadic pHGGs, including mutations in *TP53, CDKN2A, ATRX, PI3K*, and genes involved in transcription/chromatin regulation.[107,108] Furthermore, a recent study compared DNA methylation profiles of NF1-associated LGGs and HGGs in children and adults to those of sporadic gliomas from the Cancer Genome Atlas (TCGA) dataset. Supervised and unsupervised hierarchical clustering of methylation profiles showed that NF1-associated gliomas resemble a subgroup of sporadic gliomas (LGm6 *IDH* wild-type gliomas).[28,107] Thus, despite NF1-pHGGs experiencing a distinct (*NF1* heterozygous) tumor microenvironment, they share many molecular features of sporadic pHGGs and to date are treated similarly.

SECONDARY RADIATION-INDUCED PHGG

The majority of secondary pHGG have been reported in patients with a previous diagnosis of malignancy (survivors of high-risk acute lymphoblastic leukemia or CNS malignancies who received cranial radiation) and in patients with CPS including NF1 or retinoblastoma (RB).[109] These tumors develop within prior radiation fields with the interval from radiotherapy to secondary pHGG diagnosis ranging from 6 to 14 years.[110] Survival outcomes remain poor. A small series reported that *IDH1/2, H3*, and *TERT* mutations are absent while biallelic inactivation of *TP53*,

CDKN2A homozygous deletion, and amplifications or rearrangements involving RTK and MAPK pathway genes are detected at a higher frequency in secondary pHGGs, demonstrating their distinct molecular profiles when compared to primary pHGGs.[111]

TREATMENT

Unfortunately, despite improvement in neurosurgical techniques, radiation therapy delivery, and trials of various chemotherapy agents, the survival of children with HGG has not significantly changed in the past several decades. Independent of molecular features, event free survival (EFS) rates at 2 years from diagnosis range between 5% and 25% and are influenced by tumor grade, location, and extent of resection.[112,113]

SURGERY

Maximal safe resection is the preferred approach for initial diagnosis and management. Unfortunately, complete removal of HGG is rarely accomplished because these tumors are highly infiltrative and local recurrences are common even in patients who have had a gross total resection (GTR) of the tumor. pHGGs are characterized by poorly defined tumor margins with neoplastic infiltration along perivascular spaces and white matter fibers. Tumor infiltration extends beyond the tumor margin as defined by MRI and the neurosurgeon.

The goals of surgery include obtaining tissue for pathologic diagnosis and achieving a maximal safe resection. Biopsy alone is used in situations where the lesion is not amenable to resection, for example with deeper midline location such as thalamic DMG or when tumors infiltrate or are immediately adjacent to eloquent cortex and white matter pathways. While neuroimaging is generally considered sufficient for diagnosis in typical cases of DIPG, stereotactic biopsy risks are considered minimal, may be diagnostically useful in cases where imaging findings are unclear, and can aid research directed at discerning tumor biology and development of novel therapies.[114,115] Therefore, efforts at disease stratification and targeted therapies in future clinical studies may warrant revisiting the role of biopsy for DIPG patients.[116]

Depending on tumor location, the extent of surgery must be balanced with preservation of neurologic function. Preoperative MRI sequences such as diffusion tensor imaging (DTI) or functional MRI (fMRI) as well as intraoperative image guidance navigation can assist in safely achieving a greater extent of resection while preserving neurologic function for the patient. Greater extent of resection is generally associated with longer survival.[117]

RADIATION THERAPY

RADIATION THERAPY IN NON-BRAINSTEM pHGG

Because of pHGG's infiltrative nature, adjuvant radiotherapy is necessary to sterilize tumor cells that persist even after GTR.[118] Children with pHGG typically receive postoperative radiotherapy with a total dose of 54–60 Gy in daily fractions of 1.8 or 2 Gy over 6 weeks.[119] Here we discuss evolving standards for optimal radiation fractionation and dose in children with newly diagnosed pHGG (see Figure 18.5).

> Children with pHGG typically receive postoperative radiotherapy with a total dose of 54–60 Gy in daily fractions of 1.8 or 2 Gy over 6 weeks.

Findings from a series of randomized trials in adults with HGG confirmed a survival advantage with postoperative radiotherapy and support its use in pediatric HGG.[120-123] The first prospective randomized trial involving children with pHGG compared surgical resection with either adjuvant radiotherapy followed by pCV chemotherapy (prednisone, chloroethylcyclohexyl nitrosourea [CCNU] and vincristine) or radiotherapy alone.[124] Children who received chemotherapy in addition to radiotherapy had a markedly improved 5-year PFS (46%) when compared to children who received radiotherapy alone (18%). Subsequent studies sought to improve outcomes achieved with conventionally fractionated radiation using hyperfractionated schedules[125] or dose escalation[126,127]

in children and adults with high-grade gliomas but did not demonstrate a survival benefit compared to conventional fractionation.

While the role of re-irradiation (or "salvage" radiotherapy) is better established in adults with recurrent HGG,[128] to date there are limited data to support its use in pHGG. A recent retrospective analysis from the German HIT-HGG study group identified eight children with previously irradiated pHGG who received salvage re-irradiation with 24.2–55.8 Gy.[129] Three patients experienced temporary improvement in symptoms, and none developed significant acute toxicity. However, given the dearth of prospective data combined with increased risk for radiation-related toxicity, including brainstem necrosis, the use of salvage re-irradiation in children with HGG in clinical practice remains extremely limited.

RADIATION THERAPY IN DIPG

By virtue of their location in the brainstem, DIPGs are not amenable to surgical resection. Instead, patients are treated with definitive conformal radiation therapy with a total dose of 54 Gy in daily fractions of 1.8 or 2 Gy over 6 weeks.[130,131] Radiotherapy is well tolerated, improves neurological symptoms in at least two-thirds of children with DIPG, and reduces steroid dependence.[132] Since brainstem tumors were first treated with radiation therapy nearly eight decades ago,[133] studies have investigated optimal radiation dose and fractionation, as well as the role of reirradiation in recurrent disease.

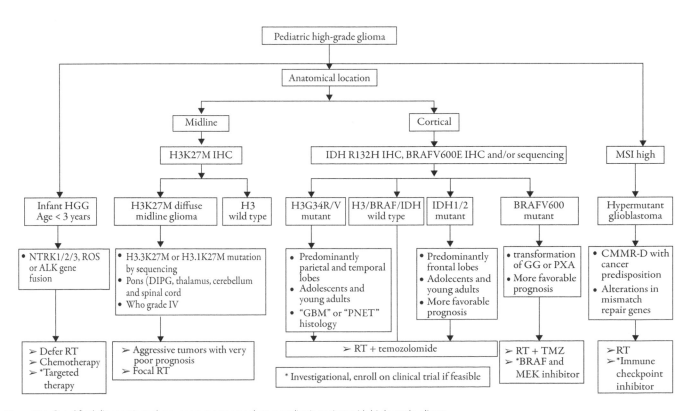

Figure 18.6 Simplified diagnostic and management approach to a pediatric patient with high grade glioma.

> Patients are treated with definitive conformal radiation therapy with a total dose of 54 Gy in daily fractions of 1.8 or 2 Gy over 6 weeks. Radiotherapy is well tolerated, improves neurological symptoms in at least two-thirds of children with DIPG, and reduces steroid dependence.

Evidence for relatively high radiation doses in DIPG comes from an early retrospective study among adult and pediatric patients with unresected infratentorial tumors, which demonstrated a marked radiation dose threshold for survival of 50 Gy to the primary tumor.[134] Subsequent dose escalation studies in children with DIPG sought to extend these initial findings by exploiting hyperfractionated radiation schedules designed to increase tumor-cell killing while limiting normal tissue toxicity. Although initially promising, these trials ultimately did not show a clinical benefit above that of conventionally fractionated radiotherapy.[135-139] More recently, interest has emerged in hypofractionated radiation schemes in DIPG, which, in contrast to the earlier hyperfractionated trials, are aimed toward decreasing treatment burden in a patient population with limited life expectancy.[140-142] A recent trial from Egypt randomized 71 children with DIPG to receive either standard radiotherapy with 54 Gy in 30 fractions or hypofractionated radiotherapy with 39 Gy in 13 fractions. At 18 months, the PFS and OS differences between the two patient groups were 1.1% and 2.2%, respectively, although the hypofractionated group did not satisfy the non-inferiority assumption.[142] Findings from this trial and others suggest similar results with hypofractionated regimens; however, standard fractionation remains the standard of care at most institutions.

DIPGs almost always recur within the high-dose radiation volume. Findings show that salvage re-irradiation for recurrent DIPG improves symptoms, may provide a modest survival benefit,[143] and should be considered in children who are older than 6 months beyond their first course of radiotherapy. Patients typically receive focal reirradiation with 30–36 Gy in daily fractions of 2 or 3 Gy,[143-146] although in rare cases of disseminated disease, patients may benefit from larger treatment volumes, including whole-brain and/or craniospinal irradiation. The optimal dose and fractionation for focal salvage re-irradiation in DIPG remains underexplored, although a recent phase I/II dose escalation study suggests that lower doses may be similarly effective for symptom palliation.[147]

Pediatric cranial irradiation is well tolerated with minimal acute toxicities and, among patients with limited life expectancy, its long-term toxicities, including cerebrovascular disease and cognitive deficits, are of lesser consideration. An exception is brainstem necrosis, a rare but potentially devastating complication that typically manifests with ataxia and/or lower cranial nerve palsies. Retrospective analyses among pediatric patients treated with photon or proton irradiation for posterior fossa tumors estimate rates of brainstem injury ranging from 2% to 10% within 2 years.[148-151] Younger age and higher radiation dose are associated with an elevated risk of symptomatic brainstem injury.

MEDICAL THERAPY

Despite numerous prospective clinical trials for pHGG either at initial diagnosis or recurrence, there has been little improvement in patient outcome, leading some to question the practice of giving chemotherapy to these patients. Nevertheless, tremendous efforts are undertaken to develop improved combinatorial and targeted treatment strategies for these patients.

CHEMOTHERAPY

The Children's Cancer Group CCG-943 study reported a significant improvement in survival outcomes with the addition of pCV chemotherapy following radiotherapy.[124] A subsequent CCG study randomized patients to receive an intensive "8-drugs-in-one-day" regimen versus pCV chemotherapy and observed no difference in 5-year PFS.[56] However, the survival rates in both studies are superior to those reported in contemporary trials. A subsequent retrospective central review demonstrated that a large number of LGGs were erroneously included[56,152]; explaining the favorable outcomes. The German cooperative group study also reported improved survival with intensive chemotherapy administered during and after radiotherapy.[140] However, the absence of molecular profiling makes it hard to interpret these results and limits the impact of these findings.

Single-agent TMZ, administered during and after RT in the Children's Oncology Group (COG) study ACNS0126 did not improve outcome compared with historical controls.[112] The subsequent COG HGG trial, ACNS0423, demonstrated that the addition of CCNU to TMZ during maintenance (to overcome MGMT-mediated resistance) resulted in improved OS and EFS compared with adjuvant TMZ alone in the ACNS0126 study. However, this was not a randomized comparison, molecular data including *IDH1/2* status were limited, and significant myelosuppression occurred.[153]

The most recent completed COG study (ACNS0822) was a "pick the winner" phase II trial that compared two different experimental arms with vorinostat (a histone de-acetylase inhibitor) or bevacizumab (a vascular endothelial growth factor [VEGF] monoclonal antibody) during radiotherapy with a control arm receiving TMZ during radiotherapy followed in a maintenance phase by TMZ/bevacizumab. This study closed when the stopping rule was met; neither of the first two arms were found to be statistically better than the radiotherapy/TMZ arm.[154] Similarly, the HERBY trial, a phase II randomized study, failed to demonstrate improvement in EFS with the addition of bevacizumab to radiation therapy and TMZ for patients with newly diagnosed non-brainstem pHGG.[155] The role of high-dose myeloablative chemotherapy with autologous hematopoietic stem cell rescue (ASCR) in pHGG remains unconfirmed.[156]

In summary, although alkylator chemotherapy including TMZ and/or CCNU appears to benefit at least a subset of pHGG patients, a standard of care has not been established and children are enrolled in clinical trials whenever possible.

MOLECULAR TARGETED THERAPY

An international phase I trial in pediatric patients with recurrent *BRAFV600E*-mutant tumors (including 23 gliomas) demonstrated impressive preliminary efficacy of dabrafenib (first-generation BRAF inhibitor) in HGG, however, responses were short lived.[157] Subsequently, a combination of dabrafenib (BRAF inhibitor) and trametinib (MEK inhibitor) is currently being evaluated in *BRAFV600*-mutant pHGG in both the newly diagnosed (NCT03919071) and recurrent/refractory settings (NCT02684058).

> Although alkylator chemotherapy including TMZ and/or CCNU appears to benefit at least a subset of pHGG patients, a standard of care has not been established and children are enrolled in clinical trials whenever possible.

Figure 18.6 provides an overview over potential management strategies for pediatric LGGs.

SPECIAL CONSIDERATIONS

DIPG

Numerous strategies including high-dose myeloablative chemotherapy with ASCR, neo-adjuvant and/or adjuvant chemotherapy including TMZ, as well as radiosensitization in DIPG have failed to improve survival when compared to radiotherapy alone.[113,158–174] Presently, adjuvant chemotherapy is not recommended for newly diagnosed DIPG outside of a clinical trial.

INFANT HGGs

HGG patients younger than 3 years are typically treated with chemotherapy regimens, such as carboplatin/etoposide or the "Baby POG" protocol, and radiotherapy is generally avoided.[175–181] Infant HGGs resemble LGGs genomically,[52,60,74,182] which likely explains their more favorable response to chemotherapy and improved outcome. Oncogenic gene fusions including *NTRK1/2/3* (neurotrophic tropomyosin-related kinase), *ROS* (protein tyrosine kinase encoded by the ROS1 gene), or *ALK* (anaplastic lymphoma kinase)[74,182] are commonly observed, and molecular targeted approaches are currently being tested in clinical trials.[183]

> HGG patients younger than 3 years are typically treated with chemotherapy regimens, such as carboplatin/etoposide or the "Baby POG" protocol, and radiotherapy is generally avoided.

SURVIVORSHIP CONSIDERATIONS

There is a paucity of studies specifically addressing the long-term outcome of pHGG patients given the relatively few survivors.[184] The COG L991 study investigated the outcomes after treatment on CCG-945 with survivors demonstrating lower scores in several domains including neuropsychological, social-emotional, behavioral, and quality of life (QoL). Midline or posterior fossa tumor location, female sex, and young age at treatment were identified as higher risk patient cohorts who should be targeted for early interventions.[185]

ACKNOWLEDGMENTS

We would like to thank Dr. Tejus Bale (neuropathology) for providing histology slides and Joe Olechnowicz for editorial assistance.

FLASHCARD

This tumor represent approximately 10% of all pediatric CNS lesions.	Pediatric high-grade glioma (pHGG)
Three common CNS locations for pHGG are:	Cerebral hemispheres, midline, and posterior fossa
What is the usual prognosis of *BRAF*-mutant gliomas?	Favorable
Surgical biopsy in DIPG should be considered for which reasons?	Atypical presentation, imaging, or for genetic testing
In pHGGs, the most common *BRAF* alteration is:	BRAF V600E
In pHGG distant neuraxial dissemination can be seen both at diagnosis and at what other time point?	Postmortem evaluation
In pHGG, most studies show maximal surgical resection is associated with improved:	Patient survival
BRAF-mutant gliomas are commonly located as:	Cortical tumors
What is the clinical utility for MGMT promoter methylation in pHGG?	Neither predictive nor prognostic
H3K27 mutant glioma is WHO grade ___ despite histology	WHO grade 4
What is the most common IDH mutation in pHGG?	*IDH1 R132H*
In pHGG, what is the goal for surgery?	Maximal safe resection (limited with deep midline tumors such as DIPG)

In pHGG, what is the goal for radiation?	Localized field irradiation standard (most combine medical therapy)
In pHGG, what is the goal for chemo/biologic therapy?	There is no established "standard" adjuvant chemotherapy regimen
Which chemotherapy is most frequently used in pHGG and would be considered closest to a "standard" therapy?	Temozolomide (ACNS0126)
Which tumors are associated with deep midline locations (including DIPG)?	*H3K27*-mutant gliomas
Diagnosis of DIPG could be determined based on:	Neuroimaging
Treatment considerations for high-grade glioma, *H3K27, IDH1/2, BRAF* wildtype include	Clinica trials; alternatively, RT with w/concurrent and adjuvant TMZ (10 cycles per ACNS0126)
CMMRD is an acronym for:	Constitutional (or biallelic) mismatch repair deficiency syndrome
CMMRD tumors have what level of microsatellite instability (MSI)?	High
This treatment modality is *always* included in the treatment of DIPG	Radiation therapy (no chemo/biologic therapy has demonstrated benefit)
This treatment modality is *always* included in the treatment of high-grade glioma, *H3K27*-mutated	Radiation therapy (no chemo/biologic therapy has demonstrated benefit)
Treatment considerations for high grade glioma, *BRAF V600E*-mutated include:	On study ACNS 1723, alternatively, RT + TMZ followed by BRAF and MEK inhibitor combination
Treatment considerations for hypermutant high grade glioma include:	RT and consider adjuvant immune checkpoint inhibitor

Treatment considerations for "infant high-grade glioma" include:	Radiation avoided, "Baby POG" chemotherapy regimens (carboplatin/etoposide), second-line targeted therapies if NTRK/ALK/ROS fusion
BRAF-mutant gliomas are typically secondary pHGG, and commonly arise from what?	Low grade tumors (i.e., gangliogliomas or pleomorphic xanthoastrocytoma)

QUESTIONS

1. A 9-year-old girl is referred to an ophthalmologist after her pediatrician noted that she was having difficulty turning her left eye outward for the past week. Physical examination is normal with no neurocutaneous stigmata evident, and she has a left VI cranial nerve palsy on neurological exam. An MRI is obtained that demonstrates diffuse enlargement of the pons with no contrast enhancement post gadolinium administration. T2/FLAIR sequences demonstrate high signal in the pons and encasement of the basilar artery. You suspect a diagnosis of DIPG based on classical radiographic appearance and discuss the role of surgical biopsy. Prior to initiating treatment, your recommendation is
   a. No further staging is required, biopsy maybe considered in cases of atypical presentation.
   b. Biopsy is required for histopathological and molecular confirmation.
   c. Further staging is required, including MRI spine to exclude neuroaxis dissemination.
   d. Further staging is required, including MRI spine and lumbar puncture for cerebrospinal fluid (CSF) cytology.

2. You are scheduled to meet with the parents of the preceding patient to discuss the prognosis. What will you tell them?
   a. DIPGs are exquisitely sensitive to radiation, and, following treatment, long term disease control is expected.
   b. Given the absence of contrast enhancement, this is likely to be a low-grade tumor, which tends to respond more favorably to treatment, with long-term disease control expected.
   c. Survival longer than 2 years is extremely unlikely.
   d. Without histological and molecular testing results, the prognosis cannot be determined with confidence.

3. Parents request a neurosurgery referral, and a stereotactic biopsy is obtained. The most likely molecular abnormality is
   a. *BRAF V600E* mutation
   b. *H3 K27M* mutation
   c. *BRAF-KIAA1549* fusion
   d. *IDH1 R132H* mutation

4. A 4-year-old boy is referred by his primary pediatrician because on a well-child visit the child is noted to have a subtle cranial nerve VII palsy. A MRI brain demonstrates a focal, exophytic, contrast-enhancing mass in the pons. The pons appears to be pushed aside. What is the next step in management?
   a. Diagnosis is consistent with DIPG and biopsy is not required.
   b. Biopsy for suspected dorsally exophytic low-grade glioma
   c. MRI spine and lumbar puncture to stage the neuroaxis
   d. Focal radiation therapy to the pontine lesion

5. A 14-year-old girl presents with a 4-week history of progressively worsening right-sided facial weakness. She was initially diagnosed with Bell's palsy in the emergency room and received steroids with mild improvement. However, her symptoms have now progressed, including a new right hemiparesis. MRI demonstrates a 4 × 3.5 cm mass within the left thalamic region with mild surrounding edema and patchy enhancement. Given the acute onset of symptoms and imaging appearance, you suspect a high-grade glioma. The *most* appropriate next step in management is:
   a. Craniospinal radiation therapy with focal boost
   b. Focal radiation therapy
   c. Maximal safe surgical resection
   d. Neoadjuvant chemotherapy
   e. Palliative care alone

6. A 14-year-old boy who received 12 Gy whole-brain radiation for high-risk acute lymphoblastic leukemia (ALL) at 2 years of age is evaluated in a survivor clinic and reports severe headaches and vomiting over the past week. MRI reveals a new 2.9 cm × 3 cm mass in the left frontal lobe which is hypointense on T1-weighted images, hyperintense on T2-weighted images, and demonstrates heterogeneous enhancement after contrast administration. Of the following, the *most* likely diagnosis is
   a. Cavernoma
   b. Secondary pediatric high-grade glioma
   c. Meningioma
   d. Radiation necrosis

7. A 1-year-old girl undergoes gross total resection for a newly diagnosed lesion of the left frontal lobe. Pathology reveals glioblastoma (WHO grade 4). What is the next best step in management?
   a. Radiochemotherapy, including focal radiation therapy and temozolomide
   b. Radiochemotherapy, including craniospinal radiation therapy
   c. Genomic testing and administration of molecular targeted therapy
   d. Chemotherapy only

8. Molecular analysis of the tumor will most likely demonstrate
   a. *IDH1 R132H* mutation
   b. *BRAF-KIAA1549* fusion
   c. *NTRK*, *ALK*, or *ROS* fusion
   d. *H3 K27M* mutation

9. A 4-year-old boy with recurrent DIPG previously treated with standard definitive radiation therapy is scheduled to undergo focal salvage radiation. What factors put him at increased risk for symptomatic brainstem radionecrosis?
   a. Young age
   b. Tumor location in the posterior fossa
   c. Radiation dose
   d. All of the above

10. An 8-year-old girl who is the product of a consanguineous marriage is diagnosed with a left parietal glioblastoma. Her physical exam demonstrates several café-au-lait macules. The tumor is gross totally resected, and she subsequently receives focal irradiation to a total of 59.4 Gy. Whole-exome sequencing results from the tumor demonstrate a very high mutational burden (22,680 mutations per exome). What underlying germline mutation and cancer predisposition syndrome do you suspect?
    a. *P53* germline mutation, Li-Fraumeni syndrome
    b. *NF1* germline mutation, neurofibromatosis type 1
    c. Mismatch repair gene mutation (*PMS2*), constitutional mismatch repair deficiency
    d. CDKN2A tumor suppressor gene germline alteration, familial melanoma astrocytoma syndrome

11. A 17-year-old boy presented with left-sided focal seizures and headaches. T2 weighted MRI demonstrates a hyperintense right parieto-temporal lesion. The contrast enhancing portion of the tumor is near-totally resected, and pathology reveals features consistent with a predominant primitive neuroectodermal component with Ki-67 and MIB-1 index of 30%. Next-generation sequencing demonstrates the following alterations: *Histone 3 G34/35 (p.G35R H3F3A)*, *TP53* Frameshift Deletion *H214Qfs*7 (c.642_643del) exon 6*, *ATRX* nonsense mutation *K183* (c.547A>T) exon 7*, and *CDKN2A* loss. There is no *1p/19q* co-deletion. Based on these pathologic and molecular findings, what diagnosis do you suspect?
    a. Primitive embryonal tumor
    b. Hemispheric high-grade glioma (H3 G34 mutant)
    c. *RELA* fused ependymoma
    d. Anaplastic oligodendroglioma

12. The preceding patient is discussed at tumor board. What additional treatment would you recommend?
    a. Cranio-spinal radiation therapy and chemotherapy because of the significant primitive embryonal tumor component noted on pathology
    b. Focal radiation therapy and chemotherapy
    c. High-dose chemotherapy with stem cell rescue
    d. Second-look surgery to obtain a gross total resection of the enhancing tumor

13. A 19-year-old man presents with a seizure and a MRI brain demonstrates a frontal lobe mass. The tumor is resected and pathology demonstrates a WHO grade 3 anaplastic astrocytoma. Molecular testing reveals an *IDH1R132H* mutation, *TP53* missense mutation *R248W*, and *ATRX* mutation. Focal radiation therapy is recommended by the radiation oncologist. What additional treatment would you recommend?
    a. No adjuvant chemotherapy is recommended
    b. Adjuvant chemotherapy with temozolomide including maintenance temozolomide
    c. High-dose chemotherapy (thiotepa, carboplatin, and etoposide) with stem cell rescue
    d. Carboplatin and etoposide chemotherapy

14. A 6-year-old girl presents with seizures. MRI demonstrates a left temporal lesion which is highly infiltrative and heterogeneously contrast enhancing. Pathology demonstrates a high-grade neuroepithelial neoplasm with astrocytic components consistent with anaplastic pleomorphic xanthoastrocytoma WHO grade 3. Molecular testing will most likely demonstrate a
    a. *BRAF-KIAA1549* fusion
    b. *FGFR3-TACC3* fusion
    c. *BRAF V600E* mutation
    d. *QKI-RAF1* fusion

15. The preceding patient is discussed at tumor board. Next-generation sequencing demonstrates a *BRAF* exon15 *p.V600E (c.1799T>A)*, *CDKN2Ap16INK4A* deletion, and *CDKN2Ap14ARF* deletion. Focal radiation therapy is recommended, and you discuss the role of chemotherapy. The parents are concerned about the toxicities associated with alkylator chemotherapy, and its limited efficacy in published pHGG trials. What alternative treatment would you consider?
    a. Molecular targeted therapy with combined BRAF inhibitor and MEK inhibitor
    b. Immune checkpoint inhibitor therapy
    c. High-dose chemotherapy with stem cell rescue
    d. Craniospinal radiation therapy

ANSWERS

1. c
2. c
3. b
4. b
5. c
6. b
7. d
8. c
9. d
10. c
11. b
12. b
13. b
14. c
15. c

REFERENCES

1. Louis DN, Perry A, Reifenberger G, et al. The 2016 World Health Organization Classification of Tumors of the Central Nervous System: A summary. *Acta Neuropathologica*. 2016;131(6):803–820.
2. Ostrom QT, de Blank PM, Kruchko C, et al. Alex's Lemonade Stand Foundation infant and childhood primary brain and central nervous system tumors diagnosed in the united states in 2007-2011. *Neuro-Oncol*. 2015;16 Suppl 10:x1–x36.
3. Freeman CR, Farmer JP. Pediatric brain stem gliomas: A review. *Int J Radiat Oncol Biol Physics*.1998;40(2):265–271.
4. Ostrom QT, Gittleman H, Truitt G, et al. CBTRUS Statistical Report: Primary brain and other central nervous system tumors diagnosed in the United States in 2011-2015. *Neuro-Oncol*. 2018;20(suppl_4):iv1–iv86.
5. Johung TB, Monje M. Diffuse intrinsic pontine glioma: New pathophysiological insights and emerging therapeutic targets. *Curr Neuropharmacol*. 2017;15(1):88–97.
6. Pettorini BL, Park YS, Caldarelli M, et al. Radiation-induced brain tumours after central nervous system irradiation in childhood: A review. *Childs Nerv Syst*. 2008;24(7):793–805.
7. Michaeli O, Tabori U. Pediatric high grade gliomas in the context of cancer predisposition syndromes. *J Korean Neurosurg Soc*. 2018;61(3):319–332.
8. Bandopadhayay P, Bergthold G, London WB, et al. Long-term outcome of 4,040 children diagnosed with pediatric low-grade gliomas: An analysis of the Surveillance Epidemiology and End Results (SEER) database. *Pediatr Blood Cancer*. 2014;61(7):1173–1179.
9. Donaldson SS, Laningham F, Fisher PG. Advances toward an understanding of brainstem gliomas. *J clinical oncology*. 2006;24(8):1266–1272.
10. Schroeder KM, Hoeman CM, Becher OJ. Children are not just little adults: Recent advances in understanding of diffuse intrinsic pontine glioma biology. *Pediatr Res*. 2014;75(1-2):205–209.
11. Tinat J, Bougeard G, Baert-Desurmont S, et al. 2009 version of the Chompret criteria for Li Fraumeni syndrome. *J Clin Oncol*. 2009;27(26):e108-109; author reply e10.
12. Ferner RE, Huson SM, Thomas N, et al. Guidelines for the diagnosis and management of individuals with neurofibromatosis 1. *J Med Gen*. 2007;44(2):81–88.
13. Herkert JC, Niessen RC, Olderode-Berends MJ, et al. Paediatric intestinal cancer and polyposis due to bi-allelic PMS2 mutations: Case series, review and follow-up guidelines. *Eur J Cancer*. 2011;47(7):965–982.
14. Jasperson KW, Samowitz WS, Burt RW. Constitutional mismatch repair-deficiency syndrome presenting as colonic adenomatous polyposis: Clues from the skin. *Clin Genet*. 2011;80(4):394–397.
15. Benesch M, Wagner S, Berthold F, Wolff JE. Primary dissemination of high-grade gliomas in children: Experiences from four studies of the Pediatric Oncology and Hematology Society of the German Language Group (GPOH). *J Neuro-Oncol*. 2005;72(2):179–183.
16. Wagner S, Benesch M, Berthold F, et al. Secondary dissemination in children with high-grade malignant gliomas and diffuse intrinsic pontine gliomas. *Br J Cancer*. 2006;95(8):991–997.
17. Sethi R, Allen J, Donahue B, et al. Prospective neuraxis MRI surveillance reveals a high risk of leptomeningeal dissemination in diffuse intrinsic pontine glioma. *J Neuro-Oncol*. 2011;102(1):121–127.
18. Fisher PG, Breiter SN, Carson BS, et al. A clinicopathologic reappraisal of brain stem tumor classification. Identification of pilocystic astrocytoma and fibrillary astrocytoma as distinct entities. *Cancer*. 2000;89(7):1569–1576.
19. Abrigo JM, Fountain DM, Provenzale JM, et al. Magnetic resonance perfusion for differentiating low-grade from high-grade gliomas at first presentation. *Cochrane Database Syst Rev*. 2018;1:cd011551.
20. Patel P, Baradaran H, Delgado D, et al. MR perfusion-weighted imaging in the evaluation of high-grade gliomas after treatment: A systematic review and meta-analysis. *Neuro-Oncol*. 2017;19(1):118–127.
21. Guzmán-De-Villoria JA, Mateos-Pérez JM, Added value of advanced over conventional magnetic resonance imaging in grading gliomas and other primary brain tumors. *Cancer Imaging*. 2014;14(1):35.
22. Zukotynski K, Fahey F, Kocak M, et al. 18F-FDG PET and MR imaging associations across a spectrum of pediatric brain tumors: A report from the pediatric brain tumor consortium. *J Nucl Med*. 2014;55(9):1473–1480.
23. la Fougère C, Suchorska B, Bartenstein P, et al. Molecular imaging of gliomas with PET: Opportunities and limitations. *Neuro-Oncol*. 2011;13(8):806–819.
24. Louis DN, Ohgaki H, Wiestler OD, et al. The 2007 WHO classification of tumours of the central nervous system. *Acta Neuropathologica*. 2007;114(2):97–109.
25. Braunstein S, Raleigh D, Bindra R, et al. Pediatric high-grade glioma: Current molecular landscape and therapeutic approaches. *J Neuro-Oncology*. 2017;134(3):541–549.
26. Pollack IF, Finkelstein SD, Woods J, et al. Expression of p53 and prognosis in children with malignant gliomas. *N Engl J Med*. 2002;346(6):420–427.
27. Castel D, Philippe C, Calmon R, et al. Histone H3F3A and HIST1H3B K27M mutations define two subgroups of diffuse intrinsic pontine gliomas with different prognosis and phenotypes. *Acta Neuropathologica*. 2015;130(6):815–827.
28. Ceccarelli M, Barthel FP, Malta TM, et al. Molecular profiling reveals biologically discrete subsets and pathways of progression in diffuse glioma. *Cell*. 2016;164(3):550–563.
29. Buczkowicz P, Bartels U, Bouffet E, et al. Histopathological spectrum of paediatric diffuse intrinsic pontine glioma: Diagnostic and therapeutic implications. *Acta Neuropathologica*. 2014;128(4):573–581.
30. Cage TA, Samagh SP, Mueller S, et al. Feasibility, safety, and indications for surgical biopsy of intrinsic brainstem tumors in children. *Childs Nerv Syst*. 2013;29(8):1313–1319.
31. Jones C, Baker SJ. Unique genetic and epigenetic mechanisms driving paediatric diffuse high-grade glioma. *Nat Rev Cancer*. 2014;14(10).
32. Broniscer A, Chamdine O, Hwang S, et al. Gliomatosis cerebri in children shares molecular characteristics with other pediatric gliomas. *Acta Neuropathologica*. 2016;131(2):299–307.
33. Sturm D, Witt H, Hovestadt V, et al. Hotspot mutations in H3F3A and IDH1 define distinct epigenetic and biological subgroups of glioblastoma. *Cancer Cell*. 2012;22(4):425–437.
34. Sturm D, Pfister SM, Jones DTW. Pediatric gliomas: Current concepts on diagnosis, biology, and clinical management. *J Clinical Oncol*. 2017;35(21):2370–2377.
35. Korshunov A, Schrimpf D, Ryzhova M, et al. H3-/IDH-wild type pediatric glioblastoma is comprised of molecularly and prognostically distinct subtypes with associated oncogenic drivers. *Acta Neuropathologica*. 2017;134(3):507–516.
36. Mackay A, Burford A, Molinari V, et al. Molecular, pathological, radiological, and immune profiling of non-brainstem pediatric high-grade glioma from the HERBY Phase II randomized trial. *Cancer Cell*. 2018;33(5):829–42.e5.
37. Wick W, Weller M, van den Bent M, et al. MGMT testing: The challenges for biomarker-based glioma treatment. *Nat Rev Neurol*. 2014;10(7):372–385.
38. Bax DA, Mackay A, Little SE, et al. A distinct spectrum of copy number aberrations in pediatric high-grade gliomas. *Clin Cancer Res*. 2010;16(13):3368–3677.
39. Faury D, Nantel A, Dunn SE, et al. Molecular profiling identifies prognostic subgroups of pediatric glioblastoma and shows increased YB-1 expression in tumors. *J Clin Oncol*. 2007;25(10):1196–1208.
40. Paugh BS, Qu C, Jones C, et al. Integrated molecular genetic profiling of pediatric high-grade gliomas reveals key differences with the adult disease. *J Clin Oncol*. 2010;28(18):3061–3068.
41. Paugh BS, Broniscer A, Qu C, et al. Genome-wide analyses identify recurrent amplifications of receptor tyrosine kinases and cell-cycle regulatory genes in diffuse intrinsic pontine glioma. *J Clin Oncol*. 2011;29(30):3999–4006.
42. Puget S, Philippe C, Bax DA, et al. Mesenchymal transition and PDGFRA amplification/mutation are key distinct oncogenic events in pediatric diffuse intrinsic pontine gliomas. *PLoS One*. 2012;7(2):e30313.
43. Zarghooni M, Bartels U, Lee E, et al. Whole-genome profiling of pediatric diffuse intrinsic pontine gliomas highlights platelet-derived growth factor receptor alpha and poly (ADP-ribose) polymerase as potential therapeutic targets. *J Clin Oncol*. 2010;28(8):1337–1344.
44. Schwartzentruber J, Korshunov A, Liu XY, et al. Driver mutations in histone H3.3 and chromatin remodelling genes in paediatric glioblastoma. *Nature*. 2012;482(7384):226–231.
45. Wu G, Broniscer A, McEachron TA, et al. Somatic histone H3 alterations in pediatric diffuse intrinsic pontine gliomas and non-brainstem glioblastomas. *Nat Genet*. 2012;44(3):251–253.
46. Korshunov A, Capper D, Reuss D, et al. Histologically distinct neuroepithelial tumors with histone 3 G34 mutation are molecularly similar and comprise a single nosologic entity. *Acta Neuropathologica*. 2016;131(1):137–46.
47. Mackay A, Burford A, Carvalho D, et al. Integrated molecular meta-analysis of 1,000 pediatric high-grade and diffuse intrinsic pontine glioma. *Cancer Cell*. 2017;32(4):520–537.e5.
48. Dubois, F.P.B., Shapira, O., Greenwald, N.F. et al. Structural variants shape driver combinations and outcomes in pediatric high-grade glioma. *Nat Cancer* (2022). https://doi.org/10.1038/s43018-022-00403-z
49. Buczkowicz P, Hoeman C, Rakopoulos P, et al. Genomic analysis of diffuse intrinsic pontine gliomas identifies three molecular subgroups and recurrent activating ACVR1 mutations. *Nat Genet*. 2014;46(5):451–456.

50. Fontebasso AM, Papillon-Cavanagh S, Schwartzentruber J, et al. Recurrent somatic mutations in ACVR1 in pediatric midline high-grade astrocytoma. *Nat Genet.* 2014;46(5):462–466.

51. Taylor KR, Mackay A, Truffaux N, et al. Recurrent activating ACVR1 mutations in diffuse intrinsic pontine glioma. *Nat Genet.* 2014;46(5):457–461.

52. Wu G, Diaz AK, Paugh BS, et al. The genomic landscape of diffuse intrinsic pontine glioma and pediatric non-brainstem high-grade glioma. *Nat Genet.* 2014;46(5):444–450.

53. Sturm D, Bender S, Jones DT, et al. Paediatric and adult glioblastoma: Multiform (epi)genomic culprits emerge. *Nat Rev Cancer.* 2014;14(2):92–107.

54. Nakamura M, Shimada K, Ishida E, et al. Molecular pathogenesis of pediatric astrocytic tumors. *Neuro-Oncol.* 2007;9(2):113–123.

55. Nicholson HS, Kretschmar CS, Krailo M, et al. Phase 2 study of temozolomide in children and adolescents with recurrent central nervous system tumors: A report from the Children's Oncology Group. *Cancer.* 2007;110(7):1542–1550.

56. Finlay JL, Boyett JM, Yates AJ, et al. Randomized phase III trial in childhood high-grade astrocytoma comparing vincristine, lomustine, and prednisone with the eight-drugs-in-1-day regimen. Childrens Cancer Group. *J Clin Oncol.* 1995;13(1):112–123.

57. Mueller S, Phillips J, Onar-Thomas A, et al. PTEN promoter methylation and activation of the PI3K/Akt/mTOR pathway in pediatric gliomas and influence on clinical outcome. *Neuro-Oncol.* 2012;14(9):1146–1152.

58. Pollack IF, Hamilton RL, Burger PC, et al. Akt activation is a common event in pediatric malignant gliomas and a potential adverse prognostic marker: A report from the Children's Oncology Group. *J Neuro-Oncol.* 2010;99(2):155–163.

59. Snuderl M, Fazlollahi L, Le LP, et al. Mosaic amplification of multiple receptor tyrosine kinase genes in glioblastoma. *Cancer Cell.* 2011;20(6):810–817.

60. Korshunov A, Ryzhova M, Hovestadt V, et al. Integrated analysis of pediatric glioblastoma reveals a subset of biologically favorable tumors with associated molecular prognostic markers. *Acta Neuropathologica.* 2015;129(5):669–678.

61. Nikbakht H, Panditharatna E, Mikael LG, et al. Spatial and temporal homogeneity of driver mutations in diffuse intrinsic pontine glioma. *Nat Commun.* 2016;7:11185.

62. Fuller CE, Jones DTW, Kieran MW. New classification for central nervous system tumors: Implications for diagnosis and therapy. *Am Soc Clin Oncol Educ Book.* 2017;37:753–763.

63. Jones C, Karajannis MA, Jones DTW, et al. Pediatric high-grade glioma: Biologically and clinically in need of new thinking. *Neuro-Oncol.* 2017;19(2):153–161.

64. Bechet D, Gielen GG, Korshunov A, et al. Specific detection of methionine 27 mutation in histone 3 variants (H3K27M) in fixed tissue from high-grade astrocytomas. *Acta Neuropathologica.* 2014;128(5):733–741.

65. Venneti S, Santi M, Felicella MM, et al. A sensitive and specific histopathologic prognostic marker for H3F3A K27M mutant pediatric glioblastomas. *Acta Neuropathologica.* 2014;128(5):743–753.

66. Bender S, Tang Y, Lindroth AM, et al. Reduced H3K27me3 and DNA hypomethylation are major drivers of gene expression in K27M mutant pediatric high-grade gliomas. *Cancer Cell.* 2013;24(5):660–672.

67. Hoeman CM, Cordero FJ, Hu G, et al. ACVR1 R206H cooperates with H3.1K27M in promoting diffuse intrinsic pontine glioma pathogenesis. *Nat Commun.* 2019;10(1):1023.

68. Korshunov A, Capper D, Reuss D, et al. Histologically distinct neuroepithelial tumors with histone 3 G34 mutation are molecularly similar and comprise a single nosologic entity. *Acta Neuropathologica.* 2016;131(1):137–146.

69. Khuong-Quang DA, Buczkowicz P, et al. K27M mutation in histone H3.3 defines clinically and biologically distinct subgroups of pediatric diffuse intrinsic pontine gliomas. *Acta Neuropathologica.* 2012;124(3):439–447.

70. Pollack IF, Hamilton RL, Sobol RW, et al. IDH1 mutations are common in malignant gliomas arising in adolescents: A report from the Children's Oncology Group. *Childs Nerv Syst.* 2011;27(1):87–94.

71. Mistry M, Zhukova N, Merico D, et al. BRAF mutation and CDKN2A deletion define a clinically distinct subgroup of childhood secondary high-grade glioma. *J Clin Oncol.* 2015;33(9):1015–1022.

72. Lassaletta A, Zapotocky M, Mistry M, et al. Therapeutic and prognostic implications of BRAF V600E in pediatric low-grade gliomas. *J Clin Oncol.* 2017;35(25):2934–2941.

73. Qaddoumi I, Sultan I, Gajjar A. Outcome and prognostic features in pediatric gliomas: A review of 6212 cases from the Surveillance, Epidemiology, and End Results database. *Cancer.* 2009;115(24):5761–5770.

74. Stücklin AG, Ryall S, Fukuoka K, et al. HGG-19: Molecular analysis uncovers 3 distinct subgroups and multiple targetable gene fusions in infant gliomas. *Neuro-Oncol.* 2019;21(Suppl 2):ii90–ii1.

75. Zhang J, Wu G, Miller CP, et al. Whole-genome sequencing identifies genetic alterations in pediatric low-grade gliomas. *Nat Genet.* 2013;45(6):602–612.

76. Jones DT, Hutter B, Jager N, et al. Recurrent somatic alterations of FGFR1 and NTRK2 in pilocytic astrocytoma. *Nat Genet.* 2013;45(8):927–932.

77. Frattini V, Trifonov V, Chan JM, et al. The integrated landscape of driver genomic alterations in glioblastoma. *Nat Genet.* 2013;45(10):1141–1149.

78. Zhang J, Walsh MF, Wu G, et al. Germline Mutations in Predisposition Genes in Pediatric Cancer. *N Engl J Med.* 2015;373(24):2336–2346.

79. Kyritsis AP, Bondy ML, Rao JS, Sioka C. Inherited predisposition to glioma. *Neuro-Oncol.* 2010;12(1):104–113.

80. Laithier V, Grill J, Le Deley MC, et al. Progression-free survival in children with optic pathway tumors: Dependence on age and the quality of the response to chemotherapy: Results of the first French prospective study for the French Society of Pediatric Oncology. *J Clin Oncol.* 2003;21(24):4572–4578.

81. Opocher E, Kremer LC, Da Dalt L, et al. Prognostic factors for progression of childhood optic pathway glioma: A systematic review. *Eur J Cancer.* 2006;42(12):1807–1816.

82. Offit K. *Clinical Cancer Genetics: Risk Counseling and Management.* New York: Wiley-Liss; 1998: xvii.

83. Walsh MF, Kennedy J, Harlan M, et al. Germ line BRCA2 mutations detected in pediatric sequencing studies impact parents' evaluation and care. *Cold Spring Harb Mol Case Stud.* 2017.

84. Evans DG, Birch JM, Ramsden RT, et al. Malignant transformation and new primary tumours after therapeutic radiation for benign disease: Substantial risks in certain tumour prone syndromes. *J Med Gen.* 2006;43(4):289–294.

85. Fangusaro J, Onar-Thomas A, Young Poussaint T, et al. Selumetinib in paediatric patients with BRAF-aberrant or neurofibromatosis type 1-associated recurrent, refractory, or progressive low-grade glioma: A multicentre, phase 2 trial. *Lancet Oncol.* 2019;20(7):1011–1022.

86. Schulmann K, Brasch FE, Kunstmann E, et al. HNPCC-associated small bowel cancer: Clinical and molecular characteristics. *Gastroenterology.* 2005;128(3):590–599.

87. Barrow E, Robinson L, Alduaij W, et al. Cumulative lifetime incidence of extracolonic cancers in Lynch syndrome: A report of 121 families with proven mutations. *Clin Genet.* 2009;75(2):141–149.

88. Bakry D, Aronson M, Durno C, et al. Genetic and clinical determinants of constitutional mismatch repair deficiency syndrome: Report from the constitutional mismatch repair deficiency consortium. *Eur J Cancer.* 2014;50(5):987–996.

89. Felton KE, Gilchrist DM, Andrew SE. Constitutive deficiency in DNA mismatch repair. *Clin Genet.* 2007;71(6):483–498.

90. Wimmer K, Etzler J. Constitutional mismatch repair-deficiency syndrome: Have we so far seen only the tip of an iceberg? *Human genetics.* 2008;124(2):105–122.

91. Van Meir EG. "Turcot's syndrome": Phenotype of brain tumors, survival and mode of inheritance. *Int J Cancer.* 1998;75(1):162–164.

92. Lusis EA, Travers S, Jost SC, Perry A. Glioblastomas with giant cell and sarcomatous features in patients with Turcot syndrome type 1: A clinicopathological study of 3 cases. *Neurosurgery.* 2010;67(3):811–817; discussion 7.

93. Ripperger T, Beger C, Rahner N, et al. Constitutional mismatch repair deficiency and childhood leukemia/lymphoma: Report on a novel biallelic MSH6 mutation. *Haematologica.* 2010;95(5):841–844.

94. Wimmer K, Kratz CP. Constitutional mismatch repair-deficiency syndrome. *Haematologica.* 2010;95(5):699–701.

95. Bouffet E, Larouche V, Campbell BB, et al. Immune checkpoint inhibition for hypermutant glioblastoma multiforme resulting from germline biallelic mismatch repair deficiency. *J Clin Oncol.* 2016;34(19):2206–2211.

96. Malkin D, Li FP, Strong LC, et al. Germ line p53 mutations in a familial syndrome of breast cancer, sarcomas, and other neoplasms. *Science.* 1990;250(4985):1233–1238.

97. Vahteristo P, Tamminen A, Karvinen P, et al. p53, CHK2, and CHK1 genes in Finnish families with Li-Fraumeni syndrome: Further evidence of CHK2 in inherited cancer predisposition. *Cancer Res.* 2001;61(15):5718–5722.

98. Olivier M, Goldgar DE, Sodha N, et al. Li-Fraumeni and related syndromes: Correlation between tumor type, family structure, and TP53 genotype. *Cancer Res.* 2003;63(20):6643–6650.

99. Kony SJ, de Vathaire F, Chompret A, et al. Radiation and genetic factors in the risk of second malignant neoplasms after a first cancer in childhood. *Lancet.* 1997;350(9071):91–95.

100. Heymann S, Delaloge S, Rahal A, et al. Radio-induced malignancies after breast cancer postoperative radiotherapy in patients with Li-Fraumeni syndrome. *Radiation Oncol (London)*. 2010;5:104.

101. Talwalkar SS, Yin CC, Naeem RC, et al. Myelodysplastic syndromes arising in patients with germline TP53 mutation and Li-Fraumeni syndrome. *Arch Pathol Lab Med*. 2010;134(7):1010–1015.

102. Villani A, Tabori U, Schiffman J, et al. Biochemical and imaging surveillance in germline TP53 mutation carriers with Li-Fraumeni syndrome: A prospective observational study. *The lancet oncology*. 2011;12(6):559–567.

103. Shen MH, Harper PS, Upadhyaya M. Molecular genetics of neurofibromatosis type 1 (NF1). *J medical genetics*. 1996;33(1):2–17.

104. Gutmann DH, Donahoe J, Brown T, et al. Loss of neurofibromatosis 1 (NF1) gene expression in NF1-associated pilocytic astrocytomas. *Neuropathol Applied Neurobiol*. 2000;26(4):361–367.

105. Weiss B, Bollag G, Shannon K. Hyperactive Ras as a therapeutic target in neurofibromatosis type 1. *Am J Med Genet*. 1999;89(1):14–22.

106. Huttner AJ, Kieran MW, Yao X, et al. Clinicopathologic study of glioblastoma in children with neurofibromatosis type 1. *Pediatr Blood Cancer*. 2010;54(7):890–896.

107. D'Angelo F, Ceccarelli M, Tala, et al. The molecular landscape of glioma in patients with Neurofibromatosis 1. *Nat Med*. 2019;25(1):176–187.

108. Gutmann DH, James CD, Poyhonen M, et al. Molecular analysis of astrocytomas presenting after age 10 in individuals with NF1. *Neurology*. 2003;61(10):1397–1400.

109. Broniscer A, Ke W, Fuller CE, et al. Second neoplasms in pediatric patients with primary central nervous system tumors. 2004;100(10):2246–2252.

110. Carret A-S, Tabori U, Crooks B, et al. Outcome of secondary high-grade glioma in children previously treated for a malignant condition: A study of the Canadian Pediatric Brain Tumour Consortium. *Radiother Oncol*. 2006;81(1):33–38.

111. López GY, Van Ziffle J, Onodera C, et al. The genetic landscape of gliomas arising after therapeutic radiation. *Acta Neuropathologica*. 2019;137(1):139–150.

112. Cohen KJ, Pollack IF, Zhou T, et al. Temozolomide in the treatment of high-grade gliomas in children: A report from the Children's Oncology Group. *Neuro-Oncol*. 2011;13(3):317–323.

113. Cohen KJ, Heideman RL, Zhou T, et al. Temozolomide in the treatment of children with newly diagnosed diffuse intrinsic pontine gliomas: A report from the Children's Oncology Group. *Neuro-Oncol*. 2011;13(4):410–416.

114. Pincus DW, Richter EO, Yachnis AT. Brainstem stereotactic biopsy sampling in children. *J Neurosurg*. 2006;104(2 Suppl):108–114.

115. Roujeau T, Machado G, Garnett MR, et al. Stereotactic biopsy of diffuse pontine lesions in children. *J Neurosurg*. 2007;107(1 Suppl):1–4.

116. Walker DA, Liu J, Kieran M, et al. A multi-disciplinary consensus statement concerning surgical approaches to low-grade, high-grade astrocytomas and diffuse intrinsic pontine gliomas in childhood (CPN Paris 2011) using the Delphi method. *Neuro-Oncol*. 2013;15(4):462–468.

117. Wisoff JH, Boyett JM, Berger MS, et al. Current neurosurgical management and the impact of the extent of resection in the treatment of malignant gliomas of childhood: A report of the Children's Cancer Group trial no. CCG-945. *J Neurosurg*. 1998;89(1):52–59.

118. MacDonald TJ, Aguilera D, Kramm CM. Treatment of high-grade glioma in children and adolescents. *Neuro-Oncology*. 2011;13(10):1049–1058.

119. MacDonald SM, Bindra RS, Sethi R, Ladra M. Principles of radiation oncology. In Gajjar A, Reaman GH, Racadio JM, Smith FO, eds., *Brain Tumors in Children*. New York: Springer; 2018:33–64.

120. Shapiro WR, Young DF. Treatment of malignant glioma. A controlled study of chemotherapy and irradiation. *Arch Neurol*. 1976;33(7):494–450.

121. Walker MD, Alexander E Jr, Hunt WE, et al. Evaluation of BCNU and/or radiotherapy in the treatment of anaplastic gliomas. A cooperative clinical trial. *J Neurosurg*. 1978;49(3):333–343.

122. Walker MD, Green SB, Byar DP, et al. Randomized comparisons of radiotherapy and nitrosoureas for the treatment of malignant glioma after surgery. *N Engl J Med*. 1980;303(23):1323–1329.

123. Kristiansen K, Hagen S, Kollevold T, et al. Combined modality therapy of operated astrocytomas grade III and IV. Confirmation of the value of postoperative irradiation and lack of potentiation of bleomycin on survival time: A prospective multicenter trial of the Scandinavian Glioblastoma Study Group. *Cancer*. 1981;47(4):649–652.

124. Sposto R, Ertel IJ, Jenkin RD, et al. The effectiveness of chemotherapy for treatment of high grade astrocytoma in children: Results of a randomized trial. A report from the Childrens Cancer Study Group. *J Neuro-Oncol*. 1989;7(2):165–177.

125. Fallai C, Olmi P. Hyperfractionated and accelerated radiation therapy in central nervous system tumors (malignant gliomas, pediatric tumors, and brain metastases). *Radiother Oncol*. 1997;43(3):235–246.

126. Biswas T, Okunieff P, Schell MC, et al. Stereotactic radiosurgery for glioblastoma: Retrospective analysis. *Radiat Oncol*. 2009;4:11.

127. Shrieve DC, Alexander E, 3rd, Black PM, et al. Treatment of patients with primary glioblastoma multiforme with standard postoperative radiotherapy and radiosurgical boost: Prognostic factors and long-term outcome. *J Neurosurg*. 1999;90(1):72–77.

128. Nieder C, Adam M, Molls M, Grosu AL. Therapeutic options for recurrent high-grade glioma in adult patients: Recent advances. *Crit Rev Oncol Hematol*. 2006;60(3):181–193.

129. Müller K, Scheithauer H, Pietschmann S, et al. Reirradiation as part of a salvage treatment approach for progressive non-pontine pediatric high-grade gliomas: Preliminary experiences from the German HIT-HGG study group. *Radiat Oncol*. 2014;9:177.

130. Warren KE. Diffuse intrinsic pontine glioma: Poised for progress. *Front Oncol*. 2012;2:205.

131. Gallitto M, Lazarev S, Wasserman I, et al. Role of radiation therapy in the management of diffuse intrinsic pontine glioma: A systematic review. *Adv Radiat Oncol*. 2019;4(3):520–531.

132. Fangusaro J. Pediatric high grade glioma: A review and update on tumor clinical characteristics and biology. *Front Oncol*. 2012;2:105.

133. Peirce CB, Bouchard J. Role of radiation therapy in the control of malignant neoplasms of the brain and brain stem. *Radiology*. 1950;55(3):337–343.

134. Lee F. Radiation of infratentorial and supratentorial brain-stem tumors. *J Neurosurg*. 1975;43(1):65–68.

135. Packer RJ, Boyett JM, Zimmerman RA, et al. Hyperfractionated radiation therapy (72 Gy) for children with brain stem gliomas: A Childrens Cancer Group Phase I/II Trial. *Cancer*. 1993;72(4):1414–1421.

136. Freeman CR, Krischer JP, Sanford RA, et al. Final results of a study of escalating doses of hyperfractionated radiotherapy in brain stem tumors in children: A Pediatric Oncology Group study. *Int J Radiat Oncol Biol Physics*. 1993;27(2):197–206.

137. Edwards MS, Wara WM, Urtasun RC, et al. Hyperfractionated radiation therapy for brain-stem glioma: A phase I-II trial. *J Neurosurg*. 1989;70(5):691–700.

138. Packer RJ, Boyett JM, Zimmerman RA, et al. Outcome of children with brain stem gliomas after treatment with 7800 cGy of hyperfractionated radiotherapy. A Childrens Cancer Group Phase I/II Trial. *Cancer*. 1994;74(6):1827–1834.

139. Mandell LR, Kadota R, Freeman C, et al. There is no role for hyperfractionated radiotherapy in the management of children with newly diagnosed diffuse intrinsic brainstem tumors: Results of a Pediatric Oncology Group phase III trial comparing conventional vs. hyperfractionated radiotherapy. *Int J Radiat Oncol Biol Physics*. 1999;43(5):959–964.

140. Janssens GO, Gidding CE, Van Lindert EJ, et al. The role of hypofractionation radiotherapy for diffuse intrinsic brainstem glioma in children: A pilot study. *Int J Radiat Oncol Biol Physics*. 2009;73(3):722–726.

141. Janssens GO, Jansen MH, Lauwers SJ, et al. Hypofraction vs conventional radiation therapy for newly diagnosed diffuse intrinsic pontine glioma: A matched-cohort analysis. *Int J Radiat Oncol Biol Physics*. 2013;85(2):315–320.

142. Zaghloul MS, Eldebawy E, Ahmed S, et al. Hypofractionated conformal radiotherapy for pediatric diffuse intrinsic pontine glioma (DIPG): A randomized controlled trial. *Radiother Oncol*. 2014;111(1):35–40.

143. Lassaletta A, Strother D, Laperriere N, et al. Reirradiation in patients with diffuse intrinsic pontine gliomas: The Canadian experience. *Pediatr Blood Cancer*. 2018;65(6):e26988.

144. Fontanilla HP, Pinnix CC, Ketonen LM, et al. Palliative reirradiation for progressive diffuse intrinsic pontine glioma. *Am J Clin Oncol*. 2012;35(1):51–57.

145. Janssens GO, Gandola L, Bolle S, et al. Survival benefit for patients with diffuse intrinsic pontine glioma (DIPG) undergoing re-irradiation at first progression: A matched-cohort analysis on behalf of the SIOP-E-HGG/DIPG working group. *Eur J Cancer*. 2017;73:38–47.

146. Massimino M, Biassoni V, Miceli R, et al. Results of nimotuzumab and vinorelbine, radiation and re-irradiation for diffuse pontine glioma in childhood. *J Neuro-Oncol*. 2014;118(2):305–312.

147. Amsbaugh MJ, Mahajan A, Thall PF, et al. A phase 1/2 trial of reirradiation for diffuse intrinsic pontine glioma. *Int J Radiat Oncol Biol Physics*. 2019;104(1):144–148.

148. Indelicato DJ, Flampouri S, Rotondo RL, et al. Incidence and dosimetric parameters of pediatric brainstem toxicity following proton therapy. *Acta Oncol*. 2014;53(10):1298–1304.

149. Gentile MS, Yeap BY, Paganetti H, et al. Brainstem injury in pediatric patients with posterior fossa tumors treated with proton beam

therapy and associated dosimetric factors. *Int J Radiat Oncol Biol Phys.* 2018;100(3):719–729.

150. Devine CA, Liu KX, Ioakeim-Ioannidou M, et al. Brainstem injury in pediatric patients receiving posterior fossa photon radiation. *Int J Radiat Oncol Biol Phys.* 2019;105(5):1034–1042.

151. Haas-Kogan D, Indelicato D, Paganetti H, et al. National Cancer Institute Workshop on Proton Therapy for Children: Considerations Regarding Brainstem Injury. *Int J Radiat Oncol Biol Phys.* 2018;101(1):152–168.

152. Pollack IF, Boyett JM, Yates AJ, et al. The influence of central review on outcome associations in childhood malignant gliomas: Results from the CCG-945 experience. *Neuro-Oncol.* 2003;5(3):197–207.

153. Jakacki RI, Cohen KJ, Buxton A, et al. Phase 2 study of concurrent radiotherapy and temozolomide followed by temozolomide and lomustine in the treatment of children with high-grade glioma: A report of the Children's Oncology Group ACNS0423 study. *Neuro-Oncol.* 2016;18(10):1442–1450.

154. Hoffman LM, Geller J, Leach J, et al. TR-14: A feasibility and randomized phase ii study of vorinostat, bevacizumab, or temozolomide during radiation followed by maintenance chemotherapy in newly-diagnosed pediatric high-grade glioma: Children's Oncology Group study ACNS0822. *Neuro-Oncol.* 2015;17(Suppl 3):iii39–iii40.

155. Grill J, Massimino M, Bouffet E, et al. Phase II, Open-label, randomized, multicenter trial (HERBY) of bevacizumab in pediatric patients with newly diagnosed high-grade glioma. *J Clin Oncol.* 2018;36(10):951–958.

156. Marachelian A, Butturini A, Finlay J. Myeloablative chemotherapy with autologous hematopoietic progenitor cell rescue for childhood central nervous system tumors. *Bone Marrow Transplant.* 2008;41(2):167–172.

157. Kieran MW, Hargrave DR, Cohen KJ, et al. Phase 1 study of dabrafenib in pediatric patients (pts) with relapsed or refractory BRAF V600E high- and low-grade gliomas (HGG, LGG), Langerhans cell histiocytosis (LCH), and other solid tumors (OST). *J Clinical Oncology.* 2015;33(15_suppl):10004.

158. Michalski A, Bouffet E, Taylor RE, et al. The addition of high-dose tamoxifen to standard radiotherapy does not improve the survival of patients with diffuse intrinsic pontine glioma. *J Neuro-Oncol.* 2010;100(1):81–88.

159. Warren K, Bent R, Wolters PL, et al. A phase 2 study of pegylated interferon alpha-2b (PEG-Intron((R))) in children with diffuse intrinsic pontine glioma. *Cancer.* 2012;118(14):3607–3613.

160. Jennings MT, Sposto R, Boyett JM, et al. Preradiation chemotherapy in primary high-risk brainstem tumors: Phase II study CCG-9941 of the Children's Cancer Group. *J Clin Oncol.* 2002;20(16):3431–3437.

161. Kretschmar CS, Tarbell NJ, Barnes PD, et al. Pre-irradiation chemotherapy and hyperfractionated radiation therapy 66 Gy for children with brain stem tumors. A phase II study of the Pediatric Oncology Group, Protocol 8833. *Cancer.* 1993;72(4):1404–1413.

162. Bernier-Chastagner V, Grill J, Doz F, et al. Topotecan as a radiosensitizer in the treatment of children with malignant diffuse brainstem gliomas: Results of a French Society of Paediatric Oncology Phase II Study. *Cancer.* 2005;104(12):2792–2797.

163. Marcus KJ, Dutton SC, Barnes P, et al. A phase I trial of etanidazole and hyperfractionated radiotherapy in children with diffuse brainstem glioma. *Int J Radiat Oncol Biol Physics.* 2003;55(5):1182–1185.

164. Turner CD, Chi S, Marcus KJ, et al. Phase II study of thalidomide and radiation in children with newly diagnosed brain stem gliomas and glioblastoma multiforme. *J Neuro-Oncol.* 2007;82(1):95–101.

165. Wolff JE, Westphal S, Molenkamp G, et al. Treatment of paediatric pontine glioma with oral trophosphamide and etoposide. *Br J Cancer.* 2002;87(9):945–949.

166. Allen J, Siffert J, Donahue B, et al. A phase I/II study of carboplatin combined with hyperfractionated radiotherapy for brainstem gliomas. *Cancer.* 1999;86(6):1064–1069.

167. Walter AW, Gajjar A, Ochs JS, et al. Carboplatin and etoposide with hyperfractionated radiotherapy in children with newly diagnosed diffuse pontine gliomas: A phase I/II study. *Med Pediatr Oncol.* 1998;30(1):28–33.

168. Sirachainan N, Pakakasama S, Visudithbhan A, et al. Concurrent radiotherapy with temozolomide followed by adjuvant temozolomide and cis-retinoic acid in children with diffuse intrinsic pontine glioma. *Neuro-Oncol.* 2008;10(4):577–582.

169. Hall WA, Doolittle ND, Daman M, et al. Osmotic blood-brain barrier disruption chemotherapy for diffuse pontine gliomas. *J Neuro-Oncol.* 2006;77(3):279–284.

170. Riina HA, Knopman J, Greenfield JP, et al. Balloon-assisted superselective intra-arterial cerebral infusion of bevacizumab for malignant brainstem glioma. A technical note. *Intervent Neuroradiol.* 2010;16(1):71–76.

171. Bouffet E, Raquin M, Doz F, et al. Radiotherapy followed by high dose busulfan and thiotepa: A prospective assessment of high dose chemotherapy in children with diffuse pontine gliomas. *Cancer.* 2000;88(3):685–692.

172. Broniscer A, Baker SD, Wetmore C, et al. Phase I trial, pharmacokinetics, and pharmacodynamics of vandetanib and dasatinib in children with newly diagnosed diffuse intrinsic pontine glioma. *Clin Cancer Res.* 2013;19(11):3050–3058.

173. Cohen KJ, Gibbs IC, Fisher PG, et al. A phase I trial of arsenic trioxide chemoradiotherapy for infiltrating astrocytomas of childhood. *Neuro-Oncol.* 2013;15(6):783–787.

174. Wagner S, Warmuth-Metz M, Emser A, et al. Treatment options in childhood pontine gliomas. *J Neuro-Oncol.* 2006;79(3):281–287.

175. Sanders RP, Kocak M, Burger PC, et al. High-grade astrocytoma in very young children. *Pediatr Blood Cancer.* 2007;49(7):888–893.

176. Geyer JR, Finlay JL, Boyett JM, et al. Survival of infants with malignant astrocytomas. A Report from the Childrens Cancer Group. *Cancer.* 1995;75(4):1045–1050.

177. Dufour C, Grill J, Lellouch-Tubiana A, et al. High-grade glioma in children under 5 years of age: A chemotherapy only approach with the BBSFOP protocol. *Eur J Cancer.* 2006;42(17):2939–2945.

178. Duffner PK, Horowitz ME, Krischer JP, et al. Postoperative chemotherapy and delayed radiation in children less than three years of age with malignant brain tumors. *N Engl J Med.* 1993;328(24):1725–1731.

179. Duffner PK, Horowitz ME, Krischer JP, et al. The treatment of malignant brain tumors in infants and very young children: An update of the Pediatric Oncology Group experience. *Neuro-Oncol.* 1999;1(2):152–161.

180. Duffner PK, Krischer JP, Burger PC, et al. Treatment of infants with malignant gliomas: The Pediatric Oncology Group experience. *J Neuro-Oncol.* 1996;28(2-3):245–256.

181. MacY ME, Birks DK, Barton VN, et al. Clinical and molecular characteristics of congenital glioblastoma. *Neuro-Oncol.* 2012;14(7):931–941.

182. Clarke MT, Jones DTW, Mackay A, et al. HGG-25. Infant gliomas comprise multiple biological and clinicopathological subgroups. *Neuro-Oncol.* 2018;20(suppl_2):i94–i.

183. Robinson G, Desai A, Gauvain K, et al. PDCT-13. Entrectinib in children and adolescents with recurrent or refractory solid tumors including primary CNS tumors. *Neuro-Oncol.* 2019;21(Supplement_6):vi186–vi.

184. Warren KE. Pediatric high-grade gliomas: Survival at what cost? *Transl Pediatr.* 2012;1(2):116–117.

185. Sands SA, Zhou T, O'Neil SH, et al. Long-term follow-up of children treated for high-grade gliomas: Children's oncology group L991 final study report. *J Clin Oncol.* 2012;30(9):943–949.

PART IV. | MANAGEMENT OF NEURO-ONCOLOGIC DISEASE

19 | NEUROSURGICAL MANAGEMENT OF ADULT CENTRAL NERVOUS SYSTEM TUMORS

ANDREW J. GOGOS, RAMIN A. MORSHED, AND SHAWN L. HERVEY-JUMPER

INTRODUCTION

With more than 100 histologically distinct primary central nervous system (CNS) tumors in addition to metastatic disease, tumors within the brain and spine each have their own distinct symptom profile and outcomes. The Central Brain Tumor Registry of the United States (CBTRUS) statistical report of primary brain and other CNS tumors diagnosed in the United States reviewed data from 388,786 brain and spinal cord samples.[1] Furthermore, the 2016 World Health Organization (WHO) classification of CNS tumors sorts tumors into the following categories: diffuse astrocytic and oligodendroglial tumors, other astrocytic tumors (pilocytic astrocytomas, subependymal giant cell astrocytomas, pleomorphic xanthoastrocytomas), ependymal tumors (subependymoma, myxopapillary ependymoma), other gliomas (chordoid gliomas of the third ventricle, astroblastoma, and angiocentric glioma), neuronal and mixed neuronal-glial tumors (dysembryoplastic neuroepithelial tumor, ganglioglioma, dysplastic cerebellar gangliocytoma, central neurocytoma, paraganglioma), tumors of the pineal region (pineocytoma, pineoblastoma, papillary tumor of the pineal region), embryonal tumors (medulloblastoma, CNS neuroblastoma, atypical teratoid rhabdoid tumor [ATRT]), and tumors of the cranial and paraspinal nerves (schwannoma).[2] Neurosurgical management of CNS tumors has evolved in tandem with advances in medical and radiation oncology. Over the past 20 years, there has been a rapid expansion in techniques which have led to improved safety for patients undergoing surgical treatment. The goal of this chapter is to explain the rationale, indications, methods, outcomes, and limitations of surgery for adult patients with tumors involving the brain and spinal cord. The surgical management of pediatric tumors is discussed in Chapter 15.

RATIONALE FOR SURGERY

In general, the goal of surgery in neuro-oncology is to provide (1) an accurate histological diagnosis, (2) cytoreduction, and (3) symptom control, including the treatment of seizures, relief of mass effect, relief of hydrocephalus, reduction of cerebral edema, and spinal stabilization. Individual patient factors, tumor type and location, and presenting symptoms all inform the selection of surgical procedures for each patient.

> The goal of surgery in neuro-oncology is to provide (1) an accurate histological diagnosis, (2) cytoreduction, and (3) symptom control.

ESTABLISHING THE DIAGNOSIS THROUGH AN OPEN OR STEREOTACTIC BIOPSY

While radiographic imaging techniques such as magnetic resonance imaging (MRI) generate a differential diagnosis, they are often not sufficient to establish a diagnosis. The gold standard for the diagnosis of most brain and spine tumors is direct tissue sampling. There are instances in which cerebrospinal fluid (CSF) sampling (primary CNS lymphoma), ophthalmology evaluation (primary CNS lymphoma), endocrine hormone assessment (pituitary macroadenoma), and serum marker assessment (germ cell tumors) may establish a diagnosis. Biopsy procedures for tissue sampling may be performed via either open or minimally invasive surgical procedures. Minimally invasive options include (1) stereotactic-guided biopsy of superficial or deep brain lesions, (2) an open biopsy for superficial cortically based tumors, and (3) computed tomography (CT)-guided biopsies for spinal column tumors. Although the approach selected must be tailored to each specific patient, there are a few considerations based on tumor location.

If tumor resection is anticipated based on neuroimaging, then a craniotomy exposing the entire lesion is needed and resection can proceed after frozen section confirms the presumptive diagnosis. For more superficial, cortically based lesions, neurosurgeons may opt for either a stereotactic biopsy using MRI navigation or an open biopsy to obtain tissue. The chosen approach may vary by surgeon preference and anatomic considerations, including the presence of cortical veins overlying a diagnostic target, which may pose a higher risk of hemorrhage for a stereotactic approach.

For deep-seated lesions in the subcortical white matter, basal ganglia, or brainstem, a framed or frameless stereotactic biopsy is used (Figure 19.1). Tumors within the deep cerebellar hemispheres or brainstem may be approached via stereotactic

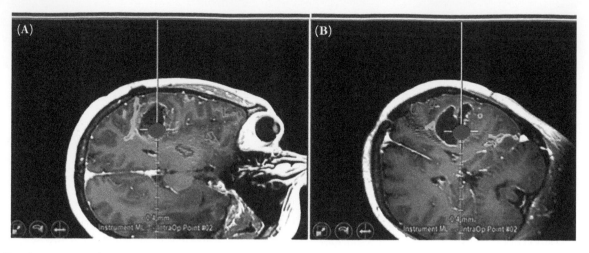

Figure 19.1 *Frameless stereotactic brain biopsy for a contrast-enhancing parietal mass. A stereotactic trajectory is selected within the T1 post gadolinium-enhancing region using axial (A) and coronal (B) MRI series.*

biopsy through a transcerebellar approach (via the middle cerebellar peduncle) to obtain tissue. Whenever considering a stereotactic approach, tumor vascularity should be assessed using preoperative MR imaging. Stereotactic biopsies of vascular lesions (e.g., hemangioblastomas) may result in postoperative hemorrhage and should therefore be avoided. Brainstem biopsies are associated with increased complication rates compared to other regions, with high rates of facial weakness, sensory changes, and respiratory compromise.[3] Pathology within the sella, suprasellar region, or clivus may be biopsied through an endonasal transsphenoidal approach. Patients with pineal masses or posterior third ventricle lesions are best biopsied using either an interhemispheric, supracerebellar infratentorial, or transcortical trans-ventricular approach.

Several factors may influence the diagnostic yield of tumor tissue. Lesion diameter has been demonstrated to be associated with diagnostic yield, with smaller lesions at risk of producing non-diagnostic tissue.[4] Tumor heterogeneity may risk obtaining non-diagnostic tissue or under sampling of a tumor region which may represent lower grade features than the remainder of the tumor. For example, patients with diffuse isocitrate dehydrogenase (IDH) wildtype gliomas had lower rates of WHO grade 4 diagnosis with smaller sample sizes, suggesting a potential risk of a sampling error.[5] Another unique entity is primary CNS lymphoma. Diagnosis of CNS lymphoma increases the risk of a non-diagnostic biopsy especially for smaller lesions and for patients who have received steroids preoperatively. When primary CNS lymphoma is included in the differential diagnosis, corticosteroids should be held, if at all possible, in order to increase the diagnostic yield of brain tissue obtained.

CYTOREDUCTION

Another major indication for brain tumor surgery is cytoreduction (i.e., maximally safe resection of tumor tissue) to improve patient survival. Recommendations regarding surgical goals for cytoreduction vary between different tumor types. In many disease contexts, more extensive resection leads

to an improvement in progression-free survival (PFS) and overall survival (OS) (e.g., diffuse low- and high-grade gliomas [HGG]) while for other slower growing tumors, subtotal resection (STR) with adjuvant stereotactic radiosurgery (SRS) has been employed for the purposes of functional preservation (e.g., vestibular schwannomas). Cytoreductive surgery is not indicated in a few particular circumstances, including primary CNS lymphoma, small cell lung cancer, germ cell tumors (unless refractory to chemotherapy), and gliomatosis cerebri. Recently, using large longitudinal datasets, the interactive effects of maximal resection combined with clinical and molecular features have enhanced our understanding of the role of cytoreduction. Younger patients with newly diagnosed glioblastoma benefit from maximal resection of non-enhancing tumor regardless of IDH status.[6] For intra-axial tumors, craniotomies may be performed asleep or awake, with intraoperative direct cortical and subcortical stimulation in an effort to identify and preserve eloquent language and motor areas. Intraoperative stimulation is the gold standard for detecting function and may be supplemented with (but not replaced by) other noninvasive techniques including tractography, functional MRI, and magnetoencephalography.[7–9]

> Another major indication for brain tumor surgery is cytoreduction (i.e., maximally safe resection of tumor tissue) to improve patient survival.

SYMPTOMATIC CONTROL

Another potential indication for surgery is to reduce mass effect and associated neurological impairments. Many tumors can elicit neurological deficits due to disruption of eloquent brain or spinal cord regions due to tumor invasion or the effects of peritumoral edema on neural networks. Alternatively, tumors may compress CSF drainage pathways, leading to symptoms of obstructive hydrocephalus or an entrapped ventricle. For example, tumors such as brain metastases, hemangioblastoma, or pineal region lesions within the posterior fossa may lead to cerebral aqueduct or fourth ventricular obstruction. Furthermore, tectal gliomas may lead to cerebral aqueduct obstruction and obstructive hydrocephalus. When brain tumors arise from within deep, eloquent regions and are not amenable to resection (i.e., diffuse intrinsic pontine glioma or tectal gliomas), a third ventriculostomy or ventriculoperitoneal shunt may be performed for relief of symptoms related to hydrocephalus. Special consideration should be made for patients with brain tumors within primary motor, sensory, or language regions. Depending on the underlying tumor type, lesion resection may relieve neurological impairments. This point is particularly important for patients with gliomas or brain metastases greater than 3 cm.[10,11]

Patients with CNS tumors may present with significant mass effect and midline shift resulting in severe neurological impairments including lethargy and weakness. In conjunction with hyperosmolar therapy, a hemicraniectomy with initial tumor debulking may be performed urgently for preservation of life, with a subsequent staged surgery to complete the resection of any residual disease (pending neurological improvements).

> A third ventriculostomy or ventriculoperitoneal shunt may be performed for relief of symptoms related to hydrocephalus.

SEIZURE CONTROL

Primary brain tumors, both intra- and extra-axial, can lead to seizures due to cortical network disruption from the tumor itself or from tumor-associated edema. Slower growing tumors such as low-grade gliomas (LGGs), gangliogliomas, and meningiomas appear to have a predilection for epileptogenesis.[12,13] Tumor resection can improve seizure control in a variety of brain tumors.[14-17] Furthermore, similar to survival outcomes, greater extent of resection for some tumors, such as LGG and HGG, is associated with higher rates of seizure freedom.[15,18,19] For example, patients with low-grade temporal lobe brain tumors have a 43% incidence of seizure freedom with STR while 79% are seizure free following gross-total lesionectomy.[18] Several studies have advocated for the use of intraoperative electrocorticography during tumor resection as a means of identifying epileptogenic cortical areas outside of classically defined lesional tissue.[20]

> Tumor resection can improve seizure control in a variety of brain tumors.

REDUCTION OF CEREBRAL EDEMA

Patient with substantial peritumoral edema (typically >1 cm) often require corticosteroid use as a means of symptom control. However, despite this medical therapy, peritumoral vasogenic edema may lead to elevated intracranial pressure, midline shift, and disruption of critical eloquent regions. Tumor debulking may help decrease the dose and duration of corticosteroids

required. Cytoreduction often results in faster resolution of peritumoral edema than treatment with SRS.[21] The use of corticosteroids is often important in the management of brain metastases; however, there is evidence that corticosteroids can reduce the efficacy of novel immunotherapies and should therefore be used judiciously.[22]

SPINAL COLUMN STABILIZATION

Although primary and metastatic tumors to the spinal column are often considered extradural, they often warrant neurosurgical interventions and multidisciplinary management with oncologists and radiation oncologists. Important factors in the management of spinal metastases include the neurological status of the patient, systemic disease control (which often requires restaging), mechanical stability of involved vertebrae, and the ability of the patient to tolerate surgery based on medical comorbidities and systemic disease status. Such considerations have been formulated by the group at Memorial Sloan-Kettering Cancer Center into the Neurologic, Oncologic, Mechanical, and Systemic (NOMS) decision-making framework for electing for SRS, external beam radiotherapy (EBRT), tumor resection, and spinal stabilization.[23]

Within this framework, mechanical instability represents an independent indication for surgery regardless of the tumor type or neurologic status. To assess this, the Spinal Instability Neoplastic Score[24] was developed to provide guidance on the need for surgical stabilization (Table 19.1). This scoring system involves assessing pathology location, associated pain, character of the bone lesion (lytic vs. blastic), spinal alignment, degree of vertebral body collapse, and posterolateral spine involvement. For total scores of 13 or greater, the involved segment is considered unstable and warrants surgical stabilization, usually via instrumentation.

As part of the NOMS framework, "separation surgery" is a consideration for the management of the spinal tumor itself. This technique involves tumor debulking (as opposed to complete removal) to increase the distance between residual tumor and the spinal cord, thus allowing for higher doses (i.e., more aggressive postoperative spinal column radiotherapy). This permits optimal radiation dosing to the tumor while decreasing the dose to neurological structures, thereby lowering the risk of treatment failure. Often separation surgery can be performed in conjunction with instrumentation for stabilization purposes.

> The NOMS decision making framework is used for electing for spinal SRS, EBRT, tumor resection, and spinal stabilization.

TUMOR-SPECIFIC NEUROSURGICAL CONSIDERATIONS

LOW- AND HIGH-GRADE GLIOMAS

Maximal extent of resection (EOR) with preservation of language, sensorimotor, and cognitive functions is the surgical goal for patients with low- and high-grade gliomas. Greater

TABLE 19.1 Spinal instability neoplastic score (SINS)

COMPONENT	SINS
Location	
Junctional (O–C2; C7–T2; T11–L1; L5–S1)	3
Mobile spine (C3–C6; L2–L4)	2
Semirigid (T3–T10)	1
Rigid (S2–S5)	0
Pain	
Mechanical	3
Oncologic	2
Pain-free lesion	1
Bone lesion	
Lytic	2
Mixed (blastic/lytic)	1
Blastic	0
Vertebral body collapse	
>50% collapse	3
<50% collapse	2
No collapse with >50% body involvement	1
None of the above	0
Radiographic alignment	
Subluxation/translation	4
Deformity (kyphosis/scoliosis)	2
Normal	0
Posterolateral involvement	
Bilateral	3
Unilateral	1
None of the above	0

≤6 = Stable, 7–12, = Indeterminant, ≥13 = Unstable.
From Fisher et al.[24]

extent of resection has been shown in multiple retrospective studies, large meta-analyses, and randomized controlled trials investigating surgical adjuncts to improve OS and PFS for newly as well as many recurrent low- and high-grade gliomas. The maximal EOR goal often requires intraoperative tools and techniques such as neuronavigation, awake or asleep intraoperative brain mapping, and intraoperative MRI, as described here.

For LGG, resection should be considered as soon as the lesion is identified, as "watchful waiting" (with or without biopsy) is associated with shorter OS.[25] There is stepwise lengthening of OS with increased EOR of the MRI fluid-attenuated inversion recovery (FLAIR) signal. Patients who have an EOR of 100%, greater than 90%, or less than 90% have 8-year PFS rates of 98%, 91%, and 76%, respectively.[26] EOR is associated with improved OS even after adjusting for other known clinical and molecular risk factors such as patient age, performance status, tumor location, or molecular subtype.[26] Recently, some surgeons have advocated for the surgical goal of achieving a "supra-maximal" resection for LGG, extending the area of tissue removal to functional boundaries, beyond the visually and radiological identifiable tumor. At present, published data are limited and demonstrated reduced rates of malignant transformation following supra-maximal resection, but no differences in OS.[27] Please refer to Chapter 17 on, LGG.

> Maximal extent of resection (EOR) with preservation of language, sensorimotor, and cognitive functions is the surgical goal.

For HGG (WHO grades 3 and 4), EOR is most commonly calculated using contrast enhanced T1-weighted MRI sequences. Similar to LGG, there is a stepwise improvement in OS with EOR, with the benefit most apparent when extent of resection exceeds 80%.[6,28] However, it is well recognized that tumor cells exist well beyond the contrast enhancing region, and recently other resection margins have been considered. It has recently been demonstrated in large cohorts that greater extent of FLAIR abnormality resection is associated with improved OS.[29] The method of tumor resection may also be important, as peri-lesional (rather than intra-lesional)[30] and anatomical[31] (i.e., temporal lobectomy) techniques have been associated with greater EOR and OS.

The importance of EOR also applies to recurrent glioma.[28,32,33] In the setting of recurrent disease, re-resection has been associated with improved survival in multiple retrospective studies,[33] although this is only appropriate in select patients. Indications for reoperation included new focal deficits, symptomatic raised intracranial pressure, increasing seizure frequency, or radiological progression. Advanced age should not preclude consideration of reoperation; however, a Karnofsky Performance Status score of 70 or greater and a time interval of at least 6 months are predictive of a survival benefit.[33]

BRAIN METASTASES

Cytoreduction also has a role in the management of brain metastases. Surgical resection may be appropriate for (1) local control of a single brain metastasis, (2) addressing mass effect from a dominant tumor even in the presence of distant CNS metastases, (3) diagnostic purposes, and (4) tumor enlargement despite prior treatment with focal radiation therapy such as SRS. However, indications for surgery as opposed to SRS, WBRT, new targeted small-molecule inhibitors, or immunotherapy remain controversial, and optimal management requires a multidisciplinary approach.

National neurosurgery organizations have provided guidelines regarding the role of surgery in management of brain metastases.[34] Patients with a single brain metastasis greater than 3 cm should be considered for surgery followed by focal brain irradiation (e.g., SRS) which is superior to focal or whole brain irradiation (WBRT) alone.[35] However, given the cognitive and health-related quality of life consequences of WBRT, post resection SRS to the surgical cavity is the standard of care for local disease control,[36] and SRS alone can be considered for small (<2 cm) brain metastasis.[34] Surgical technique and extent of tumor resection may both impact local disease control rates as well as OS. En bloc tumor resection (as opposed to piecemeal resection) reduces the risk of postoperative leptomeningeal disease when resecting single brain metastases.[37-39] Gross total resection (GTR) is recommended over STR to improve OS and prolong time to recurrence.[40,41] Although immunotherapy is revolutionizing the treatment of patients with brain metastases from immunoresponsive primary tumors such as melanoma or lung cancer, recent trials have excluded patients with symptomatic lesions or significant mass effect. Therefore, surgery followed by SRS remains the standard of care and may in fact be used as a bridge to adjuvant immunotherapy.[42]

> Surgery followed by SRS remains the standard of care.

CENTRAL NEUROCYTOMAS

Central neurocytomas are typically found intraventricularly, associated with the septum pellucidum. The main focus of treatment is surgical resection, with a low risk of recurrence with GTR.[43,44] In the setting of recurrence, repeat resection may be attempted although other adjuvant therapies including SRS and chemotherapy have proved to have limited efficacy.[45,46]

ADULT PILOCYTIC ASTROCYTOMAS

Adult pilocytic astrocytomas are non-infiltrative LGGs characterized by their sharp tumor margins and minimal infiltrate into surrounding brain parenchyma. The aim of surgical treatment for adult pilocytic astrocytomas should be GTR where possible as this can be curative. STR is associated with worse OS and the need for adjuvant treatments.[47,48]

GANGLIOGLIOMAS

Gangliogliomas are cortically based lesions that typically present with seizures and are treated with maximal resection. GTR is associated with improved recurrence-free survival with an 5-year OS rate of 98.1%.[49] However, anaplastic transformation may occur and leads to 5-year OS and recurrence rates of 100% and 24.9%, respectively.[50]

> GTR is associated with improved recurrence-free survival with an 5-year OS rate of 98.1%.

ADULT EPENDYMOMAS

Ependymomas are rare neuroepithelial tumors that arise from the ependymal lining at any point along the ventricular system. Although these lesions are typically found within the spinal cord in adults or within the fourth ventricle in pediatric patients, they can occur anywhere along the neuraxis. The mainstay of treatment for large, growing, or symptomatic cranial ependymomas is surgical resection, with greater extent of resection associated with improved survival.[51-53] Fourth ventricular ependymomas are approached via a suboccipital craniotomy. Either a telovelar approach or a midline vermis splitting approach to the fourth ventricle allows for a high extent of resection and low rate of permanent morbidity.[54] Ependymomas may be adherent to the floor of the fourth ventricle, precluding complete removal without inducing cranial nerve deficits. In these cases, focal brain irradiation can provide a management option for residual or recurrent disease.[55] These lesions are also prone to forming drop metastases, and it is therefore recommended to evaluate the entire brain and spine (total brain and spine MRI with and without gadolinium) when a posterior fossa ependymoma is considered in the differential diagnosis.

Spinal ependymomas are the most common intradural intramedullary spinal cord tumors found in adults. These tumors are usually well-defined and can be separated from the surrounding spinal cord using micro-neurosurgical techniques. GTR is considered the first choice in treatment. A laminectomy and durotomy are performed. The intraoperative ultrasound may be used to localize the tumor because the dorsal spinal cord may appear normal. A midline myelotomy through the dorsal columns minimizes the risk of permanent deficits, although almost all patients will have transient light touch and proprioceptive deficits due to dorsal column manipulation. Myxopapillary ependymomas occur in the region of the conus medullaris, and therefore postoperative bowel and bladder dysfunction are common. Most patients with perioperative neurological deficits improve with time and rehabilitation; however, 6-month postoperative neurological deficits occur in 6–29% of patients.[56-57]

> Ependymomas may be adherent to the floor of the fourth ventricle, precluding complete removal without inducing cranial nerve deficits.

MENINGIOMAS

Meningiomas are the most common benign primary brain tumor seen in adults. Indications for treatment include symptomatic mass effect, seizures, diagnostic uncertainty, and growth. Patients presenting without symptoms should be managed with observation. If treatment is indicated, meningiomas are treated with surgery as the first option. Focal radiation (e.g., SRS) may be the initial treatment options in small WHO grade 1 meningiomas in high-risk locations. Patients with incompletely resected WHO grade 2 meningiomas should receive fractionated radiotherapy. There are few systemic therapies available, even in the setting of advanced disease. The presenting symptoms, surgical approach, and specific surgical risks are dependent on the location of the tumor and are discussed later for the most common tumor locations. It has increasingly become apparent that the mutational landscape of meningiomas varies by location and that this may drive their divergent clinical behaviors, thereby impacting surgical goals.[58] Meningiomas may be multiple in up to 8% of patients with increased risk for multiple meningiomas (or meningiomatosis) most commonly seen in patients with a history of neurofibromatosis type 2 (NF2) or prior exposure to ionizing radiation.

Meningiomas can be highly vascular; therefore, preoperative embolization may be considered in select situations. The risks and success of embolization depend on tumor location. Embolization of middle meningeal or transosseous superficial temporal artery supply for convexity meningiomas may be performed with minimal risk. However, the vascular supply to olfactory groove meningiomas is from the anterior and posterior ethmoidal arteries and should not be treated with preoperative embolization given risk to the ophthalmic artery (which might share a vascular ethmoidal artery supply). Overall, the risks of embolization are low,[59] and the benefits include reduced operative duration, blood loss, and transfusion requirements. Surgical risks of meningioma resection increase with subsequent operations, which poses important considerations, particularly for recurrent disease. Focal adjuvant treatments such as brachytherapy should be considered for multiply recurrent and higher grade tumors after the failure of surgery and radiation treatment.[60] Although metastases are uncommon, screening with DOTA-TATE positron emission tomography (PET) should be performed in patients with more than two recurrences prior to surgical intervention. Systemic body metastases have been identified in approximately 1 in 3 patients using this criterion.[61]

> Meningiomas can be highly vascular; therefore, preoperative embolization may be considered in select situations.

Extent of resection for meningiomas is assessed using the Simpson grading scale (Table 19.2), which correlates with the risk of recurrence,[62] although molecular determinants of recurrence are being increasingly recognized.[58] Complete surgical resection is indicated whenever possible, and the addition of adjuvant SRS is associated with 90% PFS at 10 years for patients with WHO grade 1 meningiomas.[63] Adjuvant radiation therapy is most commonly considered in higher grade meningiomas. Even for atypical and anaplastic meningioma, more extensive cytoreduction is associated improved OS.[64]

CONVEXITY

This is the most common location for meningiomas, and tumors may present with seizures or focal neurological signs related to the functional contributions of the underlying cortex. Complete (Simpson grade 1) resection may be achieved in most cases. Although most vascular supply is derived from meningeal vessels, tumors may parasitize pial vessels, increasing the risk of ischemic injury to the underlying cortex as a consequence of tumor resection.

OLFACTORY GROOVE

Meningiomas in this location are often asymptomatic or present with anosmia, headaches, personality change, or seizures. Classically, these lesions are associated with Foster-Kennedy syndrome: the triad of anosmia, ipsilateral optic atrophy, and contralateral papilledema. Surgical approach depends on the size of the lesion and surgeon preference. Endoscopic endonasal resection may be considered for smaller olfactory meningiomas without significant lateral extension. This approach minimizes brain retraction and allows early tumor devascularization, but it increases the risk of postoperative CSF leak (see later discussion). Open approaches include the bicoronal subfrontal, pterional, or anterior interhemispheric corridors.

> Foster-Kennedy syndrome is the triad of anosmia, ipsilateral optic atrophy, and contralateral papilledema.

PARASAGITTAL

Focal symptoms in these locations are caused by compression or irritation of the medial hemispheric surface, causing, from anterior to posterior, personality change, lower limb weakness or seizures, or hemisensory neglect or visual field changes. Surgical

TABLE 19.2 Simpsons grading scale for meningioma resection

GRADE	INTRADURAL TUMOR	DURAL ATTACHMENT/EXTRADURAL[a] TUMOR
I	Macroscopically complete resection	All excised, abnormal bone removed
II	Macroscopically complete resection	Dural attachment in situ, diathermy. Extradural tumor removed.
III	Macroscopically complete resection	In situ
IV	Partial removal	In situ
V	Decompression, with or without biopsy	In situ

[a]Including tumor located within venous sinuses.

From Simpson et al.[62]

management of superior sagittal sinus tumor invasion depends on factors such as patient age, tumor location, and the degree of sinus occlusion. During resection, tumors in this location may be associated with significant blood loss or the risk of air embolism. If the sinus is completely occluded preoperatively, then consideration may be given to removing the involved portion of the sinus as alternate venous drainage pathways have been established. If only one wall of the sinus is involved, resection of the infiltrated tumor may be performed with primary repair of the sinus wall. Attempts at complete resection with superior sagittal sinus reconstruction or bypass may be performed; however, STR with adjuvant radiosurgery can achieve similar rates of tumor control with significantly lower morbidity.

SPHENOID WING

Although the surgical risks of lateral sphenoid wing meningiomas are similar to that of convexity tumors, medial sphenoid wing lesions can be challenging to manage surgically. Meningiomas in this location may encase the carotid and proximal anterior and middle cerebral arteries and their perforating vessels. They may cause optic nerve compression either directly or because of hyperostosis of the anterior clinoid and optic canal. A subset of sphenoid wing meningiomas are predominantly intraosseous and present with exophthalmos, extraocular muscle dysfunction, or visual failure from optic nerve compression or exposure keratopathy. Surgery is indicated for progressive cosmetic deformity or vision loss and involves resection of the involved bone, including the orbital roof, lateral wall, and optical canal. Reconstruction requires multidisciplinary care with an experienced skull base neurosurgeon and ophthalmologist to achieve a satisfactory cosmetic outcome and prevent complications such as optic nerve injury and extraocular muscle entrapment.[65]

INTRACRANIAL SOLITARY FIBROUS TUMOR/ HEMANGIOPERICYTOMA

Intracranial solitary fibrous tumors are rare mesenchymal neoplasms originating from the meninges. They comprise a heterogenous group of spindle cell tumors, of which hemangiopericytoma is a variant. Hemangiopericytomas are commonly located along the convexity or parasagittal region and present with headache, seizure, or focal neurological signs. They have irregular borders and bony erosion as opposed to the hyperostosis commonly seen in meningioma. Surgical management considerations are similar to meningiomas, although hemangiopericytomas commonly have increased vascularity. GTR is associated with improved OS and should be followed by SRS.[66] In the setting of recurrent disease, patients should be screened for systemic metastases, which can occur in up to two-thirds of patients, even many years after their initial presentation.[67]

> Hemangiopericytomas are commonly located along the convexity or parasagittal region and present with headache, seizure, or focal neurological signs.

VESTIBULAR SCHWANNOMAS

Vestibular schwannomas may occur sporadically or in association with NF2. Although the most common symptoms at presentation are hearing loss, tinnitus, and disequilibrium, an increasing number of tumors are discovered incidentally.[68] The Koos Classification for vestibular schwannomas has been used to stratify tumors based on extra-meatal extension (Table 19.3).[69,70] Grade 1 vestibular schwannomas are intracanalicular only; grade 2 tumors display minimal extension into the cerebellopontine angle; grade 3 tumors occupy the CPA; grade 4 tumors cause brain stem compression. Preoperative assessment includes a bedside examination of facial nerve function as well as a pure tone audiogram. "Serviceable hearing" is defined as a pure tone audiogram value of less than 50 dB and a speech discrimination score of greater than 50%. The House-Brackmann grading scale has been a mainstay of rating facial nerve function both in the pre- and postoperative settings[71] (Table 19.4). During vestibular schwannoma resection facial nerve function as well as hearing function are both at risk given the proximity of these tumors to cranial nerves VII and VIII. Tumor resection may be achieved by the translabyrinthine, retro-sigmoid, or middle fossa approach. Hearing preservation is only possible with the latter two approaches. The middle fossa approach is only suitable for small tumors, many of which are now treated with SRS. The translabyrinthine approach sacrifices any residual hearing, although it minimizes cerebellar retraction. There is conflicting evidence regarding the superiority of the translabyrinthine or retrosigmoid approach for preservation of facial nerve function; however, for both approaches the outcome is worse with larger tumors.[72] In general, the surgical approach is determined by the patient's age, hearing status, tumor size, and the surgical team's experience with each approach.

In the past, surgical resection of vestibular schwannomas favored GTR at times at the expense of facial nerve function. However, the pendulum has swung from aggressive GTR to a focus on facial nerve and hearing preservation with STR supplemented with adjuvant SRS (i.e., functional preservation surgery).[73,74] With this approach, the neurosurgeon performs intraoperative stimulation to identify and protect the facial nerve during the course of the operation. If the tumor is adherent to nervous system structures, then residual disease is left behind and treated with SRS. There is controversy as to whether this approach is associated with lower PFS compared to GTR,[75–77] but the functional outcomes of functional preservation

TABLE 19.3 Koos grading system for vestibular schwannomas

GRADE	TUMOR LOCATION
I	Intracanalicular only
II	Protrusion into the cerebellopontine angle
III	Extending to, but not displacing, the brainstem
IV	Brainstem displacement

From Koos et al.[70]

TABLE 19.4 House-Brackman grading scale for facial nerve function

GRADE	DESCRIPTION	CHARACTERISTICS
I	Normal	Normal
II	Mild dysfunction	Slight weakness on close inspection; symmetrical at rest
III	Moderate dysfunction	Obvious weakness +/- asymmetry; complete eye closure with effort
IV	Moderately severe dysfunction	Obvious weakness and disfiguring asymmetry; incomplete eye closure
V	Severe dysfunction	Barely perceptible motion with asymmetry at rest
VI	Total Paralysis	No movement

From House-Brackman et al.[71]

surgery remain superior. Hearing preservation is possible in up to 80%[78] of patients with serviceable hearing, and favorable facial nerve outcomes (as defined by House-Brackman grades 1 or 2) have been reported in between 78% and 100% of patients, respectively.[78,79]

"Serviceable hearing" is defined as a pure tone audiogram value less than 50 dB and a speech discrimination score of greater than 50%.

CHORDOMAS

Chordomas are primary malignant bone tumors occurring anywhere along the neuraxis, from the base of the skull to the sacrum. Chordomas are thought to arise from cellular remnants of the embryonic notochord and most commonly occur at its ventral and dorsal ends. Although "en bloc" or radical resection is the goal of surgery, this is often difficult to achieve given their proximity to the cranial nerve and vasculature of the skull base. STR is associated with worse PFS.[80]

PITUITARY ADENOMAS

Pituitary adenomas are extra-axial tumors which occur within the pituitary gland. They present with endocrinopathies or symptoms related to mass effect, such as headaches or visual disturbance. Many pituitary tumors are found incidentally. Micro- and macro-adenomas are defined as those smaller and larger than 1 cm, respectively. Surgical indications and outcomes differ for hormonally functional and non-functional tumors. Almost all tumors can be resected via endonasal techniques utilizing the operative microscope or endoscopic techniques. The exceptions are very large tumors with anterior or temporal extension or where anatomical factors make the endonasal corridor unfavorable. In general the perioperative

complication rate following trans-sphenoidal surgery is low, with a less than 2% incidence of major complications.[81]

Almost all pituitary tumors can be resected via endonasal techniques utilizing the operative microscope or endoscopic techniques.

NON-FUNCTIONAL ADENOMAS

Non-functional pituitary adenomas may present with symptomatic mass effect including headaches, bitemporal hemianopia, or hypopituitarism. In otherwise well patients, symptomatic tumors should be removed because operative morbidity is low. Incidentally found adenomas require thorough investigation including endocrine hormone evaluation, visual field examination, and optic nerve assessment using optical coherence tomography. Most centers advocate for close radiological, hormonal, and clinical observation of small, asymptomatic, hormonally inactive adenomas.[82]

The surgical goal is to relieve mass effect including optic chiasm compression, preserve endocrine function, and remove as much tumor as possible to prevent recurrence. In many cases, intra-cavernous tumor is not resected as the risk of cranial neuropathies or catastrophic carotid injury increases, and residual tumor in this location may be treated with radiosurgery.[83] When GTR is achieved, long-term recurrence rates are low (5- and 10-year recurrence in 3.9% and 4.7%, respectively).[84]

FUNCTIONAL ADENOMAS

The role of surgery for hormonally active pituitary adenomas depends on the hormone produced. Prolactinomas account for up to half of all pituitary tumors, and medical therapy with dopamine agonists is effective in most patients.[85] Surgery for prolactinomas is reserved for rare situations in which the tumor persists despite the use of dopamine agonists or when medication side effects prove intolerable for the patient. In this group, surgery can achieve biochemical remission in up to 85% of patients with microadenomas and 40% with macroadenomas.[86] Although medical treatments exist for both Cushing's disease and acromegaly, surgery remains the first-line treatment of choice for achieving hormonal remission. At high-volume pituitary centers hormonal remission can be achieved in 60–90% of patients.[85,87] Recurrence rates are up to 20% for Cushing's disease[85] and 8% for acromegaly.[85] Repeat transsphenoidal surgery for recurrent hormonally active adenomas is able to achieve disease control in approximately 50% of patients.[88]

Surgery can achieve biochemical remission in up to 85% of patients with microadenomas and 40% with macroadenomas.

PITUITARY APOPLEXY

Apoplexy results from ischemia or hemorrhage into the pituitary gland, which usually occurs in patients with undiagnosed pituitary adenomas. The typical presentation is a sudden-onset headache, endocrine dysfunction (particularly corticotropic deficiency which may be life-threatening), and cranial neuropathies; most commonly a third nerve palsy or visual failure (reduction of acuity or fields). Severe cases may cause altered mental status or coma, and subarachnoid spread may cause hydrocephalus. First-line management includes patient resuscitation and corticosteroid replacement. Early surgical decompression is indicated for patients with a reduced level of consciousness or visual failure. Although visual symptoms often improve with conservative management, this finding is confounded by case selection bias in the published literature.[89] Patients with headache only or ophthalmoplegia may be managed conservatively. Symptomatic third cranial neuropathies almost always resolve, with or without decompression.[90]

> First-line management includes patient resuscitation and corticosteroid replacement.

CRANIOPHARYNGIOMAS

Craniopharyngiomas are thought to arise from epithelial remnants of Rathke's pouch and can often be distinguished from pituitary adenomas by the presence of cysts, calcification, and often a normal sella size. Hypopituitarism is common, and corticosteroid and thyroid hormone replacement are often needed prior to surgery. Craniopharyngiomas present specific surgical challenges because of their deep location and close proximity to the pituitary gland, stalk and the optic nerves, and chiasm. Craniopharyngiomas may be accessed via subfrontal, pterional, interhemispheric, or transsphenoidal approaches. The choice of surgical approach is dictated by the tumor size, its relationship to the optic nerves, and the amount of tumor in the third ventricle and sella. For retrochiasmatic tumors, the subfrontal approach requires the surgeon to open the lamina terminalis to access the tumor. This membrane forms the anterior wall of the third ventricle, between the optic chiasm and anterior commissure, and represents the rostral end of the neural tube. Although GTR of craniopharyngiomas is associated with improved survival, it also increases the risks of postoperative neurological and endocrine dysfunction. Postoperative diabetes insipidus may occur in more than half of all patients and can be life-threatening.[91] Almost all patients have some degree of postoperative pituitary disfunction.[91] Hypothalamic obesity occurs in up to 70% of patients and can be extremely difficult to treat and may require bariatric surgery.[92] Most patients have improved vision postoperatively; however, disruption of the blood supply to the optic nerve, chiasm, or optic tracts can cause visual deterioration. Recently, BRAF and MEK inhibitors have shown promise in treating papillary craniopharyngiomas.[93] Improved medical treatment may allow for more limited resections, decreasing the risk of postoperative complications.

HEMANGIOBLASTOMAS

Hemangioblastomas may occur sporadically, or as part of Von Hippel-Lindau (VHL) syndrome. Most occur within the cerebellum or spinal cord. Other locations are uncommon and are very suggestive of underlying VHL syndrome. Patients presenting with imaging that is suspicious for hemangioblastoma should be screened for VHL. Additionally, patients with known VHL should undergo screening for pheochromocytoma (serum metanephrines, 24-hour urine catecholamine levels, and abdominal imaging) prior to surgery to prevent perioperative hypertensive crises.[94] Symptomatic sporadic tumors should be resected for symptom control and to confirm the diagnosis. In the largest natural history study of VHL-associated hemangioblastomas, most lesions (51%) did not grow; however, those that did exhibited a saltatory growth pattern—that is, quiescence interspersed with periods of growth.[95] Therefore, resection is reserved for symptomatic lesions. Operative management involves wide bony exposure (because of perilesional edema), and the nodule should not be entered during resection to avoid catastrophic hemorrhage. The cyst wall does not need to be surgically removed. Spinal tumors are most commonly associated with the dorsal root entry zone and so sensory symptoms are a common presentation. GTR is curative, and, postoperatively, symptoms are stable or improved in 98% of patients with cerebellar lesions[96] and 94% with spinal tumors.[97]

> Hemangioblastomas may occur sporadically or as part of Von Hippel-Lindau (VHL) syndrome.

PINEAL REGION TUMORS

Although many differing pathologies may occur within the pineal region, most lesions are either of germ cell, glial, or pineal cell origin and the relative incidence of these lesions is related to age and genetic background of the patient. Most tumors present with hydrocephalus and/or Parinaud's syndrome (compression of the midbrain causing up-gaze palsy, convergence-retraction nystagmus, lid retraction, and a pseudo-Argyll Roberts pupil). The benefit of surgical resection depends on the underlying pathology and therefore biopsy is often undertaken, although in rare cases germ cell tumors may be diagnosed using serum or CSF markers. CSF must not be taken via lumbar puncture in the presence of obstructive hydrocephalus, but it may be obtained during shunting or endoscopic third ventriculostomy.

Biopsy of a pineal region mass may be performed by an endoscopic transventricular approach, stereotactic needle biopsy, or via open craniotomy. Most centers prefer the transventricular approach when possible as this allows for simultaneous treatment of hydrocephalus with a low rate of complications. Indications for resection are controversial. Biopsy followed by adjuvant treatment is preferable for germinomas, whereas benign lesions (such as teratomas, low-grade pineocytomas, or meningiomas) may be best treated with surgical resection. Although there may be a survival benefit with greater extent of resection for malignant lesions, this must be balanced with the increased morbidity associated with open approaches. The most common approaches to the pineal region are the midline or paramedian supracerebellar infratentorial, occipital transtentorial or posterior interhemispheric transcallosal corridors. The choice of approach depends on surgeon experience and anatomical factors, such as the steepness of the tentorium, whether the tumor is predominantly supra- or infra-tentorial, and the position of the deep cerebral veins. The supracerebellar approaches are facilitated by performing the operation with the patient in the sitting position, although this is associated with a risk of air embolism and subsequent stroke in patients with patent foramen ovale or other right-to-left shunt pathologies. However, modern microsurgical techniques have reduced the operative risk for deep tumor locations and tumors with proximity to eloquent brain and essential vasculature. Although transient worsening of ocular symptoms is common, the risk of major permanent morbidity is less than 3% in most series.[98]

SURGICAL TECHNIQUES

NEURO-NAVIGATION

The evolution of neuro-navigation has occurred over a century and is now an essential component of surgical neuro-oncology practice. Clarke and Horsley described the principles of stereotaxy using Cartesian co-ordinates in 1906, in rhesus monkeys[99]; however, it wasn't until the 1940s that the technique was first reported in humans.[100] The first systems utilized ventriculography, angiography, or standardized brain atlases for localization and were predominantly used for functional lesioning in patients with movement disorders, rather than oncological indications. The convergence of advances in neuroimaging, computing power, and three-dimensional registration allowed for development of the systems currently in use. Because initial versions required a rigid frame to be attached to the patient's skull, modern registration systems are referred to as *frameless stereotaxy*. During the operation, the patient's head is rigidly fixated with a clamp to the operative table and a reference array is attached. The patient's head is then co-registered with volumetric preoperative neuroimaging by mapping the position of landmarks on the patient's head in relation to the reference array. The landmarks may be *fiducials*—adhesive markers that are attached to the patient's head prior to neuroimaging—or facial characteristics that are mapped to a three-dimensional representation of the patient derived from neuroimaging.

Additional information may be overlaid onto the navigation screens by merging divergent imaging sources in three-dimensional space, such as diffusion tensor-based tractography, magnetoencephalography, CT or MRI angiography, or PET data. These data allow the surgeon to minimize the risk to important structures during craniotomy. Although

the accuracy of navigation is within a few millimeters before durotomy, CSF drainage and brain shift occur during resection that can make navigation inaccurate. Toward the end of resection, structures may move more than 1 cm from the location predicted by neuro-navigation, and the direction of this shift can be difficult to predict.[9]

INTRAOPERATIVE IMAGING

Intraoperative MRI is a newer surgical adjunct that allows the surgeon to both assess the degree of resection intraoperatively and re-register neuro-navigation to mitigate the effect of brain shift. First introduced in the 1990s,[101] earlier versions incorporated low-field MRI. Most systems are now 1.5 or 3.0 Tesla and "dual entry," meaning that there is a second route of access to the machine so that it may be used for diagnostic purposes when not required for intraoperative imaging. Intraoperative MRI is particularly useful for the surgical resection of low- and high-grade gliomas when the tumor margins are difficult to distinguish from normal brain. Although a large number of prospective and retrospective studies have shown improved extent of resection for patients with glioma, there has been only one published randomized trial of intraoperative MRI. Although this trial showed no benefit, it utilized older ultra-low field technology and had only recruited 14 patients at the time of publication.

> Intraoperative MRI is particularly useful for the surgical resection of low- and high-grade gliomas.

Intraoperative ultrasound (US) predates MRI by many decades and was used commonly prior to the advent of neuro-navigation. Improvements in resolution, reduction in probe size, and co-registration of US and MRI data have led to a resurgence of interest in the technique. The major benefit of US is real-time data acquisition, but at the cost of image quality. The technique is particularly useful to directly visualize pathology that is underneath normal-appearing cortex or spinal cord. Ultrasound can also be utilized to account for brain shift at the end of resection when neuro-navigation has become inaccurate. Similarly, the position of spinal cord tumors in relation to bony anatomy can vary with patient position (i.e., prone on the operative table with outstretched hands vs. supine during diagnostic MRI), making real-time localization particularly important. Although US has been demonstrated to show tumor margins,[102] air and blood introduced during resection can create acoustic artifact that can make residual tumor difficult to distinguish toward the end of resection, thus limiting the utility of US to improve extent of resection.[103]

STEREOTACTIC BRAIN BIOPSY AND STEREOTACTIC TREATMENT DELIVERY

Histological diagnosis is still required for the management of most entities in neuro-oncology. Where resection is not feasible (i.e., multifocal disease) or indicated (i.e., germ cell tumors), tissue may be sampled by stereotactic biopsy. Stereotactic systems may be frame-based or frameless and rely on navigation systems described earlier. Even in high-risk locations such as the brainstem, stereotactic brain biopsy is diagnostic in more than 95% of patients, with a less than 1% chance of permanent neurological deficit or death.[104]

Adaptions of this technique allow for the stereotactic application of local treatments, such as laser interstitial thermal therapy (LITT), convection-enhanced drug delivery, or infusion of vaccine or viral vectors. Of these techniques, only LITT has passed beyond the investigational stage and will be discussed further. LITT was first described in 1990 using CT guidance[105]; however, it wasn't until MR thermography improved that the technique gained popularity. A laser probe is placed stereotactically into the target and emits photons (Figure 19.2). These enter surrounding tissue, where their energy is transformed into thermal energy and results in tissue damage. Intraoperative MRI allows for confirmation of the catheter position, and MR thermography provides real-time monitoring of the ablation effect.

LITT has been utilized most commonly for tumor recurrence in patients with glioblastoma or brain metastases after the failure of conventional therapies to achieve local control.[106] It has also been used for the treatment of radiation necrosis and for the primary treatment of glioblastoma when tumor morphology or location makes resection difficult.[107] Ventricular and cisternal CSF and large vessels can act as heat sinks, limiting the effectiveness of the technique near these structures.[106] Large tumors or those with complicated shapes may not be amenable to the technique.

Published data demonstrate improved patient survival; however, this was compared with historical controls and these results may be confounded by patient selection factors.[108] Median length of stay is less than 2 days and the procedure is relatively well-tolerated[109]; neurological complications occur in up to 13% of patients and are permanent in 3%.[109] The rate of hemorrhage has been estimated at 2.5%[110] and often requires craniotomy for treatment.

> LITT has been utilized most commonly for tumor recurrence in patients with glioblastoma or brain metastases after the failure of conventional therapies.

NEURO-ENDOSCOPY

Endoscopic approaches are designed to minimize trauma by providing minimally invasive access to deep structures. The endoscope allows for light and magnification to be brought directly to the target within a deep cavity. The primary uses in neuro-oncology are to biopsy intraventricular lesions or treat hydrocephalus, or during endonasal skull base approaches. Additionally, the endoscope may be used to assist during microscopic procedures, using angled scopes to see areas that are not directly visible during open surgery.

The use of an endoscope to access the ventricle was described as early as 1920 by Lespinasse and Dandy and used to coagulate the choroid plexus to treat hydrocephalus.[111] This procedure fell out of favor as ventricular shunt technology improved, but has more recently been revived as a treatment in resource-poor settings where shunt blockage is likely to result in death.[112] Modern ridged endoscopes have one or more working channels that allow for the passage of biopsy forceps, scissors, diathermy, and other instruments during intraventricular surgery.

In contemporary neuro-oncology practice, transventricular endoscopy is most commonly used to biopsy unresectable lesions or treat hydrocephalus. Thalamic, pineal, and tectal plate lesions are often exophytic into the third ventricle and can be biopsied endoscopically, via an approach that traverses the lateral ventricle and foramen of Munroe. As many pathologies

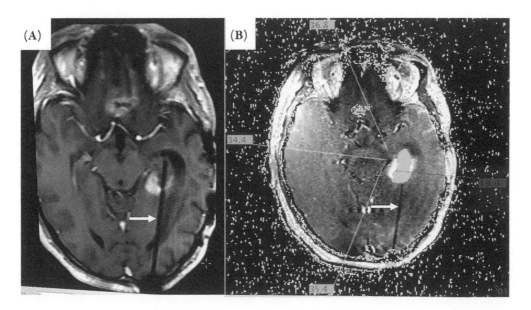

Figure 19.2 MRI showing a recurrent hippocampal glioblastoma treated with focused laser interstitial thermal therapy (LITT). (A) Intraoperative coronal T1-weighted MRI with contrast showing the probe targeting the tumor. (B) During LITT, a damage zone of tissue achieving temperatures sufficient for ablation is represented by orange pixels.

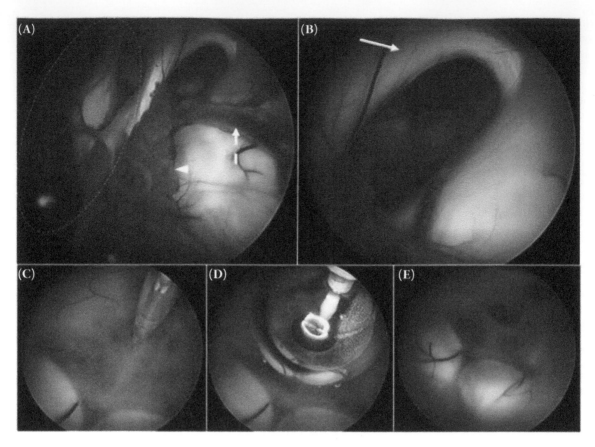

Figure 19.3 *Endoscopic third ventriculostomy intraoperative images. (A) After entry into the right lateral ventricle, it is important to identify key anatomical structures to help with orientation. The choroid plexus can be traced anteriorly as it enters the foramen of Monro (arrowhead). The thalamostriate vein is another key landmark to ensure that the correct lateral ventricle has been entered (dashed arrow). In this case, the patient had absence of a complete septum pellucidum (dashed circle). (B) The endoscope is then passed through the foramen of Monro into the third ventricle. The fornix composes the roof of the foramen (arrow) and is at risk of injury with excessive movements with the endoscope. (C) The floor of the third ventricle is identified with the mamillary bodies seen posteriorly in the endoscope's view. A Fogarty balloon is passed through the thin membrane of the floor of the third ventricle (tuber cinereum). (D and E) The balloon is then inflated, increasing the caliber of the opening to the basal cisterns and allowing for cerebrospinal fluid diversion.*

in this region (such as tectal plate glioma and pineal region germ cell tumors) are better treated without resection, the endoscopic approach allows for safe and minimally invasive acquisition of tissue for diagnosis. The approach also allows for simultaneous treatment of hydrocephalus via endoscopic third ventriculostomy (ETV) (Figure 19.3). In some cases, tumors may be resected via an intraventricular endoscopic approach, particularly for small and relatively hypovascular lesions such as colloid cysts.[113]

> Transventricular endoscopy is most commonly used to biopsy unresectable lesions or to treat hydrocephalus.

ETV treats hydrocephalus by creating a direct communication between the third ventricle and basal cisterns. This bypasses an obstructive lesion distal to the third ventricle, allowing for resolution of hydrocephalus without the need for shunting. The rate of complications is low and although subsequent blockage may occur, this is much less common than after ventricular shunting.[114] Technical factors, such as a small foramen of Munro or insufficient space between the clivus and basilar artery, may make the procedure impossible.

> ETV treats hydrocephalus by creating a direct communication between the third ventricle and basal cisterns.

ENDOSCOPIC ENDONASAL SKULL-BASE SURGERY

The trans-nasal corridor can provide excellent access to the central base of skull without brain retraction. Pituitary adenomas are the most common and well-studied tumors treated by this approach. Although surgeons can achieve comparable outcomes using microscopic or endoscopic techniques for pituitary tumors, extended endoscopic approaches allow access to midline tumors from the cribriform plate to foramen magnum. It is particularly useful for craniopharyngiomas, chordomas, chondrosarcomas, and midline meningiomas such as tuberculum, planum, or olfactory groove locations. The major advantages of endoscopic skull base approaches are the avoidance of brain or optic nerve retraction and early access to tumor blood supply. Although modern endoscopes provide excellent visualization, the narrow and long operative corridor can make microsurgery more difficult than open approaches.

A major limitation of extended endonasal approaches is the risk of CSF leak. However, the probability of this complication has been substantially reduced by the use of a nasal septal flap during closure. The mucosa of one or both sides of the nasal septum is harvested and mobilized to cover the deficit, pedicled on the sphenopalatine artery. Vascularized repair has resulted in a reduction in the risk of postoperative CSF leak from 30% to around 7%.[115]

> The major advantages of endoscopic skull base approaches are the avoidance of brain or optic nerve retraction and early access to tumor blood supply.

AWAKE CRANIOTOMY WITH CNS MAPPING AND MONITORING

For most brain tumors, the aim is to resect as much as of the tumor as possible while preventing decline in neurological function. The second aim can be facilitated by awake craniotomy,[116] where function can be both monitored and mapped. This technique remains necessary because preoperative methods (such as functional MRI, tractography, or magnetoencephalography) are insufficiently accurate to localize function or exclude function within the region of the tumor. Many perceived contraindications to awake surgery can now be overcome (Table 19.5) Surgery is performed under local anesthetic with mild sedation during non-mapping periods. *Mapping* refers to intraoperative testing of cortical and subcortical areas during electrical stimulation. Current is applied, which either activates (e.g., primary motor area or visual cortex, corticospinal tract) or inhibits (e.g., speech areas or supplementary motor area) functional tissue (Figure 19.4). Mapping practices have evolved from performing a large craniotomy to identify all relevant functional areas (positive mapping) to performing a smaller exposure and relying on the negative predictive power of the technique to exclude functional tissue. Using this technique, the approach and extent of resection can then be tailored to preserve functional areas.

Although awake craniotomy with mapping is the gold standard (and necessary for mapping language function), motor function can be monitored and mapped in an anesthetized patient. Subcortical motor mapping using a monopolar stimulator affords the surgeon the additional benefit of being able to estimate the distance to the corticospinal tract based on the current required for motor responses. In addition to mapping, motor monitoring may be performed for some extra-axial lesions, for example sphenoidal meningiomas where the vascular supply to motor (and other) cortex may be at risk. Monitoring and mapping are also used extensively during spinal tumor surgery or during peripheral nerve tumor resection, such as for vestibular schwannomas.

> Motor function can be monitored and mapped in an anesthetized patient.

INTRAOPERATIVE MOLECULAR IMAGING AND FLUORESCENCE-GUIDED SURGERY

Gliomas infiltrate normal brain and often have ill-defined margins. This can make it difficult to distinguish tumor from

TABLE 19.5 Relative contraindications and solutions for awake craniotomy patients

PRIOR CONCERNS	CURRENT SOLUTIONS
Significant mass effect (>2cm midline shift) despite preoperative diuretics and steroid	Staged internal debulking (asleep) using functional imaging (MEG/MSI) followed by reoperation w/ awake mapping
Obese patient (BMI >30)/obstructive apnea	LMA before and after mapping (limits subcortical mapping during resection if LMA is used)
Psychiatric history/emotional instability	Treated mood disorders no longer a contraindication
Age (yrs) >10 <10	 Awake 2-stage procedure w/ implanted grid
Intraoperative seizures	Iced Ringers solution, propofol IV 6 inches from vein
Smoker	Cough suppressants w/ or w/o light sedation
Intraoperative nausea	Preop medication w/ antiemetic drugs (ondansetron hydrochloride, scopolamine) and high-dose dexamethasone (10 mg)
Severely impaired preoperative function*	Attempt to improve function w/ up to 5 days of preoperative high-dose steroids w/ or w/o diuretics
Tumor location presumed to be w/in functional cortical or subcortical pathways on preop imaging	The decision to offer surgery is not made based on preop anatomical or functional imaging (attempt is always made to map, identify, and preserve)

BMI, body mass index; IV, intravenous; MEG, magnetoencephalography; MSI, magnetic source imaging.
Motor function <2/5 or baseline naming/reading errors.
Hervey-Jumper SL, Berger MS. Technical nuances of awake brain tumor surgery and the role of maximum safe resection. *J Neurosurg Sci.* 2015;59(4):351–360.

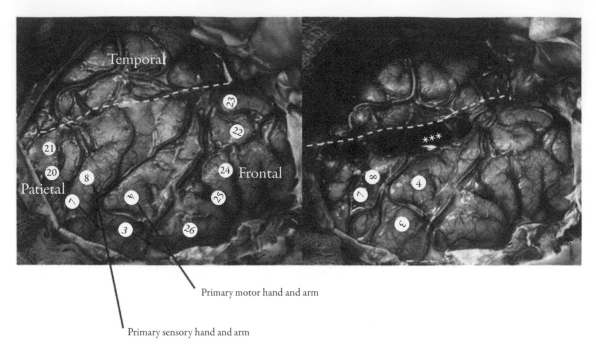

Primary motor hand and arm

Primary sensory hand and arm

Figure 19.4 Intraoperative language and motor mapping reveal cortical sites for primary motor hand (#4) and arm (#3) in addition to primary sensory hand (#8) and arm (#7). All cortical language sites (# 20–26) mapped negative. Glioma resection was performed using a surgical corridor (***) through face motor and sensory cortices.

normal brain during resection, resulting in incomplete resection. Interoperative molecular imaging leverages biological differences between tumor and normal brain to make visualization easier. Although multiple agents have been investigated (including indocyanine green and fluorescein, which rely on disruption of the blood–brain barrier), the most well studied agent is 5-aminolevulenic acid (5-ALA). After oral administration, 5-ALA is metabolized into the fluorophore protoporphyrin IX preferentially in tumor. This can then be visualized using violet-blue light for excitation and a 400–410 nm optical filter. For HGG, the intensity of fluorescence correlates with the degree of tumor cellularity.[117] Unfortunately, most LGGs do not fluoresce with 5-ALA. In a landmark randomized controlled trial of 5-ALA for resection of presumed HGG, 5-ALA–guided surgery was associated with higher rates of GTR (65% vs. 36%) and longer PFS.[118] 5-ALA is administered orally 3 hours prior to surgery. It can cause a severe photosensitive rash; however, this can be avoided by shielding the patient from UVA exposure for 24 hours postoperatively. Other adverse effects include mild, self-limiting cytopenias and derangement of liver enzymes. 5-ALA was approved for use in Europe in 2007, Australia in 2013, and the United States in 2017, and has now become standard of care for HGG where GTR is attempted.

5-ALA guided surgery was associated with higher rates of GTR (65% vs. 36%) and longer PFS.

CONCLUSION

Neurosurgical intervention remains the primary method for definitive diagnosis and the first line of treatment for many tumors within the brain and spinal cord. The goals of surgery are to obtain a tissue diagnosis, relieve mass effect, and improve survival through cytoreduction. Numerous intraoperative tools and techniques have been established to ensure maximal resection while minimizing perioperative morbidity.

FLASHCARD

Indications for neurosurgical intervention in neuro-oncology include:

Histological diagnosis

Cytoreduction

Symptom control, including, treatment of seizures, relief of mass effect, edema or hydrocephalus, and spinal stabilization

---

Biopsy may be performed via open craniotomy, stereotactic needle biopsy, or by transventricular or endonasal endoscopy. Selecting the approach depends on what?

Tumor type, location, associated features (such as hydrocephalus), and if an open resection is planned in addition to biopsy

---

Emerging evidence suggests that resection of non-contrast enhancing GBM is associated with improved:

Median overall survival

While studies are evaluating the role for preoperative SRS, the current paradigm recommends surgery (followed by SRS) in patients with isolated metastases larger than 3 cm for:

Dominant lesion symptom control tissue diagnosis

After the failure of other therapies

For benign tumors such as most meningiomas, pituitary tumors and schwannomas, surgery can be curative; however, gross total resection should not be pursued if there is significant risk of:

Neurological injury

The risks and success of resection for meningiomas are highly dependent on:

Tumor location

Subtotal resection with facial nerve (and hearing) preservation followed by SRS can achieve excellent functional and oncological outcomes for patients with:

Vestibular schwannoma

Awake craniotomy with mapping and monitoring is the gold standard to prevent:

Neurological injury during resection of intrinsic brain tumors

---

What additional steps could improve the safety of resection during surgery for brain, cranial nerve, or spinal cord lesions?

Neuromonitoring

What is a minimally invasive technique that may be indicated for patients with high-grade glioma or metastases after the failure of conventional therapies?	LITT
Intraventricular neuroendoscopy may be used to:	Biopsy select tumors To treat associated hydrocephalus (w/o need for ventricular shunting)
Endoscopic endonasal techniques allow for direct access without retraction to tumors in these locations:	Midline tumors from the cribriform plate to foramen magnum
The rate of CSF leak after extended endoscopic resection has been significantly reduced by the use of a:	Vascularized naso-septal flap during repair
5-ALA guided resection allows for improved _ _____ and is associated with improved ___ _____ in patients with high-grade glioma	Tumor visualization Progression-free survival

QUESTIONS

1. For pineal regions tumors, surgical management may involve
   a. Endoscopic third ventriculostomy and biopsy
   b. Stereotactic needle biopsy
   c. Open suboccipital transtentorial resection
   d. All of the above

2. Which of the following statements is false regarding pituitary tumors?
   a. Surgical resection is never indicated for prolactinomas.
   b. Surgical decompression improves visual acuity outcomes for patients with pituitary apoplexy.
   c. Surgical treatment is the first-line treatment for Cushing disease.
   d. Residual tumor within the cavernous sinus is common.

3. There is evidence from a randomized controlled trial that which of the following is associated with improved progression-free survival for patients with malignant glioma?
   a. Greater extent of resection
   b. The use of neuronavigation
   c. The use of intraoperative MRI
   d. Fluorescent guided resection using 5-ALA

4. Which of the following are contraindications to awake craniotomy with language mapping?
   a. Obesity
   b. Severe perioperative language deficits that are unresponsive to steroids
   c. Preoperative seizures
   d. Age younger than 18 years

5. Which of the following lesions is least accessible by an endoscopic endonasal approach?
   a. Clival chordoma
   b. Olfactory groove meningioma
   c. Pituitary adenoma
   d. Tectal plate glioma

For questions 6–8, select the answer that is true.

6. Regarding extent of resection in neuro-oncology:
   a. Greater extent of abnormal FLAIR resection is associated with improved outcome for patients with glioblastoma.
   b. Intracavernous sinus tumor should be resected in patients with non-functioning pituitary adenoma.
   c. The cyst wall of a hemangioblastoma must be resected to prevent recurrence.
   d. Gross total resection should be achieved for most pineal region tumors.

7. Regarding pituitary apoplexy:
   a. Third nerve palsy is does not recover without surgery.
   b. Sixth nerve palsies are common because this nerve is closest to the pituitary gland within the cavernous sinus.
   c. Surgery is required in all cases.
   d. Early corticosteroid replacement is mandatory.

8. Regarding surgery for craniopharyngiomas:
   a. Resection of tumors from a subfrontal approach may require opening of the lamina papyracea.
   b. An endoscopic endonasal approach may be used for resection.
   c. Postoperative weight loss is very common.
   d. Usually biopsy is all that is required.

9. All of the following are true regarding hemangioblastomas *except*
   a. Extracapsular resection is preferable to avoid significant blood loss.
   b. It is important to identity patients with pheochromocytoma preoperatively.
   c. Supratentorial tumors are almost always associated with VHL syndrome.
   d. Early surgery is preferable once lesions are identified, especially in patients with VHL syndrome.

10. Which of the following statements is true regarding neuronavigation?
    a. Intraoperative MRI is required for neuronavigation.
    b. Multiple different imaging types may be co-registered and overlaid to provide information to the surgeon during resection.
    c. The patients must be imaged in a stereotactic frame.
    d. There is no rolc for neuronavigation in anatomical exposures, such as during pituitary surgery.

11. During transventricular neuroendoscopy
    a. Complete tumor resection is never possible.
    b. Hydrocephalus can be treated by third ventriculostomy.
    c. Tumor resection or biopsy requires multiple port sites.
    d. The third ventricle is entered directly, after traversing the white matter.

12. Regarding awake craniotomy for tumor resection:
    a. Electrical stimulation inhibits motor responses in the primary motor area.
    b. Electrical stimulation inhibits motor responses in the corticospinal tract.
    c. Electrical stimulation inhibits speech production in the peri-sylvian area of the dominant hemisphere.
    d. Electrical stimulation never causes seizures.

13. Which of the following is not associated with tectal plate lesions?
    a. Obstructive hydrocephalus
    b. Parinaud's syndrome
    c. Foster-Kennedy syndrome
    d. Glial pathology

14. Which of the following grading scales is used to assess meningioma resection?
    a. Koo
    b. Simpson
    c. House-Brackman
    d. Hunt and Hess

15. Which of the following is false regarding re-resection?
    a. Screening for metastases should be performed in patients with hemangiopericytoma before re-resection.
    b. Screening for metastases should be performed in patients with greater than 2 meningioma recurrences prior to resection.
    c. Age should not be considered an absolute contradiction to re-resection for patients with glioblastoma.
    d. Re-resection for Cushing disease can achieve hormonal control in only 10% of patients.

ANSWERS

1. d
2. a
3. d
4. b
5. d
6. a
7. d
8. b
9. d
10. b
11. b
12. c
13. c
14. b
15. d

REFERENCES

1. Ostrom QT, Gittleman H, Truitt G, Boscia A, Kruchko C, Barnholtz-Sloan JS. CBTRUS statistical report: Primary brain and other central nervous system tumors diagnosed in the United States in 2011-2015. *Neuro Oncol.* 2018. doi:10.1093/neuonc/noy131
2. Louis DN, Perry A, Reifenberger G, et al. The 2016 World Health Organization Classification of Tumors of the Central Nervous System: A summary. *Acta Neuropathol.* 2016. doi:10.1007/s00401-016-1545-1
3. Cheng G, Yu X, Zhao H, et al. Complications of stereotactic biopsy of lesions in the sellar region, pineal gland, and brainstem: A retrospective, single-center study. *Medicine (Baltimore).* 2020;99(8):e18572. doi:10.1097/MD.0000000000018572
4. Maragkos GA, Penumaka A, Ahrendsen JT, et al. Factors affecting the diagnostic yield of frame-based stereotactic intracranial biopsies. *World Neurosurg.* 2020;135:e695–e701. doi:10.1016/j.wneu.2019.12.102
5. Gutt-Will M, Murek M, Schwarz C, et al. Frequent diagnostic undergrading in isocitrate dehydrogenase wild-type gliomas due to small pathological tissue samples. *Neurosurgery.* 2019;85(5):689–694. doi:10.1093/neuros/nyy433
6. Molinaro AM, Hervey-Jumper S, Morshed RA, et al. Association of maximal extent of resection of contrast-enhanced and non-contrast-enhanced tumor with survival within molecular subgroups of patients with newly diagnosed glioblastoma. *JAMA Oncol.* February 2020:10.1001/jamaoncol.2019.6143. doi:10.1001/jamaoncol.2019.6143
7. Tarapore PE, Tate MC, Findlay AM, et al. Preoperative multimodal motor mapping: A comparison of magnetoencephalography imaging, navigated transcranial magnetic stimulation, and direct cortical stimulation: Clinical article. *J Neurosurg.* 2012;117(2):354–362. doi:10.3171/2012.5.JNS112124
8. Wu JS, Zhou LF, Tang WJ, et al. Clinical evaluation and follow-up outcome of diffusion tensor imaging-based functional neuronavigation: A prospective, controlled study in patients with gliomas involving pyramidal tracts. *Neurosurgery.* 2007. doi:10.1227/01.neu.0000303189.80049.ab
9. Nimsky C, Ganslandt O, Hastreiter P, et al. Intraoperative diffusion-tensor MR imaging: Shifting of white matter tracts during neurosurgical procedures: Initial experience. *Radiology.* 2005. doi:10.1148/radiol.2341031984
10. Southwell DG, Riva M, Jordan K, et al. Language outcomes after resection of dominant inferior parietal lobule gliomas. *J Neurosurg.* 2017;127(4):781–789. doi:10.3171/2016.8.JNS16443
11. Magill ST, Han SJ, Li J, Berger MS. Resection of primary motor cortex tumors: Feasibility and surgical outcomes. *J Neurosurg.* 2018;129(4):961–972. doi:10.3171/2017.5.JNS163045
12. Leighton C, Fisher B, Bauman G, et al. Supratentorial low-grade glioma in adults: An analysis of prognostic factors and timing of radiation. *J Clin Oncol Off J Am Soc Clin Oncol.* 1997;15(4):1294–1301. doi:10.1200/JCO.1997.15.4.1294
13. Lote K, Stenwig AE, Skullerud K, Hirschberg H. Prevalence and prognostic significance of epilepsy in patients with gliomas. *Eur J Cancer.* 1998;34(1):98–102. doi:10.1016/s0959-8049(97)00374-2
14. Englot DJ, Magill ST, Han SJ, et al. Seizures in supratentorial meningioma: A systematic review and meta-analysis. *J Neurosurg.* 2016;124(6):1552–1561. doi:10.3171/2015.4.JNS142742
15. Wang DD, Deng H, Hervey-Jumper SL, et al. Seizure outcome after surgical resection of insular glioma. *Neurosurgery.* 2018;83(4):709–718. doi:10.1093/neuros/nyx486
16. Faramand AM, Barnes N, Harrison S, et al. Seizure and cognitive outcomes after resection of glioneuronal tumors in children. *Epilepsia.* 2018;59(1):170–178. doi:10.1111/epi.13961
17. Bonney PA, Glenn CA, Ebeling PA, et al. Seizure freedom rates and prognostic indicators after resection of gangliogliomas: A review. *World Neurosurg.* 2015;84(6):1988–1996. doi:10.1016/j.wneu.2015.06.044
18. Still MEH, Roux A, Huberfeld G, et al. Extent of resection and residual tumor thresholds for postoperative total seizure freedom in epileptic adult patients harboring a supratentorial diffuse low-grade glioma. *Neurosurgery.* 2019;85(2):E332-E340. doi:10.1093/neuros/nyy481
19. Chang EF, Potts MB, Keles GE, et al. Seizure characteristics and control following resection in 332 patients with low-grade gliomas. *J Neurosurg.* 2008;108(2):227–235. doi:10.3171/JNS/2008/108/2/0227
20. Yao P-S, Zheng S-F, Wang F, et al. Surgery guided with intraoperative electrocorticography in patients with low-grade glioma and refractory seizures. *J Neurosurg.* 2018;128(3):840–845. doi:10.3171/2016.11.JNS161296
21. Shimony N, Shofty B, Harosh C, et al. Surgical resection of cerebral metastases leads to faster resolution of peritumoral edema than stereotactic radiosurgery: A volumetric analysis. *Ann Surg Oncol.* 2017;24(5):1392–1398. doi:10.1245/s10434-016-5709-y
22. Alvarez-Breckenridge C, Giobbie-Hurder A, Gill CM, et al. Upfront surgical resection of melanoma brain metastases provides a bridge toward immunotherapy-mediated systemic control. *Oncologist.* 2019;24(5):671–679. doi:10.1634/theoncologist.2018-0306
23. Laufer I, Rubin DG, Lis E, et al. The NOMS framework: Approach to the treatment of spinal metastatic tumors. *Oncologist.* 2013;18(6):744–751. doi:10.1634/theoncologist.2012-0293
24. Fisher CG, DiPaola CP, Ryken TC, et al. A novel classification system for spinal instability in neoplastic disease: An evidence-based approach and expert consensus from the Spine Oncology Study Group. *Spine (Phila Pa 1976).* 2010;35(22):E1221-9. doi:10.1097/BRS.0b013e3181e16ae2
25. Jakola AS, Skjulsvik AJ, Myrmel KS, et al. Surgical resection versus watchful waiting in low-grade gliomas. *Ann Oncol.* 2017. doi:10.1093/annonc/mdx230
26. Smith JS, Chang EF, Lamborn KR, et al. Role of extent of resection in the long-term outcome of low-grade hemispheric gliomas. *J Clin Oncol.* 2008. doi:10.1200/JCO.2007.13.9337
27. Duffau H. Long-term outcomes after supratotal resection of diffuse low-grade gliomas: A consecutive series with 11-year follow-up. *Acta Neurochir (Wien).* 2016;158(1):51–58. doi:10.1007/s00701-015-2621-3
28. Oppenlander ME, Wolf AB, Snyder LA, et al. An extent of resection threshold for recurrent glioblastoma and its risk for neurological morbidity. *J Neurosurg.* 2014;120(4):846–853. doi:10.3171/2013.12.JNS13184

29. Li YM, Suki D, Hess K, Sawaya R. The influence of maximum safe resection of glioblastoma on survival in 1229 patients: Can we do better than gross-total resection? *J Neurosurg*. 2016. doi:10.3171/2015.5.JNS142087

30. Al-Holou WN, Hodges TR, Everson RG, et al. Perilesional resection of glioblastoma is independently associated with improved outcomes. *Neurosurgery*. 2020. doi:10.1093/neuros/nyz008

31. Glenn CA, Baker CM, Conner AK, et al. An examination of the role of supramaximal resection of temporal lobe glioblastoma multiforme. *World Neurosurg*. 2018. doi:10.1016/j.wneu.2018.03.072

32. Bloch O, Han SJ, Cha S, et al. Impact of extent of resection for recurrent glioblastoma on overall survival: Clinical article. *J Neurosurg*. 2012;117(6):1032–1038. doi:10.3171/2012.9.JNS12504

33. Hervey-Jumper SL, Berger MS. Reoperation for recurrent high-grade glioma: A current perspective of the literature. *Neurosurgery*. 2014. doi:10.1227/NEU.0000000000000486

34. Nahed B V, Alvarez-Breckenridge C, Brastianos PK, et al. Congress of Neurological Surgeons systematic review and evidence-based guidelines on the role of surgery in the management of adults with metastatic brain tumors. *Neurosurgery*. 2019;84(3):E152–E155. doi:10.1093/neuros/nyy542

35. Rades D, Kieckebusch S, Haatanen T, et al. Surgical resection followed by whole brain radiotherapy versus whole brain radiotherapy alone for single brain metastasis. *Int J Radiat Oncol Biol Phys*. 2008;70(5):1319–1324. doi:10.1016/j.ijrobp.2007.08.009

36. Mahajan A, Ahmed S, McAleer MF, et al. Post-operative stereotactic radiosurgery versus observation for completely resected brain metastases: A single-centre, randomised, controlled, phase 3 trial. *Lancet Oncol*. 2017;18(8):1040–1048. doi:10.1016/S1470-2045(17)30414-X

37. Patel AJ, Suki D, Hatiboglu MA, et al. Factors influencing the risk of local recurrence after resection of a single brain metastasis. *J Neurosurg*. 2010;113(2):181–189. doi:10.3171/2009.11.JNS09659

38. Suki D, Hatiboglu MA, Patel AJ, et al. Comparative risk of leptomeningeal dissemination of cancer after surgery or stereotactic radiosurgery for a single supratentorial solid tumor metastasis. *Neurosurgery*. 2009;64(4):664–666. doi:10.1227/01.NEU.0000341535.53720.3E

39. Hassaneen W, Suki D, Salaskar AL, et al. Surgical management of lateral-ventricle metastases: Report of 29 cases in a single-institution experience. *J Neurosurg*. 2010;112(5):1046–1055. doi:10.3171/2009.7.JNS09571

40. Lee C-H, Kim DG, Kim JW, et al. The role of surgical resection in the management of brain metastasis: A 17-year longitudinal study. *Acta Neurochir (Wien)*. 2013;155(3):389–397. doi:10.1007/s00701-013-1619-y

41. Quigley MR, Bello N, Jho D, et al. Estimating the additive benefit of surgical excision to stereotactic radiosurgery in the management of metastatic brain disease. *Neurosurgery*. 2015;76(6):703–707. doi:10.1227/NEU.0000000000000707

42. Alvarez-Breckenridge C, Giobbie-Harder A, Gill CM, et al. Upfront surgical resection of melanoma brain metastases provides a bridge toward immunotherapy-mediated systemic control. *Oncologist*. 2019. doi:10.1634/theoncologist.2018-0306

43. Brat DJ, Scheithauer BW, Eberhart CG, Burger PC. Extraventricular neurocytomas: Pathologic features and clinical outcome. *Am J Surg Pathol*. 2001;25(10):1252–1260. doi:10.1097/00000478-200110000-00005

44. Imber BS, Braunstein SE, Wu FY, et al. Clinical outcome and prognostic factors for central neurocytoma: Twenty year institutional experience. *J Neurooncol*. 2016;126(1):193–200. doi:10.1007/s11060-015-1959-y

45. Park H, Steven D C. Stereotactic radiosurgery for central neurocytoma: A quantitative systematic review. *J Neurooncol*. 2012;108(1):115–121. doi:10.1007/s11060-012-0803-x

46. Brandes AA, Amistà P, Gardiman M, et al. Chemotherapy in patients with recurrent and progressive central neurocytoma. *Cancer*. 2000;88(1):169–174. doi:10.1002/(sici)1097-0142(20000101)88:1<169::aid-cncr23>3.0.co;2-7

47. Bond KM, Hughes JD, Porter AL, et al. Adult pilocytic astrocytoma: An institutional series and systematic literature review for extent of resection and recurrence. *World Neurosurg*. 2018;110:276–283. doi:10.1016/j.wneu.2017.11.102

48. Yahanda AT, Patel B, Sutherland G, et al. A multi-institutional analysis of factors influencing surgical outcomes for patients with newly diagnosed grade I gliomas. *World Neurosurg*. 2020;135:e754–e764. doi:10.1016/j.wneu.2019.12.156

49. Haydon DH, Dahiya S, Smyth MD, Limbrick DD, Leonard JR. Greater Extent of Resection Improves Ganglioglioma Recurrence-Free Survival in Children: A Volumetric Analysis. *Neurosurgery*. 2014;75(1):37–42. doi:10.1227/NEU.0000000000000349

50. Terrier L-M, Bauchet L, Rigau V, et al. Natural course and prognosis of anaplastic gangliogliomas: A multicenter retrospective study of 43 cases from the French Brain Tumor Database. *Neuro Oncol*. 2017;19(5):678–688. doi:10.1093/neuonc/now186

51. Spagnoli D, Tomei G, Ceccarelli G, et al. Combined treatment of fourth ventricle ependymomas: Report of 26 cases. *Surg Neurol*. 2000;54(1):19–26; discussion 26. doi:10.1016/s0090-3019(00)00272-x

52. Healey EA, Barnes PD, Kupsky WJ, et al. The prognostic significance of postoperative residual tumor in ependymoma. *Neurosurgery*. 1991;28(5):662–666. doi:10.1097/00006123-199105000-00005

53. Nazar GB, Hoffman HJ, Becker LE, et al. Infratentorial ependymomas in childhood: Prognostic factors and treatment. *J Neurosurg*. 1990;72(3):408–417. doi:10.3171/jns.1990.72.3.0408

54. Winkler EA, Birk H, Safaee M, et al. Surgical resection of fourth ventricular ependymomas: Case series and technical nuances. *J Neurooncol*. 2016;130(2):341–349. doi:10.1007/s11060-016-2198-6

55. Kano H, Su Y-H, Wu H-M, et al. Stereotactic radiosurgery for intracranial ependymomas: An international multicenter study. *Neurosurgery*. 2019;84(1):227–234. doi:10.1093/neuros/nyy082

56. Boström A, Von Lehe M, Hartmann W, et al. Surgery for spinal cord ependymomas: Outcome and prognostic factors. *Neurosurgery*. 2011. doi:10.1227/NEU.0b013e3182004c1e

57. Nagasawa DT, Smith ZA, Cremer N, et al. Complications associated with the treatment for spinal ependymomas. *Neurosurg Focus*. 2011. doi:10.3171/2011.7.FOCUS11158

58. Youngblood MW, Duran D, Montejo JD, et al. Correlations between genomic subgroup and clinical features in a cohort of more than 3000 meningiomas. *J Neurosurg*. 2019. doi:10.3171/2019.8.jns191266

59. Raper DMS, Starke RM, Henderson F, et al. Preoperative embolization of intracranial meningiomas: Efficacy, technical considerations, and complications. *Am J Neuroradiol*. 2014. doi:10.3174/ajnr.A3919

60. Magill ST, Lau B, Raleigh DR, et al. Surgical resection and interstitial iodine-125 brachytherapy for high-grade meningiomas: A 25-year series. *Neurosurgery*. 2017. doi:10.1227/NEU.0000000000001262

61. Dalle Ore CL, Magill ST, Yen AJ, et al. Meningioma metastases: Incidence and proposed screening paradigm. *J Neurosurg*. 2019. doi:10.3171/2019.1.jns181771

62. Simpson, D. The recurrence of intracranial meningiomas after surgical treatment. *J Neurol Neurosurg Psychiatry*. 1957;20(1):22–39. doi:10.1136/jnnp.20.1.22

63. Faramand A, Kano H, Niranjan A, et al. Tumor control and cranial nerve outcomes after adjuvant radiosurgery for low-grade skull base meningiomas. *World Neurosurg*. 2019;127:e221–e229. doi:10.1016/j.wneu.2019.03.052

64. Aizer AA, Bi WL, Kandola MS, et al. Extent of resection and overall survival for patients with atypical and malignant meningioma. *Cancer*. 2015;121(24):4376–4381. doi:10.1002/cncr.29639

65. Dalle Ore CL, Magill ST, Rodriguez Rubio R, et al. Hyperostosing sphenoid wing meningiomas: Surgical outcomes and strategy for bone resection and multidisciplinary orbital reconstruction. *J Neurosurg*. 2020. doi:10.3171/2019.12.jns192543

66. Ghose A, Guha G, Kundu R, et al. CNS hemangiopericytoma: A systematic review of 523 patients. *Am J Clin Oncol*. 2017. doi:10.1097/COC.0000000000000146

67. Jääskeläinen J, Servo A, Haltia M, et al. Intracranial hemangiopericytoma: Radiology, surgery, radiotherapy, and outcome in 21 patients. *Surg Neurol*. 1985. doi:10.1016/0090-3019(85)90087-4

68. Stangerup SE, Caye-Thomasen P, Tos M, Thomsen J. The natural history of vestibular schwannoma. *Otol Neurotol*. 2006. doi:10.1097/00129492-200606000-00018

69. Erickson NJ, Schmalz PGR, Agee BS, et al. Koos classification of vestibular schwannomas: A reliability study. *Neurosurgery*. 2019;85(3):409–414. doi:10.1093/neuros/nyy409

70. Koos WT, Day JD, Matula C, Levy DI. Neurotopographic considerations in the microsurgical treatment of small acoustic neurinomas. *J Neurosurg*. 1998. Mar;88(3):506–512.

71. House JW, Brackmann DE. Facial nerve grading system. *Otolaryngol Head Neck Surg*. 1985. doi:10.1177/019459988509300202

72. Bloch O, Sughrue ME, Kaur R, et al. Factors associated with preservation of facial nerve function after surgical resection of vestibular schwannoma. *J Neurooncol*. 2011. doi:10.1007/s11060-010-0315-5

73. Raftopoulos C, Abu Serieh B, Duprez T, et al. Microsurgical results with large vestibular schwannomas with preservation of facial and cochlear nerve function as the primary aim. *Acta Neurochir (Wien)*. 2005;147(7):697–706. doi:10.1007/s00701-005-0544-0

74. Theodosopoulos P V, Pensak ML. Contemporary management of acoustic neuromas. *Laryngoscope*. 2011;121(6):1133–1137. doi:10.1002/lary.21799

75. Monfared A, Corrales CE, Theodosopoulos P V, et al. Facial nerve outcome and tumor control rate as a function of degree of resection in treatment of large acoustic neuromas: Preliminary report of the Acoustic Neuroma Subtotal Resection Study (ANSRS). *Neurosurgery*. 2016;79(2):194–203. doi:10.1227/NEU.0000000000001162

76. Sughrue ME, Kaur R, Rutkowski MJ, et al. Extent of resection and the long-term durability of vestibular schwannoma surgery. *J Neurosurg.* 2011;114(5):1218–1223. doi:10.3171/2010.11.JNS10257

77. Anaizi AN, Gantwerker EA, Pensak ML, Theodosopoulos PV. Facial nerve preservation surgery for koos grade 3 and 4 vestibular schwannomas. *Neurosurgery.* 2014;75(6):671–677. doi:10.1227/NEU.0000000000000547

78. Daniel RT, Tuleasca C, Rocca A, et al. The changing paradigm for the surgical treatment of large vestibular schwannomas. *J Neurol Surgery, Part B Skull Base.* 2018. doi:10.1055/s-0038-1668540

79. Porter RG, Larouere MJ, Kartush JM, et al. Improved facial nerve outcomes using an evolving treatment method for large acoustic neuromas. *Otol Neurotol.* 2013. doi:10.1097/MAO.0b013e31827d07d4

80. Bakker SH, Jacobs WCH, Pondaag W, et al. Chordoma: A systematic review of the epidemiology and clinical prognostic factors predicting progression-free and overall survival. *Eur Spine J.* 2018;27(12):3043–3058. doi:10.1007/s00586-018-5764-0

81. Agam MS, Wedemeyer MA, Wrobel B, et al. Complications associated with microscopic and endoscopic transsphenoidal pituitary surgery: Experience of 1153 consecutive cases treated at a single tertiary care pituitary center. *J Neurosurg.* 2019. doi:10.3171/2017.12.JNS172318

82. Karavitaki N, Collison K, Halliday J, et al. What is the natural history of nonoperated nonfunctioning pituitary adenomas? *Clin Endocrinol (Oxf).* 2007. doi:10.1111/j.1365-2265.2007.02990.x

83. Little AS, Chicoine MR, Kelly DF, et al. Evaluation of surgical resection goal and its relationship to extent of resection and patient outcomes in a multicenter prospective study of patients with surgically treated, nonfunctioning pituitary adenomas: A case series. *Oper Neurosurg (Hagerstown, Md).* 2020;18(1):26–33. doi:10.1093/ons/opz085

84. Gerges MM, Rumalla K, Godil SS, et al. Long-term outcomes after endoscopic endonasal surgery for nonfunctioning pituitary macroadenomas. *J Neurosurg.* January 2020:1–12. doi:10.3171/2019.11.JNS192457

85. Molitch ME. Diagnosis and treatment of pituitary adenomas: A review. *JAMA.* 2017. doi:10.1001/jama.2016.19699

86. Gillam MP, Molitch ME, Lombardi G, Colao A. Advances in the treatment of prolactinomas. *Endocr Rev.* 2006. doi:10.1210/er.2005-9998

87. Dabrh AMA, Mohammed K, Asi N, et al. Surgical interventions and medical treatments in treatment-naïve patients with acromegaly: Systematic review and meta-analysis. *J Clin Endocrinol Metab.* 2014. doi:10.1210/jc.2014-2900

88. Ram Z, Nieman LK, Cutler GB, et al. Early repeat surgery for persistent Cushing's disease. *J Neurosurg.* 1994. doi:10.3171/jns.1994.80.1.0037

89. Barkhoudarian G, Kelly DF. Pituitary apoplexy. *Neurosurg Clin N Am.* 2019. doi:10.1016/j.nec.2019.06.001

90. Briet C, Salenave S, Bonneville JF, et al. Pituitary apoplexy. *Endocr Rev.* 2015. doi:10.1210/er.2015-1042

91. Karavitaki N, Brufani C, Warner JT, et al. Craniopharyngiomas in children and adults: Systematic analysis of 121 cases with long-term follow-up. *Clin Endocrinol (Oxf).* 2005. doi:10.1111/j.1365-2265.2005.02231.x

92. Ni W, Shi X. Interventions for the treatment of craniopharyngioma-related hypothalamic obesity: A systematic review. *World Neurosurg.* 2018. doi:10.1016/j.wneu.2018.06.121

93. Juratli TA, Jones PS, Wang N, et al. Targeted treatment of papillary craniopharyngiomas harboring BRAF V600E mutations. *Cancer.* 2019;125(17):2910–2914. doi:10.1002/cncr.32197

94. Wind JJ, Lonser RR. Management of von Hippel-Lindau disease-associated CNS lesions. *Expert Rev Neurother.* 2011. doi:10.1586/ern.11.124

95. Lonser RR, Butman JA, Huntoon K, et al. Prospective natural history study of central nervous system hemangioblastomas in von Hippel-Lindau disease: Clinical article. *J Neurosurg.* 2014. doi:10.3171/2014.1.JNS131431

96. Jagannathan J, Lonser RR, Smith R, et al. Surgical management of cerebellar hemangioblastomas in patients with von Hippel-Lindau disease. *J Neurosurg.* 2008. doi:10.3171/JNS/2008/108/2/0210

97. Mehta GU, Asthagiri AR, Bakhtian KD, et al. Functional outcome after resection of spinal cord hemangioblastomas associated with von Hippel-Lindau disease: Clinical article. *J Neurosurg Spine.* 2010. doi:10.3171/2009.10.SPINE09592

98. Sonabend AM, Bowden S, Bruce JN. Microsurgical resection of pineal region tumors. *J Neurooncol.* 2016. doi:10.1007/s11060-016-2138-5

99. Clarke R, Horsley V. On a method of investigating the deep ganglia and tracts of the central nervous system. *Br Med J.* 1906;2:1799–1800.

100. Spiegel EA, Wycis HT, Marks M, Lee AJ. Stereotaxic apparatus for operations on the human brain. *Science.* 1947 (80). doi:10.1126/science.106.2754.349

101. Black PML, Moriarty T, Alexander E, et al. Development and implementation of intraoperative magnetic resonance imaging and its neurosurgical applications. *Neurosurgery.* 1997. doi:10.1097/00006123-199710000-00013

102. Hammoud MA, Ligon BL, Elsouki R, et al. Use of intraoperative ultrasound for localizing tumors and determining the extent of resection: A comparative study with magnetic resonance imaging. *J Neurosurg.* 1996. doi:10.3171/jns.1996.84.5.0737

103. Gerganov VM, Samii A, Giordano M, et al. Two-dimensional high-end ultrasound imaging compared to intraoperative MRI during resection of low-grade gliomas. *J Clin Neurosci.* 2011. doi:10.1016/j.jocn.2010.08.017

104. Hamisch C, Kickingereder P, Fischer M, et al. Update on the diagnostic value and safety of stereotactic biopsy for pediatric brainstem tumors: A systematic review and meta-analysis of 735 cases. *J Neurosurg Pediatr.* 2017. doi:10.3171/2017.2.PEDS1665

105. Sugiyama K, Sakai T, Fujishima I, et al. Stereotactic interstitial laser-hyperthermia using Nd-YAG laser. *Stereotact Funct Neurosurg.* 1990. doi:10.1159/000100263

106. Ashraf O, Patel NV, Hanft S, Danish SF. Laser-induced thermal therapy in neuro-oncology: A review. *World Neurosurg.* 2018. doi:10.1016/j.wneu.2018.01.123

107. Thomas JG, Rao G, Kew Y, Prabhu SS. Laser interstitial thermal therapy for newly diagnosed and recurrent glioblastoma. *Neurosurg Focus.* 2016. doi:10.3171/2016.7.FOCUS16234

108. Sloan AE, Ahluwalia MS, Valerio-Pascua J, et al. Results of the NeuroBlate system first-in-humans phase I clinical trial for recurrent glioblastoma. *J Neurosurg.* 2013. doi:10.3171/2013.1.JNS1291

109. Patel P, Patel NV, Danish SF. Intracranial MR-guided laser-induced thermal therapy: Single-center experience with the Visualase thermal therapy system. *J Neurosurg.* 2016. doi:10.3171/2015.7.JNS15244

110. Medvid R, Ruiz A, Komotar RJ, et al. Current applications of MRI-guided laser interstitial thermal therapy in the treatment of brain neoplasms and epilepsy: A radiologic and neurosurgical overview. *Am J Neuroradiol.* 2015. doi:10.3174/ajnr.A4362

111. Abbott R. History of neuroendoscopy. *Neurosurg Clin N Am.* 2004. doi:10.1016/S1042-3680(03)00065-2

112. Warf BC. Comparison of endoscopic third ventriculostomy alone and combined with choroid plexus cauterization in infants younger than 1 year of age: A prospective study in 550 African children. *J Neurosurg.* 2005. doi:10.3171/ped.2005.103.6.0475

113. Chowdhry SA, Cohen AR. Intraventricular neuroendoscopy: Complication avoidance and management. *World Neurosurg.* 2013. doi:10.1016/j.wneu.2012.02.030

114. Lu L, Chen H, Weng S, Xu Y. Endoscopic third ventriculostomy versus ventriculoperitoneal shunt in patients with obstructive hydrocephalus: Meta-analysis of randomized controlled trials. *World Neurosurg.* 2019. doi:10.1016/j.wneu.2019.04.255

115. Harvey RJ, Parmar P, Sacks R, Zanation AM. Endoscopic skull base reconstruction of large dural defects: A systematic review of published evidence. *Laryngoscope.* 2012. doi:10.1002/lary.22475

116. Gogos AJ, Young JS, Morshed RA, et al. Awake glioma surgery: Technical evolution and nuances. *J Neurooncol.* 2020. doi:10.1007/s11060-020-03482-z

117. Lau D, Hervey-Jumper SL, Chang S, et al. A prospective Phase II clinical trial of 5-aminolevulinic acid to assess the correlation of intraoperative fluorescence intensity and degree of histologic cellularity during resection of high-grade gliomas. *J Neurosurg.* 2016. doi:10.3171/2015.5.JNS1577

118. Stummer W, Pichlmeier U, Meinel T, et al. Fluorescence-guided surgery with 5-aminolevulinic acid for resection of malignant glioma: A randomised controlled multicentre phase III trial. *Lancet Oncol.* 2006. doi:10.1016/S1470-2045(06)70665-9

MOLLY HAVARD BLAU AND LIA M. HALASZ

INTRODUCTION

Radiation therapy (RT) has been a cornerstone of brain tumor treatment since it was first introduced in the early 1900s.[1] Originally born out of radiology departments, the field of radiation oncology has developed to involve multiple specialists. Physicians evaluate patients, explain recommendations, design individualized RT plans, and address side effects. Nurses educate patients about their course of treatment and address side effects. Radiation therapists position patients for treatment and deliver the radiation. Medical physicists ensure the accuracy of dose delivered and oversee the technical aspects of therapy machines. Dosimetrists create radiation plans with specialized software under the supervision of the physicians and medical physicists.

As imaging capabilities and technology have improved, the precision of RT has increased. This has allowed for improvement of the *therapeutic index*, the ratio of the probability of tumor control to the probability of normal tissue complication. Increasing radiation dose allows for increased tumor control; however, higher doses are associated with higher risk of injury to brain and surrounding organs. The allowable dose depends on multiple factors, especially the location and volume treated. Thus, scientific efforts over the past several decades have concentrated on optimizing delivery as well as studying the effects of combining RT with systemic therapy.

RADIATION BIOLOGY

Radiation biology is the study of the effect of ionizing radiation on living things, particularly the acute and long-term effects of radiation exposure on humans.

Several types of electromagnetic and particulate radiation are used for therapy. *Photons* (x-rays) are a form of electromagnetic radiation and are *indirectly ionizing*. When photons are absorbed in tissue, energy is transferred to create fast-moving electrons that in turn produce biologic damage through the creation of free radicals. *Free radicals* cause chemical changes leading to breaks in DNA, which eventually leads to cell death. *Electrons* are negatively charged particles that do not penetrate tissue deeply and are used for skin cancers or other superficial targets.

> When photons are absorbed in tissue, energy is transferred to create fast-moving electrons that in turn produce biologic damage through the creation of free radicals.

Protons are charged particles with mass roughly 2,000 times that of an electron and are accelerated to 40–70% of the speed of light for cancer therapy. *Alpha-particles* are emitted during the decay process of heavy radionuclides like radium and are a major source of background radiation for the general public. Heavy charged particles (e.g., carbon) must be produced in specialized facilities to be used for radiation therapy and they are uncommon. Charged particles are *directly ionizing*, with enough kinetic energy to cause nuclear damage without an intermediary step.

Radiation cell killing is predominantly through DNA damage, including base damage, single strand breaks (SSB), and double-strand breaks (DSB). SSBs can be easily repaired with the opposite strand as a template. DSBs are believed to be most responsible for cell killing and carcinogenesis. DSBs are repaired via non-homologous end joining and homologous recombination. Similar to the mechanism of chemotherapeutic agents, radiation therapy preferentially affects dividing tumor cells over normal cells.

The dose prescribed for therapeutic radiation varies depending on the goals of treatment, type of cancer, and numerous other considerations. The international unit of radiation dose is expressed in terms of the absorbed energy per unit mass of tissue. The *gray (Gy)* is the derived unit of radiation dose. 1 Gy = 1 Joule/kg and is equivalent to 100 Rad. Standard definitive treatments are typically delivered in 1.8–2 Gy daily fractions, to a total dose of 50.4–60 Gy for most central nervous system (CNS) malignancies. Hypofractionated treatments have been increasingly utilized as technology allows for precise delivery. For example, stereotactic radiosurgery delivers 15–22 Gy in a single fraction, and stereotactic body RT delivers 25–35 Gy in 3–5 fractions.

> The *gray (Gy)* is the derived unit of radiation dose. 1 Gy = 1 Joule/kg and is equivalent to 100 Rad.

Injury to normal tissue depends on many factors, including total radiation dose, fraction size (dose delivered in a single treatment), treated volume, concurrent systemic therapy, past therapies, and anatomic location. Some organs such as optic chiasm, pituitary, retina, lacrimal gland, lenses, and cochleae are more sensitive to radiation than others. Side effects from RT can be acute or late. Historical "tolerance" values for organs at risk have been established based on past experience, clinical trials, and preclinical data. Smaller fraction sizes are associated with less risk of late effects, but larger fraction sizes are well tolerated when the treated volume is limited.

TREATMENT MODALITIES

Today, RT is most often delivered by complex machines based on plans that are created using anatomic data obtained from computed tomography (CT). Planning CTs are fused with magnetic resonance imaging (MRI) so that the physicians can delineate the targets (generally the residual tumor or tumor bed, with a margin) and normal organs. Computer algorithms are then utilized to model the radiation dose to be delivered, and measurements are made on the machines to verify these algorithms. This process takes anywhere from a few hours to several days depending on the complexity of the plan. Custom masks are made for patients undergoing intracranial radiation to facilitate reproducible set up for daily treatment, with precision ranging from 1 to 5 mm. Verification of the set-up is most often performed by imaging, including x-ray plain films or CT imaging on the machine. MRI for verification on the machines is being investigated as well. Figure 20.1 shows a patient in a standard Aquaplast mask.

Photon (x-ray)-based radiation is the most widely available RT modality used for CNS treatments, delivered with linear accelerators (LINAC). 3D conformal, *intensity modulated radiation therapy* (IMRT), and *volumetric modulated arc therapy* (VMAT) are different methods of shaping the beam to deliver photon radiation. 3D conformal planning is typically used for palliative whole-brain radiation plans that require less normal tissue sparing. IMRT is a more advanced form of treatment planning in which several beam angles are used to achieve higher dose at the target and spare dose to normal tissues in each beam path. Each beam is modulated by metal leaves in the treatment head that move to shape the beam and create a more conformal

radiation plan. VMAT delivers radiation continuously as the treatment machine rotates 360 degrees around the patient. As the machine rotates around the patient, the beam is dynamically shaped to create a highly conformal dose distribution.

Proton therapy is a form of particle radiation treatment. Protons deposit the majority of their dose within the tumor because of a unique physical property called the *Bragg peak*. Rather than continuing past the target and exiting the patient (as with photon radiation), proton radiation stops at a defined range, which is beneficial for normal tissue sparing. Proton and photon therapy both work by damaging cellular DNA and are equally effective in cancer cell killing. Thus, the advantage of proton therapy is in reducing side effects of treatment. This is an important consideration in the CNS patient population, and particularly with pediatric patients whose nervous systems are still developing. As a result, proton therapy is frequently used in pediatric patients. See Figure 20.2 for a comparison between a proton and photon plan.

> Proton therapy is frequently used in pediatric patients.

Stereotactic radiosurgery (SRS) is a non-invasive procedure delivering highly conformal radiation to ablative doses in single or a small number of sessions. Multiple platforms have been developed to deliver SRS. These systems are complex given the difficulty of calculating and delivering dose for small targets. Colbalt-60–based SRS utilizes 192 beams to deliver gamma radiation to small brain lesions with either a frame- or mask-based system. LINAC systems use circular cutouts or small leaves to shape the beam delivered from many angles. Immobilization techniques are more robust for single-fraction SRS. A rigid frame with a 3-D coordinate system is often attached to the patient's skull with screws under local anesthesia. Masks with movement tracking devices are increasingly

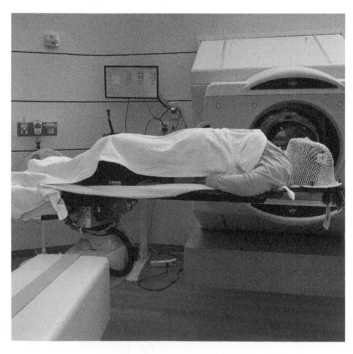

Figure 20.1 *A patient is set up in treatment position with customized mask for immobilization before undergoing radiation therapy.*

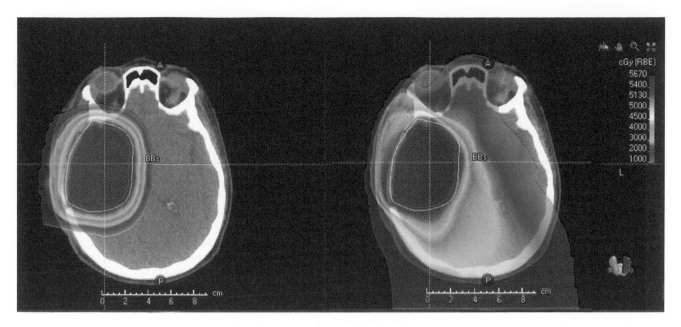

Figure 20.2 The dose map on the left shows a proton therapy plan for a patient with a low grade glioma. The dose map on the right shows a 3D conformal photon plan. The advantage of proton therapy is that it eliminates the exit dose. This allows for sparing of normal brain and contra-lateral hippocampus.

utilized for single and 3–5 fraction treatments. Depending on the size and number of lesions treated, treatment can take 20 minutes to a few hours to deliver a single fraction.

Brachytherapy is a form of radiotherapy in which a radiation source is placed in or very near the area requiring treatment. Temporary or permanent brachytherapy implants may be placed at the time of tumor resection, and several isotopes have been used for this purpose including iodine-125 and cesium-131.

GLIOBLASTOMA

Multiple trials in the 1960s and 1970s established RT's influence on the survival of patients with malignant glioma and a dose-effect relationship.[2] Those who received 60 Gy had improved survival compared to those who received 45 or 50 Gy.[3, 4] Initially RT was delivered as whole-brain RT; however, as CT became available, targeting the tumor more precisely became possible. Despite its diffuse nature, the vast majority of recurrences are at the original site.[5] Margins were typically added based on data that 78% of recurrences were within 2 cm of the margin of the initial tumor bed.[6,7] Multiple trials then showed that decreasing the size of the treatment fields did not lead to worse outcomes.[8,9]

Currently, the Radiation Therapy Oncology Group (RTOG) contouring guidelines describe the initial target volume including the surgical cavity + residual enhancing tumor and surrounding edema with a 2 cm margin treated to 46 Gy/23 fractions. Margins are routinely edited for anatomical barriers. An additional 14 Gy/7 fractions is then delivered to a smaller volume encompassing the surgical cavity + residual enhancing tumor with a 2 cm margin. Targeting the T2 extent comes from biopsy data showing isolated tumor infiltration extending as far as the T2 changes on MRI.[10] The European Organisation for Research and Treatment of Cancer (EORTC) contouring guidelines do not include the surrounding edema in the target volume, and the entire 60 Gy is delivered to one volume (surgical resection cavity + residual enhancing tumor with a 2 cm margin). Additional planning target volume (PTV) margin is added in all cases to account for patient movement on the treatment table. Comparison of these two approaches in combined clinical trials shows no difference in overall survival (OS) outcomes.[11,12]

In 2005, Stupp and colleagues published the landmark study, that showed that adding concurrent and adjuvant temozolomide (TMZ) to maximal safe resection and adjuvant radiation therapy to 60 Gy improved OS.[13] TMZ is thought to act as a radiosensitizer as well as directly affecting the tumor. More recently, Stupp and colleagues showed that adding tumor treating fields during the adjuvant TMZ part of treatment additionally improved OS by nearly 5 months.[14]

Progress in glioblastoma (GBM) treatment has been limited, and there are a number of ongoing trials evaluating systemic therapy and radiation dose escalation. NRG BN-001 is an ongoing randomized phase II trial studying dose-escalated IMRT or proton therapy (75 Gy/30 fractions) with TMZ compared to standard dose RT (60 Gy/30 fractions) in patients with newly diagnosed GBM (https://clinicaltrials.gov/ct2/show/NCT02179 086). Multiple previous trials have tested radiation dose escalation to a smaller volume centered at the tumor bed without demonstrating improved outcomes. Various techniques were utilized in these trials, including SRS, brachytherapy, and proton therapy, but none of these trials was done in the era of TMZ.

In patients who are elderly or have poor performance status, the standard course of RT may be poorly tolerated. A French trial randomized patients older than 70 to 50.4 Gy/ 28 fractions plus supportive care or supportive care alone. RT plus supportive care was associated with longer OS compared to supportive care alone (median, 6.7 months vs. 3.9 months), with no significant differences in quality of life or in cognition.[10] A Canadian trial of patients older than 60 randomly assigned patients after surgery to standard radiation (60 Gy/ 30 fx) alone versus an abbreviated course (40 Gy/15 fractions). There was no difference in survival outcomes (median, 5.1 vs. 5.6 months), similar Karnofsky Performance Scale (KPS) scores, and decreased steroid requirement in the abbreviated course of RT, establishing this as the recommendation for older patients with GBM.[15] Subsequent trials showed similar results for hypofractionated regimens.[16,17] Most recently, an international trial randomized patients who were 65 or older years to hypofractionated RT (40 Gy in 15 fractions) alone or hypofractionated RT with concurrent and adjuvant TMZ. The OS was longer with TMZ (median 9.3 months vs. 7.6 months).[18]

Pseudoprogression is a common phenomenon following RT for malignant glioma. Radiation increases capillary permeability, leading to edema and observation of a radiographic increase in contrast enhancement on MRI, falsely suggesting tumor progression. Though pseudoprogression occurs after RT alone, the addition of TMZ appears to increase rates.[19] In a study by Brandes et al., nearly 50% of tumors appear larger on MRI obtained 1 month following completion of chemoradiation treatment. Of the tumors that appeared larger on imaging 1 month after RT, 64% appeared stable or reduced at 3 months and were determined to represent pseudoprogression, while 36% continued to enlarge due to early progression. The study further showed that two-thirds of pseudoprogression cases had O6-methylguanine DNA methyltransferase (MGMT) methylation whereas 90% of early progression had unmethylated MGMT.[20] Patients with pseudoprogression had improved OS compared with patients with no concerning imaging findings, though it is unclear if pseudoprogression is actually a marker for better prognosis. The Response Assessment in Neuro-Oncology (RANO) criteria were established to assist in determination of tumor progression. Progression within 3 months of RT may be called if there is new enhancement beyond the 80% isodose line or if there is unequivocal pathologic evidence of viable tumor.[21] Generally, pseudoprogression is distinguished as an early phenomenon after RT, in contrast with radiation necrosis, which occurs several months to years after RT.

> Generally, *pseudoprogression* is distinguished as an early phenomenon after RT, in contrast with *radiation necrosis*, which occurs several months to years after RT.

ANAPLASTIC GLIOMAS

In 2016, the WHO updated the glioma classification system to put greater emphasis on molecular markers (isocitrate dehydrogenase [IDH] mutation, 1p/19q codeletion status) rather than histopathologic features. In this chapter, given that published trials categorized lower grade gliomas based on grade and did not all have data on molecular markers, we will consider WHO grade 2 and 3 gliomas separately, discussing the implications of the molecular classification.

For WHO grade 3 anaplastic astrocytoma, the RT principles are similar to those applied to GBM. Since grade 3 tumors may be predominantly non-enhancing, in general, trials such as CATNON (which established the role of adjuvant TMZ in addition to RT for these tumors) have targeted the T2 extent with a 1.5–2.0 cm margin (edited for anatomical barriers) to a total dose of 59.4 Gy in 33 fractions.[22] The difference between 60 Gy in 30 fractions and 59.4 Gy in 33 fractions is minor. Radiobiological principles predict that delivering similar total dose in a greater number of fractions decreases the risk of long-term late effects such as optic neuropathy and neurocognitive decline. The two dose schedules, however, have not been compared in a randomized trial.

For WHO grade 3 oligodendroglioma and oligoastrocytoma, two trials (RTOG 9402 and EORTC 26951) have established up-front treatment with RT and chemotherapy, in this case procarbazine, lomustine [CCNU] and vincristine (PCV), given either before or after RT.[23,24] For RTOG 9402, radiation therapy was delivered to 50.4 Gy in 28 fractions to the T2-weighted abnormality plus a 2-cm margin, followed by an additional 9 Gy in 5 fractions to the enhanced T1-weighted abnormality plus a 1-cm margin.[23,24] As oligodendroglial tumors are often quite extensive, this approach allows for decreased dose to a large volume of brain tissue. Overall, with molecular data suggesting that IDH mutation and 1p19q codeletion are more indicative of prognosis than grade, there is controversy about whether to decrease the total dose for WHO grade 3 glioma with IDH mutation based on trial results for patients with WHO grade 2 glioma. These trials are discussed in the next section.

In an effort to avoid up-front radiation, the NOA-04 trial randomized patients with WHO grade 3 glioma (52% anaplastic astrocytoma) to receive standard radiation treatment versus chemotherapy with either PCV or TMZ in a 2:1:1 ratio.[25] There was no difference in OS between chemotherapy and RT. However, since multiple trials including RTOG 9402 and EORTC 26951 have established that adding chemotherapy to RT improves survival versus RT alone for anaplastic oligodendroglioma/oligoastrocytoma, enthusiasm for monotherapy with chemotherapy has lessened.[23,24,26]

LOW-GRADE GLIOMAS

Patients with LGG have a more favorable prognosis, and treatment should balance optimization of local control with long-term toxicity. Due to concern regarding the toxicity of radiation, early trials asked whether postoperative radiation can be avoided for these patients. EORTC 22845 randomized patients with WHO grade 2 astrocytoma, oligodendroglioma, or oligoastrocytoma after surgery to immediate postoperative RT (54 Gy/30 fractions) versus observation.[27] Early RT improved median progression-free survival (PFS) by 2 years compared with observation (5.3 years vs. 3.4 years), and seizures were better controlled at 1 year in the early RT arm. There was no significant difference in OS between the two arms. In the observation arm, 62% went on to have RT as salvage therapy.

In the mid-1990s, EORTC 22844 demonstrated that dose escalation from 45 Gy to 59.4 Gy did not improve survival and was associated with worse psychological depression.[28] The INT/NCCTG 867251 trial randomized patients with LGG to 50.4 versus 64.8 Gy. More grade 3 or 4 toxicity was seen with the higher dose, with no difference in OS. Importantly, 92% of the patients failed in field.[29] Thus, dose recommendations for LGG are variable by organization. The RTOG recommends 54 Gy/30 fractions to the surgical cavity + T2/fluid-attenuated inversion recovery (FLAIR) signal on postoperative MRI, with 1cm CTV margin edited for anatomical barriers. The EORTC recommends 50.4 Gy/28 fractions with similar target volumes. The ongoing CODEL trial does incorporate an additional boost to a total of 59.4 Gy to enhancing disease on postoperative MRI.

> EORTC 22844 demonstrated that dose escalation from 45 Gy to 59.4 Gy did not improve survival and was associated with worse psychological depression.

Given the relatively young patient population, EORTC 22033-26033 asked whether patients with high-risk LGG (age >40, progressive disease, tumor >5 cm, tumor crossing midline, neurologic symptoms) could be treated with chemotherapy alone to avoid the long-term risks of RT. Patients were randomized postoperatively to RT alone (50.4 Gy/28 fractions) versus dose-dense TMZ alone (12 cycles). There was no significant difference in PFS between the two arms (46 months vs. 39 months).[30] Given that RTOG 9802 has shown that patients with high risk LGG (defined as subtotal resection and/or age ≥40 years) treated to 54 Gy in 30 fractions benefited from the addition of PCV (median survival improved from 7.8 to 13.3 years), monotherapy with chemotherapy or RT is not typically recommended as initial treatment for high-risk patients.[26] However, whether patients can be observed without any adjuvant treatment (thus delaying radiation therapy and its side effects for several years) is currently debated.

Radiation techniques used to mitigate long-term neurocognitive effects include using hippocampal and/or overall brain-sparing techniques, such as IMRT or proton therapy. NRG BN-005 is an ongoing trial randomizing patients with IDH-mutant grade 2 or 3 glioma to radiation with proton therapy (54 Gy/30 fx) + TMZ vs IMRT (54 Gy/30 fx) + TMZ, with primary outcome measuring cognitive change. Patients are stratified by baseline cognitive function, 1p19q co-deletion status, and extent of surgical resection (https://clinicaltrials.gov/ct2/show/NCT03180502).

BRAIN METASTASES

The incidence of brain metastases is increasing as systemic therapies and imaging modalities improve. Early reports of whole-brain radiation therapy (WBRT) for brain metastases include a 1954 manuscript,[31] which reported 63% of patients achieving symptom relief. RTOG performed several randomized studies in the 1970s and 1980s comparing dose fractionation schemes.[32] Response rates were equivalent across treatment arms, though faster treatment schedules led to more rapid symptom response. 30 Gy in 10 fractions has become a standard regimen in the United States, though 20 Gy in 5 fractions can be considered in patients with poor prognosis.

To mitigate neurocognitive effects, memantine may be used concurrently with WBRT based on the RTOG trial suggesting a longer time to cognitive decline with memantine compared to placebo, as well as decreased rates of cognitive failure at 24 weeks (53.8% vs. 64.9%; p = 0.059).[33] The NRG Oncology phase III trial CC001 recently demonstrated further decreases in risk of cognitive failure with hippocampal-sparing WBRT techniques plus memantine versus standard WBRT plus memantine. Patients in whom hippocampal avoidance was used demonstrated less decline in executive function at 4 months and learning and memory at 6 months. Patients reported less fatigue, less difficulty with memory, and less interference of symptoms with daily activity.[34]

> To mitigate neurocognitive effects, memantine may be used concurrently with WBRT based on the RTOG trial suggesting a longer time to cognitive decline with memantine compared to placebo.

Given the side effects of WBRT, its utility has been increasingly questioned as alternatives such as SRS, systemic therapy alone, or supportive care have been further studied. The QUARTZ trial randomized patients with brain metastases from non-small cell lung cancer who were not amenable to SRS or surgical resection to WBRT to 20 Gy in 5 fractions or supportive care and found no difference in survival or quality of life for these patients.[35]

In 1951, SRS was first reported as a more precise form of radiation for skull-base tumors and has become widely used on various available platforms for brain tumors. SRS dose for brain metastases is generally based on size or volume of the targeted metastases. The RTOG 9005 was a dose escalation study that established 15 Gy for 3–4 cm diameter, 18 Gy for 2–3 cm, and 24 Gy for less than 2 cm.[36] Given risk of radionecrosis and lack of data showing improved control with the higher dose, many will treat metastases of less than 2 cm with 20 Gy. Stereotactic hypofractionated regimens over 2–5 treatments are being increasingly used for larger metastases in attempts to improve local control and decrease risk of radionecrosis.

A number of trials have investigated the addition of targeted SRS +/− WBRT for patients with a limited number of brain metastases.[37,38] Following these trials, the American Society for Radiation Oncology has made a strong recommendation against routinely adding WBRT and SRS, though SRS may now be used alone for patients with limited brain metastases. SRS significantly decreases local recurrence following surgical resection or may be used as the primary treatment modality in patients for whom surgery is not desired or recommended.[39] Surveillance is important in patients treated with SRS, as some patients develop asymptomatic intracranial recurrence that may fare better with early salvage. By treating limited brain metastases with SRS, WBRT may be saved for salvage therapy at a later time or eliminated, thereby delaying the associated neurocognitive toxicity.

BENIGN BRAIN TUMORS

MENINGIOMA

Non-malignant meningiomas are typically slow growing and have imaging characteristics such that histopathologic confirmation may not be necessary. Eighty-one percent of meningiomas are classified as WHO grade 1, though there is significant heterogeneity in cell type, molecular characteristics, and growth rate among them. WHO grade 2 meningiomas (17%) are termed "atypical" and are characterized by hypercellularity, frequent mitoses, sheeting cells, brain invasion, and increased growth rates.[40] These may be asymptomatic and incidentally identified on imaging or may cause significant morbidity by compressing nearby structures (e.g., cranial nerves).

The risk of morbidity and mortality caused by tumor growth must be weighed against the morbidity of treatment-related toxicity. For patients with imaging-defined asymptomatic meningiomas, observation may be appropriate. If intervention is needed, surgery has long been established as the first-line therapy for presumed grade 1 meningioma. This is an effective means of relieving symptoms rapidly and provides pathologic confirmation. However, achieving a gross total resection (GTR) is often difficult due to tumor location (particularly in the skull base).[41] In patients who are not surgical candidates or wish to avoid invasive procedures, RT has emerged as an effective alternative. A multi-institutional study of 4,565 consecutive patients with 5,300 benign meningiomas with average volume less than 5cm^3 were treated with SRS resulting in 5- and 10-year PFS rates of 95.2% and 88.6%, respectively.[42] In the case of a STR of a grade 1 meningioma, there is controversy regarding whether to observe or give adjuvant radiation.

SRS dose and fractionation depends on tumor grade, size, and location. For unresectable or recurrent grade 1 meningioma, SRS may be delivered to 12–15 Gy in a single fraction for smaller tumors. Hypofractionated stereotactic RT to 25 Gy in 5 fractions may decrease toxicity for patients in whom surrounding structures are dose-limiting or tumors are large. External beam RT for benign meningioma is given to 45–54 Gy in 1.8–2 Gy fractions if a stereotactic approach is not feasible either due to size or proximity to a dose-limiting structure such as the optic nerve.

The role of adjuvant radiation has been better established in the case of atypical meningioma following STR, though controversy remains regarding adjuvant therapy following GTR.[43,44] Given the slow-growing nature of these tumors, older patients may never have a symptomatic recurrence following GTR, and the long-term effects of radiation may be avoided by reserving RT for salvage therapy. Adjuvant radiation to 54 Gy following GTR for intermediate-risk meningioma led to 3-year PFS of 93.8% and OS of 96% with no high-grade toxicity on RTOG 0539.[45] If the patient underwent STR, the radiation dose delivered was increased to 59.4–60 Gy. These findings support the use of postoperative radiotherapy for WHO grade 2 meningioma, regardless of the extent of resection, but do not establish an impact on survival. NRG BN-003 is a current phase III trial that randomizes patients with grade 2 meningioma after GTR to observation versus RT to 59.4 Gy to determine whether early RT improves OS and how it impacts quality of life (NCT03180268).

WHO grade 3 meningiomas (2%) are considered malignant. Dose escalation above 60 Gy has been shown to improve local control and OS with a mixed approach using photon and proton therapy.[46] However, there is increasing risk of radionecrosis with dose escalation that must be weighed against these benefits. EORTC 22042-26042 aims to help answer the dose escalation question and has completed accrual. Patients with atypical or malignant meningioma received radiation to 60 Gy following GTR, and an additional 10 Gy boost was added following STR.

VESTIBULAR SCHWANNOMA

Schwannomas predominantly affect cranial nerve (CN) VIII and are typically slow growing tumors with well-circumscribed margins; they cause displacement of local structures and smooth displacement of osseous foramina. These may be asymptomatic and incidentally identified or may cause symptoms such as hearing loss, tinnitus, imbalance, facial or trigeminal nerve palsies, or brainstem compression. There is controversy regarding the best treatment strategy for small vestibular schwannomas, including observation, surgery, or RT.

A meta-analysis of studies comprising 1,345 patients who underwent observation for vestibular schwannoma found that 57% of tumors demonstrated no growth or tumor regression. Hearing loss occurred in 51% of patients (subset), and 20% eventually failed conservative management.[47] Patients requiring treatment may undergo microsurgery, though morbidity may include high risk of facial nerve palsy, and hearing preservation is variable.

SRS is an appropriate treatment option for many patients, with effective local control rates of greater than 90% at relatively low doses of 12–13 Gy in a single fraction. Damage to CN V or VII occurs in fewer than 10% of patients, and serviceable hearing is maintained in 50–75%.[48] There is risk of vestibular dysfunction, post-treatment tumor expansion, and, rarely, cystic degeneration or malignant transformation.[49] Fractionated RT to 54 Gy/30 fx or 25 Gy/5 fx has also been pursued based on radiobiologic principles that predict decreased cochlear toxicity with more prolonged courses of RT. However, longer term and comparative studies are needed to truly compare the outcomes of these different approaches. Similarly, multiple studies assessing quality of life following microsurgery versus SRS have reported mixed results. Patients with vestibular schwannoma benefit from a multidisciplinary approach to determine the most appropriate approach depending on the patient's priorities.

> SRS is an appropriate treatment option for many patients with vestibular schwannoma, with effective local control rates of greater than 90% at relatively low doses of 12–13 Gy in a single fraction.

CRANIOPHARYNGIOMA

Craniopharyngiomas are benign tumors that arise from Rathke's pouch. These are often solid and cystic tumors, diagnosed in patients with a bimodal age distribution, with the first peak at 5–14 years old and second peak at 50–75 years.[50] The location of these tumors in the sellar/suprasellar region leads to morbidity caused by tumor growth as well as any intervention. GTR was considered the optimal treatment for several years, but an aggressive surgical approach is often associated with endocrine and behavioral side effects. There is now controversy regarding treatment algorithms for these tumors. Yang et al. published a meta-analysis of 442 patients treated with GTR, STR, or STR + adjuvant RT. PFS rates were not significantly different between GTR and STR + RT, and there was no statistically significant difference in rate of neurologic deficits across treatment groups in univariate analysis. However, they felt that toxicity was underreported.[51] Tumor progression following STR can be associated with visual or endocrine compromise, so adjuvant radiation therapy to 50.4–54 Gy is often recommended.

PREDOMINANTLY PEDIATRIC TUMORS

MEDULLOBLASTOMA

Medulloblastoma is the most common CNS malignancy of childhood, and patients are stratified into average- or high-risk groups. Average-risk patients are 3 years old or older, have no evidence of disease metastasis, and achieved GTR/near total resection (NTR) (no more than 1.5 cm^3 of residual disease) following maximal safe resection. Patients are classified as high risk if they have metastatic disease, greater than 1.5 cm^2 of residual disease, or diffuse anaplasia (COG ACNS 0332 protocol).

For average-risk patients, resection is followed by craniospinal irradiation (CSI) to 23.4 Gy in 13 fractions, beginning within 31 days of surgery (CCG-9892).[52] CSI includes the whole brain and spinal CSF space, including nerve roots and the thecal sac. This is followed by an involved field boost to the resection bed plus a margin to a total dose of 54 Gy in an additional 17 fractions. COG ACNS0331 established that an involved field boost is non-inferior to a full posterior fossa boost for average-risk patients, allowing radiation oncologists to treat a smaller volume of normal tissue. This also established 23.4 Gy as the standard CSI dose, with inferior 5-year event-free survival and OS in patients treated to a reduced dose of 18 Gy. RT is given with concurrent weekly vincristine, followed by adjuvant vincristine, cisplatin, and cyclophosphamide or CCNU/(lomustine).

High-risk medulloblastoma patients undergo maximal safe resection followed by CSI to 36–39.6 Gy, depending on extent of resection. For high-risk patients, the whole posterior fossa is treated to a total dose of 55.8 Gy though involved field boost is under investigation. This is followed by adjuvant chemotherapy. Four prospective randomized trials have evaluated altering the sequence of chemo and RT (SIOP II, SIOP III, POG 9031, and HIT 91), and all except SIOP III demonstrated no improvement in outcomes with chemo immediately following surgery.[53-55] SIOP III demonstrated improved 3-year OS (84.1% vs 70.9%) with RT delivered within 50 days of surgery, reinforcing sequencing of RT prior to chemotherapy.

Radiation toxicity is increasingly significant for younger patients, so a number of studies have attempted to do away with radiation completely in children younger than 3 years.[56] Baby POG#1 was a prospective randomized trial that demonstrated postoperative chemotherapy is acceptable to delay radiation, with 5-year OS of 40%.[57]

As survivors of childhood cancers are increasing in number, there are special considerations for the late effects of RT in pediatric patients. Neurocognitive testing is recommended, as there may be a spectrum of subtle to profound neurocognitive deficits following brain irradiation. Special consideration is also paid to secondary malignancy and late vascular events. CSI with photon therapy is quite toxic and difficult for patients to tolerate. With proton therapy, dose to the esophagus, heart, stomach, bowel, kidneys, and reproductive organs is much lower and minimizes both acute and long-term toxicity in these organs. Patients experience myelosuppression due to vertebral bodies in the radiation field, which may be decreased in patients who have reached their full growth potential, given the ability to spare some of the vertebral column. See Figure 20.3 for a sample of a proton craniospinal plan.

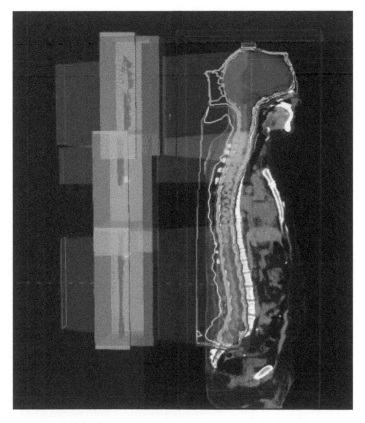

Figure 20.3 This dose map of a proton craniospinal plan illustrates the use of three beams with gradients to allow for safe matching.

Medulloblastoma is rare in adult populations so management of adult patients is largely extrapolated from pediatric studies. Adults with medulloblastoma undergo surgical resection followed by CSI to 30–36 Gy with boost to the primary site to 54–55.8 Gy. The role of chemotherapy is unknown in adults, and there is significant variation in treatment across centers.[58] Brown et al. completed a retrospective review of adult patients with medulloblastoma treated at MD Anderson Cancer Center with either proton or photon therapy; median CSI dose and total dose were 30.6 Gy and 54 Gy, respectively. Patients treated with proton therapy experienced less gastrointestinal and hematologic toxicity, though survival outcomes were not assessed.[59]

> Adults with medulloblastoma undergo surgical resection followed by CSI to 30–36 Gy with boost to the primary site to 54–55.8 Gy.

Studies of molecular variants in medulloblastoma have identified four variants in pediatric populations: WNT, SHH, group 3, and group 4. Remke et al. demonstrated that adult tumors comprise only three variants: SHH, WNT, and group 4.[60] Although molecular classifications are guiding ongoing studies, these factors are not yet guiding radiation treatment algorithms.

EPENDYMOMA

Initial management for ependymoma is surgical resection. Though historically all patients received CSI, in 2002 Merchant et al. established limited-field RT as the standard because the majority of ependymoma failures occur locally.[61] In limited-field radiation, RT is delivered locally to the postoperative bed with a 0.5–1.0 cm margin to 54 Gy–59.4 Gy. If there is evidence of metastatic disease in patients 3 years or older, CSI to 36 Gy is recommended with boost to the postoperative bed. While radiation is recommended for most pediatric patients with ependymoma, the role of radiation is controversial in grade 1 myxopapillary ependymoma, which most frequently appears in the spine.

> The role of radiation is controversial in grade 1 myxopapillary ependymoma, which most frequently appears in the spine.

Ependymomas are also rare in adult populations, thus there are few trials to direct treatment decisions and the use of radiation therapy remains controversial. Similar to pediatrics, maximal safe resection is the standard of care. For WHO grade 3 ependymoma, this is typically followed by radiation to the resection bed with a 0.5–1.0 cm margin to 54–59.4 Gy in standard fractionation. In patients with metastatic disease, CSI to 36 Gy is recommended with boost to the postoperative bed. For patients with WHO grade 2 ependymoma in the brain after GTR, it is unclear whether patients should be observed or undergo adjuvant radiation therapy. For patients with spinal WHO grade 2 ependymoma, observation is recommended after GTR. With STR, adjuvant radiation therapy to 45–54 Gy in 1.8 Gy fractions is considered. New understanding of the molecular classification of ependymomas will likely lead to further refinements in stratification for adjuvant treatment recommendations.

DIFFUSE INTRINSIC PONTINE GLIOMA

> DIPGs are the most common brainstem gliomas in children and are associated with poor prognosis.

Diffuse intrinsic pontine gliomas (DIPGs) are the most common brainstem gliomas in children and are associated with poor prognosis. Radiation therapy alone to 54 Gy/30 fractions is the standard of care and should be started as quickly as possible. Other radiation approaches that could be completed in a shorter time period (e.g., hyperfractionation, I-125 brachytherapy, and SRS) have not shown benefit over standard fractionation.[62-64] Many patients show initial clinical improvement, with time to progression 5–6 months following RT. In patients with relatively longer response to radiation, palliative re-irradiation to lower doses may be considered for symptom management with limited toxicity.[65]

RADIATION TOXICITY

RT can cause both acute and late toxicity. Side effects depend on the location and size of the treatment field. Acute side effects may develop while the patient is still on treatment and generally improve several days following completion of the treatment course. RT most commonly causes fatigue, which is not typically profound unless combined with systemic therapy or additional comorbidities. Other common acute effects include headache, worsening of presenting neurologic deficits, alopecia within the radiation portals, nausea, or localized edema.

Late effects may develop months to years following completion of treatment. These may include cognitive changes, vascular anomalies, radiation necrosis, hypopituitarism, cataracts, vision loss, or hearing loss (depending on location of the radiation field). Exposure of the lacrimal gland to high doses can cause long-term dry eye, which can impact vision. The threshold dose for cataract formation is quite low; these can be treated with an outpatient surgical intervention. Radiation-induced optic neuropathy typically presents with painless rapid visual loss, typically 10–20 months following radiation. There is no treatment for this, so care is taken to meet dose constraints during radiation planning. Radiation-induced retinopathy may occur particularly in patients with comorbid risks for retinopathy like diabetes, hypertension, concurrent chemotherapy, or pregnancy. Treatments for RT-induced retinopathy include laser therapy or anti-vascular endothelial growth factor (VEGF) medication injections. Damage to the cochlea may lead to early hearing loss, particularly in the high-frequency range.

> Late effects may develop months to years following completion of treatment. These may include cognitive changes, vascular anomalies, radiation necrosis, hypopituitarism, cataracts, vision loss, or hearing loss (dependent on location of the radiation field).

Neurocognitive changes associated with RT are difficult to quantify. The executive functioning, psychomotor functioning, working memory, and attention domains are most affected in long-term studies. Radiation appears to have less of an effect on verbal memory or information processing speed.[66] Memantine is an N-methyl-D-aspartic acid (NMDA) antagonist used for dementia that may be given to patients receiving WBRT to help mitigate neurocognitive effects. Patients may be given 10 mg twice daily during and after WBRT for 24 weeks. Hippocampal sparing planning techniques are becoming more commonly adopted to minimize these neurocognitive effects.

There is a small risk of secondary malignancy caused by radiation. If secondary malignancy occurs, it is typically 15–20 years following completion of treatment and develops within the treatment field. The most common tumor developed following CNS radiation is meningioma but malignant tumors are also possible.

> If secondary malignancy occurs, it is typically 15–20 years following completion of treatment and develops within the treatment field.

CONCLUSION

Radiation therapy has been a vital part of treatment for brain tumors since it was first used more than 100 years ago. Advances in imaging and technology have allowed for more precise targeting with fewer resultant side effects. More recently, clinical trials have established the benefit of concurrent chemotherapy with radiation therapy. Future directions include still greater precision in delivery, with more specific imaging and advancement of technology, as well as combined treatments with drugs designed to improve tumor control and minimize toxicity.

What is the predominant way that radiation causes cell damage?	Via DNA double strand breaks
What is the international unit of radiation dosing?	Gray (Gy) [1 Gy = 1 J/kg]
What are four commonly used photon delivery methods?	1. 3D conformal 2. IMRT 3. VMAT 4. SRS
What is standard treatment for glioblastoma (GBM) after maximal safe surgical resection?	RT to 60 Gy in 30 fractions (fx) with concurrent TMZ, then adjuvant TMZ for 6 months. The addition of tumor-treating fields to adjuvant TMZ also improves overall survival
For elderly or poor performance status patients with glioblastoma, what radiation dose/schedule has similar survival outcomes to the standard 6-week schedule and should be considered?	A hypofractionated course of 40 Gy in 15 fx
What is a common MRI finding following chemo-RT for GBM and is more commonly associated with MGMT methylated tumors?	Pseudoprogression
What radiation dose is most commonly given for anaplastic glioma?	59.4 Gy in 33 fx, though lower doses may be appropriate in light of newer molecular classifications
Given their relatively better prognosis, what concern should be considered in treatment planning for patients with low-grade glioma (LGG), and what are two strategies for doing so?	Long-term toxicity Proton therapy or hippocampal sparing techniques may be used to minimize neurocognitive effects
What are the RTOG and EORTC recommendations for radiation of LGG?	*RTOG:* Radiation to 54 Gy in 30 fx to the surgical cavity + T2/FLAIR signal on postoperative MRI, with 1 cm clinical target volume (CTV) margin *EORTC:* 50.4 Gy in 28 fx, with similar target volumes as that of the RTOG

What radiation technique may be used for palliation of brain metastases, and what are two commonly used dose regimens?	Whole-brain RT (WBRT) 30 Gy in 10 fx for patients with good functional status 20 Gy in 5 fx for patients with poor functional status
What are two methods to mitigate neurocognitive effects when giving WBRT?	Concurrent memantine Use of hippocampal avoidance techniques
For patients with limited brain metastases, in what situations may SRS be used, and with what dose/schedule?	SRS may be delivered either as definitive treatment or as postoperative treatment Treatment is delivered in 1–5 fractions, with dose fractionation depending on tumor volume (generally 15–24 Gy)
RT is an effective alternative to surgery for benign meningioma (WHO grade 1) when treatment is required. What is its 5-year PFS?	5-year PFS is 95.2%
What are three potential doses and schedules of RT for benign meningioma?	Single fraction SRS to 12-15 Gy Fractionated SRS to 25 Gy in 5 fx Conventional fractionation to 50.4–54 Gy
For atypical meningioma (WHO grade 2), what are two treatment options following GTR?	Consider adjuvant RT to 54 Gy, though observation may be appropriate for older patients with slow-growing tumors
What is recommended for atypical meningioma following STR?	Adjuvant RT, to 59.4–60 Gy
What is the recommended adjuvant treatment for malignant meningioma (WHO grade 3)?	RT to 59.4–60 Gy (Ongoing studies are assessing further dose escalation for patients who undergo STR)
What radiation regimen is used for vestibular schwannomas, and what is the disease control rate?	Single fraction SRS to 12–13 Gy, with local control >90%

How well does it work for hearing retention?	Hearing is maintained in 50–75% of patients
What radiation regimen and timing is recommended for average-risk medulloblastoma patients?	Craniospinal radiation (CSI) to 23.4 Gy in 13 fx within 31 days of surgery, followed by focal radiation to the resection bed plus a margin to a total dose of 54 Gy. Protons are often used Concurrent weekly vincristine is given with RT
What radiation regimen is recommended for high-risk medulloblastoma patients?	CSI to 36–39.6 Gy, depending on the extent of resection, followed by RT to a total dose of 55.8 Gy to the whole posterior fossa
What radiation regimen is recommended for patients with ependymoma?	RT to 54–59.4 Gy to the resection bed plus a margin
RT is a critical component of therapy for DIPG. What is the recommended dose and timing?	RT should be started as quickly as possible. It is delivered to 54 Gy, typically with photons instead of protons
On what five factors does radiation toxicity depend?	1. Total dose 2. Fraction size 3. Volume treated 4. Anatomic location 5. Past and concurrent therapies

QUESTIONS

1. The risk of long-term radiation toxicity depends on:
   a. Radiation dose
   b. Volume treated
   c. Fraction size
   d. All of the above

2. The radiation target for treating localized malignant glioma is:
   a. Whole brain
   b. Craniospinal axis
   c. Tumor bed with a margin
   d. Residual disease only

3. Radiation for treatment of medulloblastoma should cover
   a. Whole brain
   b. Craniospinal axis with a boost to the tumor bed
   c. Tumor bed with a margin
   d. Residual disease only

4. All of following are used for therapeutic radiation therapy, *except*
   a. Photons
   b. Uranium
   c. Cesium
   d. Protons
   e. Electrons

5. Which of the following is a method of delivering stereotactic radiosurgery (SRS)?
   a. Electrons
   b. I-125 brachytherapy
   c. Gamma knife
   d. 3D conformal photons
   e. Protons

6. Which of the following may be used to mitigate the neurocognitive effects of WBRT?
   a. Memantine
   b. Entacapone
   c. Selegiline
   d. Rivastigmine

7. What is the recommended management for a presumed WHO grade 1 meningioma?
   a. Observation
   b. Surgical resection
   c. Stereotactic radiation
   d. Any of the above

8. What is a widely practiced dose fractionation for WBRT?
   a. 8 Gy/1 fraction
   b. 12 Gy/4 fractions
   c. 24 Gy/6 fractions
   d. 30 Gy/10 fractions

9. What is the standard dose radiation given concurrently with temozolomide following a gross total resection for glioblastoma?
   a. 50 Gy
   b. 54 Gy
   c. 60 Gy
   d. 74 Gy

10. Which of the following has been shown to improve survival when given with adjuvant temozolomide for glioblastoma following GTR and standard chemo-RT?
    a. Proton therapy
    b. Tumor-treating fields
    c. Cesium brachytherapy
    d. Neutron therapy

11. Which tumor feature is associated with higher risk for pseudoprogression on surveillance imaging following chemoradiation for glioblastoma?
    a. MGMT methylation
    b. IDH mutation
    c. Patient age
    d. Tumor hemorrhage

12. Which of the following is a potential long-term risk for pediatric patients who receive craniospinal irradiation?
    a. Meningioma resulting from radiation exposure
    b. Growth hormone deficiency
    c. Sleep/wake cycle disturbance
    d. Stroke within 20 years
    e. All of the above

13. What is the primary biologic mechanism of cell killing in radiation therapy?
    a. Mitochondrial damage
    b. Double-strand DNA damage
    c. Mitotic arrest, resulting in DNA breakdown and apoptosis
    d. Direct damage to the cell wall causing lysis and cell death

14. Which of the following is true regarding proton and photon therapy?
    a. Protons have improved rates of tumor control.
    b. Protons reduce low-dose exposure to normal tissues, thus decreasing side effects of treatment.
    c. Protons and photons are equally available in radiation therapy centers around the United States.
    d. Protons and photons have the same radiobiologic mechanism of causing cell damage.

15. True or False? Re-irradiation is never considered for intracranial disease due to the significant risk of radionecrosis.
    a. True
    b. False

ANSWERS

1. d
2. c
3. b
4. b
5. c
6. a
7. d
8. d
9. c
10. b
11. a
12. e
13. b
14. b
15. b

REFERENCES

1. Tice GM, Irving NW. Roentgen therapy supplementing surgery in the treatment of gliomas. *J Neurosurg*. Nov 1950;7(6):509–520. doi:10.3171/jns.1950.7.6.0509
2. Walker MD, Alexander E, Jr., Hunt WE, et al. Evaluation of BCNU and/or radiotherapy in the treatment of anaplastic gliomas. A cooperative clinical trial. *J Neurosurg*. Sep 1978;49(3):333–343. doi:10.3171/jns.1978.49.3.0333
3. Walker MD, Strike TA, Sheline GE. An analysis of dose-effect relationship in the radiotherapy of malignant gliomas. *Int J Radiat Oncol Biol Phys*. Oct 1979;5(10):1725–1731. doi:10.1016/0360-3016(79)90553-4
4. Bleehen NM, Stenning SP. A Medical Research Council trial of two radiotherapy doses in the treatment of grades 3 and 4 astrocytoma. The Medical Research Council Brain Tumour Working Party. *Br J Cancer*. Oct 1991;64(4):769–774. doi:10.1038/bjc.1991.396
5. Sahm F, Capper D, Jeibmann A, et al. Addressing diffuse glioma as a systemic brain disease with single-cell analysis. *Arch Neurol*. Apr 2012;69(4):523–526. doi:10.1001/archneurol.2011.2910
6. Hochberg FH, Pruitt A. Assumptions in the radiotherapy of glioblastoma. *Neurology*. Sep 1980;30(9):907–911. doi:10.1212/wnl.30.9.907
7. Wallner KE, Galicich JH, Krol G, Arbit E, Malkin MG. Patterns of failure following treatment for glioblastoma multiforme and anaplastic astrocytoma. *Int J Radiat Oncol Biol Phys*. Jun 1989;16(6):1405–1409. doi:10.1016/0360-3016(89)90941-3
8. Shapiro WR, Green SB, Burger PC, et al. Randomized trial of three chemotherapy regimens and two radiotherapy regimens and two radiotherapy regimens in postoperative treatment of malignant glioma. Brain Tumor Cooperative Group Trial 8001. *J Neurosurg*. Jul 1989;71(1):1–9. doi:10.3171/jns.1989.71.1.0001
9. Sharma RR, Singh DP, Pathak A, et al. Local control of high-grade gliomas with limited volume irradiation versus whole brain irradiation. *Neurol India*. Dec 2003;51(4):512–517.
10. Kelly PJ, Daumas-Duport C, Scheithauer BW, et al. Stereotactic histologic correlations of computed tomography- and magnetic resonance imaging-defined abnormalities in patients with glial neoplasms. *Mayo Clin Proc*. Jun 1987;62(6):450–459. doi:10.1016/s0025-6196(12)65470-6
11. Gilbert MR, Wang M, Aldape KD, et al. Dose-dense temozolomide for newly diagnosed glioblastoma: A randomized phase III clinical trial. *J Clin Oncol*. Nov 10 2013;31(32):4085–4091. doi:10.1200/JCO.2013.49.6968
12. Stupp R, Hegi ME, Gorlia T, et al. Cilengitide combined with standard treatment for patients with newly diagnosed glioblastoma with methylated MGMT promoter (CENTRIC EORTC 26071-22072 study): A multicentre, randomised, open-label, phase 3 trial. *Lancet Oncol*. Sep 2014;15(10):1100–1108. doi:10.1016/S1470-2045(14)70379-1
13. Stupp R, Hegi ME, Mason WP, et al. Effects of radiotherapy with concomitant and adjuvant temozolomide versus radiotherapy alone on survival in glioblastoma in a randomised phase III study: 5-year analysis of the EORTC-NCIC trial. *Lancet Oncol*. May 2009;10(5):459–466. doi:10.1016/S1470-2045(09)70025-7
14. Stupp R, Taillibert S, Kanner A, et al. Effect of tumor-treating fields plus maintenance temozolomide vs maintenance temozolomide alone on survival in patients with glioblastoma: A randomized clinical trial. *JAMA*. Dec 19 2017;318(23):2306–2316. doi:10.1001/jama.2017.18718
15. Roa W, Brasher PM, Bauman G, et al. Abbreviated course of radiation therapy in older patients with glioblastoma multiforme: A prospective randomized clinical trial. *J Clin Oncol*. May 1 2004;22(9):1583–1588. doi:10.1200/JCO.2004.06.082
16. Roa W, Kepka L, Kumar N, et al. International Atomic Energy Agency randomized phase III study of radiation therapy in elderly and/or frail patients with newly diagnosed glioblastoma multiforme. *J Clin Oncol*. Dec 10 2015;33(35):4145–4150. doi:10.1200/JCO.2015.62.6606
17. Malmstrom A, Gronberg BH, Marosi C, et al. Temozolomide versus standard 6-week radiotherapy versus hypofractionated radiotherapy in patients older than 60 years with glioblastoma: The Nordic randomised, phase 3 trial. *Lancet Oncol*. Sep 2012;13(9):916–926. doi:10.1016/S1470-2045(12)70265-6
18. Perry JR, Laperriere N, O'Callaghan CJ, et al. Short-course radiation plus temozolomide in elderly patients with glioblastoma. *N Engl J Med*. Mar 16 2017;376(11):1027–1037. doi:10.1056/NEJMoa1611977
19. Chamberlain MC, Glantz MJ, Chalmers L, et al. Early necrosis following concurrent Temodar and radiotherapy in patients with glioblastoma. *J Neurooncol*. Mar 2007;82(1):81–83. doi:10.1007/s11060-006-9241-y
20. Brandes AA, Franceschi E, Tosoni A, et al. MGMT promoter methylation status can predict the incidence and outcome of pseudoprogression after concomitant radiochemotherapy in newly diagnosed glioblastoma patients. *J Clin Oncol*. May 1 2008;26(13):2192–2197. doi:10.1200/JCO.2007.14.8163
21. Wen PY, Macdonald DR, Reardon DA, et al. Updated response assessment criteria for high-grade gliomas: Response assessment in neuro-oncology working group. *J Clin Oncol*. Apr 10 2010;28(11):1963–1972. doi:10.1200/JCO.2009.26.3541
22. van den Bent MJ, Baumert B, Erridge SC, et al. Interim results from the CATNON trial (EORTC study 26053-22054) of treatment with concurrent and adjuvant temozolomide for 1p/19q non-co-deleted anaplastic glioma: A phase 3, randomised, open-label intergroup study. *Lancet*. Oct 7 2017;390(10103):1645–1653. doi:10.1016/S0140-6736(17)31442-3
23. Cairncross G, Wang M, Shaw E, et al. Phase III trial of chemoradiotherapy for anaplastic oligodendroglioma: Long-term results of RTOG 9402. *J Clin Oncol*. Jan 20 2013;31(3):337–343. doi:10.1200/JCO.2012.43.2674
24. van den Bent MJ, Brandes AA, Taphoorn MJ, et al. Adjuvant procarbazine, lomustine, and vincristine chemotherapy in newly diagnosed anaplastic oligodendroglioma: Long-term follow-up of EORTC brain tumor group study 26951. *J Clin Oncol*. Jan 20 2013;31(3):344–350. doi:10.1200/JCO.2012.43.2229
25. Wick W, Roth P, Hartmann C, et al. Long-term analysis of the NOA-04 randomized phase III trial of sequential radiochemotherapy of anaplastic glioma with PCV or temozolomide. *Neuro Oncol*. Nov 2016;18(11):1529–1537. doi:10.1093/neuonc/now133
26. Buckner JC, Shaw EG, Pugh SL, et al. Radiation plus procarbazine, CCNU, and vincristine in low-grade glioma. *N Engl J Med*. Apr 7 2016;374(14):1344–1355. doi:10.1056/NEJMoa1500925
27. van den Bent MJ, Afra D, de Witte O, et al. Long-term efficacy of early versus delayed radiotherapy for low-grade astrocytoma and oligodendroglioma in adults: The EORTC 22845 randomised trial. *Lancet*. Sep 17-23 2005;366(9490):985–990. doi:10.1016/S0140-6736(05)67070-5
28. Karim AB, Maat B, Hatlevoll R, et al. A randomized trial on dose-response in radiation therapy of low-grade cerebral glioma: European Organization for Research and Treatment of Cancer (EORTC) Study 22844. *Int J Radiat Oncol Biol Phys*. Oct 1 1996;36(3):549–556. doi:10.1016/s0360-3016(96)00352-5
29. Shaw E, Arusell R, Scheithauer B, et al. Prospective randomized trial of low- versus high-dose radiation therapy in adults with supratentorial low-grade glioma: Initial report of a North Central Cancer Treatment Group/Radiation Therapy Oncology Group/Eastern Cooperative Oncology Group study. *J Clin Oncol*. May 1 2002;20(9):2267–2276. doi:10.1200/JCO.2002.09.126
30. Baumert BG, Hegi ME, van den Bent MJ, et al. Temozolomide chemotherapy versus radiotherapy in high-risk low-grade glioma (EORTC 22033-26033): A randomised, open-label, phase 3 intergroup study. *Lancet Oncol*. Nov 2016;17(11):1521–1532. doi:10.1016/S1470-2045(16)30313-8
31. Chao JH, Phillips R, Nickson JJ. Roentgen-ray therapy of cerebral metastases. *Cancer*. Jul 1954;7(4):682–689. doi:10.1002/1097-0142(195407)7:4<682::aid-cncr2820070409>3.0.co;2-s
32. Borgelt B, Gelber R, Kramer S, et al. The palliation of brain metastases: Final results of the first two studies by the Radiation Therapy Oncology Group. *Int J Radiat Oncol Biol Phys*. Jan 1980;6(1):1–9. doi:10.1016/0360-3016(80)90195-9
33. Brown PD, Pugh S, Laack NN, et al. Memantine for the prevention of cognitive dysfunction in patients receiving whole-brain

radiotherapy: A randomized, double-blind, placebo-controlled trial. *Neuro Oncol.* Oct 2013;15(10):1429–1437. doi:10.1093/neuonc/not114

34. Brown PD, Gondi V, Pugh S, et al. Hippocampal avoidance during whole-brain radiotherapy plus memantine for patients with brain metastases: Phase III trial NRG Oncology CC001. *J Clin Oncol.* Apr 1 2020;38(10):1019–1029. doi:10.1200/JCO.19.02767

35. Mulvenna P, Nankivell M, Barton R, et al. Dexamethasone and supportive care with or without whole brain radiotherapy in treating patients with non-small cell lung cancer with brain metastases unsuitable for resection or stereotactic radiotherapy (QUARTZ): Results from a phase 3, non-inferiority, randomised trial. *Lancet.* Oct 22 2016;388(10055):2004–2014. doi:10.1016/S0140-6736(16)30825-X

36. Shaw E, Scott C, Souhami L, et al. Single dose radiosurgical treatment of recurrent previously irradiated primary brain tumors and brain metastases: Final report of RTOG protocol 90-05. *Int J Radiat Oncol Biol Phys.* May 1 2000;47(2):291–298. doi:10.1016/s0360-3016(99)00507-6

37. Kocher M, Soffietti R, Abacioglu U, et al. Adjuvant whole-brain radiotherapy versus observation after radiosurgery or surgical resection of one to three cerebral metastases: Results of the EORTC 22952-26001 study. *J Clin Oncol.* Jan 10 2011;29(2):134–141. doi:10.1200/JCO.2010.30.1655

38. Brown PD, Jaeckle K, Ballman KV, et al. Effect of radiosurgery alone vs radiosurgery with whole brain radiation therapy on cognitive function in patients with 1 to 3 brain metastases: A randomized clinical trial. *JAMA.* Jul 26 2016;316(4):401–409. doi:10.1001/jama.2016.9839

39. Mahajan A, Ahmed S, McAleer MF, et al. Post-operative stereotactic radiosurgery versus observation for completely resected brain metastases: A single-centre, randomised, controlled, phase 3 trial. *Lancet Oncol.* Aug 2017;18(8):1040–1048. doi:10.1016/S1470-2045(17)30414-X

40. Louis DN, Ohgaki H, Wiestler OD, et al. The 2007 WHO classification of tumours of the central nervous system. *Acta Neuropathol.* Aug 2007;114(2):97–109. doi:10.1007/s00401-007-0243-4

41. Pettersson-Segerlind J, Orrego A, et al. Long-term 25-year follow-up of surgically treated parasagittal meningiomas. *World Neurosurg.* Dec 2011;76(6):564–571. doi:10.1016/j.wneu.2011.05.015

42. Santacroce A, Walier M, Regis J, et al. Long-term tumor control of benign intracranial meningiomas after radiosurgery in a series of 4565 patients. *Neurosurgery.* Jan 2012;70(1):32–39; discussion 39. doi:10.1227/NEU.0b013e31822d408a

43. Aizer AA, Arvold ND, Catalano P, et al. Adjuvant radiation therapy, local recurrence, and the need for salvage therapy in atypical meningioma. *Neuro Oncol.* Nov 2014;16(11):1547–1553. doi:10.1093/neuonc/nou098

44. Zhu H, Bi WL, Aizer A, et al. Efficacy of adjuvant radiotherapy for atypical and anaplastic meningioma. *Cancer Med.* Jan 2019;8(1):13–20. doi:10.1002/cam4.1531

45. Rogers L, Zhang P, Vogelbaum MA, Mehta MP. Erratum. Intermediate-risk meningioma: Initial outcomes from NRG Oncology RTOG 0539. *J Neurosurg.* Dec 1 2018;129(6):1650. doi:10.3171/2018.8.JNS161170a

46. Boskos C, Feuvret L, Noel G, et al. Combined proton and photon conformal radiotherapy for intracranial atypical and malignant meningioma. *Int J Radiat Oncol Biol Phys.* Oct 1 2009;75(2):399–406. doi:10.1016/j.ijrobp.2008.10.053

47. Smouha EE, Yoo M, Mohr K, Davis RP. Conservative management of acoustic neuroma: A meta-analysis and proposed treatment algorithm. *Laryngoscope.* Mar 2005;115(3):450–454. doi:10.1097/00005537-200503000-00011

48. Watanabe S, Yamamoto M, Kawabe T, et al. Stereotactic radiosurgery for vestibular schwannomas: Average 10-year follow-up results focusing on long-term hearing preservation. *J Neurosurg.* Dec 2016;125(Suppl 1):64–72. doi:10.3171/2016.7.GKS161494

49. Niu NN, Niemierko A, Larvie M, et al. Pretreatment growth rate predicts radiation response in vestibular schwannomas. *Int J Radiat Oncol Biol Phys.* May 1 2014;89(1):113–119. doi:10.1016/j.ijrobp.2014.01.038

50. Bunin GR, Surawicz TS, Witman PA, et al. The descriptive epidemiology of craniopharyngioma. *J Neurosurg.* Oct 1998;89(4):547–551. doi:10.3171/jns.1998.89.4.0547

51. Yang I, Sughrue ME, Rutkowski MJ, et al. Craniopharyngioma: A comparison of tumor control with various treatment strategies. *Neurosurg Focus.* Apr 2010;28(4):E5. doi:10.3171/2010.1.FOCUS09307

52. Packer RJ, Goldwein J, Nicholson HS, et al. Treatment of children with medulloblastomas with reduced-dose craniospinal radiation therapy and adjuvant chemotherapy: A Children's Cancer Group Study. *J Clin Oncol.* Jul 1999;17(7):2127–2136. doi:10.1200/JCO.1999.17.7.2127

53. Bailey CC, Gnekow A, Wellek S, et al. Prospective randomised trial of chemotherapy given before radiotherapy in childhood medulloblastoma. International Society of Paediatric Oncology (SIOP) and the (German) Society of Paediatric Oncology (GPO): SIOP II. *Med Pediatr Oncol.* Sep 1995;25(3):166–178. doi:10.1002/mpo.2950250303

54. Kortmann RD, Kuhl J, Timmermann B, et al. Postoperative neoadjuvant chemotherapy before radiotherapy as compared to immediate radiotherapy followed by maintenance chemotherapy in the treatment of medulloblastoma in childhood: Results of the German prospective randomized trial HIT '91. *Int J Radiat Oncol Biol Phys.* Jan 15 2000;46(2):269–279. doi:10.1016/s0360-3016(99)00369-7

55. Tarbell NJ, Friedman H, Polkinghorn WR, et al. High-risk medulloblastoma: A pediatric oncology group randomized trial of chemotherapy before or after radiation therapy (POG 9031). *J Clin Oncol.* Aug 10 2013;31(23):2936–2941. doi:10.1200/JCO.2012.43.9984

56. Fouladi M, Gilger E, Kocak M, et al. Intellectual and functional outcome of children 3 years old or younger who have CNS malignancies. *J Clin Oncol.* Oct 1 2005;23(28):7152–7160. doi:10.1200/JCO.2005.01.214

57. Duffner PK, Horowitz ME, Krischer JP, et al. The treatment of malignant brain tumors in infants and very young children: An update of the Pediatric Oncology Group experience. *Neuro Oncol.* Apr 1999;1(2):152–161. doi:10.1093/neuonc/1.2.152

58. Lassaletta A, Ramaswamy V. Medulloblastoma in adults: They're not just big kids. *Neuro Oncol.* Jul 2016;18(7):895–897. doi:10.1093/neuonc/now110.

59. Brown AP, Barney CL, Grosshans DR, et al. Proton beam craniospinal irradiation reduces acute toxicity for adults with medulloblastoma. *Int J Radiat Oncol Biol Phys.* Jun 1 2013;86(2):277–284. doi:10.1016/j.ijrobp.2013.01.014.

60. Remke M, Hielscher T, Northcott PA, et al. Adult medulloblastoma comprises three major molecular variants. *J Clin Oncol.* Jul 1 2011;29(19):2717–2123. doi:10.1200/JCO.2011.34.9373.

61. Merchant TE, Li C, Xiong X, et al. Conformal radiotherapy after surgery for paediatric ependymoma: A prospective study. *Lancet Oncol.* Mar 2009;10(3):258–266. doi:10.1016/s1470-2045(08)70342-5

62. Mandell LR, Kadota R, Freeman C, et al. There is no role for hyperfractionated radiotherapy in the management of children with newly diagnosed diffuse intrinsic brainstem tumors: Results of a Pediatric Oncology Group phase III trial comparing conventional vs. hyperfractionated radiotherapy. *Int J Radiat Oncol Biol Phys.* Mar 15 1999;43(5):959–964. doi:10.1016/s0360-3016(98)00501-x

63. Chuba PJ, Zamarano L, Hamre M, et al. Permanent I-125 brain stem implants in children. *Childs Nerv Syst.* Oct 1998;14(10):570–577. doi:10.1007/s003810050274

64. Fuchs I, Kreil W, Sutter B, et al. Gamma knife radiosurgery of brainstem gliomas. *Acta Neurochir Suppl.* 2002;84:85–90. doi:10.1007/978-3-7091-6117-3_10

65. Fontanilla HP, Pinnix CC, Ketonen LM, et al. Palliative reirradiation for progressive diffuse intrinsic pontine glioma. *Am J Clin Oncol.* Feb 2012;35(1):51–57. doi:10.1097/COC.0b013e318201a2b7

66. Douw L, Klein M, Fagel SS, et al. Cognitive and radiological effects of radiotherapy in patients with low-grade glioma: Long-term follow-up. *Lancet Neurol.* Sep 2009;8(9):810–818. doi:10.1016/S1474-4422(09)70204-2

21 | PRINCIPLES OF SYSTEMIC THERAPY IN NEURO-ONCOLOGY

NIKOLAOS ANDREATOS AND DAVID M. PEEREBOOM

INTRODUCTION

OVERVIEW

Among adults, tumors of the central nervous system (CNS) are most commonly metastatic in origin.[1] On the other hand, while relatively infrequent (1.4% of new cancer diagnoses in 2019), primary malignancies of the CNS are also responsible for considerable morbidity and mortality with aggregate 5-year survival rates estimated at approximately 33%.[2] Tumors of the meninges (39% of cases) and the neuroepithelium (gliomas, ependymal, and choroid plexus tumors [28% of cases]) are the most common primary CNS malignancies encountered in clinical practice.[3] While the biologic behavior of different CNS primary tumors exhibits fascinating variability, anatomical proximity to vital structures and unique therapeutic obstacles imposed by CNS physiology render these neoplasms uniformly challenging to treat. A multidisciplinary approach, which often includes surgery, radiation therapy (RT), tumor-treating fields (TTF), (see Chapters 19, 20, and 22) and systemic therapy, is central to the treatment of CNS tumors. Limited management options and a paucity of high-quality evidence to guide many everyday clinical decisions emphasize the importance of offering a clinical trial to each patient whenever possible.[4] This chapter discusses the fundamental principles underlying the use of systemic therapy in patients with CNS malignancies and describes their implementation in the setting of the evolving contemporary standard of care.

GENERAL PRINCIPLES OF SYSTEMIC THERAPY

"Systemic therapy" is an umbrella term used to describe different types of treatment that aim to eradicate cancer cells systemically, in contrast with local therapies—such as surgery, RT, and TTF—which affect only the site at which they are targeted. Several terms deserve mention. The term "chemotherapy" refers to any drug used to treat cancer regardless of the mechanism of action and therefore is synonymous with systemic therapy. "Cytotoxic chemotherapy" refers to agents that are directly cytotoxic, in contrast, for example, to "targeted" therapies and immunotherapies (discussed later). Cytotoxic agents include drug classes such as alkylating agents, antimetabolites, taxanes, vinca alkaloids, and topoisomerase

inhibitors, all of which have in common disruption of cell division by means of interference with DNA or RNA replication or mitosis. These drugs, which preferentially target dividing cells, were the first group of systemic therapy agents to be employed against cancer. Cytotoxic agents demonstrated considerable success in the treatment of some hematologic malignancies and solid tumors.[5] While still widely employed (especially in CNS malignancies),[6-8] cytotoxic chemotherapy is highly effective against only a minority of neoplasms and is associated with multiple adverse effects due to its relatively non-selective action on rapidly proliferating cells. Mitotically active cellular populations are commonly encountered in the bone marrow, gastrointestinal epithelium, and hair follicles, resulting in corresponding toxicities such as myelosuppression, diarrhea, nausea, and alopecia.

> Cytotoxic agents include drug classes such as alkylating agents, antimetabolites, taxanes, vinca alkaloids, and topoisomerase inhibitors, all of which have in common disruption of cell division by means of interference with DNA or RNA replication or mitosis.

Better understanding of tumor biology led to the development of so-called *targeted therapies* (generally small molecules or monoclonal antibodies) aimed at specific molecular targets known to be overexpressed in tumors or important in neoplastic proliferation.[5] In general, small molecules carry the ending "-inib" (e.g., osimertinib, trametinib) and are most often oral agents. Monoclonal antibodies carry the ending "-mab" (e.g., bevacizumab, pembrolizumab) and are large proteins that need to be given intravenously. While impressive results have been achieved by such approaches in some malignancies (e.g., imatinib in chronic myeloid leukemia[9] or a variety of targeted inhibitors in lung cancer[10]), most tumors (including CNS malignancies) exhibit such complex molecular aberrations that effective targeted therapies still elude our grasp. Immunotherapies, on the other hand, are novel and highly promising approaches that aim to harness the body's immune system against the tumor, either by blocking important molecular "brakes" (checkpoints) which normally prevent immune activation[11] or by modifying T-cells or natural killer

(NK) cells to enhance their activity against tumor antigens.[12] Such immune and cellular therapeutics are increasingly employed in other malignancies and will hopefully introduce a paradigm-shift in the management of CNS tumors in the future.

> Small molecules carry the ending "-ib," while monoclonal antibodies carry the ending "-mab."

At present, systemic therapy in CNS malignancies consists largely of traditional cytotoxic chemotherapy; a summary of currently approved agents and their mechanisms of action can be found in Table 21.1. In general, systemic therapy can be administered with a curative intent or with a palliative intent, in which case prolongation of survival and maintenance of quality of life via inhibition of tumor growth are the main objectives. While highly desirable, cure is so far possible for only a minority of patients and tumor types. A prominent example of a potentially curable CNS tumor is primary CNS lymphoma (PCNSL) (see Chapter 11) which, like other hematologic malignancies, exhibits rapid proliferation; this property renders a large fraction of tumor cells vulnerable to chemotherapy to the point where complete eradication of the tumor may be possible

TABLE 21.1 Systemic therapy agents commonly used in the treatment of primary central nervous system (CNS) malignancies

AGENT	MECHANISM OF ACTION	ADMINISTRATION	SELECTED TOXICITIES
Temozolomide	Methylation of guanine residues leading to inhibition of DNA, RNA, and protein synthesis	Oral	Myelosuppression Nausea/vomiting Rash
Carmustine (BCNU)	Production of chloroethyl metabolites which interfere with DNA, RNA, and protein synthesis	Intravenous	Myelosuppression generally 4–6 weeks after therapy Facial flushing Hepatoxicity, with veno-occlusive disease noted in high-dose regimens Sterility Pulmonary fibrosis Renal toxicity Secondary malignancies
Lomustine (CCNU)	Alkylating activity that interferes with DNA, RNA, and protein synthesis and function	Oral	Myelotoxicity generally 4–6 weeks after therapy Sterility Pulmonary fibrosis Renal toxicity Neurotoxicity notably confusion, lethargy, dysarthria and ataxia Secondary malignancies
Procarbazine	Unclear mechanism of action, but is thought to inhibit DNA, RNA, and protein synthesis possibly via alkylating activity	Oral	Sympathetic overactivation if co-administered with tricyclic antidepressants, tyramine-containing foods, levodopa, etc. given procarbazine's inhibition of monoamine oxidase Myelosuppression, most pronounced being thrombocytopenia approximately 4 weeks after ingestion. Flu-like symptoms can be noted with initial therapy. Neurotoxicity such as paresthesias, neuropathy, ataxia, lethargy, or seizures Sterility Secondary malignancies
Vincristine	Disruption of microtubule formation during mitosis leading to arrest of cellular division and cell death	Intravenous	Neurotoxicity, most frequently peripheral neuropathy; cranial nerve palsies, dysautonomia, ataxia, cortical blindness, and seizures have also been reported Decreased gut motility leading to constipation and occasionally paralytic ileus Alopecia Myelosuppression (generally mild) Sterility SIADH Hypersensitivity reactions
Etoposide	Inhibition of topoisomerase II leading to arrest of DNA unwinding necessary for DNA replication	Oral/Intravenous	Myelosuppression generally 10–14 days after therapy Nausea/vomiting and anorexia Alopecia Mucositis and diarrhea Secondary malignancies

(continued)

TABLE 21.1 Continued

AGENT	MECHANISM OF ACTION	ADMINISTRATION	SELECTED TOXICITIES
Carboplatin	DNA cross-linkage leading to inhibition of DNA synthesis and transcription	Intravenous	Myelosuppression with platelets most affected; nadir approximately 21 days after therapy Renal toxicity Peripheral neuropathy Allergic reactions which uncommonly may involve bronchospasm and hypotension
Bevacizumab	Inhibition of VEGF leading to reduced angiogenesis and tumor blood vessel permeability.	Intravenous	Gastrointestinal perforation and delayed wound healing Increased risk of bleeding Increased risk of thromboembolic events both arterial (myocardial infarction and stroke) and venous (deep vein thrombosis and pulmonary embolism) Hypertension Proteinuria and, more rarely, nephrotic syndrome Posterior reversible encephalopathy syndrome
Methotrexate	Inhibition of dihydrofolate reductase leading to folate depletion and, ultimately, inhibition of purine synthesis	Intravenous	Myelotoxicity with nadir noted within 4–7 days of treatment Mucositis Acute renal failure which in turn leads to delayed drug clearance and medication accumulation; glucarpidase can be used as an antidote in this setting. Transient hepatotoxicity Pneumonitis Acute arachnoiditis with intrathecal administration; demyelinating encephalopathy can be seen with chronic use. Acute neurotoxicity with paresis, aphasia, and seizures in those receiving high-dose therapy; dementia can be seen as a late complication. Can induce abortion in pregnant women; reversible effect on spermatogenesis
Thiotepa	Alkylation of guanine leading to inhibition of DNA, RNA, and protein synthesis	Intravenous	Myelosuppression (leukocyte nadir at 7–10 days, platelet at 21 days) Mucositis Hypersensitivity reactions Cystitis Skin desquamation, bronze discoloration Teratogenic Secondary malignancies
Cytarabine (cytosine arabinoside, Ara-C)	Incorporation into DNA leading to termination of replication; inhibition of DNA polymerase	Intravenous	Myelosuppression generally on days 7–10; megaloblastic anemia can sometimes be noted Cerebellar ataxia, generally reversible Hepatic dysfunction (generally transient) Ara-C syndrome (mostly in pediatric patients); hypersensitivity reaction with fever, myalgia, malaise, maculopapular rash, and conjunctivitis Non-cardiogenic pulmonary edema Skin erythema, in more rare cases hand-foot syndrome Conjunctivitis, keratitis Seizures, altered mental status with intrathecal administration
Cyclophosphamide	Formation of DNA cross-links which inhibit replication and function	Intravenous	Myelosuppression (nadir 7–14 days) Hemorrhagic cystitis Alopecia Sterility Cardiotoxicity Secondary malignancies SIADH
Busulfan	Promotes cross-linking between DNA molecules and DNA with proteins thus preventing DNA replication and expression	Oral/Intravenous	Myelosuppresion Mucositis Hyperpigmentation Sterility Pulmonary fibrosis Adrenal insufficiency Hepatotoxicity, including veno-occlusive disease Secondary malignancies

TABLE 21.1 Continued

AGENT	MECHANISM OF ACTION	ADMINISTRATION	SELECTED TOXICITIES
Pemetrexed	Inhibition of thymidylate synthase, dihydrofolate reductase, and purine synthesis thus preventing DNA replication	Intravenous	Myelosuppression Mucositis, diarrhea Transient hepatotoxicity Hand-foot syndrome
Lenalidomide	Stimulation of T-cell antitumor activity and anti-angiogenic effects via as yet unclear mechanisms	Oral	Myelosuppression Secondary malignancies Teratogenicity Nausea, vomiting, diarrhea
Rituximab	Binding to CD20 leading to inhibition of cell cycle progression as well as direct cell death via complement and antibody-mediated cytotoxicity	Intravenous	Hypersensitivity reactions Tumor lysis syndrome Pemphigus, Stevens-Johnson, toxic epidermal necrolysis, and lichenoid dermatitis have been described. Reactivation of chronic infections such as tuberculosis or hepatitis B
Ibrutinib	Inhibition of Bruton's tyrosine kinase, which is important in B-cell proliferation	Oral	Bleeding Myelosuppression Renal failure Secondary malignancies

[a]Neurological toxicities of systemic agents are also covered in the Chapter 23 "Neurologic Complications of Cancer."

From Chu E, DeVita VT. *Physicians' Cancer Chemotherapy Drug Manual 2019*. 19th ed. New York: Jones & Bartlett Learning; 2019.

prior to the development of treatment resistance, especially with the use of combination chemotherapy as predicted by Skipper's classic log kill model.[5,8,13,14] In most other CNS tumor types (e.g., gliomas), delay of disease progression and death without undue interference in quality of life is the main goal of therapy.

Important concepts from tumor kinetics help to illustrate why cure is much more challenging to achieve in less rapidly proliferating tumors and suggest how therapy may be structured to maximize efficacy. In a seminal series of publications during the late 1970s, Norton and Simon showed that solid tumors behave in a radically different way from the leukemia models which had been used to develop the log kill hypothesis; only a minority of tumor cells are actively dividing (and therefore vulnerable to cytotoxic agents) at any one time and, importantly, this "growth fraction" is inversely correlated to tumor size.[15] As such, not only is the potential efficacy of a single chemotherapy cycle much diminished, thus requiring multiple cycles to achieve the same effect (while increasing the risk that resistance mutations will emerge in the interim), but successful treatment is ultimately self-defeating; as a tumor shrinks the growth fraction increases and proliferation accelerates, threatening to nullify any benefit achieved during prior therapy. On the basis of this hypothesis, Norton and Simon predicted that "dose-dense" regimens which minimize the interval between treatments would improve outcomes by taking advantage of the transient increase in the growth fraction that occurs between therapy cycles. Clinical trials based on these principles in, for example, breast[16] and colorectal cancer[17] did indeed provide evidence that dose-dense regimens may improve outcomes; however, this has so far not proved to be the case in gliomas,[18] possibly due to the inherent chemoresistance of most gliomas.

In a similar vein, the use of chemotherapy in combination with another treatment modality such as surgery or RT that reduces tumor burden would be expected to produce superior outcomes based on kinetic considerations alone; in the case of chemoradiation especially, synergistic antineoplastic effects have been described which would be expected to augment therapeutic efficacy still further.[19] Indeed concurrent and adjuvant (i.e., therapy as an adjunct to initial treatment) therapy with temozolomide (TMZ) and RT following initial surgical resection is commonly used in gliomas; interestingly, while the CATNON trial (described in detail later) established the benefit of adjuvant TMZ, it failed to do the same for concurrent TMZ.[20,21] Of course, combined modality therapy results not only in synergistic efficacy but also in cumulative toxicity, which needs to be considered; such concerns have, for example, led to abandonment of combined RT and chemotherapy for primary CNS lymphoma in spite of evidence of delayed disease progression with this approach.[8] A comparable theoretical framework addressing the effects of targeted, immune, and cellular therapies has not yet emerged but will be crucial in guiding their rational utilization and the formulation of combination approaches.

PHARMACOKINETICS: OVERCOMING THE BLOOD–BRAIN BARRIER

Beyond the challenges inherent in CNS tumor kinetics and biology, further complications are added by the unique properties of the blood–brain barrier (BBB). This structure consists mainly of tight junctions between endothelial cells of neuronal capillaries and multiple drug efflux transporters which pump drugs from the brain back out to the capillaries. While the BBB protects the CNS from toxic exposures, it also limits substantially the concentration of systemically administered agents that reach tumor cells in the CNS.[22] Therefore, most chemotherapeutic drugs do not cross the BBB in concentrations high enough to be effective. Agents that can cross the BBB in sufficient quantities are generally limited to lipid-soluble drugs (e.g., lomustine) or small molecules, generally less than 500 Daltons. Examples of such agents include TMZ and many of the small-molecule targeted agents such as osimertinib (effective against non-small cell lung cancer [NSCLC] brain metastases) and dabrafenib and trametinib, both of which have efficacy against melanoma brain metastases.[23,24]

> Agents that can cross the BBB in sufficient quantities are generally limited to lipid-soluble drugs (e.g., lomustine) or small molecules (generally less than 500 Daltons).

The importance of the BBB is illustrated by recent molecular studies of medulloblastoma. While sonic hedgehog (SHH)-medulloblastoma has an intact BBB and is resistant to treatment, wingless (WNT)-medulloblastoma is supplied by fenestrated vasculature with relatively high BBB permeability, responds well to chemotherapy, and has an excellent prognosis.[25] Primary CNS and metastatic lesions have variable BBB permeability, as evidenced by variable contrast enhancement because contrast only "leaks" into the brain at sites of BBB disruption. However, this effect is often not sufficient to allow drug penetration.[22] Furthermore, non-enhancing brain surrounding enhancing tumor harbors malignant cells but generally has an intact BBB. Thus, while some amount of a drug could perhaps penetrate enhancing tumor, a much smaller amount, if any, can cross the intact BBB that exists in non-enhancing regions known to harbor tumor cells. Interestingly, an older report assessing the penetration of etoposide in a mixed cohort of patients with primary and metastatic CNS tumors suggested that concentration of the drug was much higher in lesions than in the surrounding parenchyma and decreased gradually as distance from the lesion increased; in turn, this may imply that micrometastatic foci are relatively protected from systemic therapy by the BBB and in turn give rise to recurrence.[22]

Circumvention of the BBB is a complex challenge unique to cancers in the CNS. Many strategies have sought to circumvent the BBB. Several examples include (1) development of agents able to cross it in sufficient quantities, (2) administration of high doses such as the use of high-dose methotrexate (HD-MTX), (3) intra-arterial therapy with osmotic BBB disruption, (4) "Trojan horse" strategies using nanoparticles or receptor ligands to transport drugs across the BBB, (5) inhibition of drug efflux pumps that are central to BBB function, and (6) focused ultrasound to cause transient BBB disruption. These and other strategies to circumvent the BBB are the subject of clinical trials for which eligible patients should be referred whenever possible.

Some systemic agents do not require transit across the BBB to achieve their desired effect. For example, bevacizumab inhibits the formation of new tumor vessels ("neovasculature") and thus functions "outside" of the BBB (albeit with possible restoration of BBB physiology which has been posited to impact the penetration of other treatments at least

theoretically).[26] Similarly, immunotherapies in primary CNS malignancies increase the recruitment of T cells from the periphery, which subsequently cross the BBB and eliminate tumor cells.[27]

SYSTEMIC THERAPY IN THE MANAGEMENT OF GLIOMAS

CLASSIFICATION

The classification of gliomas was originally based on histologic characteristics, but the most recent taxonomy proposed by the World Health Organization (WHO) in 2016 incorporated molecular parameters.[28] A detailed discussion of these changes can be found in the respective Chapter 1 of this volume; importantly, while histologic grading was retained, astrocytomas were further subdivided according to the presence of isocitrate dehydrogenase-1/2 (IDH1/2) mutations, with the mutant phenotype conferring a more favorable prognosis.[28] In the 2016 WHO classification, the diagnosis of oligodendroglioma now requires the presence of IDH mutation and 1p/19q co-deletion.[28] This classification has implications for the use of chemotherapy. Oligodendrogliomas tend to respond well to chemotherapy, while tumors that appear to be oligodendrogliomas histologically but lack IDH mutations or 1p/19q co-deletions do not respond as well and, in fact, are now classified as astrocytomas. Patients with those tumors at the time of initial treatment require radiation with chemotherapy, but true oligodendrogliomas can sometimes be treated with chemotherapy alone. Thus, refinements in the classification scheme can guide the use of systemic therapy for patients with brain tumors.

Another biomarker that deserves mention is O6-methylguanine-DNA methyltransferase (MGMT). This DNA-repair enzyme repairs damage caused by alkylating agents, most notably TMZ, and serves as a predictive marker for response to the latter.[29] Patients whose tumors have methylation of the MGMT gene promoter have decreased MGMT expression, which in turn allows alkylating agents to work more effectively. Thus, genetic markers have a direct impact on the utility of systemic agents for CNS malignancies.

Systemic therapy is central to the management of grade 2–4 gliomas and is employed in multiple different roles, including radio-sensitization, adjuvant treatment after locoregional intervention, and as primary therapy aiming to curtail tumor growth in more advanced disease.[6,7] *Radio-sensitization* refers to the use of an agent to increase the efficacy of RT therapy. The best example in neuro-oncology is TMZ, which acts as a radiosensitizer in the treatment of gliomas.[30] In this context, TMZ is usually given concurrently with RT on a low-dose daily schedule such that the drug is present in the tumor when the daily radiation dose is delivered. While prognosis varies widely based on grade and molecular subtype, systemic therapy is unfortunately not curative in this setting.[6,7] In the next section, we briefly review landmark trials that established the main treatment paradigms for systemic therapy among patients with gliomas. Overall, for many subtypes of grade 2–4 gliomas, RT plus chemotherapy prolongs survival when compared to RT alone.

Overall, for many subtypes of grade 2–4 gliomas, RT plus chemotherapy prolongs survival when compared to RT alone.

DIFFUSE (GRADE 2) AND ANAPLASTIC (GRADE 3) ASTROCYTOMAS AND OLIGODENDROGLIOMAS

The utility of chemotherapy added to RT following resection of high-risk grade 2 astrocytomas/oligodendrogliomas (Chapter 4) was established by two large randomized trials: RTOG 9802[31] and RTOG 0424.[32] In the former, the addition of six 8-week cycles of procarbazine, lomustine, and vincristine (PCV) after RT resulted in a significant overall survival (OS) benefit over RT alone. In a subgroup analysis by histologic subtype, OS differences remained statistically significant among patients with oligodendrogliomas, but not those with astrocytomas, while a molecular subgroup analysis of patients whose tumors had IDH1 R132H mutation showed that they also retained a significant OS benefit with combination therapy.[31] While RTOG 0424 lacked an active comparator arm, it similarly showed that RT and concurrent TMZ (daily during RT) followed by a maximum of 12 28-day cycles of adjuvant TMZ was associated with promising 3-year OS of 73% compared to a historical rate of 54% with RT alone.[32] These results established the use of combination RT and chemotherapy in this setting. However, given the additive neurotoxicity of combined modality therapy, the EORTC 22033-26033 trial assessed whether dose-dense TMZ could potentially substitute for RT.[33] Progression-free survival (PFS) did not differ between the two arms, while a subgroup analysis suggested an advantage of RT over TMZ among patients with IDH mutations but without 1p/19q co-deletions. Even though direct head-to-head comparison of chemotherapy versus chemoradiotherapy was not performed, taken together, these findings do suggest that combined modality therapy is likely a superior strategy.

For patients with anaplastic astrocytomas, the CATNON trial investigated the efficacy of concurrent TMZ and RT versus RT alone, as well that of adjuvant TMZ versus post-radiation surveillance.[20,21] The initial report of the study showed an OS advantage for adjuvant TMZ versus post-radiation surveillance[20]; in a more updated report this benefit was shown to stem from the IDH mutant population which also enjoyed a superior prognosis overall.[21] Interestingly, a benefit from concurrent TMZ could not be proved conclusively, with only a non-significant trend noted among IDH mutant cases, although more mature data are awaited.[21] Unlike grade 2 disease, a head-to-head comparison of TMZ with nitrosoureas (albeit not PCV) was performed among patients with grade 3 astrocytomas in the NRG RTOG 9813 trial.[34] The study assessed concurrent RT plus either TMZ or nitrosourea (lomustine or carmustine). No significant difference in efficacy was noted, but TMZ was better tolerated, which provided the rationale for wide adoption of this agent in practice.[34]

The role of chemotherapy both prior to and following RT in grade 3 oligodendrogliomas was assessed by RTOG 9402[35] and EORTC 26951[36]; the former compared the addition of four cycles of PCV prior to RT and the latter of six cycles of PCV after RT to RT alone. In RTOG 9402, a marked OS benefit in the intervention arm (median OS: 14.7 vs. 7.3 years, P = 0.03) was noted only among patients with 1p/19q co-deletion (a requirement for the diagnosis of oligodendroglioma under the 2016 WHO classification[28]).[35] The EORTC 26951 trial showed a significant OS benefit following PCV for the entire cohort, but that appeared more pronounced among patients whose tumors had 1p/19q co-deletion, IDH mutation, or MGMT promoter methylation.[36] These trials established the role of chemoradiotherapy among patients with oligodendrogliomas, while evidence from the early CODEL study solidified this further by suggesting that chemotherapy alone (TMZ) leads to worse survival compared to either RT or a combination strategy.[37] Comparing RT/PCV and RT/TMZ is the logical next step; the revised CODEL study aims to investigate this question.[37] In summary, patients with grade 3 gliomas appear to benefit from the addition of chemotherapy to RT compared to radiation alone.

GLIOBLASTOMA

While gliomas are not particularly sensitive to chemotherapy in general, the outcomes among patients with glioblastoma (GBM) (Chapter 3) are especially grim, and limited progress has been made in developing effective new treatments.[6] The current standard of care for first-line therapy consists of surgical resection followed by radiation and both concurrent and adjuvant TMZ[6]; this was established by Stupp et al. in the EORTC-NCIC trial, which assessed the benefit of administering TMZ concomitant with RT followed by six cycles of adjuvant TMZ over RT alone.[38,39] While a statistically significant OS benefit was indeed noted, its magnitude was limited (2.5 months for the overall cohort) and largely driven by patients whose glioblastoma demonstrated methylation of the MGMT promoter.[38,39] Similar results were seen in older patients, for whom the combination of hypofractionated RT with TMZ was superior to hypofractionated RT alone in spite of reasonable concerns about the risk of cumulative toxicity with advancing age.[40] Nonetheless, assuming combined modality therapy proves not to be an option for some frail elderly patients, data from the Nordic and NOA-08 trials suggest that adjuvant TMZ monotherapy (e.g., without radiation) is at least non-inferior to RT alone and possibly superior for patients with MGMT methylated tumors.[41,42]

Attempts to improve outcomes by increasing the dose-density of adjuvant TMZ in this setting (75–100 mg/m^2 for 21 of 28-cycle days) have been unsuccessful.[18] Moreover, while six cycles of adjuvant TMZ was the standard established by the EORTC-NCIC trial, it is reasonable to examine whether additional cycles may offer benefit to responders per the established paradigm in grade 2–3 disease. While this question has not been studied prospectively, retrospective analysis of prior trials suggests that administering more than six cycles of TMZ cycles does not correlate with improved OS, despite a small PFS benefit.[43] In summary, the addition of chemotherapy to radiation offers superior survival compared to RT alone for patients with newly diagnosed glioblastoma.

Attempts to combine the RT/TMZ standard in the first-line setting with additional treatment strategies have shown mixed results. The addition of bevacizumab to concurrent and adjuvant TMZ demonstrated a small PFS benefit but no OS benefit in both the RTOG 0825[44] and AVAglio[45] trials. Therefore, bevacizumab does not improve outcomes in the initial management of patients with glioblastoma. A recent small trial also demonstrated that, among patients with MGMT promoter methylation, a lomustine-TMZ combination regimen may offer an OS advantage over the current TMZ standard of care; however, the treatment groups were significantly imbalanced and statistical significance of the findings was borderline, so additional data are needed prior to implementing this approach in clinical practice.[46] To date, no addition of systemic therapy to standard radiation plus TMZ has improved outcomes for glioblastoma patients. Interestingly, the combination of TTF, a portable electronic device that is thought to inhibit tumor mitosis, with adjuvant TMZ following standard RT and concomitant TMZ was associated with a significant OS benefit (20.9 vs. 16.0 months, P < 0.001) in a recent trial, results that constitute an important development in the first-line setting.[47]

While systemic therapy remains the cornerstone in the management of recurrent or progressive disease, outcomes in the second-line setting and beyond are poor and the evidence supporting the efficacy of employed therapies is less robust. Single-agent chemotherapy is the most frequently used approach. TMZ rechallenge has shown activity when administered in varying schedules (e.g., 7 out of 14 cycle-days, or 21 out of 28 cycle-days, or daily continuous) and is frequently employed.[48,49] Other chemotherapy agents with anti-GBM activity that may be employed in this setting include the nitrosoureas lomustine/carmustine,[50–52] carboplatin,[53,54] and etoposide.[55] The introduction of bevacizumab was originally thought to hold much promise for patients with recurrent disease; however, the universally reported improvement in PFS associated with bevacizumab use has yet to be linked with a significant OS benefit.[50,56,57] The effects of bevacizumab on peritumoral edema and consequently on imaging assessment of response may be responsible for this imbalance; however, they also provide a rationale for employing the agent in cases where reduction of cerebral edema is desirable, either alone or in combination with chemotherapy.[6] Furthermore, bevacizumab often reduces the requirement for corticosteroids in the management of cerebral edema and offers a meaningful improvement in neurological symptoms.[58]

> Given the overall paucity of treatment options for gliomas, clinical trials play a critical role in advancing the current standard of care and should be integrated into routine practice.

Given this overall paucity of treatment options, clinical trials play a critical role in advancing the current standard of care and should be integrated into routine practice. In fact, clinical trials should be considered the treatment of choice at every juncture in a patient's disease trajectory (e.g., initial diagnosis or at progression) rather than as an option only after standard therapies have failed. It may be hoped that novel agents such as, for example, checkpoint inhibitors will help to expand our therapeutic armamentarium in the near future.[59]

INTRACRANIAL AND SPINAL EPENDYMOMAS

These rare tumors are generally managed most effectively by surgery with or without the addition of radiation; systemic therapy currently has no established role in the first-line setting and has only been used for recurrent disease.[60] Even in that context, data are relatively sparse and mostly based on retrospective reports. In adults, platinum-based regimens have been used most frequently as they may be associated with higher response rates, albeit without a survival advantage.[61] TMZ has shown some efficacy after progression on platinum-based therapy,[62,63] and the activity of bevacizumab may also be promising.[64] Interestingly, the discovery that ependymomas (Chapter 6) are characterized by constitutive activation of the ERBB pathway[65] and only infrequently exhibit MGMT promoter methylation[66] led to the hypothesis that a combination strategy of ERBB blockade and dose-dense chemotherapy to overcome the capacity of MGMT to repair DNA damage may lead to synergistic efficacy. Indeed, a small trial which assessed response to the combination of TMZ and lapatinib demonstrated encouraging results which will need to be validated in larger studies.[67]

> Systemic therapy currently has no established role in the first-line setting for treatment of ependymomas.

PRIMARY CENTRAL NERVOUS SYSTEM LYMPHOMA

As with other lymphomas encountered outside the CNS, PCNSL (Chapter 11) is highly sensitive to and potentially curable by systemic chemotherapy, at least in a minority of patients.[8] Nonetheless, its anatomic location and the properties of the BBB pose unique challenges.[8] After diagnosis is established by surgery, chemotherapy is initiated as soon as possible and constitutes the main therapeutic intervention; first-line bimodality therapy with chemotherapy and whole-brain radiation therapy (WBRT) has gradually fallen out of favor given the high incidence of neurotoxicity with this approach and the lack of clearly demonstrated OS benefit over chemotherapy alone.[68] Similar to well-established leukemia/lymphoma treatment paradigms, the therapeutic approach in PCNSL consists of three phases: induction, in which rapid reduction of tumor burden and achievement of remission is the goal; consolidation, in which the eradication of microscopic remnant disease is attempted; and, ultimately, a maintenance phase which aims to preserve remission for the long term.[8,69] A summary of employed regimens during these phases as well as following disease relapse is presented in Table 21.2. No consensus on the optimal chemotherapy strategy exists at present; we attempt to present fundamental principles underlying contemporary

TABLE 21.2 Chemotherapy regimens commonly employed in primary central nervous system (CNS) lymphoma

INDUCTION THERAPY	CONSOLIDATION THERAPY	RELAPSE/REFRACTORY DISEASE
Methotrexate monotherapy	Carmustine, thiotepa with stem cell rescue	Rechallenge with methotrexate-containing regimen
MTR (methotrexate, temozolomide, rituximab)	TBC (thiotepa, busulfan, cyclophosphamide) with stem cell rescue	Ibrutinib
R-MPV (rituximab, methotrexate, procarbazine, vincristine)	High-dose cytarabine and etoposide	Lenalidomide (or pomalidomide)
R-MBVP (rituximab, methotrexate, carmustine, teniposide, prednisone)	High-dose cytarabine	Temozolomide (or pemetrexed)
MATRIX (methotrexate, cytarabine, thiotepa, rituximab)		High-dose cytarabine

From NCCN Clinical Practice Guidelines in Oncology[4]; Ferreri et al.[71]; Grommes et al.[70]

approaches in the following paragraphs. For a more in-depth discussion, we refer the reader to the respective Chapter 11 of this volume, as well as the following recent reviews.[70,71]

> Chemotherapy constitutes the main therapeutic intervention for PCNSL; first-line bimodality therapy with chemotherapy and WBRT has gradually fallen out of favor.

As most cases of PCNSL are of B-cell origin, variations of the cyclophosphamide, doxorubicin, vincristine and prednisone (CHOP) regimen, which has been successful in B-cell lymphomas outside the CNS, were initially employed, but with poor results.[72,73] Research subsequently turned to agents able to penetrate the BBB in sufficient quantities to deliver effective results; pharmacokinetic studies demonstrated that MTX can in fact achieve adequate concentrations in the cerebrospinal fluid (CSF) if administered at very high intravenous doses (commonly between 3 and 8 mg/m^2 in clinical practice).[74-77] In addition, infusion over 4 hours or less is required to achieve the "spike" in serum MTX concentration that enables a sufficient dose to cross the BBB.[78] HD-MTX would have prohibitive systemic toxicity if not for the fact that leucovorin, an agent that can mitigate the effects of MTX, does not adequately penetrate the CSF and can therefore provide peripheral "salvage" from MTX toxicity without affecting its antineoplastic activity in the CNS (though toxicity is still a concern for patients with renal impairment).[8] These theoretical considerations were confirmed in clinical studies which demonstrated the superiority of HD-MTX over previously used regimens and cemented its place as the cornerstone of induction therapy in PCNSL.[79,80] In line with the accepted paradigm in other hematologic malignancies, evidence suggests that combining HD-MTX with other chemotherapy agents leads to superior outcomes; however, the optimal induction regimen has not been determined and practices vary.[8,13]

In addition to cytotoxic chemotherapy, the use of the anti-CD20 antibody rituximab has efficacy in the induction setting in both retrospective reports[81,82] and the phase II IELSG32 trial.[83] In the latter, addition of rituximab to HD-MTX and cytarabine was associated with improved response rate. Based on these results, many practitioners now incorporate rituximab as part of induction therapy.[8] The management of patients with evidence of ocular or leptomeningeal involvement is less clear; despite the anticipated pharmacokinetic challenges associated with these sites of disease, high-dose intravenous (8 mg/m^2) MTX may still achieve sufficient concentration in the CSF and vitreous to provide effective therapy.[84] Of note, the entry of systemic therapy into various components of the CNS—brain parenchyma, CSF, or ocular compartment—varies depending on the site as each has its own barrier—e.g., BBB, blood–meningeal barrier, and blood–retinal barrier, respectively.[85]

> The phase II IELSG32 trial demonstrated that the addition of rituximab to HD-MTX and cytarabine was associated with improved response rate.

The primary strategies employed for consolidation and maintenance therapy include nonmyeloablative chemotherapy, high-dose chemotherapy with stem cell rescue (to enable the administration of otherwise myeloablative doses of chemotherapy which can better penetrate the CSF[8]), and WBRT with or without concomitant chemotherapy; however, the optimal approach is unclear and multiple different regimens have been employed (Table 21.2).[8] For example, reduced-dose WBRT in addition to cytarabine appeared to have encouraging results with median PFS of 7.7 years in a small cohort[86]; comparable outcomes were reported in single-arm trials assessing high-dose chemotherapy with stem-cell rescue.[87,88] More recently, the IELSG32 trial did not demonstrate a clear difference between consolidation WBRT and carmustine/thiotepa chemotherapy with stem-cell rescue, although there was a slight trend in favor of the former.[89] Data from larger studies with long-term follow-up (especially given the neurotoxicity associated with WBRT) are needed before more conclusive recommendations can be made. Similarly, management of refractory or recurrent disease is based on limited evidence; various strategies, such as rechallenge with HD-MTX–containing regimens, WBRT, chemotherapy with or without stem cell rescue, and, more recently, use of lenalidomide[90,91] and ibrutinib[92,93] have been employed either alone or in combination and may successfully induce remissions in some cases.[8] Intriguingly, a small series reported that the intraventricular administration of rituximab resulted in a complete response rate of 43% even in the brain parenchyma[94]; the authors attributed these impressive results to complement activation and complex immunomodulatory effects that transcend the traditional mechanism of action of rituximab and will hopefully be confirmed in future studies.[95]

MENINGIOMAS

Meningiomas are infrequently managed by neuro-oncologists as surgical resection and RT (if feasible) are efficacious even at recurrence.[96] However, in cases where anatomic and functional considerations do not permit the use of localized treatment, systemic therapy may be attempted. Cytotoxic chemotherapy has not demonstrated appreciable efficacy in this setting and is not employed; while the quality of the respective evidence is limited, targeted inhibitors of angiogenesis (possibly in combination with mTOR inhibitors), somatostatin-analogues, and interferon-alpha have demonstrated modest activity against meningiomas and may be employed.[96]

More specifically, patients treated with interferon-alpha therapy demonstrated a median time to tumor progression of 7 months and OS of 8 months in a phase II study at the cost of considerable toxicity.[97] Sustained-release somatostatin achieved comparable response and survival results in another small trial but with a more favorable toxicity profile.[98] More recently sunitinib, a tyrosine kinase inhibitor that targets the vascular endothelial growth factor (VEGF) pathway demonstrated some efficacy in heavily pretreated patients with high-grade disease that was more pronounced for tumors expressing VEGFR2, compared to those who did not.[99] Small retrospective reports with bevacizumab similarly suggested a median PFS of about 6 months,[100,101] while a recent prospective trial combining bevacizumab with mTOR inhibitor everolimus reported an encouraging median PFS of 22 months.[102] Given the differences in baseline prognostic factors among the treated populations, the results of these reports are not directly comparable. However, they do point at the relatively limited effectiveness of systemic therapy in a condition with otherwise favorable prognosis, thus highlighting the need for novel approaches.

ADULT MEDULLOBLASTOMAS AND GERM CELL TUMORS

While common in children, these tumor types are exceedingly rare in adults; as a result, management is largely guided by extrapolation from pediatric treatment paradigms supplemented by limited data from adult populations.[103,104] In the case of medulloblastoma, systemic therapy is generally used in conjunction with RT following maximal safe resection, especially in patients with high-risk disease.[103] The employed regimens vary between reports, and there is no generally accepted standard of care. Neoadjuvant chemotherapy followed by RT was shown to result in limited response rates in a small study,

and, as a result, many practitioners opt for adjuvant chemotherapy after radiation is completed.[103,105] Concurrent chemotherapy with vincristine during RT was associated with high rates of peripheral neurotoxicity in another small trial and is infrequently employed in practice.[106] Management of recurrent disease is similarly based on limited evidence; re-resection, RT, and systemic therapy are generally used, with a possible role for high-dose chemotherapy and autologous stem cell rescue in selected cases.[103] Vismodegib, an SHH pathway inhibitor, has also shown promising activity in SHH-medulloblastoma and may be considered in this setting.[107]

After diagnosis is established by surgery, systemic therapy with platinum-based regimens and RT are the primary treatment modalities employed among patients with intracranial germ cell tumors; specific therapeutic strategies vary based on tumor histology and institutional practice.[104] Additional information on the biology and management of medulloblastomas and germ cell tumors of the CNS can be found in the respective Chapter 10 of this volume.

PRIMARY NEOPLASMS OF THE SPINAL CORD

Surgery and radiation are the main tools employed in the management of these tumors. There is currently no evidence regarding the role of systemic therapy, and the National Comprehensive Cancer Network guidelines recommend that all patients in whom the use of systemic therapy is contemplated should be enrolled in a clinical trial.[4]

NOVEL SYSTEMIC THERAPIES IN THE MANAGEMENT OF METASTATIC DISEASE TO THE CNS

The role of systemic therapy in the management of metastatic disease to the CNS (most commonly from lung cancer, breast cancer, and melanoma) has developed substantially in recent years with the advent of effective targeted agents and immunotherapies with meaningful activity in the CNS.[108] A brief survey of selected regimens for some of the most common causes of brain metastases can be found in Table 21.3. We briefly review the evidence supporting the efficacy of immunotherapy and selected targeted agents in brain metastases given the possible extension of these therapies to the management of primary CNS malignancies.

Therapy with checkpoint inhibitors has revolutionized oncologic practice and has also shown efficacy in the treatment of brain metastases. For example, a small phase II study assessing the effect of PD-1 inhibitor pembrolizumab in patients with brain metastases from melanoma or NSCLC showed response rates of 22% and 33%, respectively.[109] The combination of another PD-1 inhibitor, nivolumab, with the CTLA-4 inhibitor ipilimumab, a standard regimen in metastatic melanoma, demonstrated even more impressive response rates in patients with brain metastases, with 26% of patients achieving a complete response and 57% deriving some clinical benefit

TABLE 21.3 Selected therapies used against metastatic disease to the central nervous system (CNS)

PRIMARY TUMOR	PARENCHYMAL METASTASES	LEPTOMENINGEAL DISEASE
Melanoma	BRAF and checkpoint inhibitors (see text)	
Non-small cell lung cancer	EGFR, ALK or NTRK inhibitors for patients with these mutations (see text) Checkpoint inhibitors for PD-L1 positive tumors (see text)	For EGFR positive patients, osimertinib or weekly pulsed erlotinib may be effective
Small cell lung cancer	Topotecan	
HER2/neu positive breast cancer	Capecitabine and lapatinib/neratinib Capecitabine Paclitaxel and neratinib	Intrathecal trastuzumab Intrathecal or high-dose methotrexate
HER2/neu negative breast cancer	Cisplatin and etoposide Cisplatin Etoposide High-dose methotrexate	Intrathecal or high-dose methotrexate
Lymphoma	High-dose methotrexate	Intrathecal rituximab

From NCCN Clinical Practice Guidelines in Oncology.[4]

in the Checkmate 204 study[110]; somewhat lower but still clinically significant response rates were reported in an Australian trial.[111] An earlier report also showed activity for ipilimumab monotherapy in patients with melanoma and brain metastases, particularly with limited disease.[112] Taken together, these results provide proof of concept that checkpoint inhibitors are active in CNS disease. Of note, pseudoprogression can occur with these treatments, as the immune response can disrupt the BBB to increase contrast enhancement and edema. This false progression can last months.

> Therapy with checkpoint inhibitors has revolutionized oncologic practice and has specifically shown efficacy in the treatment of brain metastases.

Evidence of BBB penetration and activity of targeted inhibitors in the CNS largely stem from trials in metastatic melanoma and lung cancer. Combined BRAF/MEK inhibition for BRAF-mutated tumors with the standard melanoma regimen dabrafenib/trametinib showed considerable efficacy in the COMBI-MB study although responses were not durable.[24] In lung cancer, novel ALK and EGFR inhibitors are thought to have better CNS penetration than earlier agents and show promising activity in intracranial disease[113,114]; for example, treatment with the ALK inhibitor alectinib resulted in a CNS response rate of 64% in patients with ALK-positive NSCLC metastatic to the brain,[115] and treatment with the EGFR inhibitor osimertinib among patients with T790M EGFR mutations demonstrated a response rate of 54%.[23] Last, exciting new results have emerged with TRK inhibitors larotrectinib and entrectinib: a small report in a mixed cohort of patients with primary and metastatic CNS disease harboring NTRK fusions showed universal disease control with larotrectinib with a minimum response duration of 9 months,[116] while a pooled analysis of patients with CNS metastases eligible to receive entrectinib (ROS1-positive NSCLC or NTRK-positive solid

tumor) also demonstrated robust and durable response rates.[117] More mature data are eagerly awaited.

The presence of leptomeningeal disease heralds much worse prognosis than parenchymal brain metastasis, and there are few data to guide management with systemic therapy.[114] While direct administration of chemotherapy into the CSF via the intrathecal or intraventricular route has a role in several tumor types, systemic therapy can show efficacy in some cases, suggesting that systemically administered drugs can reach the CSF in therapeutic concentrations. In addition, systemic therapy has a few potential advantages over CSF administration.[118] First, unlike intra-CSF therapy, systemic therapy can reach areas of bulky leptomeningeal disease and achieve more uniform drug distribution. In addition, it can be used safely in the presence of a CSF obstruction.[118] Examples of potentially effective systemic therapies for leptomeningeal disease include HD-MTX, osimertinib, and pembrolizumab.[118,119]

> Examples of potentially effective systemic therapies for leptomeningeal disease include HD-MTX, osimertinib, and pembrolizumab.

CONCLUSION AND FUTURE DIRECTIONS

The development of new systemic therapies for both primary and metastatic CNS tumors remains challenging despite advances in decoding disease biology and the development of novel therapies. Intrinsic biologic aggressiveness of these tumors and the singularly unfavorable environment of the CNS, which not only complicates treatment delivery but also increases potential toxicities and magnifies the impact of disease progression on quality of life and survival, are responsible for these suboptimal outcomes. Given the rarity of primary CNS malignancies and the tendency of many investigators to exclude patients with brain metastases from clinical trial populations due to their adverse prognosis, more clinical evidence to guide treatment decisions is needed. This will require coordinated conduct of clinical trials and innovative design approaches so that the maximum number of clinical questions can be addressed from a given patient sample. Significant gaps in our understanding of disease biology, especially with respect to primary CNS tumors, remain and must be transcended before more effective systemic therapies can be developed. We refer the reader to a recent consensus statement by thought leaders in the field for a more comprehensive discussion of outstanding issues and possible solutions.[120]

In spite of these obstacles, however, there is room for cautious optimism. Multiple promising therapeutic approaches from immunotherapy to CAR T and CAR NK cells, targeted agents, and even more innovative solutions such as recombinant viral vectors[121] are under development and will hopefully have a measurable impact on the outcomes of patients suffering from these devastating conditions in the near future. To this end, clinical trials serve a fundamental role in the optimal management of patients with CNS malignancies.

For targeted therapies, what do the suffixes "-ib" and "-mab" correspond to, respectively?

In general, small molecules carry the ending "-ib" (e.g., osimertinib, trametinib) and are most often oral agents, while monoclonal antibodies carry the ending "-mab" (e.g., bevacizumab, pembrolizumab) and are large proteins that need to be given intravenously

What type of treatment did Norton and Simon predict would improve outcomes in solid tumors, and why?

They predicted that "dose-dense" regimens which minimize the interval between treatments would improve outcomes in solid tumors by taking advantage of the transient increase in the growth fraction that occurs between therapy cycles

What two types of agents are likely to cross the BBB in sufficient quantities?

Lipid-soluble drugs

or

Small molecules (generally <500 Daltons)

What general treatment paradigm is effective for many subtypes of grade 2–4 gliomas?

RT plus chemotherapy (vs. RT alone)

For PCNSL, for what two reasons has first-line bimodality therapy with chemotherapy and whole-brain radiation therapy (WBRT) gradually fallen out of favor?

The high incidence of neurotoxicity with this approach and the lack of clearly demonstrated OS benefit over chemotherapy alone

Why is leucovorin an important component of HD-MTX therapy for brain tumors?

Leucovorin mitigates the effects of MTX, but does not adequately penetrate the CSF. Therefore, it can provide peripheral "salvage" from MTX toxicity without affecting its antineoplastic activity in the CNS

In addition to revolutionizing oncologic practice, what class of drugs has demonstrated efficacy in treatment of brain metastases?

Checkpoint inhibitors

What are three examples of potentially effective systemic therapies for leptomeningeal disease?

HD-MTX

Osimertinib

Pembrolizumab

QUESTIONS

1. Each of the following factors impedes delivery of chemotherapeutic drugs to the CNS *except*
   a. Drug efflux pumps
   b. High lipid solubility
   c. High protein binding of the drug
   d. Concurrent use of corticosteroids
   e. Concurrent use of hepatic enzyme inducing antiepileptic drugs

2. Which of the following agents used in the treatment of CNS malignancies would be considered "targeted therapy"?
   a. Temozolomide
   b. Lomustine
   c. Nivolumab
   d. Bevacizumab
   e. Methotrexate

3. The study of tumor kinetics provides useful conceptual tools to aid in the design of chemotherapy regimens. Which of the following statements is true?
   a. Solid tumors demonstrate an exponential growth pattern that is largely unaffected by tumor size.
   b. The Norton-Simon hypothesis explains the lack of additional benefit from dose-dense temozolomide in glioblastoma.
   c. The log kill hypothesis is applicable in primary CNS lymphoma because of its relatively indolent growth rate.
   d. The slow growth rate noted in anaplastic gliomas is related to the low growth fractions of these tumors and underlies the rationale for prolonged adjuvant therapy in this setting.

4. Which of the following is true regarding the use of alkylating agents?
   a. For GBM patients on adjuvant temozolomide, dose intense treatment (e.g., given 21 of 28 days) improves outcomes when compared to standard dosing (i.e., 5 of 28 days).
   b. The risk of pneumonitis represents a contraindication to temozolomide for patients with severe chronic obstructive pulmonary disease (COPD).
   c. Patients who receive procarbazine should avoid selective serotonin reuptake inhibitors (SSRIs) and foods high in tyramine.
   d. Patients who develop neutropenia on temozolomide should receive concurrent filgrastim (G-CSF; Neupogen) with subsequent cycles of temozolomide.

5. Which of the following is true regarding the management of patients with anaplastic gliomas?
   a. Level I evidence demonstrates that the addition of chemotherapy with PCV to radiotherapy offers a statistically significant overall survival benefit over radiotherapy alone among patients with oligodendrogliomas; similar trends were observed among patients with astrocytomas.
   b. Temozolomide demonstrated superior efficacy and side-effect profile compared to PCV in the adjuvant treatment of anaplastic glioma following surgery and radiation therapy in two recent phase III trials; these data led to its widespread adoption.
   c. The CATNON trial showed no benefit for the use of adjuvant temozolomide in grade 3 astrocytomas.
   d. Bevacizumab in combination with an alkylating agent adds a survival benefit compared to chemotherapy alone following resection of anaplastic oligodendrogliomas.

6. Mr. Brown is a 61-year-old man with a right frontal glioblastoma with symptomatic progressive disease associated with substantial vasogenic edema. For which of the following scenarios would bevacizumab be a reasonable option?
   a. Deep venous thrombosis (DVT) managed with IVC filter due to contraindication for anticoagulation
   b. Petechial hemorrhage on magnetic resonance imaging (MRI) of the brain
   c. Transient ischemic attack (TIA) 3 weeks ago
   d. Poorly controlled hypertension
   e. Two weeks postoperatively from appendectomy.

7. Ms. Young was originally diagnosed with a left parietal glioblastoma with methylation of the MGMT promoter at the age of 65. She underwent surgical resection followed by radiation with concurrent and adjuvant temozolomide which she completed 3 months ago with no significant toxicities. MRI today demonstrates progressive disease at the surgical site. Consultation with a neurosurgeon and a radiation oncologist indicates that localized treatment for the recurrence is not technically feasible. There is mild peritumoral edema. The patient has good performance status and is interested in further therapy. If the patient is not eligible for a clinical trial, which of the following agents would be most appropriate in this setting?
   a. Lomustine
   b. Rechallenge with temozolomide
   c. Etoposide
   d. Carboplatin
   e. Bevacizumab

8. Which of the following is true regarding the management of primary CNS lymphoma?
   a. A wide surgical resection leads to a durable survival advantage and increases the likelihood of response to adjuvant therapy.
   b. The combination of WBRT and induction chemotherapy has synergistic activity and is associated with increased overall survival and

minimal cognitive toxicity; as such, it is the treatment of choice for young, fit patients.

c. If a complete response is achieved with induction therapy, close surveillance is generally an appropriate next step.

d. The R-MPV regimen has been consistently shown to be superior to other induction therapies and is preferred by most practitioners.

e. A methotrexate dose of 8 mg/m^2 may reach sufficient concentrations in the vitreous and CSF to achieve response without the need for local therapy.

9. In addition to adequate antiemetics, proper adjunctive measures for high-dose cytarabine must include
   a. Peg-filgrastim given on day 1
   b. Filgrastim given on day 1
   c. Dexamethasone 8 mg at the time of antiemetics
   d. Oral leucovorin rescue for 4 days
   e. Dexamethasone eye drops for 4 days

10. Which of the following is the correct mechanism of action for the agent listed?
    a. Vincristine: Formation of DNA adducts
    b. Cytarabine: Anti-folate antimetabolite
    c. Carboplatin: Anti-microtubule agent
    d. Erlotinib: Anti-VEGF tyrosine kinase inhibitor
    e. Lomustine: Alkylating agent

11. Which of the following toxic effects are associated with the agent listed?
    a. Ibrutinib: Decreased wound healing
    b. Bevacizumab: Hypertension
    c. Temozolomide: Peripheral neuropathy
    d. Pemetrexed: Hemorrhagic cystitis
    e. Lomustine: Hypotension after rapid infusion

12. Which of the following measures can help reduce neurotoxicity associated with chemotherapy (more than one answer possible)?
    a. Dexamethasone with intrathecal cytarabine
    b. Avoidance of concurrent radiation therapy and methotrexate
    c. Glucarpidase for high-dose cytarabine
    d. Control of blood pressure in patients on bevacizumab
    e. Dose cap on vincristine

13. Several agents used for systemic malignancies have shown activity in brain metastases. All of the following statements are true *except*
    a. Ipilimumab, a CTLA4 inhibitor, can cause hypopituitarism.
    b. Therapy with immune active agents such as nivolumab can result in pseudoprogression, which can include the appearance of new enhancement and which can sometimes last for months.

c. Vemurafenib and dabrafenib are inhibitors of MGMT with activity in subsets of patients with melanoma.

d. Trametinib inhibits MEK, a component of the MAP kinase pathway.

14. All of the following are true regarding the treatment of brain metastases *except*
    a. Treatment with BRAF/MEK inhibition has shown clinical activity among patients with brain metastases from BRAF-mutant melanoma.
    b. Osimertinib penetrates the blood–brain barrier and has shown efficacy among patients with EGFR-mutated, non-small cell lung cancer that has metastasized to the brain.
    c. Checkpoint inhibitors have demonstrated activity among patients with brain metastases stemming from melanoma and non-small cell lung cancer.
    d. Larotrectinib is highly efficacious in the treatment of brain metastases from ALK-positive, non-small cell lung cancer.

15. Which of the following statements regarding the management of leptomeningeal disease is false?
    a. A phase III trial showed promising efficacy for intrathecal methotrexate for patients with leptomeningeal involvement from breast cancer.
    b. Prognosis is uniformly poor and symptom management is the main goal of therapy.
    c. Penetration of intrathecal chemotherapy in bulky leptomeningeal disease is limited to a few mm.
    d. Intrathecal targeted therapies such as rituximab in lymphoma and trastuzumab in HER2/neu-positive breast cancer may be of benefit, but additional data are needed.

ANSWERS

1. b
2. d
3. d
4. c
5. a
6. b
7. a
8. e
9. e
10. e
11. b
12. a, b, d, e
13. c
14. d
15. a

REFERENCES

1. Villano JL, Durbin EB, Normandeau C, et al. Incidence of brain metastasis at initial presentation of lung cancer. *Neuro Oncol.* Jan 2015;17(1):22–28. doi:10.1093/neuonc/nou099
2. National Cancer Institute. Brain and other nervous system cancer: Cancer Stat Facts. Mar 7 2020. https://seer.cancer.gov/statfacts/html/brain.html
3. Ostrom QT, Cioffi G, Gittleman H, et al. CBTRUS statistical report: Primary brain and other central nervous system tumors diagnosed in the United States in 2012–2016. *Neuro Oncol.* Nov 2019;21(5):v1–v100. doi:10.1093/neuonc/noz150
4. NCCN Clinical Practice Guidelines in Oncology. Mar 7 2020. https://www.nccn.org/professionals/physician_gls/default.aspx#cns
5. DeVita VT, Chu E. A history of cancer chemotherapy. *Cancer Res.* Nov 2008;68(21:8643–8653. doi:10.1158/0008-5472.CAN-07-6611
6. Alexander BM, Cloughesy TF. Adult glioblastoma. *J Clin Oncol.* Jul 2017;35(21):2402–2409. doi:10.1200/JCO.2017.73.0119
7. Van Den Bent MJ, Smits M, Kros JM, Chang SM. Diffuse infiltrating oligodendroglioma and astrocytoma. *J Clin Oncol.* Jul 2017;35(21):2394–2401. doi:10.1200/JCO.2017.72.6737
8. Grommes C, DeAngelis LM. Primary CNS lymphoma. *J Clin Oncol.* Jul 2017;35(21):2410–2418. doi:10.1200/JCO.2017.72.7602
9. Hochhaus A, Larson RA, Guilhot F, et al. Long-term outcomes of imatinib treatment for chronic myeloid leukemia. *N Engl J Med.* Mar 2017;376(10):917–927. doi:10.1056/NEJMoa1609324
10. Arbour KC, Riely GJ. Systemic therapy for locally advanced and metastatic non-small cell lung cancer: A review. *JAMA.* Aug 2019;322(8):764–774. doi:10.1001/jama.2019.11058
11. Darvin P, Toor SM, Sasidharan Nair V, Elkord E. Immune checkpoint inhibitors: Recent progress and potential biomarkers. *Exp Mol Med.* Dec 2018;50(12):1–11. doi:10.1038/s12276-018-0191-1
12. Rezvani K. Adoptive cell therapy using engineered natural killer cells. *Bone Marrow Transplant.* Aug 2019;54(2:785–788. doi:10.1038/s41409-019-0601-6
13. Ferreri AJ, Reni M, Foppoli M, et al. High-dose cytarabine plus high-dose methotrexate versus high-dose methotrexate alone in patients with primary CNS lymphoma: A randomised phase 2 trial. *Lancet.* 2009;374(9700):1512–1520. doi:10.1016/S0140-6736(09)61416-1
14. Skipper HE. Laboratory models: Some historical perspective. *Cancer Treat Rep.* Jan 1986;70(1):3–7.
15. Simon R, Norton L. The Norton-Simon hypothesis: Designing more effective and less toxic chemotherapeutic regimens. *Nat Clin Pract Oncol.* Aug 2006;3(8):406–407. doi:10.1038/ncponc0560
16. Bonadonna G, Zambetti M, Valagussa P. Sequential or alternating doxorubicin and CMF regimens in breast cancer with more than three positive nodes: Ten-year results. *JAMA.* Feb 1995;273(7):542–547. doi:10.1001/jama.1995.03520310040027
17. de Gramont A, Bosset JF, Milan C, et al. Randomized trial comparing monthly low-dose leucovorin and fluorouracil bolus with bimonthly high-dose leucovorin and fluorouracil bolus plus continuous infusion for advanced colorectal cancer: A French intergroup study. *J Clin Oncol.* 1997;15(2):808–815. doi:10.1200/JCO.1997.15.2.808
18. Gilbert MR, Wang M, Aldape KD, et al. Dose-dense temozolomide for newly diagnosed glioblastoma: A randomized phase III clinical trial. *J Clin Oncol.* Nov 2013;31(32):4085–4091. doi:10.1200/JCO.2013.49.6968
19. Herscher LL, Cook JA, Pacelli R, et al. Principles of chemoradiation: Theoretical and practical considerations. *Oncology.* 1999;13(10 Suppl. 5):11–22.
20. van den Bent MJ, Baumert B, Erridge SC, et al. Interim results from the CATNON trial (EORTC study 26053-22054) of treatment with concurrent and adjuvant temozolomide for 1p/19q non-co-deleted anaplastic glioma: A phase 3 randomised open-label intergroup study. *Lancet.* Oct 2017;390(10103):1645–1653. doi:10.1016/S0140-6736(17)31442-3
21. Van Den Bent MJ, Erridge S, Vogelbaum MA, et al. Second interim and first molecular analysis of the EORTC randomized phase III intergroup CATNON trial on concurrent and adjuvant temozolomide in anaplastic glioma without 1p/19q codeletion. *J Clin Oncol.* May 2019;37(15_Suppl):2000. doi:10.1200/jco.2019.37.15_suppl.2000
22. Deeken JF, Löscher W. The blood-brain barrier and cancer: Transporters, treatment, trojan horses. *Clin Cancer Res.* Mar 2007;13(6):1663–1674. doi:10.1158/1078-0432.CCR-06-2854
23. Goss G, Tsai C-M, Shepherd FA, et al. CNS response to osimertinib in patients with T790M-positive advanced NSCLC: Pooled data from two phase II trials. *Ann Oncol.* 2018;29(3):687–693. doi:10.1093/annonc/mdx820
24. Davies MA, Saiag P, Robert C, et al. Dabrafenib plus trametinib in patients with BRAFV600-mutant melanoma brain metastases (COMBI-MB) a multicentre multicohort open-label phase 2 trial. *Lancet Oncol.* Jul 2017;18(7):863–873. doi:10.1016/S1470-2045(17)30429-1
25. Phoenix TN, Patmore DM, Boop S, et al. Medulloblastoma genotype dictates blood brain barrier phenotype. *Cancer Cell.* Apr 2016;29(4):508–522. doi:10.1016/j.ccell.2016.03.002
26. Thompson EM, Neuwelt EA, Frenkel EP. The paradoxical effect of bevacizumab in the therapy of malignant gliomas. *Neurology.* Jan 2011;76(1):87–93. doi:10.1212/WNL.0b013e318204a3af
27. Ratnam NM, Gilbert MR, Giles AJ. Immunotherapy in CNS cancers: The role of immune cell trafficking. *Neuro Oncol.* 2019;21(1):37–46. doi:10.1093/neuonc/noy084
28. Louis DN, Perry A, Reifenberger G, et al. The 2016 World Health Organization Classification of Tumors of the Central Nervous System: A summary. *Acta Neuropathol.* Jun 2016;131(6):803–820. doi:10.1007/s00401-016-1545-1
29. Hegi ME, Diserens A-C, Gorlia T, et al. MGMT gene silencing and benefit from temozolomide in glioblastoma. *N Engl J Med.* Mar 2006;352(10):997–1003. doi:10.1056/NEJMoa043331
30. van Nifterik KA, van den Berg J, Stalpers LJA, et al. Differential radiosensitizing potential of temozolomide in MGMT promoter methylated glioblastoma multiforme cell lines. *Int J Radiat Oncol Biol Phys.* Nov 2007;69(4):1246–1253. doi:10.1016/j.ijrobp.2007.07.2366
31. Buckner JC, Shaw EG, Pugh SL, et al. Radiation plus procarbazine. CCNU, vincristine in low-grade glioma. *N Engl J Med.* Apr 2016;374(14):1344–1355. doi:10.1056/NEJMoa1500925
32. Fisher BJ, Hu C, Macdonald DR, et al. Phase 2 study of temozolomide-based chemoradiation therapy for high-risk low-grade gliomas: Preliminary results of Radiation Therapy Oncology Group 0424. *Int J Radiat Oncol Biol Phys.* Mar 2015;91(3):497–504. doi:10.1016/j.ijrobp.2014.11.012
33. Baumert BG, Hegi ME, van den Bent MJ, et al. Astro II high risk temozolomide vs RT in high-risk low-grade glioma (EORTC 22033-26033), phase 3 intergroup study. *Lancet Oncol.* Nov 2016;17(11):1521–1532. doi:10.1016/S1470-2045(16)30313-8
34. Chang S, Zhang P, Cairncross JG, et al. Phase III randomized study of radiation and temozolomide versus radiation and nitrosourea therapy for anaplastic astrocytoma: Results of NRG Oncology RTOG 9813. *Neuro Oncol.* 2017;19(2):252–258. doi:10.1093/neuonc/now236
35. Cairncross G, Wang M, Shaw E, et al. Phase III trial of chemoradiotherapy for anaplastic oligodendroglioma: Long-term results of RTOG 9402. *J Clin Oncol.* Jan 2013;31(3):337–343. doi:10.1200/JCO.2012.43.2674
36. Van Den Bent MJ, Brandes AA, Taphoorn MJB, et al. Adjuvant procarbazine, lomustine, vincristine chemotherapy in newly diagnosed anaplastic oligodendroglioma: Long-term follow-up of EORTC brain tumor group study 26951. *J Clin Oncol.* Jan 2013;31(3):344–350. doi:10.1200/JCO.2012.43.2229
37. Jaeckle K, Vogelbaum M, Ballman K, et al. CODEL (Alliance-N0577; EORTC-26081/22086; NRG-1071; NCIC-CEC-2). Phase III randomized study of RT vs. RT+TMZ vs. TMZ for newly diagnosed 1p/19q-codeleted anaplastic oligodendroglial tumors: Analysis of patients treated on the original protocol design. *Neurology.* 2015;17(Suppl 5): v4.4–v5.
38. Stupp R, Mason WP, Van Den Bent MJ, et al. Radiotherapy plus concomitant and adjuvant temozolomide for glioblastoma. *N Engl J Med.* Mar 2005;352(10):987–996. doi:10.1056/NEJMoa043330
39. Stupp R, Hegi ME, Mason WP, et al. Effects of radiotherapy with concomitant and adjuvant temozolomide versus radiotherapy alone on survival in glioblastoma in a randomised phase III study: 5-year analysis of the EORTC-NCIC trial. *Lancet Oncol.* 2009;10(5):459–466. doi:10.1016/S1470-2045(09)70025-7
40. Perry JR, Laperriere N, O'Callaghan CJ, et al. Short-course radiation plus temozolomide in elderly patients with glioblastoma. *N Engl J Med.* Mar 2017;376(11):1027–1037. doi:10.1056/NEJMoa1611977
41. Wick W, Platten M, Meisner C, et al. Temozolomide chemotherapy alone versus radiotherapy alone for malignant astrocytoma in the elderly: The NOA-08 randomised, phase 3 trial. *Lancet Oncol.* Jul 2012;13(7):707–715. doi:10.1016/S1470-2045(12)70164-X
42. Malmström A, Grønberg BH, Marosi C, et al. Temozolomide versus standard 6-week radiotherapy versus hypofractionated radiotherapy in patients older than 60 years with glioblastoma: The Nordic randomised, phase 3 trial. *Lancet Oncol.* Sep 2012;13(9):916–926. doi:10.1016/S1470-2045(12)70265-6
43. Blumenthal DT, Gorlia T, Gilbert MR, et al. Is more better? The impact of extended adjuvant temozolomide in newly diagnosed glioblastoma: A secondary analysis of EORTC and NRG Oncology/RTOG. *Neuro Oncol.* Aug 2017;19(8):1119–1126. doi:10.1093/neuonc/nox025

44. Gilbert MR, Dignam JJ, Armstrong TS, et al. A randomized trial of bevacizumab for newly diagnosed glioblastoma. *N Engl J Med.* Feb 2014;370(8):699–708. doi:10.1056/NEJMoa1308573

45. Chinot OL, Wick W, Mason W, et al. Bevacizumab plus radiotherapy-temozolomide for newly diagnosed glioblastoma. *N Engl J Med.* 2014;370(8):709–722. doi:10.1056/NEJMoa1308345

46. Herrlinger U, Tzaridis T, Mack F, et al. Lomustine-temozolomide combination therapy versus standard temozolomide therapy in patients with newly diagnosed glioblastoma with methylated MGMT promoter (CeTeG/NOA-09): A randomised, open-label, phase 3 trial. *Lancet.* Feb 2019;393(10172):678–688. doi:10.1016/S0140-6736(18)31791-4

47. Stupp R, Taillibert S, Kanner A, et al. Effect of tumor-treating fields plus maintenance temozolomide vs maintenance temozolomide alone on survival in patients with glioblastoma: A randomized clinical trial. *JAMA.* Dec 2017;318(23):2306–2316. doi:10.1001/jama.2017.18718

48. Weller M, Tabatabai G, Kästner B, et al. MGMT promoter methylation is a strong prognostic biomarker for benefit from dose-intensified temozolomide rechallenge in progressive glioblastoma: The DIRECTOR Trial. *Clin Cancer Res.* May 2015;21(9):2057–2064. doi:10.1158/1078-0432.CCR-14-2737

49. Perry JR, Bélanger K, Mason WP, et al. Phase II trial of continuous dose-intense temozolomide in recurrent malignant glioma: RESCUE study. *J Clin Oncol.* Apr 2010;28(12):2051–2057. doi:10.1200/JCO.2009.26.5520

50. Wick W, Gorlia T, Bendszus M, et al. Lomustine and bevacizumab in progressive glioblastoma. *N Engl J Med.* Nov 2017;377(20):1954–1963. doi:10.1056/NEJMoa1707358

51. Wick W, Puduvalli VK, Chamberlain MC, et al. Phase III study of enzastaurin compared with lomustine in the treatment of recurrent intracranial glioblastoma. *J Clin Oncol.* Mar 2010;28(7):1168–1174. doi:10.1200/JCO.2009.23.2595

52. Brandes AA, Tosoni A, Amistà P, et al. How effective is BCNU in recurrent glioblastoma in the modern era? A phase II trial. *Neurology.* Oct 2004;63(7):1281–1284. doi:10.1212/01.WNL.0000140495.33615.CA

53. Thompson EM, Dosa E, Kraemer DF, Neuwelt EA. Treatment with bevacizumab plus carboplatin for recurrent malignant glioma. *Neurosurgery.* Jul 2010;67(1):87–93. doi:10.1227/01.NEU.0000370918.51053.BC

54. Mrugala MM, Crew LK, Fink JR, Spence AM. Carboplatin and bevacizumab for recurrent malignant glioma. *Oncol Lett.* Nov 2012;4(5):1082–1086. doi:10.3892/ol.2012.839

55. Fulton D. Phase II study of prolonged oral therapy with etoposide (VP16) for patients with recurrent malignant glioma. *J Neurooncol.* 1996;27(2):149–155. doi:10.1007/BF00177478

56. Brandes AA, Gil-Gil M, Saran F, et al. A randomized phase II trial (TAMIGA) evaluating the efficacy and safety of continuous bevacizumab through multiple lines of treatment for recurrent glioblastoma. *Oncologist.* Apr 2019;24(4):521–528. doi:10.1634/theoncologist.2018-0290

57. Taal W, Oosterkamp HM, Walenkamp AME, et al. Single-agent bevacizumab or lomustine versus a combination of bevacizumab plus lomustine in patients with recurrent glioblastoma (BELOB trial). A randomised controlled phase 2 trial. *Lancet Oncol.* Aug 2014;15(9):943–953. doi:10.1016/S1470-2045(14)70314-6

58. Schiff D, Lee EQ, Nayak L, et al. Medical management of brain tumors and the sequelae of treatment. *Neuro Oncol.* 2015;17(4):488–504. doi:10.1093/neuonc/nou304

59. McGranahan T, Therkelsen KE, Ahmad S, Nagpal S. Current state of immunotherapy for treatment of glioblastoma. *Curr Treat Options Oncol.* Mar 2019;20(3). doi:10.1007/s11864-019-0619-4

60. Wu J, Armstrong TS, Gilbert MR. Biology and management of ependymomas. *Neuro Oncol.* Jul 2016;18(7):902–913. doi:10.1093/neuonc/now016

61. Brandes AA, Cavallo G, Reni M, et al. A multicenter retrospective study of chemotherapy for recurrent intracranial ependymal tumors in adults by the Gruppo Italiano Cooperativo di Neuro-Oncologia. *Cancer.* Jul 2005;104(1):143–148. doi:10.1002/cncr.21110

62. Chamberlain MC, Johnston SK. Temozolomide for recurrent intracranial supratentorial platinum-refractory ependymoma. *Cancer.* Oct 2009;115(20):4775–4482. doi:10.1002/cncr.24524

63. Rehman S, Brock C, Newlands ES. A case report of a recurrent intracranial ependymoma treated with temozolomide in remission 10 years after completing chemotherapy. *Am J Clin Oncol.* Feb 2006;29(1):106–107. doi:10.1097/01.coc.0000158891.09531.11

64. Green RM, Cloughesy TF, Stupp R, et al. Bevacizumab for recurrent ependymoma. *Neurology.* Nov 2009;73(20):1677–1680. doi:10.1212/WNL.0b013e3181c1df34

65. Gilbertson RJ, Bentley L, Hernan R, et al. ERBB receptor signaling promotes ependymoma cell proliferation and represents a potential novel therapeutic target for this disease. *Clin Cancer Res.* Oct 2002;8(10):3054–3064.

66. Buccoliero AM, Castiglione F, Rossi Degl'Innocenti D, et al. O6-methylguanine-DNA-methyltransferase in recurring anaplastic ependymomas: PCR and immunohistochemistry. *J Chemother.* Apr 2008;20(2):263–268. doi:10.1179/joc.2008.20.2.263

67. Gilbert M, Yuan Y, Wani K, et al. A phase II study of lapatinib and dose-dense temozolomide (TMZ) for adults with recurrent ependymoma: Patient reported outcomes (PRO) from a CERN clinical trial. *Neuro Oncol.* 2021;23(3):468–477. doi:10.1093/neuonc/noaa240. PMID: 33085768; PMCID: PMC7992893.

68. Thiel E, Korfel A, Martus P, et al. High-dose methotrexate with or without whole brain radiotherapy for primary CNS lymphoma (G-PCNSL-SG-1): A phase 3 randomised non-inferiority trial. *Lancet Oncol.* Nov 2010;11(11):1036–1047. doi:10.1016/S1470-2045(10)70229-1

69. Freireich EJ, Wiernik PH, Steensma DP. The leukemias: A half-century of discovery. *J Clin Oncol.* 2014;32(31):3463–3469. doi:10.1200/JCO.2014.57.1034

70. Grommes C, Rubenstein JL, DeAngelis LM, et al. Comprehensive approach to diagnosis and treatment of newly diagnosed primary CNS lymphoma. *Neuro Oncol.* 2019;21(3):296–305. doi:10.1093/neuonc/noy192

71. Ferreri AJM, Holdhoff M, Nayak L, Rubenstein JL. Evolving treatments for primary central nervous system lymphoma. *Am Soc Clin Oncol Educ B.* May 2019(39):454–466. doi:10.1200/edbk_242547

72. Schultz C, Scott C, Sherman W, et al. Preirradiation chemotherapy with cyclophosphamide, doxorubicin, vincristine, dexamethasone for primary CNS lymphomas: Initial report of Radiation Therapy Oncology Group protocol 88-06. *J Clin Oncol.* Feb 1996;14(2):556–564. doi:10.1200/JCO.1996.14.2.556

73. Mead GM, Bleehen NM, Gregor A, et al. A medical research council randomized trial in patients with primary cerebral non-Hodgkin lymphoma: Cerebral radiotherapy with and without cyclophosphamide, doxorubicin, vincristine, prednisone chemotherapy. *Cancer.* Sep 2000;89(6):1359–1370. doi:10.1002/1097-0142(20000915)89:6<1359::AID-CNCR21>3.0.CO;2-9

74. Shapiro WR, Young DF, Mehta BM. Methotrexate: Distribution in cerebrospinal fluid after intravenous, ventricular and lumbar injections. *N Engl J Med.* Jul 1975;293(4):161–166. doi:10.1056/NEJM197507242930402

75. Borsi JD, Moe PJ. A comparative study on the pharmacokinetics of methotrexate in a dose range of 0.5 g to 33.6 g/m2 in children with acute lymphoblastic leukemia. *Cancer.* Jul 1987;60(1):5–13. doi:10.1002/1097-0142(19870701)60:1<5::aid-cncr2820600103>3.0.co;2-d

76. Gavrilovic IT, Hormigo A, Yahalom J, et al. Long-term follow-up of high-dose methotrexate-based therapy with and without whole brain irradiation for newly diagnosed primary CNS lymphoma. *J Clin Oncol.* Oct 2006;24(28):4570–4574. doi:10.1200/JCO.2006.06.6910

77. Batchelor T, Carson K, O'Neill A, et al. Treatment of primary CNS lymphoma with methotrexate and deferred radiotherapy: A report of NABTT 96-07. *J Clin Oncol.* Mar 2003;21(6):1044–1049. doi:10.1200/JCO.2003.03.036

78. Hiraga S, Arita N, Ohnishi T, et al. Rapid infusion of high-dose methotrexate resulting in enhanced penetration into cerebrospinal fluid and intensified tumor response in primary central nervous system lymphomas. *J Neurosurg.* Aug 1999;91(2):221–230. doi:10.3171/jns.1999.91.2.0221

79. Kasenda B, Ferreri AJM, Marturano E, et al. First-line treatment and outcome of elderly patients with primary central nervous system lymphoma (PCNSL): A systematic review and individual patient data meta-analysis. *Ann Oncol.* Jul 2015;26(7):1305–1313. doi:10.1093/annonc/mdv076

80. Ferreri AJM, Reni M, Villa E. Therapeutic management of primary central nervous system lymphoma: Lessons from prospective trials. *Ann Oncol.* 2000;11(8):927–937. doi:10.1023/A:1008376412784

81. Gregory G, Arumugaswamy A, Leung T, et al. Rituximab is associated with improved survival for aggressive B cell CNS lymphoma. *Neuro Oncol.* Aug 2013;15(8):1068–1073. doi:10.1093/neuonc/not032

82. Holdhoff M, Ambady P, Abdelaziz A, et al. High-dose methotrexate with or without rituximab in newly diagnosed primary CNS lymphoma. *Neurology.* Jul 2014;83(3):235–239. doi:10.1212/WNL.0000000000000593

83. Ferreri AJM, Cwynarski K, Pulczynski E, et al. Chemoimmunotherapy with methotrexate, cytarabine, thiotepa, rituximab (MATRix regimen) in patients with primary CNS lymphoma: Results of the first randomisation of the International Extranodal Lymphoma Study Group-32 (IELSG32) phase 2 trial. *Lancet Haematol.* May 2016;3(5):e217–e227. doi:10.1016/S2352-3026(16)00036-3

84. Henson JW, Yang J, Batchelor T. Intraocular methotrexate level after high-dose intravenous infusion. *J Clin Oncol.* Apr 1999;17(4):1329. doi:10.1200/JCO.1999.17.4.1326c

85. Keep RF, Jones HC, Drewes LR. This was the year that was: Brain barriers and brain fluid research in 2019. *Fluids Barriers CNS.* Dec 2020;17(1):20. doi:10.1186/s12987-020-00181-9

86. Morris PG, Correa DD, Yahalom J, et al. Rituximab, methotrexate, procarbazine, vincristine followed by consolidation reduced-dose whole-brain radiotherapy and cytarabine in newly diagnosed primary CNS lymphoma: Final results and long-term outcome. *J Clin Oncol*. Nov 2013;31(31):3971–3979. doi:10.1200/JCO.2013.50.4910

87. Illerhaus G, Kasenda B, Ihorst G, et al. High-dose chemotherapy with autologous haemopoietic stem cell transplantation for newly diagnosed primary CNS lymphoma: A prospective, single-arm, phase 2 trial. *Lancet Haematol*. Aug 2016;3(8):e388–e397. doi:10.1016/S2352-3026(16)30050-3

88. Omuro A, Correa DD, DeAngelis LM, et al. R-MPV followed by high-dose chemotherapy with TBC and autologous stem-cell transplant for newly diagnosed primary CNS lymphoma. *Blood*. Feb 2015;125(9):1403–1410. doi:10.1182/blood-2014-10-604561

89. Ferreri AJM, Cwynarski K, Pulczynski E, et al. Whole-brain radiotherapy or autologous stem-cell transplantation as consolidation strategies after high-dose methotrexate-based chemoimmunotherapy in patients with primary CNS lymphoma: Results of the second randomisation of the International Extranodal Lymphoma Study Group-32 phase 2 trial. *Lancet Haematol*. Nov 2017;4(11):e510–e523. doi:10.1016/S2352-3026(17)30174-6

90. Houillier C, Choquet S, Touitou V, et al. Lenalidomide monotherapy as salvage treatment for recurrent primary CNS lymphoma. *Neurology*. Jan 2015;84(3):325–326. doi:10.1212/WNL.0000000000001158

91. Ghesquieres H, Chevrier M, Laadhari M, et al. Lenalidomide in combination with intravenous rituximab (REVRI) in relapsed/refractory primary CNS lymphoma or primary intraocular lymphoma: A multicenter prospective "proof of concept": Phase II study of the French Oculo-Cerebral lymphoma (LOC) Network and the Lymphoma Study Association (LYSA). *Ann Oncol*. 2019;30(4):621–628. doi:10.1093/annonc/mdz032

92. Lionakis MS, Dunleavy K, Roschewski M, et al. Inhibition of B cell receptor signaling by ibrutinib in primary CNS lymphoma. *Cancer Cell*. Jun 2017;31(6):833–843. doi:10.1016/j.ccell.2017.04.012

93. Grommes C, Tang SS, Wolfe J, et al. Phase 1b trial of an ibrutinib-based combination therapy in recurrent/refractory CNS lymphoma. *Blood*. Jan 2019;133(5):436–445. doi:10.1182/blood-2018-09-875732

94. Rubenstein JL, Li J, Chen L, et al. Multicenter phase 1 trial of intraventricular immunochemotherapy in recurrent CNS lymphoma. *Blood*. Jan 2013;121(5):745–751. doi:10.1182/blood-2012-07-440974

95. Kadoch C, Li J, Wong VS, et al. Complement activation and intraventricular rituximab distribution in recurrent central nervous system lymphoma. *Clin Cancer Res*. Feb 2014;20(4):1029–1041. doi:10.1158/1078-0432.CCR-13-0474

96. Apra C, Peyre M, Kalamarides M. Current treatment options for meningioma. *Expert Rev Neurother*. Mar 2018;18(3):241–249. doi:10.1080/14737175.2018.1429920

97. Chamberlain MC, Glantz MJ. Interferon-α for recurrent world health organization grade 1 intracranial meningiomas. *Cancer*. Oct 2008;113(8):2146–2151. doi:10.1002/cncr.23803

98. Chamberlain MC, Glantz MJ, Fadul CE. Recurrent meningioma: Salvage therapy with long-acting somatostatin analogue. *Neurology*. Sep 2007;69(10):969–973. doi:10.1212/01.wnl.0000271382.62776.b7

99. Kaley TJ, Wen P, Schiff D, et al. Phase II trial of sunitinib for recurrent and progressive atypical and anaplastic meningioma. *Neuro Oncol*. Jan 2015;17(1):116–121. doi:10.1093/neuonc/nou148

100. Nayak L, Iwamoto FM, Rudnick JD, et al. Atypical and anaplastic meningiomas treated with bevacizumab. *J Neurooncol*. Aug 2012;109(1):187–193. doi:10.1007/s11060-012-0886-4

101. Lou E, Sumrall AL, Turner S, et al. Bevacizumab therapy for adults with recurrent/progressive meningioma: A retrospective series. *J Neurooncol*. Aug 2012;109(1):63–70. doi:10.1007/s11060-012-0861-0

102. Shih KC, Chowdhary S, Rosenblatt P, et al. A phase II trial of bevacizumab and everolimus as treatment for patients with refractory, progressive intracranial meningioma. *J Neurooncol*. Sep 2016;129(2):281–288. doi:10.1007/s11060-016-2172-3

103. Majd N, Penas-Prado M. Updates on management of adult medulloblastoma. *Curr Treat Options Oncol*. Aug 2019;20(8):64. https://doi.org/10.1007/s11864-019-0663-0

104. Mascarin M, Coassin E, Franceschi E, et al. Medulloblastoma and central nervous system germ cell tumors in adults: Is pediatric experience applicable? *Child Nerv Syst*. Dec 2019;35(12):2279–2287. doi:10.1007/s00381-019-04340-8

105. Moots PL, O'neill A, Londer H, et al. Preradiation chemotherapy for adult high-risk medulloblastoma. *Am J Clin Oncol Cancer Clin Trials*. 2018;41(6):588–594. doi:10.1097/COC.0000000000000326

106. Beier D, Proescholdt M, Reinert C, et al. Multicenter pilot study of radiochemotherapy as first-line treatment for adults with medulloblastoma (NOA-07). *Neuro Oncol*. Feb 2018;20(3):400–410. doi:10.1093/neuonc/nox155

107. Robinson GW, Orr BA, Wu G, et al. Vismodegib exerts targeted efficacy against recurrent sonic hedgehog—Subgroup medulloblastoma: Results from phase II Pediatric Brain Tumor Consortium studies PBTC-025B and PBTC-032. *J Clin Oncol*. Aug 2015;33(24):2646–2654. doi:10.1200/JCO.2014.60.1591

108. Boire A, Brastianos PK, Garzia L, Valiente M. Brain metastasis. *Nat Rev Cancer*. Jan 2020;20(1):4–11. doi:10.1038/s41568-019-0220-y

109. Goldberg SB, Gettinger SN, Mahajan A, et al. Pembrolizumab for patients with melanoma or non-small-cell lung cancer and untreated brain metastases: Early analysis of a non-randomised, open-label, phase 2 trial. *Lancet Oncol*. Jul 2016;17(7):976–983. doi:10.1016/S1470-2045(16)30053-5

110. Tawbi HA, Forsyth PA, Algazi A, et al. Combined nivolumab and ipilimumab in melanoma metastatic to the brain. *N Engl J Med*. Aug 2018;379(8):722–730. doi:10.1056/NEJMoa1805453

111. Long GV, Atkinson V, Lo S, et al. Combination nivolumab and ipilimumab or nivolumab alone in melanoma brain metastases: A multicentre randomised phase 2 study. *Lancet Oncol*. May 2018;19(5):672–681. doi:10.1016/S1470-2045(18)30139-6

112. Margolin K, Ernstoff MS, Hamid O, et al. Ipilimumab in patients with melanoma and brain metastases: An open-label, phase 2 trial. *Lancet Oncol*. May 2012;13(5):459–465. doi:10.1016/S1470-2045(12)70090-6

113. Aizer AA, Lee EQ. Brain metastases. *Neurol Clin*. Aug 2018;36(3):557–577. doi:10.1016/j.ncl.2018.04.010

114. Wang N, Bertalan MS, Brastianos PK. Leptomeningeal metastasis from systemic cancer: Review and update on management. *Cancer*. Jan 2018;124(1):21–35. doi:10.1002/cncr.30911

115. Gandhi L, Ignatius Ou SH, Shaw AT, et al. Efficacy of alectinib in central nervous system metastases in crizotinib-resistant ALK-positive non–small-cell lung cancer: Comparison of RECIST 1.1 and RANO-HGG criteria. *Eur J Cancer*. Sep 2017;82:27–33. doi:10.1016/j.ejca.2017.05.019

116. Drilon AE, DuBois SG, Farago AF, et al. Activity of larotrectinib in TRK fusion cancer patients with brain metastases or primary central nervous system tumors. *J Clin Oncol*. May 2019;37(15_Suppl):2006. doi:10.1200/jco.2019.37.15_suppl.2006

117. Siena S, Doebele RC, Shaw AT, et al. Efficacy of entrectinib in patients (pts) with solid tumors and central nervous system (CNS) metastases: Integrated analysis from three clinical trials. *J Clin Oncol*. May 2019;37(15_Suppl):3017. doi:10.1200/jco.2019.37.15_suppl.3017

118. Glantz MJ, Cole BF, Recht L, et al. High-dose intravenous methotrexate for patients with nonleukemic leptomeningeal cancer: Is intrathecal chemotherapy necessary? *J Clin Oncol*. Apr 1998;16(4):1561–1567. doi:10.1200/JCO.1998.16.4.1561

119. Le Rhun E, Preusser M, van den Bent M, et al. How we treat patients with leptomeningeal metastases. *ESMO Open*. 2019;4(Suppl 2):e000507. doi:10.1136/esmoopen-2019-000507

120. Aldape K, Brindle KM, Chesler L, et al. Challenges to curing primary brain tumours. *Nat Rev Clin Oncol*. Aug 2019;16(8):509–520. doi:10.1038/s41571-019-0177-5

121. Desjardins A, Gromeier M, Herndon JE, et al. Recurrent glioblastoma treated with recombinant poliovirus. *N Engl J Med*. Jul 2018;379(2):150–161. doi:10.1056/NEJMoa1716435

22 | DEVICE-BASED TREATMENTS IN NEURO-ONCOLOGY

EKOKOBE FONKEM, AMIR AZADI, AND RAMYA TADIPATRI

INTRODUCTION

Glioblastoma heterogeneity has posed significant challenges in developing therapies. A major limitation of many cancer treatments is poor therapeutic index given the side-effect profile of many chemotherapeutic agents. In addition, GBM is an aggressive tumor that can have debilitating symptoms including seizures, headaches, and focal neurological deficits, which can result in significant limitations in quality of life. This is compounded by the difficulty in identifying therapeutic targets for drug development. On the other hand, although it is a diffusely infiltrative tumor, it almost never metastasizes and is therefore potentially suitable for regional therapy.

> GBM is a diffusely infiltrative tumor that almost never metastasizes and is therefore potentially suitable for regional therapy.

For these reasons, GBM has been an ideal target for developing therapeutic devices. Devices that provide regional therapy include tumor-treating fields (TTFields, Optune), carmustine wafers (Gliadel), GammaTile, Nativis Voyager, laser interstitial thermal therapy devices (NeuroBlate, Visualase), and Tumor Monorail. TTFields, Nativis Voyager, NeuroBlate, and Tumor Monorail rely on physical rather than biological or chemical mechanisms, so they are less likely to be dependent on a particular cellular feature.

These devices have shown much promise overall and in some cases have significantly improved survival in glioblastoma patients.

TUMOR-TREATING FIELDS

Tumor treating fields (TTFields, Optune) are low intensity alternating electric fields which disrupt mitosis and inhibit tumor growth (Figure 22.1). They were approved by the US Food and Drug Administration (FDA) for recurrent GBM in 2011[1] and newly diagnosed GBM in 2015.[2] TTFields have demonstrated significant benefit in overall survival (OS) and progression-free survival (PFS) when combined with concurrent radiation and temozolomide (TMZ).[3]

Electric fields have been demonstrated to affect cellular and tissue function in various ways depending on field frequency. Direct current and low-frequency alternating fields (<1 kHz) alter membrane polarization and induce either excitatory or inhibitory effects on neuronal and muscle tissue. High-frequency alternating fields (MHz range) are more disruptive and instead cause friction, characterized by fast oscillation of polar molecules, leading to tissue heating. These high-frequency fields have traditionally been utilized for diathermy and tissue ablation. Intermediate-frequency alternating fields (several hundred kHz), which are too fast to stimulate or inhibit neuronal and muscle tissue and too slow to induce significant heating, had not been considered for medical applications until recently.[4-6]

Since the early 2000s, studies have shown that intermediate-frequency electric fields disrupt cell division in cancer cells. In 2004, a study by Kirson et al. showed that 24-hour exposure of 11 cancer cell lines to a frequency of 100 kHz and intensities of 1.0–1.4 V/cm caused significant mitotic inhibition which was observed up to 72 hours post-treatment, while noncancerous kidney cells were unaffected, suggesting selectivity for cells undergoing rapid cellular division. Fields were generated by pairs of insulated wires fixed to the bottom of culture dishes and connected to an oscillator and high-voltage amplifier. It was further demonstrated that there is an optimal frequency for maximal inhibition which is inversely related to cell size, established to be 200 kHz across all malignant glioma cell lines. Cell growth rates begin to decrease when the field intensity exceeds approximately 1 V/cm and achieve complete growth arrest at approximately 2.5 V/cm. TTFields were thus defined as alternating electric fields in the frequency range of 100–500 kHz and intensities ranging from 1 to 3 V/cm.[7]

Additional studies investigating the mechanism of mitotic disturbance have shown that TTFields lead to prolonged mitosis, formation of abnormal mitotic figures, and mitotic cell death. During telophase, dividing cells have an hourglass shape which is theorized to disrupt the uniformity of the intrinsic cellular electric field, resulting in dielectrophoretic (DEP) forces. This may result in proteins with large dipole moments, such as tubulin and septin, aligning with the electric field, thus disrupting microtubule polymerization and interfering with chromosome segregation. This effect is likened to drugs such as paclitaxel or vinca alkaloids which directly interfere with microtubule polymerization. Failure of septin to migrate to the cell mid-zone is thought to lead to violent membrane blebbing during telophase, resulting in formation of abnormal daughter cells and induction of cell death during the following interphase. However, an in-depth analysis by Tuszynski et al. found

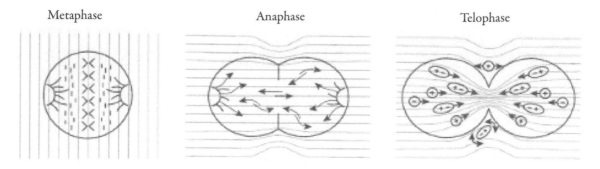

Metaphase   Anaphase   Telophase

Figure 22.1 Tumor-treating fields (TTFields) mechanism of action. TTFields act on rapidly dividing cancer cells by disrupting the mitotic spindles that assemble during the metaphase/anaphase of mitosis. TTFields also induce disruptive electric fields within cancer cells that affect intracellular organelles and macromolecules, causing abnormal chromosomal segregation and multinucleation (telophase) affecting further replication of daughter cells.

that although DEP forces are strong enough to interfere with mitosis, the forces and torques generated by electric field effect on tubulin dipoles were too small to significantly affect tubulin alignment.[4,8]

> TTFields lead to prolonged mitosis, formation of abnormal mitotic figures, and mitotic cell death.

TTFields exert numerous other secondary antitumor effects. In vitro studies using wound healing and Boyden chamber assays have demonstrated significant reduction in human glioma cell migration and invasion. TTFields have also been found to suppress angiogenesis by down-regulating vascular endothelial growth factor (VEGF), HIF1alpha, and matrix metalloproteinases 2 and 9,[9] and to inhibit DNA repair by down-regulating BRCA1.[10] Irradiating non-small cell lung cancer (NSCLC) cells in the presence of TTFields resulted in an increased number of double-strand breaks, chromatid aberrations, and radical oxygen species. Furthermore, TTFields have been shown to facilitate immunogenic cell death in lung and ovarian cancer cells by increasing cell surface calreticulin expression, decreasing intracellular adenosine triphosphate (ATP) levels, and promoting HMGB1 secretion.[11] Combining TTFields with immune checkpoint inhibitors significantly decreased tumor volume compared with either therapy alone,[12] and synergistic effects have also been demonstrated with cytotoxic chemotherapeutic agents including paclitaxel, doxorubicin, and dacarbazine.[3]

Cell orientation was also found to be a factor in determining susceptibility to TTFields. An in vitro study by Kirson et al. testing different angles of cellular orientation relative to the electric field at different stages of mitosis revealed that alignment parallel to the field resulted in a significantly higher fraction of damaged cells at all stages of mitosis.[7] Periodically switching the field between two orthogonal field directions was found to be 20% more effective than applying a single-direction field.[4]

> For TTFields, periodically switching the field between two orthogonal field directions was found to be 20% more effective than applying a single-direction field.

The first-generation Optune system, known as NovoTTF-100A, was developed by Novocure in Haifa, Israel. It is an external and transportable TTField therapeutic medical device comprised of an electric field generator and insulated ceramic transducer array with a total weight of approximately 6 pounds. Transducer arrays are placed on the patient's shaved scalp and allow the patient to proceed with usual daily activities during use. A second-generation system known as NovoTTF-200A was later developed, with a reduced weight of 2.7 pounds and the battery incorporated into the device (Figure 22.2). The improved portability and convenience of the second-generation device improved compliance from 70% of patients with greater than 75% compliance to 90% of patients with greater than 75% compliance.[3,8,13,14]

The first human pilot study was conducted between 2004 and 2007 using the NovoTTF-100A system (later known as Optune) developed by Novocure. It was tested in 10 patients with recurrent glioblastoma, and subjects had a median OS of 62.2 weeks and a median time to progression of 26.1 weeks.[15] Subsequently, the EF-11 phase III trial for recurrent glioblastoma was conducted between 2006 and 2009 comparing NovoTTF-100A to best physician's choice chemotherapy, which included bevacizumab, irinotecan, BCNU/CCNU, carboplatin, TMZ, and procarbazine, CCNU, and vincristine (PCV). Patients receiving NovoTTF-100A had a similar OS of 6.6 months, compared with 6 months for other treatments, but had a significantly more favorable safety profile. This led to FDA approval of the NovoTTF-100A system for recurrent glioblastoma in 2011.[1]

The EF-14 phase III trial was conducted in newly diagnosed glioblastoma patients following initial treatment with concurrent radiation and TMZ. After completion of radiochemotherapy, patients were randomized to receive either TTFields with adjuvant TMZ or TMZ monotherapy. Median OS was 20.9 months from randomization for the TTFields plus TMZ arm compared with 16 months for the TMZ monotherapy arm (p < 0.001). Median PFS was 6.7 months from randomization for the TTFields plus TMZ arm compared with 4 months for the TMZ monotherapy arm (p < 0.001). This led to FDA approval of the NovoTTF-100A system for newly diagnosed glioblastoma.[16] TTFields has also been FDA approved for treatment of malignant mesothelioma and is under investigation in a number of other solid tumors as well as in brain metastases.

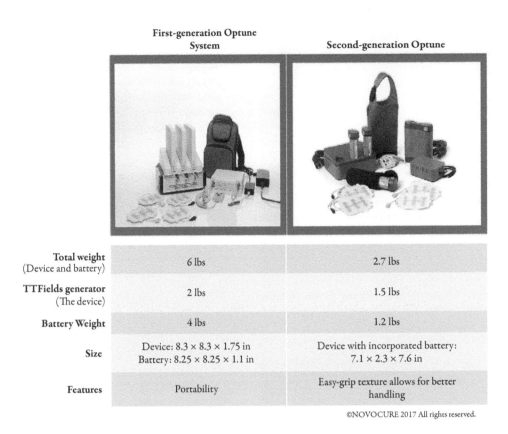

	First-generation Optune System	Second-generation Optune
Total weight (Device and battery)	6 lbs	2.7 lbs
TTFields generator (The device)	2 lbs	1.5 lbs
Battery Weight	4 lbs	1.2 lbs
Size	Device: 8.3 × 8.3 × 1.75 in Battery: 8.25 × 8.25 × 1.1 in	Device with incorporated battery: 7.1 × 2.3 × 7.6 in
Features	Portability	Easy-grip texture allows for better handling

Figure 22.2 Comparison of first- and second- generation Optune systems for glioblastoma.

> Median OS was 20.9 months from randomization for the TTFields plus TMZ arm compared with 16 months for the TMZ monotherapy arm (p < 0.001).

Although improved efficacy and low rate of systemic toxicities were observed in the EF-14 trial, 43% of patients experienced mild to moderate skin irritation, with 2% experiencing severe skin reactions. Prophylactic management was proposed in order to minimize these reactions, including frequent shifting of transducer array locations, avoidance of placing arrays on surgical scars, and maximizing transducer array–skin contact.[17]

The NovoTAL system was developed in an effort to optimize treatment array layouts based on tumor location and has been FDA approved. Using this platform, the physician first inputs 20 head and tumor measurements taken from T1 postcontrast MRI images. The NovoTAL system then chooses the layout most applicable to the patient from a selection of multiple stored precalculated array layouts. It allows for remapping and modification of the array layout with changes in tumor size, and it has been demonstrated to be reliable and reproducible.[18–20]

CARMUSTINE WAFERS

Carmustine (1,3-bis[2-chloroethyl]-1-nitrosourea [BCNU]) is an FDA-approved medication for recurrent glioblastoma (Gliadel). It exerts its effects through alkylating nucleoproteins

and interfering with DNA synthesis and repair.[21] It has been used as early as the 1960s with reported clinical response rates of up to 30%. A retrospective review of 35 patients treated with intravenous BCNU on days 1 to 3 every 8 weeks showed a median PFS of 11 weeks and median OS of 22 weeks, comparable to historical data on recurrent glioblastoma showing a median PFS of 9 weeks and a median OS of 25 weeks. Observed toxicities included thrombocytopenia, leukopenia, anemia, infection, pulmonary embolism, and interstitial lung fibrosis.[22,23]

Carmustine wafers are biodegradable polymers containing 3.85% BCNU. They were developed in the 1990s to overcome the limitations of blood–brain barrier impermeability to antineoplastic agents. BCNU was selected as the best candidate for incorporation into the polymer due to its documented efficacy. Gliadel wafers employ a controlled-release delivery method and are implanted into the resection cavity (Figures 22.3 and 22.4). Each wafer typically supplies 7.7 mg BCNU over the course of 5 days.[21,24]

A phase III clinical trial with 222 patients with recurrent glioblastoma compared carmustine wafers to placebo wafers and demonstrated an increase in median OS from 23 to 31 weeks (p = 0.006). This was followed by a phase III trial with 32 patients investigating use of carmustine wafers in newly diagnosed glioblastoma that demonstrated an increase in median OS from 39.9 to 58.1 weeks (p = 0.012). A larger phase III trial with 240 patients confirmed this finding, with median OS increased from 11.6 to 13.9 months (p = 0.03). This led to FDA approval of carmustine wafers for treatment of recurrent glioblastoma in 1997 and newly diagnosed

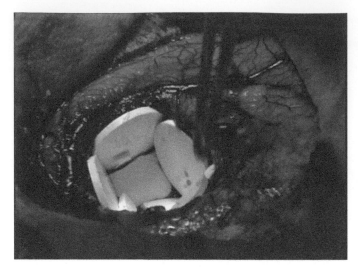

Figure 22.3 *Surgical implantation of Gliadel wafers. Up to eight wafers may be placed to cover as much of the resection cavity as possible.*

Courtesy of Henry Brem, MD, Johns Hopkins School of Medicine.

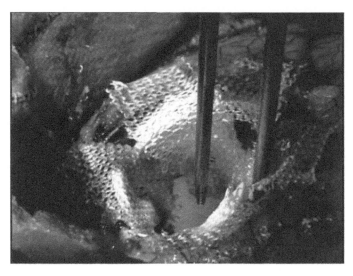

Figure 22.4 *Surgical placement of Surgicel to secure wafers against the cavity surface.*

Courtesy of Henry Brem MD, Johns Hopkins School of Medicine.

grade 3 and grade 4 glioma in 2003. A systematic review of 11 clinical trials supported the use of multimodal therapy combining carmustine wafers with radiotherapy and adjuvant TMZ, with a median OS of 18.2 months and weighted mean of PFS of 9.7 months, with no significant increase in toxicity.[24]

Carmustine wafers are FDA approved for both newly diagnosed and recurrent GBM. Neuro-oncologists should carefully evaluate each patient for potential use of this therapy, keeping in mind side-effect profile and future clinical trial eligibility. Lack of systemic toxicity makes this treatment useful for patients with chronic neutropenia and thrombocytopenia.

GAMMATILE

Brachytherapy is a method of using radioactive isotopes to deliver ionizing radiation directly to the tumor bed. Unstable nuclei break down into more stable forms, releasing high-energy gamma rays into surrounding tissue. Through the Compton and photoelectric effects, electrons are released and atomic bonds are disrupted. Isotopes used most frequently in treatment of glioblastoma are I-125 and 192-Ir. Low-dose rate brachytherapy delivers 5–20 cGy/hr, most commonly with I-125, and minimizes toxicity to normal brain tissue, allowing repair of sublethal damage even during radiation. High-dose rate brachytherapy, which may utilize I-125 or 192-Ir, delivers at least 30 cGy/hr, leading to shorter procedure times and less patient discomfort, but this typically results in greater damage to normal brain tissue and more adverse events. There have been variable outcomes with each of these techniques, but the majority of studies reported survival advantages over standard of care. High-dose brachytherapy appears to offer better local tumor control and patient outcomes, although risk of radiation-related complications such as brain necrosis increases.[25]

GammaTile, also known as *surgically targeted radiation therapy* (STaRT), was developed by GT Medical Technologies. It is a permanent brachytherapy implant which improves upon previous brachytherapy methods by optimizing interseed spacing, minimizing source-to-brain contact, and functioning as a multiseed carrier, thus hastening the implant process. Each tile contains four encapsulated radioactive Cs-131 seeds embedded in collagen (Figure 22.5). In a prospective trial with 79 recurrent previously irradiated tumors, including 40 high-grade gliomas, patients were implanted with GammaTile. Median treatment site local control and median OS were each 12 months for high-grade gliomas. The rate of adverse surgical events was minimal, ranging from 1.3% to 2.5%, and symptomatic radiation brain changes occurred in 7.6% of cases.[26] This led to FDA approval of GammaTile for recurrent glioblastoma in 2019.

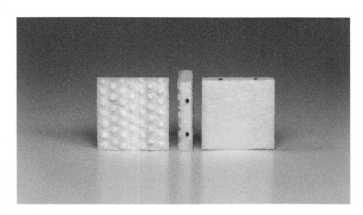

Figure 22.5 *GammaTile implants.*

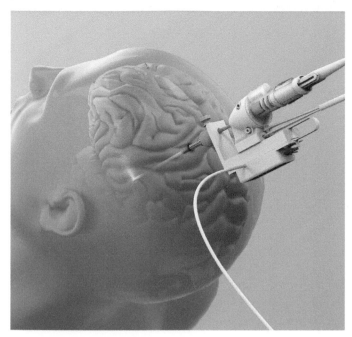

Figure 22.6 NeuroBlate system.

Used with permission. © 2020 Monteris Medical.

LASER INTERSTITIAL THERMAL THERAPY

Evidence has suggested that aggressive surgical treatment in glioblastoma patients improves outcomes, with extent of resection correlating with survival.[27] However, feasibility of extensive surgical resection is often limited by tumor location and invasion. Laser interstitial thermal therapy (LITT), also known as *stereotactic laser ablation* (SLA), is a minimally invasive alternative to open surgery developed in the 1980s and has been used to remove epileptogenic zones, deep-seated intracranial tumors, and recurrent metastases.[28]

LITT involves use of high-intensity laser light to induce thermocoagulative necrosis. The probe is constructed from an optical fiber tube or flexible catheter with a light-diffusing tip. The target tissue is identified stereotactically, a hole is drilled into the skull at that location, and the probe is placed over the tissue. The energy is converted from light to heat within the tissue and induces enzymes leading to protein denaturation, membrane dissolution, and vessel sclerosis.[28] LITT has been in use as an ablative treatment for glioma and other tumors for more than two decades.[29]

> LITT involves use of high-intensity laser light to induce thermocoagulative necrosis.

The NeuroBlate System was developed by Monteris Medical, Inc. and allows for more accurate prediction of thermal tissue damage in real time based on temperature and duration of thermal exposure. It utilizes a side-firing laser probe equipped with software that performs these calculations (Figures 22.6 and 22.7).[29] The Visualase system, developed by Visualase, Inc., is a similar system that also predicts thermal tissue damage in real time. It uses a 15 W, 980 nm diode laser; a 1.6 mm diameter probe with silicon fiberoptic core and light-diffusing tip surrounded by an outer cooling sheath, and an image-processing workstation.[30]

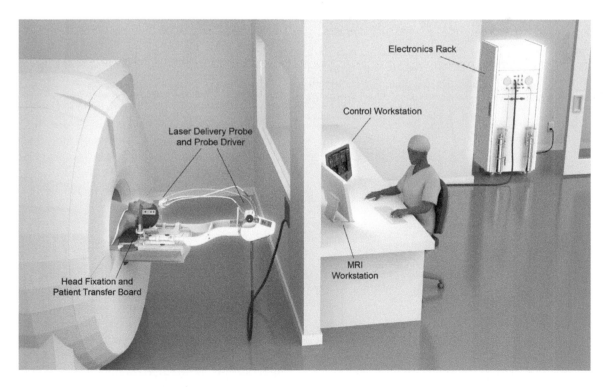

Figure 22.7 NeuroBlate system workflow.

Used with permission. © 2020 Monteris Medical.

A phase I study at Case Comprehensive Cancer Center tested the NeuroBlate System in 10 patients with recurrent glioblastoma and demonstrated a median survival of 316 days; three patients had grade 3 adverse events at the highest dose.[29] A review of survival outcomes in newly diagnosed glioblastoma compared to a matched cohort of biopsy-only patients showed comparable survival effects, and it further demonstrated that extent of tumor ablation by thermal damage threshold lines was prognostic.[31] The NeuroBlate system has also been combined with minimally invasive transsulcal resection using a tubular retracting system for large and difficult to access brain tumors, although conclusions on survival impact could not be drawn.[32]

EXPERIMENTAL APPROACHES

VOYAGER

The Voyager system was developed by EMulate Therapeutics (formerly known as Nativis) for potential uses in cancer, chronic pain, and inflammatory diseases and is specifically being investigated for use in glioblastoma treatment. It is a noninvasive nonthermal, nonionizing portable medical device that uses localized ultra-low (0–22 kHz) radiofrequency energy (u/RFE). It consists of a battery-operated controller, an electromagnetic coil, and a battery charger. The electromagnetic coil is worn on the patient's head and connected to the controller, and the system is designed for the patient to proceed with daily activities during use, much like the Optune device. However, the Voyager device is much lighter, with the controller weighing only 2.7 ounces and approximately the size of a pager (Figures 22.8 and 22.9).[33]

The physics underlying the mechanism of action involves the ability of a time-varying magnetic field to exert force on a point charge through a process known as *magnetic induction* (Lorentz force). The u/RFE signal, referred to as a "cognate," is obtained from solvated molecules using a direct-current superconducting quantum interference device. A sample of the solvated molecule of interest is placed in a magnetically

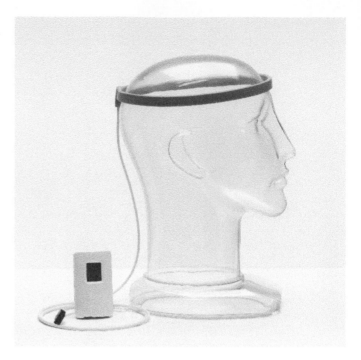

Figure 22.9 Voyager device as worn by a patient.

shielded Faraday cage, centered within the gradiometer, in order to produce the cognate. Two u/RFE cognates in particular have been studied. The cognate A1A acts on the distribution of charge within the beta-tubulin monomer through magnetic induction, forcing a conformational change that strengthens bonds between monomers and dimers, thus leading to multinucleation and disrupting mitotic spindle activity during metaphase. The cognate A2HU is derived from siRNA sequences known to inhibit expression of CTLA-4 and PD-1, so it can create magnetic fields that reduce the expression of these proteins.[33]

An early feasibility study using the A1A cognate in 11 patients with recurrent glioblastoma demonstrated median OS of 16 months for Voyager alone and 11 months for Voyager combined with standard of care, concluding that the device was safe and feasible.[33] An Australian feasibility study with 15 patients with recurrent glioblastoma showed median OS of 8.04 months in the A1A treatment arm and 6.89 months in the A2HU treatment arm and also concluded that the device was safe and feasible.[34]

CONVECTION-ENHANCED DELIVERY

Convection-enhanced delivery was developed in 1994 as another method of overcoming the blood–brain barrier. It involves stereotactic intratumoral insertion of a cannula or catheter for delivery of therapeutics. It relies on bulk flow kinetics and pressure gradients, as opposed to concentration gradients utilized in diffusion-based therapies, thus allowing for delivery to the tumor in higher quantities with less toxic doses. Clinical trial results have been variable due to differences in choice of agent, cannula design, and cannula placement. Other limitations include tumor heterogeneity

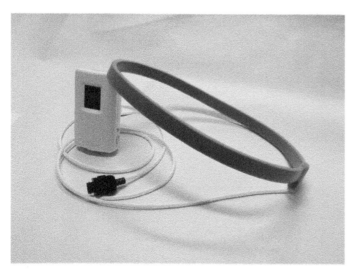

Figure 22.8 Voyager device components, including electromagnetic coil (headband), controller, and cable.

resulting in physical and physiological barriers preventing full tumor distribution, as well as infusate reflux, which occurs when the pressure gradient equalizes. These technical challenges have yet to be addressed prior to translation into successful clinical trials.[35,36]

TUMOR MONORAIL

Glioblastoma cells tend to invade and migrate along white matter tracts and blood vessels. In 2014, a group of researchers at Georgia Tech and Emory University developed a device designed to mimic these white matter tracts and blood vessels in order to guide invasive tumor cells away from the primary tumor site to an extracortical location that can easily be evacuated. A 2.4 mm diameter conduit was constructed using polycaprolactone (PCL)/polyurethane and contained PCL nanofibers aligned to mimic the topography of white matter tracts and blood vessels. These nanofibers were then coated with laminin. The conduit was attached to a "sink" consisting of a collagen hydrogel conjugated with cyclopamine in order to exploit overexpression of the sonic hedgehog (SHH) pathway in glioblastoma cells and exert cytotoxic effect.[37]

When implanted in rat brains that had been inoculated with glioblastoma cells, the PCL nanofiber film conduit contained more tumor cells than the smooth PCL film conduit or the empty conduit, suggesting that it effectively promoted tumor migration. It also resulted in significantly decreased tumor volume inside the brain compared with either the smooth PCL film conduit or the empty conduit. The cytotoxic effect of the cyclopamine-conjugated collagen hydrogel was demonstrated in vitro, with increased cell death compared to collagen alone.[37]

This device was adapted for human use at Duke University and was dubbed the "Tumor Monorail." Although it has not yet been approved by the FDA, it has been designated as a "breakthrough device" for expedited review.

What frequency of electric fields are used in TTFields?

Intermediate frequency (100–500 kHz)

What physical effect on cells does TTFields have?

Primarily disrupt cells undergoing mitosis through disruption of microtubules and a variety of other mechanisms

What was the efficacy impact of the addition of the TTFields device to initial chemoradiation for newly diagnosed glioblastoma patients?

Improvement in overall survival of newly diagnosed patients from 16 months to 20.9 months ($p < 0.001$), and improvement in progression-free survival from 4 months to 6.7 months ($p < 0.001$)

What was the efficacy impact of carmustine wafer placement for newly diagnosed glioblastoma patients?

Improvement in overall survival from 11.6 to 13.9 months ($p = 0.03$)

What is GammaTile?

A form of brachytherapy using Cs-131 seeds embedded in collagen

What is the clinical impact of laser interstitial therapy?

It has demonstrated comparable survival in newly diagnosed glioblastoma patients when compared with patients who undergo biopsy only

How does the Voyager system work?

It uses ultra-low (0–22 kHz) radiofrequency signals known as "cognates," which are derived from particular molecules, to exert targeted force on a point charge and induce conformational changes

QUESTIONS

1. What is the frequency range of TTFields?
   a. <1 kHz
   b. 1–22 kHz
   c. 100–500 kHz
   d. 1–22 MHz
   e. 100–500 MHz

2. What is the intensity range of TTFields?
   a. <1 V/cm
   b. 1–3 V/cm
   c. 3–5 V/cm
   d. 5–7 V/cm
   e. 7–10 V/cm

3. TTFields have been theorized to exert their effects through all the following mechanisms *except*
   a. Disrupting microtubule polymerization and interfering with chromosome segregation
   b. Down-regulating VEGF, HIF1alpha, and matrix metalloproteinases 2 and 9
   c. Inhibiting DNA repair by down-regulating BRCA1
   d. Alkylating nucleoproteins and interfering with DNA synthesis and repair
   e. Facilitating immunogenic cell death by increasing cell surface calreticulin expression, decreasing intracellular ATP levels, and promoting HMGB1 secretion

4. Which method was demonstrated to maximize susceptibility to tumor-treating fields?
   a. Maintaining a single direction field
   b. Periodically switching between two parallel field directions
   c. Periodically switching between two orthogonal fields directions
   d. Periodically switching the field on and off
   e. Simultaneously applying fields in two orthogonal field directions

5. What is an advantage of the second-generation Optune system?
   a. Improved portability
   b. Improved efficacy
   c. Decreased time of use required to achieve similar results
   d. Fewer side effects
   e. Decreased cost

6. With the second-generation Optune system, what is the percentage of patients who are >75% compliant?
   a. 60%
   b. 70%
   c. 80%
   d. 90%
   e. 100%

7. What is the median overall survival of glioblastoma patients who are treated with the Stupp regimen followed by TTFields combined with adjuvant temozolomide?
   a. 4 months
   b. 7 months
   c. 10 months
   d. 15 months
   e. 20 months

8. What is the median progression-free survival of glioblastoma patients who are treated with the Stupp regimen followed by TTFields combined with adjuvant temozolomide?
   a. 4 months
   b. 7 months
   c. 10 months
   d. 15 months
   e. 20 months

9. What challenge was the Gliadel wafer primarily designed to overcome?
   a. Blood–brain barrier impermeability
   b. Systemic toxicity
   c. Adverse effects of radiation
   d. Impaired quality of life
   e. High cost of care

10. What was the rationale behind selecting BCNU for use in development of the Gliadel wafer?
    a. Improved efficacy compared with temozolomide
    b. Improved safety profile compared with temozolomide
    c. Improved drug availability compared with temozolomide
    d. Compatibility with polymer drug delivery system
    e. Documented efficacy due to early use

11. What radioactive agent is used in GammaTile?
    a. I-125
    b. Ir-192
    c. Cs-131
    d. Pd-103
    e. Co-60

12. Which physics principle underlies the mechanism of action of the Voyager device?
    a. Strong nuclear force
    b. Weak nuclear force
    c. Gravitational force
    d. Electromotive force
    e. Lorentz force

13. What is one difference between the Optune and Voyager devices?
    a. Optune uses intermediate frequency (100–500 kHz) waves while Voyager uses low frequency (0–22 kHz) waves.

b. Optune uses low frequency (0–22 kHz) waves while Voyager uses intermediate frequency (100–500 kHz) waves.

c. Optune uses intermediate frequency (100–500 kHz) waves while Voyager uses high frequency (MHz range) waves.

d. Optune uses high frequency (MHz range) waves while Voyager uses intermediate frequency (100–500 kHz) waves.

e. Optune uses low frequency (0–22 kHz) waves while Voyager uses high frequency (MHz range) waves.

14. NeuroBlate was developed based on which previously used surgical technology?
a. Electrocauterization
b. Cryoablation
c. Radiofrequency ablation
d. Laser interstitial thermal therapy
e. Ultrasonic devices

15. What is the Tumor Monorail conduit designed to mimic?
a. Brain parenchyma
b. Blood vessels and white matter tracts
c. Neuronal axons and dendrites
d. Meninges
e. Ventricles and cisternae

ANSWERS

1. c
2. b
3. d
4. c
5. a
6. d
7. e
8. b
9. a
10. e
11. c
12. e
13. a
14. d
15. b

REFERENCES

1. Stupp R, Wong ET, Kanner AA, et al. NovoTTF-100A versus physician's choice chemotherapy in recurrent glioblastoma: A randomised phase III trial of a novel treatment modality. *Eur J Cancer.* 2012;48(14):2192–2202.
2. Stupp R, Taillibert S, Kanner AA, et al. Maintenance therapy with tumor-treating fields plus temozolomide vs temozolomide alone for glioblastoma: A randomized clinical trial. *JAMA.* 2015;314(23):2535–2543.
3. Zhu P, Zhu JJ. Tumor treating fields: A novel and effective therapy for glioblastoma: Mechanism, efficacy, safety and future perspectives. *Chin Clin Oncol.* 2017;6(4):41.
4. Wenger C, Miranda PC, Salvador R, et al. A review on tumor-treating fields (TTFields): Clinical implications inferred from computational modeling. *IEEE Rev Biomed Eng.* 2018;11:195–207.
5. Markx GH. The use of electric fields in tissue engineering: A review. *Organogenesis.* 2008;4(1):11–17.
6. Chu KF, Dupuy DE. Thermal ablation of tumours: Biological mechanisms and advances in therapy. *Nat Rev Cancer.* 2014;14(3):199–208.
7. Kirson ED, Gurvich Z, Schneiderman R, et al. Disruption of cancer cell replication by alternating electric fields. *Cancer Res.* 2004;64(9):3288–3295.
8. Mittal S, Klinger NV, Michelhaugh SK, et al. Alternating electric tumor treating fields for treatment of glioblastoma: Rationale, preclinical, and clinical studies. *J Neurosurg.* 2018;128(2):414–421.
9. Kim EH, Song HS, Yoo SH, Yoon M. Tumor treating fields inhibit glioblastoma cell migration, invasion and angiogenesis. *Oncotarget.* 2016;7(40):65125–65136.
10. Karanam NK, Srinivasan K, Ding L, et al. Tumor-treating fields elicit a conditional vulnerability to ionizing radiation via the downregulation of BRCA1 signaling and reduced DNA double-strand break repair capacity in non-small cell lung cancer cell lines. *Cell Death Dis.* 2017;8(3):e2711.
11. Voloshin T, Kaynan N, Davidi S, et al. Tumor-treating fields (TTFields) induce immunogenic cell death resulting in enhanced antitumor efficacy when combined with anti-PD-1 therapy. *Cancer Immunol Immunother.* 2020 Jul;69(7):1191–1204. doi:10.1007/s00262-020-02534-7. Epub 2020 Mar 6.
12. Wang Y, Pandey M, Ballo MT. Integration of tumor-treating fields into the multidisciplinary management of patients with solid malignancies. *Oncologist.* 2019;24(12):e1426–e1436.
13. Fonkem E, Wong ET. NovoTTF-100A: A new treatment modality for recurrent glioblastoma. *Expert Rev Neurother.* 2012;12(8):895–899.
14. Kinzel A, Ambrogi M, Varshaver M, Kirson ED. Tumor treating fields for glioblastoma treatment: Patient satisfaction and compliance with the second-generation Optune® system. *Clin Med Insights Oncol.* 2019;13:1179554918825449.
15. Kirson ED, Dbaly V, Tovarys F, et al. Alternating electric fields arrest cell proliferation in animal tumor models and human brain tumors. *Proc Natl Acad Sci U S A.* 2007;104(24):10152–10157.
16. Stupp R, Taillibert S, Kanner A, et al. Effect of tumor-treating fields plus maintenance temozolomide vs maintenance temozolomide alone on survival in patients with glioblastoma: A randomized clinical trial. *JAMA.* 2017;318(23):2306–2316.
17. Branter J, Basu S, Smith S. Tumour treating fields in a combinational therapeutic approach. *Oncotarget.* 2018;9(93):36631–36644.
18. Trusheim J, Dunbar E, Battiste J, et al. A state-of-the-art review and guidelines for tumor treating fields treatment planning and patient follow-up in glioblastoma. *CNS Oncol.* 2017;6(1):29–43.
19. Connelly J, Hormigo A, Mohilie N, et al. Planning TTFields treatment using the NovoTAL system-clinical case series beyond the use of MRI contrast enhancement. *BMC Cancer.* 2016;16(1):842.
20. Chaudhry A, Benson L, Varshaver M, et al. NovoTTF-100A System (Tumor Treating Fields) transducer array layout planning for glioblastoma: A NovoTAL system user study. *World J Surg Oncol.* 2015;13:316.
21. Xing WK, Shao C, Qi ZY, et al. The role of Gliadel wafers in the treatment of newly diagnosed GBM: A meta-analysis. *Drug Des Devel Ther.* 2015;9:3341–3348.
22. Reithmeier T, Graf E, Piroth T, et al. BCNU for recurrent glioblastoma multiforme: Efficacy, toxicity and prognostic factors. *BMC Cancer.* 2010;10:30.
23. Wong ET, Hess KR, Gleason MJ, et al. Outcomes and prognostic factors in recurrent glioma patients enrolled onto phase II clinical trials. *J Clin Oncol.* 1999;17(8):2572–2578.
24. Ashby LS, Smith KA, Stea B. Gliadel wafer implantation combined with standard radiotherapy and concurrent followed by adjuvant temozolomide for treatment of newly diagnosed high-grade glioma: A systematic literature review. *World J Surg Oncol.* 2016;14(1):225.
25. Barbarite E, Sick JT, Berchmans E, et al. The role of brachytherapy in the treatment of glioblastoma multiforme. *Neurosurg Rev.* 2017;40(2):195–211.
26. Nakaji P YE, Dardis C, et al. Surgically targeted radiation therapy: A prospective trial in 79 recurrent, previously irradiated intracranial neoplasms. American Association of Neurological Surgeons Annual Scientific Meeting. San Diego, CA: April 13–17, 2019. *Journal of Neurosurgery JNS,* 131(1):2–116. Retrieved Dec 12, 2021, from https://thejns.org/view/journals/j-neurosurg/131/1/article-p2.xml
27. Sanai N, Berger MS. Glioma extent of resection and its impact on patient outcome. *Neurosurgery.* 2008;62(4):753–764; discussion 264–266.
28. Williams D, Loshak H. Laser interstitial thermal therapy for epilepsy and/or brain tumours: A review of clinical effectiveness and cost-effectiveness

[Internet]. Ottawa (ON): Canadian Agency for Drugs and Technologies in Health; 2019 Jun 17. PMID: 31449372.

29. Sloan AE, Ahluwalia MS, Valerio-Pascua J, et al. Results of the NeuroBlate System first-in-humans Phase I clinical trial for recurrent glioblastoma: Clinical article. *J Neurosurg*. 2013;118(6):1202–1219.

30. Riordan M, Tovar-Spinoza Z. Laser induced thermal therapy (LITT) for pediatric brain tumors: Case-based review. *Transl Pediatr*. 2014;3(3):229–235.

31. Mohammadi AM, Sharma M, Beaumont TL, et al. Upfront magnetic resonance imaging-guided stereotactic laser-ablation in newly diagnosed glioblastoma: A multicenter review of survival outcomes compared to a matched cohort of biopsy-only patients. *Neurosurgery*. 2019;85(6):762–772.

32. Wright J, Chugh J, Wright CH, et al. Laser interstitial thermal therapy followed by minimal-access transsulcal resection for the treatment of large and difficult to access brain tumors. *Neurosurg Focus*. 2016;41(4):E14.

33. Cobbs C, McClay E, Duic JP, et al. An early feasibility study of the Nativis Voyager® device in patients with recurrent glioblastoma: First cohort in US. *CNS Oncol*. 2019;8(1):CNS30.

34. Murphy M, Dowling A, Thien C, et al. A feasibility study of the Nativis Voyager® device in patients with recurrent glioblastoma in Australia. *CNS Oncol*. 2019;8(1):CNS31.

35. Halle B, Mongelard K, Poulsen FR. Convection-enhanced drug delivery for glioblastoma: A systematic review focused on methodological differences in the use of the convection-enhanced delivery method. *Asian J Neurosurg*. 2019;14(1):5–14.

36. Jahangiri A, Chin AT, Flanigan PM, et al. Convection-enhanced delivery in glioblastoma: A review of preclinical and clinical studies. *J Neurosurg*. 2017;126(1):191–200.

37. Jain A, Betancur M, Patel GD, et al. Guiding intracortical brain tumour cells to an extracortical cytotoxic hydrogel using aligned polymeric nanofibres. *Nat Mater*. 2014;13(3):308–316.

PART V. | COMPLICATIONS OF SYSTEMIC AND CENTRAL NERVOUS SYSTEM CANCERS

23 | NEUROLOGIC COMPLICATIONS IN CANCER PATIENTS

KATHERINE B. PETERS

INTRODUCTION

Cancer patients can develop neurological complications of their malignancy and its treatments. These complications can lead to the diagnosis of underlying cancer or occur during the disease trajectory. Moreover, these complications can manifest directly from cancer itself or from the treatments that the patients are receiving. This chapter highlights how cancer can cause neurological complications, whether it is from direct extension of cancer into the nervous system, via a paraneoplastic disorder, or complications of cancer therapeutics.

NEUROLOGICAL COMPLICATIONS: DIRECTLY RELATED TO UNDERLYING CANCER

BRAIN METASTASES

Brain metastases are the most common neurological complication in cancer patients, with upward of 30% of all cancer patients having to contend with this issue.[1] Certain cancers can have a propensity to spread to the brain, and these include lung cancer, breast cancer, colorectal cancer, melanoma, and renal cell cancers. As cancer therapeutics improve and cancer patients get older, the chance of developing brain metastases becomes more prevalent. These observations, along with improved access to advanced brain imaging, are likely responsible for the rising incidence of brain metastases.

> As cancer therapeutics improve and cancer patients get older, the chance of developing brain metastases becomes more prevalent.

Imaging can detect asymptomatic brain metastases at the time of staging or inclusion into clinical trials; more commonly, patients with cancer manifest symptoms of focal neurological dysfunction, seizures, headaches, and signs of increased intracranial pressure leading to imaging. The most common tumor types associated with brain metastases are lung cancer, breast cancer, melanoma, and renal cell cancer.[2] Of course, it is essential to consider metastatic disease in any cancer patient who presents with a brain mass on imaging. Table 23.1 highlights the features of the most common primary solid tumors associated with brain metastases and factors related to resultant brain metastases.

TABLE 23.1 Factors related to brain metastases for specific solid tumor

CANCER	FACTORS
Lung	Can be multiple lesions or be a solitary lesion For small-cell lung cancer, diagnosis of brain metastases can come before the definitive diagnosis of lung cancer
Breast	Can be multiple lesions or be a solitary lesion Has a propensity to leptomeningeal disease Occurs more frequently in younger breast cancer patients
Renal cell	Presents generally as a solitary mass lesion Bleeding can occur
Melanoma	Exhibits the highest propensity to the development of metastatic brain disease Commonly presents as multiple brain metastases Bleeding can occur

From Boire.[3]

The spread of the primary tumor to the brain is mediated via the vasculature. Common areas involved in the brain parenchyma are along the gray–white junction.

Imaging of brain metastases can include head computed tomography (CT) and magnetic resonance imaging (MRI). The standard is MRI with and without contrast because it is superior to head CT in the detection of small lesions and lesions in the posterior fossa. Figure 23.1 shows the axial T1+ contrast MRI image from a patient with metastatic melanoma. Figure 23.2 demonstrates axial T1+ contrast MRI image with a solitary brain metastases from endometrial cancer. To diagnose brain metastases, patients may require a brain biopsy, particularly in situations where the primary is not yet identified or if one is concerned about another diagnosis, such as brain abscess or radiation necrosis.

Treatment is multimodal and rapidly advancing as new targeted therapeutics and immunotherapies emerge to treat systemic cancers. The utility of surgery depends on the number of lesions and surgical accessibility of the lesions. In general, if there is a solitary to three surgically accessible metastatic lesions, the recommendation is the best surgical resection followed by radiation therapy (RT). For more abundant metastases, surgery is usually deferred except for diagnostic biopsy.

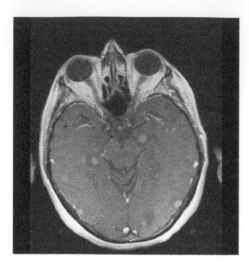

Figure 23.1 *Axial T1 + contrast MRI brain demonstrating multiple enhancing lesions at gray–white junction consistent with metastatic melanoma in a 56-year-old woman.*

RT with and without neurosurgical resection has a vital role in the treatment of brain metastases. In particular, for patients with 1–3 brain metastases, the use of stereotactic radiosurgery (SRS) is particularly key given the results of NCCTG N0574 (Alliance) study, which showed that the overall survival after SRS alone versus SRS with whole-brain RT (WBRT) is no different. Moreover, cognitive outcomes measured 3 months after treatment revealed that patients who received only SRS had better outcomes than SRS with WBRT.[4,5] With the positive results of N0574, it is now common practice to treatment upward of 10 brain metastases with SRS and avoid the use of WBRT when possible. WBRT is still utilized in the treatment of brain metastases, particularly in widespread disease and as prophylaxis in small-cell lung cancer patients.

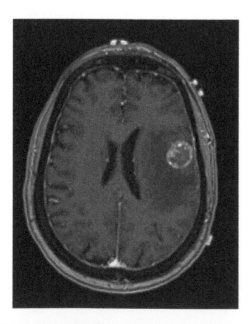

Figure 23.2 *Axial T1 + contrast MRI brain demonstrating solitary brain metastases in a 72-year-old woman with advanced endometrial cancer.*

Systemic therapies for the treatment of brain metastases are rapidly evolving. Understanding the genetics of the underlying primary malignancy and targetable mutations is critical in planning systemic therapeutic approaches. More information about brain metastases can be found in Chapter 12.

SPINAL METASTASES

For metastatic disease that affects the spine, the disease usually involves the spinal column rather than the intrinsic spinal cord. For roughly 10% of cancer patients, particularly with prostate, lung, and breast cancers, metastases to the bones of the spine will occur.

Metastatic spinal cancer typically involves the spinal column rather than spinal cord itself.

These patients often present with back pain that can be severe and localizes to a dermatomal pattern. Weakness and sensory deficits can emerge if the tumor grows further into the spinal canal, and the development of sexual dysfunction, urinary incontinence, and fecal incontinence can progress or develop depending on the extent of disease and location of the disease. Initial testing can be an x-ray evaluation, but the standard recommendation is MRI spine with and without contrast. Treatment for spinal metastasis involves prompt neurosurgical assessment and intervention. It is vital to utilize multidisciplinary providers in neurosurgery, neuro-oncology, neurology, radiation oncology, medical oncology, and palliative care medicine to manage the symptoms and signs that these patients face.

Intramedullary spinal cord metastases are rare and present in fewer than 0.01% of patients. In a manuscript by Payer and colleagues, the authors postulated that the incidence of intramedullary spinal cord metastases is rising, with primary cancers being from the lung, brain, and breast.[6] Common presenting symptoms were dysesthesia, paresis, and, less commonly, urinary retention.

LEPTOMENINGES

Cancer patients with solid tumors (primary brain and other systemic cancers) and hematological malignancies can develop leptomeningeal metastasis. Depending on the primary cancer, the incidence of leptomeningeal disease is 5–15% and most frequently occurs in advanced cancers. Common tumors that lead to leptomeningeal disease are breast cancer, lung cancer (particularly small-cell lung cancer), and melanoma. Unfortunately, survival remains poor at 2–4 months after diagnosis with leptomeningeal disease. The presentation of leptomeningeal disease depends on the location of involvement. Common sites involved include the brainstem, cranial nerves, and spinal column. When the brain parenchyma is involved, patients can have global delirium/confusion, headaches, and symptoms of increased intracranial pressure. Symptoms and signs associated with multiple cranial neuropathies, including but not limited to new-onset binocular diplopia, point to the brain-stem and cranial nerve involvement. New onset of back pain, bladder/bowel dysfunction, and weakness, mainly referred to nerve roots, indicates spinal cord or nerve roots leptomeningeal spread.

Evaluation for leptomeningeal disease includes lumbar puncture with an assessment of cerebrospinal fluid cell count, protein (usually elevated), glucose (traditionally decreased), cytology (solid tumors), and cytometry (hematologic malignancies). Imaging, as seen in Figure 23.3 may show enhancement of the leptomeninges on T1 contrasted MRI of the brain and spine. For more information regarding leptomeningeal disease see Chapter 12.

Treatment is generally palliative rather than with curative intent and can include RT and systemic therapy. Systemic treatment is guided by the underlying primary malignancy.

PLEXUS

Metastatic plexopathy is a rare occurrence that presents in patients with advanced metastatic primary cancers.[7] Depending on the location of disease, the associated primary cancers and presenting symptoms can vary.

Metastatic plexopathy is a rare complication that presents in patients with advanced metastatic primary cancers and is frequently associated with pain.

Table 23.2 shows the characteristics and symptoms of cancer involvement of the cervical, brachial, lumbar, and sacral plexuses.

The critical presenting symptom for all of metastatic cancer-related plexopathies is pain. This symptom is in contrast to radiation-induced plexopathy that is usually painless and shows myokymia on electromyography/nerve conduction study (EMG/NCS) evaluation; therefore, appropriate neuro-diagnostic testing is warranted if one suspects metastatic plexopathy. Providers should perform imaging of the involved areas with MRI or CT/positron emission tomography (PET) to evaluate for the extent of disease. The mainstay of treatment is to control pain, and, given that this phenomenon is associated with advanced cancers, local RT and systemic therapy are treatment considerations that can help alleviate pain.

PERIPHERAL NERVE

Cancer cells can spread and surround the peripheral nerve sheath, leading to neurological symptoms.[7] This condition is termed *perineural spread* or *perineural invasion of tumors*. The most commons tumors associated with perineural spread are skin cancers, including basal cell cancers, squamous cell cancers, and melanoma. Other commonly implicated cancers are cancers of the head and neck.

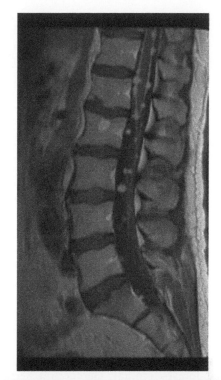

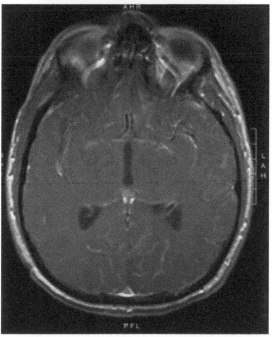

Figure 23.3 Axial T1 + contrast MRI lumbar spine demonstrating nodular enhancement at the leptomeninges in a 47-year-old woman with metastatic breast cancer (upper panel) and axial T1+ contrast MRI brain demonstrating fine widespread enhancement in the leptomeninges of the brain in a 43-year-old man with lung cancer (lower panel).

The most commons tumors associated with perineural spread are skin cancers, including basal cell cancers, squamous cell cancers, and melanoma.

This phenomenon has been documented in patients with breast cancer, prostate cancer, lymphoma, GI cancers,

PLEXUS	ASSOCIATED PRIMARY CANCERS	PRESENTING SYMPTOMS/SIGNS	OTHER POINTS
Cervical	Head and neck cancers, lymphoma	Pain at the neck region Palpable mass Dysesthesias to C2–C7 dermatomes Pain is worsened by coughing, swallowing, or moving	Rare Associated with direct extension of the primary tumor
Brachial	Lung, breast, lymphoma, sarcoma	Lower plexus → more common, pain in the C8/T1 dermatome with weakness in intrinsic hand muscles, Horner's syndrome can be present Upper plexus → pain in the shoulder with weakness in deltoid, biceps, and triceps	Invasion from below → Pancoast's tumor, associated with lung cancers in the apex Invasion from above → from head and neck cancers extending to the upper plexus
Lumbar	Colorectal cancer, cervical cancer, uterine cancer, prostate cancer, lymphoma, sarcoma	L1–L4 → Pain in the anterior thigh, numbness in the groin and thigh, weakness in quadriceps and iliopsoas L4–L5→ pain in the lower leg/foot, footdrop	Most common of the plexopathies, but still rare
Sacral	Prostate cancer, cervical cancer, uterine cancer, anorectal cancer	Pain in the sacrum, buttock, and perianal area Weakness in foot flexors and hamstrings	Lower plexus only (S1–S4)

cervical cancers, bladder cancers, and primary cancers of the muscle (rhabdomyosarcoma). Garcia and Serra identified 76 skin cancer patients who had perineural invasion.[8] The most common sites of initial cancer involvement were the skin of the maxilla, nasolabial fold, and lips, and the first symptom was skin dysesthesia followed by pain, numbness, or even motor deficits if the spread was not untreated or detected earlier. Peripheral cranial nerves are usually the most affected, with trigeminal nerve followed by the facial nerve. One can use imaging to add in the diagnosis of this complication, and this can include CT and MRI. A biopsy can confirm perineural invasion. Treatment involves surgical evaluation for diagnosis, followed by local RT and treatment of the underlying primary malignancy with systemic treatment.[7]

NEUROLOGICAL COMPLICATIONS: PARANEOPLASTIC NEUROLOGICAL SYNDROMES

OVERVIEW OF PARANEOPLASTIC NEUROLOGIC SYNDROMES

Paraneoplastic neurologic syndromes represent a rare autoimmune indirect complication of systemic cancer that occurs in fewer than 1% of all cancer patients.[9] One should consider a paraneoplastic syndrome in a cancer patient who develops new neurological symptoms. Still, it is critical to note that paraneoplastic syndromes can be the first presentation of cancer. Moreover, paraneoplastic syndromes can even occur even if the underlying malignancy cannot be detected by advanced imaging modalities. The phenomenon of paraneoplastic disorders can involve all components of the central nervous and peripheral nervous systems. These syndromes are well characterized in lung cancer, in particular small-cell lung cancer and thymomas,

but a myriad of underlying cancers (and non-neoplastic conditions) can be associated with these syndromes. Box 23.1 presents a summary of the common paraneoplastic neurological syndromes, commonly associated cancers, symptoms, and autoantibodies. These syndromes can occur in isolation or as a combination of syndromes. The mechanism by which cancers lead to paraneoplastic neurological syndromes involves the observation that cancer cells and healthy neural tissues can share antigens. Antibodies then can cross-react with healthy neural tissue, leading to neurological dysfunction.

It is vital in the diagnosis of paraneoplastic neurologic syndromes that providers rule out other causes of neurological complications in these patients, including the direct effects of cancer or the therapies that are used to treat the underlying malignancy.

> Before considering the diagnosis of paraneoplastic syndrome, other causes of neurologic complications in cancer patients should be ruled out.

Detection of high levels of characterized antibodies in the serum and cerebrospinal fluid aids in the diagnosis of paraneoplastic neurological syndromes, but it is important to note that these antibodies may not be present. Other cerebrospinal fluid findings can include pleocytosis and hyperproteinorachia. Treatment of paraneoplastic neurological syndromes entails supportive care of the neurological symptoms, such as pain, delirium, seizures, and rigidity; treatment of the underlying malignancy; and use of therapies such as IV immunoglobin, plasma exchange, corticosteroids, rituximab, or cyclophosphamide. For more information about paraneoplastic syndromes see Chapter 24.

BOX 23.1 COMMON PARANEOPLASTIC NEUROLOGIC SYNDROMES—KEY FEATURES AND ASSOCIATED ANTIBODIES

CENTRAL NERVOUS SYSTEM

Paraneoplastic cerebellar degeneration

One of the most frequent paraneoplastic neurological syndromes that involves subacute, insidious onset of cerebellar ataxia (limb and gait), dysarthria, nystagmus. MRI brain shows cerebellar atrophy.
Common involved cancers: breast cancer, ovarian cancer, Hodgkin's lymphoma, small-cell lung cancer
Common autoantibodies: anti-Yo, anti-PCA-2, anti-mGluR1

Stiff person syndrome

Rigidity that fluctuates involving usually the axial musculature in agonist and antagonist muscle groups. Can be very painful and accompanied by spasms.
EMG/NCS → continuous activity of motor units in the stiffened muscles that considerably improve after treatment with benzodiazepines.
Common involved cancers: breast cancer, ovarian cancer
Common autoantibodies: anti-amphiphysin (can also be associated with anti-GAD65 antibodies, but associated condition is classically type 1 diabetes and not cancer)

Limbic encephalitis

Progressively encephalopathy that can begin with mood changes, insomnia, behavioral changes, memory dysfunction leading to progressive dementia.
Common involved cancers: small cell lung cancer, breast cancer, Hodgkin's lymphoma, colorectal cancers
Common autoantibodies: anti-Ma, anti-Hu

Paraneoplastic encephalomyelitis

Rapid onset of neurological dysfunction that effects higher cortex, brainstem, and spinal cord in varying degrees leading to encephalitis, brainstem dysfunction, and spinal cord dysfunction.
Common involved cancers: testicular cancer, lung cancer
Common autoantibodies: anti-Ma2, anti-Hu, anti-Ri

Anti-NMDAR encephalitis

Commonly presents as a mood and behavioral changes in young females patients that can escalate to severe psychiatric symptoms suggestive of bipolar disorder, schizophrenia, or catatonia. Notably, patients can have central hypoventilation requiring ventilator support. Can recover after removal of teratoma.
Common involved cancers: ovarian teratomas
Common autoantibodies: anti-NMDAR

Cancer-associated retinopathy

Progressive, painless visual loss
Common involved cancers: endometrial cancer, ovarian cancer, breast cancer, cervical cancer, small cell lung cancer
Common autoantibodies: anti-recoverin

NEUROMUSCULAR JUNCTION/PERIPHERAL NERVE

Lambert-Easton myasthenic syndrome

Weakness and fatigue that improves with brief periods of exercise, tends to involve proximal muscle groups and lower extremities. Can have symptoms of autonomic dysfunction and can include dry mouth. Can be treated with 3,4-diaminopyridine.
EMG/NCS → repetitive stimulation at >20 Hertz or after exercise, facilitation occurs and incremental response >100%
Common involved cancers: small cell lung cancer
Common autoantibodies: anti-VGCC

Myasthenia gravis

Classic fatigable weakness involving face, limbs, and respiratory muscles
Common involved cancers: thymomas
Common autoantibodies: anti-acetylcholine receptor, anti-MuSK

BOX 23.1 CONTINUED

Paraneoplastic sensory neuronopathy

Progressive syndrome leading to pain, numbness, and paraesthesia that starts unilaterally and then spreads bilaterally. Thought to be due to immune-mediated damage to neurons on the dorsal root ganglia.
Common involved cancers: small cell lung cancer, many other cancers
EMG/NCS → low amplitude sensory nerve action potentials; motor action potentials and F-wave studies are usually normal
Common autoantibodies: anti-Hu

Autoimmune autonomic neuropathy

Insidiously progressive autonomic dysfunction including hypotension, dry mouth and eyes, GI/GU autonomic dysfunction. Can have pupillary involvement.
Common involved cancers: adenocarcinomas
Common autoantibodies: anti-ganglionic acetylcholine receptors

MUSCLE

Inflammatory myopathy

Commonly seen with dermatomyositis with proximal muscle weakness, fatigue, elevated levels of CPK. Look for skin sequelae of dermatomyositis (heliotropic rash of eyelids, cheek, and chest, Gottron's papules, nail bed changes).
Common involved cancers: adenocarcinomas of different origins
Common autoantibodies: anti-Jo

CPK, creatine phosphokinase; GAD65, glutamic acid decarboxylase 65; mGluR1, metabotropic glutamate receptor 1; MuSK, muscle-specific tyrosine kinase; NMDAR, N-methyl-D-aspartate receptor; PCA-2, Purkinje cell antibody type 2; VGCC, voltage-gated calcium channel.

From Lancaster.[9]

NEUROLOGICAL COMPLICATIONS DUE TO TREATMENT

CHEMOTHERAPY

Neurological complications remain a prominent cause of dose-limiting toxicity and unpleasant symptoms for many chemotherapeutic agents.[10] Toxicity can occur at any part of the neural axis: brain, spinal cord, and peripheral nerves. The most common dose-limiting toxicities are polyneuropathy and acute encephalopathy. Some factors can contribute to the development of neurotoxicity of chemotherapy. These can include patient age, the dose of chemotherapy (intensity and cumulative dose), route of administration (intrathecal can be more neurotoxic), underlying preexisting conditions (neurological conditions, diabetes, hepatic dysfunction, and renal dysfunction), and concomitant effects from other therapies (concurrent or tandem immunotherapy, stem-cell transplantation, and RT).

> The most common dose-limiting toxicities associated with chemotherapy are polyneuropathy and acute encephalopathy.

CHEMOTHERAPY-INDUCED PERIPHERAL NEUROPATHY

This common dose-limiting toxicity usually is a sensory or sensorimotor neuropathy, but can involve the autonomic nervous system. Chemotherapy-induced peripheral neuropathy (CIPN) can appear immediately, shortly after medication is received, or after a long delay, often termed "coasting." The degree and type of neuropathy depend on the kind of agent, duration of treatment, and cumulative dosage. Most cases of CIPN are partly reversible, but in certain circumstances the effects can be long-lasting and irreversible. Table 23.3 details commonly implicated chemotherapeutics and associated factors involved in CIPN. EMG/NCS can be helpful to discern the extent and type of neuropathy. Mainstays of management are cessation of the neurotoxic chemotherapeutic agent and symptomatic treatment of neuropathic symptoms and pain.

SPECIFIC CENTRAL NERVOUS SYSTEM DYSFUNCTION

Acute encephalopathy can present in patients receiving chemotherapy. The symptoms and signs can vary but can include delirium, seizures, and altered mental status. Ifosfamide, an analog cyclophosphamide and alkylating agents used for the treatment of sarcoma, lymphoma, and germ cell cancer, can elicit an acute encephalopathy in as many as 40% of patients.[10]

> Ifosfamide can cause acute encephalopathy in more than 40% of patients.

Patients with concurrent electrolyte abnormalities, renal insufficiency, hepatic impairment, and previous exposure to cisplatin are more likely to develop this condition. Within 24 hours to a few days after ifosfamide infusion, patients can experience delirium, behavioral and personality changes, lethargy, seizures, hallucinations, and myoclonus. Once this is identified, patients should not be rechallenged with this medication as encephalopathy can reoccur and be severe. Methylene

TABLE 23.3 Chemotherapy-induced peripheral neuropathy (CIPN) and associated agents

CHEMOTHERAPY	CLINICAL FINDINGS	TYPE OF NEUROPATHY	PROGNOSIS/OUTCOME
Bortezomib	Small-fiber symptoms predominate with numbness and paresthesia. Pain is a common manifestation. Of note, can have autonomic dysfunction.	Sensory neuropathy, rate autonomic neuropathy	Reversible after cessation of agent
Cisplatin	Since large fibers are affected, patients develop numbness, loss of proprioception and vibration sense, and exhibit areflexia on examination. Note: Commonly causes ototoxicity.	Sensory neuronopathy	Reversible after cessation of the agent, but can worsen after removal in a delayed fashion (coasting phenomenon)
Oxaliplatin	Acute: Leads to peripheral nerve hyperexcitability characterized by transient perioral dysesthesia with subjective dysphagia and dyspnea. This can be very severe and exacerbated by cold temperatures. Chronic: Similar to cisplatin.	Sensory neuronopathy	Acute: Reversible after cessation of agent Chronic: Similar to cisplatin
Taxanes: paclitaxel, docetaxel	Distal symmetrical paresthesia, loss of proprioception. Can manifest with Lhermitte's sign, painful dysesthesias. Can develop an acute pain syndrome within 1–2 days after RX, which then resolves after several days.	Sensory/sensorimotor axonal polyneuropathy	Cessation of agent → can be reversible
Thalidomide	Small fiber symptoms predominate with numbness and paresthesia. Reflexes are intact.	Sensory neuropathy	Reversible after cessation of the agent but can worsen after removal in a delayed fashion (coasting phenomenon)
Vincristine	Starts as pain and paresthesia distally and can lead to motor weakness. Autonomic symptoms can be severe and include GI/GU dysfunction with paralytic ileus and urogenital dysfunction. It can lead to postural hypotension.	Sensorimotor neuronopathy, autonomic neuropathy	Reversible after cessation of agent

From Nolan, DeAngelis.[10]

blue and thiamine are helpful for both treatment and prophylaxis. Other agents associated with acute encephalopathy can include procarbazine, methotrexate, cisplatin, vincristine, and high-dose IV nitrosoureas.[10]

> Acute encephalopathy can be associated with use of the following agents: procarbazine, methotrexate, cisplatin, vincristine, and high-dose IV nitrosoureas.

Methotrexate, the primary agent given for systemic and primary central nervous lymphoma, can cause CNS toxicity. The severity of neurotoxicity from methotrexate can vary and depends on the use of concurrent chemotherapy and RT, the dose of methotrexate, delivery route of methotrexate (more toxic if delivered intrathecally), and age of the patient. Similar to variations in severity, the presentation of methotrexate neurotoxicity ranges from acute encephalopathy to leukoencephalopathy to long-standing dementia. Studies have demonstrated that methotrexate disrupts adaptive myelination

and likely is responsible for the long-term neurotoxicity of this drug.[11,12] If neurotoxicity occurs acutely, methotrexate can be discontinued and leucovorin can be used as a rescue agent. The leukoencephalopathy caused by methotrexate can occur at the time of the administration of the drug or develop weeks to months after completion of therapy. MRI brain demonstrates bilateral symmetric white matter hyperintensities on T2 weighted imaging with no associated perfusion abnormalities. Figure 23.4 shows an MRI brain scan from a 70-year-old patient before methotrexate infusion (on the left) and 3 years after methotrexate infusion (on the right): notable are the white matter abnormalities and global atrophy on the image on the right.

Both cytarabine, an anti-metabolite used commonly in leukemias and lymphomas, and 5-fluorouracil, a thymidylate synthase inhibitor widely used in gastrointestinal cancers, can lead to specific neurotoxicity in the cerebellum. After infusion of either of these agents, an acute cerebellar dysfunction can present with gait and limb ataxia, nystagmus, and dysarthria. Patients receiving these agents

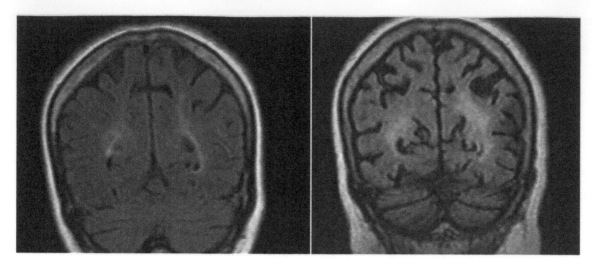

Figure 23.4 *Coronal fluid-attenuated inversion recovery (FLAIR) MRI brain in a woman with primary CNS lymphoma before methotrexate infusion (left) and coronal fluid-attenuated inversion recovery (FLAIR) MRI brain in a woman with primary CNS lymphoma 3 years after methotrexate treatment (right).*

are monitored closely for symptoms, and, if signs develop, infusions can be discontinued. MRI of the brain can reveal, in some cases, T2 hyperintensities in the cerebellum that can resolve over time.[10]

> Cytarabine and 5-fluorouracil are associated with cerebellar toxicity.

Posterior reversible encephalopathy is the described condition associated with the onset of headaches, lethargy, seizures, and visual dysfunction (including cortical blindness). The key to diagnosing this condition is MRI that shows distinctive vasogenic edema, indicated by T2/fluid-attenuated inversion recovery (FLAIR) hyperintensities, prominently in the occipital and parietal lobes bilaterally. More importantly, the condition is reversible on the treatment of causative factors, such as the removal of the offending agent in question. The literature points to a myriad of agents linked to posterior reversible encephalopathy. Notably, this can include but is not limited to traditional chemotherapeutics such as cyclophosphamide, ifosfamide, and gemcitabine and targeted agents such as bevacizumab, tacrolimus, sorafenib, and sunitinib.

Seizures can occur in the setting of chemotherapy administration. One of the most commonly associated agents is busulfan, an alkylating agent used in conditioning regimens in leukemia. Busulfan, when given in high doses in conditioning regimens for allogeneic stem cell transplant, can lower the seizure threshold and cause seizures in patients without a known history of seizures. Other agents implicated in lowering the seizure threshold include bevacizumab, carmustine, cisplatin, cyclosporine, etoposide, and methotrexate.[13]

> Busulfan can lower seizure threshold and can lead to seizures, especially when given at high doses.

Both ischemic and hemorrhagic stroke can occur in cancer patients. Cancer patients can have a propensity to hypercoagulability that can lead to ischemic stroke. Acute focal neurological deficits and subsequent finding of intracranial hemorrhage can manifest in severely leukemic patients and in patients on myelosuppressive chemotherapeutic regimens with severe thrombocytopenia. Therapeutic agents that can be responsible for ischemic and hemorrhagic cerebrovascular events can include the antiangiogenetic agent bevacizumab and platinated compounds such as cisplatin.

Of note, chemotherapeutic agents delivered intrathecally can lead to aseptic meningitis. Intrathecal agents that have been shown to be responsible for this include intrathecally administered cytarabine and methotrexate. It is crucial to note that intrathecal injection of vincristine should never be done and is fatal.

> Intrathecal administration of vincristine is fatal and it is absolutely contraindicated.

CANCER-RELATED COGNITIVE IMPAIRMENT

Cognitive impairment can occur in patients with non-CNS associated cancers that are not as severe as frank chemotherapy-induced encephalopathy. Previously referred to as "chemobrain" or "chemofog," the more acceptable term for this phenomenon is a *cancer-related cognitive impairment* (CRCI).[14] CRCI, best characterized and studied in breast cancer patients, is encountered during chemotherapy or hormonal therapy and involves mild to moderate impairment of memory, attention/concentration, processing speed, and executive functions. Cancer types other than breast cancer have been described as associated with CRCI, and it can occur in the survivorship period, with as many as of 35% of survivors endorsing symptoms of CRCI. Proper consideration of CRCI should be given when patients exhibit complaints and evaluation with formal neuropsychological testing should be undertaken. Time and research need to continue to evaluate the appropriate diagnosis and management of CRCI.

> Cancer-related cognitive impairment is common and can affect patients for many years after the diagnosis and treatment of cancer.

RADIATION THERAPY
BRAIN

RT is essential in the treatment of a myriad of different cancers, including primary brain tumors and metastatic brain tumors. Unfortunately, RT can cause damage to healthy brain tissues, leading to early and delayed neurological complications.[10] The mechanism by which RT damages tissue is via the generation of reactive oxygen species, which in turn leads to oxidative stress. The oxidative stress is not only responsible for damaging tumor cell DNA and killing these cells but also leads to damage in the white matter. CNS toxicity from RT is defined as acute, early delayed, and late delayed.

> Radiation toxicity to the CNS can present at three different phases: acute, early delayed, and late delayed.

The acute form can occur during RT and is more apparent with doses greater than 60 Gy. Symptoms are secondary to increased brain edema and increased intracranial pressure. Given better modern parameters allowing lower total dose of RT and the use of dexamethasone for acute symptoms, this dysfunction is less prevalent. Early delayed encephalopathy is characterized clinically by somnolence, attention deficits, and challenges with short-term memory. This occurs between 1 and 6 months after RT and is thought to be due to transient demyelination. Late delayed encephalopathy occurs months to years after RT, and, clinically, patients demonstrate a pattern of subcortical dementia (short-term memory loss, problems with gait, and attention). Mechanism of action involves damage to the supporting vasculature, which in turn leads to demyelination. MRI of the brain can show cerebral atrophy with periventricular white matter hyperintensities on T2/FLAIR sequences. The impact to patients is cognitive impairment and reduction in quality of life. In fact, 50–90% of brain tumor patients who received RT demonstrated cognitive impairment if they survived longer than 6 months after RT.

> A significant proportion of brain tumor patients who receive radiation-therapy experience cognitive impairment more than 6 months after completion of radiotherapy.

Severe late delayed leukoencephalopathy can be accompanied by hydrocephalus. In these cases, one can consider ventriculoperitoneal (VP) shunting, but it is unlikely to lead to lasting positive reversible outcomes. Because of concerns about the toxicity of RT to critical structures such as the hippocampus, researchers and providers have made recent advances in the development of RT techniques that allow for hippocampal sparing. Another consideration to prevent cognitive dysfunction is prophylaxis with memantine, an N-methyl-D-aspartic acid (NMDA) receptor antagonist used in Alzheimer's disease, which showed an improvement in cognitive performance in patients with brain metastases who received standard RT. For cancer survivors with cognitive deficits secondary to cranial RT, providers can consider using psychostimulants such as methylphenidate or armodafinil to improve attention and alertness and anti-Alzheimer's medications like donepezil.

Two other conditions that can be late manifestations of brain RT include radiation necrosis and *stroke-like migraine attacks after RT* (SMART) syndrome. Focal radiation necrosis can develop months to years after RT and can look like enhancing recurrent tumor on brain MRI. Symptoms of radiation necrosis can range from asymptomatic (incidental finding on imaging) to focal neurological deficits. Advanced imaging, including MRI perfusion imaging, PET imaging, and MR spectroscopy (MRS), can be helpful to determine the difference between recurrent tumor or radiation necrosis. Still, the results are not always definitive, and biopsy should be considered given the fact that recurrent tumor and radiation necrosis can appear similar. Treatment can include dexamethasone, vitamin E with pentoxifylline, bevacizumab, and laser interstitial thermal therapy (LITT). Hyperbaric oxygen is reserved for severe refractory cases.

SMART represents a rare late neurological complication of cranial RT. The syndrome consists of episodes of migraines headaches with associated focal neurological symptoms that are reversible. One can see transient T2/FLAIR changes and even changes in enhancement on MRI imaging. Sometimes seizures can occur, and electroencephalogram (EEG) can be useful to characterize this. Treatment is mainly supportive, and attempted remedies have included verapamil, corticosteroids, aspirin, and various anticonvulsants.

While direct damage to the brain parenchyma can lead to neurological complications, RT can also indirectly cause neurological complications by damaging intracranial vasculature. Cerebrovascular disease is more common in patients who received brain or head/neck RT because radiation caused accelerated atherosclerosis. The risk of stroke for patients who received head and neck RT is 10 times greater than the general population.

> The risk of stroke in patients who received radiotherapy to the head and neck is 10 times greater than in general population.

One should consider the use of screening carotid ultrasound to evaluate for carotid stenosis in head/neck cancer survivors who received RT. RT can promote aberrant vasculature proliferation. Therefore survivors of cranial radiation can develop moyamoya disease, telangiectasias, cavernomas, and even small microhemorrhages in the brain parenchyma. These can bleed and lead to intracranial hemorrhage.

For survivors of brain cancer or leukemia that was treated with cranial RT (in particular survivors of pediatric cancers),

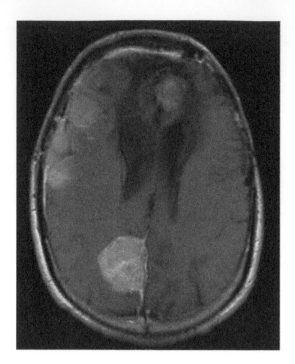

Figure 23.5 Axial T1 + contrast MRI brain demonstrating multiple meningiomas in a 46-year-old man with a history of craniospinal therapy for childhood leukemia.

secondary tumors of the CNS can manifest as a consequence of cranial RT. The most common types to develop are meningiomas, sarcomas, and gliomas.

> Cancer survivors who were treated with radiotherapy to the head as part of their initial therapy are at risk for developing meningioma, sarcoma, and glioma.

Figure 23.5 shows multiple meningiomas in a 46-year-old male survivor of childhood leukemia treated with craniospinal RT. Important factors to consider when making a diagnosis of a secondary tumor include an extended period between the detection of the secondary tumor and RT (years to decades), location of the secondary tumor in the RT treatment field, and a histology for the secondary tumor that differs from the initial cancer.

SPINE

Similar to the brain, RT can damage spinal cord tissue. The type of damage can occur acutely (early delayed myelopathy) or late (late delayed myelopathy). For the early delayed myelopathy, the symptoms of this presentation depend on the location of the RT and occur roughly weeks to months after the RT. For example, patients receiving cervical spine radiation can manifest with Lhermitte's phenomenon, whereas thoracic spine RT might experience a sensation of band-like tightness in the associated dermatomal regions. Months to years after RT, patients can develop late delayed myelopathy. The presentation is usually progressive, with worsening sensory changes and weakness in the lower extremities. Depending on the location of the original RT, there might be pain and dysesthesias

in a dermatomal pattern. MRI of the affected area can demonstrate cord enlargement with hyperintensity on T2 weighted imaging with or without enhancement. This is similar in pathology to late radiation necrosis, and therapies for radiation necrosis, such as anti-inflammatory agents and hyperbaric oxygen, have been explored. Unfortunately, the management is mainly supportive.

PLEXUS/PERIPHERAL NERVES

Plexopathy can occur secondary to RT, but it remains a rare complication ranging in frequency, particularly at the brachial plexus, from 1.8% to 4.9%.[15,16] The presentation in terms of location, sensory-related symptoms, and patterns of weakness is similar to metastatic cancer–induced plexopathy. The two defining factors in favor of radiation-induced plexopathy are lack of pain and the presence of myokymia on EMG/NCS. Of course, one should perform a full history and physical to rule out other causes of plexopathy.

> Radiation-induced plexopathy is typically painless, and EMG studies may show myokymia.

Imaging is helpful if there are concerns about cancer invading the plexus. Again, utilization of EMG/NCS is critical in the diagnosis of this condition because myokymia (>60% of patients have this sign) is pathognomic for radiation-induced plexopathy. Imaging is useful because a dedicated MRI of the affected area can exhibit increased T2 signal at the affected areas with no associated enhancement that would be indicative of cancer. Treatment is mostly supportive.

For a more in-depth review of radiation-induced plexopathy and radiation-induced neuropathy in cancer patients, please see the excellent manuscript by Delanian and colleagues.[15] Depending on the clinical examination and localization of the peripheral nerves involved, it is useful to obtain a history of radiation dose and map of radiation treatments to the associated affected areas.

Similar to the CNS, RT can lead to secondary tumors in the peripheral nervous system. This can occur with schwannomas and plexiform neurofibromas, causing the development of secondary sarcomas or transformation to malignant nerve sheath tumors.

IMMUNOTHERAPIES

Cancer therapy is advancing to develop more efficacious therapies, and immunotherapy is at the forefront of this change. With this advancement in therapies comes a new understanding of novel toxicities, including neurotoxicity. Immune checkpoint inhibitors are now commonly used for the treatment of cancer, such as melanoma and lung cancer, but come with the potential for neurotoxicity, occurring in 1–14% of patients.[17,18] Table 23.4 summarizes the common immune checkpoint inhibitors and associated severe neurological complications.

It is important to note that most neurotoxicity is mild to moderate and involves headaches and peripheral sensory

TABLE 23.4 Summary of immune checkpoint inhibitors and reported neurological complications

IMMUNE CHECKPOINT INHIBITOR	REPORTED NEUROLOGICAL COMPLICATIONS
Ipilimumab, CTLA-4 inhibitor	Inflammatory myopathy Vasculitis Autoimmune encephalitis Optic neuropathy Multiple sclerosis Guillain-Barré syndrome Aseptic meningitis Transverse myelitis Myasthenia gravis
Nivolumab, PD-1 inhibitor	Myasthenia gravis Guillain-Barré syndrome Inflammatory myopathy Multiple sclerosis
Pembrolizumab, PD-1 inhibitor	Myasthenia gravis Inflammatory myopathy Guillain-Barré syndrome Autoimmune encephalitis Multiple sclerosis
Atezolizumab, PD-L1 inhibitor	Encephalitis

TABLE 23.5 Summary of common neurological complications for cancer patients treated with stem cell transplantation

TIMING	COMMON NEUROLOGICAL COMPLICATION
Pre-stem cell transplantation conditioning	Neurotoxicity from chemotherapy
First month post stem cell transplantation	Posterior reversible encephalopathy caused by tacrolimus or cyclosporine Human herpesvirus 6 infection leading to limbic encephalitis
Second through sixth month post stem cell transplantation	Opportunistic infections of the nervous system by virus, fungi, and parasites
Late survivorship post stem cell transplantation	Chronic graft versus host disease leading to dermatomyositis, polymyositis, inflammatory demyelinating polyradiculopathy, myasthenia gravis

neuropathy.[19] Treatment recommendations include cessation of the agent at once even if mild neurotoxicity develops. With moderate symptoms, one can administer corticosteroids, in particular 1–2 mg/kg per day methylprednisolone or prednisone weaned over 4 weeks, and in more severe cases consider IV immunoglobin or plasma exchange.[20]

> Neurologic complications associated with checkpoint inhibitors are usually mild to moderate and frequently include headaches and sensory neuropathy.

Use of chimeric antigen receptor T-cell therapy (CAR-T) has changed outcomes for pediatric and adults patients with acute lymphoblastic leukemia, non-Hodgkin's lymphoma, and chronic lymphocytic leukemia. Neurological complications are a common side effect of this necessary therapy and more commonly manifests as an acute encephalopathy.[21] Symptoms can include delirium, confusion, lethargy, headaches, and seizures, and presents roughly 4–5 days after CAR-T infusion. Symptoms can last from 1 to 2 weeks, and there are rare instances of severe life-threatening brain edema leading to brain death. It is important to note that this acute encephalopathy is different from the more common constellation of symptoms known as *cytokine release syndrome* (fever, tachycardia, and hypotension caused by cytokines released by infused CAR-T). Depending on the severity of the neurotoxicity, dexamethasone (usually 10 mg IV bid) can be administered. This can be done in concert with tocilizumab, a humanized anti-IL-6 receptor monoclonal antibody, for the treatment of cytokine release syndrome.

STEM CELL TRANSPLANTATION

Stem cell transplantation has revolutionized the treatment of both pediatric and adult advanced cancer, in particularly for patients with leukemia. At all stages of the stem cell transplantation process patients are at risk for the development of neurological complications. Table 23.5 summarizes the common neurological complications that can manifest for the stem cell transplantation throughout the illness trajectory. For neurology providers and consultants, understanding the timing and development of these neurological complications is vital to identify, diagnose, and treat these neurological complications.[22]

CONCLUSION

Neurological complications in cancer patient stem from the direct consequence of the malignancy and the treatments that the patients receive. It is critical to identify neurological complications quickly to mitigate further morbidity and ultimately mortality. Moreover, these neurological symptoms and signs, in particularly for paraneoplastic disorder, can herald the presence of a yet-undiagnosed cancer. Even as our therapeutics evolve from RT to now cutting-edge immunotherapies, toxicities continue to challenge the central and peripheral nervous systems. Remaining aware of the neurological complications that can develop in cancer patients will allow providers from all specialties to provide the best care to patients and caregivers.

What is the most common direct neurologic complication in cancer?	Brain metastasis
When may neurologic complications of cancer occur?	Before the diagnosis of the primary disease or throughout the course of the disease
The two most common complications from chemotherapy are:	Peripheral neuropathy Acute encephalopathy
The most common tumors associated with perineural spread are:	Skin cancers, including basal cell cancers, squamous cell cancers, and melanoma
Ifosfamide can frequently cause:	Acute encephalopathy (in >40% of patients)
Agents associated with acute encephalopathy include:	Procarbazine, methotrexate, cisplatin, vincristine, and high-dose IV nitrosoureas
Cerebellar toxicity is typically seen with:	Cytarabine and 5-fluorouracil
Busulfan is frequently associated with:	Seizures
Which chemotherapy drug should never be given intrathecally?	Vincristine
What are the phases of radiation toxicity to CNS?	Acute, early delayed, and delayed
Radiation-induced plexopathy is typically:	Painless
Meningioma, glioma, and sarcoma are the most common malignancies following which treatment modality?	Radiotherapy

Neurologic complications of checkpoint inhibitors are:	Usually mild and include headaches and sensory neuropathy
Following radiotherapy to the head and neck, what is the risk of stroke?	Ten times greater than in general population
Myokymia on EMG may be the feature of what disorder?	Radiation-induced plexopathy
Cancer-related cognitive impairment is:	Common and may affect patients for many years after the diagnosis and treatment
Calcium leucovorin should be given to all patients receiving what treatment?	High-dose methotrexate
Ototoxicity is commonly seen in patients receiving which chemotherapy agent?	Cisplatin
Posterior reversible encephalopathy and human herpesvirus 6 infection leading to limbic encephalitis are usually when?	Within the first month after stem-cell transplantation
Anti-NMDAR encephalitis typically presents with what symptoms?	Mood and behavioral changes in young women

QUESTIONS

1. 67-year-old man presents for treatment for primary CNS lymphoma. He acutely develops confusion during methotrexate infusion. What is the next step in management?
   a. Increase dose of methotrexate
   b. Start dexamethasone
   c. Administer methylene blue
   d. Administer leucovorin

2. 65-year-old man presents with focal seizures involving the left upper extremity and left face. MRI reveals a 2 cm enhancing mass in the right frontal lobe. Of note, he is a heavy smoker, and chest CT shows large mass at the left lower lobe of his lungs. What is the most likely diagnosis?
   a. Glioblastoma
   b. Lung cancer metastasis
   c. Anaplastic oligodendroglioma
   d. Melanoma metastases

3. The patient from Question 2 has the primary tumor removed and is treated systemically. He also received stereotactic radiosurgery to the brain. Six months later, an MRI reveals a new enhancing lesion in the same area as before. A biopsy is performed, and pathology is radiation necrosis. Which is not a therapy for radiation necrosis?
   a. Bevacizumab
   b. Cytarabine
   c. Dexamethasone
   d. Laser interstitial thermal therapy

4. The patient from Question 2 has the primary tumor removed and is treated systemically. He also received stereotactic radiosurgery to the brain. If he would also have whole-brain radiation therapy, what would be a likely consequence?
   a. Development of more brain metastases
   b. Reduction in blood counts
   c. Development of cognitive dysfunction
   d. Peripheral neuropathy

5. Which primary cancer of women is most commonly responsible for the development of leptomeningeal disease?
   a. Breast cancer
   b. Cervical cancer
   c. Ovarian cancer
   d. Uterine cancer

6. What is required to classify a tumor as a secondary tumor due to cranial radiation therapy?
   a. Short interval between radiation therapy and the development of secondary tumor
   b. Long interval between radiation therapy and the development of secondary tumor
   c. Concomitant chemotherapy
   d. Concomitant stereotactic radiosurgery with whole-brain radiation therapy

7. What cancer most commonly leads to spinal metastasis?
   a. Prostate cancer
   b. Germ cell cancers
   c. Colorectal cancers
   d. Brain cancers

8. A 36-year-old woman with a newly diagnosed sarcoma undergoes chemotherapy in the inpatient oncology unit. After the infusion of chemotherapy, she develops confusion, agitation, hallucinations, and seizures. What is likely responsible for this phenomenon?
   a. New brain metastasis
   b. Leptomeningeal disease
   c. Infusion of ifosfamide
   d. Depression

9. The patient from Question 8 continues to have neurological symptoms. How do you next proceed?
   a. Take her to the neurosurgical suite for debulking
   b. Insert an Ommaya for intrathecal infusion
   c. Administer methylene blue
   d. Give her sertraline

10. A 25-year-old woman with a history of medulloblastoma who received craniospinal radiation therapy in the past develops headaches with focal neurological symptoms. MRI imaging is negative for recurrence, and the episodes come and go. What is the likely diagnosis?
    a. Moyamoya disease
    b. SMART syndrome
    c. Early delayed encephalopathy
    d. Radiation necrosis

11. What is the most common tumor associated with NMDAR autoantibodies?
    a. Chondrosarcoma
    b. Rhabdomyosarcoma
    c. Ovarian teratoma
    d. Yolk sac tumor

12. Which one of the following has not been identified as a neurological complication of nivolumab treatment?
    a. Moyamoya disease
    b. Guillain-Barré syndrome
    c. Myasthenia gravis
    d. Encephalitis

13. What infection is associated with limbic encephalitis for cancer patients during the first month post stem cell transplantation?
    a. COVID-19
    b. Cytomegalovirus
    c. Human herpesvirus 6
    d. Varicella

14. A 59-year-old woman female with ovarian cancer develops oral dysesthesias during the first chemotherapy infusion. What is the likely causative agent?
    a. Carboplatin
    b. Cisplatin
    c. Cyclophosphamide
    d. Oxaliplatin

15. This finding on EMG/NCS study aids in the determination of radiation-induced plexopathy.
    a. Presence of F-wave
    b. Myokymia
    c. Decrement on repetitive nerve stimulation
    d. Prolonged distal motor latency of compound muscle action potentials.

ANSWERS

1. d
2. b
3. b
4. c
5. a
6. b
7. a
8. c
9. c
10. b
11. c
12. a
13. c
14. d
15. b

REFERENCES

1. Pruitt AA. Epidemiology, treatment, and complications of central nervous system metastases. *Continuum (Minneap Minn)*. 2017;23(6):1580–1600.
2. Ostrom QT, Wright CH, Barnholtz-Sloan JS. Brain metastases: Epidemiology. *Handb Clin Neurol*. 2018;149:27–42.
3. Boire A. Metastasis to the central nervous system. *Continuum (Minneap Minn)*. 2020;26(6):1584–1601.
4. Brown PD, Jaeckle K, Ballman KV, et al. Effect of radiosurgery alone vs radiosurgery with whole brain radiation therapy on cognitive function in patients with 1 to 3 brain metastases: A randomized clinical trial. *JAMA*. 2016;316(4):401–409.
5. Qie S, Li Y, Shi HY, et al. Stereotactic radiosurgery (SRS) alone versus whole brain radiotherapy plus SRS in patients with 1 to 4 brain metastases from non-small cell lung cancer stratified by the graded prognostic assessment: A meta-analysis (PRISMA) of randomized control trials. *Medicine (Baltimore)*. 2018;97(33):e11777.
6. Payer S, Mende KC, Westphal M, Eicker SO. Intramedullary spinal cord metastases: An increasingly common diagnosis. *Neurosurg Focus*. 2015;39(2):E15.
7. Jaeckle KA. Metastases involving spinal cord, roots, and plexus. *Continuum (Minneap Minn)*. 2011;17(4):855–871.
8. Garcia-Serra A, Hinerman RW, Mendenhall WM, et al. Carcinoma of the skin with perineural invasion. *Head Neck*. 2003;25(12):1027–1033.
9. Lancaster E. Paraneoplastic disorders. *Continuum (Minneap Minn)*. 2017;23(6):1653–1679.
10. Nolan CP, DeAngelis LM. Neurologic complications of chemotherapy and radiation therapy. *Continuum (Minneap Minn)*. 2015;21(2):429–451.
11. Geraghty AC, Gibson EM, Ghanem RA, et al. Loss of adaptive myelination contributes to methotrexate chemotherapy-related cognitive impairment. *Neuron*. 2019;103(2):250–265e8.
12. Gibson EM, Nagaraja S, Ocampo A, et al. Methotrexate chemotherapy induces persistent tri-glial dysregulation that underlies chemotherapy-related cognitive impairment. *Cell*. 2019;176(1–2):43–55 e13.
13. Gonzalez Castro LN, Milligan TA. Seizures in patients with cancer. *Cancer*. 2020;126(7):1379–1389.
14. Janelsins MC, Kesler SR, Ahles TA, Morrow GR. Prevalence, mechanisms, and management of cancer-related cognitive impairment. *Int Rev Psychiatry*. 2014;26(1):102–113.
15. Delanian S, Lefaix JL, Pradat PF. Radiation-induced neuropathy in cancer survivors. *Radiother Oncol*. 2012;105(3):273–282.
16. Fathers E, Thrush D, Huson SM, Norman A. Radiation-induced brachial plexopathy in women treated for carcinoma of the breast. *Clin Rehabil*. 2002;16(2):160–165.
17. Haugh AM, Probasco JC, Johnson DB. Neurologic complications of immune checkpoint inhibitors. *Expert Opin Drug Saf*. 2020:1–10.
18. Johnson DB, et al. Neurologic toxicity associated with immune checkpoint inhibitors: A pharmacovigilance study. *J Immunother Cancer*. 2019;7(1):134.
19. Puzanov I, Diab A, Abdallah K, Bingham CO 3rd, et al. Managing toxicities associated with immune checkpoint inhibitors: Consensus recommendations from the Society for Immunotherapy of Cancer (SITC) Toxicity Management Working Group. *J Immunother Cancer*. 2017;5(1):95.
20. Reid PD, Cifu AS, Bass AR. Management of immunotherapy-related toxicities in patients treated with immune checkpoint inhibitor therapy. *JAMA*. 2021;325(5):482–483.
21. Gust J, Taraseviciute A, Turtle CJ. Neurotoxicity associated with CD19-targeted CAR-T cell therapies. *CNS Drugs*. 2018;32(12):1091–1101.
22. Pruitt AA. Neurologic complications of transplantation. *Continuum (Minneap Minn)*. 2017;23(3):802–821.

24 | PARANEOPLASTIC NEUROLOGICAL SYNDROMES

CRISTINA VALENCIA-SANCHEZ AND MACIEJ M. MRUGALA

INTRODUCTION

Paraneoplastic neurological syndromes (PNS) are a group of disorders associated with cancer that can affect any area of the central or peripheral nervous system. They result from auto-immune responses triggered by the ectopic expression of neuronal proteins in cancer cells. The antitumor immune response is misdirected against the nervous system.[1]

The neurological presentation is often the first clue to the existence of an underlying tumor. Sometimes cancer remains undetectable for long intervals after neurological symptom onset. In patients with a previous history of cancer, the development of PNS may indicate tumor recurrence.[2]

The presentation is often multifocal, affecting multiple areas in the central and peripheral nervous systems, with a subacute onset and rapid progression over days to a few months.[1] The recognition that a neurologic presentation is paraneoplastic allows earlier diagnosis of a new or recurrent cancer. The identification of various paraneoplastic antibodies and their target neural antigens that can be tested for has substantially improved our ability to make an early diagnosis. Detection of one or more paraneoplastic neural autoantibodies in serum or cerebrospinal fluid (CSF) strongly supports the clinical suspicion and directs the search for cancer (Tables 24.1 and 24.2). There is considerable overlap in the syndromes that these antibodies are associated with, but each antibody is typically associated with a restricted group of cancers only.[1,3]

PNS are rare, occurring in fewer than 1% of patients with cancer[4] and are most commonly associated with small-cell lung cancer (SCLC), thymoma, gynecologic cancers (ovarian carcinoma or teratoma, endometrial, fallopian tube, or breast carcinoma), seminoma, and hematologic malignancies.[3,4]

> Paraneoplastic syndromes are most commonly associated with small-cell lung cancer, thymoma, and gynecologic and hematologic malignancies.

IMMUNOLOGIC MECHANISMS

PNS reflect immune responses directed against autoantigens expressed in tumors. Some antigens expressed by the tumor are identical or similar to antigens expressed in the nervous system. The immune system identifies the tumor antigen as foreign and initiates an attack to control the growth of the cancer; however, the immune response triggered by the tumor also leads to attacks against these self-antigens in the nervous system.[1,2]

In general, neural autoantibodies serving as biomarkers of autoimmune neurological disorders can be classified into two categories based on the antigen location: antibodies targeting intracellular antigens or antigens located on the plasma membrane.

> Paraneoplastic antibodies belong to two main categories: those targeting neuronal intracellular antigens and those targeting neuronal cell surface antigens.

In paraneoplastic disorders, neural autoantibodies more frequently are directed against intracellular antigens (nuclear, nucleolar, or cytoplasmic) and the nerve cell damage is mediated by CD8 cytotoxic T cells. In this case, peptides derived from intracellular proteins are displayed on MHC class-I molecules and are recognized by peptide-specific cytotoxic T cells. The antibodies targeting intracellular antigens are markers of a T-cell–mediated injury but not directly pathogenic.[2] These antibodies are also known as "onconeural" antibodies, and their detection in serum and/or CSF almost always indicates the presence of an underlying cancer.[5] Some examples in this group include antineuronal antibody, type 1 (ANNA-1) and Purkinje cerebellar antibody type 1 (PCA-1) (Table 24.1).

In contrast, antibodies targeting neural cell surface antigens (such as receptors, ion channels, and water channels) interact with the neural antigen and have direct pathogenic effects. The mechanisms of injury may include agonist or antagonist effects on the receptors, activation of Fc receptors on immune cells (leading to antibody-dependent cell-mediated cytotoxicity), complement cascade activation, and internalization of the antigen that reduces the antigen density on the cell surface.[6] These autoantibodies can occur in patients with or without cancer.[2,7] Some examples include N-methyl-D-aspartate receptor (NMDA-R) and alpha-amino-3-hydroxy-5-methyl-4-isoxazolepropionic acid receptor (AMPA-R) (Table 24.2).

TABLE 24.1 Antibodies directed against intracellular antigens with their most common neurological manifestations and associated malignancies

ANTIBODY	NEUROLOGICAL MANIFESTATIONS	ASSOCIATED CANCER
Amphiphysin	Encephalomyelopathy, stiff-person, neuropathy	Breast carcinoma, SCLC
ANNA-1 (Hu)	Limbic encephalitis, encephalomyelitis, sensory neuronopathy, dysautonomia, ataxia	SCLC
ANNA-2 (Ri)	Opsoclonus-myoclonus, jaw dystonia, laryngospasm, brainstem encephalitis	SCLC, breast carcinoma
ANNA-3	Encephalomyelitis, polyneuropathy	SCLC
AGNA (SOX1)	LEMS	SCLC
AP3B2	Cerebellar axatia, myelopathy, neuropathy	Renal cell carcinoma
CRMP-5	Encephalomyelitis, retinitis, chorea, cranial neuropathies, radiculoplexopathy	SCLC, thymoma
GAD65	Stiff-person, cerebellar ataxia, encephalitis and seizures, myelopathy	Thymoma, SCLC
GFAP	Meningoencephalomyelitis, papilledema	Ovarian teratoma, diverse adenocarcinomas
GRAF	Cerebellar ataxia	Ovarian carcinoma
ITPR-1	Cerebellar ataxia, neuropathy	Lung adenocarcinoma
KLHL-11	Brainstem encephalitis, cerebellar ataxia	Seminoma (testicular germ cell tumor)
Ma2	Brainstem and limbic encephalitis	Seminoma (testicular germ cell tumor)
Neurochondrin	Cerebellar ataxia, brainstem, myelopathy	Uterine carcinoma
NIF	Cerebellar ataxia, encephalopathy, myelopathy	Neuroendocrine tumors (SCLC, Merkel cell carcinoma)
PCA-1 (Yo)	Cerebellar ataxia	Gynecologic carcinomas (breast, ovary, fallopian tube, uterus)
PCA-2 (MAP1B)	Encephalitis, cerebellar ataxia, neuropathy	SCLC
PDE10A	Encephalopathy, movement disorders	Renal cell and lung adenocarcinoma
TRIM9, TRIM67	Cerebellar ataxia	Lung adenocarcinoma
TRIM46	Encephalitis, cerebellar ataxia	SCLC
ZIC4	Cerebellar ataxia	SCLC

ANNA, Antineuronal nuclear antibody; AGNA, Antiglial neuronal nuclear antibody; AP3B2, Adaptor related protein complex 3 subunit beta 2; CRMP-5, collapsin response mediator protein-5; GAD65, 65 kDa isoform of glutamic acid decarboxylase; GFAP, glial fibrillary acidic protein; GRAF, GTPase regular associated with focal adhesion kinase; ITPR, Inositol 1,4,5- triphosphate receptor; KLHL-11, Kelch-like protein 11; MAP microtubule associated protein; NIF, neuronal intermediate filament; PCA, Purkinje cytoplasmic antibody; PDE, phosphodiesterase, TRIM, tripartite motif-containing, ZIC, Zinc finger protein.

CLINICAL PRESENTATION OF PARANEOPLASTIC NEUROLOGICAL SYNDROMES

Diagnostic criteria for PNS were proposed by Graus et al. in 2004. Based on clinical phenotypes, PNS were subclassified according to clinical phenotypes. Thus, the term "classical PNS" was reserved for those neurological syndromes that are typically associated with cancer. These include encephalomyelitis, limbic encephalitis, subacute cerebellar degeneration, opsoclonus-myoclonus, subacute sensory neuronopathy, chronic gastrointestinal pseudo-obstruction, Lambert-Eaton myasthenic syndrome (LEMS), and dermatomyositis. In these patients, a thorough workup for underlying malignancy is essential even if no onconeural antibody is found.[5]

Alternatively, PNS can be classified by antibody type (i.e., intracellular vs. cell-surface antigen target). They can also be classified anatomically by the level of the neuroaxis affected (i.e., cortex, diencephalon, basal ganglia, brainstem, cerebellum, spinal cord, peripheral nerve, neuromuscular junction, muscle); however, this type of classification can be challenging as PNS are often multifocal. In this chapter, we therefore review PNS according to the classification based on neurological syndromes. The paraneoplastic antibodies commonly associated with these syndromes are outlined in Table 24.3.

TABLE 24.2 Antibodies directed against neural membrane antigens with their most common neurological manifestations and associated malignancies

ANTIBODY	NEUROLOGICAL MANIFESTATIONS	ASSOCIATED CANCER
AChR	Myasthenia gravis	Thymoma, carcinoma (lung, prostate, ovary, breast)
AChR, α3 ganglionic type	Dysautonomia, encephalopathy, peripheral neuropathy	Adenocarcinoma (breast, prostate, lung, gut), thymoma, B-cell neoplasia
AMPA-R	Encephalitis, seizures	Thymoma, SCLC, breast carcinoma
CASPR-2	Peripheral nerve hyperexcitability, encephalitis, dysautonomia, neuropathy	Thymoma
DPPX	Encephalitis, dysautonomia with gastrointestinal hypermotility, psychiatric, myoclonus, rigidity, exaggerated startle	B-cell neoplasia
GABA-A receptor	Limbic encephalitis	Thymoma, lymphoma
GABA-B receptor	Limbic encephalitis	SCLC, thymoma
GlyRα1	Progressive encephalomyelitis with rigidity and myoclonus, stiff-person	Thymoma, lymphoma, breast cancer
IgLON5	Sleep disorder, brainstem dysfunction	No cancer association
LGI-1	Limbic encephalitis, faciobrachial dystonic seizures, hypothalamitis/hyponatremia	Thymoma
mGluR1	Cerebellar ataxia	Hodgkin lymphoma
mGluR5	Limbic encephalitis	Hodgkin lymphoma
MUSK	Myasthenia gravis	Thymoma
NMDA-R	Psychosis, catatonia, dyskinesias, seizures, encephalitis, dysautonomia, central hypoventilation	Ovarian teratoma
Septin 5	Cerebellar ataxia	No cancer association
PCA-Tr (DNER)	Cerebellar ataxia, brainstem encephalitis	Hodgkin lymphoma
VGCC,P/Q type	LEMS, cerebellar ataxia	SCLC

AChR, Acetylcholine receptor; AMPA-R, 2-amino-3-hydroxy-5-methyl-4-isoxazole-propionic acid receptor; CASPR, contactin-associated protein; DNER, delta notch—like epidermal growth factor –related receptor; DPPX,dipeptidyl-peptidase-like protein 6; GABA, γ-aminobutyric acid; GlyRα1, Glycine receptor α1; LGI, leucine-rich, glioma-inactivated; mGluR, metabotropic glutamate receptor; MUSK, muscle specific tyrosine kinase; NMDA-R, N-methyl-D-aspartate receptor; PCA-Tr, Purkinje cell antibody-Trotter; VGCC, voltage-gated calcium channel.

PARANEOPLASTIC ENCEPHALOMYELITIS

This syndrome involves multiple areas of the nervous system including the limbic system, brainstem, cerebellum, spinal cord, dorsal root ganglia, and myenteric plexuses.[8] The response to immunosuppressive therapy of these syndromes is poor. ANNA-1 (anti-Hu) is the antibody most frequently associated with this syndrome, and these patients have a high risk for SCLC.[9] Chest computed tomography (CT) typically is the first step in the cancer workup, followed by positron emission tomography (PET)-CT, if negative.[10]

Anti-Ma2 (anti-Ta)-associated encephalitis characteristically involves the limbic system, diencephalon, or upper brainstem. Patients may also develop hypothalamic dysfunction. The most commonly associated malignancy is testicular germ cell tumor.[11] A screening testicular ultrasound, followed by CT of the pelvis if the ultrasound is negative, is recommended. It is worth mentioning here that a novel autoantibody,

anti-KLHL11 (Kelch-like protein 11), was recently identified in men with paraneoplastic brainstem encephalitis associated with testicular cancer.[12] Clinical presentation and long-term outcomes are similar to Ma2 encephalitis, although ataxia, vertigo, hearing loss, and tinnitus are more frequent in patients with KHLH11 encephalitis.[13]

Other antibodies associated with paraneoplastic encephalomyelitis include collapsin response mediator protein-5 (CRMP5) antibody, which is associated with SCLC and thymoma,[14] and amphyphisin[15] and ANNA-2 (anti-Ri)[16] antibodies associated with breast carcinoma and SCLC.

LIMBIC ENCEPHALITIS

This syndrome is characterized by subacute onset of short-term memory loss, confusion, seizures, and psychiatric symptoms suggesting involvement of the limbic system. Magnetic resonance imaging (MRI) characteristically shows T2 signal abnormalities involving the hippocampus and amygdala bilaterally.[5] Even though limbic encephalitis was initially described as a PNS, in 60% of patients it is not associated with cancer.[17] The type of autoantibody indicates the likelihood of cancer association. Onconeural autoantibodies associated with limbic encephalitis include ANNA-1[18] and Ma2.[19] The most frequent tumor is SCLC, followed by testicular germ cell tumors and Hodgkin lymphoma.[20]

In addition, multiple neural surface antibodies can cause limbic encephalitis, and, in these cases, the prognosis is typically better than in cases associated with onconeural antibodies, possibly because of the more favorable response to immunosuppressive therapies.

- AMPA-R antibody encephalitis may present with limbic involvement, prominent psychiatric symptoms, and diffuse encephalopathy. It is associated with thymoma, lung carcinoma, and breast cancer.[21]

- Gamma-aminobutyric-acid-type-B (GABA-B) receptor antibodies typically cause limbic encephalitis with prominent seizures. It has been associated with SCLC.[22]

- Metabotropic-glutamate-receptor-5 (mGluR5) antibodies are associated with a neuropsychiatric disorder known as "Ophelia syndrome," characterized by encephalitis with confusion. It is associated with Hodgkin lymphoma.[23]

- Anti-NMDA-R encephalitis and leucine-rich, glioma-inactivated 1 (LGI-1) encephalitis can be included in this section, but these antibodies have very characteristic clinical manifestations beyond limbic encephalitis and are discussed in more detail later.

ANTI-N-METHYL D-ASPARTATE RECEPTOR ENCEPHALITIS

Anti-NMDA-R encephalitis affects mainly children and young adults, with female predominance. The neurological manifestations evolve in stages, with prominent psychiatric symptoms, short-term memory deficits, orofacial and limb dyskinesias, seizures, decreased level of consciousness, autonomic instability (with fluctuations in blood pressure and heart rate), and central hypoventilation.[24] MRI of the brain is frequently normal, but it may show increased T2 signal involving the cortical, subcortical, or cerebellar regions in 30% of cases.[24,25]

In women of reproductive age, there is high risk for ovarian teratoma. MRI of the pelvis with contrast and transvaginal ultrasound are useful tests. Pelvic tumors may not be apparent on initial screening, so periodic imaging should be considered.[25]

Most patients recover after immunosuppressive therapy and tumor removal, although recovery may take many months, with mild memory and psychiatric symptoms being the most persistent.[24,25]

NMDA-R encephalitis is a severe form of paraneoplastic encephalitis affecting mostly young women; it has a prolonged clinical course but generally good prognosis.

LEUCINE-RICH, GLIOMA INACTIVATED-1 ENCEPHALITIS AND CONTACTIN-ASSOCIATED PROTEIN-LIKE 2 ASSOCIATED SYNDROMES

Antibodies directed against LGI1 and CASPR2 are the two primary antigens that account for positive responses on the voltage-gated potassium channel (VGKC) complex antibody assay. LGI1 and CASPR2 antibodies have been associated with clinical syndromes involving both the peripheral and central nervous systems. They affect predominantly late-middle-aged men.[26]

Anti-LGI-1 associated encephalitis presents with seizures, often characteristic faciobrachial dystonic seizures (brief episodic ipsilateral arm and hemiface posturing that last a few seconds) that occur multiple times per day. This is followed by memory loss and neuropsychiatric manifestations. Brain MRI is normal in 50% of cases, or it may show the classical uni- or bilateral abnormal T2 signal in the hippocampus. This disorder is particularly steroid responsive.[26,27]

Morvan's syndrome is characterized by an overlap of peripheral and central nervous system manifestations, including peripheral nerve hyperexcitability, seizures, movement disorders, sleep disturbance, and serum hyponatremia.[26] Some patients have an underlying thymoma. Patients with both LGI-1 and CASPR2 antibodies have a higher likelihood of cancer. Chest CT to rule out thymoma, followed by cancer workup appropriate for age and risk factors is recommended.[26,27]

PARANEOPLASTIC CEREBELLAR DEGENERATION

PCD presents with a rapidly evolving and severe pan-cerebellar syndrome due to widespread loss of cerebellar Purkinje cells. Initial brain MRI is usually normal but cerebellar atrophy becomes evident with progression over several months. The outcome of these patients is usually poor. The most common associated tumors are breast and ovarian cancer, Hodgkin lymphoma, and SCLC.[28]

Purkinje-cerebellar-antibody-type-1 (PCA-1) or anti-Yo predicts the presence of adenocarcinoma of the ovary, uterus, fallopian tube, peritoneum, or breast with up to 90% certainty.[29] Therefore, pelvic MRI with contrast, mammogram, and Pap smear are useful initial studies. Breast MRI should be done if the mammogram is negative. If initial tests are negative, PET/CT may be appropriate, and in some cases, exploratory laparoscopy/laparotomy might be considered.[30,31]

Purkinje cell cytoplasmic antibody, type Tr (PCA-Tr) antibodies are directed against the delta/notch-like epidermal growth factor-related receptor (DNER) on the cerebellar Purkinje cell membrane.[32] The risk of Hodgkin lymphoma in these patients is very high (90%) and therefore extensive studies to rule out lymphoma are indicated, including PET, consideration of lymph node biopsy, and repeat imaging if no tumor is found. Although DNER is a surface protein, patients with cerebellar degeneration and PCA-Tr antibodies often have suboptimal response to immunological or oncological therapies.[33]

NEUROLOGICAL SYNDROME	INTRACELLULAR ANTIGENS	CELL-SURFACE ANTIGENS
Limbic encephalitis	ANNA-1, Ma2, KLHL11, CRMP-5, amphiphysin	AMPA-R, GABA$_B$-R, LGI-1, CASPR2, mGluR5, NMDA-R, DPPX
Movement disorders	CRMP-5, ANNA-1, ANNA-2, PDE10A, GAD65	IgLON5, NMDA-R, GlyRα1, DPPX
Brainstem encephalitis	Ma2, KLHL11, ANNA-2, ANNA-1, PCA-1, PCA-2, neurochondrin	IgLON5, DPPX
Cerebellar ataxia	PCA-1, PCA-2, amphiphysin, GAD65, NIF, ANNA-1, ANNA-2, ANNA-3, CRMP-5, Ma2,KLHL-11, NIF, GRAF, ITPR1,ZIC4, AP3B2, neurochondrin, TRIM9, TRIM67, TRIM46	mGluR1, PCA-Tr, VGCC, CASPR2, septin5
Myelopathy	CRMP-5, amphiphysin, ANNA-1, ANNA-2, ANNA-3, PCA-1, PCA-2, GAD65, NIF, AP3B2, neurochondrin	GlyRα1
Sensory neuronopathy and neuropathy	ANNA-1, CRMP-5, PCA-2, amphiphysin	CASPR2 (hyperexcitability)
Dysautonomia	ANNA-1	AchR ganglionic type
Neuromuscular junction	AGNA	VGCC, AchR muscle type, MUSK

> In patients with PCA-Tr antibodies the risk of harboring Hodgkin's lymphoma is very high.

The number of antibodies associated with autoimmune cerebellar ataxias has grown significantly in recent years (Table 24.3). The likelihood of finding an underlying malignancy varies depending on the antibody found. For example, antibodies directed against metabotropic glutamate receptor 1 (mGLuR1) are described in patients who present with subacute ataxia and history of Hodgkin's disease, although many cases have no associated malignancy.[34]

Of note, about 30% of patients with PCD and SCLC do not have detectable onconeural autoantibodies.[35]

PARANEOPLASTIC MOVEMENT DISORDERS

Movement disorders, both hyper- and hypokinetic, may occur in the context of PNS. Chorea has been reported most commonly in association with CRMP-5[14] and ANNA-1 antibodies.[36] Phosphodiesterase 10A, an antibody reported in association with diverse malignancies, may present with hyperkinetic movement disorders, with T2 basal ganglia hyperintensities on brain MRI.00.[37] Orofacial dyskinesias and dystonic posture of the limbs are common in NMDA-R encephalitis, and catatonia may also occur.[38]

Opsoclonus–myoclonus syndrome (OMS) is characterized by multidirectional saccadic eye movements, usually accompanied by limb myoclonus, tremor, dysarthria, and gait ataxia. This syndrome is frequently post-infectious or idiopathic. In children, the most common tumor association is neuroblastoma. In adults, the most common antibody found is ANNA-2 (anti-Ri). SCLC and breast cancer are the most common associated tumors.[39] ANNA-2 brainstem encephalitis may also characteristically present with jaw dystonia.[40]

Stiff-person syndrome (SPS) and progressive encephalomyelitis with rigidity and myoclonus can also be included in this movement disorders section.

STIFF-PERSON SYNDROME

SPS manifestations include exaggerated startle response, limb and truncal stiffness, and spasms. Symptoms are frequently precipitated by loud noise or other startling phenomena. Physical exam characteristically shows hyperlordotic spinal deformities from long-standing rigidity that do not reduce on lying supine or flexing the spine forward. There are also limited forms of this syndrome, including "stiff-limb" and "stiff-trunk" syndromes. Antibodies involved in this condition target inhibitory interneurons in the spinal cord and brainstem, leading to hyperexcitability.[41]

The majority of patients with SPS have glutamic acid decarboxylase (GAD65) antibodies, usually with coexisting autoimmune disorders, and rarely have an associated neoplasm, particularly thymoma. It is worth noting that only high titers of GAD65 are associated with neurological autoimmunity. Besides stiff-person syndrome, other clinical presentations of GAD65 neurological autoimmunity include epilepsy and cerebellar degeneration.[42]

> Anti-GAD65-mediated neurological autoimmunity can be associated with stiff-person syndrome, epilepsy, and cerebellar degeneration.

Other antibodies associated with SPS are directed against amphiphysin and glycine receptor-alpha, subunit 1 (GlyRα1), respectively. Amphiphysin antibodies account for most of the true paraneoplastic cases of SPS, albeit representing less than 5% of all SPS, and are associated with breast cancer and SCLC.[41] GlyRα1 is a neural surface antigen, and thus patients have a more favorable response to immunosuppressive therapy.[43]

PROGRESSIVE ENCEPHALOMYELITIS WITH RIGIDITY AND MYOCLONUS

Progressive encephalomyelitis with rigidity and myoclonus (PERM) is a related disorder that extends beyond the classic SPS, also referred to as *SPS-plus phenotypes*. Neurological manifestations are more severe and widespread with encephalopathy, eye and bulbar dysfunction, myelopathy, and dysautonomia. GlyRα1 antibodies and dipeptidyl peptidase-like protein 6 (DPPX) antibodies have been found in these patients. Thymoma, lymphoma, and breast cancer have been associated with GlyRα1 antibodies.[43] DPPX manifestations typically include a prodrome of diarrhea and/or weight loss, followed by encephalopathy, prominent central hyperexcitability (tremor, myoclonus, rigidity, exaggerated startle), and brainstem or cerebellar dysfunction. Few patients may have an underlying malignancy, usually a B-cell neoplasm.[44]

PARANEOPLASTIC MYELOPATHIES

Paraneoplastic myelopathies occur most often in the context of multifocal neurologic involvement, with encephalopathy, peripheral neuropathy, or cerebellar dysfunction. They are typically associated with onconeural autoantibodies such as ANNA-1,[9] amphiphysin,[15] ANNA-2,[16] and collapsing response-mediator protein-5 (CRMP-5).[14]

Some patients may present with a subacute, usually severe, and isolated myelopathy. Spinal MRI shows longitudinally extensive tract- or gray matter–specific T2 signal abnormalities with or without enhancement after gadolinium administration. SCLC and breast cancer are the most commonly associated tumors.[45]

SENSORY NEURONOPATHY AND OTHER PERIPHERAL NERVOUS SYSTEM MANIFESTATIONS

Patients with sensory neuronopathy present with subacute sensory deficits, frequently with an asymmetric onset. The upper extremities may be affected first, and, over time, all extremities are involved. Patients develop sensory ataxia and may have pseudoathetosis in the deafferented limbs. Patients may also have weakness, autonomic dysfunction, and symptoms suggestive of brain or spinal cord involvement. SCLC is the most commonly found tumor, in many cases with ANNA-1 antibodies. Other antibodies include CRMP5,[46] amphiphysin,[47] and PCA-2.[48] This syndrome is rarely responsive to immunosuppressive therapy.[18,49]

Other peripheral nervous system manifestations in patients with PNS include polyradiculoneuropathy, which is typically painful and asymmetric with CRMP5 antibody.[46] PCA-2[48] and amphiphysin have also been associated with a polyradiculoneuropathy phenotype.[47]

Antibodies directed against CASPR2 have been associated with PNS manifestations including neuromyotonia due to peripheral nerve hyperexcitability that results in cramps, stiffness, and fasciculations (Isaac's syndrome).[26,27]

LAMBERT-EATON MYASTHENIC SYNDROME

LEMS is a neuromuscular junction disorder caused by P/Q-type voltage-gated calcium channel (VGCC) autoantibodies that interfere with the release of acetylcholine at the presynaptic terminal.[50] Patients present with proximal muscle weakness and autonomic dysfunction (dry mouth, erectile dysfunction). Nerve conduction studies reveal low-amplitude compound muscle action potentials (CAMPs) with a characteristic increment following high-frequency supramaximal repetitive nerve stimulation. Diagnosis is confirmed by detection of P/Q-type VGCC autoantibodies in the serum. Approximately 50% of the patients with LEMS have underlying malignancy, usually SCLC.[50] Detection of serum antibodies against the developmental transcription factor SOX1 occurs frequently in patients with paraneoplastic LEMS and only rarely in patients with idiopathic LEMS.[51]

Cases of LEMS and concurrent cerebellar ataxia associated with P/Q-type VGCC antibodies have been described, often paraneoplastic and related to SCLC.[52]

OTHER NEUROLOGICAL SYNDROMES

GLIAL FIBRILLARY ACIDIC PROTEIN ANTIBODY-ASSOCIATED ASTROCYTOPATHY

In glial fibrillary acid protein (GFAP) antibody-associated astrocyopathy, patients present with symptoms of meningitis, encephalitis, and myelitis or a combination of these syndromes. Optic disc papillitis is common. MRI of the brain characteristically shows radial periventricular, leptomeningeal, and punctate or periependymal T1 post-gadolinium enhancement. Spinal MRI may show subtle T2 signal change and predominantly central post-gadolinium enhancement. CSF studies reveal lymphocytic pleocytosis. GFAP-IgG detection is more reliable in CSF than in serum. The most frequently associated malignancy is ovarian teratoma. Para-infectious autoimmunity is suspected in some other patients. This syndrome is characteristically steroid responsive.[53]

PARANEOPLASTIC NEUROLOGICAL SYNDROMES ASSOCIATED WITH IMMUNE CHECKPOINT INHIBITORS

Immune checkpoint inhibitors (ICIs) are novel immunotherapies that enhance anti-tumor immune responses. They have become standard treatments for many malignancies, and their use is likely to continue to increase. Currently approved ICIs include CTLA-4 inhibitors, which promote expansion of tumor-specific effector T cells, and PD1/PD-L1 inhibitors, which increase cytotoxic tumor immune response.[54]

ICIs may trigger immune-related adverse events that can affect any organ. Neurological immune-related adverse events have been reported early after initiating treatment (in the first days or weeks), but sometimes the onset is delayed and may occur even following treatment cessation.[55] Neurological immune-related adverse events associated with ICI can be reviewed in Chapter 23.

ICIs have also been associated with increased incidence of PNS.[55] In these cases, aberrant expression of neural antigens by a tumor, in conjunction with the augmented immune response after treatment with ICIs, has the potential to enhance and misdirect anti-tumor immune responses against the nervous system, leading to the development of a PNS. Interestingly, PNS associated with ICIs have also arisen in patients with cancers not commonly associated with spontaneous PNS, such as melanoma.[56,57]

Patients may present with classical PNS, such as limbic encephalitis, after ICI treatment. Encephalitis involving the brainstem, diencephalon, and cases of paraneoplastic cerebellar ataxia have also been described. Onconeural autoantibodies, such as ANNA-1 and Ma2 may be detected.[57,58] In fact, an increase in the incidence of some PNS, such as Ma2-associated encephalitis, has been observed since introduction of cancer immunotherapy with ICIs.[59]

Peripheral nervous system PNS have also been reported after ICI treatment, such as Lambert-Eaton syndrome associated with associated with P/Q VGCC antibodies[60] and sensory neuronopathy associated with ANNA-1 antibody.[61]

Preexisting PNSs can be worsened by ICIs. Patients with known CNS PNS may develop severe deterioration of their neurological symptoms, and outcomes are usually poor.[57] Patients with serological evidence of onconeural antibodies prior to treatment with ICI have the potential risk of triggering the PNS. It has been demonstrated that preexisting anti-acetylcholine receptor autoantibodies are associated with the development of myositis in patients with thymoma treated with ICI.[62]

Further research is needed to identify patients who are at risk of developing PNS when treated with ICIs, perhaps by determining a patient's baseline serological profile to decide whether these patients can be selected for treatment with ICIs and to increase surveillance for autoimmune complications, especially when treating cancers that are frequently associated with neurological autoimmune complications.[56,37]

Early diagnosis and treatment of PNS triggered by ICIs are essential because these syndromes are frequently T cell–mediated and thus cause irreversible neuronal loss and neurological deficits.[54] Treatment includes steroids and discontinuation of ICI therapy.[63] In severe cases, additional therapies such as intravenous immunoglobulin (IVIG) and plasma exchange might be necessary. Second-line therapies such as rituximab and cyclophosphamide might be considered in cases with severe CNS involvement or in cases that are refractory to treatment.[64] The potential deleterious effect of discontinuation of ICIs and immunosuppressive therapy on cancer progression is a concern that needs to be discussed on a case-by-case basis, taking into consideration the severity of the neurological symptoms and the treatment options available for advanced malignancies.

> It is critical to recognize the association between PNS and many novel immune therapies for cancer.

DIAGNOSIS OF PARANEOPLASTIC NEUROLOGIC DISORDER

CLINICAL PRESENTATION

Recognition of the clinical syndrome is essential to diagnose a paraneoplastic disorder. There is considerable overlap in the syndromes that these antibodies are associated with. For example, limbic encephalitis can be associated with a number of different antibodies. Other paraneoplastic neurological manifestations are more specific and highly suggest presence of a particular antibody (e.g., presence of faciobrachial dystonic seizures in LGI-1-associated encephalitis).

CENTRAL NERVOUS SYSTEM IMAGING

MRI most often is not specific to a particular underlying syndrome, although some imaging patterns may provide clues to a particular paraneoplastic diagnosis. For example, increased T2 signal in the medial temporal lobes is suggestive of limbic encephalitis (Figure 24.1).[28] Characteristic post-contrast enhancement of GFAP-enriched brain regions can be seen in GFAP astrocytopathy.[53] MRI of the spine might demonstrate T2 signal changes in patients with paraneoplastic myelopathy (Figure 24.2).[45]

LABORATORY WORKUP

CSF analysis should include tests for markers of CSF inflammation such as pleocytosis, elevated protein, CSF unique oligoclonal bands, and elevated IgG index and synthesis rate.[65] CSF analysis is also required to exclude infection and leptomeningeal dissemination of the malignancy.

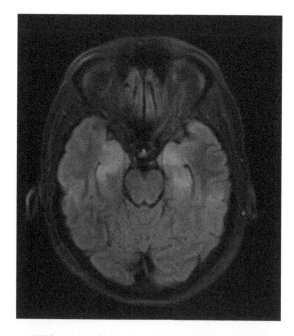

Figure 24.1 MRI brain, axial fluid attenuation inversion recovery (FLAIR) sequence showing T2 hyperintense signal in mesial temporal lobes bilaterally in patient with limbic encephalitis associated with Ma2 antibodies.

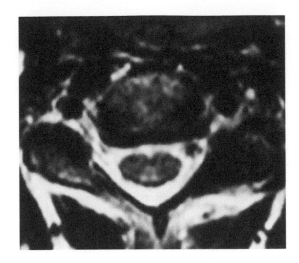

Figure 24.2 *MRI of the spine, axial T2 sequence, showing T2 hyperintensity involving the dorsal columns in a patient with CRMP-5 myelopathy.*

Neural autoantibodies should be tested in both serum and CSF to increase the diagnostic yield, especially if the clinical suspicion is high.[66] Some antibodies such as anti-NMDA-R[24] may be missed when only the serum is tested. GFAP-IgG has a higher specificity when detected in the CSF.[53] LGI-1 IgG[27] and aquaporin-4,[66] in contrast, are better detected in serum.

> Paraneoplastic antibodies should always be measured in both serum and CSF to increase diagnostic yield.

Finding a neural antibody supports the diagnosis of PNS, but negative testing does not exclude the diagnosis if the clinical suspicion is high. Some patients may have novel antibodies for which the antigen has not been discovered yet or for which testing is not yet commercially available. It is also important to keep in mind that a positive antibody has to be interpreted in the context of the patient's clinical presentation and should not replace clinical judgment.[67]

Low positive VGKC-complex antibody titers with negative anti-LGI1 and anti-CASPR2 results are of doubtful clinical significance, and, rather than testing for VGKC antibodies, the current recommendation is to directly test for LGI1 and CASPR2 antibodies, respectively.[68]

OTHER DIAGNOSTIC STUDIES

Electroencephalography (EEG) findings are varied in different PNS and can include rhythmic patterns, seizures, and new-onset refractory status epilepticus. In NMDA receptor encephalitis, the characteristic EEG pattern "extreme delta brush" may be seen (Figure 24.3).[69]

In patients with neuromuscular and peripheral nerve syndromes, electromyography and nerve conduction studies (EMG/NCS) may support diagnoses of LEMS, myasthenia gravis, sensory neuronopathy and others.

OCCULT MALIGNANCY WORKUP

The workup should include appropriate tumor screening based on age, sex, and risk factors.[10] The frequency and type of cancer vary according to the autoantibody. The detection of a specific antibody can guide the search for the underlying malignancy. Coexistence of multiple paraneoplastic autoantibodies in the same patient can also predict cancer pathology.[3] If the tumor found is different from the histological type expected, the possibility of a second, occult tumor should be considered. For example, PCA-1 is detected almost exclusively in women and has a 90% positive predictive value of ovarian cancer or breast adenocarcinoma. ANNA-1 is found almost exclusively in patients with pulmonary or extra-pulmonary small-cell carcinoma. In patients with antibodies directed against cell-surface antigens, the likelihood of finding an underlying malignancy is lower, but workup for known associated tumors is recommended. For example, NMDA-R antibody is highly specific for ovarian teratoma.[2]

Diagnostic tests may include CT scan of chest, abdomen, pelvis, mammography, testicular ultrasound and pelvic ultrasound.[10,70]

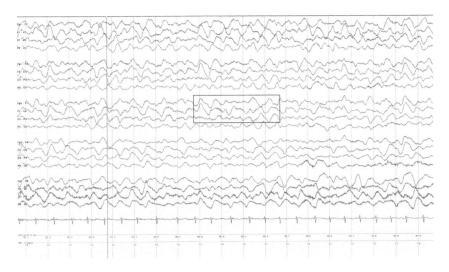

Figure 24.3 *Electroencephalogram (EEG) demonstrating extreme delta brush pattern in N-methyl-D-aspartic acid (NMDA) encephalitis.*

Whole-body PET co-registered with CT may permit higher sensitivity for detection of certain cancers.[71] In many cases, the underlying malignancy is not initially evident, and these patients should be monitored closely with follow up imaging.

In selected cases where suspicion for a specific underlying malignancy is high and diagnostic testing is not revealing, exploratory surgery may be necessary. This can be particularly relevant in cases of occult ovarian tumors.[31]

TREATMENT OF PARANEOPLASTIC NEUROLOGICAL DISORDERS

The primary principles of treatment of PNS include removal of the source of the antigen by treatment of the underlying tumor and suppression of the immune response.

TREATMENT OF THE UNDERLYING CANCER

Cancer treatment (surgery, chemotherapy, radiation therapy) may aid in the stabilization or improvement of the neurological syndrome.[65,72] For example, in anti-NMDA-R encephalitis, removal of ovarian teratoma combined with immunosuppressive therapy is associated with substantial improvement and a decreased rate of relapse.[25]

IMMUNOSUPPRESSIVE THERAPY

The type of autoantibodies may predict the response to immunosuppressive therapy. PNS associated with autoantibodies against neuronal cell surface antigens are directly mediated by the autoantibodies and often respond to oncological treatment and immunosuppressive therapy. In contrast, PNS associated with autoantibodies targeting intracellular antigens often have limited responsiveness to treatment. Early treatment is associated with a better neurological outcome. Immunosuppressive therapy can be divided into acute and maintenance phases. Treatment recommendations are primarily based on case series and expert recommendations.[65,70,72]

Acute Immunosuppressive Treatment
First-line (acute) therapy usually includes intravenous corticosteroids, IVIG, or plasmapheresis.[70] The typical treatment regimen consists of 1,000 mg IV methylprednisolone daily or 0.4 g/kg of IVIG daily for 3–5 consecutive days.[65,70] For patients with partial or no response, plasma exchange every other day for 5–7 treatments may be of benefit. In general, weekly infusions of IV steroids or IVIG (monthly or weekly) are continued for 5–11 additional weeks.[65,70] In severe cases, or if there is no improvement, rituximab (often 1,000 mg IV for 2 doses separated by 2 weeks) or cyclophosphamide (500–1,000 mg/m² IV monthly for 3–6 months) are increasingly considered.[70]

Chronic or Maintenance Immunosuppressive Treatment
The duration of treatment depends on the clinical syndrome and associated neural antibodies. If there is clinical improvement, the initial treatment trial is followed by a slow taper over several months to avoid early relapses, with gradually increasing time intervals between IV treatments, or a taper of oral steroids over a period of 3–6 months.[65,67,72]

Some autoimmune encephalitis can be monophasic, and prolonged initial treatment can be sufficient.

If there is concern for relapse, maintenance immunosuppressive therapy with a steroid-sparing agent may be considered. The relapse rates for each antibody and the severity of the initial presentation need to be taken into consideration The initiation of a steroid-sparing agent usually overlaps with the gradual tapering of steroids or IVIG for 3–6 months.[65,67,72]

It is important to note that prolonged steroid use may cause side effects such as gastrointestinal ulcers, hyperglycemia, opportunistic infections, avascular necrosis of the hip, osteopenia, and psychosis among others. In an effort to minimize the risk of these, prophylactic treatment for *Pneumocystis jirovecii*, gastrointestinal ulcer prophylaxis, and osteoporosis is recommended for patients treated with steroid-sparing for more than 1 month.[65]

Commonly used steroid-sparing agents used as long-term treatments include azathioprine, mycophenolate mofetil, and rituximab.[65,67,72] Cyclophosphamide, oral or IV monthly for 3–6 months, can be used in severe cases and in classic paraneoplastic T-cell–mediated diseases.[73]

There is no established duration for chronic immunosuppressive therapy. In autoimmune encephalitis, it has been suggested that after 3 years without relapse, withdrawal of therapy may be considered.[67,73] However, in patients with onconeural antibodies and an underlying malignancy, long-term immunosuppression is generally avoided given that the relapse rate is low once the tumor has been treated, response to immunotherapy may be limited, and it could potentially increase the risk of progression of the underlying malignancy.[72] In case of relapse, IV steroids and cyclophosphamide can be used.[72]

MONITORING OF TREATMENT RESPONSE

Serum antibody titers usually do not correlate with the course of the disease and may remain detectable after clinical recovery,[7] so clinical response is a more important outcome measure than change in antibody titers. It is recommended to obtain objective measures of treatment response, such as MRI, EEG, and video before and after treatment.[73] In case of suspected relapse, CSF pleocytosis or increasing abnormalities on brain imaging can support the clinical diagnosis of relapse.[72]

> Serum antibody titers usually do not correlate with the course of the disease and may remain detectable after clinical recovery.

That said, a substantial rise in antibody values at a remote time from initial attack with new neurological symptoms may indicate relapse of neurological autoimmunity and sometimes of the underlying cancer.[73]

CONCLUSION

Since the description of a classical PNS, a growing number of neural antigen-specific antibodies have been identified. Neurological manifestations are highly variable and frequently involve multiple parts of the nervous system. Finding a neural antigen-specific antibody supports the diagnosis of a PNS and guides the search for an underlying tumor. Early recognition of the neurological syndrome as a possible paraneoplastic disorder is essential to investigate for an underlying malignancy and to initiate treatment early on in an effort to prevent irreversible neurological damage.

More recently, an increased incidence of neurological autoimmune syndromes has been recognized in patients undergoing cancer treatment with ICI.

How can paraneoplastic neurological disorders be defined immunologically?	Paraneoplastic neurological disorders reflect immune responses directed against shared autoantigens expressed in tumors and the nervous system
Which parts of the nervous system are affected, and what is the typical clinical course?	Paraneoplastic neurological disorders typically affect multiple neuroaxis levels, with subacute onset and rapid progression
Which paraneoplastic syndromes have the strongest association with an underlying malignancy?	Classical PNS such as limbic encephalitis, subacute cerebellar degeneration, sensory neuronopathy opsoclonus-myoclonus syndrome, and Lambert-Eaton syndrome, are highly suggestive of an underlying malignancy
How can paraneoplastic antibodies be classified?	Paraneoplastic antibodies belong to two main categories: targeting neuronal intracellular antigens or neuronal cell surface antigens
Which class of paraneoplastic antibodies is commonly associated with an underlying malignancy? How does this affect response to treatment?	Antibodies against intracellular antigens are more commonly associated with an underlying malignancy, whereas antibodies against neural cell surface antigens can occur in patients with or without cancer. Responses to therapy are better in cases associated with neural surface antibodies
This class of paraneoplastic antibodies can be detected in both serum and CSF	Paraneoplastic neural antibodies can be detected and therefore should be tested for in both, serum and CSF
What is the clinical implication in a patient who presents with a PNS?	The development of a PNS may herald development of a new cancer or recurrence of a known tumor
What are the principles of therapy in patients with paraneoplastic disorders?	Treatment of PNS includes immunosuppressive therapies in conjunction with treatment of the underlying tumor. Response to therapy may be limited in cases associated with antibodies directed against intracellular antigens

ANNA-1 is most commonly associated with which PNS? What is the most likely tumor association?	ANNA-1 most commonly associated with a sensory neuronopathy. However, ANNA-1 can also cause a variety of other paraneoplastic neurological disorders. ANNA-1 is most strongly associated with SCLC, although other tumors can occur
PCA-1 is classically associated with which PNS? What is the most likely tumor association?	In women, PCA-1 is classically associated with paraneoplastic cerebellar degeneration. PCA-1 is strongly associated with breast cancer and tumors of the female reproductive tract
PCA-Tr is associated with which PNS? What is the most likely tumor association?	PCA-Tr is associated with paraneoplastic cerebellar degeneration. PCA-Tr is strongly associated with Hodgkin lymphoma
Anti-Ma2 is associated with which PNS? What is the most likely tumor association?	Anti-Ma1 is associated with encephalitis involving the limbic system, diencephalon, or upper brainstem. Patients should be evaluated for germ cell testicular tumors
A young woman with anti-NMDA-R encephalitis is at high risk for which tumor?	A young woman with anti-NMDA-R encephalitis has a high risk of ovarian teratoma
What life-threatening complications can be seen with anti-NMDA-R encephalitis and, therefore, patients require close monitoring?	Patients with anti-NMDA-R encephalitis should be closely monitored for autonomic instability and central hypoventilation during the acute phase of the illness
What about paraneoplastic neurological disorders in the era of tumor-targeted therapy with immune checkpoint inhibitors?	Immune checkpoint inhibitors have been associated with a range of neurological immune-related adverse effects, some of which are PNS. The diagnosis is aided by the recognition of distinct clinical syndromes and/or the presence of autoantibodies

1. A 32-year-old man is brought to the hospital with 3 weeks of progressive confusion and abnormal behavior. He also developed dysphagia, dysarthria, and decreased level of consciousness. Brain MRI shows increased T2 signal of the brainstem and medial temporal lobes bilaterally. Which of the following tests is most likely to identify an underlying malignancy?
   a. CT scan of the chest
   b. CT scan of the abdomen
   c. Thyroid ultrasound
   d. Testicular ultrasound
   e. CT scan of the pelvis

2. A 25-year-old woman presented with 2 weeks of paranoia and abnormal behavior and required psychiatry hospitalization. MRI of the brain was unremarkable. Over the following week, she became less responsive, developed orofacial dyskinesias, and eventually required transfer to the ICU due to low level of consciousness, blood pressure variability, and respiratory failure. Which of the following antibodies are most likely to be associated with this syndrome?
   a. LGI-1
   b. Ma2
   c. NMDA-R
   d. P/Q VGCC
   e. PCA-1

3. For the patient in Question 2, which of the following tests is more likely to reveal the underlying malignancy?
   a. Transvaginal ultrasound
   b. CT scan of the chest
   c. Mammogram
   d. CT scan of the abdomen
   e. Thyroid ultrasound

4. A 55-year-old man presents with subacute cerebellar degeneration. He is found to have PCA-Tr antibody. Malignancy workup included CT with contrast of the chest, abdomen, and pelvis, which were unremarkable. Which of the following tests is indicated?
   a. PET/CT to rule out Hodgkin lymphoma
   b. Testicular ultrasound to rule out seminoma
   c. Thyroid ultrasound to rule out thyroid cancer
   d. Rectal ultrasound to rule out prostate adenocarcinoma
   e. No further malignancy workup is necessary

5. A 2-year-old boy presents with irregular rapid eye movements in all directions and truncal and limb jerks. Which of the following tumors is associated with this condition?
   a. Medulloblastoma
   b. Neuroblastoma
   c. Pilocytic astrocytoma
   d. Ependymoma
   e. Choroid plexus papilloma

6. A 60-year-old man presents with 3 weeks of confusion, short-term memory difficulties, and seizures. MRI of the brain showed abnormal T2 signal of bilateral medial temporal lobes. Which of the following antibodies associated with limbic encephalitis has a lower risk for an underlying malignancy?
   a. LGI-1
   b. AMPA-R
   c. GABA type B
   d. ANNA-1
   e. Ma2

7. Which of the following tumor and paraneoplastic antibody association is incorrect?
   a. SCLC—ANNA-1
   b. Hodgkin lymphoma—PCA-Tr
   c. Testicular germ cell tumor—PCA-1
   d. Ovarian teratoma—NMDA-R
   e. Breast adenocarcinoma—Amphiphysin

8. Which of the following paraneoplastic syndromes is paired with an incorrect antibody?
   a. Cerebellar degeneration—PCA-1
   b. Sensory neuronopathy—ANNA-1
   c. Limbic encephalitis—GABA B receptor
   d. Brainstem encephalitis—Ma2
   e. Lambert-Eaton myasthenic syndrome—GAD65

9. Which of the following clinical features is typically seen in the course of LGI-1 encephalitis?
   a. Orofacial dyskinesias
   b. Faciobrachial dystonic seizures
   c. Autonomic dysfunction
   d. Optic neuritis
   e. Opsoclonus-myoclonus

10. Which of the following autoantibodies has not been associated with stiff-person syndrome and/or PERM?
    a. DPPX
    b. GAD65
    c. Amphiphysin
    d. Glycine receptor
    e. PCA-1

11. A 54-year-old man with history of SCLC treated 2 years ago presents with 8 weeks of progressive numbness and sensory ataxia. He also has gastroparesis. He is found to have ANNA-1 antibodies. Which of the following is the most appropriate next step in the management of this patient?
    a. Screening for melanoma
    b. Symptomatic treatment for small-fiber neuropathy secondary to chemotherapy
    c. Watchful waiting
    d. Testicular ultrasound
    e. The patient requires workup to rule out recurrent SCLC

12. A 64-year-old woman presents with 4 weeks of ataxia, diplopia, and dysarthria. MRI of the brain was unremarkable. CSF analysis revealed increased white cell count. CT of the abdomen and pelvis showed an ovarian mass. Which of the following antibodies are most likely to be associated with this syndrome?
    a. PCA-Tr
    b. PCA-1 (anti-Yo)
    c. Ma2
    d. Glutamic acid decarboxylase
    e. Amphiphysin

13. Which of the following tumors is most commonly associated with Lambert-Eaton syndrome?
    a. Prostate adenocarcinoma
    b. Breast carcinoma
    c. Hodgkin lymphoma
    d. Thymoma
    e. SCLC

14. Which of the following treatments is not considered an acute immunotherapy treatment?
    a. Oral methotrexate
    b. IV cyclophosphamide
    c. IV methylprednisolone
    d. Rituximab
    e. IVIG

15. Which of the following syndromes is more likely to have a favorable outcome after immunotherapy?
    a. Subacute cerebellar degeneration associated with PCA-1
    b. LGI-1 encephalitis
    c. Sensory neuronopathy associated with ANNA-1
    d. Encephalomyelopathy associated with amphiphysin
    e. Paraneoplastic myelopathy associated with CRMP-5

ANSWERS

1. d
2. c
3. a
4. a
5. b
6. a
7. c
8. e
9. b
10. e
11. e
12. b
13. e
14. a
15. b

REFERENCES

1. Darnell RB, Posner JB. Paraneoplastic syndromes involving the nervous system. *N Engl J Med.* 2003;349`:1543–1554.
2. McKeon A, Pittock SJ. Paraneoplastic encephalomyelopathies: Pathology and mechanisms. *Acta neuropathologica.* 2011;122(4):381.
3. Pittock SJ, Kryzer TJ, Lennon VA. Paraneoplastic antibodies co-exist and predict cancer, not neurological syndrome. *Ann Neurol.* 2004;56(5):715–719.
4. Vogrig A, Gigli GL, Segatti S, et al. Epidemiology of paraneoplastic neurological syndromes: A population-based study. *J Neurol.* 2020;267(1):26–35.
5. Graus F, Delattre JY, Antoine JC, et al. Recommended diagnostic criteria for paraneoplastic neurological syndromes. *J Neurol Neurosurg Psychiatry.* 2004;75(8):1135–1140.
6. Diamond B, Huerta PT, Mina-Osorio P, et al. Losing your nerves? Maybe it's the antibodies. *Nat Rev Immunol.* 2009;9(6):449–456.
7. Dalmau J, Graus F. Antibody-mediated encephalitis. *N Engl J Med.* 2018;378(9):840–851.
8. Henson RA, Hoffman HL, Urich H. Encephalomyelitis with carcinoma. *Brain.* 1965;88(3):449–464.
9. Graus F, Keime-Guibert F, Reñe R, et al. Anti-Hu-associated paraneoplastic encephalomyelitis: Analysis of 200 patients. *Brain.* 2001;124(Pt 6):1138–1148.
10. Titulaer MJ, Soffietti R, Dalmau J, et al. Screening for tumours in paraneoplastic syndromes: Report of an EFNS task force. *Eur J Neurol.* 2011;18(1):19–e3.
11. Dalmau J, Graus F, Villarejo A, et al. Clinical analysis of anti-Ma2-associated encephalitis. *Brain.* 2004;127(Pt 8):1831–1844.
12. Mandel-Brehm C, Dubey D, Kryzer TJ, et al. Kelch-like protein 11 antibodies in seminoma-associated paraneoplastic encephalitis. *N Engl J Med.* 2019;381(1):47–54.
13. Dubey D, Wilson MR, Clarkson B, et al. Expanded Clinical Phenotype, Oncological Associations, and Immunopathologic Insights of Paraneoplastic Kelch-like Protein-11 Encephalitis. *JAMA Neurol.* 2020 Nov 1;77(11):1420–1429.
14. Yu Z, Kryzer TJ, Griesmann GE, et al. CRMP-5 neuronal autoantibody: Marker of lung cancer and thymoma-related autoimmunity. *Ann Neurol.* 2001;49(2):146–154.
15. Pittock SJ, Lucchinetti CF, Parisi JE, et al. Amphiphysin autoimmunity: Paraneoplastic accompaniments. *Ann Neurol.* 2005;58(1):96–107.
16. Pittock SJ, Lucchinetti CF, Lennon VA. Anti-neuronal nuclear autoantibody type 2: Paraneoplastic accompaniments. *Ann Neurol.* 2003;53(5):580–587.
17. Graus F, Escudero D, Oleaga L, et al. Syndrome and outcome of antibody-negative limbic encephalitis. *Eur J Neurol.* 2018;25(8):1011–1016.
18. Graus F, Keime-Guibert F, Rene R, et al. Anti-Hu-associated paraneoplastic encephalomyelitis: Analysis of 200 patients. *Brain.* 2001;124(6):1138–1148.
19. Dalmau J, Graus F, Villarejo A, et al. Clinical analysis of anti-Ma2-associated encephalitis. *Brain.* 2004;127(8):1831–1844.
20. Gultekin SH, Rosenfeld MR, Voltz R, et al. Paraneoplastic limbic encephalitis: Neurological symptoms, immunological findings and tumour association in 50 patients. *Brain.* 2000;123 (Pt 7):1481–1494.
21. Höftberger R, van Sonderen A, Leypoldt F, et al. Encephalitis and AMPA receptor antibodies: Novel findings in a case series of 22 patients. *Neurology.* 2015;84(24):2403–2412.
22. Lancaster E, Lai M, Peng X, et al. Antibodies to the GABAB receptor in limbic encephalitis with seizures: Case series and characterisation of the antigen. *Lancet Neurol.* 2010;9(1):67–76.
23. Lancaster E, Martinez-Hernandez E, Titulaer M, et al. Antibodies to metabotropic glutamate receptor 5 in the Ophelia syndrome. *Neurology.* 2011;77(18):1698–1701.
24. Dalmau J, Lancaster E, Martinez-Hernandez E, et al. Clinical experience and laboratory investigations in patients with anti-NMDAR encephalitis. *Lancet Neurol.* 2011;10(1):63–74.
25. Titulaer MJ, McCracken L, Gabilondo I, et al. Treatment and prognostic factors for long-term outcome in patients with anti-NMDA receptor encephalitis: An observational cohort study. *Lancet Neurol.* 2013;12(2):157–165.
26. Binks SNM, Klein CJ, Waters P, et al. LGI1, CASPR2 and related antibodies: A molecular evolution of the phenotypes. *J Neurol Neurosurg Psychiatry.* 2018;89(5):526–534.
27. Gadoth A, Pittock SJ, Dubey D, et al. Expanded phenotypes and outcomes among 256 LGI 1/CASPR 2-I g G–positive patients. *Ann Neurol.* 2017;82(1):79–92.

28. Graus F, Dalmau J. Paraneoplastic neurological syndromes: Diagnosis and treatment. *Curr Opin Neurol.* 2007;20(6):732–737.

29. McKeon A, Tracy JA, Pittock SJ, et al. Purkinje cell cytoplasmic autoantibody type 1 accompaniments: The cerebellum and beyond. *Arch Neurol.* 2011;68(10):1282–1289.

30. Lancaster E. Paraneoplastic Disorders. Continuum (Minneap Minn). 2017 Dec;23(6, Neuro-oncology):1653-1679.

31. Zaborowski MP, Spaczynski M, Nowak-Markwitz E, Michalak S. Paraneoplastic neurological syndromes associated with ovarian tumors. *J Cancer Res Clin Oncol.* 2015;141(1):99–108.

32. Greene M, Lai Y, Baella N, et al. Antibodies to Delta/notch-like epidermal growth factor-related receptor in patients with anti-Tr, paraneoplastic cerebellar degeneration, and Hodgkin lymphoma. *JAMA Neurol.* 2014;71(8):1003–1008.

33. Bernal F, Shams'Ili S, Rojas I, et al. Anti-Tr antibodies as markers of paraneoplastic cerebellar degeneration and Hodgkin's disease. *Neurology.* 2003;60(2):230–234.

34. Lopez-Chiriboga AS, Komorowski L, Kümpfel T, et al. Metabotropic glutamate receptor type 1 autoimmunity: Clinical features and treatment outcomes. *Neurology.* 2016;86(11):1009–1013.

35. Sabater L, Höftberger R, Boronat A, et al. Antibody repertoire in paraneoplastic cerebellar degeneration and small cell lung cancer. *PLoS One.* 2013;8(3):e60438.

36. O'Toole O, Lennon VA, Ahlskog JE, et al. Autoimmune chorea in adults. *Neurology.* 2013 Mar 19;80(12):1133–44.

37. Zekeridou A, Lennon VA. Neurologic autoimmunity in the era of checkpoint inhibitor cancer immunotherapy. *Mayo Clin Proc.* 2019;94(9):1865–1878.

38. Mohammad SS, Sinclair K, Pillai S, et al. Herpes simplex encephalitis relapse with chorea is associated with autoantibodies to N-Methyl-D-aspartate receptor or dopamine-2 receptor. *Mov Disord.* 2014 Jan;29(1):117–122. doi:10.1002/mds.25623. Epub 2013 Oct 1.

39. Klaas JP, Ahlskog JE, Pittock SJ, et al. Adult-onset opsoclonus-myoclonus syndrome. *Arch Neurol.* 2012;69(12):1598–1607.

40. Pittock SJ, Parisi JE, McKeon A, et al. Paraneoplastic jaw dystonia and laryngospasm with antineuronal nuclear autoantibody type 2 (anti-Ri). *Arch Neurol.* 2010 Sep;67(9):1109–1115. doi:10.1001/archneurol.2010.209

41. McKeon A, Robinson MT, McEvoy KM, et al. Stiff-man syndrome and variants: Clinical course, treatments, and outcomes. *Arch Neurol.* 2012;69(2):230–238.

42. Budhram A, Sechi E, Flanagan EP, et al. Clinical spectrum of high-titre GAD65 antibodies. *J Neurol Neurosurg Psychiatry.* 2021 Feb 9;92(6):645–54.

43. McKeon A, Martinez-Hernandez E, Lancaster E, et al. Glycine receptor autoimmune spectrum with stiff-man syndrome phenotype. *JAMA Neurol.* 2013;70(1):44–50.

44. Tobin WO, Lennon VA, Komorowski L, et al. DPPX potassium channel antibody: Frequency, clinical accompaniments, and outcomes in 20 patients. *Neurology.* 2014;83(20):1797–1803.

45. Flanagan E, McKeon A, Lennon VA, et al. Paraneoplastic isolated myelopathy: Clinical course and neuroimaging clues. *Neurology.* 2011;76(24):2089–2095.

46. Dubey D, Lennon VA, Gadoth A, et al. Autoimmune CRMP5 neuropathy phenotype and outcome defined from 105 cases. *Neurology.* 2018;90(2):e103–e110.

47. Dubey D, Jitprapaikulsan J, Bi H, et al. Amphiphysin-IgG autoimmune neuropathy: A recognizable clinicopathologic syndrome. *Neurology.* 2019 Nov 12;93(20):e1873–e1880

48. Jitprapaikulsan J, Klein C, Pittock SJ, et al. Phenotypic presentations of paraneoplastic neuropathies associated with MAP1B-IgG. *J Neurol Neurosurg Psychiatry.* 2020;91(3):328–330.

49. Rudnicki SA, Dalmau J. Paraneoplastic syndromes of the peripheral nerves. *Curr Opin Neurol.* 2005;18(5):598–603.

50. Lennon VA, Kryzer TJ, Griesmann GE, et al. Calcium-channel antibodies in the Lambert-Eaton syndrome and other paraneoplastic syndromes. *N Engl J Med.* 1995 Jun 1;332(22):1467–74

51. Sabater L, Titulaer M, Saiz A, et al. SOX1 antibodies are markers of paraneoplastic Lambert–Eaton myasthenic syndrome. *Neurology.* 2008;70(12):924–928.

52. Zalewski N, Lennon VA, Pittock SJ, McKeon A. Calcium channel autoimmunity: Cerebellar ataxia and lambert-eaton syndrome coexisting. *Muscle Nerve.* 2017.

53. Flanagan EP, Hinson SR, Lennon VA, et al. Glial fibrillary acidic protein immunoglobulin G as biomarker of autoimmune astrocytopathy: Analysis of 102 patients. *Ann Neurol.* 2017;81(2):298–309.

54. Pardoll DM. The blockade of immune checkpoints in cancer immunotherapy. *Nat Rev Cancer.* 2012;12(4):252–264.

55. Johnson DB, Manouchehri A, Haugh AM, et al. Neurologic toxicity associated with immune checkpoint inhibitors: A pharmacovigilance study. *J Immunother Cancer.* 2019;7(1):134.

56. Graus F, Dalmau J. Paraneoplastic neurological syndromes in the era of immune-checkpoint inhibitors. *Nat Rev Clin Oncol.* 2019;16(9):535–548.

57. Sechi E, Markovic SN, McKeon A, et al. Neurologic autoimmunity and immune checkpoint inhibitors: Autoantibody profiles and outcomes. *Neurology.* 2020;95(17):e2442–e2452.

58. Vogrig A, Muñiz-Castrillo S, Joubert B, et al. Central nervous system complications associated with immune checkpoint inhibitors. *J Neurol Neurosurg Psychiatry.* 2020;91(7):772–778.

59. Vogrig A, Fouret M, Joubert B, et al. Increased frequency of anti-Ma2 encephalitis associated with immune checkpoint inhibitors. *Neurol Neuroimmunol Neuroinflamm.* 2019;6(6).

60. Agrawal K, Agrawal N. Lambert-Eaton myasthenic syndrome secondary to nivolumab and ipilimumab in a patient with small-cell lung cancer. *Case Rep Neurol Med.* 2019;2019:5353202.

61. Mongay-Ochoa N, Vogrig A, et al. Anti-Hu-associated paraneoplastic syndromes triggered by immune-checkpoint inhibitor treatment. *J Neurol.* 2020;267(7):2154–2156.

62. Mammen AL, Rajan A, Pak K, et al. Pre-existing antiacetylcholine receptor autoantibodies and B cell lymphopaenia are associated with the development of myositis in patients with thymoma treated with avelumab, an immune checkpoint inhibitor targeting programmed death-ligand 1. *Ann Rheum Dis.* 2019;78(1):150–152.

63. Brahmer JR, Lacchetti C, Schneider BJ, et al. Management of immune-related adverse events in patients treated with immune checkpoint inhibitor therapy: American Society of Clinical Oncology clinical practice guideline. *J Clin Oncol.* 2018;36(17):1714–1768.

64. Sechi E, Zekeridou A. Neurologic complications of immune checkpoint inhibitors in thoracic malignancies. *J Thorac Oncol.* 2021;16(3):381–394.

65. McKeon A. Immunotherapeutics for autoimmune encephalopathies and dementias. *Curr Treat Options Neurol.* 2013;15(6):723–737.

66. McKeon A, Pittock SJ, Lennon VA. CSF complements serum for evaluating paraneoplastic antibodies and NMO-IgG. *Neurology.* 2011;76(12):1108–1110.

67. López-Chiriboga AS, Flanagan EP. Diagnostic and therapeutic approach to autoimmune neurologic disorders. *Semin Neurol.* 2018;38(3):392–402.

68. Michael S, Waters P, Irani SR. Stop testing for autoantibodies to the VGKC-complex: Only request LGI1 and CASPR2. *Pract Neurol.* 2020;20(5):377–384.

69. Moise AM, Karakis I, Herlopian A, et al. Continuous EEG findings in autoimmune encephalitis. *J Clin Neurophysiol.* 2021;38(2):124–129.

70. Abboud H, Probasco JC, Irani S, et al. Autoimmune encephalitis: Proposed best practice recommendations for diagnosis and acute management. *J Neurol Neurosurg Psychiatry.* 2021.

71. McKeon A, Apiwattanakul M, Lachance DH, et al. Positron emission tomography-computed tomography in paraneoplastic neurologic disorders: Systematic analysis and review. *Arch Neurol.* 2010;67(3):322–329.

72. Abboud H, Probasco J, Irani SR, et al. Autoimmune encephalitis: Proposed recommendations for symptomatic and long-term management. *J Neurol Neurosurg Psychiatry.* 2021.

73. McKeon A, Zekeridou A. Autoimmune encephalitis management: MS centers and beyond. Mult Scler. 2020;26(13):1618–1626.

25 | NEURO-ONCOLOGIC EMERGENCIES

MAYA HRACHOVA, DAVID GRITSCH, SIMON GRITSCH, AND MACIEJ M. MRUGALA

INTRODUCTION

Neuro-oncologic emergencies are serious complications of primary and secondary central nervous system (CNS) malignancies that significantly impact the mortality and morbidity rates of cancer patients. Expedited diagnostic workup is imperative because presenting symptoms could stem from various pathological processes necessitating different management strategies. In fact, the acuity of presenting symptoms often leads to emergent evaluation.

Status epilepticus (SE), ischemic and hemorrhagic stroke, and metastatic spinal cord compression are the most common causes of morbidity due to the direct tumor effect. Importantly, advances in diagnostic and treatment options outlined in this chapter provide opportunities to improve outcomes in patients with these particular complications. Evaluation of recent guidelines shows encouraging trends when management decisions are guided and developed on a case-by-case bases rather than by applying automatic paradigms that disqualify cancer patients from potential interventions.

Neuro-oncologists face severe complications affecting their patients in daily out-patient and in-patient practice. Therefore, working closely with Emergency Room (ER) physicians is critical because it may expedite diagnostic workup and multidisciplinary decision-making. It is worthwhile to invest in building a good relationship with the ER and other services that commonly take care of the acute needs of neuro-oncology patients (neurology, neurosurgery, internal medicine, oncology). Recent introduction of chimeric antigen receptor (CAR)-T cell therapy led to development of multidisciplinary "CAR-T cell care teams" at many hospitals. These teams are able to promptly recognize systemic toxicity and neurotoxicity associated with this treatment and implement appropriate therapeutic measures. This particular experience shows that patient outcomes can be significantly improved when timely and well-organized care is provided.

Adverse effects of chemotherapy, such as coagulopathy, pulmonary embolism, thrombocytopenia, and neutropenia, are common systemic complications encountered in brain cancer patients. A high level of suspicion is required because these conditions can be indolent at onset but eventually lead to life-threatening complications. Thus, it is imperative to recognize signs and symptoms of neuro-oncological emergencies in a timely manner to prevent serious and irreversible complications.

This chapter reviews the most common neuro-oncologic emergencies and provides a framework for their diagnostic workup and management.

STATUS EPILEPTICUS

EPIDEMIOLOGY AND PATHOPHYSIOLOGY

SE is the most serious manifestation of epilepsy that is frequently seen in patients with brain tumors and metastatic lesions to the brain; SE has long-term mortality rates as high as 22% in children and 57% in adults.[1]

Brain tumors are the underlying etiology of SE in 3–12% of cases.[2] Although the risk of seizures is 70–90% in low-grade gliomas, patients with high-grade gliomas were found to have the highest risk of developing SE, attributed to the rapid tumor growth, cortical invasion, and surrounding edema.[3] SE secondary to glioma has been shown to respond relatively well to antiepileptic treatment when compared to SE due to other causes.[3] Thus, SE in this patient population should be treated aggressively regardless of the prognosis.

> Patients with high-grade gliomas have the highest risk of developing SE. Short-term mortality associated with SE is higher in brain tumor patients.

CLASSIFICATION OF STATUS EPILEPTICUS

The International League Against Epilepsy (ILAE) defines SE as a condition resulting either from the failure of seizure termination or the initiation of a mechanism that leads to the prolonged seizure.[2] The time beyond which the seizure is likely to be prolonged, leading to continuous seizure activity, and the time of seizure activity after which there is a risk of long-term consequences are the two major operational dimensions of SE (Table 25.1).[2]

Seizure semiology, etiology, electroencephalography (EEG) correlates, and age comprise four axes in the classification of SE.[2] Based on clinical presentation, SE is stratified into SE with prominent motor and without prominent motor symptoms (nonconvulsive SE [NCSE]). SE with prominent motor symptoms is further subdivided into convulsive SE (CSE) (including generalized CSE [GCSE]), myoclonic SE, focal motor, tonic status, and hyperkinetic SE. NCSE has been

TABLE 25.1 Operational dimensions of status epilepticus

TYPE OF SE	TIME WHEN A SEIZURE IS LIKELY LEAD TO CONTINUOUS SEIZURE ACTIVITY	TIME WHEN A SEIZURE IS LIKELY TO CAUSE LONG TERM CONSEQUENCES
Tonic-clonic SE	5 minutes	30 minutes
Focal SE with impaired consciousness	10 minutes	>60 minutes
Absence SE	10–15 minutes	Unknown

Adapted from Trinca E, et al.[2]

classified into NCSE with coma and NCSE without coma (Figure 25.1).[2] GCSE has the highest risk of morbidity and mortality and constitutes a neurological emergency. A prospective clinical study identified that the majority of patients with glioma had SE with prominent motor symptoms.[3] Specifically, 48% of patients had convulsive SE with focal onset, 26% had focal SE with impaired consciousness, and 26% had focal SE without impaired consciousness.[3] However, more information is needed to draw any definitive conclusions.[2]

> A prospective clinical study identified that the majority of patients with glioma have SE with prominent motor symptoms.

DIAGNOSIS AND TREATMENT

GCSE is diagnosed clinically, and treatment should not be delayed to obtain an EEG or imaging studies. The American Epilepsy Society (AES) recommends beginning the treatment with benzodiazepines after the stabilization phase.[4] Subsequently, use of the longer acting antiseizure drugs (ASD) such as fosphenytoin, valproic acid, and levetiracetam should be initiated at a sufficient dose.[4,5] A recent randomized clinical trial concluded that fosphenytoin, valproic acid, and levetiracetam were equally effective in achieving seizure cessation in half the patients with benzodiazepine-refractory CSE.[6] In patients with brain tumors, first-line treatment was successful in 48%, while 23% of patients responded to the second ADS.[3] Importantly, these medications should be administered promptly and in adequate doses.[7]

If seizure activity continues despite the initial treatment with benzodiazepine followed by another ASD, it is defined as a *refractory SE* (RSE), which occurs in approximately 23% of SE.[5,8] A retrospective study identified that 57.9% of patients with brain metastases developed refractory and super-refractory SE.[9] However, unlike patients with glioma who most commonly develop focal SE with secondary generalization, patients with brain metastases had NCSE.[9]

A randomized clinical trial established that the efficacy of the second ADS in aborting CSE was 7.0% and of the third ADS was only 2.3%; therefore clinicians commonly proceed with a continuous infusion of anesthetic agents (midazolam, pentobarbital, propofol) in patients with refractory SE.[10] The duration and intensity of treatment is directed by continuous EEG with the goal of cessation of electrographic seizures or burst suppression.[5]

SE that continues despite the use of anesthetic agents is called *super-refractory SE* (SRSE) and has no established treatment guidelines. Immunosuppressive therapy, barbiturate and benzodiazepine taper, ketogenic diet, repetitive transcranial magnetic stimulation, surgical intervention, and ketamine infusion have been evaluated in the past. However, randomized controlled trials (RCTs) are needed to compare

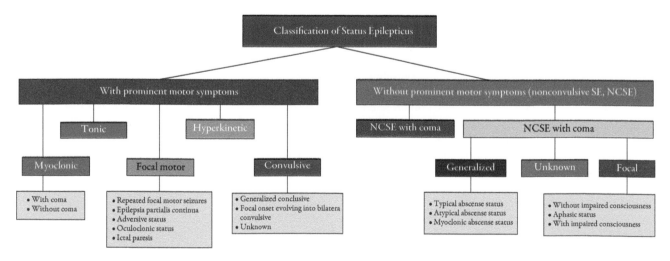

Figure 25.1 Classification of status epilepticus.
Based on Trinca E, et al.[2]

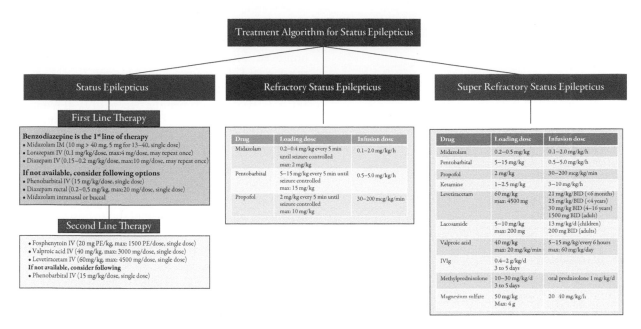

Figure 25.2 Treatment algorithm for status epilepticus.*

Based on Glauser T, et al.[4]; Brophy GM, et al.[5]; Rai S, et al.[7]; Vossler DG, et al.[11]

the effectiveness of anesthetizing and nonanesthetizing ADS to establish effectiveness.[11] The most recent retrospective study showed that high-dose ketamine was associated with a decrease in seizure burden and vasopressor requirements without increase in intracranial pressure (ICP) in patients with SRSE.[12] A treatment algorithm based on the most recent recommendations proposed is shown in Figure 25.2.[4–12]

The clinical outcome after SE appears to be primarily dictated by the underlying disease process, and short-term mortality has been described as higher in brain tumor–related SE compared to SE secondary to other causes.

ACUTE STROKE IN CANCER PATIENTS

EPIDEMIOLOGY

In the United States, stroke constitutes the fifth leading cause of death and is associated with substantial morbidity.[13] Every year, more than 800,000 patients are diagnosed with a stroke; every 3 minutes and 42 seconds someone dies from stroke.[14] Ischemic strokes comprise 87% of all strokes, while intracerebral hemorrhages (ICH) account for 10%, with the remaining 3% attributed to subarachnoid hemorrhages (SAH).[15] Approximately 10% of stroke patients have a comorbid cancer.[16,17] Lung, gastrointestinal, and breast are the most common cancers seen in patients with strokes.[18] The risk of a fatal stroke in cancer patients is two times higher than in the general population and is highest among patients with brain and gastrointestinal malignancies.[17]

ETIOLOGY

Clinical presentation of an ischemic event depends greatly on the underlying etiology; however, encephalopathy, hemiparesis, and seizures have been commonly seen in cancer patients with strokes.[19,20]

Even though the majority of strokes in cancer patients are cryptogenic, atherosclerosis is the most commonly identified mechanism of stroke.[17] Prior radiation, chemotherapy, surgery, recurrent infections, sepsis, invasive procedures, direct tumor invasion, thrombocytosis, leukopenia, disseminated intravascular coagulation, and advanced cancers among other causes that have been linked to an increased risk of stroke in cancer patients (Box 25.1).[18] In fact, it is not uncommon to see asymptomatic small strokes in the resection region on postoperative imaging (Figure 25.3). Randomized studies also highlighted the increased risk of arterial thromboembolic events, including transient ischemic attack or ischemic stroke in bevacizumab-treated patients.[21]

Imaging studies commonly show multifocal-appearing infarcts, while serum workup often reveals increased D-dimer and fibrin degradation products. In fact, high D-dimer levels are associated with early neurological deterioration and ischemic stroke in cancer patients.[22]

PATHOPHYSIOLOGY

Pathophysiology of cancer-related strokes is likely secondary to the combination of direct tumor invasion, coagulation disorders, or sequelae of infections. On the molecular level, production of mucin, and release of tissue factors and procoagulants such as tumor necrosis factor-alpha (TNF-α), interleukin (IL)-1, and IL-6 have been linked to cancer.[23,24] An ongoing prospective study is aiming to evaluate the role of hypercoagulability and cardio-embolism in cancer-associated strokes.[25]

DIAGNOSIS

Patients with signs and symptoms of acute stroke typically undergo immediate general assessment and stabilization in the emergency department followed by neurological evaluation that includes the patient's history, determination of the last known well time, and the stroke severity rating scale. Noncontrast computed tomography (NCCT) of the head should be obtained in all cases before initiating any specific therapy to exclude intracerebral hemorrhage.[26] Additional imaging is recommended for certain cases outlined later.

TREATMENT

Since the publication of the National Institute of Neurological Disorders and Stroke rt-PA Stroke Study (NINDS) in 1995, which showed that the administration of intravenous tissue plasminogen activator (IV tPA) within 3 hours of stroke onset improved clinical outcomes at 3 months, IV tPA has become the standard of care for qualified patients.[23]

In 2008, the European Cooperative Acute Stroke Study III (ECASS III) demonstrated the benefit of IV tPA administered within 4.5 hours of stroke onset in patients without a prior history of stroke and concomitant diabetes, severe stroke scale, warfarin use, and younger than 80 years old.[25] In 2018, the WAKE-UP trial (Efficacy and Safety of MRI-based Thrombolysis in Wake-Up Stroke) showed that the treatment with IV tPA resulted in significantly better functional outcomes in patients with unknown time of stroke onset who had a mismatch between diffusion weighted imaging (DWI) and fluid-attenuated inversion recovery (FLAIR) images in the region of ischemia.[26]

Since patients with malignancies were excluded from these clinical trials, and current guidelines on the early management of patients with acute ischemic stroke indicate that the safety and efficacy of IV tPA with concurrent malignancy are not well established.[27] However, guidelines indicate that patients with systemic malignancy, with the exception of gastrointestinal malignancy, and a reasonable (>6 months) life expectancy might benefit from IV tPA if there are no other contraindications, such as coagulation abnormalities, recent surgery, or systemic bleeding.[27]

Limited data exist on the use of IV tPA in patients with brain tumors. Retrospective case series included 12 patients with meningiomas, acoustic schwannoma, glioblastomas, and astrocytoma who received IV tPA and showed that 2 out of 3 patients with meningioma had favorable outcome while 1 patient with glioblastoma experienced intraparenchymal hemorrhage.[28] Therefore, it is not surprising that current guidelines indicate that IV tPA is contraindicated and thought

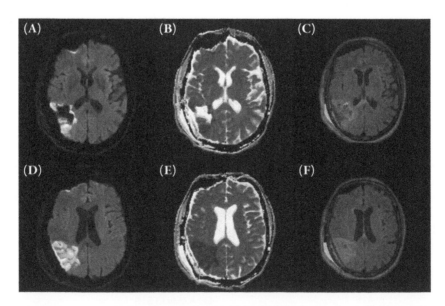

Figure 25.3 MRI brain with and without contrast in a patient who underwent right posterior temporal craniotomy. A 76-year-old right-handed man with glioblastoma underwent redo right posterior temporal craniotomy complicated by acute infarction superior to the resection cavity. (A and D) Diffusion weighted imaging (DWI) shows area of the restricted diffusion surrounding the resection cavity. (B and E) Apparent diffusion coefficient (ADC) maps delineate decreased signal around the resection cavity. (C and F) T2/fluid-attenuated inversion recovery (FLAIR) hyperintense signal in the same region indicative of an acute infarction.

to be potentially harmful in patients who harbor an intra-axial intracranial neoplasm.[27] No official recommendations exist for treatment of patients with extra-axial intracranial neoplasms.

A recent study evaluated 9.5 million acute ischemic stroke hospitalizations from 1998 to 2015, including 0.5 million cancer patients. This study showed that patients with cancer received IV tPA about two-thirds as often as patients without cancer. IV tPA use among cancer patients increased from 0.01% in 1998 to 4.91% in 2015, while IV tPA among patients without cancer increased from 0.02% in 1998 to 7.22% in 2015.[29]

In 2015, multiple independently conducted clinical trials demonstrated the benefit of mechanical thrombectomy with stent retrievers when performed less than 6 hours from stroke onset in patients with proximal arterial occlusion in the anterior circulation (Figures 25.4 and 25.5).[27]

In 2018, clinical trials DAWN (Clinical Mismatch in the Triage of Wake Up and Late Presenting Strokes Undergoing Neurointervention with Trevo) and DIFUSE 3 (Diffusion and Perfusion Imaging Evaluation for Understanding Stroke Evolution) that used clinical-core mismatch as an eligibility criterion to select patients with large anterior circulation vessel occlusion for endovascular thrombectomy between 6 and 24 hours from the last known well time demonstrated that the outcome for disability at 90 days was better with thrombectomy plus standard care than with standard care alone.[27] Patients with cancers were excluded from these trials.

The use of endovascular therapy in cancer patients has not been evaluated on a large scale. Nevertheless, small case series suggest some benefit for endovascular therapy in cancer patients with good premorbid status.[30] Interestingly, use of endovascular therapy in ischemic stroke patients with cancer increased from 0.05% in 2006 to 1.90% in 2015, which was similar to non-cancer patients who received endovascular treatments.[29]

> Given the paucity of data on the best management of ischemic stroke in brain cancer patients, a case-by-case multidisciplinary approach is recommended.

Recent developments for acute stroke care has expanded treatment options for patients with cancer (IV tPA and endovascular thrombectomy). However, further evaluation is necessary to create guidelines and ensure treatment for all qualified patients.

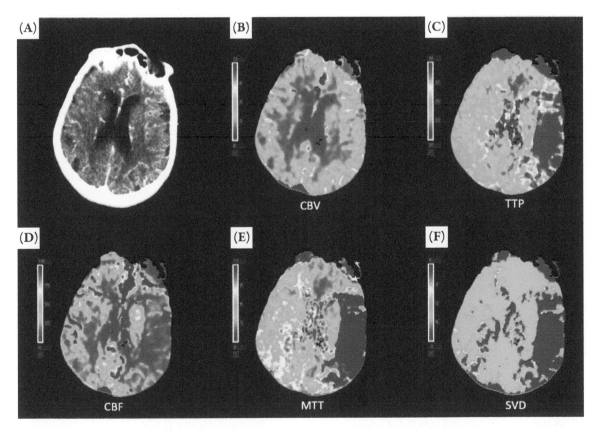

Figure 25.4 CT perfusion in a patient with acute ischemic stroke demonstrating ischemic penumbra. A 63-year-old right-handed woman with stage III breast cancer presents with an acute onset of aphasia and right-sided hemiparesis. (A) Non-contrast CT shows no evidence of acute infarction. (B) CT perfusion cerebral blood volume (CBV) map demonstrates no abnormality. (C) TTP map shows prolongation in the left middle cerebral artery (MCA) territory. (D) Cerebral blood flow (CBF) map shows a region of decreased perfusion in the left MCA region. (E) Mean transit time (MTT) map shows a corresponding prolongation within the same region therefore representing a CBV/MTT mismatch of ischemic penumbra. (F) Singular value deconvolution (SVD) map.

Abbreviations: CBF, cerebral blood flow; CBV, cerebral blood volume; MTT, mean transit time; TTP, time to peak; MCA, middle cerebral artery; SVD, singular value deconvolution.

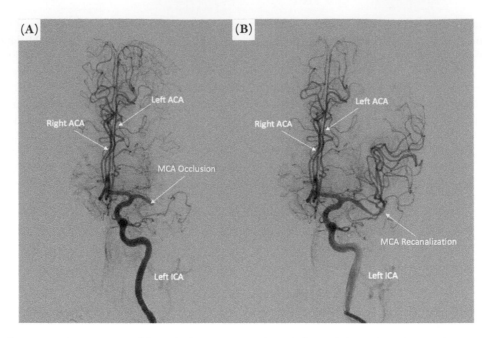

Figure 25.5 *Conventional angiogram demonstrating middle cerebral artery (MCA) occlusion before and after endovascular thrombectomy. A 52-year-old right-handed man with glioblastoma on bevacizumab presented with an acute onset of aphasia and right-sided hemiparesis. (A) Conventional angiogram shows the left M1 MCA occlusion. (B) Conventional angiogram shows recanalization of the M1 MCA.*

Abbreviations: ICA, internal carotid artery; ACA, anterior cerebral artery; MCA, middle cerebral artery.

INTRACEREBRAL HEMORRHAGE IN CANCER PATIENTS

EPIDEMIOLOGY

Spontaneous non-traumatic ICH, accounts for 10% of all strokes in the general population and nearly half of the cerebrovascular events in cancer patients; it has a median case fatality of 40.4% at 1 month.[31-34] Age, severity of neurological impairment, ICH volume, and antithrombotic therapy are main predictors of early mortality.[35] Recently, distant metastatic cancer has been identified as an independent predictor of a poor outcome following ICH.[36] Patients with non-metastatic hematologic tumors and those with metastatic disease fared the worst.[37]

The incidence of cancer in patients with ICH ranges from 1% to 10% and is mainly attributed to metastatic solid tumors.[37-39] Primary brain tumors associated with ICH have an incidence ranging from 7% to 35%.[40,21] Not surprisingly, cancer patients on anticoagulation for treatment of atrial fibrillation have an increased incidence rate of ICH.[41] ICH commonly occurs later in the disease course with only 15% of ICH cases leading to the initial diagnosis of cancer.[31,42]

In cancer patients, intraparenchymal hemorrhage (IPH) is the most common type of ICH, followed by subdural (SDH), subarachnoid (SAH), and epidural hemorrhages.[40]

ETIOLOGY AND PATHOPHYSIOLOGY

The underlying mechanism of IPH depends on the cancer type, coagulation status, anticoagulation use, and chemotherapy.[31] A retrospective study showed that intra-tumoral hemorrhage (61%), coagulopathy (46%), head trauma (6%), hypertension (5%), hemorrhagic conversion of an ischemic stroke (4%), and venous thrombosis (1%) are predisposed to ICH in cancer patients.[38] Intratumoral hemorrhage is commonly observed in patients with vascularized tumors (glioblastoma, melanoma, renal cell carcinoma, thyroid cancer, and choriocarcinoma) while coagulopathy or leukostasis are commonly seen in hematological malignancies.[31,38]

Glioblastoma is the most common malignant primary brain tumor associated with ICH due to its highly invasive and angiogenic nature.[40] Low-grade gliomas could also cause hemorrhage as they contain fragile retiform capillaries.[40,43] Moreover, intratumor hemorrhage has been seen in patients with benign brain tumors such as meningioma.[40]

> Glioblastoma is the most common malignant primary brain tumor associated with ICH due to its highly invasive and angiogenic biological features.

The risk of ICH as a consequence of chemotherapy is relatively low and most commonly occurs in the acute setting.[31,44] L-asparaginase, cisplatin, 5-flourouracil, methotrexate, trastuzumab, and bevacizumab are the most commonly implicated agents.[31] The incidence of ICH in glioblastoma patients on bevacizumab ranges from 0% to 4% based the clinical trials data.[21] However, a recent meta-analysis identified that bevacizumab does not significantly increase the risk of ICH in patients with metastatic solid tumors.[45] Moreover, a retrospective study suggested that bevacizumab use was safe in patients with recurrent high-grade glioma following IPH for whom no other meaningful treatment options exists.[46]

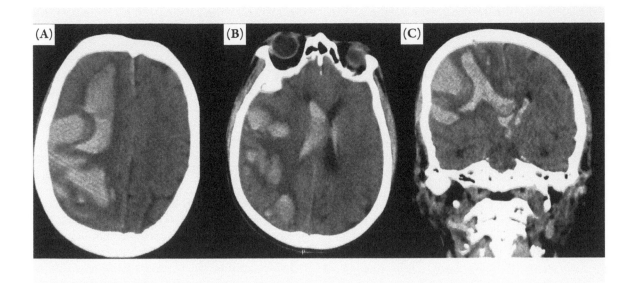

Figure 25.6 *Intraparenchymal hemorrhage with intraventricular extension and brain herniation. A 76-year-old man on anti-coagulation for management of deep venous thromboses (DVTs) and metastatic lung cancer was found down and unresponsive by his family. (A and B) Axial non-contrast CT shows acute massive intracerebral hemorrhage (ICH) in the right hemisphere with surrounding edema and intraventricular extension. (C) Coronal non-contrast CT shows the right hemispheric ICH with subfalcine brain herniation.*

DIAGNOSIS

The majority (94%) of cancer patients with ICH are symptomatic at presentation and commonly experience hemiparesis, headache, encephalopathy, nausea, vomiting, seizure, or coma (Figure 25.6).[38] No difference in location, hemorrhage volume, or Glasgow Coma Scales (GCS) scores was seen in cancer patients with ICH in comparison to the general population.[31]

TREATMENT

Guidelines for Management of Spontaneous Intraparenchymal Hemorrhage highlight the importance of early diagnosis and aggressive care (Box 25.2).[47,48] Seizure prophylaxes in asymptomatic patients is not recommended. Patients with cerebellar

BOX 25.2 CLASS I RECOMMENDATIONS FOR MANAGEMENT OF SPONTANEOUS INTRACEREBRAL HEMORRHAGE (ICH)

Rapid neuroimaging with CT or MRI to distinguish ischemic stroke from ICH

Determination of the baseline severity score

Correction of severe coagulation factors deficiency and thrombocytopenia

Normalization of systolic blood pressure to 140 mm Hg

Initial monitoring and management in the intensive care or stroke units

Maintenance of normoglycemia

Initiation of antiseizure medications in patients with clinical or subclinical seizures

From Hamphill JC, et al.[46]

hemorrhage and worsening neurological examination or those with brainstem compression and/or hydrocephalus, should be considered for urgent surgical intervention.[47]

Current guidelines indicate that intracranial monitoring might be considered for patients with GCS of 8 or lower and for patients with transtentorial herniation, significant intraventricular hemorrhage, or hydrocephalus, with the goal of maintaining a cerebral perfusion pressure (CPP) of 50–70 mm Hg based on the status of cerebral autoregulation (Class IIb).[47] Importantly, steroids should not be administered for treatment of elevated ICP in ICH patients.[47]

VENOUS THROMBOEMBOLISM

EPIDEMIOLOGY

Brain tumor patients have an increased risk of venous thromboembolism (VTE) due to a variety of factors including cancer-associated hypercoagulability, decreased mobility, lower limb paresis, surgical intervention, and antiangiogenic therapy. The risk for VTE is especially increased in patients with high-grade brain tumors compared to benign tumors or low-grade gliomas.[49] Primary outpatient thromboprophylaxis is not generally recommended in brain tumor patients. However, brain tumor patients should be offered pharmacologic thromboprophylaxis in the perioperative settings.[50]

DIAGNOSIS

Accurate diagnosis of VTE in brain cancer patients is important because systemic complications could be detrimental. The diagnostic algorithm is based on the pretest probability (PTP) for individual patients who are stratified into low, intermediate, and high PTP groups.[51] The American Society of Hematology (ASH) recommends initiating diagnostic workup with D-dimer followed by lower extremity ultrasound for patients with low PTP/prevalence (≤10%) of VTE.[51] In a patient with intermediate PTP/prevalence (~25%) of VTE, the guideline suggests starting with an ultrasound of the lower extremity. Patients in the high PTP/prevalence (≥50%) group should also be evaluated with lower extremity ultrasound initially, and, if negative, this should be followed by serial ultrasounds.[51]

TREATMENT

The basic principles of treatment of acute VTE also apply in patients with brain tumors, but the need for anticoagulation has to be balanced with the increased risk of ICH in this patient population. Malignant brain tumors have generally a higher propensity to intratumoral hemorrhage than do benign tumors. In primary brain tumors, bleeding risk additionally increases with tumor grade, with glioblastoma having a significantly higher risk of intratumoral hemorrhage compared to low-grade gliomas.[52] Brain metastases from melanoma, renal cell carcinoma, choriocarcinoma, and thyroid carcinoma carry the highest bleeding risk.[53] Other brain tumor–specific factors that increase the risk for intracerebral hemorrhage include recent neurosurgical intervention, prior tumor-associated hemorrhage, and antiangiogenic therapy with bevacizumab.[54]

> Brain metastases from melanoma, renal cell carcinoma, choriocarcinoma, and thyroid carcinoma carry the highest bleeding risk.

ANTICOAGULATION

In most brain tumor patients, the increased risk for ICH is not prohibitive to therapeutic anticoagulation.[55] Additionally, untreated VTE carries a high risk for serious morbidity and mortality. Therefore, brain tumor-associated VTE generally shares the same treatment approach and absolute contraindications as VTE in other patient populations. Prohibitive to anticoagulation are acute serious bleeding (including ICH), uncontrolled malignant hypertension, uncompensated coagulopathy, severe platelet dysfunction, severe thrombocytopenia, and a high-risk invasive procedure in a critical side of the brain within the last 7–14 days.[50] Relative contraindications specific to brain tumor patients are a history of prior tumor-associated hemorrhage or high-risk tumor type (metastases from melanoma, renal cell, and thyroid carcinomas). In those cases, the benefit of anticoagulation has to be weighed against the bleeding risk on a case-by-case basis.

Brain tumor patients who are deemed appropriate candidates for anticoagulation are preferably treated with low-molecular-weight heparin (LMWH) due to its superior effectiveness in preventing recurrent VTE in cancer patients when compared to vitamin K antagonists.[50] Direct oral anticoagulants (DOACs) are also increasingly used in the treatment of cancer patients with VTE. However, there is insufficient data regarding their efficacy and safety profile in brain tumor patients, and their role remains less clear. To prevent recurrence of VTE, anticoagulation should be continued for at least 6 months. Anticoagulation beyond 6 months should be considered in select patients with high risk of recurrence, especially patients with recurrent VTE, metastatic active cancer, glioblastoma, and patients receiving chemotherapy.[50]

FEBRILE NEUTROPENIA

Cancer patients are at risk for myelosuppression from their underlying disease and as a consequence of antineoplastic therapy. Severe hematologic toxicity is less common in the treatment of brain tumors when compared to systemic malignancies. When it does occur however, it poses a substantial risk to the patient and can result in treatment delays or discontinuation.

Fever is a common complication in neutropenic patients and can be indicative of a potentially severe underlying infection or occur in isolation. The National Cancer Institute's Common Terminology Criteria for Adverse Events (CTCAE) v.5.0 currently define neutropenic fever as a grade 3–4 complication characterized by an absolute neutrophil count (ANC) of less than 1,000/mm³ and a single temperature of greater than 38.3°C(101°F) or a sustained temperature of ≥38°C (100.4°F) for more than 1 hour.[56] Neutropenia in brain tumor patients is most commonly observed with nitrosoureas and other alkylating agents but less frequently with temozolomide.[57]

Lymphopenia is more commonly seen with temozolomide, especially with concomitant corticosteroid therapy, and can predispose to certain infections including *Pneumocystis jiroveci* pneumonia (PCP) due to selective CD4⁺ T-cell depletion.[57,58] Armstrong et al. performed a retrospective analysis of 680 patients with malignant glioma and found that severe myelotoxicity with temozolomide was almost twice as common in women when compared to men (p = 0.015).[58] The current National Comprehensive Cancer Network (NCCN) clinical practice guidelines for prevention and treatment of cancer-related infections recommend empiric broad-spectrum antimicrobial treatment in all patients with neutropenic fever while a careful workup for infection is completed. Inpatient admission and IV antibiotic treatment is recommended for all patients with high-risk features.[59]

> Neutropenia in brain tumor patients is most commonly seen when nitrosoureas and other alkylating agents are used.

THROMBOCYTOPENIA

Thrombocytopenia is another potentially severe complication in brain tumor patients undergoing cytotoxic chemotherapy. Thrombocytopenia in adults is commonly defined as a platelet count of less than 150,000/μL and severe thrombocytopenia as a platelet count of less than 50,000/μL.[60]

In patients with glioblastoma undergoing radiochemotherapy with temozolomide, thrombocytopenia has been reported in 11% of patients in the adjuvant phase and 3% in the concomitant phase of treatment.[61] American Society of Clinical Oncology (ASCO) guidelines currently recommend prophylactic platelet transfusion in patients with solid tumors and a platelet count of less than 10,000/μL; however, a lower threshold will be appropriate in patients with necrotic or hemorrhagic tumors and those undergoing neurosurgical intervention, those on anti-coagulation, actively bleeding, and those with high risk of seizures.[62]

> Per American Society of Clinical Oncology Guidelines, prophylactic platelet transfusion in oncologic patients should be considered when platelet counts drops below 10,000/μL unless other risk factors exist.

Importantly, concomitant therapy with bevacizumab significantly increased the risk of both neutropenia and thrombocytopenia in a randomized trial in patients with newly diagnosed glioblastoma.[62] Overall, hematologic toxicities are common in patients with brain tumors and the correct diagnosis and treatment of these potentially severe complications is an integral part of neuro-oncological practice.

BOWEL PERFORATION IN PATIENTS RECEIVING ANTI-VEGF AND CORTICOSTEROID THERAPY

Inhibitors of angiogenesis have been found to be effective in the treatment of several advanced solid malignancies by limiting blood supply and inhibiting tumor growth. There are currently several classes of angiogenesis inhibitors available, including monoclonal antibodies directed against vascular endothelial growth factor (VEGF) or its receptor and multiple orally active tyrosine kinase inhibitors. Bevacizumab, a monoclonal antibody that binds to VEGF, has been approved in the United States for the treatment of recurrent high-grade gliomas.[63-66]

The use of bevacizumab in newly diagnosed high-grade gliomas is limited as randomized trials failed to show a significant effect on overall survival and demonstrated increased treatment-related toxicity.[54,67] Nevertheless, bevacizumab and oral corticosteroids both have important roles in the treatment of tumor-related edema, radiation necrosis, and associated neurological symptoms. When using these therapies it is, however, important to be aware of potential treatment-related side effects and complications. VEGF-pathway inhibitors particularly have been associated with a number of unique side effects that are not typically observed with conventional cytotoxic chemotherapy. These include cardiovascular side effects such as arterial and venous thrombosis and left ventricular dysfunction, as well as non-cardiovascular side effects involving the gastrointestinal, genitourinary, hematologic, endocrine, respiratory, and nervous systems. Gastrointestinal side effects are common and can include abdominal pain, decreased appetite, diarrhea, nausea, and stomatitis. In addition, rare but severe and occasionally fatal reactions have been observed with

bevacizumab therapy, including GI perforation, hemorrhage, and thromboembolism.[68]

GI perforation is a life-threatening but potentially reversible complication that demands a high level of vigilance from the treating physician. Patients with ovarian cancer and malignancies of the GI tract appear to be at increased risk for GI perforations, but cases of bowel perforation have also been reported in other malignancies. Hapani et al. performed a literature review of prospective RCTs published between 1966 and 2008 comparing bevacizumab with standard therapy. Among 12,294 patients with various types of solid tumors, the incidence of GI perforation with bevacizumab was found to be 0.9% (95% confidence interval [CI] 0.7–1.2) with a mortality of 21.7% (11.5–37.0) and relative risk (RR) of 2.14 (95% CI 1.19–3.85; p = 0.011) when compared to controls.[69] Norden et al. performed a review of 244 glioma patients who were treated with anti-angiogenic drugs between 2003 and 2008 and found six cases (2.5%) with GI perforation.[70] Importantly, all six patients had received dexamethasone, 2 mg or more, for at least 2 weeks.[70]

Corticosteroid therapy is a well-known risk factor for GI perforation with an incidence of close to 3% in retrospective case series of patients treated with 16 mg/day or more of dexamethasone.[71,72] Other proposed risk factors for GI perforation with bevacizumab include local factors affecting the GI tract such as diverticulosis, bowel metastasis, history of prior abdominopelvic radiation, and abdominal carcinomatosis.[73] Early recognition is crucial in the management of GI perforation, and initial management depends on clinical factors such as severity and performance status. Badgwell et al. reported a retrospective series of 24 patients with systemic malignancies who had been treated with bevacizumab and developed bowel perforation. In the study, 79% of patients were initially managed conservatively and 21% underwent surgical repair with an overall 30-day mortality rate of 12.5%.[74]

In summary, GI perforation is a rare but severe complication of anti-VEGF and corticosteroid therapy that demands a high degree of vigilance and prompt treatment to avoid further complications or death.

> Brain cancer patients frequently receive bevacizumab and corticosteroids – both associated with potentially severe GI complications. Clinical vigilance is critical in this patient population.

MALIGNANT SPINAL CORD COMPRESSION

EPIDEMIOLOGY

Malignant spinal cord compression (MSCC) is considered to be one of the most devastating complications of cancer that could result in an irreversible neurological impairment if not diagnosed and managed promptly.[75] MSCC is defined as a compression of the spinal cord or cauda equina by metastatic tumor or direct spread of cancer to the vertebral bodies.[75,76] MSCC occurs in up to 5% of all cancer patients and is most commonly seen with breast, lung, and prostate cancers,

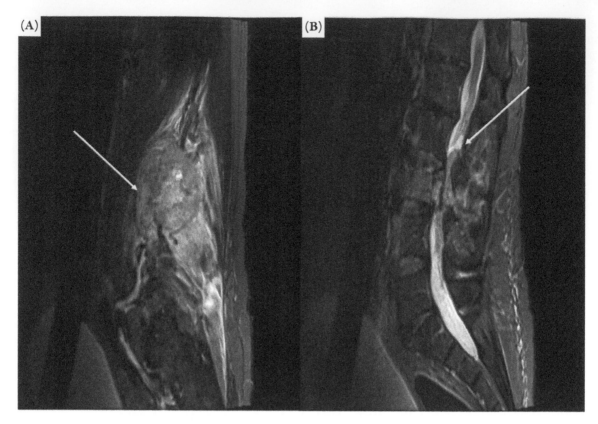

Figure 25.7 *Metastatic spinal cord lesion seen in the thoracolumbar region. A 52-year-old man presented with back pain and bilateral lower extremities weakness. (A and B) MRI short tau inversion recovery (STIR) T2 shows spinal cord compression without visible cerebral spinal fluid.*

comprising together 61% of all MSCC cases.[77] About 20% of MSCC cases represent the new manifestation of cancer.[77]

ETIOLOGY AND PATHOPHYSIOLOGY

Metastatic lesions are most commonly seen in the thoracic spine (70%) followed by the lumbar (20%) and cervical spine (10%).[78,79] Hematogenous dissemination of malignant cells from solid tumors that express tropism for the vertebral body is the major mechanism of metastases to the spine.[80,81] MSCC could be due to the collapse of the vertebral body or by epidural spinal cord compression (ESCC).[82]

Clinical presentation may be insidious in onset and initially manifest as a localized or generalized back pain in more than 95% of patients.[80,83] With disease progression, sensory-motor deficits occur, followed by the loss of sphincter control and paraplegia.[75]

Malignant spinal cord compression must be recognized and treated promptly to avoid permanent neurologic damage.

DIAGNOSIS

The initial evaluation of patients with suspected MSCC should be comprehensive to include history; neurological examination to evaluate strength, sensation, reflexes, and sphincter function; and imaging studies. Magnetic resonance imaging (MRI) is the imaging modality of choice and provides sensitivity of 93% and specificity of 98% (Figure 25.7).[75] Evaluation with CT and

myelography is used in cases when MRI is contraindicated.[75] The ESCC score is calculated based on imaging findings and utilized in the determination of the treatment options (Box 25.3).[84]

TREATMENT

Initial management includes glucocorticoid use that provides analgesia and preserves neurological function.[84] A systematic review concluded that an initial 10 mg intravenous bolus of dexamethasone followed by 16 mg oral daily dose was associated with fewer complications compared with 100 mg bolus and 96 mg daily dose.[85] Pain management medications (opioids),

---

BOX 25.3 EPIDURAL SPINAL CORD COMPRESSION (ESCC) SCALE

0: Tumor confined to bone
1: Tumor extension into the epidural space without deformation of the spinal cord
    1a: Epidural impingement but no deformation of the thecal sac
    1b: Deformation of the thecal sac but without spinal cord abutment
    1c: Deformation of the thecal sac but without spinal cord abutment
2: Spinal cord compression with visible cerebral spinal fluid
3: Spinal cord compression without visible cerebral spinal fluid

Adapted from Lawton AJ, et al.[82]

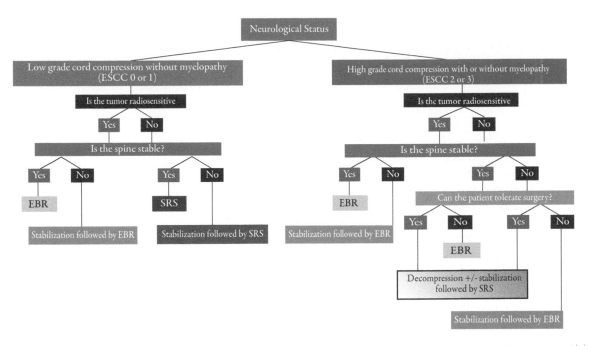

Figure 25.8 *Spinal cord metastases treatment decision framework. Patients with neurological impairment should undergo symptomatic treatment with high-dose steroids to reduce inflammation and pain. Proposed regimen: loading dose of dexamethasone 10 mg followed by 4 mg every 6 hours.*

Abbreviations: ESCC, epidural spinal cord compression scale; EBR, external beam radiation; SRS, stereotactic radiation. Adapted from Lawton AJ, et al.[82]; Laufer I, et al.[86]

neuropathic pain adjuvants (gabapentin, pregabalin, amitriptyline, nortriptyline), bone pain adjuvants (zoledronic acid, pamidronate, acetaminophen), and bowel regimen medications are commonly utilized for symptomatic management.[84]

Surgical intervention and radiation therapy (RT) are two major treatment modalities commonly used in MSCC patients. Spinal stability, the extent of neurological impairment, and the patient's prognosis determine the indication for surgery before RT.[84] Studies indicate that surgery improved neurological function, resulted in immediate and sustained pain relief, and improved quality of life.[84-88] In 2005, a randomized controlled clinical trial determined that in selected patients with solid tumors decompressive surgery followed by RT was superior to RT alone.[89] However, in 2010, matched pair analysis showed no difference between patients who regained ambulatory function and underwent either surgery and RT or RT alone (Figure 25.8).[90,91] Thus, additional investigations are warranted to delineate and specify patients who are likely to benefit from each approach.

ACUTE TOXICITIES FROM CAR-T CELL THERAPY

Diffuse gliomas are the most common primary brain tumors. In the absence of effective therapies for these incurable malignancies, there is a tremendous medical need for new therapeutic concepts. Selective immunological targeting of glioma cells is an attractive therapeutic option for these highly heterogeneous tumors. Recently, there has been remarkable clinical success with immunotherapeutic approaches that use chimeric antigen receptor (CAR) T cells in hematological B-cell malignancies.[92,93] CAR-T cells allow targeting of tumor-specific antigens without the need for MHC expression or co-stimulation.

First experiences with CAR-T cells in diffuse gliomas have shown evidence for antitumor activity in a subset of patients, including complete tumor regression in one patient.[94-97] However, response rates compared to hematological malignancies have been relatively low and neurotoxicity remains an important concern.[98]

CYTOKINE RELEASE SYNDROME

Three commercially manufactured CD-19–directed CAR-T cell preparations (tisagenlecleucel, axicabtagene ciloleucel, and, most recently, brexucabtagene autoleucel) are currently approved by the FDA for treatment of advanced acute lymphoblastic leukemia (ALL) and non-Hodgkin lymphoma (NHL). A unique and common side effect of CAR-T cell therapy is cytokine release syndrome (CRS). CRS is caused by the excessive release of pro-inflammatory cytokines by CAR-T cells after binding to the target antigen. Cytokines involved include TNF-α and interleukins such as IL-2, IL-8, and IL-10.[99] This in turn triggers production of IL-6 and IL-1 by components of the host's innate immune system, as well as other proinflammatory chemokines and cytokines.

Clinical manifestations of CRS include constitutional symptoms such as a fever, malaise, fatigue, myalgias, and arthralgias in mild cases and a shock-like picture that can progress to cardiovascular collapse and multisystem organ failure in severe cases.[100] The CAR T-cell Therapy-Associated Toxicity (CARTOX) Working Group and American Society for Transplantation and Cellular Therapy (ASTCT) have proposed standardized grading systems to assess CRS severity based on vital signs and organ toxicity.[101,102]

NEUROTOXICITY

Neurotoxicity is common with CAR-T cell therapy, and its manifestations range from mild headaches to severe symptoms that can lead to coma and death. A distinct syndrome of T-cell therapy-associated neurotoxicity has been described based on clinical characteristics and is termed *immune effector cell-associated neurotoxicity syndrome* (ICANS). ICANS typically occurs 4–5 days following CAR-T cell infusion and resolves within 3–8 weeks (median duration of 5–12 days); however, a delayed form with onset in the third to fourth week following treatment has been described.[101,103] High tumor burden, higher CAR T-cell expansion, earlier and/or severe CRS, preexisting neurological conditions, and younger age have all been associated with a higher risk of ICANS.[104–106]

> ICANS typically occurs 4–5 days following CAR-T cell infusion and resolves within 3–8 weeks, with median duration of 5–12 days.

Classic early/mild symptoms of ICANS consist of altered mental status and changes in handwriting and expressive aphasia, and these can occur either during, after, or independently of CRS. This can then rapidly progress to cerebral edema, seizures, coma, and possibly death if treatment is not administered rapidly.[107] The ASTCT suggested a 10-point IEC-associated encephalopathy (ICE) score that includes cognitive tests as well as testing of writing abilities and speech and that can be used to grade the severity and as a screening tool for early recognition of ICANS. While the diagnosis is clinical, cranial neuroimaging via CT or MRI brain and lumbar puncture may be indicated to diagnose ICANS and associated cerebral edema.

The first-line therapy of ICANS is corticosteroids. Tocilizumab has been used successfully in the treatment of CRS but has shown limited effectiveness in the treatment of CAR-T cell–related neurotoxicity and should therefore not be used in cases of isolated ICANS.[105,108] Fatal neurotoxicity has been observed in about 3% of patients treated with CD-19–directed CART-T cell therapy and typically occurs in the setting of rapidly progressive cerebral edema[101-103]. Neurotoxicity of other immunotherapies is discussed in Chapter 21.

HYPONATREMIA

Sodium homeostasis is essential for life and is a highly regulated process in which the CNS plays an integral role.[109] Not surprisingly, patients with CNS insults such as brain tumors commonly present with hyponatremia. Hyponatremia is defined as serum sodium concentration of less than 135 mEq/L and is seen in approximately 15% of brain tumor patients.[110] The most recent study identified that 9.3% patients with brain tumors also had concomitant hyponatremia.[111] The study concluded that brain tumor patients with obstructive hydrocephalus, hypertension, and diabetes were more likely to develop perioperative hyponatremia.[111]

> Hyponatremia is common in patients with brain tumors.

Spasovski et al. provided classification of hyponatremia that correlated the severity of the condition with symptom constellations.[112] In fact, patients with mild hyponatremia typically exhibit problems with concentration; those with moderate condition may complain of headache, confusion, or nausea; while severe hyponatremia presents with vomiting, cardiorespiratory distress, somnolence, seizures, or coma.[112] Chronic hyponatremia leads to cognitive impairment, falls, gait instability, fractures and osteoporosis, and calcium-forming kidney stones.[113]

The majority of hyponatremias arise from the imbalance of the electrolyte free water intake and loss.[113] Osmolality, tonicity, and volume status provide the diagnostic framework for hyponatremia classification.[113] Brain tumor patients commonly present with either euvolemic hypotonic hyponatremia indicative of the syndrome of inappropriate antidiuretic hormone secretion (SIADH) or hypovolemic hyponatremia commonly seen with cerebral salt wasting syndrome (CSWS).[113,114] To confirm volume status, fractional sodium excretion (FE_{NA}), fractional uric acid excretion (FE_{UA}), and fractional urea excretion (FE_{urea}) are calculated. Importantly, glucocorticoid deficiency, severe forms of hypothyroidism, thiazides diuretics, and use of nonsteroidal anti-inflammatory drugs (NSAIDs) could also lead to the euvolemic state and must be ruled out before establishing the diagnosis of SIADH.[114, 115] Treatment of hyponatremia is based on underlying etiology.

CEREBRAL EDEMA

Cerebral edema is commonly seen in neuro-oncological patients and categorized into ether vasogenic, cellular, osmotic, or interstitial.[116] Vasogenic cerebral edema results from the disruption of the blood–brain barrier, causing an increased concentration of ions and proteins in the extravascular space leading to an increased fluid content within the brain interstitium via osmosis.[116] Vasogenic edema is predominantly seen in brain tumor patients.

Clinical presentation of cerebral edema ranges from asymptomatic findings on imaging to life-threatening manifestations secondary to increased ICP. Management greatly depends on the extent of the edema and includes positioning, oxygenation/ventilation, hemodynamic support, medical therapy with corticosteroids, and osmotherapy.[117,118] Surgical interventions are indicated in severe cases with mass effect and increased ICP.[117]

CONCLUSION

Neurological emergencies frequently arise in patients with primary brain tumors or with systemic malignancies. Clinical history and examination findings play an essential role in delineating an underlying etiology of the neurological syndrome. Clinicians should be aware that patients with high-grade glioma are at increased risk of developing focal SE with secondary generalization, while patients with brain metastases commonly present with NCSE. Management of an acute ischemic stroke in cancer patients should be addressed on a case-by-case basis as recent developments have expanded available treatment options. ICH is commonly observed in patients with vascular tumors such as glioblastoma, melanoma, renal cell carcinoma, thyroid cancer, and choriocarcinoma. The treatment decision becomes challenging as these patients often require anticoagulation for management of VTE/PE. Myelosuppression could lead to life-threatening conditions such as febrile neutropenia, leukopenia, and thrombocytopenia. Moreover, physicians must be aware that bevacizumab and corticosteroids increase the risk of severe gastrointestinal complications including bowel perforation. Acute neuro-toxicity due to the CAR-T cell therapy manifests with a wide variety of neurological syndromes and must be considered in patients who develop symptoms while undergoing treatment. A high index of suspicion is essential to diagnose hyponatremia and cerebral edema as these conditions could present in mild forms but could lead to rapid deterioration and even death.

Status epilepticus in high-grade glioma patients:	Is more common than in patients with low grade glioma Is associated with high risk of short-term mortality
A study evaluating status epilepticus in patients with glioma found that:	These patients frequently have SE with prominent motor symptoms
The American Epilepsy Society (AES) recommends that:	Treatment of SE with benzodiazepines starts promptly and should not be delayed by obtaining EEG and imaging
Stroke in brain tumor patients:	1. The risk of fatal stroke is high 2. Asymptomatic small strokes adjacent to the resection cavity are common following resection 3. Acute ischemic stroke should be treated on a case-by-case basis by a multidisciplinary team
IV tPA in brain cancer patients:	Is generally not recommended in patients with intra-axial neoplasms (multidisciplinary evaluation is highly recommended) May benefit stroke patients with systemic malignancy with the exception of gastrointestinal malignancy and reasonable (>6 months) life expectancy if there are no other contraindications such as coagulation abnormalities, recent surgery, or systemic bleeding
What is the incidence of intracerebral hemorrhage (ICH) in patients with primary brain tumors?	From 7% to 35%; most hemorrhages occur in the later stages of the disease; patients with glioblastoma are at the highest risk
Is the incidence of ICH in glioblastoma patients receiving bevacizumab high or low?	Low (0–4%)
Venous thromboembolism in brain tumor patients:	Is common; clinical suspicion should be high Patients who are candidates for anticoagulation are preferably treated with low-molecular-weight heparin (LMWH)

Per American Society of Clinical Oncology Guidelines, prophylactic platelet transfusion in oncologic patients should be considered when platelet count drops below what level?	<10,000/μL unless other risk factors exist (i.e., tumors with high risk for ICH, seizures, risk of falls due to neurologic deficits)
Brain metastases from which primary cancers have the highest risk of bleeding?	Melanoma, renal cell carcinoma, choriocarcinoma, and thyroid carcinoma
Immune effector cell-associated neurotoxicity syndrome (ICANS) typically occurs when?	About 4–5 days following CAR-T cell infusion and resolves within 3–8 weeks with median duration of 5–12 days

QUESTIONS

1. The incidence of status epilepticus is highest in:
   a. Low-grade glioma
   b. High-grade glioma
   c. Brain metastases
   d. Benign brain tumors

2. A 53-year-old woman with the right parietal glioblastoma on chemotherapy with temozolomide presented with decreased level of consciousness. Non-contrast head CT showed no acute abnormality. Continuous EEG showed rhythmical epileptogenic discharges in the right temporoparietal region. She received IV lorazepam 0.1 mg/kg/dose twice with no improvement. What would be the next best step in management?

   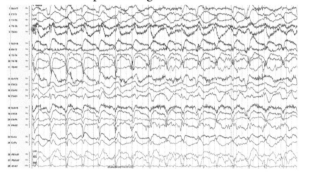

   a. Midazolam (0.2 mg/kg every 5 minutes until seizure control)
   b. Levetiracetam IV (60 mg/kg)
   c. Ketamine (3 mg/kg)
   d. Magnesium sulfate (10 mg/kg)

3. A 72-year-old man with multiple metastatic lung cancer lesions was found down, unresponsive with a GCS of 5. Non-contrast head CT showed left temporal ICH without intraventricular involvement.

   Continuous EEG showed rhythmical epileptogenic discharges in the left temporoparietal region. No clinical or electrographic changes were seen after first- and second-line therapy. However, burst suppression was achieved after he was initiated on the third agent. How do you define this continuous seizure activity?

   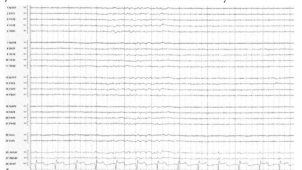

   a. Super-refractory status epilepticus
   b. Epilepsia partialis continua
   c. Status epilepticus
   d. Refractory status epilepticus

4. The following statements about status epilepticus in brain tumor patients are true *except*
   a. Generalized convulsive status epilepticus is a clinical diagnosis.
   b. Status epilepticus secondary to glioma is especially treatment-resistant.
   c. Status epilepticus is operationally defined as continuous seizure lasting for more than 5 minutes or multiple seizures without a return to baseline consciousness between seizures.
   d. The clinical outcome of status epilepticus is primarily dictated by the underlying disease process.

5. Primary outpatient thromboprophylaxis is generally recommended in brain tumor patients in the following scenarios:
   a. In the perioperative setting
   b. For all brain tumor patients
   c. During treatment with antiangiogenic therapy
   d. During chemotherapy

6. Brain tumor patients who require anticoagulation due to VTE are preferably treated with
   a. Warfarin
   b. Rivaroxaban
   c. Dabigatran
   d. Low-molecular-weight heparin

7. Intracranial monitoring in patients with ICH could be considered in following situations:
   a. GCS ≤8
   b. Transtentorial herniation
   c. Intraventricular hemorrhage
   d. Hydrocephalus
   e. All of the above

8. The following Class I recommendations for management of ICH are true *except*
   a. Rapid neuroimaging
   b. Determination of the baseline severity score
   c. Normalization of systolic blood pressure to 160 mm Hg
   d. Maintenance of normoglycemia
   e. Initiation of antiseizure medications in patients with clinical or subclinical seizures

9. Based on the CTCAE v. 5.0, neutropenic fever defined as
   a. ANC of less than 500/mm^3 and a single temperature of greater than 38.0°C (100.4°F)
   b. ANC of less than 1,000/mm^3 and a single temperature of greater than 38.0°C (100.4°F)
   c. ANC of less than 1,000/mm^3 and a single temperature of greater than 38.3°C (101°F)
   d. sustained temperature of 38.3°C (101°F) or higher

10. In a patient with a radiosensitive tumor and unstable low-grade metastatic spinal cord compression without myelopathy, the optimal treatment modality is
    a. External beam radiation

b. Stabilization followed by external beam radiation
c. SRS
d. Stabilization followed by SRS
e. Decompression followed by stabilization and SRS

11. What is the first-line therapy for ICANS?
    a. Tocilizumab
    b. Corticosteroids
    c. IVIG
    d. Plasmapheresis

12. You are reviewing imaging of a GBM patient who recently underwent gross total resection. You see a thin rim of diffusion restriction at the margin of a resection cavity and the radiology report suggests acute stroke. Your next steps are
    a. Call stroke code and evaluate the patient for antithrombotic therapy.
    b. Put the patient on low-dose aspirin.
    c. Call neurosurgery for urgent consult.
    d. Order follow up MRI in 2–4 weeks.

13. A 65-year-old woman with anaplastic astrocytoma comes to the ED with fever (102°F), chills, and shortness of breath. Her absolute neutrophil count is 500/mm³. You are reviewing her oncologic history. The drug that *most likely* led to her current condition is
    a. Bevacizumab
    b. Levetiracetam
    c. Lomustine
    d. Vincristine

14. Seizure prophylaxis in asymptomatic patients with tumor-related intracerebral hemorrhage is always recommended.
    a. True
    b. False

15. A 70-year-old man with progressive GBM presents with acute abdominal pain. KUB shows free air under the diaphragm. You don't have access to his medical records, the patient is confused, and family is not available. The surgeon consulting on the case asks you about possible treatments that the patient could have received recently and if there are any concerns about potential surgical intervention. You suspect
    a. Bowel perforation secondary to bevacizumab, and you educate the surgeon about potential post-surgical wound healing complications.
    b. Severe constipation from ondansetron; you disagree with the surgeon that the patient needs laparotomy.
    c. Appendicitis unrelated to patient's primary diagnosis, and you notify the surgeon that you will hold chemotherapy until the patient is stable postoperatively.
    d. Bowel perforation caused by temozolomide, and you educate the surgeon about possible neutropenia.

ANSWERS

1. b
2. b
3. d
4. b
5. a
6. d
7. e
8. c
9. c
10. b
11. b
12. d
13. c
14. b
15. a

REFERENCES

1. Sculier C, Gaínza-Lein M, Sánchez Fernández I, Loddenkemper T. Long-term outcomes of status epilepticus: A critical assessment. *Epilepsia*. 2018;59(Suppl 2):155–169. doi:10.1111/epi.14515
2. Trinka E, Cock H, Hesdorffer D, et al. A definition and classification of status epilepticus: Report of the ILAE Task Force on Classification of Status Epilepticus. *Epilepsia*. 2015;56(10):1515–1523. doi:10.1111/epi.13121
3. Knudsen-Baas KM, Power KN, Engelsen BA, et al. Status epilepticus secondary to glioma. *Seizure*. 2016;40:76–80. doi:10.1016/j.seizure.2016.06.013
4. Glauser T, Shinnar S, Gloss D, et al. Evidence-based guideline: Treatment of convulsive status epilepticus in children and adults: Report of the Guideline Committee of the American Epilepsy Society. *Epilepsy Curr*. 2016;16(1):48–61. doi:10.5698/1535-7597-16.1.48
5. Brophy GM, Bell R, Claassen J, et al. Guidelines for the evaluation and management of status epilepticus. *Neurocrit Care*. 2012;17(1):3–23. doi:10.1007/s12028-012-9695-z
6. Kapur J, Elm J, Chamberlain JM, et al. Randomized trial of three anticonvulsant medications for status epilepticus. *N Engl J Med*. 2019;381(22):2103–2113. doi:10.1056/NEJMoa1905795
7. Rai S, Drislane FW. Treatment of refractory and super-refractory status epilepticus. *Neurotherapeutics*. 2018;15(3):697–712. doi:10.1007/s13311-018-0640-5
8. Novy J, Logroscino G, Rossetti AO. Refractory status epilepticus: A prospective observational study. *Epilepsia*. 2010;51(2):251–256. doi:10.1111/j.1528-1167.2009.02323.x
9. Fox J, Ajinkya S, Greenblatt A, et al. Clinical characteristics, EEG findings and implications of status epilepticus in patients with brain metastases. *J Neurol Sci*. 2019;407:116538. doi:10.1016/j.jns.2019.116538
10. Treiman DM, Meyers PD, Walton NY, et al. A comparison of four treatments for generalized convulsive status epilepticus: Veterans Affairs Status Epilepticus Cooperative Study Group. *N Engl J Med*. 1998;339(12):792–798. doi:10.1056/NEJM199809173391202
11. Vossler DG, Bainbridge JL, Boggs JG, et al. Treatment of refractory convulsive status epilepticus: A comprehensive review by the American Epilepsy Society Treatments Committee. *Epilepsy Curr*. 2020;20(5):245–264. doi:10.1177/1535759720928269
12. Alkhachroum A, Der-Nigoghossian CA, Mathews E, et al. Ketamine to treat super-refractory status epilepticus. *Neurology*. 2020;95(16):e2286–e2294. doi:10.1212/WNL.0000000000010611
13. Heron M. Deaths: Leading causes for 2017. *Natl Vital Stat Rep*. 2019;68(6):1–77.
14. Virani SS, Alonso A, Benjamin EJ, et al. Heart disease and stroke statistics-2020 update: A report from the American Heart Association. *Circulation*. 2020;141(9):e139–e596. doi:10.1161/CIR.0000000000000757
15. Caplan LR. Stroke classification: A personal view. *Stroke*. 2011;42(1 Suppl):S3–S6. doi:10.1161/STROKEAHA.110.594630
16. Zaorsky NG, Zhang Y, Tchelebi LT, et al. Stroke among cancer patients. *Nat Commun*. 2019;10(1):5172. doi:10.1038/s41467-019-13120-6
17. Sanossian N, Djabiras C, Mack WJ, Ovbiagele B. Trends in cancer diagnoses among inpatients hospitalized with stroke. *J Stroke Cerebrovasc Dis*. 2013;22(7):1146–1150. doi:10.1016/j.jstrokecerebrovasdis.2012.11.016

18. Navi BB, Iadecola C. Ischemic stroke in cancer patients: A review of an underappreciated pathology. *Ann Neurol.* 2018;83(5):873-883. doi:10.1002/ana.25227

19. Dardiotis E, Aloizou AM, Markoula S, et al. Cancer-associated stroke: Pathophysiology, detection and management (Review). *Int J Oncol.* 2019;54(3):779-796. doi:10.3892/ijo.2019.4669

20. Nguyen T, DeAngelis LM. Stroke in cancer patients. *Curr Neurol Neurosci Rep.* 2006;6(3):187-192. doi:10.1007/s11910-006-0004-0

21. Brandes AA, Bartolotti M, Tosoni A, et al. Practical management of bevacizumab-related toxicities in glioblastoma. *Oncologist.* 2015;20(2):166-175. doi:10.1634/theoncologist.2014-0330

22. Hacke W, Kaste M, Bluhmki E, et al. Thrombolysis with alteplase 3 to 4.5 hours after acute ischemic stroke. *N Engl J Med.* 2008;359(13):1317-1329. doi:10.1056/NEJMoa0804656

23. National Institute of Neurological Disorders and Stroke rt-PA Stroke Study Group. Tissue plasminogen activator for acute ischemic stroke. *N Engl J Med.* 1995;333(24):1581-1587.

24. Adams HP Jr. Cancer and cerebrovascular disease. *Curr Neurol Neurosci Rep.* 2019;19(10):73. doi:10.1007/s11910-019-0985-0

25. Mechanism of ischemic Stroke in Cancer patients (MOST—Cancer) (clinicaltrials.gov ID NCT02604667). https://clinicaltrials.gov/ct2/show/NCT02604667

26. Thomalla G, Simonsen CZ, Boutitie F, et al. MRI-guided thrombolysis for stroke with unknown time of onset. *N Engl J Med.* 2018;379(7):611-622. doi:10.1056/NEJMoa1804355

27. Warner JJ, Harrington RA, Sacco RL, Elkind MSV. Guidelines for the early management of patients with acute ischemic stroke: 2019 update to the 2018 guidelines for the early management of acute ischemic stroke. *Stroke.* 2019;50(12):3331-3332. doi:10.1161/STROKEAHA.119.027708

28. Etgen T, Steinich I, Gsottschneider L. Thrombolysis for ischemic stroke in patients with brain tumors. *J Stroke Cerebrovasc Dis.* 2014;23:361-366.

29. Chatterjee A, Merkler AE, Murthy SB, et al. Temporal trends in the use of acute recanalization therapies for ischemic stroke in patients with cancer. *J Stroke Cerebrovasc Dis.* 2019;28(8):2255-2261. doi:10.1016/j.jstrokecerebrovasdis.2019.05.009

30. Merkler AE, Marcus JR, Gupta A, et al. Endovascular therapy for acute stroke in patients with cancer. *Neurohospitalist.* 2014;4:133-135.

31. Weinstock MJ, Uhlmann EJ, Zwicker JI. Intracranial hemorrhage in cancer patients treated with anticoagulation. *Thromb Res.* 2016;140 Suppl 1:S60-S65. doi:10.1016/S0049-3848(16)30100-1

32. Virani SS, Alonso A, Aparicio HJ, et al. Heart disease and stroke statistics-2021 update: A report from the American Heart Association. *Circulation.* 2021;143(8):e254-e743. doi:10.1161/CIR.0000000000000950

33. van Asch CJ, Luitse MJ, Rinkel GJ, et al. Incidence, case fatality, and functional outcome of intracerebral haemorrhage over time, according to age, sex, and ethnic origin: A systematic review and meta-analysis. *Lancet Neurol.* 2010;9(2):167-176.

34. Graus F, Rogers LR, Posner JB. Cerebrovascular complications in patients with cancer. *Medicine.* 1985;64:16-35.

35. Pinho J, Costa AS, Araújo JM, et al. Intracerebral hemorrhage outcome: A comprehensive update. *J Neurol Sci.* 2019;398:54-66. doi:10.1016/j.jns.2019.01.013

36. Gon Y, Todo K, Mochizuki H, Sakaguchi M. Cancer is an independent predictor of poor outcomes in patients following intracerebral hemorrhage. *Eur J Neurol.* 2018;25(1):128-134. doi:10.1111/ene.13456

37. Murthy SB, Shastri A, Merkler AE, et al. Intracerebral hemorrhage outcomes in patients with systemic cancer. *J Stroke Cerebrovasc Dis.* 2016;25(12):2918-2924. doi:10.1016/j.jstrokecerebrovasdis.2016.08.006

38. Navi BB, Reichman JS, Berlin D, et al. Intracerebral and subarachnoid hemorrhage in patients with cancer. *Neurology.* 2010;74(6):494-501. doi:10.1212/WNL.0b013e3181cef837

39. Yuguang L, Meng L, Shugan Z, et al. Intracranial tumoural haemorrhage: A report of 58 cases. *J Clin Neurol* 2002;9:637-639.

40. Velander AJ, DeAngelis LM, Navi BB. Intracranial hemorrhage in patients with cancer. *Curr Atheroscler Rep.* 2012;14(4):373-381. doi:10.1007/s11883-012-0250-3

41. Aspberg S, Yu L, Gigante B, et al. Risk of ischemic stroke and major bleeding in patients with atrial fibrillation and cancer. *J Stroke Cerebrovasc Dis.* 2020;29(3):104560. doi:10.1016/j.jstrokecerebrovasdis.2019.104560

42. Gon Y, Okazaki S, Terasaki Y, et al. Characteristics of cryptogenic stroke in cancer patients. *Ann Clin Transl Neurol.* 2016;3:280-287.

43. Liwnicz BH, Wu SZ, Tew JM. The relationship between the capillary structure and hemorrhage in gliomas. *J Neurosurg.* 1987;66:536-541.

44. Li SH, Chen WH, Tang Y, et al. Incidence of ischemic stroke post-chemotherapy: A retrospective review of 10,963 patients. *Clin Neurol Neurosurg.* 2006;108:150-6.

45. Yang, L., Chen, C., Guo, X. et al. Bevacizumab and risk of intracranial hemorrhage in patients with brain metastases: A meta-analysis. *J Neurooncol.* 2018;137:49-56. https://doi.org/10.1007/s11060-017-2693-4

46. Lin X, Daras M, Pentsova E, et al. Bevacizumab in high-grade glioma patients following intraparenchymal hemorrhage. *Neurooncol Pract.* 2017;4(1):24-28. doi:10.1093/nop/npw008

47. Hemphill JC 3rd, Greenberg SM, Anderson CS, et al. Guidelines for the management of spontaneous intracerebral hemorrhage: A guideline for healthcare professionals from the American Heart Association/American Stroke Association. *Stroke.* 2015;46(7):2032-2060. doi:10.1161/STR.0000000000000069

48. Hemphill JC 3rd, Bonovich DC, Besmertis L, et al. The ICH score: A simple, reliable grading scale for intracerebral hemorrhage. *Stroke.* 2001;32(4):891-897. doi:10.1161/01.str.32.4.891

49. Perry JR. Thromboembolic disease in patients with high-grade glioma. *Neuro Oncol.* 2012;14 Suppl 4(Suppl 4):iv73-iv80. doi:10.1093/neuonc/nos197

50. Key NS, Khorana AA, Kuderer NM, et al. Venous thromboembolism prophylaxis and treatment in patients with cancer: ASCO clinical practice guideline update. *J Clin Oncol.* 2020;38(5):496-520. doi:10.1200/JCO.19.01461

51. Cuker A, Arepally GM, Chong BH, et al. American Society of Hematology 2018 guidelines for management of venous thromboembolism: Heparin-induced thrombocytopenia. *Blood Adv.* 2018;2(22):3360-3392. doi:10.1182/bloodadvances.2018024489

52. Baek HJ, Kim SM, Chung SY, Park MS. Hemorrhagic recurrence in diffuse astrocytoma without malignant transformation. *Brain Tumor Res Treat.* 2014;2(2):119-123. doi:10.14791/btrt.2014.2.2.119

53. Donato J, Campigotto F, Uhlmann EJ, et al. Intracranial hemorrhage in patients with brain metastases treated with therapeutic enoxaparin: A matched cohort study. *Blood.* 2015;126(4):494-499. doi:10.1182/blood-2015-02-626788

54. Chinot OL, Wick W, Cloughesy T. Bevacizumab for newly diagnosed glioblastoma. *N Engl J Med.* 2014;370(21):2049. doi:10.1056/NEJMc1403303

55. Chai-Adisaksopha C, Linkins LA, ALKindi SY, et al. Outcomes of low-molecular-weight heparin treatment for venous thromboembolism in patients with primary and metastatic brain tumours. *Thromb Haemost.* 2017;117(3):589-594. doi:10.1160/TH16-09-0680

56. National Cancer Institute. Division of Cancer Treatment & Diagnosis. Cancer Therapy Evaluation Program. Common Terminology Criteria for Adverse Events (CTCAE) v5.0. Published online on November 27, 2017.https://ctep.cancer.gov/protocolDevelopment/electronic_applications/docs/CTCAE_v5_Quick_Reference_5x7.pdf

57. Villano JL, Letarte N, Yu JM, et al. Hematologic adverse events associated with temozolomide. *Cancer Chemother Pharmacol.* 2012;69(1):107-113. doi:10.1007/s00280-011-1679-8

58. Armstrong TS, Cao Y, Scheurer ME, et al. Risk analysis of severe myelotoxicity with temozolomide: The effects of clinical and genetic factors. *Neuro Oncol.* 2009;11(6):825-832. doi:10.1215/15228517-2008-120

59. National Comprehensive Cancer Network (NCCN). Clinical practice guidelines in oncology. Prevention and treatment of cancer-related infections. Version 2.2020. http://www.nccn.org

60. Williamson DR, Albert M, Heels-Ansdell D, et al. Thrombocytopenia in critically ill patients receiving thromboprophylaxis: Frequency, risk factors, and outcomes. *Chest.* 2013;144(4):1207-1215. doi:10.1378/chest.13-0121

61. Stupp R, Mason WP, van den Bent MJ, et al. Radiotherapy plus concomitant and adjuvant temozolomide for glioblastoma. *N Engl J Med.* 2005;352(10):987-996. doi:10.1056/NEJMoa043330

62. Schiffer CA, Bohlke K, Delaney M, et al. Platelet transfusion for patients with cancer: American Society of Clinical Oncology clinical practice guideline update. *J Clin Oncol.* 2018;36(3):283-299. doi:10.1200/JCO.2017.76.1734

63. Kreisl TN, Kim L, Moore K, et al. Phase II trial of single-agent bevacizumab followed by bevacizumab plus irinotecan at tumor progression in recurrent glioblastoma. *J Clin Oncol.* 2009;27(5):740-745. doi:10.1200/JCO.2008.16.3055

64. Friedman HS, Prados MD, Wen PY, et al. Bevacizumab alone and in combination with irinotecan in recurrent glioblastoma. *J Clin Oncol.* 2009;27(28):4733-4740. doi:10.1200/JCO.2008.19.8721

65. Taal W, Oosterkamp HM, Walenkamp AM, et al. Single-agent bevacizumab or lomustine versus a combination of bevacizumab plus lomustine in patients with recurrent glioblastoma (BELOB trial): A randomised controlled phase 2 trial. *Lancet Oncol.* 2014;15(9):943-953. doi:10.1016/S1470-2045(14)70314-6

66. Brandes AA, Finocchiaro G, Zagonel V, et al. AVAREG: A phase II, randomized, noncomparative study of fotemustine or bevacizumab for patients with recurrent glioblastoma. *Neuro Oncol.* 2016;18(9):1304-1312. doi:10.1093/neuonc/now035

67. Gilbert MR, Dignam JJ, Armstrong TS, et al. A randomized trial of bevacizumab for newly diagnosed glioblastoma. *N Engl J Med.* 2014;370(8):699–708. doi:10.1056/NEJMoa1308573

68. Ranpura V, Hapani S, Wu S. Treatment-related mortality with bevacizumab in cancer patients: A meta-analysis [published correction appears in JAMA. 2011 Jun 8;305(22):2294]. *JAMA.* 2011;305(5):487–494. doi:10.1001/jama.2011.51

69. Hapani S, Chu D, Wu S. Risk of gastrointestinal perforation in patients with cancer treated with bevacizumab: A meta-analysis. *Lancet Oncol.* 2009;10(6):559–568. doi:10.1016/S1470-2045(09)70112-3

70. Norden AD, Drappatz J, Ciampa AS, et al. Colon perforation during antiangiogenic therapy for malignant glioma. *Neuro Oncol.* 2009;11(1):92–95. doi:10.1215/15228517-2008-071

71. Fadul CE, Lemann W, Thaler HT, Posner JB. Perforation of the gastrointestinal tract in patients receiving steroids for neurologic disease. *Neurology.* 1988;38(3):348–352. doi:10.1212/wnl.38.3.348

72. Koehler PJ. Use of corticosteroids in neuro-oncology. *Anticancer Drugs.* 1995;6(1):19–33. doi:10.1097/00001813-199502000-00002

73. Heinzerling JH, Huerta S. Bowel perforation from bevacizumab for the treatment of metastatic colon cancer: Incidence, etiology, and management. *Curr Surg.* 2006;63(5):334–337. doi:10.1016/j.cursur.2006.06.002

74. Badgwell BD, Camp ER, Feig B, et al. Management of bevacizumab-associated bowel perforation: A case series and review of the literature. *Ann Oncol.* 2008;19(3):577–582. doi:10.1093/annonc/mdm508

75. Boussios S, Cooke D, Hayward C, et al. Metastatic spinal cord compression: Unraveling the diagnostic and therapeutic challenges. *Anticancer Res.* 2018;38(9):4987–4997. doi:10.21873/anticanres.12817

76. Drudge-Coates L, Rajbabu K. Diagnosis and management of malignant spinal cord compression: Part 1. *Int J Palliat Nurs.* 2008;14(3):110–116. doi:10.12968/ijpn.2008.14.3.28890

77. Loblaw DA, Laperriere NJ. Emergency treatment of malignant extradural spinal cord compression: An evidence-based guideline. *J Clin Oncol.* 1998;16(4):1613–1624. doi:10.1200/JCO.1998.16.4.1613

78. Sciubba DM, Petteys RJ, Dekutoski MB, et al. Diagnosis and management of metastatic spine disease. A review. *J Neurosurg Spine.* 2010;13:94–108.

79. Barzilai O, Laufer I, Yamada Y, et al. Integrating evidence-based medicine for treatment of spinal metastases into a decision framework: Neurologic, oncologic, mechanicals stability, and systemic disease. *J Clin Oncol.* 2017;35(21):2419–2427. doi:10.1200/JCO.2017.72.7362

80. Nair C, Panikkar S, Ray A. How not to miss metastatic spinal cord compression. *Br J Gen Pract.* 2014;64(626):e596–e598. doi:10.3399/bjgp14X681589

81. Di Martino A, Caldaria A, De Vivo V, Denaro V. Metastatic epidural spinal cord compression. *Expert Rev Anticancer Ther.* 2016;16(11):1189–1198. doi:10.1080/14737140.2016.1240038

82. Schmidt MH, Klimo P, Vrionis FD. Metastatic spinal cord compression. *J Natl Compr Cancer Netw.* 2005;3:711–719.

83. Cole JS, Patchell RA. Metastatic epidural spinal cord compression. *Lancet Neurol.* 2008;7(5):459–466. doi:10.1016/S1474-4422(08)70089-9

84. Lawton AJ, Lee KA, Cheville AL, et al. Assessment and management of patients with metastatic spinal cord compression: A multidisciplinary review. *J Clin Oncol.* 2019;37(1):61–71. doi:10.1200/JCO.2018.78.1211

85. Kumar A, Weber MH, Gokaslan Z, et al. Metastatic spinal cord compression and steroid treatment: A systematic review. *Clin Spine Surg.* 2017;30(4):156–163. doi:10.1097/BSD.0000000000000528

86. Fehlings MG, Nater A, Tetreault L, et al. Survival and clinical outcomes in surgically treated patients with metastatic epidural spinal cord compression: Results of the prospective multicenter AOSpine study. *J Clin Oncol.* 2016;34:268–276.

87. Ibrahim A, Crockard A, Antonietti P, et al. Does spinal surgery improve the quality of life for those with extradural (spinal) osseous metastases? An international multicenter prospective observational study of 223 patients. Invited submission from the Joint Section Meeting on Disorders of the Spine and Peripheral Nerves, March 2007. *J Neurosurg Spine.* 2008;8:271–278.

88. Wu J, Zheng W, Xiao JR, et al. Health-related quality of life in patients with spinal metastases treated with or without spinal surgery: A prospective, longitudinal study. *Cancer.* 2010;116:3875–3882.

89. Patchell RA, Tibbs PA, Regine WF, et al. Direct decompressive surgical resection in the treatment of spinal cord compression caused by metastatic cancer: A randomised trial. *Lancet.* 2005;366:643–648.

90. Rades D, Huttenlocher S, Dunst J, et al. Matched pair analysis comparing surgery followed by radiotherapy and radiotherapy alone for metastatic spinal cord compression. *J Clin Oncol.* 2010;28:3597–3604.

91. Laufer I, Rubin DG, Lis E, et al. The NOMS framework: Approach to the treatment of spinal metastatic tumors. *Oncologist.* 2013;18(6):744–751. doi:10.1634/theoncologist.2012-0293

92. Gill S, June CH. Going viral: Chimeric antigen receptor T-cell therapy for hematological malignancies. *Immunol Rev.* 2015;263(1):68–89. doi:10.1111/imr.12243

93. Scarfò I, Maus MV. Current approaches to increase CAR T cell potency in solid tumors: Targeting the tumor microenvironment. *J Immunother Cancer.* 2017;5:28. doi:10.1186/s40425-017-0230-9

94. Ahmed N, Brawley V, Hegde M, et al. HER2-specific chimeric antigen receptor-modified virus-specific T cells for progressive glioblastoma: A Phase 1 dose-escalation trial. *JAMA Oncol.* 2017;3(8):1094–1101. doi:10.1001/jamaoncol.2017.0184

95. Brown CE, Alizadeh D, Starr R, et al. Regression of glioblastoma after chimeric antigen receptor T-cell therapy. *N Engl J Med.* 2016;375(26):2561–2569. doi:10.1056/NEJMoa1610497

96. Jonnalagadda M, Mardiros A, Urak R, et al. Chimeric antigen receptors with mutated IgG4 Fc spacer avoid fc receptor binding and improve T cell persistence and antitumor efficacy. *Mol Ther.* 2015;23(4):757–768. doi:10.1038/mt.2014.208

97. O'Rourke DM, Nasrallah MP, Desai A, et al. A single dose of peripherally infused EGFRvIII-directed CAR T cells mediates antigen loss and induces adaptive resistance in patients with recurrent glioblastoma. *Sci Transl Med.* 2017;9(399):eaaa0984. doi:10.1126/scitranslmed.aaa0984

98. Mount CW, Majzner RG, Sundaresh S, et al. Potent antitumor efficacy of anti-GD2 CAR T cells in H3-K27M+ diffuse midline gliomas. *Nat Med.* 2018;24(5):572–579. doi:10.1038/s41591-018-0006-x

99. Titov A, Petukhov A, Staliarova A, et al. The biological basis and clinical symptoms of CAR-T therapy-associated toxicites. *Cell Death Dis.* 2018;9(9):897. Published 2018 Sep 4. doi:10.1038/s41419-018-0918-x

100. Alvi RM, Frigault MJ, Fradley MG, et al. Cardiovascular events among adults treated with chimeric antigen receptor T-cells (CAR-T). *J Am Coll Cardiol.* 2019;74(25):3099–3108. doi:10.1016/j.jacc.2019.10.038

101. Neelapu SS, Tummala S, Kebriaei P, et al. Chimeric antigen receptor T-cell therapy: Assessment and management of toxicities. *Nat Rev Clin Oncol.* 2018;15(1):47–62. doi:10.1038/nrclinonc.2017.148

102. Lee DW, Santomasso BD, Locke FL, et al. ASTCT consensus grading for cytokine release syndrome and neurologic toxicity associated with immune effector cells. *Biol Blood Marrow Transplant.* 2019;25(4):625–638. doi:10.1016/j.bbmt.2018.12.758

103. Hunter BD, Jacobson CA. CAR T-cell associated neurotoxicity: Mechanisms, clinicopathologic correlates, and future directions. *J Natl Cancer Inst.* 2019;111(7):646–654. doi:10.1093/jnci/djz017

104. Gust J, Hay KA, Hanafi LA, et al. Endothelial activation and blood-brain barrier disruption in neurotoxicity after adoptive immunotherapy with CD19 CAR-T cells. *Cancer Discov.* 2017;7(12):1404–1419. doi:10.1158/2159-8290.CD-17-0698

105. Santomasso BD, Park JH, Salloum D, et al. Clinical and biological correlates of neurotoxicity associated with CAR T-cell therapy in patients with B-cell acute lymphoblastic leukemia. *Cancer Discov.* 2018;8(8):958–971. doi:10.1158/2159-8290.CD-17-1319

106. Schuster SJ, Bishop MR, Tam CS, et al. Tisagenlecleucel in adult relapsed or refractory diffuse large B-cell lymphoma. *N Engl J Med.* 2019;380(1):45–56. doi:10.1056/NEJMoa1804980

107. Varadarajan I, Lee DW. Management of T-cell engaging immunotherapy complications. *Cancer J.* 2019;25(3):223–230. doi:10.1097/PPO.0000000000000377

108. Neelapu SS, Locke FL, Bartlett NL, et al. Axicabtagene ciloleucel CAR T-cell therapy in refractory large B-cell lymphoma. *N Engl J Med.* 2017;377(26):2531–2544. doi:10.1056/NEJMoa1707447

109. Sterns RH. Disorders of plasma sodium: Causes, consequences, and correction. *N Engl J Med.* 2015;372(1):55–65. doi:10.1056/NEJMra1404489

110. Human T, Cook AM, Anger B, et al. Treatment of hyponatremia in patients with acute neurological injury. *Neurocrit Care.* 2017;27(2):242–248. doi:10.1007/s12028-016-0343-x

111. Patel S, Chiu RG, Rosinski CL, et al. Risk factors for hyponatremia and perioperative complications with malignant intracranial tumor resection in adults: An analysis of the nationwide inpatient sample from 2012 to 2015. *World Neurosurg.* 2020;144:e876–e882. doi:10.1016/j.wneu.2020.09.097

112. Spasovski G, Vanholder R, Allolio B, et al. Clinical practice guideline on diagnosis and treatment of hyponatraemia [published correction appears in Nephrol Dial Transplant. 2014 Jun;40(6):924. *Nephrol Dial Transplant.* 2014;29 Suppl 2:i1–i39. doi:10.1093/ndt/gfu040

113. Seay NW, Lehrich RW, Greenberg A. Diagnosis and management of disorders of body tonicity-hyponatremia and hypernatremia: Core Curriculum 2020. *Am J Kidney Dis.* 2020;75(2):272–286. doi:10.1053/j.ajkd.2019.

114. Mrozek S, Rousset D, Geeraerts T. Pharmacotherapy of sodium disorders in neurocritical care. *Curr Opin Crit Care.* 2019;25(2):132–137. doi:10.1097/MCC.0000000000000589

115. Farrokh S, Cho SM, Suarez JI. Fluids and hyperosmolar agents in neurocritical care: An update. *Curr Opin Crit Care.* 2019;25(2):105–109. doi:10.1097/MCC.0000000000000585

116. Nehring SM, Tadi P, Tenny S. Cerebral edema. Updated Nov 20, 2020. StatPearls. Treasure Island (FL): StatPearls Publishing. https://www.ncbi.nlm.nih.gov/books/NBK537272/

117. Malbari F, Staggers KA, Minard CG, et al. Provider views on perioperative steroid use for patients with newly diagnosed pediatric brain tumors. *J Neurooncol.* 2020;147(1):205–212. doi:10.1007/s11060-020-03416-9

118. Kaal EC, Vecht CJ. The management of brain edema in brain tumors. *Curr Opin Oncol.* 2004;16(6):593–600. doi:10.1097/01.cco.0000142076.52721.b3

PART VI. | GENETICS AND NEURO-ONCOLOGIC DISEASE

26 | FAMILIAL SYNDROMES IN NEURO-ONCOLOGY

RADHIKA DHAMIJA, JOSEPH M. HOXWORTH, AND ASHOK R. ASTHAGIRI

INTRODUCTION

Advances in genetics and genetic diagnosis have led to the identification of a number of familial cancer syndromes. Many of these syndromes increase the risk for central nervous system (CNS) tumors. Identification of the molecular basis for these tumor predisposition syndromes has made early diagnosis and surveillance possible for at-risk patients. Genetic diagnosis has not only led to improved knowledge about tumor biology but has also modified treatment and surveillance recommendations in some cases.

This chapter describes the following genetic disorders associated with CNS tumors:

1. Cowden syndrome (CS)

2. Tuberous sclerosis (TSC)

3. Li-Fraumeni syndrome (LFS)

4. Turcot syndrome

5. Gorlin syndrome

6. Von Hippel Lindau (VHL) syndrome

Neurofibromatosis types 1 and 2 and schwannomatosis are covered in Chapter 27.

COWDEN SYNDROME

CS (also known as *multiple hamartoma syndrome* (Online Mendelian Inheritance in Man [OMIM] 158350) is a rare autosomal dominant familial cancer syndrome characterized by multiple hamartomas of ectodermal, mesodermal, and endodermal origin. It is caused by loss of function mutations in the phosphatase and tensin homolog (*PTEN*) gene located on chromosome 10q23.[1] CS is now considered broadly as part of a spectrum of disorders termed *PTEN* hamartoma tumor syndrome.[2] Loss of function of this gene contributes to overgrowth and risk for a variety of benign and malignant tumors of breast, thyroid, endometrium, skin, kidneys, and colon. Clinical manifestations are seen by the second decade in more than 90% of patients.[1] Diagnostic criteria were updated and are available online through National Comprehensive Cancer Network (https://www.nccn.org/about/news/ebulletin/ebul

letindetail.aspx?ebulletinid=535).[2] Two CNS tumors described in this syndrome are *Lhermitte-Duclos disease* (LDD) and *meningiomas*.

> Cowden syndrome is associated with Lhermitte-Duclos disease and meningiomas.

LHERMITTE-DUCLOS DISEASE

LDD is a major criterion for the diagnosis of CS.[2] It is a slow-growing tumor, containing dysplastic cells in the cerebellum and is also referred to as a dysplastic gangliocytoma. It is currently classified with neuronal and mixed neuronal-glial tumors in the most recent World Health Organization (WHO) classification of tumors of the CNS.[3] It has been suggested by some that LDD may be considered a hypertrophic cellular growth phenomenon superimposed on a developmental malformation.[4] Immunohistochemical analysis of LDD indicates activation of the PTEN/AKT/mTOR pathway, suggesting a central role for mammalian target of rapamycin (mTOR) in the pathogenesis of LDD.[4] LDD is histologically characterized by thickening and abnormal myelination of the molecular layer in the cerebellum, attenuated or absent Purkinje cells, infiltration of the granular cell layer by abnormal dysplastic ganglion cells, and variable vacuolization of white matter.[4,5]

MRI is the imaging modality of choice for LDD and shows a characteristic striated or laminar appearance of the mass. T1-weighted MRI will typically show a hypointense lesion, and T2-weighted MRI will demonstrate alternating hyperintensity and hypointensity with infrequent contrast enhancement (Figure 26.1).[6-8]

In most patients it presents as an insidious unilateral mass, although bilateral masses have also been reported.[9] Patients may present with cerebellar signs and headaches. Patients with larger lesions could have signs and symptoms of elevated intracranial pressure, such as headache, cranial nerve palsy, and papilledema secondary to hydrocephalus. Surgical resection is the mainstay of treatment.

MENINGIOMA

A meta-analysis of 109 patients with CS and confirmed *PTEN* mutation found a meningioma frequency of 8.25%, which was similar to the 9.17% frequency of LDD.[10] Another case series

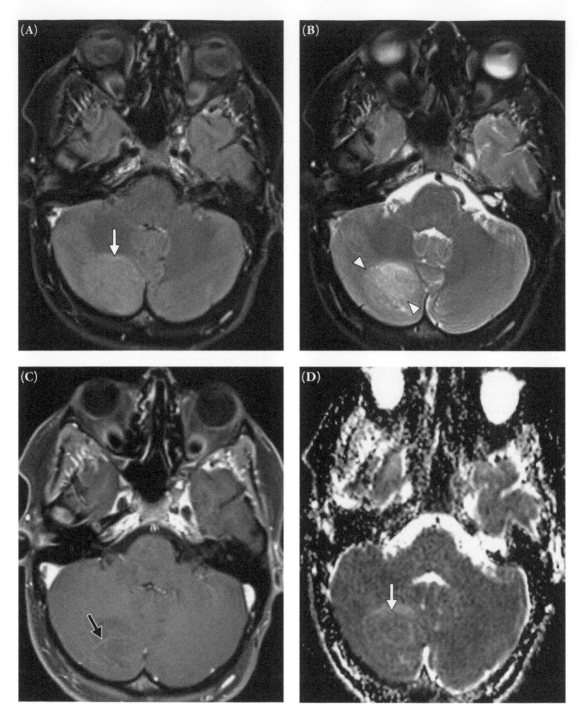

Figure 26.1 *Cowden syndrome with Lhermitte-Duclos disease. A 37-year-old woman with Cowden syndrome and right cerebellar Lhermitte-Duclos disease. (A) Axial fluid attenuated inversion recovery (FLAIR) MRI demonstrates a rounded mildly hyperintense lesion in the posterior right cerebellum (arrow). (B) Axial T2-weighted MRI illustrates a characteristic striated pattern with alternating bands of hyperintensity and isointensity (relative to gray matter) running parallel to the arrowheads. (C) On axial T1-weighted MRI following intravenous contrast administration, there is no significant solid or nodular enhancement, though note is made of a small enhancing vein (arrow) traversing the lesion. (D) Axial apparent diffusion coefficient (ADC) map demonstrates that the lesion (arrow) has mildly elevated ADC values compared with contralateral normal cerebellum.*

presented intracranial imaging findings in 22 patients with CS, of which 4 (18.2%) were found to have a meningioma.[11] On imaging, meningiomas present as dural-based extra-axial masses that can variably enhance. There are no unique imaging features of CS-associated meningiomas as opposed to sporadic cases. Symptoms of meningioma depend on the location of the tumor. Surgical resection is the mainstay of treatment.

TUBEROUS SCLEROSIS COMPLEX

TSC is an autosomal dominant neurocutaneous disorder characterized by development of benign tumors in multiple organs. It is caused by a heterozygous pathogenic variant in *TSC1* gene on 9q34.13 (OMIM 191100) (25% of cases) or *TSC2* gene 16p13.3 (OMIM 613254) (70% of cases). *TSC1* and

TSC2 genes encode for hamartin (TSC1) and tuberin (TSC2), respectively, which form a regulatory complex responsible for limiting the activity of an important intracellular regulator of cell growth and metabolism known as mTOR complex 1 (mTORC1) via inhibition of the small GTPase ras homolog enriched in brain (Rheb). This functional relationship between TSC1/TSC2 and mTORC1 is the basis of the use of mTOR inhibitors for the treatment of several clinical manifestations of TSC, including cerebral subependymal giant cell astrocytoma (SEGA), discussed later.

The diagnostic criteria were updated in 2012 and are available online through international Tuberous Sclerosis Complex Consensus Conference guidelines (http://www.tscinternational.org/international-tsc-consensus-guidelines/).[12]

The lesions in different organs that can develop over the lifetime of an affected individual include skin (hypomelanotic macules, angiofibromas, ungual fibromas), brain (subependymal nodules, cortical dysplasias, and subependymal giant cell astrocytomas [SEGAs]); kidney (angiomyolipomas, cysts, renal cell carcinomas); heart (rhabdomyomas); and lungs (lymphangioleiomyomatosis). Clinical manifestations are highly variable in affected individuals.

SUBEPENDYMAL GIANT CELL ASTROCYTOMA

The CNS tumor seen in TSC is SEGA. It is one of the major features in the clinical diagnostic criteria and is seen in 10–15% of patients with TSC.[12] These tumors can be unilateral or bilateral and arise from subependymal nodules (hamartomas) most commonly at the foramen of Monro. The risk for these tumors is highest in the first two decades of life. They are typically slow-growing glial neuronal tumors. Subependymal nodules larger than 5 mm, located near foramen of Monro and those with incomplete calcification have the highest risk of changing to SEGAs. They remain asymptomatic until they are large enough to block cerebrospinal fluid (CSF) flow and can then cause symptoms related to hydrocephalous (Figure 26.2).

Screening for tumors is essential to be able to intervene in a timely manner and provide the best quality of life to affected individuals. Brain magnetic resonance imaging (MRI) every 1–3 years in asymptomatic individuals with TSC younger than 25 years is recommended to monitor for new occurrence of SEGA. Those with asymptomatic SEGA in childhood should continue to be imaged periodically in adulthood.[13]

> SEGA is a slow-growing tumor that develops in patients with TSC, typically in the first two decades of life.

Surgery is considered standard of care. mTOR inhibitor therapy (everolimus) is indicated in patients older than 3 years when surgery cannot be complete or for certain locations like the bilateral fornix, where complication rates may be high. In a recent meta-analysis mTOR inhibitors significantly reduced tumor volume in SEGA (≥50% reduction in tumor volume relative to the baseline). The most common dose studied has been 4.5 mg/m², and median duration of treatment studied has been up to 34.2 months. Stomatitis, upper respiratory tract infections, and nasopharyngitis are the most common side effects.[14]

LI-FRAUMENI SYNDROME

LFS is an autosomal dominant cancer predisposition syndrome associated with high risk for a number of childhood- and adult-onset malignancies. The diagnosis of LFS is established in a proband who meets *all three* classic clinical criteria and/or has a heterozygous germline pathogenic variant in *TP53* on 17p13.1. (OMIM 151623).

The classic clinical criteria are:

- A patient with a sarcoma diagnosed before age 45 years
- A first-degree relative with any cancer diagnosed before age 45 years
- A first- or second-degree relative with any cancer diagnosed before age 45 years or a sarcoma diagnosed at any age

TP53 encodes for the protein p53, a transcription factor triggered as a protective cellular mechanism. Loss of p53 function renders affected individuals highly susceptible to a broad range of solid and hematologic cancers. Cancer types that account for the majority of LFS tumors are adrenocortical carcinomas (50%), CNS tumors (2–10%), osteosarcomas (2–3%), and soft-tissue sarcomas (8–9%).[15] It is a highly penetrant disorder; the lifetime risk of cancer in individuals with LFS is 70% or greater for men and 90% or greater for women.

> LFS is a highly penetrant genetic disorder with a very high lifetime risk of developing cancer: 70% or greater for men and 90% or greater for women.

CNS tumors account for 2–10% of LFS cancers. In one series, the cumulative incidence of brain cancer by age 70 was 6% for women and 19% for men. The age of onset of brain tumors is before age 40 years in most cases. Infiltrative astrocytoma is the most common CNS tumor types, although other CNS tumor types have also been reported, including ependymomas, choroid plexus carcinomas, oligodendroglioma, and supratentorial primitive neuroectodermal tumors.[15–18]

Recent gene sequencing studies have shown that LFS is responsible for about 40% of children with choroid plexus tumors (Figure 26.3)[17] and more than 10% of children with sonic hedgehog (SHH) medulloblastoma.[19]

For screening of CNS tumors, annual neurological examination and brain MRI is recommended. Patients who follow surveillance recommendations do have improved survival in this syndrome.[18]

> CNS tumors most commonly associated with LFS include diffuse astrocytoma, choroid plexus tumors, and medulloblastoma.

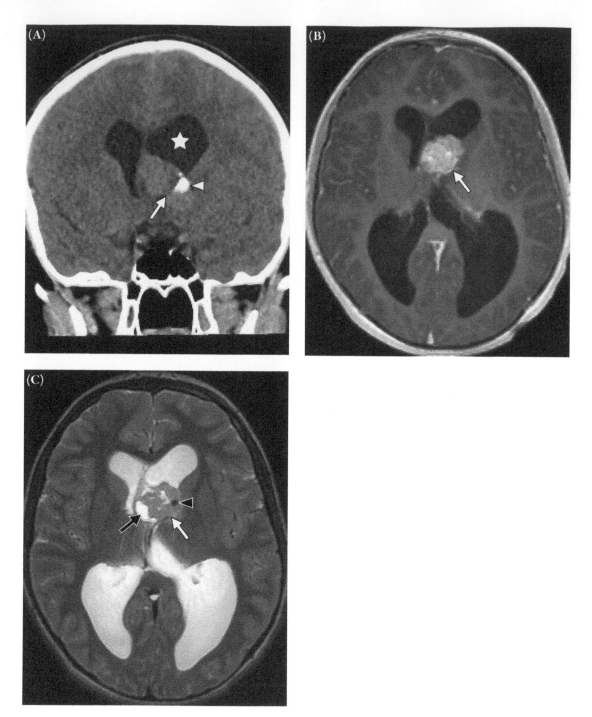

Figure 26.2 *Tuberous sclerosis with subependymal giant cell astrocytoma. A 13-year-old boy with tuberous sclerosis and subependymal giant cell astrocytoma. (A) Coronal reconstruction from non-contrast head CT reveals a lobulated mass (arrow) arising from the region of left foramen of Monro and abutting the septum pellucidum. Coarse calcification is present in the superolateral aspect of the mass (arrowhead). Note the presence of obstructive hydrocephalus (star). (B) On axial T1-weighted post-contrast MRI, the mass (arrow) avidly enhances. (C) Most of the mass demonstrates intermediate T2-weighted MRI signal (white arrow) with smaller interspersed foci of T2 hyperintensity (black arrow) consistent with cystic change. A small focus of hypointensity (arrowhead) corresponds to the calcification seen on CT.*

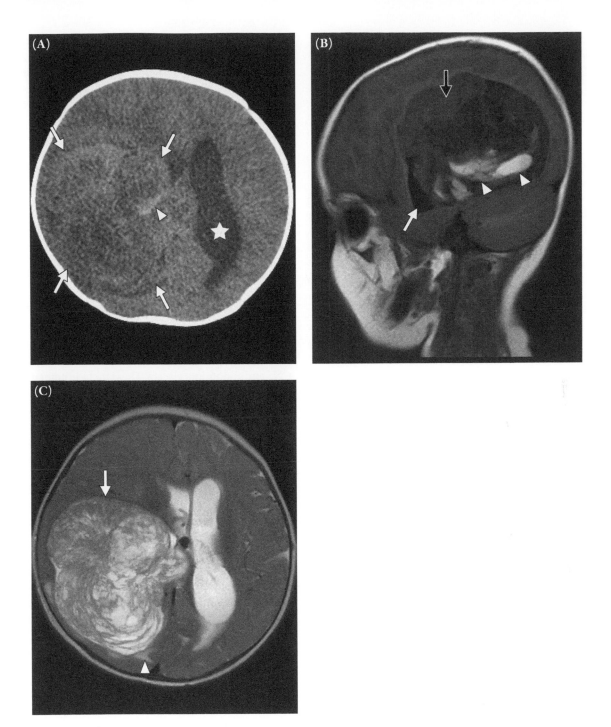

Figure 26.3 Li-Fraumeni syndrome with choroid plexus carcinoma. A 9-month-old boy with Li-Fraumeni syndrome and choroid plexus carcinoma. (A) Axial non-contrast head CT reveals a large heterogeneous tumor in the right cerebral hemisphere (arrows) with small interspersed foci of high density compatible with minimal intratumoral hemorrhage (arrowhead). In addition to significant right-to-left midline shift, obstructive hydrocephalus (star) is present. (B) Sagittal T1-weighted MRI illustrates that the tumor (black arrow) is splaying the temporal horn of the right lateral ventricle (white arrow), confirming its intraventricular location. Multiple foci of T1 hyperintensity (arrowheads) further confirm the presence of hemorrhage. (C) Axial T2-weighted MRI demonstrates heterogeneous mixed signal characteristics within the tumor (arrow) along with a small amount of peritumoral edema (arrowhead).

TURCOT SYNDROME (COLONIC POLYPOSIS AND CENTRAL NERVOUS SYSTEM TUMORS)

Turcot syndrome, first described in 1959 in two siblings, refers to the co-occurrence of a primary CNS tumor and colorectal polyposis.[20] Turcot syndrome has been linked to both familial adenomatous polyposis (FAP) and hereditary nonpolyposis colorectal cancer syndrome (HNPCC or Lynch syndrome).[21]

FAP is an autosomal dominant cancer syndrome caused by a germline mutation in the *APC* gene, a tumor suppressor gene located on chromosome 5q21 (OMIM 175100).[22] It is highly penetrant and has variable expressivity. It is characterized by numerous adenomatous polyps, which progress to colorectal carcinoma. More than 70% of patients with FAP develop extraintestinal manifestations, which can be benign or malignant.[22] The combination of colonic polyposis and CNS tumors was historically designated as Turcot syndrome, but this terminology is no longer preferred. It is now known that all individuals with FAP are at increased risk for brain tumors, and FAP patients with extraintestinal manifestations are now referred as *FAP spectrum* patients. Genotype-phenotype correlations have been observed in FAP, and the severity of extraintestinal manifestations corresponds to specific regions of *APC* gene mutation. FAP patients with *APC* gene mutations between codons 697 and 1224 are at an increased risk of brain tumors in general and have a 13-fold increased risk of medulloblastoma when compared with FAP patients with other APC gene mutations. The incidence of medulloblastomas in patients with FAP is greatest before the age of 10 years.[23,24] Anaplastic astrocytomas and ependymomas have also been described.[21]

In contrast, HNPCC (Lynch syndrome) is attributable to mutations in mismatch repair genes (*MLH1, MSH2, MSH6, PMS2*) where the major associated CNS tumor is glioblastoma. In most patients it presents before the age of 30.[21]

> Patients with Turcot syndrome have very high risk of developing medulloblastoma, particularly before the age of 10.

Careful neurological examination is recommended for colonic polyposis families with a member affected by a CNS tumor due to evidence of familial clustering. A periodic brain MRI scan can be considered. Though a set frequency for screening has not been established, intervals of 1–3 years starting in the first decade of life is considered reasonable by most providers.[25] Even when screening is offered and completed, there are no studies to suggest that this improves survival (Figure 26.4).[21]

NEVOID BASAL CELL CARCINOMA SYNDROME (GORLIN SYNDROME)

Nevoid basal cell carcinoma syndrome (NBCCS), also known as Gorlin syndrome, is an autosomal dominant syndrome characterized by facial dysmorphism (macrocephaly, frontal bossing, coarse facial features), multiple jaw keratocysts, and basal cell carcinomas (OMIM 109400). Pathogenic variants in *PTCH1* (Protein patched homolog 1) on 9q22.32 and *SUFU* (suppressor of fused homolog) at 10q24.32 are associated with this syndrome. Approximately 5% of all children with NBCCS develop medulloblastoma, typically between age 1 and 2. The tumor tends to be of desmoplastic histology and has a favorable prognosis. The risk of developing medulloblastoma is significantly higher (20 times) in individuals with an *SUFU* pathogenic variant (33%) than in those with a *PTCH1* pathogenic variant (<2%).[26-28]

Annual brain MRI surveillance for medulloblastoma is suggested for up to age 8 years. For those patients positive for the *SUFU* mutation, more frequent contrast-enhanced MR imaging until age 3 years can be justified due to increased medulloblastoma occurrence (Figure 26.5).[29]

VON HIPPEL-LINDAU SYNDROME

VHL syndrome is a highly penetrant, autosomal dominant tumor predisposition syndrome characterized by lesions in the CNS and abdominal viscera. These include hemangioblastomas of the brain, spinal cord, and retina; endolymphatic sac tumors; renal cysts and renal cell carcinoma; pheochromocytoma and paraganglioma; pancreatic cysts and neuroendocrine tumors; and cystadenomas of the reproductive adnexal organs (epididymal and broad ligament). It is caused by a pathogenic variant in the *VHL* gene at 3p25.3.[30]

CNS hemangioblastoma (80% in brain and 20% spine) is the hallmark lesion of VHL syndrome. They are often multiple.[31] Hemangioblastomas are benign tumors composed of vessels and stromal component.[32] Within the brain, the vast majority are infratentorial, primarily localized to the cerebellar hemispheres. The pituitary stalk is the most common site for the development of supratentorial hemangioblastomas in individuals with VHL syndrome.[33] Spinal hemangioblastomas are most commonly intramedullary, although some may be associated with the nerve root alone.

> CNS hemangioblastomas most commonly occurring in cerebellum are hallmark lesions of the VHL syndrome.

The primary treatment for most CNS hemangioblastomas is surgical resection when they become symptomatic.[34] Often, the cause for symptoms is development of a peritumoral cyst or adjacent edema, as opposed to growth of the solid tumor itself. Because hemangioblastomas in VHL may demonstrate stuttering patterns of growth with many years of relative senescence, asymptomatic tumors, regardless of their location, are generally not treated.[33] Endolymphatic sac tumors (ELST), even in VHL, are identified less frequently but may present with sudden onset of hearing loss or vertigo due to intralabyrinthine hemorrhage or progressive hearing loss and vertigo due to development of endolymphatic hydrops. Therefore, a more prophylactic approach to surgical resection of ELST upon identification or with early symptoms may be a better approach for hearing preservation (Figure 26.6).[35,36]

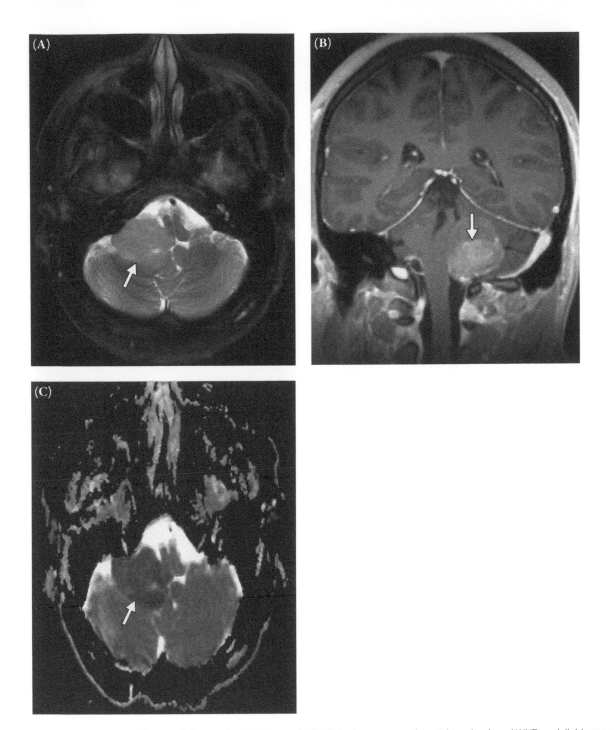

Figure 26.4 Turcot syndrome. A 22-year-old man with history of total colectomy for familial adenomatous polyposis later developed WNT medulloblastoma. (A) Axial T2-weighted MRI demonstrates an intra-axial mass (arrow) involving the ventral right cerebellum and right inferior cerebellar peduncle with exophytic extension into the cerebellopontine angle. T2 signal characteristics are similar to gray matter. (B) On coronal T1-weighted MRI following intravenous contrast administration, the mass (arrow) diffusely enhances. (C) Axial apparent diffusion coefficient (ADC) map demonstrates that the mass (arrow) has decreased ADC values compared with normal cerebellum, which is characteristic of the high nuclear-to-cytoplasmic ratio seen with small round blue cell tumors.

Life expectancy has improved due to surveillance.[37] Age-appropriate screening guidelines are available online through the VHL alliance (https://www.vhl.org/wp-content/uploads/2017/07/Active-Surveillance-Guidelines.pdf). Recently, Food and Drug Administration (FDA) approved Hypoxia-Inducible Factor 2-Alpha (HIF-2-alpha) inhibitor, belzutifan for the treatment of patients with certain types of VHL-associated tumors, including CNS hemangioblastomas.[38,39]

GENETIC COUNSELING

All cancer syndromes discussed here are autosomal dominant in inheritance. Each child of an individual with any of these discussed cancer syndromes has a 50% chance of inheriting the pathogenic variant. The risk to the siblings of the proband depends on the genetic status of the proband's parents. If a parent of the proband is affected,

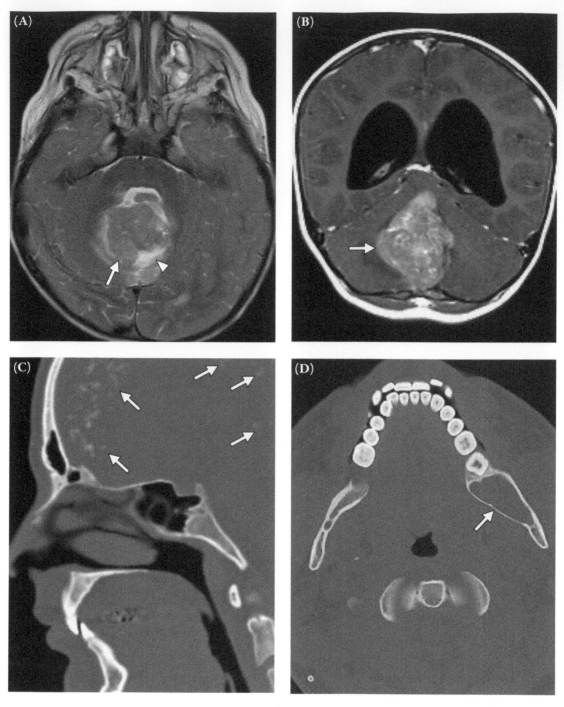

Figure 26.5 *Gorlin syndrome. A 2-year-old boy with Gorlin syndrome and nodular desmoplastic SHH-activated medulloblastoma. (A) On axial T2-weighted MRI, a mass (arrow) is identified dorsal to the fourth ventricle lateralizing more toward the right. Although the mass is slightly heterogeneous, overall T2 characteristics are similar to gray matter, with note made of some adjacent peritumoral edema (arrowhead). (B) Coronal T1-weighted post-contrast MRI reveals a heterogeneous pattern of enhancement within the tumor (arrow). In a different patient (20-year-old man), additional clues for the diagnosis of Gorlin syndrome are seen on non-contrast CT. (C) Sagittal CT reconstruction reveals numerous dural calcifications along the falx (arrows). (D) A lytic expansile lesion in the posterior left mandible with cortical thinning (arrow) was found to represent a keratocystic odontogenic tumor on resection.*

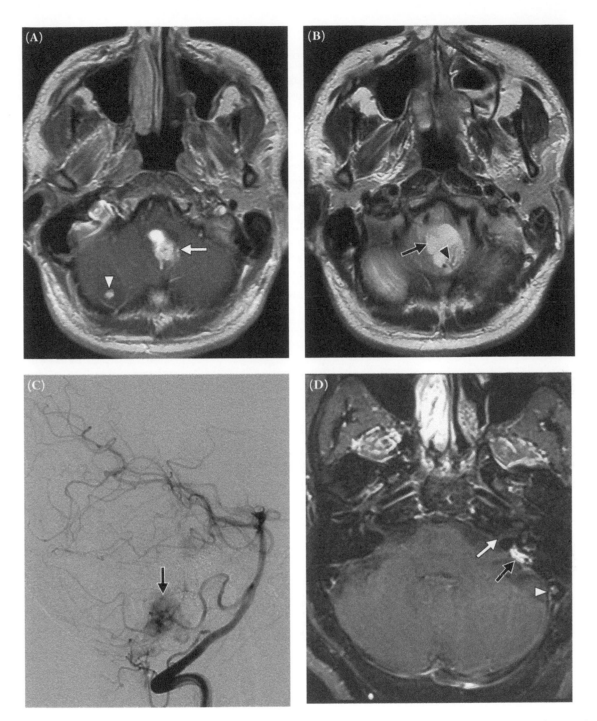

Figure 26.6 *Von Hippel-Lindau syndrome. A 26-year-old man with Von Hippel-Lindau syndrome and cerebellar hemangioblastomas. (A) Axial T1-weighted post-contrast MRI reveals a large midline cerebellar mass with avid contrast enhancement (arrow). A second smaller mass is present in the posterior right cerebellum (arrowhead). (B) More inferiorly, axial T2-weighted MRI depicts a large cyst (arrow) associated with the dominant mass, and a cluster of abnormally prominent vascular flow voids is apparent posteriorly (arrowhead). (C) Lateral projection of the posterior fossa during digital subtraction angiography was acquired during selective contrast injection into the left vertebral artery. The abnormal vascularity (arrow) of the dominant mass is readily apparent angiographically. (D) In a different patient (47-year-old man), an additional clue for the diagnosis of Von Hippel-Lindau syndrome is evident on axial T1-weighted post-contrast MRI with fat saturation. A small enhancing mass (black arrow) along the posterior left temporal bone is compatible with an endolymphatic sac tumor. For anatomic reference, the internal auditory canal (white arrow) and sigmoid sinus (arrowhead) are also annotated. The region of the endolymphatic sac should be closely scrutinized in all patients with a known diagnosis of Von Hippel-Lindau syndrome.*

SYNDROME	GENE MUTATION	CNS TUMORS	NOTES
Cowden syndrome	*PTEN*	Lhermitte-Duclos disease (LDD), meningiomas	LDD also known as dysplastic gangliocytoma; characteristic MRI appearance; surgical treatment often needed.
Tuberous sclerosis complex	*TSC1 and TSC2*	Subependymal giant cell astrocytomas (SEGA)	Be aware of diagnostic criteria and associated skin, brain, renal, pulmonary, and cardiac lesions. SEGA responds to mTOR inhibitors.
Li-Fraumeni syndrome	*P53*	Astrocytoma (most common); ependymoma, choroid plexus tumors, medulloblastoma, oligodendroglioma	Very high risk of developing cancer. Frequent screening for CNS tumors is recommended (annual exam and MRI).
Turcot syndrome	*APC*	Medulloblastoma, glioblastoma	Very high risk for childhood onset medulloblastoma. MRI of the brain every 1-3 years in the first decade of life is suggested.
Nevoid Basal Cell Carcinoma syndrome (Gorlin syndrome)	*PTCH1 and SUFU*	Medulloblastoma	Be aware of facial dysmorphism and basal cell carcinomas. Frequent MRI surveillance for medulloblastoma up to age of 8 years old.
Von Hippel-Lindau syndrome	*VHL*	Hemangioblastoma	Posterior fossa location of most hemangioblastomas. Be aware of endolymphatic sac tumor and associated sudden hearing loss and vertigo.

the risk to the siblings is 50%. Intra- and interfamilial variation in expression typically exists. It is important to offer genetic counseling (including discussion of potential risks to offspring and reproductive options) to young adults who are affected or at risk. In some syndromes genotype-phenotype correlation may exist. Genetic testing can be performed by either issuing concurrent gene testing or a multigene panel.

What is the cause of familial cancer syndromes?	Inherited mutations in tumor suppressor genes; most commonly autosomal dominant in inheritance
What are familial cancer syndromes known to increase the risk of CNS tumors?	Neurofibromatosis type 1 and 2, Cowden syndrome, Tuberous sclerosis complex (TSC), Li-Fraumeni syndrome, Turcot syndrome, Gorlin syndrome, and Von Hippel-Lindau syndrome
What are the causative mutations in Cowden syndrome?	Loss of function mutations in the PTEN gene
Which CNS neuro-oncologic conditions are associated with Cowden syndrome?	Lhermitte-Duclos disease and meningiomas
Slow-growing cerebellar tumor containing dysplastic cells, also called dysplastic gangliocytoma, are found in what disease?	Lhermitte-Duclos disease
Lhermitte-Duclos disease appears on MRI as:	A mass with striated laminar appearance
What are the inheritance and clinical manifestations of TSC?	Autosomal dominant neurocutaneous disorder; benign tumor development in multiple organs
These brain lesions can develop in TSC:	Subependymal nodules (SENs), cortical dysplasias, and subependymal giant cell astrocytomas (SEGAs)
These slow-growing CNS tumors are found in patients with TSC and develop typically in the first two decades of life	SEGAs
When surgical resection of SEGA is incomplete or not recommended due to high-risk tumor location, this treatment is recommended	mTOR inhibitor therapy (in patients >3 years of age)

This is a highly penetrant genetic disorder with a very high lifetime risk of developing cancer (≥70% for men and ≥90% for women)	Li-Fraumeni syndrome
Which CNS tumors are most commonly associated with Li-Fraumeni syndrome?	Diffuse astrocytoma, choroid plexus tumors, and medulloblastoma
The combination of colonic polyposis and CNS tumors was historically called this syndrome, but it is now known that all individuals with familial adenomatous polyposis are at increased risk of brain tumors; the disorder is now referred to by this name	Turcot syndrome; familial adenomatous polyposis (FAP) spectrum
Turcot syndrome has been linked to these colonic cancer syndromes	FAP, hereditary nonpolyposis colorectal cancer syndrome (also called Lynch syndrome)
Patients with Turcot syndrome have a very high risk of developing this type of CNS tumor?	Medulloblastoma, particularly before the age of 10
Approximately 5% of all children with Gorlin syndrome develop this CNS malignancy	Medulloblastoma, typically between ages 1 and 2
What is the most common CNS tumor in Von Hippel-Lindau syndrome?	Hemangioblastoma, most commonly in the cerebellum

QUESTIONS

1. Which of the following CNS tumors are most commonly seen with Turcot syndrome?
   a. Glioma
   b. Ependymoma
   c. Meningioma
   d. Medulloblastoma

2. Which of the following CNS tumors is seen in patients with Gorlin syndrome?
   a. Glioma
   b. Ependymoma
   c. Meningioma
   d. Medulloblastoma

3. Most familial cancer syndromes are autosomal dominant in nature.
   a. True
   b. False

4. Which of the following CNS tumors is seen most commonly in patients with Li-Fraumeni syndrome (LFS)?
   a. Infiltrative astrocytoma
   b. Ependymoma
   c. Meningioma
   d. Medulloblastoma

5. Subependymal nodules that have the highest risk of developing into SEGAs have the following characteristics:
   a. Size >5 mm
   b. Located near foramen of Monro
   c. Incomplete calcification
   d. All the above

6. Which of the following is an incorrect association.
   a. Cowden syndrome: PTEN gene
   b. Tuberous sclerosis complex: TS1 gene
   c. Gorlin syndrome: mismatch repair genes
   d. Turcot syndrome: APC gene

7. CNS tumors may develop is roughly what percentage of patients with Li-Fraumeni syndrome?
   a. 25%
   b. 100%
   c. 1%
   d. 10%

8. In Von Hippel Lindau syndrome, what is the most common CNS site for hemangioblastomas?
   a. Cerebellum
   b. Cortex
   c. Spinal cord
   d. Pituitary stalk

9. mTOR inhibitors have shown most promise in which tumor syndrome?
   a. Tuberous sclerosis complex

   b. Neurofibromatosis type 1
   c. Neurofibromatosis type 2
   d. Turcot syndrome

10. Cowden syndrome is caused by germline mutation in which gene?
    a. Neurofibromatosis type 1 NF-1
    b. Tuberous sclerosis complex TS1
    c. PTCH1
    d. PTEN

11. Endolymphatic sac tumors associated with Von Hippel Lindau syndrome are known to cause hearing loss through a variety of mechanisms including intralabyrinthine hemorrhage, development of endolymphatic hydrops, and direct invasion of the otic capsule.
    a. True
    b. False

12. In addition to CNS and retinal hemangioblastomas, Von Hippel Lindau syndrome is a multiple neoplasia predisposition syndrome associated with which of the following conditions?
    a. Breast adenocarcinoma
    b. Renal cell carcinoma
    c. Melanoma
    d. Cholangiocarcinoma
    e. Lymphoma

13. A 6-month-old boy is brought to the clinic for spells suspicious for infantile spasms. His medical record notes that he has had a heart murmur since birth. A dermatological exam shows three areas of hypopigmentation on his body that are each 1 2 cm in size. A brain MRI reveals four periventricular nodules that distort the normally smooth ventricular margins. What is this patient's most likely diagnosis?
    a. Tuberous sclerosis complex
    b. Neurofibromatosis type 1
    c. Neurofibromatosis type 2
    d. Turcot syndrome

14. A 26-year-old man presents with hematuria. Imaging shows bilateral renal cyst. His family history is significant for a brother with retinal hemangioblastomas and mother with renal cell carcinoma. What is this patient's most likely diagnosis?
    a. Von Hippel Lindau syndrome
    b. Neurofibromatosis type 1
    c. Turcot syndrome
    d. Tuberous sclerosis complex

15. All individuals with familial adenomatous polyposis (FAP) syndrome are at decreased risk of developing a brain tumor.
    a. True
    b. False

ANSWERS

1. d
2. d
3. a
4. a
5. d
6. c
7. d
8. a
9. a
10. d
11. a
12. b
13. a
14. a
15. b

REFERENCES

1. Eng C. PTEN: One gene, many syndromes. *Hum Mutat.* 2003;22(3):183–198.
2. Pilarski R, Burt R, Kohlman W, et al. Cowden syndrome and the PTEN hamartoma tumor syndrome: Systematic review and revised diagnostic criteria. *J Natl Cancer Inst.* 2013;105(21):1607–1616.
3. Komori T. The 2016 WHO classification of tumours of the central nervous system: The major points of revision. *Neurologia Medico-Chirurgica.* 2017;57(7):301–311.
4. Abel TW, Baker SJ, Fraser MM, et al. Lhermitte-Duclos disease: A report of 31 cases with immunohistochemical analysis of the PTEN/AKT/mTOR pathway. *J Neuropathol Exp Neurol.* 2005;64(4):341–349.
5. Wei G, Zhang W, Li Q, et al. Magnetic resonance characteristics of adult-onset Lhermitte-Duclos disease: An indicator for active cancer surveillance? *Mol Clin Oncol.* 2014;2(3):415–420.
6. Meltzer CC, Smirniotopoulos JG, Jones RV. The striated cerebellum: An MR imaging sign in Lhermitte-Duclos disease (dysplastic gangliocytoma). *Radiology.* 1995;194(3):699–703.
7. Kulkantrakorn K, Awwad EE, Levy B, et al. MRI in Lhermitte-Duclos disease. *Neurology.* 1997;48(3):725–731.
8. Dhamija R, Wood CP, Porter AB, et al. Updated imaging features of dysplastic cerebellar gangliocytoma. *J Comput Assist Tomogr.* 2019;43(2):277–281.
9. Khandpur U, Huntoon K, Smith-Cohn M, et al. Bilateral recurrent dysplastic cerebellar gangliocytoma (Lhermitte-Duclos disease) in Cowden syndrome: A case report and literature review. *World Neurosurg.* 2019;127:319–325.
10. Yakubov E, Ghoochani A, Buslei R. Hidden association of Cowden syndrome, PTEN mutation and meningioma frequency. *Oncoscience.* 2016;3(5–6):149–155.
11. Dhamija R, Weindling SM, Porter AB, et al. Neuroimaging abnormalities in patients with Cowden syndrome: Retrospective single-center study. *Neurol Clin Pract.* 2018;8(3):207–213.
12. Northrup H, Krueger DA, International Tuberous Sclerosis Complex Consensus. Tuberous sclerosis complex diagnostic criteria update: Recommendations of the 2012 International Tuberous Sclerosis Complex Consensus Conference. *Pediatr Neurol.* 2013;49(4):243–254.
13. Krueger DA, Northrup H, International Tuberous Sclerosis Complex Consensus. Tuberous sclerosis complex surveillance and management: Recommendations of the 2012 International Tuberous Sclerosis Complex Consensus Conference. *Pediatr Neurol.* 2013;49(4):255–265.
14. Jozwiak S, Nabbout R, Curatolo P, et al. Management of subependymal giant cell astrocytoma (SEGA) associated with tuberous sclerosis complex (TSC): Clinical recommendations. *Eur J Paediatr Neurol.* 2013;17(4):348–352.
15. Orr BA, Clay MR, Pinto EM, Kesserwan C. An update on the central nervous system manifestations of Li-Fraumeni syndrome. *Acta Neuropathol.* 2020 Apr;139(4):669–687.
16. Mai PL, Malkin D, Garber JE, et al. Li-Fraumeni syndrome: Report of a clinical research workshop and creation of a research consortium. *Cancer Genet.* 2012;205(10):479–487.
17. Bougeard G, Renaux-Petel M, Flaman JM, et al. Revisiting Li-Fraumeni syndrome from TP53 mutation carriers. *J Clin Oncol.* 2015;33(21):2345–2352.
18. Valdez JM, Nichols KE, Kesserwan C. Li-Fraumeni syndrome: A paradigm for the understanding of hereditary cancer predisposition. *Br J Haematol.* 2017;176(4):539–552.
19. Kool M, Jones DT, Jager N, et al., IPT Project. Genome sequencing of SHH medulloblastoma predicts genotype-related response to smoothened inhibition. *Cancer Cell.* 2014;25(3):393–405.
20. Turcot J, Despres JP, St Pierre F. Malignant tumors of the central nervous system associated with familial polyposis of the colon: Report of two cases. *Dis Colon Rectum.* 1959;2:465–468.
21. Hamilton SR, Liu B, Parsons RE, et al. The molecular basis of Turcot's syndrome. *N Engl J Med.* 1995;332(13):839–847.
22. Galiatsatos P, Foulkes WD. Familial adenomatous polyposis. *Am J Gastroenterol.* 2006;101(2):385–398.
23. Attard TM, Giglio P, Koppula S, et al. Brain tumors in individuals with familial adenomatous polyposis: A cancer registry experience and pooled case report analysis. *Cancer.* 2007;109(4):761–766.
24. Novelli M. The pathology of hereditary polyposis syndromes. *Histopathology.* 2015;66(1):78–87.
25. Provenzale D, Gupta S, Ahnen DJ, et al. Genetic/familial high-risk assessment: Colorectal version 1.2016, NCCN Clinical Practice Guidelines in Oncology. *J Natl Compr Canc Netw.* 2016;14(8):1010–1030.
26. Evans DG, Ladusans EJ, Rimmer S, et al. Complications of the naevoid basal cell carcinoma syndrome: Results of a population based study. *J Med Genet.* 1993;30(6):460–464.
27. Evans DG, Oudit D, Smith MJ, et al. First evidence of genotype-phenotype correlations in Gorlin syndrome. *J Med Genet.* 2017;54(8):530–536.
28. Amlashi SF, Riffaud L, Brassier G, Morandi X. Nevoid basal cell carcinoma syndrome: Relation with desmoplastic medulloblastoma in infancy. A population-based study and review of the literature. *Cancer.* 2003;98(3):618–624.
29. Smith MJ, Beetz C, Williams SG, et al. Germline mutations in SUFU cause Gorlin syndrome-associated childhood medulloblastoma and redefine the risk associated with PTCH1 mutations. *J Clin Oncol.* 2014;32(36):4155–4161.
30. Maher ER, Yates JR, Harries R, et al. Clinical features and natural history of von Hippel-Lindau disease. *Q J Med.* 1990;77(283):1151–1163.
31. Lonser RR, Glenn GM, Walther M, et al. Von Hippel-Lindau disease. *Lancet.* 2003;361:2059–2067.
32. Vortmeyer AO, Gnarra JR, Emmert-Buck MR, et al. von Hippel-Lindau gene deletion detected in the stromal cell component of a cerebellar hemangioblastoma associated with von Hippel-Lindau disease. *Hum Pathol.* 1997;28(5):540–543.
33. Lonser RR, Butman JA, Kiringoda R, et al. Pituitary stalk hemangioblastomas in von Hippel-Lindau disease. *J Neurosurg.* 2009;110(2):350–353.
34. Lonser RR, Butman JA, Huntoon K, et al. Prospective natural history study of central nervous system hemangioblastomas in von Hippel-Lindau disease. *J Neurosurg.* 2014;120(5):1055–1062.
35. Butman JA, Kim HJ, Baggenstos M, et al. Mechanisms of morbid hearing loss associated with tumors of the endolymphatic sac in von Hippel-Lindau disease. *JAMA.* 2007;298(1):41–48.
36. Butman JA, Nduom E, Kim HJ, Lonser RR. Imaging detection of endolymphatic sac tumor-associated hydrops. *J Neurosurg.* 2013;119(2):406–411.
37. Wilding A, Ingham SL, Lalloo F, et al. Life expectancy in hereditary cancer predisposing diseases: An observational study. *J Med Genet.* 2012;49(4):264–269.
38. https://www.fda.gov/drugs/resources-information-approved-drugs/fda-approves-belzutifan-cancers-associated-von-hippel-lindau-disease
39. Jonasch E, Donskov F, Iliopoulos O, et al. Belzutifan for Renal Cell Carcinoma in von Hippel-Lindau Disease. *N Engl J Med.* 2021 Nov 25;385(22):2036–2046. doi: 10.1056/NEJMoa2103425. PMID: 34818478; PMCID: PMC9275515.

27 | THE NEUROFIBROMATOSES

Neurofibromatosis 1, Neurofibromatosis 2, and Schwannomatosis

KUN-WEI SONG AND SCOTT R. PLOTKIN

INTRODUCTION

Neurofibromatosis type 1 (NF1), neurofibromatosis type 2 (NF2), and schwannomatosis are genetically distinct tumor suppressor syndromes that affect the nervous system. Together, these three syndromes are termed the neurofibromatoses. They exhibit autosomal dominant inheritance and predispose to central and peripheral nervous system tumors.

Although NF1 and NF2 are commonly confused by clinicians, these two disorders have distinct genetic pathophysiology and manifestations. The hallmark of NF1 is the early skin findings of café-au-lait macules, intertriginous freckling, and neurofibromas. The common neuro-oncology manifestations include low-grade gliomas (most commonly pilocytic astrocytomas), high-grade gliomas, and malignant nerve sheath tumors. In contrast, NF2 is characterized by vestibular schwannomas, meningiomas, and ependymomas. Schwannomatosis represents yet another genetically distinct syndrome characterized by multiple schwannomas and, less commonly, meningiomas.

This chapter highlights these lesions' pathophysiology, clinical manifestations, and neuroimaging characteristics as well as standard and experimental management strategies relevant to the practicing neuro-oncologist.

NEUROFIBROMATOSIS 1

EPIDEMIOLOGY

NF1 is a common neurogenetic disorder with a birth incidence of 1:2,000 to 3,000.[1-3] It has an autosomal dominant inheritance with 100% penetrance. While all individuals with the affected gene show disease manifestations, affected individuals have variable clinical disease severity. Approximately 42% of NF1 patients have no family history and carry a de novo pathogenic variant in the NF1 gene. NF1 affects all racial groups and genders equally. Population studies suggest that patients with NF1 have reduced lifespan compared with the general population (median of 71.5 years vs 80 years),[4,5] mostly due to increased rates of malignancy and vascular disease.

> While all individuals with the affected NF1 gene show disease manifestations, affected individuals have variable clinical disease severity.

GENETICS AND PATHOGENESIS

A pathogenic variant in the NF1 gene on chromosome 17 can be identified in more than 95% of NF1 patients. The NF1 gene product is neurofibromin, a 220–280kD cytoplasmic protein that functions as a tumor suppressor. Neurofibromin is in the family of GTPase-activating proteins[6] that serves as negative regulators of the RAS oncogene, an important regulator of cell proliferation. A large number of distinct variants in the NF1 gene have been identified, including nonsense (37%), splice-site (28%), frameshift (18%), and missense (9%) mutations.[7] This finding is consistent with its role as a tumor suppressor gene in which inactivation due to pathogenic variants leads to loss of protein function. Despite the large number of pathogenic NF1 gene variants, only a few genotype–phenotype correlations have been elucidated.[8] These correlations include deletion of the entire NF1 gene (1.4Mkb), which is associated with a severe phenotype with less cutaneous fibromas but more dysmorphisms, cognitive impairment, and increased rates of malignancy[9]; codon 1809 mutation variants, which are associated with café-au-lait macules, short stature, pulmonic stenosis, but no plexiform or cutaneous neurofibromas[10]; and a 3-bp in-frame deletion in exon 17 of the NF1, which is associated with mild disease.[11]

DIAGNOSTIC CRITERIA

The diagnostic criteria for NF1 should be viewed in context of its lifetime disease manifestations. Nearly all patients with NF1 develop clinical signs within the first decade of life. The most common childhood presenting feature is multiple café au lait macules, which commonly occur before age 1.[12] Axillary and inguinal freckling as well as Lisch nodules also develop during childhood, and cutaneous neurofibromas commonly develop in adolescence. While optic pathway gliomas (OPGs) and plexiform neurofibromas can be congenital lesions, symptomatic lesions commonly manifest in early childhood.

> Nearly all patients with NF1 develop clinical signs within the first decade of life.

The US National Institutes of Health (NIH) Consensus Conference established the NF1 diagnostic criteria in 1987.[13]

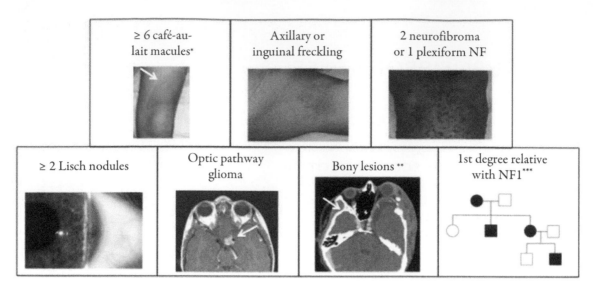

| ≥ 6 café-au-lait macules* | Axillary or inguinal freckling | 2 neurofibroma or 1 plexiform NF |
| ≥ 2 Lisch nodules | Optic pathway glioma | Bony lesions ** | 1st degree relative with NF1*** |

Figure 27.1 *National Institutes of Health diagnostic criteria for neurofibromatosis type 1. Patients must have at least two of these criteria to be diagnosed with NF1.*

At least two of the following criteria:

* Café au lait spots with size ≥5mm in diameter before puberty or ≥1.5 mm after puberty.

** A distinctive bony lesion, such as sphenoid wing dysplasia (shown here) or cortical thinning of long bones.

*** First-degree relative such as parent, sibling, or offspring.

From Gutmann DH, et al.[13]

Approximately 50% of patients with NF1 will meet diagnostic criteria by age 1, 97% of patients by age 8, and virtually all NF1 patients will fulfill diagnostic criteria by age 20.[12] (Figure 27.1). Therefore, patients who do not meet diagnostic criteria by age 20 are very unlikely to have NF1. While the NIH diagnostic criteria perform well overall, one study showed that sensitivity can be low in infancy since approximately 46% of sporadic cases may not meet criteria by age 1.[12] This weakness is particularly true for sporadic patients who lack a family history and have not developed skin fold freckling. When evaluating a new patient, it is important to be aware of other conditions that may mimic NF1 and that can also present with pigmented lesions that can be resemble café au lait spots or cutaneous tumors that can be mistaken for neurofibromas (Box 27.1).

> Approximately 50% of patients with NF1 will meet diagnostic criteria by age 1, 97% of patients by age 8, and virtually all NF1 patients will fulfill diagnostic criteria by age 20.

While genetic testing is not part of the diagnostic criteria for NF1, it can be helpful to clarify difficult cases. For example, patients with Legius syndrome carry a germline pathogenic variant in the *SPRED1* gene,[14] which also presents with multiple café-au-lait spots and axillary freckling. However, these patients do not have neurofibromas, optic tract gliomas, and are at lower risk for nerve sheath tumors and other malignancies.[15] Genetic testing is necessary for prenatal and preimplantation genetic diagnosis and can be helpful for family planning. As noted earlier, genetic testing (genotype) cannot reliably predict disease severity (phenotype) and is not used for prognosis.

LOW-GRADE GLIOMAS

NF1 patients have an increased rate of both low-grade and high-grade gliomas.[16] OPGs are the most common intracranial tumor associated with NF1 and part of the diagnostic criteria. Pathologically, OPGs are mostly pilocytic astrocytomas, which are World Health Organization (WHO) grade 1 tumors. On microscopic examination, these tumors have low cellularity

---

BOX 27.1 CONDITIONS THAT RESEMBLE NF1

Other neurofibromatoses (associated genes)

Neurofibromatosis 2 (NF2)

Schwannomatosis (SMARCB1, LZTR1)

Conditions with pigmented skin lesions (associated genes)

Noonan syndrome (multiple including PTPN11, SOS1, RAF1, RIT1)

Cardiofaciocutaneous syndrome (multiple, including RAF, MAP2K1, MAP2K2, or KRAS)

Legius syndrome (SPRED1)

McCune-Albright syndrome (GNAS1)

Congenital mismatch repair syndromes (MLH1, MSH2, MSH6, or PMS2)

Watson syndrome (NF1)

Noonan syndrome with multiple lentigines (formerly LEOPARD syndrome, PTPN11)

Neurocutaneous melanosis (NRAS)

Peutz-Jegher syndrome (SKT11)

Piebaldism (KIT, SNAI2)

Conditions with neurofibromas-like growths

Lipomatosis

Multiple endocrine neoplasia type 2B

Fibromatoses

Adapted with permission of MedReviews, LLC. From Lu-Emerson, Plotkin SR.[45]

with a biphasic pattern that includes compact areas with piloid cells and Rosenthal fibers and loose areas with microcystic features. A minority of OPGs are low-grade astrocytomas (WHO grade 2).[17]

> OPGs are the most common intracranial tumor associated with NF1.

OPGs are identified in approximately 15% of patients with NF1 and comprise the majority (66%) of CNS tumors.[17] While OPGs can involve any part of the optic nerve, chiasm, and tract, as well as the adjacent hypothalamus, the most common location is the anterior optic tract (Figure 27.2A). Two-thirds of OPGs are asymptomatic and non-progressive or self-limited in their progression. However, a small percentage (~4%) are symptomatic,[12] which can cause visual symptoms such as decreased visual acuity, proptosis, and nystagmus. Precocious puberty, caused by involvement of the adjacent hypothalamus, is seen in 12–30% of patients with OPGs and can be the presenting symptom of symptomatic OPGs.[18] Thus,

careful monitoring of growth curves is recommended for children with NF1. Most symptomatic lesions are diagnosed before 6 years of age, but they can rarely become symptomatic in older adolescents and adults.[19]

Routine screening of NF1 patients with magnetic resonance imaging (MRI) is not recommended for asymptomatic patients since the majority of OPGs are asymptomatic and are unlikely to progress. There is no clear evidence that early detection and treatment of asymptomatic lesions leads to reduced rates of vision loss.[18] However, screening ophthalmologic examinations are recommended annually for children between the ages of 2 and 7 to identify symptomatic OPGs since the first 6 years of life are highest risk for development of OPGs. Visual evoked potentials are not routinely recommended due to increased detection of asymptomatic lesions.

Symptomatic OPGs should be followed closely, generally at 3-month intervals in the first year, with therapy reserved for progressive lesions. Surgical decompression may be indicated for treatment of painful proptosis and blindness or for hydrocephalus due to ventricular compression. In contrast to non-NF1 patients, radiation is generally avoided in NF1

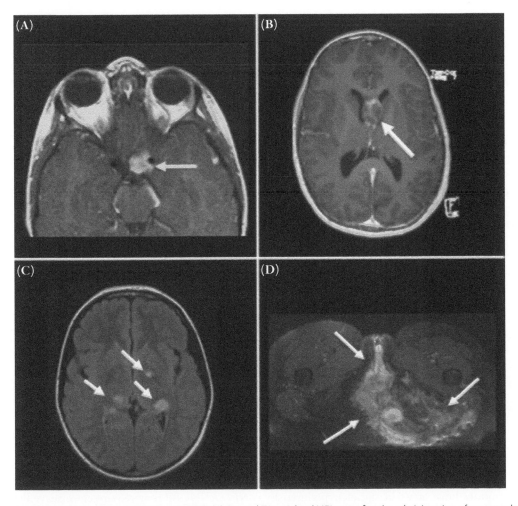

Figure 27.2 Neuroimaging findings in neurofibromatosis type 1 (NF1). (A) Coronal T1-weighted MRI scan after the administration of contrast demonstrating an optic pathway glioma expanding the optic chiasm. (B) Axial T1-weighted MRI scan after the administration of contrast demonstrating a non-optic pathway glioma arising from the septum pellucidum. (C) Fluid-attenuated inversion recovery (FLAIR) sequence on MRI scan demonstrating multiple unidentified bright objects (UBO), which can resemble low-grade gliomas. (D) FLAIR sequence on MRI scan demonstrating T2-hyperintense lesion consistent with plexiform neurofibroma diffusely involving the left buttock and perineum.

patients given the high risk for neurovascular complications, such as moyamoya syndrome, endocrine complications, and malignant transformation.[20] Chemotherapy can also be considered for progressive symptomatic lesions with a combination carboplatin/vincristine, vinblastine, temozolomide, or bevacizumab.

> Radiation to treat CNS disease is generally avoided in NF1 patients given the high risk for neurovascular complications, such as moyamoya syndrome, endocrine complications, and secondary malignancies.

Non-optic gliomas also occur at increased frequency in NF1. After the optic pathway, the brainstem is the most common location, followed by cerebral hemispheres, basal ganglia, and cerebellum[17] (Figure 27.2B). Asymptomatic non-optic tract lesions should be followed closely to establish a growth pattern. Stable lesions do not require treatment. and biopsy or resection can be considered for progressive disease. Again, radiation is avoided if possible due to complications similar to those with OPGs. Clinical trials are investigating therapeutic agents such as selumetinib, a MEK inhibitor, for low-grade gliomas. A phase I trial showed that 20% of patients achieved partial response and 37% had stable disease.[21] The phase II trial showed that 40% had sustained partial response,[22] and the phase III trial comparing selumetinib to carboplatin/vincristine is ongoing (NCT03871257).

HIGH-GRADE GLIOMAS

High-grade gliomas represent a minority of intracranial tumors in NF1 patients.[23] High-grade gliomas in NF1 patients can include anaplastic astrocytoma (WHO grade 3) and glioblastoma (WHO grade 4).[17] Aggressive tumors are most commonly associated with a non-optic location and diagnosis in adulthood.[17] NF1 patients with glioblastoma may have improved survival compared with sporadic patients in one small study.[24] However, given the rarity of these tumors, the outcome is generally not well-described, and gliomas remain the second most common cause of mortality in NF1 patients.[23] Treatment includes multimodality therapy with surgery, radiation, and chemotherapy similar to sporadic tumors. Given the poor prognosis with high-grade gliomas, radiation is generally indicated, unlike with low-grade gliomas.

> Given the poor prognosis with high-grade gliomas, radiation is generally indicated, unlike with low-grade gliomas.

UNIDENTIFIED BRIGHT OBJECTS/FOCAL AREAS OF SIGNAL INTENSITY

NF1 patients commonly have areas of signal hyperintensity on MRI T2-weighted sequences termed NF-associated bright spots, unidentified bright objects (UBOs), or focal areas of signal intensity (FASIs) (Figure 27.2C). UBOs can be mistaken for low-grade gliomas. Radiographically, UBOs are identified in up to 92% of NF1 patients on MRI brain.[25] While a common finding, they are not part of the diagnostic criteria for NF1. They most commonly occur in the cerebellum, basal ganglia, brainstem, and subcortical white matter and may be due to dysplastic glial proliferation.[26] One study found that lesions representing tumors were more commonly found in the brainstem and basal ganglia, while UBOs occurred more frequently in the cerebellum, medial temporal lobes, and thalamus.[25] UBOs have no documented clinical significance and are not associated with increased rates of epilepsy or cognitive dysfunction.[27]

> UBOs are identified in up to 92% of NF1 patients, they have no documented clinical significance, and are not associated with increased rates of epilepsy or cognitive dysfunction.

NEUROFIBROMAS

Neurofibromas are benign multicellular tumors derived from the nerve sheath that are composed of Schwann cells, perineurium-like cells, fibroblasts, and mast cells.[28] They grow in nerve bundles and are generally well-circumscribed, but not encapsulated. Histology shows spindle cells with short, elongated, and curved nuclei embedded in a matrix, which routinely expresses S-100. As the most common tumor in NF1, more than 80% of NF1 patients develop neurofibromas by puberty.[12] Neurofibromas can develop anywhere on the body and can be cutaneous, subcutaneous, deep in the spinal root, or in the nerve plexus. Cutaneous neurofibromas usually present in early adulthood, with no difference between genders. Subcutaneous neurofibromas that present as breast lumps may need extra evaluation since women with NF1 are at higher risk for breast carcinoma.[29] Plexiform neurofibromas are a subset of neurofibromas that involve multiple nerve fascicles and develop in approximately 50% of NF1 patients[30] (Figure 27.2D). Spinal neurofibromas are relatively common on MRI, but rarely symptomatic (<2%) in one large observational study.[31] Head and neck neurofibromas can lead to disfigurement, visual impairment, dysphagia, and respiratory issues.[32,33]

> Plexiform neurofibromas are a subset of neurofibromas that involve multiple nerve fascicles and develop in approximately 50% of NF1 patients.

Some symptomatic neurofibromas show atypical histology with hypercellularity and atypical nuclei with few mitoses and no necrosis.[34] These lesions are termed *atypical neurofibromatous neoplasms of uncertain biologic potential* (ANNUBP), and may be premalignant.[35] ANNUBP may harbor molecular changes such as homozygous deletion of cyclin-dependent kinase inhibitor 2A/B[36] along with loss of *NF1*. ANNUBP may require close surveillance to monitor for malignant transformation.[37]

Treatment for neurofibromas remains primarily surgical although plexiform neurofibromas are challenging given their invasive nature. Surgery is typically reserved for symptomatic or progressive tumors given risk of postoperative morbidity. However, in patients with minimal dysfunction, close surveillance may help prolong preservation of neurologic function. Radiation is typically avoided given increased risk of malignant transformation.[38] Excitingly, selumetinib was approved by the US Food and Drug Administration (FDA) in April 2020 for treatment of symptomatic plexiform neurofibromas in children older than age 2.[39] This determination was based on results from the phase I trial, which showed 71% of NF1 patients had partial response, and the phase II trial, which showed 72% of NF1 patients had partial response sustained for 6 months or longer.[40]

> Selumetinib was approved in April 2020 for treatment of symptomatic plexiform neurofibromas in children older than age 2.

Other clinical trials are under way for treatment of neurofibromas. Other MEK inhibitors such as mirdametinib (NCT02096471, NCT03962543), binimetinib (NCT03231306), and trametinib (NCT03741101) are currently in phase II trials, with preliminary results suggesting clinical activity. Other agents under investigation include pegylated interferon (NCT00396019),[41] imatinib (NCT03688568), and cabozantinib (NCT02101736).

MALIGNANT PERIPHERAL NERVE SHEATH TUMORS

Malignant peripheral nerve sheath tumors (MPNST) are sarcomas that typically develop within preexisting plexiform neurofibromas[42] but can rarely develop spontaneously. Not all neurofibromas are at risk for malignant transformation since MPNST do not appear to arise from cutaneous neurofibromas.[28] Histologically, MPNSTs are fasciculated and composed of closely packed hyperchromatic spindle cells.[28] The lifetime risk of MPNST in NF1 patients is approximately 8–13%; they tend to present typically in the third or fourth decade of life.[43] Risk factors for development of MPNST include large internal neurofibroma burden, presence of ANNUBP, previous treatment with radiation, personal or family history of MPNST, and microdeletions of the *NF1* locus.[44]

> The lifetime risk of MPNST in NF1 patients is approximately 8–13%; they tend to present typically in the third or fourth decade of life.

Since MPNST tend to arise within preexisting neurofibromas, they can be challenging to diagnose. Neurofibromas that present with persistent or nocturnal pain, rapid increase in size, change in texture, or new neurologic deficits warrant urgent evaluation.[45] Fluorodeoxyglucose (FDG)-PET is the most sensitive and specific non-invasive diagnostic tool[46] and can help guide biopsies to the site of highest FDG uptake.

> Neurofibromas that present with persistent or nocturnal pain, rapid increase in size, change in texture, or new neurologic deficits warrant urgent evaluation.

MPNST is the leading cause of mortality in NF1 patients.[23] MPNSTs are treated and staged as malignant soft tissue sarcomas. Low-grade MPNSTs may be surgically resected with favorable prognosis, but high-grade MPNSTs are aggressive and can metastasize widely. For MPNSTs, achieving local tumor control through surgery and radiation is the goal. Surgical resection aims for complete excision with negative tumor margins. Adjuvant radiotherapy is standard and achieves better control than either surgery or radiation alone.[47] Neoadjuvant chemotherapy is controversial, but some studies showed benefit with anthracycline and ifosfamide prior to surgical removal.[48,49] Prognosis is generally worse in patients with NF1 compared to general population, perhaps because NF1 patients tend to present at later stages with larger tumors.[50,51] However, the difference in mortality has been slowly improving.[52,53]

DERMATOLOGIC AND OPHTHALMOLOGIC MANIFESTATIONS

Café-au-lait macules most commonly present during the first year of life and increase in size and number during childhood and puberty. Café-au-lait spots are not pathognomonic for NF1, and even children with more than six café-au-lait macules, with no other manifestations, do not qualify for a diagnosis of NF1.[54] While approximately 95% of adults with NF1 have café-au-lait macules, they tend to fade later in life and may require a Wood's lamp for visualization.[55] Freckling in the intertriginous areas, especially in the axilla or groin, develops around age 3–5.[54]

Lisch nodules are iris hamartomas, which are visualized with slit lamp examination rather than direct ophthalmoscopy to distinguish them from iris nevi. Lisch nodules tend to develop in late childhood or early adolescence and do not impact vision.

OTHER CLINICAL FEATURES

Non-nervous system tumors that are associated with NF1 include pheochromocytomas, rhabdomyosarcomas, gastrointestinal stromal tumors, leukemia, breast cancer, and carcinoid.[45] NF1 patients also have a number of non-tumor manifestations that affect multiple organ systems.

> Non-nervous system tumors that are associated with NF1 include pheochromocytomas, rhabdomyosarcomas, gastrointestinal stromal tumors, leukemia, breast cancer, and carcinoid.

Neurologic manifestations are common, with higher incidence of cognitive issues (4–8%) compared with the general population. Intellectual abilities are average to low-average, with learning disabilities occurring in 50–75% of patients.[56] Seizures are also more twice as common as in the general population with prevalence of 4–6%.[57,58] However, screening electroencephalograms (EEGs) are not generally recommended. Peripheral neuropathy can also occur, with nerve compression in up to 4% of patients and spinal root compression in up to 3% of patients.[55] Vascular abnormalities can also be associated such as ectatic vessels, stenotic vessels, moyamoya, and aneurysms.[59]

Hypertension is more common in NF1 patients and can develop during childhood. As a result, blood pressure should be routinely monitored for all NF1 patients. A minority of cases, particularly in children and young adults, are due to renovascular complications and thus children with hypertension should be screened for renal artery stenosis.[60] Rarely is hypertension due to an underlying pheochromocytoma, but this should be considered in young adults or in the appropriate clinical scenario given its association with NF1.

> Hypertension is more common in NF1 patients and can develop during childhood. As a result, blood pressure should be routinely monitored for all NF1 patients.

Skeletal abnormalities are another common complication and part of the diagnostic criteria for NF1. Approximately 5% NF1 patients can suffer from sphenoid wing dysplasia, which can lead to orbital malformations.[61] Other bony complications include scoliosis, vertebral dysplasia, pseudoarthrosis, nonossifying fibromas of the long bones, and bone overgrowth.

NEUROFIBROMATOSIS 2

EPIDEMIOLOGY

NF2 is less common than NF1, with a prevalence of approximately 1:50,500[62] and an incidence of 1:25,00.[63] It is also an autosomal dominant disorder with full penetrance. An estimated 56% of patients have no family history and harbor a de novo pathogenic varient.[1] NF2 affects all races and genders equally. Patients with NF2 have a reduced lifespan of 69 years compared with 80 years.[4]

GENETICS AND PATHOGENESIS

The *NF2* gene is located on chromosome 22,[64] which is composed of 17 exons with a number of pathogenic variants including nonsense, splice-site, frameshift, and missense mutations.[65,66] A pathogenic variant in the NF2 gene can be identified in 70–90% of patients who meet the clinical criteria for NF2. However, in 33% of patients with bilateral vestibular schwannomas and 60% of patients with unilateral schwannoma, a pathogenic variant is not identified, likely due to somatic mosaicism.[67] One study found that 50% of de novo cases may actually be due to mosaicism.[68] Genotype–phenotype correlations for NF2 are more robust compared to NF1 and several clear examples are noted.

1. *Nonsense or frameshift mutations leading to truncated proteins* result in severely affected patients with younger age at diagnosis, increased prevalence of meningioma, spinal tumors, and non-cranial nerve VIII tumors.[69] Non-truncating mutations are associated with milder disease.

2. *Pathogenic variants in latter exons* (e.g., 14–15) are associated with milder disease (positional effect).[70]

3. *Truncating mutation in earlier exons* 2–13 are also associated with increased mortality.[71] The Manchester Genetic Severity Score can be used to predict clinical phenotype from genotype across several measures including age at diagnosis, tumor burden, and age at NF-2–related death.[72]

The predominant protein product of the *NF2* gene is merlin. Merlin links membrane-associated proteins to the actin cytoskeleton and acts as a tumor suppressor[73] regulating the growth of cells. Loss of both *NF2* alleles leads to tumor growth, and inactivation of *NF2* is seen in the majority of sporadic vestibular schwannomas[74] as well as in 50–60% of sporadic meningiomas.[75] However, the exact molecular mechanisms of tumorigenesis are not fully understood.

DIAGNOSTIC CRITERIA

The diagnostic criteria for NF2 should also be viewed in the context of lifetime presentation. NF2 is characterized by bilateral vestibular schwannomas as well as meningiomas, ependymomas, and non-vestibular schwannomas of the spinal, peripheral, and cutaneous nerves. Ninety-five percent of patients with NF2 develop vestibular schwannomas.[76] The average initial age of presentation for NF2 is around 17–24 years old.[77] Pediatric patients can present with vision problems, weakness, pain or seizures unrelated to classic vestibular schwannomas.[78] Adult patients often present with unilateral hearing loss or vestibular symptoms.[77] Malignant tumors are rare in NF2 since schwannomas do not undergo malignant transformation. However, patients who receive radiation therapy are at increased risk for MPNST and high-grade glioma.[79]

> NF2 is characterized by bilateral vestibular schwannomas as well as meningiomas, ependymomas, and non-vestibular schwannomas of the spinal, peripheral, and cutaneous nerves.

The NIH Consensus Conference on NF1 and NF2 established the diagnostic criteria for NF2 in 1987, which was revised in 1991.[80,81] The diagnostic criteria require bilateral vestibular schwannoma or a family history of NF2, which may be absent in patients with sporadic NF2. As a result, two other diagnostic criteria were proposed, the Manchester Criteria in 1992 and updated in 2017 and the Children's Tumor Foundation Criteria in 1997[82] (Box 27.2). However, while the current diagnostic criteria captures the majority of NF2 patients, some sporadic patients may still be missed.[83] In addition, some patients, especially individuals over age 70, can develop bilateral vestibular schwannomas by chance without underlying *NF2* mutation.[84] As a result, controversy still exists regarding the most suitable set of diagnostic criteria.[85] Patient with schwannomatosis due to pathogenic variants in *LZTR1* may also present with unilateral vestibular schwannomas but do not develop other tumors typical of NF2, such as ependymomas. Thus, NF2 is important to distinguish from other disorders such as NF1, sporadic vestibular schwannomas, schwannomatosis, and familial meningioma syndromes.[86]

> NF2 is important to distinguish from other disorders such as NF1, sporadic vestibular schwannomas, schwannomatosis, and familial meningioma syndromes.

Genetic testing is not part of the diagnostic criteria but may be useful for patients with sporadic NF2 whose initial presentation may not fit all the diagnostic criteria. Genetic mosaicism is common among patients without a family history and thus genetic testing is ideally conducted on tumor specimens if no variant is identified in blood. If two mutations are found, such as one genetic mutation and one allele lost, then one mutation can be assumed to be the underlying constitutional mutation.[87]

INITIAL EVALUATION AND SURVEILLANCE

Initial evaluation for patients with diagnosis of NF2 should include evaluation of auditory and vestibular function, focal neurologic deficits, and family history. MRI brain should be completed for vestibular schwannomas and MRI spine for intramedullary spinal tumors (ependymomas) and extramedullary spinal tumors (schwannomas and meningiomas). Patients should also have a baseline ophthalmologic exam (for juvenile cataracts, retinal hamartomas, and epiretinal membranes), audiology testing, and complete neurologic exam. Patients can be seen at 3- to 6-month intervals until the growth pattern of the tumor is identified and then followed annually thereafter. Surveillance should include neurologic exam, MRI brain, and MRI of any symptomatic extracranial lesions.

SCHWANNOMAS

Schwannomas are benign encapsulated tumors that are derived from Schwann cells. They grow eccentric to the nerve and normally become symptomatic due to compression rather than direct invasion.[88] Vestibular schwannomas are the most common intracranial tumor in NF2 patients. They can arise from the superior or inferior vestibular branches of cranial nerve VIII as multiple discrete nodules[89]. Nodules are also identified on the cochlear nerve, labyrinth, and semicircular canals.[89] Schwannomas typically enhance with contrast and histologically show Antoni A regions with palisading nuclei and Verocay bodies as well as hypercellular Antoni B regions. The amount of tumor growth in vestibular schwannomas and hearing loss is not highly correlated.[90] Most (~73%) of newly diagnosed patients can have stable hearing for 1–2 years after diagnosis.[91]

> Vestibular schwannomas are the most common intracranial tumor in NF2 patients.

Surgery for vestibular schwannomas is indicated for patients with brainstem or spinal cord compression and obstructive hydrocephalus.[76] If there is no significant impairment of neurologic function, watchful waiting may result in the best preservation of function.[92,93] Common complications of surgery include facial weakness, which can be deforming, and laryngeal weakness, which results in hoarseness and swallowing difficulty. Because patients with NF2 associated vestibular schwannomas may be at higher risk for malignant transformation after radiation, therapy is often reserved for older individuals or for younger individuals who do not have other good treatment options.[92,94] However, fractionated stereotactic radiotherapy may be beneficial for hearing preservation.[95] There are no standard chemotherapy agents, but several treatments are under investigation. Bevacizumab has shown some efficacy in both hearing improvement and tumor growth, with one study showing initial tumor shrinkage in 90% of patients and durable response in 40% of patients. Additionally, hearing improvement was also observed in approximately 40% and 20%, respectively, with hearing stabilization.[96] One small study showed a similar rate of tumor shrinkage of approximately 40% with bevacizumab treatment in the pediatric population as well.[97] As a result, treatment with bevacizumab has become standard for patients who develop hearing loss when they are able to hear in only one ear. Treatment with mTOR inhibitors such as everolimus has been associated with prolonged stable disease in single-arm trials, but there were no radiographic responses.[98]

Non-vestibular schwannomas can also occur in approximately one-half to one-third of NF patients,[99] most commonly on the trigeminal and occulomotor nerves.[100] Cutaneous schwannomas, subcutaneous schwannomas, and, more rarely, plexiform schwannomas can also occur.[101] Management is primarily surgical and reserved for neurologic dysfunction or rapid tumor growth.

MENINGIOMAS

Meningiomas are common in NF2 patients, with an incidence of 80% by 70 years of age.[70] Approximately 5% of patients have multiple meningiomas, but 20% of patients with multiple meningiomas have NF2[102] (Box 27.2). Meningiomas may be less common in patients with pathogenic NF2 variants after exon 13.[70] Intracranial meningiomas occur most frequent at the cerebral falx (~72%), skull base (25%), and ventricles (3%).[102] A majority of NF2 patients had fewer than three meningiomas, but a small minority (28%) had seven or more meningiomas. Most meningiomas (~66%) had minimal growth on serial imaging, but again a minority (~10%) had growth of greater than 4 mm/year.[102] In symptomatic meningiomas that were resected, 35% were grade 2 or 3. Approximately 11% of meningiomas had associated peritumoral edema; this was also associated with higher grade (WHO 2 or 3). Interestingly, skull base meningiomas are uncommon in NF2 patients and were all grade 1 in one study.[102] Spinal meningiomas also occur in an estimated 20% of NF2 patients.[103] Whether meningiomas in NF2 are more aggressive is a controversial topic, with some studies showing more aggressive tumors with higher mitotic index in NF2 patients[104] and some with no difference between NF2 and sporadic patients.[102] However, meningiomas are a marker of more severe disease and are associated with 2.5-fold higher mortality in NF2 patients.[105]

Given that NF2 patients can have multiple meningiomas, surgical resection of all lesions may not be feasible. Surgical indications include symptomatic lesions causing neurologic deficit or significant growth on imaging.[102,106] Spinal tumors may require surgical intervention, especially if they are extramedullary compared with intramedullary.[107] Radiation therapy can be considered for surgically inoperable tumors,[108] but it is not well established and there is additional concern for malignant transformation.[109,110] In addition, outcomes may be worse compared with sporadic tumors.[111] Several chemotherapy agents are under investigation for NF2-associated meningiomas including bevacizumab,[112] lapatinib[113] and sunitinib.[114]

SPINAL EPENDYMOMAS

Ependymomas are another common feature in NF2 and found in approximately 33–53% of patients.[106,107] Of the NF2 patients with ependymomas, 58% of NF2 patients may have multiple ependymomas.[115] In NF2 patients, ependymomas shows predilection for the cervicomedullary junction or cervical spinal cord[115] (Figure 27.3C) as opposed to the brain and lumbar spine, which is more common for sporadic ependymomas. The majority of ependymomas were asymptomatic, and pathology indicated they were-low grade (WHO 1 or 2).[115] Radiographic progression occurs in fewer than 10% of patients.[106,107] However, truncating mutations of the NF2 gene were found in 68% of patients with ependymomas suggesting that ependymomas may be associated with a more severe form of the disease.[115] Gliomas associated with NF2 are actually ependymomas,[116] and many have suggested revision of the diagnostic criteria.[85]

Since most spinal ependymomas in NF2 are asymptomatic, the treatment is often conservative. Approximately only 12–20% of NF2 patients require surgical intervention.[107,115] In select cases, such as in symptomatic ependymoma without overwhelming tumor load, surgery can help prevent morbidity but requires careful consideration given risk for surgical morbidity.[117] A small study showed that bevacizumab may help with neurologic or pain improvement related to a decrease in tumor cysts but had no clear radiographic response in the enhancing tumor.[118]

OTHER CLINICAL FEATURES

Other manifestations in NF2 patients include neuropathies thought to be due to compression or due to schwannoma tumorlets.[119] Ophthalmic manifestations include cataracts, posterior capsular lens opacities, retinal hamartomas, and optic sheath meningiomas.[120] Cutaneous tumors include plaque-like lesions and subcutaneous nodules, which reflect schwannomas. Despite the name "neurofibromatosis type 2," neurofibromas are a rarely identified in NF2 patients upon careful pathologic inspection.[121]

SCHWANNOMATOSIS

EPIDEMIOLOGY

Schwannomatosis is an uncommon disorder with an estimated prevalence of 1:126,315 in one UK study, which is less than ½ of NF2 prevalence.[62] The challenge in estimating prevalence of schwannomatosis is its non-specific presentation—typically pain—as opposed to the cutaneous manifestations of NF1 or the vestibular schwannomas of NF2.[88] Approximately 2–10% of patients with resected schwannomas have schwannomatosis.[122,123] Of patients with schwannomatosis, 15% are thought to be familial and 85% to be sporadic.[124]

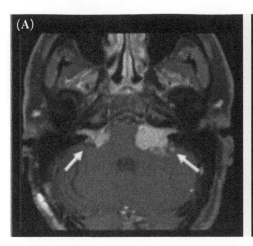
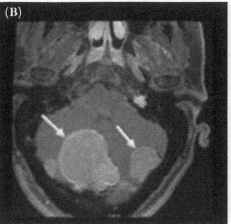
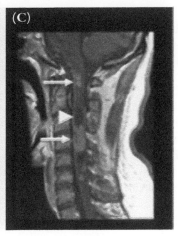

Figure 27.3 *Neuroimaging findings in neurofibromatosis type 2 (NF2). (A) Axial T1-weighted MRI scan after the administration of contrast demonstrating bilateral vestibular schwannomas. (B) Axial T1-weighted MRI scan after the administration of contrast demonstrating multiple meningiomas in the posterior fossa. (C) Sagittal T1-weighted MRI scan of the cervical spine after the administration of contrast demonstrating multiple ependymomas with enhancing tumor (arrows) and cysts (arrowhead).*

GENETICS AND PATHOGENESIS

Familial schwannomatosis is transmitted in an autosomal dominant fashion with variable penetrance. Analysis of a family with schwannomatosis led to discovery of pathogenic variants in the *SMARCB1* gene on chromosome 22,[125] which acts as a tumor suppressor gene. Mutations in *SMARCB1* appears to account for approximately 40-50% of patients with familial schwannomatosis and approximately 8–10% of patients with sporadic schwannomas.[126-129] Pathogenic variants in *SMARCB1* for affected families tend to be non-truncating, while sporadic schwannomas tend to have truncating variants.[128] The pathogenesis of schwannomas is best explained by a three-step, four-hit model with (1) germline mutation in *SMARCB1* gene (step 1); (2 and 3) mutation in chromosome 22 that contains the SMARCB1 allele and the NF2 allele (step 2); and (4) mutation in wildtype NF2 allele (step 3).[130]

Pathogenic variants in the *LZTR1* gene also cause schwannomatosis and account for approximately 37.5% of familial cases and 22% of sporadic cases in one study.[131]

DIAGNOSTIC CRITERIA

Schwannomatosis is genetically distinct from NF2 but shares a predisposition to multiple schwannomas and, less commonly, meningiomas (Box 27.3).[88] The schwannomas can affect cranial nerves, peripheral nerves, and spinal nerves but not cutaneous nerves. The median age of diagnosis is 40 years, but symptom onset typically precedes diagnosis by 10 years. Patients commonly present with pain, a mass, or both; motor deficits are an uncommon presentation.[124,132] Patients with familial schwannomatosis may present earlier compared to those with sporadic schwannomatosis.[123]

> Schwannomatosis is genetically distinct from NF2 but shares a predisposition to multiple schwannomas and less commonly meningiomas.

The diagnostic criteria for schwannomatosis were published in 2005 and specifically excluded patients with vestibular schwannomas since these individuals were thought to have NF2. These criteria permitted the diagnosis of definite, probable, or segmental schwannomatosis.[124] The criteria were later updated in 2013 to include both molecular and clinical features.[129] However, the criteria were developed before the discovery of *LZTR1* gene and before the realization that some patients with schwannomatosis can have unilateral vestibular schwannomas. As a result, revisions are in process.

The current criteria allow for a diagnosis of schwannomatosis through either clinical or molecular criteria (Box 27.3). The molecular diagnosis is confirmed by pathologically proven schwannomas and meningiomas, as well as by genetic studies. A clinical diagnosis requires at least two schwannomas, one with pathological confirmation and no bilateral vestibular schwannomas or one pathological confirmed schwannomas or intracranial meningioma and an affected first-degree relative. Patients who fulfill diagnostic criteria for NF2, have a first-degree relative with NF2, or schwannomas limited to prior radiation field were excluded from the diagnostic criteria.

However, in light of recent discoveries, the 2011 diagnostic criteria can lead to misdiagnoses between mosaic NF2 and schwannomatosis patients with estimates of 9% of mosaic NF2 misdiagnosed as schwannomatosis and 1–2% of *LZTR1* schwannomatosis patients misdiagnosed with NF2.[62] As a result, patients with multiple nonvestibular schwannomas, unilateral vestibular schwannomas, and other schwannomas may benefit from genetic testing. Bilateral vestibular schwannomas, cutaneous schwannomas, spinal ependymomas, juvenile cataracts, and epiretinal membranes currently appear unique to NF2 and are unlikely to be due to schwannomatosis.

CLINICAL MANIFESTATIONS

Schwannomas of the peripheral nerves are identified in 89% of patients, the spine in 74% of patients, and non-vestibular intracranial nerves in 9% of patients.[132] Spinal schwannomas most commonly affect the lumbar spine as opposed to the cervical spine in sporadic schwannomas.[133] As opposed to NF2, the cranial nerve most commonly affected in schwannomatosis is the trigeminal nerve,[123] but patients with schwannomatosis can rarely have unilateral vestibular schwannomas.[134] Subcutaneous schwannomas are also seen in 20–30% of patients[135] but cutaneous schwannomas have not been identified. On whole-body MRI, schwannomas are most often discrete (81%) with a minority that are plexiform (8%), and some have features of both plexiform and discrete schwannomas (11%)[135] (Figure 27.4).

> Spinal schwannomas in schwannomatosis most commonly affect the lumbar spine as opposed to the cervical spine being more commonly affected by sporadic schwannomas.

There is no pathologic difference between schwannomas from NF2 and schwannomatosis since both are composed of differentiated Schwann cells.[124] On MRI scan, schwannomas appear as multiple, well-circumscribed, rounded lesions along the course of peripheral nerves and spinal roots.[124] However, schwannomatosis-associated schwannomas tend to have more peritumoral edema, intratumoral myxoid changes, and intraneural growth patterns as opposed to sporadic schwannomas.[124] While vestibular schwannomas were initially thought to occur only in NF2, patients with and *LZTR1* pathogenic variant, and perhaps *SMARCB1*[134] pathogenic variant, have been found to have unilateral vestibular

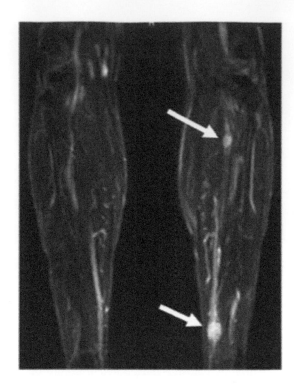

Figure 27.4 Neuroimaging finding in schwannomatosis (SWN). Coronal T1-weighted MRI scan after the administration of contrast demonstrating multiple schwannomas of the left leg.

schwannomas.[136] While there is a phenotypic overlap in NF2 and schwannomatosis, bilateral schwannomas have not been reported in schwannomatosis.

Five percent of schwannomatosis patients have meningiomas,[132] which occur most commonly in the cerebral falx.[137] One study described familial schwannomatosis with multiple meningiomas associated with the *SMARCB1* gene.[138] Malignant peripheral nerve sheath tumors have also been reported in schwannomatosis patients.[139] However, the risk of malignancy is not well-characterized. In one study, three patients with initial diagnosis of MPNST were later reclassified as having cellular schwannomas (2) and melanoma (1).[132] However, rapid growth and change in pain are concerning features for malignancy and require evaluation. Some families with *SMARCB1* or *SMARCA4* gene mutations are also predisposed to rhabdoid tumors.

MANAGEMENT

Initial evaluation of patients with concern for schwannomatosis should include evaluation to exclude NF1 and NF2. History should include review of auditory and vestibular function, visual function, and dermatologic signs as well as family history. Evaluating neurologic symptoms, pain, weakness, or myelopathy is crucial. Patients should also undergo an MRI brain with contrast including thin-cuts (<3 mm) through the internal auditory canal (IAC) to evaluate for vestibular schwannomas. MRI spine is also recommended to evaluate for spinal involvement and risk for cord impingement. Additional imaging should be guided by patient symptoms.

Treatment is primarily based on symptomatic lesions. Chronic pain is unfortunately a persistent and common problem in a majority of schwannomatosis patients.[132] Increased tumor volume may be associated with degree of pain.[140] However, pain is not always localized to the site of the schwannomas.[141] No class of pain medication has been shown to be more efficacious, and patients may benefit from referral to a pain center. A phase II clinical trial is currently investigating the effect of tanezumab for moderate to severe pain in schwannomatosis (NCT04163419).

> Chronic pain is a persistent and common problem in a majority of schwannomatosis patients.

Surgery is the mainstay of treatment for symptomatic lesions causing severe pain or neurologic deficits. Surgery can occasionally occur prophylactically if there is concern for impending spinal cord compression.[124] However, surgery does pose the risk of nerve injury and morbidity. Radiation therapy poses a theoretical risk of malignant transformation but can be considered for enlarging lesions that are inoperable. There are no established chemotherapy regimens, but case reports have described the use of bevacizumab.[142] A phase II clinical trial is investigating antigen-specific T cells (CAR-T), engineered immune effector cytotoxic T cells (EIE) modified by immunoregulatory genes, and immune-modified dendritic cell vaccine (DCvac) for schwannomatosis (NCT04085159).

CONCLUSION

NF1, NF2, and schwannomatosis are complex disorders with a wide range of neuro-oncologic manifestations. Understanding of these distinct genetic syndromes will help with early detection and proactive management of complications. Patients benefit from a multidisciplinary care approach, with the neuro-oncologist as a key member of that team. With new research and innovation, the management of these patients is still evolving with numerous new treatment options.

FLASHCARD

Genetics and Pathogenesis

	INHERITANCE	GENE AFFECTED	GENE PRODUCT	PROTEIN FUNCTION
NF1	Autosomal dominant	*NF1* (chromosome 17)	Neurofibromin	RAS pathway
NF2	Autosomal dominant	*NF2* (chromosome 22)	Merlin	Linking cell membrane to actin cytoskeleton
SWN	Autosomal dominant	*SMARCB1* and *LZTR1* (chromosome 22)	SWI/SNF protein complexes; LZTR1 protein	Chromatin remodeling; cellular control

Majority are asymptomatic, surgery is reserved for symptomatic lesions causing proptosis, blindness, or hydrocephalus, treatment otherwise is chemotherapy for progressive symptomatic lesions, radiation is avoided	Optic pathway gliomas in NF1
What is the treatment of high-grade gliomas in patients with NF1?	Multimodality treatment including radiation, modeled after sporadic gliomas
Common MRI T2 hyperintense lesions in NF1 without enhancement that can be difficult to distinguish from low-grade gliomas	Unidentified bright objects (UBOs), or focal areas of signal intensity (FASIs)
What drug was FDA-approved in 2020 for treatment of plexiform neurofibromas?	Selumetinib
Neurofibroma that may be premalignant	Atypical neurofibromatous neoplasms of uncertain biologic potential
What is an aggressive cancer that can develop within existing plexiform neurofibroma?	Malignant peripheral nerve sheath tumor, present with persistent pain, and/or rapid increase in tumor size
Which tumors are common in NF2?	Vestibular schwannomas (commonly bilateral), meningiomas, non-vestibular schwannomas, ependymomas

Which systemic therapy is shown to have some efficacy in hearing improvement and tumor growth in NF2-associated vestibular schwannomas?	Bevacizumab
This is characterized by multiple peripheral nerve, spinal, and non-vestibular nerve schwannomas with rare unilateral vestibular schwannomas	Schwannomatosis
Chronic pain is common in this form of neurofibromatosis, often without corresponding tumor/lesion	Schwannomatosis

1. What is the leading cause of mortality in NF1 patients?
   a. Malignant peripheral nerve sheath tumors
   b. Optic pathway glioma
   c. High-grade gliomas
   d. Vascular disease

2. Which of the following is *not* a criterion for NF1 diagnosis?
   a. Optic glioma
   b. First degree relative with NF1
   c. Freckling in axillary or inguinal areas
   d. Genetic analysis

3. What test is recommended for screening in asymptomatic optic pathway glioma patients?
   a. Visual evoked potentials
   b. Optic coherence tomography (OCT)
   c. Visual exam including visual field, color vision, and visual acuity
   d. MRI scan

4. A 10-year-old boy with NF1 was found to have a presumed focal area of signal intensity (FASI) in his temporal lobe on MRI brain during evaluation of a concussion. What is important to counsel the family?
   a. He needs surgical excision of the lesion since it is likely a low-grade glioma.
   b. He will likely develop epilepsy.
   c. He is unlikely to have any clinical manifestations from this lesion.
   d. The lesion is likely to develop into high-grade glioma in the future.

5. A 58-year-old woman with NF1 presents to clinic with acute worsening of chronic right arm pain that keeps her up at night. What diagnosis is important to exclude?
   a. New neurofibroma
   b. Extension of her plexiform neurofibroma
   c. Malignant peripheral nerve sheath tumor
   d. Nerve compression from neurofibroma

6. What is the best diagnostic tool to evaluate for malignant peripheral nerve sheath tumor?
   a. CT scan
   b. MRI scan
   c. Ultrasound
   d. FDG-PET

7. Which of the following is *not* a common complication of radiation therapy in NF1 patients?
   a. Moyamoya syndrome
   b. Malignant transformation of tumors
   c. Pseudoprogression
   d. Endocrinopathies

8. What is an approved chemotherapy regimen for symptomatic progressive plexiform neurofibromas in NF1 patients?
   a. Bevacizumab
   b. Selumetinib
   c. Carboplatin/Cisplatin
   d. Temozolomide

9. What symptom is *not* a complication of surgery for vestibular schwannomas in NF2?
   a. Arm weakness
   b. Hearing loss
   c. Facial weakness
   d. Hoarseness

10. A 20-year-old man presents with unilateral vestibular schwannoma and a family history of NF2. Which of the following would not be required for initial evaluation?
    a. Genetic testing
    b. MRI brain
    c. Ophthalmologic exam
    d. Audiology testing

11. Which of the following is the most common location for meningiomas in NF2?
    a. Skull base
    b. Cerebral falx
    c. Ventricles
    d. Sphenoid wing

12. A 30-year-old woman with NF2 undergoes a spine MRI with the following finding.
    What is the most likely diagnosis?
    a. Meningioma
    b. Ependymoma
    c. Astrocytoma
    d. Schwannomas

13. Which chemotherapy has been shown to improve hearing and shrink vestibular schwannomas in NF2 patients?
    a. Bevacizumab
    b. Selumetinib
    c. Temozolomide
    d. Carboplatin/Vincristine

14. Pathogenic variants in which two genes are associated with schwannomatosis?
    a. *SMARCB1* and *SPRED1*
    b. *SPRED1* and *LZTR1*
    c. *LZTR1* and *GNASI*
    d. *SMARCB1* and *LZTR1*

15. Which of the following is *not* identified in patients with schwannomatosis?
    a. Spinal ependymoma
    b. Spinal schwannoma
    c. Trigeminal schwannoma
    d. Meningioma

ANSWERS

1. a
2. d
3. c
4. c
5. c
6. d
7. c
8. b
9. a
10. a
11. b
12. b
13. a
14. d
15. a

REFERENCES

1. Evans DG, Howard E, Giblin C, et al. Birth incidence and prevalence of tumor-prone syndromes: Estimates from a UK family genetic register service. *Am J Med Genet A.* 2010;152A(2):327–332. doi:10.1002/ajmg.a.33139
2. Lammert M, Friedman JM, Kluwe L, Mautner VF. Prevalence of neurofibromatosis 1 in German children at elementary school enrollment. *Arch Dermatol.* 2005;141(1):71–74. doi:10.1001/archderm.141.1.71
3. Uusitalo E, Leppävirta J, Koffert A, et al. Incidence and mortality of neurofibromatosis: A total population study in Finland. *J Invest Dermatol.* 2015;135(3):904–906. doi:10.1038/jid.2014.465
4. Wilding A, Ingham SL, Lalloo F, Clancy T, Huson SM, Moran A, Evans DG. Life expectancy in hereditary cancer predisposing diseases: an observational study. *J Med Genet.* 2012 Apr;49(4):264–9. doi: 10.1136/jmedgenet-2011-100562. Epub 2012 Feb 23. PMID: 22362873.
5. Rasmussen SA, Yang Q, Friedman JM. Mortality in neurofibromatosis 1: An analysis using U.S. death certificates. *Am J Hum Genet.* 2001;68(5):1110–1118. doi:10.1086/320121
6. Bollag G, McCormick F. Ras regulation. NF is enough of GAP. *Nature.* 1992;356(6371):663–664. doi:10.1038/356663a0
7. Messiaen LM, Callens T, Mortier G, et al. Exhaustive mutation analysis of the NF1 gene allows identification of 95% of mutations and reveals a high frequency of unusual splicing defects. *Hum Mutat.* 2000;15(6):541–555. doi:10.1002/1098-1004(200006)15:6<541::AID-HUMU6>3.0.CO;2-N
8. Gutmann DH, Ferner RE, Listernick RH, et al. Neurofibromatosis type 1. *Nat Rev Dis Primer.* 2017;3:17004. doi:10.1038/nrdp.2017.4
9. Cnossen MH, van der Est MN, Breuning MH, et al. Deletions spanning the neurofibromatosis type 1 gene: Implications for genotype-phenotype correlations in neurofibromatosis type 1? *Hum Mutat.* 1997;9(5):458–464. doi:10.1002/(SICI)1098-1004(1997)9:5<458::AID-HUMU13>3.0.CO;2-1
10. Rojnueangnit K, Xie J, Gomes A, et al. High incidence of Noonan syndrome features including short stature and pulmonic stenosis in patients carrying NF1 missense mutations affecting p.Arg1809: Genotype-phenotype correlation. *Hum Mutat.* 2015;36(11):1052–1063. doi:10.1002/humu.22832
11. Upadhyaya M, Huson SM, Davies M, et al. An absence of cutaneous neurofibromas associated with a 3-bp inframe deletion in exon 17 of the NF1 gene (c.2970-2972 delAAT): Evidence of a clinically significant NF1 genotype-phenotype correlation. *Am J Hum Genet.* 2007;80(1):140–151. doi:10.1086/510781
12. DeBella K, Szudek J, Friedman JM. Use of the national institutes of health criteria for diagnosis of neurofibromatosis 1 in children. *Pediatrics.* 2000;105(3 Pt 1):608–614. doi:10.1542/peds.105.3.608
13. Gutmann DH, Aylsworth A, Carey JC, et al. The diagnostic evaluation and multidisciplinary management of neurofibromatosis 1 and neurofibromatosis 2. *JAMA.* 1997;278(1):51–57. doi:10.1001/jama.1997.03550010065042
14. Brems H, Chmara M, Sahbatou M, et al. Germline loss-of-function mutations in SPRED1 cause a neurofibromatosis 1-like phenotype. *Nat Genet.* 2007;39(9):1120–1126. doi:10.1038/ng2113
15. Messiaen L, Yao S, Brems H, et al. Clinical and mutational spectrum of neurofibromatosis type 1-like syndrome. *JAMA.* 2009;302(19):2111–2118. doi:10.1001/jama.2009.1663
16. Gutmann DH, Rasmussen SA, Wolkenstein P, et al. Gliomas presenting after age 10 in individuals with neurofibromatosis type 1 (NF1). *Neurology.* 2002;59(5):759–761. doi:10.1212/wnl.59.5.759
17. Guillamo J-S, Créange A, Kalifa C, et al. Prognostic factors of CNS tumours in Neurofibromatosis 1 (NF1): A retrospective study of 104 patients. *Brain J Neurol.* 2003;126(Pt 1):152–160. doi:10.1093/brain/awg016
18. Listernick R, Ferner RE, Liu GT, Gutmann DH. Optic pathway gliomas in neurofibromatosis-1: Controversies and recommendations. *Ann Neurol.* 2007;61(3):189–198. doi:10.1002/ana.21107
19. Listernick R, Charrow J, Greenwald M, Mets M. Natural history of optic pathway tumors in children with neurofibromatosis type 1: A longitudinal study. *J Pediatr.* 1994;125(1):63–66. doi:10.1016/s0022-3476(94)70122-9
20. Ullrich NJ, Robertson R, Kinnamon DD, et al. Moyamoya following cranial irradiation for primary brain tumors in children. *Neurology.* 2007;68(12):932–938. doi:10.1212/01.wnl.0000257095.33125.48
21. Banerjee A, Jakacki RI, Onar-Thomas A, et al. A phase I trial of the MEK inhibitor selumetinib (AZD6244) in pediatric patients with recurrent or refractory low-grade glioma: A Pediatric Brain Tumor Consortium (PBTC) study. *Neuro-Oncol.* 2017;19(8):1135–1144. doi:10.1093/neuonc/now282
22. Fangusaro J, Onar-Thomas A, Young Poussaint T, et al. Selumetinib in paediatric patients with BRAF-aberrant or neurofibromatosis type 1-associated recurrent, refractory, or progressive low-grade glioma: A multicentre, phase 2 trial. *Lancet Oncol.* 2019;20(7):1011–1022. doi:10.1016/S1470-2045(19)30277-3
23. Evans DGR, O'Hara C, Wilding A, et al. Mortality in neurofibromatosis 1: In North West England: An assessment of actuarial survival in a region of the UK since 1989. *Eur J Hum Genet EJHG.* 2011;19(11):1187–1191. doi:10.1038/ejhg.2011.113
24. Huttner AJ, Kieran MW, Yao X, et al. Clinicopathologic study of glioblastoma in children with neurofibromatosis type 1. *Pediatr Blood Cancer.* 2010;54(7):890–896. doi:10.1002/pbc.22462
25. Griffith JL, Morris SM, Mahdi J, et al. Increased prevalence of brain tumors classified as T2 hyperintensities in neurofibromatosis 1. *Neurol Clin Pract.* 2018;8(4):283–291. doi:10.1212/CPJ.0000000000000494
26. DiPaolo DP, Zimmerman RA, Rorke LB, et al. Neurofibromatosis type 1: Pathologic substrate of high-signal-intensity foci in the brain. *Radiology.* 1995;195(3):721–724. doi:10.1148/radiology.195.3.7754001
27. Hsieh H-Y, Fung H-C, Wang C-J, et al. Epileptic seizures in neurofibromatosis type 1 are related to intracranial tumors but not to neurofibromatosis bright objects. *Seizure.* 2011;20(8):606–611. doi:10.1016/j.seizure.2011.04.016
28. Woodruff JM. Pathology of tumors of the peripheral nerve sheath in type 1 neurofibromatosis. *Am J Med Genet.* 1999;89(1):23–30. doi:10.1002/(sici)1096-8628(19990326)89:1<23::aid-ajmg6>3.0.co;2-#
29. Uusitalo E, Kallionpää RA, Kurki S, et al. Breast cancer in neurofibromatosis type 1: Overrepresentation of unfavourable prognostic factors. *Br J Cancer.* 2017;116(2):211–217. doi:10.1038/bjc.2016.403
30. Plotkin SR, Bredella MA, Cai W, et al. Quantitative assessment of whole-body tumor burden in adult patients with neurofibromatosis. *PloS One.* 2012;7(4):e35711. doi:10.1371/journal.pone.0035711
31. Thakkar SD, Feigen U, Mautner VF. Spinal tumours in neurofibromatosis type 1: An MRI study of frequency, multiplicity and variety. *Neuroradiology.* 1999;41(9):625–629. doi:10.1007/s002340050814
32. Plotkin SR, Wick A. Neurofibromatosis and schwannomatosis. *Semin Neurol.* 2018;38(1):73–85. doi:10.1055/s-0038-1627471
33. Prada CE, Rangwala FA, Martin LJ, et al. Pediatric plexiform neurofibromas: Impact on morbidity and mortality in neurofibromatosis type 1. *J Pediatr.* 2012;160(3):461–467. doi:10.1016/j.jpeds.2011.08.051
34. Lin BT, Weiss LM, Medeiros LJ. Neurofibroma and cellular neurofibroma with atypia: A report of 14 tumors. *Am J Surg Pathol.* 1997;21(12):1443–1449. doi:10.1097/00000478-199712000-00006
35. Miettinen MM, Antonescu CR, Fletcher CDM, et al. Histopathologic evaluation of atypical neurofibromatous tumors and their transformation into malignant peripheral nerve sheath tumor in patients with neurofibromatosis-1—a consensus overview. *Hum Pathol.* 2017;67:1–10. doi:10.1016/j.humpath.2017.05.010
36. Pemov A, Hansen NF, Sindiri S, et al. Low mutation burden and frequent loss of CDKN2A/B and SMARCA2, but not PRC2, define pre-malignant neurofibromatosis type 1-associated atypical neurofibromas. *Neuro-Oncol.* Published online Feb 5, 2019. doi:10.1093/neuonc/noz028

37. Beert E, Brems H, Daniëls B, et al. Atypical neurofibromas in neurofibromatosis type 1 are premalignant tumors. *Genes Chromosomes Cancer.* 2011;50(12):1021–1032. doi:10.1002/gcc.20921

38. Evans DGR, Birch JM, Ramsden RT, et al. Malignant transformation and new primary tumours after therapeutic radiation for benign disease: Substantial risks in certain tumour prone syndromes. *J Med Genet.* 2006;43(4):289–294. doi:10.1136/jmg.2005.036319

39. FDA approves selumetinib for neurofibromatosis type 1 with symptomatic, inoperable plexiform neurofibromas. FDA. Apr 13, 2020. https://www.fda.gov/drugs/resources-information-approved-drugs/fda-approves-selumetinib-neurofibromatosis-type-1-symptomatic-inoperable-plexiform-neurofibromas

40. Gross AM, Wolters P, Baldwin A, et al. SPRINT: Phase II study of the MEK 1/2 inhibitor selumetinib (AZD6244, ARRY-142886) in children with neurofibromatosis type 1 (NF1) and inoperable plexiform neurofibromas (PN). *J Clin Oncol.* 2018;36(15_Suppl):10503–10503. doi:10.1200/JCO.2018.36.15_suppl.10503

41. Jakacki RI, Dombi E, Steinberg SM, et al. Phase II trial of pegylated interferon alfa-2b in young patients with neurofibromatosis type 1 and unresectable plexiform neurofibromas. *Neuro-Oncol.* 2017;19(2):289–297. doi:10.1093/neuonc/now158

42. Tucker T, Wolkenstein P, Revuz J, et al. Association between benign and malignant peripheral nerve sheath tumors in NF1. *Neurology.* 2005;65(2):205–211. doi:10.1212/01.wnl.0000168830.79997.13

43. Evans DGR, Baser ME, McGaughran J, et al. Malignant peripheral nerve sheath tumours in neurofibromatosis 1. *J Med Genet.* 2002;39(5):311–314. doi:10.1136/jmg.39.5.311

44. Ferner RE, Gutmann DH. International consensus statement on malignant peripheral nerve sheath tumors in neurofibromatosis. *Cancer Res.* 2002;62(5):1573–1577.

45. Lu-Emerson C, Plotkin SR. The neurofibromatoses. Part 1: NF1. *Rev Neurol Dis.* 2009;6(2):E47–53.

46. Warbey VS, Ferner RE, Dunn JT, et al. [18F]FDG PET/CT in the diagnosis of malignant peripheral nerve sheath tumours in neurofibromatosis type-1. *Eur J Nucl Med Mol Imaging.* 2009;36(5):751–757. doi:10.1007/s00259-008-1038-0

47. Yang JC, Chang AE, Baker AR, et al. Randomized prospective study of the benefit of adjuvant radiation therapy in the treatment of soft tissue sarcomas of the extremity. *J Clin Oncol Off J Am Soc Clin Oncol.* 1998;16(1):197–203. doi:10.1200/JCO.1998.16.1.197

48. Frustaci S, Gherlinzoni F, De Paoli A, et al. Adjuvant chemotherapy for adult soft tissue sarcomas of the extremities and girdles: Results of the Italian randomized cooperative trial. *J Clin Oncol Off J Am Soc Clin Oncol.* 2001;19(5):1238–1247. doi:10.1200/JCO.2001.19.5.1238

49. Kroep JR, Ouali M, Gelderblom H, et al. First-line chemotherapy for malignant peripheral nerve sheath tumor (MPNST) versus other histological soft tissue sarcoma subtypes and as a prognostic factor for MPNST: An EORTC soft tissue and bone sarcoma group study. *Ann Oncol Off J Eur Soc Med Oncol.* 2011;22(1):207–214. doi:10.1093/annonc/mdq338

50. Carli M, Ferrari A, Mattke A, et al. Pediatric malignant peripheral nerve sheath tumor: The Italian and German soft tissue sarcoma cooperative group. *J Clin Oncol Off J Am Soc Clin Oncol.* 2005;23(33):8422–8430. doi:10.1200/JCO.2005.01.4886

51. Hagel C, Zils U, Peiper M, et al. Histopathology and clinical outcome of NF1-associated vs. sporadic malignant peripheral nerve sheath tumors. *J Neurooncol.* 2007;82(2):187–192. doi:10.1007/s11060-006-9266-2

52. LaFemina J, Qin L-X, Moraco NH, et al. Oncologic outcomes of sporadic, neurofibromatosis-associated, and radiation-induced malignant peripheral nerve sheath tumors. *Ann Surg Oncol.* 2013;20(1):66–72. doi:10.1245/s10434-012-2573-2

53. Kolberg M, Høland M, Agesen TH, et al. Survival meta-analyses for >1800 malignant peripheral nerve sheath tumor patients with and without neurofibromatosis type 1. *Neuro-Oncol.* 2013;15(2):135–147. doi:10.1093/neuonc/nos287

54. Korf BR. Diagnostic outcome in children with multiple café au lait spots. *Pediatrics.* 1992;90(6):924–927.

55. Friedman JM, Birch PH. Type 1 neurofibromatosis: A descriptive analysis of the disorder in 1,728 patients. *Am J Med Genet.* 1997;70(2):138–143. doi:10.1002/(sici)1096-8628(19970516)70:2<138::aid-ajmg7>3.0.co;2-u

56. North KN, Riccardi V, Samango-Sprouse C, et al. Cognitive function and academic performance in neurofibromatosis. 1: Consensus statement from the NF1 Cognitive Disorders Task Force. *Neurology.* 1997;48(4):1121–1127. doi:10.1212/wnl.48.4.1121

57. Ostendorf AP, Gutmann DH, Weisenberg JLZ. Epilepsy in individuals with neurofibromatosis type 1. *Epilepsia.* 2013;54(10):1810–1814. doi:10.1111/epi.12348

58. Korf BR, Carrazana E, Holmes GL. Patterns of seizures observed in association with neurofibromatosis 1. *Epilepsia.* 1993;34(4):616–620. doi:10.1111/j.1528-1157.1993.tb00437.x

59. Rosser TL, Vezina G, Packer RJ. Cerebrovascular abnormalities in a population of children with neurofibromatosis type 1. *Neurology.* 2005;64(3):553–555. doi:10.1212/01.WNL.0000150544.00016.69

60. Fossali E, Signorini E, Intermite RC, et al. Renovascular disease and hypertension in children with neurofibromatosis. *Pediatr Nephrol Berl Ger.* 2000;14(8-9):806–810. doi:10.1007/s004679900260

61. Delucia TA, Yohay K, Widmann RF. Orthopaedic aspects of neurofibromatosis: Update. *Curr Opin Pediatr.* 2011;23(1):46–52. doi:10.1097/MOP.0b013e32834230ce

62. Evans DG, Bowers NL, Tobi S, et al. Schwannomatosis: A genetic and epidemiological study. *J Neurol Neurosurg Psychiatry.* 2018;89(11):1215–1219. doi:10.1136/jnnp-2018-318538

63. Evans DGR, Moran A, King A, et al. Incidence of vestibular schwannoma and neurofibromatosis 2 in the North West of England over a 10-year period: Higher incidence than previously thought. *Otol Neurotol.* 2005;26(1):93–97. doi:10.1097/00129492-200501000-00016

64. Wallace AJ, Watson CJ, Oward E, et al. Mutation scanning of the NF2 gene: An improved service based on meta-PCR/sequencing, dosage analysis, and loss of heterozygosity analysis. *Genet Test.* 2004;8(4):368–380. doi:10.1089/gte.2004.8.368

65. Ahronowitz I, Xin W, Kiely R, et al. Mutational spectrum of the NF2 gene: A meta-analysis of 12 years of research and diagnostic laboratory findings. *Hum Mutat.* 2007;28(1):1–12. doi:10.1002/humu.20393

66. Baser ME, Kuramoto L, Woods R, et al. The location of constitutional neurofibromatosis 2 (NF2) splice site mutations is associated with the severity of NF2. *J Med Genet.* 2005;42(7):540–546. doi:10.1136/jmg.2004.029504

67. Evans DGR, Ramsden RT, Shenton A, et al. Mosaicism in neurofibromatosis type 2: An update of risk based on uni/bilaterality of vestibular schwannoma at presentation and sensitive mutation analysis including multiple ligation-dependent probe amplification. *J Med Genet.* 2007;44(7):424–428. doi:10.1136/jmg.2006.047753

68. Evans DG, Hartley CL, Smith PT, et al. Incidence of mosaicism in 1055 de novo NF2 cases: Much higher than previous estimates with high utility of next-generation sequencing. *Genet Med Off J Am Coll Med Genet.* 2020;22(1):53–59. doi:10.1038/s41436-019-0598-7

69. Selvanathan SK, Shenton A, Ferner R, et al. Further genotype–phenotype correlations in neurofibromatosis 2. *Clin Genet.* 2010;77(2):163–170. doi:10.1111/j.1399-0004.2009.01315.x

70. Smith MJ, Higgs JE, Bowers NL, et al. Cranial meningiomas in 411 neurofibromatosis type 2 (NF2) patients with proven gene mutations: Clear positional effect of mutations, but absence of female severity effect on age at onset. *J Med Genet.* 2011;48(4):261–265. doi:10.1136/jmg.2010.085241

71. Hexter A, Jones A, Joe H, et al. Clinical and molecular predictors of mortality in neurofibromatosis 2: A UK national analysis of 1192 patients. *J Med Genet.* 2015;52(10):699–705. doi:10.1136/jmedgenet-2015-103290

72. Halliday D, Emmanouil B, Pretorius P, et al. Genetic Severity Score predicts clinical phenotype in NF2. *J Med Genet.* 2017;54(10):657–664. doi:10.1136/jmedgenet-2017-104519

73. Trofatter JA, MacCollin MM, Rutter JL, et al. A novel moesin-, ezrin-, radixin-like gene is a candidate for the neurofibromatosis 2 tumor suppressor. *Cell.* 1993;72(5):791–800. doi:10.1016/0092-8674(93)90406-g

74. Jacoby LB, MacCollin M, Barone R, et al. Frequency and distribution of NF2 mutations in schwannomas. *Genes Chromosomes Cancer.* 1996;17(1):45–55. doi:10.1002/(SICI)1098-2264(199609)17:1<45::AID-GCC7>3.0.CO;2-2

75. Wellenreuther R, Kraus JA, Lenartz D, et al. Analysis of the neurofibromatosis 2 gene reveals molecular variants of meningioma. *Am J Pathol.* 1995;146(4):827–832.

76. Plotkin SR, Wick A. Neurofibromatosis and schwannomatosis. *Semin Neurol.* 2018;38(1):73–85. doi:10.1055/s-0038-1627471

77. Evans DG, Huson SM, Donnai D, et al. A clinical study of type 2 neurofibromatosis. *Q J Med.* 1992;84(304):603–618.

78. Anand G, Vasallo G, Spanou M, et al. Diagnosis of sporadic neurofibromatosis type 2 in the paediatric population. *Arch Dis Child.* 2018;103(5):463–469. doi:10.1136/archdischild-2017-313154

79. Baser ME, Evans DGR, Jackler RK, et al. Neurofibromatosis 2, radiosurgery and malignant nervous system tumours. *Br J Cancer.* 2000;82(4):998. doi:10.1054/bjoc.1999.1030

80. From the Office of Medical Applications of Research, National Institutes of Health, Bethesda, Md. Neurofibromatosis. Conference statement. National Institutes of Health Consensus Development Conference. *Arch Neurol.* 1988 May; 45(5):575–578. PMID: 3128965.

81. Mulvihill JJ, Parry DM, Sherman JL, et al. NIH conference. Neurofibromatosis 1 (Recklinghausen disease) and neurofibromatosis

2 (bilateral acoustic neurofibromatosis). An update. *Ann Intern Med.* 1990;113(1):39–52. doi:10.7326/0003-4819-113-1-39

82. Children's Tumor Foundation. NF2. Accessed August 1, 2020. https://www.ctf.org/understanding-nf/nf2#nf2-diagnosis

83. Baser ME, Friedman JM, Wallace AJ, et al. Evaluation of clinical diagnostic criteria for neurofibromatosis 2. *Neurology.* 2002;59(11):1759–1765. doi:10.1212/01.wnl.0000035638.74084.f4

84. Evans DG, Freeman S, Gokhale C, et al. Bilateral vestibular schwannomas in older patients: NF2 or chance? *J Med Genet.* 2015;52(6):422–424. doi:10.1136/jmedgenet-2014-102973

85. Evans DG, King AT, Bowers NL, et al. Identifying the deficiencies of current diagnostic criteria for neurofibromatosis 2 using databases of 2777 individuals with molecular testing. *Genet Med Off J Am Coll Med Genet.* 2019;21(7):1525–1533. doi:10.1038/s41436-018-0384-y

86. Evans DGR, Watson C, King A, et al. Multiple meningiomas: Differential involvement of the NF2 gene in children and adults. *J Med Genet.* 2005;42(1):45–48. doi:10.1136/jmg.2004.023705

87. Kluwe L, Friedrich RE, Tatagiba M, Mautner VF. Presymptomatic diagnosis for children of sporadic neurofibromatosis 2 patients: A method based on tumor analysis. *Genet Med.* 2002;4(1):27–30. doi:10.1097/00125817-200201000-00005

88. Lu-Emerson C, Plotkin SR. The neurofibromatoses. Part 2: NF2 and schwannomatosis. *Rev Neurol Dis.* 2009;6(3):E81-86.

89. Stivaros SM, Stemmer-Rachamimov AO, Alston R, et al. Multiple synchronous sites of origin of vestibular schwannomas in neurofibromatosis Type 2. *J Med Genet.* 2015;52(8):557–562. doi:10.1136/jmedgenet-2015-103050

90. Fisher LM, Doherty JK, Lev MH, Slattery WH. Concordance of bilateral vestibular schwannoma growth and hearing changes in neurofibromatosis 2: Neurofibromatosis 2 natural history consortium. *Otol Neurotol.* 2009;30(6):835–841. doi:10.1097/MAO.0b013e3181b2364c

91. Masuda A, Fisher LM, Oppenheimer ML, et al., Natural History Consortium. Hearing changes after diagnosis in neurofibromatosis type 2. *Otol Neurotol.* 2004;25(2):150–154. doi:10.1097/00129492-200403000-00012

92. Maniakas A, Saliba I. Neurofibromatosis type 2 vestibular schwannoma treatment: A review of the literature, trends, and outcomes. *Otol Neurotol.* 2014;35(5):889–894. doi:10.1097/MAO.0000000000000272

93. Liu R, Fagan P. Facial nerve schwannoma: Surgical excision versus conservative management. *Ann Otol Rhinol Laryngol.* 2001;110(11):1025–1029. doi:10.1177/000348940111001106

94. Evans DGR, Birch JM, Ramsden RT, et al. Malignant transformation and new primary tumours after therapeutic radiation for benign disease: Substantial risks in certain tumour prone syndromes. *J Med Genet.* 2006;43(4):289–294. doi:10.1136/jmg.2005.036319

95. Combs SE, Volk S, Schulz-Ertner D, et al. Management of acoustic neuromas with fractionated stereotactic radiotherapy (FSRT): Long-term results in 106 patients treated in a single institution. *Int J Radiat Oncol Biol Phys.* 2005;63(1):75–81. doi:10.1016/j.ijrobp.2005.01.055

96. Plotkin SR, Stemmer-Rachamimov AO, Barker FG, et al. Hearing improvement after bevacizumab in patients with neurofibromatosis type 2. *N Engl J Med.* 2009;361(4):358–367. doi:10.1056/NEJMoa0902579

97. Hochart A, Gaillard V, Baroncini M, et al. Bevacizumab decreases vestibular schwannomas growth rate in children and teenagers with neurofibromatosis type 2. *J Neurooncol.* 2015;124(2):229–236. doi:10.1007/s11060-015-1828-8

98. Goutagny S, Raymond E, Esposito-Farese M, et al. Phase II study of mTORC1 inhibition by everolimus in neurofibromatosis type 2 patients with growing vestibular schwannomas. *J Neurooncol.* 2015;122(2):313–320. doi:10.1007/s11060-014-1710-0

99. Parry DM, Eldridge R, Kaiser-Kupfer MI, et al. Neurofibromatosis 2 (NF2): Clinical characteristics of 63 affected individuals and clinical evidence for heterogeneity. *Am J Med Genet.* 1994;52(4):450–461. doi:10.1002/ajmg.1320520411

100. Fisher LM, Doherty JK, Lev MH, Slattery WH. Distribution of nonvestibular cranial nerve schwannomas in neurofibromatosis 2. *Otol Neurotol.* 2007;28(8):1083–1090. doi:10.1097/MAO.0b013e31815a8411

101. Berg JC, Scheithauer BW, Spinner RJ, et al. Plexiform schwannoma: A clinicopathologic overview with emphasis on the head and neck region. *Hum Pathol.* 2008;39(5):633–640. doi:10.1016/j.humpath.2007.10.029

102. Goutagny S, Bah AB, Henin D, et al. Long-term follow-up of 287 meningiomas in neurofibromatosis type 2 patients: Clinical, radiological, and molecular features. *Neuro-Oncol.* 2012;14(8):1090–1096. doi:10.1093/neuonc/nos129

103. Coy S, Rashid R, Stemmer-Rachamimov A, Santagata S. An update on the CNS manifestations of neurofibromatosis type 2. *Acta Neuropathol (Berl).* 2020;139(4):643–665. doi:10.1007/s00401-019-02029-5

104. Perry A, Giannini C, Raghavan R, et al. Aggressive phenotypic and genotypic features in pediatric and NF2-associated meningiomas: A clinicopathologic

study of 53 cases. *J Neuropathol Exp Neurol.* 2001;60(10):994–1003. doi:10.1093/jnen/60.10.994

105. Baser ME, Friedman JM, Aeschliman D, et al. Predictors of the risk of mortality in neurofibromatosis 2. *Am J Hum Genet.* 2002;71(4):715–723. doi:10.1086/342716

106. Mautner VF, Tatagiba M, Lindenau M, et al. Spinal tumors in patients with neurofibromatosis type 2: MR imaging study of frequency, multiplicity, and variety. *Am J Roentgenol.* 1995;165(4):951–955. doi:10.2214/ajr.165.4.7676998

107. Patronas NJ, Courcoutsakis N, Bromley CM, et al. Intramedullary and spinal canal tumors in patients with neurofibromatosis 2: MR imaging findings and correlation with genotype. *Radiology.* 2001;218(2):434–442. doi:10.1148/radiology.218.2.r01fe40434

108. Wentworth S, Pinn M, Bourland JD, et al. Clinical experience with radiation therapy in the management of neurofibromatosis-associated central nervous system tumors. *Int J Radiat Oncol Biol Phys.* 2009;73(1):208–213. doi:10.1016/j.ijrobp.2008.03.073

109. Baser ME, Evans DG, Jackler RK, et al. Neurofibromatosis 2, radiosurgery and malignant nervous system tumours. *Br J Cancer.* 2000;82(4):998. doi:10.1054/bjoc.1999.1030

110. Thomsen J, Mirz F, Wetke R, et al. Intracranial sarcoma in a patient with neurofibromatosis type 2 treated with gamma knife radiosurgery for vestibular schwannoma. *Am J Otol.* 2000;21(3):364–370. doi:10.1016/s0196-0709(00)80046-0

111. Fuss M, Debus J, Lohr F, et al. Conventionally fractionated stereotactic radiotherapy (FSRT) for acoustic neuromas. *Int J Radiat Oncol Biol Phys.* 2000;48(5):1381–1387. doi:10.1016/s0360-3016(00)01361-4

112. Nunes FP, Merker VL, Jennings D, et al. Bevacizumab treatment for meningiomas in NF2: A retrospective analysis of 15 patients. *PloS One.* 2013;8(3):e59941. doi:10.1371/journal.pone.0059941

113. Osorio DS, Hu J, Mitchell C, et al. Effect of lapatinib on meningioma growth in adults with neurofibromatosis type 2. *J Neurooncol.* 2018;139(3):749–755. doi:10.1007/s11060-018-2922-5

114. Kaley TJ, Wen P, Schiff D, et al. Phase II trial of sunitinib for recurrent and progressive atypical and anaplastic meningioma. *Neuro-Oncol.* 2015;17(1):116–121. doi:10.1093/neuonc/nou148

115. Plotkin SR, O'Donnell CC, Curry WT, et al. Spinal ependymomas in neurofibromatosis type 2: A retrospective analysis of 55 patients. *J Neurosurg Spine.* 2011;14(4):543–547. doi:10.3171/2010.11.SPINE10350

116. Hagel C, Stemmer-Rachamimov AO, Bornemann A, et al. Clinical presentation, immunohistochemistry and electron microscopy indicate neurofibromatosis type 2-associated gliomas to be spinal ependymomas. *Neuropathol Japan.* 2012;32(6):611–616. doi:10.1111/j.1440-1789.2012.01306.x

117. Kalamarides M, Essayed W, Lejeune JP, et al. Spinal ependymomas in NF2: A surgical disease? *J Neurooncol.* 2018;136(3):605–611. doi:10.1007/s11060-017-2690-7

118. Farschtschi S, Merker VL, Wolf D, et al. Bevacizumab treatment for symptomatic spinal ependymomas in neurofibromatosis type 2. *Acta Neurol Scand.* 2016;133(6):475–480. doi:10.1111/ane.12490

119. Sperfeld AD, Hein C, Schröder JM, et al. Occurrence and characterization of peripheral nerve involvement in neurofibromatosis type 2. *Brain J Neurol.* 2002;125(Pt 5):996–1004. doi:10.1093/brain/awf115

120. Ragge NK, Baser ME, Klein J, et al. Ocular abnormalities in neurofibromatosis 2. *Am J Ophthalmol.* 1995;120(5):634–641. doi:10.1016/s0002-9394(14)72210-x

121. Mautner VF, Lindenau M, Baser ME, et al. Skin abnormalities in neurofibromatosis 2. *Arch Dermatol.* 1997;133(12):1539–1543.

122. Antinheimo j, Sankila R, Carpen O, et al. Population-based analysis of sporadic and type 2 neurofibromatosis-associated meningiomas and schwannomas. *Neurology.* 2000; 54(1):71–76. doi:10.1212/wnl.54.1.71.

123. Gonzalvo A, Fowler A, Cook RJ, et al. Schwannomatosis, sporadic schwannomatosis, and familial schwannomatosis: A surgical series with long-term follow-up. Clinical article. *J Neurosurg.* 2011;114(3):756–762. doi:10.3171/2010.8.JNS091900

124. MacCollin M, Chiocca EA, Evans DG, et al. Diagnostic criteria for schwannomatosis. *Neurology.* 2005;64(11):1838–1845. doi:10.1212/01.WNL.0000163982.78900.AD

125. Hulsebos TJM, Kenter SB, Jakobs ME, et al. SMARCB1/INI1 maternal germ line mosaicism in schwannomatosis. *Clin Genet.* 2010;77(1):86–91. doi:10.1111/j.1399-0004.2009.01249.x

126. Hadfield KD, Newman WG, Bowers NL, et al. Molecular characterisation of SMARCB1 and NF2 in familial and sporadic schwannomatosis. *J Med Genet.* 2008;45(6):332–339. doi:10.1136/jmg.2007.056499

127. Rousseau G, Noguchi T, Bourdon V, et al. SMARCB1/INI1 germline mutations contribute to 10% of sporadic schwannomatosis. *BMC Neurol.* 2011;11:9. doi:10.1186/1471-2377-11-9

128. Smith MJ, Wallace AJ, Bowers NL, et al. Frequency of SMARCB1 mutations in familial and sporadic schwannomatosis. *Neurogenetics.* 2012;13(2):141–145. doi:10.1007/s10048-012-0319-8

129. Plotkin SR, Blakeley JO, Evans DG, et al. Update from the 2011 International Schwannomatosis Workshop: From genetics to diagnostic criteria. *Am J Med Genet A.* 2013;161A(3):405–416. doi:10.1002/ajmg.a.35760

130. Sestini R, Bacci C, Provenzano A, et al. Evidence of a four-hit mechanism involving SMARCB1 and NF2 in schwannomatosis-associated schwannomas. *Hum Mutat.* 2008;29(2):227–231. doi:10.1002/humu.20679

131. Smith MJ, Isidor B, Beetz C, et al. Mutations in LZTR1 add to the complex heterogeneity of schwannomatosis. *Neurology.* 2015;84(2):141–147. doi:10.1212/WNL.0000000000001129

132. Merker VL, Esparza S, Smith MJ, et al. Clinical features of schwannomatosis: A retrospective analysis of 87 patients. *Oncologist.* 2012;17(10):1317–1322. doi:10.1634/theoncologist.2012-0162

133. Li P, Zhao F, Zhang J, et al. Clinical features of spinal schwannomas in 65 patients with schwannomatosis compared with 831 with solitary schwannomas and 102 with neurofibromatosis Type 2: A retrospective study at a single institution. *J Neurosurg Spine.* 2016;24(1):145–154. doi:10.3171/2015.3.SPINE141145

134. Smith MJ, Kulkarni A, Rustad C, et al. Vestibular schwannomas occur in schwannomatosis and should not be considered an exclusion criterion for clinical diagnosis. *Am J Med Genet A.* 2012;158A(1):215–219. doi:10.1002/ajmg.a.34376

135. Plotkin SR, Bredella MA, Cai W, et al. Quantitative assessment of whole-body tumor burden in adult patients with neurofibromatosis. *PloS One.* 2012;7(4):e35711. doi:10.1371/journal.pone.0035711

136. Gripp KW, Baker L, Kandula V, et al. Constitutional LZTR1 mutation presenting with a unilateral vestibular schwannoma in a teenager. *Clin Genet.* 2017;92(5):540–543. doi:10.1111/cge.13013

137. van den Munckhof P, Christiaans I, Kenter SB, et al. Germline SMARCB1 mutation predisposes to multiple meningiomas and schwannomas with preferential location of cranial meningiomas at the falx cerebri. *Neurogenetics.* 2012;13(1):1–7. doi:10.1007/s10048-011-0300-y

138. Bacci C, Sestini R, Provenzano A, et al. Schwannomatosis associated with multiple meningiomas due to a familial SMARCB1 mutation. *Neurogenetics.* 2010;11(1):73–80. doi:10.1007/s10048-009-0204-2

139. Carter JM, O'Hara C, Dundas G, et al. Epithelioid malignant peripheral nerve sheath tumor arising in a schwannoma, in a patient with "neuroblastoma-like" schwannomatosis and a novel germline SMARCB1 mutation. *Am J Surg Pathol.* 2012;36(1):154–160. doi:10.1097/PAS.0b013e3182380802

140. Merker VL, Bredella MA, Cai W, et al. Relationship between whole-body tumor burden, clinical phenotype, and quality of life in patients with neurofibromatosis. *Am J Med Genet A.* 2014;164A(6):1431–1437. doi:10.1002/ajmg.a.36466

141. Dhamija R, Plotkin S, Asthagiri A, et al. Schwannomatosis. In Adam MP, Ardinger HH, Pagon RA, et al., eds., *GeneReviews.* Seattle: University of Washington; 1993. http://www.ncbi.nlm.nih.gov/books/NBK487394/

142. Blakeley J, Schreck KC, Evans DG, et al. Clinical response to bevacizumab in schwannomatosis. *Neurology.* 2014;83(21):1986–1987. doi:10.1212/WNL.0000000000000997

143. Smith MJ, Bowers NL, Bulman M, et al. Revisiting neurofibromatosis type 2 diagnostic criteria to exclude LZTR1-related schwannomatosis. *Neurology.* 2017;88(1):87–92. doi:10.1212/WNL.0000000000003418

PART VII. | SPECIAL CONSIDERATIONS IN NEURO-ONCOLOGY

28 | DESIGNING AND DECIPHERING CLINICAL TRIALS

Methodological Ingredients to Nourish a Healthy Study

MICHAEL GLANTZ AND ALIREZA MANSOURI

INTRODUCTION

Turn lead into gold? Been there. Done that. In 1981.[1] The ability to transform "base metals" into "noble metals" (chrysopoeia) eluded ancient alchemists for many reasons. But the effort may not have taken nearly two millennia to accomplish if early experimenters had embraced the now widely accepted practice of "showing your work." Before 1665, experimenters were eager to share their results but jealously guarded their methods. In that year, a new concept was introduced by a small group of "natural philosophers." They proposed, in a first-of-its-kind scientific journal (Figure 28.1),[2] that scientific progress required complete transparency of experimental technique as well as a description of study results. In this chapter, we discuss the basic tenets of clinical trial design, with an emphasis on showing your work. And since the same knowledge that permits investigators to design high-quality clinical trials is also required to effectively evaluate the strength of published research, familiarity with these techniques will serve two critical purposes. In addition, time, money, and—most crucially—study participants, are precious and scarce. If a clinical trial is poorly designed, the likelihood of that study providing useful information is low, and the researcher's contract with his or her funding agencies, institution, and patients is betrayed. We will concentrate on therapeutic trials, but the same principles apply to diagnostic and prognostic studies and investigations of causal association. We will frequently refer to published studies to illustrate points, but we cannot emphasize enough that being critical of a research study in no way implies disdain. Clinical research is incredibly challenging, and all research endeavors teach us important lessons. Some studies may permit stronger (more reliable) inferences than others, but studies are never "invalid." Researchers and consumers of research must always be critical, but should not fall prey to skepticism. We will also refer to a hypothetical randomized controlled clinical trial throughout this chapter in an attempt to render theories more concrete. The topic of this hypothetical clinical trial will become evident almost immediately in what follows.

> If a clinical trial is poorly designed, the likelihood of that study providing useful information is low, and the researcher's contract with his or her funding agencies, institution, and patients is betrayed.

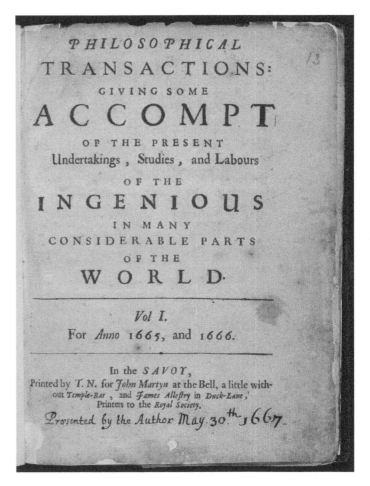

Figure 28.1 Frontispiece to volume 1 of *Philosophical Transactions*, the world's first and longest extant scientific journal. Since 1792, the journal has been managed by the Royal Society, and, since 1887, has been published as *Philosophical Transactions A and B* (physical and biological sciences, respectively).

TABLE 28.1 Structure of a PICOT-formatted research question

CHARACTERISTIC	ABBREVIATION	SAMPLE STATEMENT
Population	P	Patients with newly diagnosed glioblastoma who have not experienced a seizure
Intervention	I	Anticonvulsant prophylaxis
Comparator (co-intervention)	C	No anticonvulsant prophylaxis (placebo)
Outcome	O	Frequency of first seizures
Time	T	One year

ASKING THE RIGHT QUESTION

The essential first step in designing a clinical trial is asking a good question. Time is precious for both investigators and readers. Developing a clear, concise, focused, and answerable question directs the literature search, facilitates discussion between investigators, and provides an efficient template for protocol design. We strongly advocate the PICOT question format[3-5] (Table 28.1). Starting with a well-designed PICOT format question increases the likelihood that the ensuing trial will come to a conclusion. Similarly, if a published trial cannot be summarized with a PICOT format question, this constitutes a red flag, and suggests a potentially important flaw in the trial design.[6] At this point let us introduce a hypothetical study which we will return to throughout the chapter. Although much has been written about anticonvulsant prophylaxis in patients with brain tumors,[7-9] a conclusive trial using a new-generation antiepileptic agent remains to be conducted. A PICOT format question for such a study might read something like this: "In patients with newly diagnosed glioblastomas who have not experienced a seizure (P), does the administration of prophylactic anticonvulsant medication (I), compared to placebo (C), reduce the occurrence of first seizures after one year of treatment (O and T)." This format can accommodate a great deal of information. For example, the investigator could

specify (under "P") the age range of eligible patients, or in a different circumstance gender, tumor histology, or antecedent therapies. The specific antiepileptic drug, dose and treatment schedule, and timing of initiation of therapy can be added to "I" and, in studies where an active comparator intervention is being used, to "C." Finally, the outcome (O) and time (T) can be even more specific, and can include details such as how the outcome will be measured or adjudicated and can also include both primary and secondary outcome measures, for example time to first seizure and frequency of seizures interfering with consciousness at the end of 1 year. The PICOT formulation can be adapted to any type of study question (therapeutic, diagnostic, prognostic, or causal association) if the "I" is thought of in broader epidemiologic terms as the exposure and "C" as the comparative exposure. For example, in a study examining the ability of electroencephalography (EEG) at tumor diagnosis to predict subsequent seizures (a prognostic question), "I" might be "epileptiform activity on the pre-treatment EEG" and "C" might be "absence of epileptiform activity on the pre-treatment EEG."

> If there is uncertainty within the community of providers about the optimum approach ("collective uncertainty"), randomization of study participants is ethical.

Once a well-crafted research question has been devised, it should be vetted using a checklist to ensure that the study question is optimum (Table 28.2). One of these checklist items, "equipoise," merits some additional embellishment. For a clinical trial in which patients are randomly assigned to competing treatment arms to be ethically defensible, genuine uncertainty about the relative benefit of the competing treatments must exist. Researchers often struggle over this point.[10,11] Healthcare providers in particular will frequently have a "hunch" about which treatment arm is "best." In fact, outside of the clinical trials setting, providers are routinely called on to make decisions regarding the optimum treatment for a given patient when inadequate information exists. If, however, there is uncertainty within the community of providers about the optimum approach ("collective uncertainty"), randomization

TABLE 28.2 Asking the right research question

	YES	NO	UNCERTAIN
Is the research question presented in clear PICOT format?			
Is the question important?			
Relevant body of research or comprehensive systematic review available?			
Proposal informed by that body of research?			
Is the new treatment compared to an accepted, relevant standard?			
Does genuine uncertainty (equipoise) exist?			
Overall quality?	CIRCLE ONE		
	Good	Fair	Poor

TABLE 28.3 Relationship between study phase and study design options for therapeutic trials

STUDY PHASE	STUDY OUTCOME GOALS	STUDY DESIGN OPTIONS
Phase I	*Practicality* (Safety of the intervention; optimum drug dose; feasibility of patient accrual or data collection strategy; variance in outcome measures; suggestion of activity)	Case report, case series, case-control, prospective or retrospective cohort
Phase II	*Activity* (Is the approach worthy of further study?)	Case report, case series, case-control, prospective or retrospective cohort
Phase III	*Efficacy* (Usually compared to placebo or standard therapy)	Randomized controlled trial
Phase IV	*Confirmation of safety and efficacy* (Documentation of rare, late, or unexpected outcomes, additional data regarding efficacy)	Prospective cohort

of study participants is ethical.[12–15] We return to the issue of randomization shortly.

CONSTRUCTING A GOOD THERAPEUTIC TRIAL

Confusion in the design of therapeutic clinical trials often arises because of competing trial classification systems. On the one hand, studies are often categorized according to "phase," and, on the other, according to study design. These two classification schemes are related, but there is not a one-to-one correspondence (Table 28.3). Regardless of the type of trial, the most critical question an investigator must ask is "How can I be wrong?" The answer is deceptively simple. Investigators designing clinical trials and healthcare providers interpreting the results of published trials can be "wrong" or misled by three forces: bias, confounding, and random error. A detailed discussion of these forces is beyond the scope of this chapter, but an overview is presented in Table 28.4. The goal of this chapter is to provide a framework that allows investigators to recognize potential risks to reliability and avoid them in the design of their clinical trials. We focus on the randomized, controlled trial (phase III study), because, when well-constructed and executed, this study design provides the highest quality of evidence (the most reliable information) upon which to base treatment decisions.[4,16] But the principles discussed apply equally to each of the trial and design types included in Table 28.3 and to all

types of research questions (therapeutic, diagnostic, prognostic, causal association). The critical elements of the optimum randomized controlled trial have been worked out over decades and are meticulously expressed in the CONSORT publication and diagrams.[17] Table 28.5 provides a condensed and perhaps more approachable checklist. Each of the eight items on this condensed list merits additional discussion. Corresponding documents have been produced for the other therapeutic study designs (cohort, case-control, etc.) and for studies asking other types of questions (diagnostic, prognostic, causal association, meta-analysis) and are summarized in Table 28.6.[18,19]

> Investigators designing clinical trials and healthcare providers interpreting the results of published trials can be "wrong" or misled by three forces: bias, confounding, and random error.

RANDOMIZATION

Randomization is the quintessential component of an optimally designed study assessing treatment efficacy. Assigning study participants to treatment arms according to the play of chance constitutes the best strategy for achieving equal distribution of prognostically important features between those treatment arms and avoiding selection bias (Figure 28.2).[20] Moreover, randomization, if it is performed well and if it is not thwarted by chance, constitutes the *only* known strategy for achieving equal

TABLE 28.4 Answering the question: How can I be wrong?

THREAT TO RELIABILITY	DESCRIPTION	CAUSE	PRIMARILY CONTROLLED BY
Random error (the effect of chance)	May distort the study result in either direction (in favor of the intervention or the control)	Unrepresentative sampling	Increasing the sample size
Systematic error (bias)	Distorts the study result away from the truth (either too high or too low; toward or away from the intervention of interest) but in a consistent direction. Examples include selection bias and misclassification bias	Flaws in study design or execution	Improved study design
Confounding ("mixing of effects")	A confounder is a factor associated with both the "exposure" and the "outcome" (but not on the direct causal pathway between the two). Confounders distort the true relationship between exposure and outcome, leading to a false apparent association, or the loss of a true association	Flaws in study design or execution	Improved study design or post hoc analysis (e.g., multivariate analysis)

TABLE 28.5 Constructing a good therapeutic trial

	YES	NO	UNCERTAIN	N/A
Primary outcome clearly stated and clinically important?				
Proper sample size/power analysis?				
Are patients randomized?				
Is the randomization concealed?				
Are the treatment arms similar at baseline?				
Masked intervention and outcome assessment?				
Aside from the intervention, are all patients treated equally?				
Are all patients accounted for?				
Intention to treat analysis used?				
Are benefits *and* harms reported?				
Overall strength?	Circle One			
	Good	Fair	Poor	

distribution of both known and unknown prognostic factors.[20,21] If equal distribution of risk factors is not achieved, a difference in outcome at the conclusion of a trial may not be a consequence of treatment assignment, but might rather be the result of an imbalance in a good or bad prognostic feature between treatment arms ("confounders"). And while study design strategies (e.g., matching or stratification) and statistical techniques (e.g., multivariate regression analysis or propensity score matching) can sometimes mitigate imbalances in *known* confounders of outcome, there is no other mathematical or design strategy for remediating the effect of *unknown* confounders.

> Randomization, if it is performed well and if it is not thwarted by chance, constitutes the *only* known strategy for achieving equal distribution of both known and unknown prognostic factors.

ALLOCATION CONCEALMENT

To be effective, the strategy for randomizing study participants must remain hidden from study participants and, most importantly, must remain hidden from the investigators who are responsible for enrolling those participants, a feature called *allocation concealment.*[22-24] The reason for this harkens back to our discussion about equipoise. Investigators often form opinions about which treatment approach in a multiarm trial is best suited to individual patients. As a result, either intentionally or unintentionally, investigators may steer patients toward or away from enrollment if they are aware of what treatment arm a given study candidate will be assigned to. Lack of allocation concealment has been estimated to distort the results of studies (almost always in favor of the novel intervention) by as much as 40%—a greater diversion from the truth than even

TABLE 28.6 Guidelines for constructing and evaluating the spectrum of study questions and study designs

STUDY QUESTION/DESIGN	GUIDELINE	WEBSITE ACCESS ADDRESS
Therapeutic studies		
RCT	CONSORT	http://www.consort-statement.org/
Observational	STROBE	http://www.strobe-statement.org/
Case report	CARE	https://www.equator-network.org/reporting-guidelines/care/
N-of-1	CENT	https://www.equator-network.org/reporting-guidelines/consort-cent/
Diagnostic and prognostic studies	STARD	http://www.stard-statement.org/
Quality improvement studies	SQUIRE	https://www.equator-network.org/reporting-guidelines/squire/
Economic evaluations	CHEERS	https://www.equator-network.org/reporting-guidelines/cheers/
Meta-analysis	PRISMA	http://www.prisma-statement.org

RANDOMIZATION

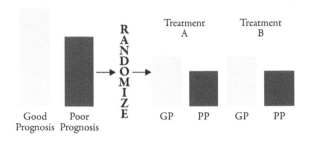

Figure 28.2 Distribution of prognostically important characteristics by randomization.
Abbreviations: GP, good prognostic characteristic; PP, poor prognostic characteristic.

a complete absence of randomization produces.[21,24] To return to our proposed study of anticonvulsant prophylaxis, if an investigator is aware of how the next participant will be randomized (e.g., if patients are alternately assigned to prophylaxis or placebo) and that investigator believes that the potential study participant is at high risk of having a seizure (because, for example, of the location of the tumor, the presence of tumor-associated hemorrhage, or persistent hyponatremia) that investigator might only enroll this patient if "prophylaxis" was the next treatment assignment. This problem often plagues surgical randomized controlled trials, and the lack of allocation concealment converts an otherwise well-designed randomized controlled trial into a poor-quality cohort study.

> Lack of allocation concealment has been estimated to distort the results of studies (almost always in favor of the novel intervention) by as much as 40%.

This problem likely accounts for the apparent efficacy, in non-randomized cohort studies, of warfarin for secondary prevention of major vascular events in patients with strokes related to intracranial arterial stenosis[25]—a finding that was clearly refuted in a subsequent randomized controlled trial.[26] Similarly, the failure of anticonvulsant therapy to reduce the risk of second seizures in patients with first unprovoked seizures in non-randomized cohort trials[27–31] was convincingly refuted once well-designed randomized controlled trials addressing this issue were conducted.[32,33] In both cases, the physicians responsible for making treatment decisions likely steered patients toward the treatment they felt was best suited to their patients. In the stroke example, older patients with poorly controlled hypertension (both important risk factors for subsequent strokes) were steered toward aspirin rather than warfarin because of the perceived increased risk of warfarin-associated bleeding. In the seizure example, patients who were believed by their physicians to be at greatest risk for subsequent seizures were steered toward anticonvulsant therapy rather than observation.

MASKED ASSESSMENT

Masked assessment of outcomes (sometimes referred to as "blinding") is the third crucial feature of a well-designed trial. Intentional falsification of study results appears, thankfully, to be rare.[34–36] However, the implicit expectations of investigators and study participants with respect to the outcomes from different treatment arms exert a profound effect on the assessment of those outcomes and can lead to *outcome assessment bias* (a type of misclassification bias).[37–39] For this reason, patients and investigators responsible for making outcome determinations must not know which treatment a study participant received.

> The implicit expectations of investigators and study participants with respect to the outcomes from different treatment arms exert a profound effect on the assessment of those outcomes and can lead to *outcome assessment bias*.

A remarkable demonstration of the potential for lack of blinding to inadvertently corrupt the results of a trial is illustrated in Figure 28.3.[40] In this randomized controlled trial, patients with progressive multiple sclerosis were assigned to one of three treatment arms: intravenous cyclophosphamide (group I), weekly plasma exchange plus

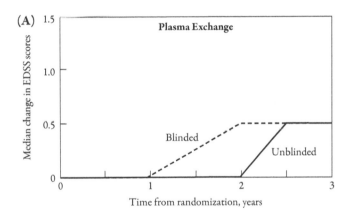

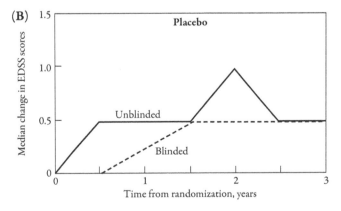

Figure 28.3 The median change in Expanded Disability Status Scale (EDSS) scores after randomization to either an active (A; plasma exchange, group II) or control (B; placebo, group III) treatment limb as recorded by the blinded, or evaluating and unblinded, treating neurologists. An increase in EDSS indicates clinical worsening.

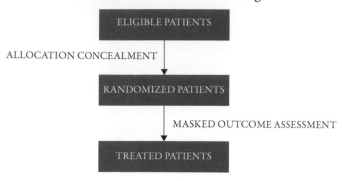

Allocation Concealment vs. Blinding

ELIGIBLE PATIENTS

ALLOCATION CONCEALMENT

RANDOMIZED PATIENTS

MASKED OUTCOME ASSESSMENT

TREATED PATIENTS

Figure 28.4 Timing of the protective effects of allocation concealment and masked outcome assessment in therapeutic trials.

oral cyclophosphamide (group II), or sham plasma exchange and placebo medication (group III). Change in the Expanded Disability Status Scale (EDSS) was the primary study endpoint (an increased score indicates worsening condition), and all patients were evaluated separately by masked and unmasked neurologists at designated study time points. When assessing patients receiving plasma exchange, a worsening EDSS score was reported 5 months later by unmasked compared to masked outcome assessors. In contrast, in the sham plasma exchange group, deterioration was identified a full year earlier in the unmasked compared to the masked assessments. These differences resulted in statistically significant 6-, 12-, and 24-month advantages of plasma exchange compared to sham exchange in the unmasked assessment study but no such differences in the parallel masked assessment study conducted on the same patients. Together with allocation concealment, masked assessment protects the integrity of randomization from the time of study entry until final outcome assessment (Figure 28.4). Two additional points about masked assessment figure prominently in decisions regarding study design. First, not all endpoints are equally susceptible to corruption by unmasked assessment. Some completely objective (e.g., blood test results) or relatively objective outcome measures (e.g., survival) are independent or at least less dependent on the imposition of masked assessment, while more subjective outcome measures (clinical deterioration or radiographic progression) are exquisitely dependent. Second, when masked assessment is impossible to build into a trial (uncommon in "medical" studies, but more frequent in surgical studies), an unmasked non-treater study investigator (who, presumably, feels less of a stake in the outcome of the trial) is likely to provide a more reliable outcome assessment than an unmasked treating investigator and should be designated as the arbiter of trial outcomes. A more labor-intensive version of this strategy, increasingly employed in large, multicenter trials (often those intended to lead to drug approval by the US Food and Drug Administration [FDA]) involves the use of independent central review committees to arbitrate pathologic diagnosis, as well as radiographic, neurocognitive, and clinical response.[41]

BASELINE PATIENT CHARACTERISTICS AND TREATMENT

As discussed earlier, the value of randomization lies in its ability to help ensure that patients in competing treatment arms have similar characteristics, especially with respect to features of potential prognostic importance. Unfortunately, randomization sometimes fails to provide well-balanced treatment arms simply because of chance. This unfortunate outcome is more common when the number of patients in the study is small (one of several reasons why small trials tend to exaggerate the reported effect of investigational interventions compared to large trials).[42] For this reason, similarity of baseline characteristics between treatment arms (typically presented in table 1 of most manuscripts) should always be assessed by consumers of clinical trial data. In this context, p-values have limited value. P-values only evaluate whether observed differences are due to chance. In randomized controlled trials, any differences between treatment groups *must* have arisen by chance (unless the randomization process was corrupted). In cohort and case-control studies, differences are likely to indicate underlying bias resulting from flaws in study design. In either instance, however, the critical question is not why the differences arose, but whether their magnitude is clinically important. P-values are entirely mute on this point.

> Similarity of baseline characteristics between treatment arms should always be assessed by consumers of clinical trial data. However, the critical question is not why the differences arose, but whether their magnitude is clinically important.

Analogous to similarity in baseline characteristics, patients assigned to different treatment arms should be managed identically except for the intervention being investigated. The frequency, content, and reporting of assessments (including laboratory tests, radiographic studies, and clinical evaluations) should be identical. If, for example, patients in one treatment arm are seen more frequently, they may appear to have reached an endpoint sooner simply by virtue of their more frequent assessments. Conversely, more frequent medical attention may forestall an undesirable outcome compared to patients in the less closely monitored treatment arm. If patients assigned to the active treatment arm of a placebo-controlled trial require frequent drug dose adjustments or laboratory studies, similar dose modifications and tests should be imposed on patients in the placebo arm, or masked assessment may be compromised.

INCLUSION AND EXCLUSION CRITERIA

Integral to the composition of treatment arms is the *a priori* establishment of detailed inclusion and exclusion criteria. These criteria must be established prior to the start of study enrollment in order to avoid *selection bias* during the recruitment phase of the trial, and they must be detailed and specific enough to ensure that patients are not found to be ineligible for study participation after they are enrolled, an outcome similar in its analytic implications to "loss to follow-up" (discussed later).[43,44] There is an important tension that investigators must navigate when establishing inclusion and exclusion criteria. The ability to demonstrate a difference between treatment arms (the aspiration of an interventional trial) is enhanced by selecting a more homogenous study cohort. At the same time, the more homogenous the study group, the less broadly applicable the study results may be to patients outside of the study setting (in other words, generalizability is reduced). The frequent underrepresentation of racial and ethnic minorities, medically underserved and economically disadvantaged populations, and children in clinical trials represents a society-level example of this problem. There is no formula which balances these competing interests, but investigators must be aware of the consequences of their decisions regarding study eligibility.[45]

ACCOUNTING FOR PATIENTS IN THE STUDY

This important feature of well-conducted clinical trials has two components. First, are all patients enrolled onto the trial followed until they reach a study outcome? Second, do patients receive the treatment to which they are assigned? When patients are enrolled and are then lost to follow-up, we cannot be certain (in fact, the assumption seems unlikely) that the loss to follow-up was random. Instead, patients in one treatment arm may drop out of the study more frequently than patients in a competing arm—for example, because of an untoward side effect or because of rapid disease progression. Conversely, patients in one treatment arm may enjoy a remarkable response and no longer feel compelled to maintain contact with the study investigators. If patients are lost to follow-up randomly, the ability of the study to demonstrate a difference between treatment arms (if a difference exists) will be reduced (a type II error). If patients are lost to follow-up non-randomly, and the patients remaining in the study are systematically different from those who dropped out, the resulting bias may distort the study result sufficiently to suggest a false association between one of the treatment arms and the study outcome (a type I error). Although numerous statistical techniques have been proposed for mitigating the consequences of loss to follow-up,[46] none is equivalent to taking aggressive measures to insure complete follow-up.[46-48] Since some loss to follow-up is sometimes unavoidable, investigators routinely increase projected enrollment onto their trials, typically by 10%. This precaution may help ameliorate the risk of at type II error; however, if loss to follow-up exceeds 20%, the study results must be questioned.[47,48] Similarly, if patients assigned to a given treatment arm fail to receive that treatment or "cross over" and receive the treatment from a competing treatment arm, the results of the study can be corrupted. Randomization only protects entire study populations. If patients (or their providers) are permitted to select their treatment arm following randomization, this practice converts a randomized controlled trial into a flawed cohort study of minimal reliability.

INTENTION TO TREAT ANALYSIS

Intention to treat means that patients are analyzed according to the treatment arm to which they are initially assigned, irrespective of whether they actually received that assigned treatment or even if they received treatment according to a competing treatment arm.

While investigators cannot control the willingness of study participants to remain in their assigned treatment arm, they can address this problem in the design of their study by insisting on an "intention to treat" model for the primary analysis of study data. *Intention to treat* means that patients are analyzed according to the treatment arm to which they are initially assigned, irrespective of whether they actually received that assigned treatment or even if they received treatment according to a competing treatment arm. This requirement often unsettles clinical researchers who naturally feel that an intervention isn't being given a "fair chance" if patients who never actually received the intervention must be analyzed along with those who did receive the treatment. As a consequence, investigators (and the editors of leading journals) routinely ignore the intention to treat mandate and potentially distort the results of their trials.[49-54]

Another example serves to illustrate the necessity of intention to treat analyses (Table 28.7A,B).[55] In this large study, 3,892 patients who had experienced a myocardial infarction were randomized to receive clofibrate or placebo. Overall, the clofibrate group experienced a small (20.0% vs. 20.9%) but statistically insignificant reduction in 5-year mortality (the primary study endpoint) when compared to the placebo group. Remarkably, however, when the treatment arms are examined according to adherence to the assigned treatment (a non-intention to treat analysis that study authors often disguise with terms such as "per protocol," "effective treatment," or "adequately treated" groups), the results are very different. The survival advantage for the clofibrate group compared to the placebo group disappears among adherent patients (15.0% vs.

TABLE 28.7 A. Coronary drug project: Five-year mortality by treatment group

TREATMENT GROUP	N	PERCENT MORTALITY
Clofibrate*	1,103	20.0
Placebo	2,789	20.9

*P = 0.55

B. Coronary drug project: Five-year mortality by treatment group and adherence

	CLOFIBRATE		PLACEBO	
ADHERENCE	N	% MORTALITY	N	% MORTALITY
<80%	357	24.6	882	28.2
≥80%	708	15.0	1,813	15.1

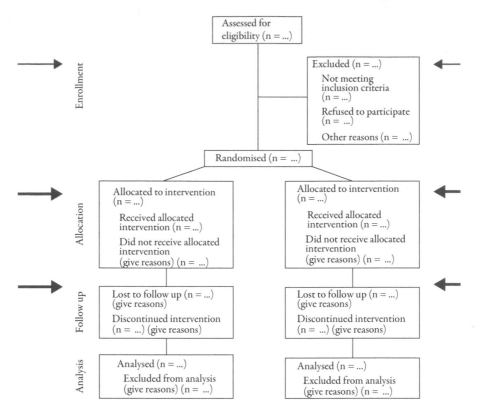

Figure 28.5 CONSORT diagram for tracking patient flow in a randomized controlled trial. Loss of patients prior to randomization (thin arrows) can threaten the generalizability ("external validity") of a trial. Loss of patients following randomization (thick arrows) threatens the reliability of study conclusions ("internal validity").

15.2%), and a dramatic survival advantage emerges between adherent and non-adherent patients irrespective of treatment assignment. While much can be said about these results, including about the "placebo effect,"[56–60] one conclusion is incontestable: patients must be analyzed according to the arm to which they were assigned in order to preserve the integrity of the trial.

The CONSORT collaborators have provided a superb flow diagram to track and summarize the disposition of patients participating in clinical trials (Figure 28.5).[17] Completion of this diagram is required for publication in high-impact journals and is essential for investigators to consider while designing their trial. The CONSORT flow diagram also highlights an important distinction between the impact of potentially eligible study participants who are evaluated for study participation but are not ultimately randomized (pre-randomization loss to follow-up) and participants who are randomized onto the trial but are then lost to follow-up or cross over to an alternative treatment (post-randomization loss to follow-up). Patients in the first category affect the generalizability ("external validity") of the study. Fortunately, study consumers can easily evaluate this concern by examining the inclusion and exclusion criteria of the study and the characteristics of the patients who were enrolled and by comparing those characteristics to the characteristics of the patient to whom one wishes to apply the study result. In contrast, patients who are lost from the study after randomization will affect the reliability ("internal validity") of

the study. If this loss is random, it will make it harder for the study to show a difference if a difference really exists (a type II error). More ominously, if the patient loss is not random (and often readers cannot discern this), it will distort the truth (potentially leading to a type I error).

PRIMARY AND SECONDARY OUTCOMES

An important feature of any clinical trial protocol is the *a priori* statement of a primary outcome. While any number of secondary outcomes can also be specified, these must be considered hypothesis-generating and are never definitive. By specifying a primary outcome, the investigator assures us that the study was intended to answer a specific question and that the analysis provided is the one the study was designed to address. When a specific primary outcome is not defined or a long list of results is presented, one cannot be certain that the investigators have not selected for presentation those outcomes which are most impressive or which support the investigators' preconceived ideas, or that the planned statistical analysis has not been modified to obtain a desired result. This kind of biased reporting appears to be quite common.[61–66] In addition, when multiple outcomes are analyzed, the risk of a type I error (detecting a difference when one doesn't really exist) increases.[67] When more than one primary outcome is identified *a priori*, there are specific statistical techniques that can reduce the risk of such errors.[68]

SAMPLE SIZE CALCULATIONS

Estimating the number of patients required to achieve a statistically significant study result, together with the actual intervention being compared, constitutes the central hypothesis of a randomized controlled trial. This sample size or "power" calculation is frequently omitted from the statistical section of therapeutic trials[69] and is overlooked by readers even more frequently. Calculating sample size is a straightforward algebraic problem with (in its simplest form) four variables: level of statistical significance (i.e., risk of a type I error, traditionally set at 0.05), power (i.e., risk of avoiding a type II error, usually 0.80), effect size, and number of patients. If three of these values are known, the fourth is easily derived. Typically investigators focus on patient number as the unknown variable and spend little time considering the other three assumptions. In the worst case, these other three variables (especially the effect size) are manipulated to produce a sample size estimate that is commensurate with available resources (eligible patients, funding, feasible study duration, etc.). Investigators particularly tend to ignore the effect size assumption. This constitutes a fatal flaw in study design because the effect size estimate represents the investigators' judgment of what a clinically meaningful study outcome would be. Consider this example. An investigator has discovered an antineoplastic agent with a novel mechanism of action, impressive efficacy against glioblastoma in non-human trials, and acceptable safety in early human studies. Based on these results, the investigator proposes a randomized trial to demonstrate the superiority of the new drug compared to the standard treatment regimen for patients with glioblastomas at first recurrence. The pre-specified primary outcome measure is the percentage of patients who are alive and free of recurrent disease at 6 months. Based on previous studies,[70] the investigator estimates that 9% of patients will fulfill these requirements. To justify the toxicity, inconvenience, and increased expense of the new agent, the investigator determines that the new agent would have to increase the frequency of good 6-month outcomes from 9% to 25%. Using 0.05 as the level of significance and 80% as the power, the investigator estimates that 161 patients in each treatment arm would be required. The study is conducted and finds that the novel agent is superior to conventional therapy (p = 0.023). Is this a positive trial? We cannot tell. More information is required. Fortunately, a journal editor requests additional information. It turns out that the novel agent resulted in good outcomes (alive and progression-free at 6 months) in 29 of 161 patients (18%) in the novel treatment arm, compared to 15 good outcomes (9.3%) in the conventional treatment arm (relative risk 1.93, 95% confidence interval 1.08–3.48, number needed to treat 11.5). Now, is this a positive trial? The short answer is "no." The study hypothesis required a 25% response rate for the investigational agent to become the new standard of care. The study failed to achieve that response rate. A more nuanced interpretation is possible. Perhaps the threshold of a 25% response rate was too high. Maybe 18% is sufficient. Perhaps for individual patients the new drug

would be preferable even if the response rate were less than 25%. Additional studies may be appropriate. But retrospectively interpreting a statistically significant result as proof of a positive study when the difference in outcomes is less than what was pre-specified as clinically meaningful is unjustified can lead to incorrect and potentially dangerous treatment decisions[69,71] and emphasizes the importance of meticulously considering every assumption of the sample size calculation during the design phase of a clinical trial. An *a priori* sample size calculation also helps to protect studies from two additional kinds of erroneous conclusion. If the sample size is too small, the demonstration of a clinically meaningful effect may constitute a type I error. In the most extreme example, consider a study with two participants. One participant receives the investigational intervention and does well, while the other participant is assigned to the control treatment arm and does poorly. The conclusion that the novel treatment is 100% effective is clearly suspect. Conversely, the failure to demonstrate a clinically meaningful difference between two treatment arms in an underpowered trial may simply reflect a type II error. In both instances, looking at the confidence interval associated with the estimate of treatment effect will disclose this study design flaw.

REPORTING BENEFITS AND HARMS

The focus of therapeutic trials is, naturally, on the primary outcome of the intervention being studied. But the ultimate value of that intervention cannot be fully assessed without considering both its benefits and associated harms. Harms associated with an intervention are notoriously underreported in papers describing the results of clinical trials, and, when data are provided, it is often incomplete and unreliable.[72-74] Details regarding the collection and analysis of harms must be incorporated into the design of therapeutic trials with as much rigor as the collection and analysis of benefits. The types of adverse outcomes, how and with what frequency they will be assessed, how they will be analyzed, and, if appropriate, when the trial should be suspended because of unexpected or unexpectedly frequent toxicity should all be pre-specified in the study protocol.

INTERPRETING THE RESULTS OF A THERAPEUTIC TRIAL

Evaluating the evidence presented in the report of a therapeutic trial comes after the trial is completed, but we have included this final rubric (Table 28.8) because investigators need to be mindful of how their results will be interpreted. The essential questions that must be answered in the affirmative if a clinical trial is to be considered "successful" are not whether the outcome was "positive" or "negative" or whether the results corroborated or refuted a preexisting belief, but rather whether the conclusions of the study are reliable, whether they are relevant to patient populations outside of the study setting, and whether they are sufficiently persuasive to change or fortify existing practice. While a

TABLE 28.8 Interpreting the results of a therapeutic trial

	YES	NO	UNCERTAIN
Is the statistical analysis appropriate and adequately described?			
What are the results?			
Are the results complete?			
Are measures of effect size, precision (confidence intervals), and the role of chance provided?			
Are the primary endpoints reported, and are they clinically meaningful?			
Are the treatment arms appropriate?			
Are the inclusion and exclusion criteria relevant?			
Are study patients similar to my patients?			
Overall relevance to my patient population (is this study useful and will it change my practice)?	CIRCLE ONE		
	High	Medium	Low

detailed discussion of the relative merits of different analytic techniques is beyond the scope of this chapter, and while considerable latitude is afforded to investigators as long as they are transparent in their calculations, general guidelines have been suggested.[71,75] The three, only slightly tongue-in-cheek, rules of thumb that we apply when analyzing the statistical techniques used in or proposed for a clinical trial are: (1) were the techniques selected *a priori* (the identical requirement applied to patient eligibility criteria and the primary outcome measure); (2) are those techniques described with sufficient clarity to allow intelligent non-statisticians to understand the techniques, the reasons they were selected, and their appropriateness; and (3) is the paragraph describing the statistical techniques shorter than the paragraph describing the primary outcome result?

CONFLICT OF INTEREST

Not surprisingly, authors who play key roles in the conception, design, analysis, interpretation, and reporting of clinical trials commonly have financial ties to the industrial sponsors of the drugs, devices, or tests those trials investigate.[76,77] Such ties pose a risk of bias at each step in the clinical trials process, from study design to reporting.[41,49,78] Like all forms of bias (and unlike random error), conflict of interest is not precisely quantifiable. For this reason we talk about the "risk of bias" rather than bias itself. The risk of conflict of interest is primarily related to two variables: the potential for an investigator to benefit from the outcome of the research and the ability of the investigator to influence that outcome through patient selection, treatment assignment, outcome assessment, data analysis, or presentation of results. This is the rationale for requiring complete disclosure of the nature and extent of investigator–sponsor relationships and the role each investigator has played

in the study.[79] When the potential for conflict of interest is made explicit, "consumers" of clinical trials can recalibrate their estimate of the persuasiveness of a research finding in a way exactly analogous to how those consumers would evaluate inadequate allocation concealment, unmasked outcome assessment, or any other threat to reliability. Professional societies and journal editors have provided specific guidance for disclosure to investigators.[80] When even the *potential* for conflict of interest exists, investigators should solicit outside guidance from an institutional review board or hospital ethics committee beginning at the design phase of the trial in order to mitigate this risk.

> The risk of conflict of interest is primarily related to two variables: the potential for an investigator to benefit from the outcome of the research and the ability of the investigator to influence that outcome through patient selection, treatment assignment, outcome assessment, data analysis, or presentation of results.

CONCLUSION

Innovative clinical trials have always been, and remain, the generators of improved patient care and the source of novel insights. The tenets of clinical trial design outlined in this chapter are intended to serve as an infrastructure but are not intended to supersede investigator experience and judgment or patient values. "Evidence-based" practice does not mean "evidence-only" practice. We hope that a new generation of clinician-scientists will master this challenging integration of clinical wisdom and evidence-based principles and will once again transform lead into gold.

The essential foundation of all research studies is a well-formulated research question. What are its five components?

Population

Intervention

Comparator

Outcome

Timing

What three key factors can distort the results of a clinical trial and lead to inaccurate conclusions?

Bias, confounding, and random error

When well-designed and executed, what type of clinical trial provides the highest quality of evidence to answer a clinical (or laboratory) question?

A randomized, double-blinded phase III clinical trial

What is the key strength of randomization, and what is its limitation?

Randomization is the only strategy that can equally distribute both known and *unknown* prognostic factors between treatment arms in a study. However, even a well-executed randomization procedure can be subverted by random error, especially if patient numbers are small

What is a key limitation of both design strategies such as stratification, case-control methodology, and propensity score matching, and analytic strategies such as multivariable analysis?

They can only help mitigate imbalances in *known* confounders

What is the function of allocation concealment?

Allocation concealment helps to reduce selection bias during patient enrollment resulting from investigator bias (whether recognized or unrecognized) in favor of one treatment arm over another. Allocation concealment operates *prior* to randomization

What is the function of blinding (e.g., masked assessment of outcome)?

To prevent outcome assessment bias, a type of misclassification bias. This strategy protects the integrity of the trial *after* randomization has occurred

What types of outcomes are less subject to outcome assessment bias even in the absence of masked outcome assessment?

Objective outcomes (e.g., survival)

How should evaluation of potential baseline differences in characteristics between treatment arms (table 1 in most manuscripts) be done in a properly conducted randomized trial?	One should assess whether any differences present between the arms are *clinically important*; use of p-values to evaluate differences is not appropriate
Why must eligibility criteria be established prior to the start of study enrollment?	To avoid selection bias
What two important mandates must be balanced when choosing eligibility criteria for a study?	The desire to detect a difference between treatment groups, which is enhanced by homogeneous treatment arms ("internal validity"), and the imperative for broad applicability to patients outside of the current study setting (generalizability or "external validity")
What is the essential question when evaluating a clinical trial?	Whether the study results are reliable and inferences based on those results are strong or weak. Trials themselves are never "valid" or "invalid"
In addition to collection and analysis of benefits, what else must be rigorously incorporated prospectively into the design of a therapeutic trial?	Details regarding the collection and analysis of harms
When assessing estimates of treatment effect, what provides more information than p-values and why?	Evaluation of confidence intervals, as doing so can help identify flaws in study design and interpretation
How should secondary study outcomes be considered?	As question-generating, not question-answering

QUESTIONS

1. The following table lists the three key threats to study reliability. Please complete the table by adding the causes of these three threats and how each can be mitigated.

THREAT TO RELIABILITY	CAUSE	PRIMARY STRATEGY FOR CONTROL
Random error (Effect of chance)		
Effect of bias (Systematic error)		
Confounding (Mixing of effects—a specific type of bias)		

2. A prospective cohort trial assessed the contribution of mobile phone use to the development of gliomas. The 5-year relative risk for the heaviest mobile phone users (cumulative lifetime duration of calls ≥896 hours) compared to participants who were not regular mobile phone users was 1.4. The 95% confidence interval was 1.02–1.85. Which p-value is most consistent with these results?
   a. 0.03
   b. 0.06
   c. 0.09
   d. 0.11
   e. 0.25

3. The three primary determinants of sample size in a clinical trial are the anticipated effect of the intervention, the required level of statistical significance (i.e., the acceptable type 1 error rate, often designated as "α"), and the desired power (i.e., 1: the type II error rate, often designated as 1-β). In the table, draw the appropriated directed arrow (up or down) to describe the effect on sample size resulting from the suggested changes in these three variables.

CHANGE IN STUDY DESIGN CHARACTERISTIC	RESULTING CHANGE IN SAMPLE SIZE (INCREASE = ↑; DECREASE = ↓)
A decrease in the anticipated improvement in response rate due to a novel intervention from 35% to 25%	
A decrease in the desired Type I error rate (α) from 0.05 to 0.01	
An increase in the power (1-β) of the study from 80% to 90%	

4. The figure depicts the results (relative risk, confidence interval, and associated p-value) for five hypothetical randomized controlled trials. The shaded background indicates the range of relative risks which are clinically important (white), marginal (light blue) The light blue shading is not visible in the figure, and unimportant (darker blue). Please complete the following table,

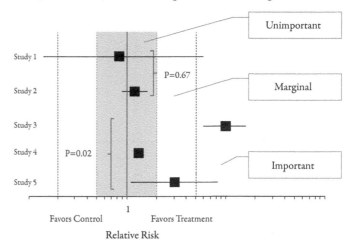

including your assessment of the statistical significance and the clinical importance of the results of each study based on the figure.

SCENARIO	STATISTICAL SIGNIFICANCE	CLINICAL IMPORTANCE	DISCUSSION
Study 1			
Study 2			
Study 3			
Study 4			
Study 5			

ANSWERS

1.

Threat to reliability	Cause	Primary strategy for control
Random error (Effect of chance)	Unrepresentative sampling	Adequate numbers of patients
Effect of bias (Systematic error)	Flaws in study design or execution	Improving study design and execution
Confounding (Mixing of effects—a specific type of bias)	Flaws in study design or execution	Improving study design and execution, or post-hoc statistical adjustment (multivariable analysis)

2. a

3.

Change in study design characteristic	Resulting change in sample size (increase = ↑, heredecrease = ↓)
A decrease in the anticipated improvement in response rate due to a novel intervention from 35% to 25%	↑
A decrease in the desired type I error rate (α) from 0.05 to 0.01	↑
An increase in the power (1-β) of the study from 80% to 90%	↑

4.

Scenario	Statistical significance	Clinical importance	Discussion
Study 1	No	Can't tell	The intervention may be great or it may be terrible. The effect size estimate is too imprecise (i.e., the confidence interval is too wide) to tell. This result provides no guidance.
Study 2	No	No	Even the upper limit of the confidence interval is not clinically important. A definitively "negative" result.
Study 3	Yes	Yes	This study is both clinically and statistically significant. The effect size is large, favors the intervention, and the confidence interval lies entirely within the "important" range. A definitively "positive" result.
Study 4	Yes	No	The effect size falls entirely within the "unimportant" range. Again, a definitively "negative" result.
Study 5	Yes	Can't tell	The confidence interval includes both clinically important and unimportant effects. The effect size estimate is too imprecise to provide any guidance.

REFERENCES

1. Aleklett K, Morrissey DJ, Loveland W, et al. Energy dependence of ^{209}Bi fragmentation in relativistic nuclear collisions. *Physical Rev C.* 1981;23:1045–1046.
2. The Royal Society Publishing. Home page. https://royalsocietypublishing.org/rstl/about
3. Richardson WS, Wilson MC, Nishikawa J, Hayward RS. The well-built clinical question: A key to evidence-based decisions. *Am Coll Physician J Club.* 1995;123:A12-13.
4. Haynes RB. Forming research questions. In Haynes RB, Sacket DL, Guyatt GH, Tugwell P, eds., *Clinical Epidemiology: How to do Clinical Practice Research*, 3rd ed. Philadelphia, PA: Lippincott Williams & Wilkins, 2006:3–14.
5. Abbade LPF, Wang M, Sriganesh K, et al. Framing of research question using the PICOT format in randomized controlled trials of venous ulcer disease: A protocol for a systematic survey of the literature. *BMJ Open.* 2016;6:1–5, e013117.
6. Rios LP, Ye C, Thabane L. Association between framing of the research question using the PICOT format and reporting quality of randomized controlled trials. *BMC Med Res Method.* 2010;10:11–18.
7. Tremont-Lukats IW, Ratilal BO, Armstrong T, Gilbert MR. Antiepileptic drugs for preventing seizures in people with brain tumors. *Cochrane Database Syst Rev.* 2008;16:CD004424. doi:10.1002/14651858.CD004424.pub2.
8. Sirven JI, Wingerchuk DM, Drazkowski JF, et al. Seizure prophylaxis in patients with brain tumors: A meta-analysis. *Mayo Clin Proc.* 2004;79:1489–1494.
9. Glantz MJ, Cole BF, Forsyth PA, et al. Practice parameter: Anticonvulsant prophylaxis in patients with newly diagnosed brain tumors [RETIRED] Report of the Quality Standards Subcommittee of the American Academy of Neurology. *Neurology* 2000;54:1886–1893; doi:10.1212/WNL.54.10.1886
10. Truog RD, Robinson W, Randolph A, Morris A. Is informed consent always necessary for randomized, controlled trials? *N Engl J Med.* 1999;340:804–807.
11. Hellman S, Hellman DS. Of mice but not men: Problems of the randomized clinical trial. *New Engl J Med.* 1991;324:1585–1589.
12. Sim J. Outcome-adaptive randomization in clinical trials: Issues of participant welfare and autonomy. *Theor Med Bioethics.* 2019;40:83–101.
13. Mhaskar R, Bercu BB, Djulbegovic B. At what level of collective equipoise does a randomized clinical trial become ethical for the members of institutional review board/ethical committees? *Acta Inform Med.* 2013;21:156–159.
14. Parsons NR, Kulikov Y, Girling A, Griffin D. A statistical framework for quantifying clinical equipoise for individual cases during randomized controlled surgical trials. *Trials.* 2011;12:258–268.
15. Johnson N, Lilford RJ, Brazier W. At what level of collective equipoise does a clinical trial become ethical? *J Med Ethics.* 1991;17:30–34.
16. Guyatt G, Drummond R, Meade M, Cook D. *The Evidence-Based-Medicine Working Group Users' Guides to the Medical Literature*, 2nd ed. Chicago: McGraw Hill; 2008.
17. Schulz KF, Altman DG, Moher D. CONSORT 2010 statement: Updated guidelines for reporting parallel group randomized trials. *BMJ.* 2010;340:c332.
18. Goodman D, Ogrinc G, Davies L, et al. Explanation and elaboration of the SQUIRE (Standards for Quality Improvement Reporting Excellence) guidelines, v.2.0: Examples of SQUIRE elements in the healthcare improvement literature. *BMJ Qual Saf.* 2016;25:e7–e30.
19. Simera I, Moher D, Hirst A, Hoey J, et al. Transparent and accurate reporting increases reliability, utility, and impact of your research: Reporting guidelines and the EQUATOR Network. *BMC Med.* 2010;8:24–29.
20. Altman DG, Bland JM. Treatment allocation in controlled trials: Why randomize? *Br Med J.* 1999;318:1209.
21. Kunz R, Vist GE, Oxman AD. Randomisation to protect against selection bias in healthcare trials. *Cochrane Database Syst Rev.* 2007(2):MR000012. doi:10.1002/14651858.MR000012.pub2.
22. Hewitt C, Hahn S, Torgerson DJ, et al. Adequacy and reporting of allocation concealment: Review of recent trials published in four general medical journals. *Br Med J.* 2005;330:1057–1058.
23. Altman DG, Schulz KF. Concealing treatment allocation in randomized trials. *Br Med J.* 2001;323:446–447.
24. Schulz KF, Chalmers I, Hayes RJ, Altman DG. Empirical evidence of bias: Dimensions of methodological quality associated with estimates of treatment effects in controlled trials. *JAMA.* 1995;273:408–412.
25. Chimowitz MI, Kokkinos J, Strong J, et al. The warfarin-aspirin symptomatic intracranial disease study. *Neurology.* 1995;45:1488–1493.
26. Chimowitz MI, Lynn MJ, Howlett-Smith H, et al. Comparison of warfarin and aspirin for symptomatic intracranial arterial stenosis. *N Engl J Med.* 2005;352:1305–1316.
27. Shinnar S, Berg AT, Moshe SL, et al. Risk of seizure recurrence following a first unprovoked seizure in childhood: A prospective study. *Pediatrics.* 1990;85:1076–1085.
28. Hauser WA, Rich SS, Annegers JF, Anderson VE. Seizure recurrence after a 1st unprovoked seizure: An extended follow-up. *Neurology.* 1990;40:1163–1170.
29. Hopkins A, Garman A, Clarke C. The first seizure in adult life. *Lancet.* 1988;1:721–726.
30. Annegers JF, Shirts SB, Hauser WA, Kurland LT. Risk of recurrence after an initial unprovoked seizure. *Epilepsia.* 1986;27:43–50.
31. Camfield PR, Camfield CS, Dooley JM, et al. Epilepsy after a first unprovoked seizure in childhood. *Neurology.* 1985;35:1657–1660.
32. Marson A, Jacoby A, Johnson A, et al. Immediate versus deferred antiepileptic drug treatment for early epilepsy and single seizures: A randomised controlled trial. *Lancet.* 2005;365:2007–2013.

33. First Seizure Trial Group. Randomized clinical trial on the efficacy of antiepileptic drugs in reducing the risk of relapse after a first unprovoked tonic-clonic seizure. *Neurology.* 1993;43:478–483.

34. Bollard MJ, Avenell A, Gamble, GD, Grey A. Systematic review and statistical analysis of the integrity of 33 randomized controlled trials. *Neurology.* 2016;87:2391–2402.

35. Sakamoto J, Buysse M. Fraud in clinical trials: Complex problem, simple solutions? *Int J Clin Oncol.* 2016;21:13–14.

36. Weiss RB, Vogelzang NJ, Peterson BA, et al. A successful system of scientific data audits for clinical trials. A report from the Cancer and Leukemia Group B. *JAMA.* 1993;270:459–464.

37. Moustgaard H, Clayton GL, Jones HE, et al. Impact of blinding on estimated treatment effects in randomised clinical trials: meta-epidemiological study. *BMJ.* 2020;368:l6802.

38. Hrobjartsson A, Emanuelsson F, Thomsen ASS, et al. Bias due to lack of patient blinding in clinical trials: A systematic review of trials randomizing patients to blind and nonblind sub-studies. *Int J Epidemiol.* 2014;43:1272–1283.

39. Day SJ, Altman DG. Blinding in clinical trials and other studies. *BMJ.* 2000;32:504.

40. Noseworthy JH, Ebers GC, Vandervoort MK, et al. The impact of blinding on the results of a randomized, placebo-controlled multiple sclerosis clinical trial. *Neurology.* 1994;44:16–20.

41. Mehta MP, Shapiro WR, Glantz MJ, et al. Lead-in phase to randomized trial of motexafin gadolinium and whole-brain radiation for patients with brain metastases: Centralized assessment of magnetic resonance imaging, neurocognitive, and neurologic end points. *J Clin Oncol.* 2002;20:3445–3453.

42. Mills EJ, Ayers D, Chou R, Thorlund K. Are current standards of reporting quality for clinical trials sufficient in addressing important sources of bias? *Contemporary Clin Trials.* 2015;45:2–7.

43. Berger VW. Quantifying the magnitude of baseline covariate imbalances resulting from selection bias in randomized clinical trials. *Biom J.* 2005;47:119–127.

44. Berger VW, Exner DV. Detecting selection bias in randomized clinical trials. *Control Clin Trials.* 1999;20:319–327.

45. Lee EQ, Weller M, Sul J, et al. Optimizing eligibility criteria and clinical trial conduct to enhance clinical trial participation for primary brain tumor patients. *Neuro-Oncology.* 2020;22:601–612.

46. Marshall A, Altman DG, Holder RL. Comparison of imputation methods for handling missing covariate data when fitting a Cox proportional hazards model: A resampling study. *BMC Medical Res Methodol.* 2010;10:112.

47. Bell ML, Fiero M, Horton NJ, Hsu C-H. Handling missing data in RCTs; a review of the top medical journals. *BMC Med Res Methodol.* 2014;14:118–125.

48. Wood AM, White IR, Thompson SG. Are missing outcome data adequately handled? A review of published randomized controlled trials in major medical journals. *Clin Trials.* 2004;1:368–376.

49. Abraha I, Cherubini A, Cozzolino F, et al. Deviation from intention to treat analysis in randomized trials and treatment effect estimates: Meta-epidemiological study. *BMJ.* 2015;350:2445–2457.

50. Montedori A, Bonacini MI, Casazza G, et al. Modified versus standard intention-to-treat reporting: Are there differences in methodological quality, sponsorship, and findings in randomized trials? A cross-sectional study. *Trials.* 2011;12:58–66.

51. Abraha I, Montedori A. Modified intention to treat reporting in randomised controlled trials: Systematic review. *Br Med J.* 2010;340:2697–2705.

52. Gravel J, Opatrny L, Shapiro S. The intention-to-treat approach in randomized controlled trials: Are authors saying what they do and doing what they say? *Clin Trials.* 2007;4:350–356.

53. Kruse RL, Alper BS, Reust C, et al. Intention-to-treat analysis: Who is in? Who is out? *J Fam Pract.* 2002;51:969–971.

54. Hollis S, Campbell F. What is meant by intention to treat analysis? Survey of published randomised controlled trials. *Br Med J.* 1999;319:670–674.

55. The Coronary Drug Project Research Group. Influence of adherence to treatment and response of cholesterol on mortality in the coronary drug project. *N Engl J Med.* 1980;303:1038–1041.

56. Munnangi S, Sundjaja JH, Singh K, et al. Placebo Effect. [Updated 2021 Aug 23]. In: StatPearls [Internet]. Treasure Island (FL): StatPearls Publishing; 2021 Jan. Available from: https://www.ncbi.nlm.nih.gov/books/NBK513296/

57. Chen JA, Papakostas GI, Youn SJ, et al. Association between patient beliefs regarding assigned treatment and clinical response: Reanalysis of data from the Hypericum Depression Trial Study Group. *J Clin Psychiatr.* 2011;72:1669–1676.

58. Sinyor M, Levitt AJ, Cheung AH, et al. Does inclusion of a placebo arm influence response to active antidepressant treatment in randomized controlled trials? Results from pooled and meta-analyses. *J Clin Psychiatry.* 2010;71:270–279.

59. Papakostas GI, Fava M. Does the probability of receiving placebo influence clinical trial outcome? A meta-regression of double-blind, randomized clinical trials in MDD. *Eur Neuropsychopharmacol.* 2009;19:34–40.

60. Rosenthal R, Fode KL. The effect of experimenter bias on the performance of the albino rat. *Behavioral Sci.* 1963;8:183–189.

61. Jones CW, Keil LG, Holland WC, et al. Comparison of registered and published outcomes in randomized controlled trials: A systematic review. *BMC Med.* 2015;13:282–293.

62. Dwan K, Altman DG, Clarke M, et al. Evidence for the selective reporting of analyses and discrepancies in clinical trials: A systematic review of cohort studies of clinical trials. *PLos Med.* 2014;11(6):1–22, e1001666. doi:10.1371/journal.pmed.1001666.

63. Page MJ, McKenzie JE, Kirkham J, et al. Bias due to selective inclusion and reporting of outcomes and analyses in systematic reviews of randomised trials of healthcare interventions. *Cochrane Database Syst Rev.* 2014(10):MR000035. doi:10.1002/14651858.MR000035.pub2.

64. Chan AW, Altman DG. Identifying outcome reporting bias in randomized trials on PubMed: Review of publications and survey of authors. *BMJ.* 2005;330:753.

65. Chan AW, Hrobjartsson A, Haahr MT, et al. Empirical evidence for selective reporting of outcomes in randomized trials: Comparison of protocols to published articles. *JAMA.* 2004;291:2457–2465.

66. Chan AW, Krleza-Jeric K, Schmidt I, Altman DG. Outcome reporting bias in randomized trials funded by the Canadian Institutes of Health Research. *Canadian Med Assoc J.* 2004;171:735–740.

67. Austin PC, Mamdani MM, Juurlink DN, Hux JE. Testing multiple statistical hypotheses resulted in spurious associations: A study of astrological signs and health. *J Clin Epidemiol.* 2006;59:964–969.

68. Wang D, Li Y, Wang X, et al. Overview of multiple testing methodology and recent development in clinical trials. *Contemporary Clin Trials.* 2015;45:13–20.

69. Bedard PL, Krzyzanowska MK, Pintilie M, Tannock IF. Statistical power of negative randomized controlled trials presented at American Society for Clinical Oncology annual meetings. *J Clin Oncol.* 2007;25:3482–3487.

70. Ballman KV, Buckner JC, Brown PD, et al. The relationship between six-month progression-free survival and 12-month overall survival end points for phase II trials in patients with glioblastoma multiforme. *Neuro-Oncology.* 2007;9:29–38.

71. Glantz M, Brandmeir N. Editorial. When can we be positive about p values? *J Neurosurg.* 2019;132:656–661.

72. Hodkinson A, Gamble C, Smith CT. Reporting of harms outcomes: A comparison of journal publications with unpublished clinical study reports of orlistat trials. *Trials.* 2016;17:207–217.

73. Chou R, Fu R, Carson S, et al. Methodological shortcomings predicted lower harm estimates in one of two sets of studies of clinical interventions. *J Clin Epidemiol.* 2007;60:18–28.

74. Ioannidis JPA, Chew P, Lau J. Standardized retrieval of side effects for meta-analysis of safety outcomes. A feasibility study in acute sinusitis. *J Clin Epidemiol.* 2002;55:619–626.

75. Gamble C, Krishan A, Stocken D, et al. Guidelines for the content of statistical analysis plans in clinical trials. *JAMA.* 2017;318:2337–2343.

76. Roseman M, Milette K, Bero LA, et al. Reporting of conflicts of interest in meta-analyses of trials of pharmacologic treatments. *JAMA.* 2011;305:1008–1017.

77. Rose SI, Krzyzanowska MK, Joffe S. Relationships between authorship contributions and authors' industry financial ties among oncology clinical trials. *J Clin Oncol.* 2010;28:1316–1321.

78. Johnson DH, Horn L. Authorship and industry financial relationships: The tie that binds. *J Clin Oncol.* 2010;28:1281–1283.

79. Garattini L, Padula A. Conflict of interest disclosure: Striking a balance? *Eur J Health Economics.* 2019;20:633–636.

80. Fontanarosa P, Bauchner H. Conflict of interest and Medical Journals. *JAMA.* 2017;17:1768–1771.

29 | PROCEDURES AND WELL-CARE CLINICS IN NEURO-ONCOLOGY

Roles for Advanced Practice Providers

ERIKA N. LEESE, ALYSSA CALLELA, AND NA TOSHA N. GATSON

INTRODUCTION

The term "advanced practice provider" (APP) most commonly includes two provider types: physician assistants (PAs) and nurse practitioners (NPs). APPs are also referred to as advance practitioners (APs), non-physician providers (NPPs), and, less commonly as physician extenders (PEs). While there are important differences between PAs and NPs related to autonomy, supervision, and legal consenting, for example, many of these practice points are state- or institution-specific. NPs receive formal training as registered nurses then add advanced-level degrees, such as a master's or doctoral degree in nursing. PAs typically complete a master's degree from an accredited institution (2 years postgraduate training after completion of a 4-year degree).[1] PAs and NPs can generally work up to the level of their supervising physician's license, with some limitations that vary from state to state.

WELL-CARE AND PROCEDURAL CLINICS IN NEURO-ONCOLOGY

WELL-CARE CLINICS

APPs add value to all subspecialties of medicine, especially neuro-oncology. Well-care clinics and procedural clinics are two such approaches to added-value. Well-care clinics are intended to offer access for routine care and surveillance of patients on active therapy or surveillance. These clinics can also provide opportunities for the patients or their caregivers to educate themselves on the diagnosis and treatment plan, identify concerns, or discuss ongoing symptoms. These clinics are not designed to care for emergent issues. Many cancer neurology issues can be addressed in the well-care clinic setting. *Cancer neurology* pertains to the diagnosis and/or treatment of neurological signs/symptoms that are secondary to cancer or cancer therapies. These conditions commonly include peripheral neuropathy; headache; seizures; stroke; weakness; tremors and other movement issues; some pain syndromes; cancer-related fatigue; changes in cognition, gait/balance, vision, hearing or sleep; some infections, and thromboembolic complications as well as side effects associated with treatments used in cancer care (chemotherapy, immunotherapy, device-based therapies).

> *Cancer neurology* pertains to the diagnosis and/or treatment of neurological signs/symptoms that are secondary to cancer or cancer therapies.

These visits often require some escalation of care, with further diagnostic testing or examination or subspecialty referrals. Subspecialty referrals commonly include palliative medicine, physical medicine and rehabilitation, cognitive or neuropsychiatry, and hospice care. However, there are instances where patients are referred for other chronic medical issues such as endocrine, cardiologic, nephrological, or dermatologic. Occasionally, an acute assessment in the emergency room or urgent care clinic is needed, and patients can be directly referred from the well-care clinic. De-escalation of therapy is sometimes warranted in patients who are identified as having issues related to polypharmacy or with cumulative neurological effects of systemic chemotherapy.

Often the well-care visit and the procedural clinics run simultaneously and can be billed concurrently with specific billing modifiers to account for the increased level of care. During these outpatient visits, APPs conduct comprehensive history and physical examinations to assess for improvement in neurological deficits or evaluate for new deficits. There is also an opportunity for the APP to uncover a variety of different medical conditions, which are outlined in Table 29.2. Well-trained APPs can identify non-neurological medical concerns in cancer patients, such as difficulties with breathing and extremity swelling, which could be signs of pulmonary embolism or deep vein thrombosis, respectively. Understanding that hypercoagulable states are common in cancer patients, along with risk for stroke, mood changes, and a host of other conditions, makes these well-care visits so valuable to our neuro-oncology practices.

APP-run well-care clinics serve an important role in care of neuro-oncology patients. Many non-urgent and semi-urgent conditions can be managed in these clinics, thus preventing unnecessary, costly, and stressful ER evaluations. Patient education is extremely important in general

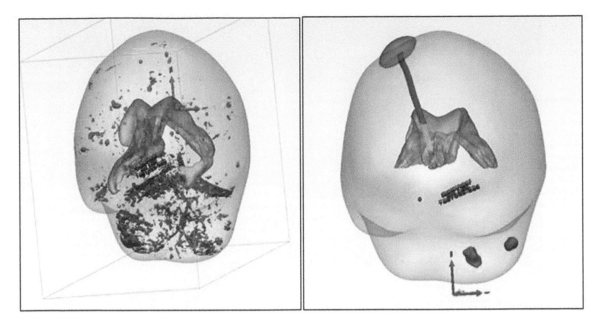

Figure 29.1 A 3D brain tumor model. An example of a patient with leptomeningeal disease prior to treatment versus after 2 months on treatment (post 5 fractions of whole brain radiation therapy, Ommaya placement, and weekly intrathecal chemotherapy).

neuro-oncology practice. It is essential for the patient to understand their diagnosis and treatment plan. Patient education through the use of 3D brain tumor models is a valuable approach that helps brain tumor patients better understand the magnetic resonance imaging (MRI) findings and neurological deficits they might be experiencing. Figure 29.1 demonstrates one example of a 3D rendering of a patient's brain MRI. Standardized or individualized informational handouts can also be utilized in these well-care visits to assist patients and caregivers in understanding their diagnosis. The addition of survivorship programs and clinics has become a staple in neuro-oncological care and offers patients and caregivers the opportunity to connect with others who have the same or similar diagnoses. Brain tumor support groups serve this purpose well.

PROCEDURAL CLINICS

APPs can obtain privileges in several different procedures for neuro-oncology, such as lumbar punctures, Ommaya reservoir taps, intrathecal chemotherapy administration via Ommaya reservoir or lumbar puncture, ventriculoperitoneal (VP) shunt interrogation/reprogramming and vagal nerve stimulator (VNS) interrogation/reprogramming. Once privileged, procedural clinics can be designed to have an APP lead who performs procedures with a varied level of supervision and access to the supervising physician. Having an APP available for these procedures in neuro-oncology clinics allows the physician to open up more patient-facing, nonprocedural clinic time.

> APPs can be credentialed in performing frequently time-consuming neuro-oncologic procedures, allowing physicians to dedicate more time to direct patient care.

Figure 29.2 shows an example of APP versus physician time utilization in a neuro-oncology procedural clinic as reported in a recent pilot study done at Geisinger Medical Center after development of the APP-led Ommaya/LP clinic.[2]

In neuro-oncology, lumbar punctures are commonly performed to evaluate for neoplastic leptomeningeal metastasis (also referred to as leptomeningeal carcinomatosis or leptomeningeal disease). In addition to collecting cerebrospinal fluid (CSF) for analysis, opening and closing pressures are frequently measured (Figure 29.3). If a patient is found to have leptomeningeal metastasis or is at high risk for leptomeningeal metastasis, they may require intrathecal (IT) chemotherapy. IT chemotherapy may be given via Ommaya reservoir (intraventricular route) or

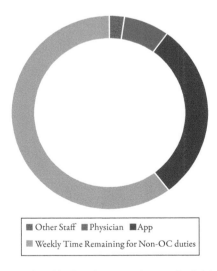

■ Other Staff ■ Physician ■ App
■ Weekly Time Remaining for Non-OC duties

Figure 29.2 Estimated weekly clinical time requirement for Geisinger Ommaya Clinic (GOC) Staff/ Providers. APP (red) spends ~12 hrs/ week compared to the physician (blue) ~4 hrs/ week. Nursing staff (gray) typically spends less than 1 hr/ week on GOC duties. The APP evaluates/ treats approximately 8 patients per week in the GOC, leaving 38 hours remaining per week to devote to other clinical duties outside of the GOC.

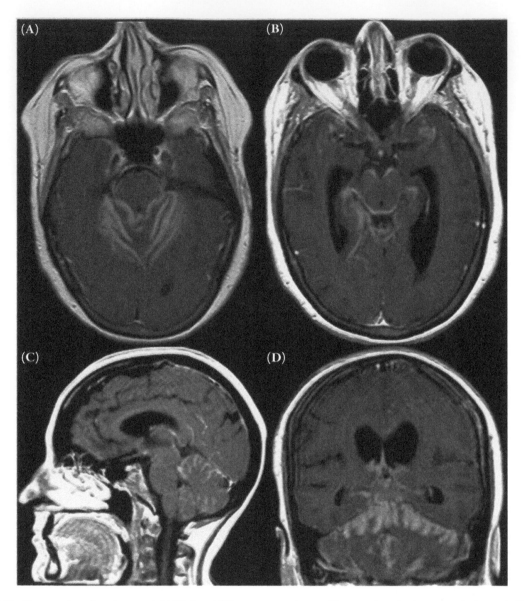

Figure 29.3 (A–D) MRI of leptomeningeal carcinomatosis (LMC). An axial T1 post-contrast image of leptomeningeal enhancement in the cerebellar folia and around the brainstem. (C) Sagittal T1 post-contrast that demonstrates cerebellar folia leptomeningeal enhancement. (D) Coronal post-contrast image that demonstrates cerebellar folia leptomeningeal enhancement.

via the spinal tap (lumbar route). Single-agent IT chemotherapy is the most common, but in some circumstances patients are given multidrug IT chemotherapy. The most common primary malignancies leading to leptomeningeal metastasis and the most common IT chemotherapies used in therapy of this condition are outlined in Table 29.1.[3-5] Common side effects of IT chemotherapy include nausea, vomiting, fever, headache, neck stiffness, seizures, fatigue, MRI brain imaging abnormalities, and cognitive changes.[6] Neuro-oncology patients may require VP shunt placement, which may require interrogation and reprogramming, depending on the model, after each brain MRI. Less commonly, brain tumor patients may have refractory epilepsy that may require a VNS that also requires interrogation and reprogramming.

In neuro-oncology, lumbar punctures are commonly performed to evaluate for neoplastic leptomeningeal metastasis.

TABLE 29.1 Most common primary cancer types and types of intrathecal (IT) chemotherapy for LMD

PRIMARY CANCER TYPES	EXAMPLES OF FREQUENTLY USED IT CHEMOTHERAPY
Breast	Methotrexate, thiotepa, trastuzumab, cytarabine
Lung	Methotrexate, topotecan
Melanoma	Methotrexate
GI	Methotrexate, topotecan
Hematological	Methotrexate, cytarabine, etoposide, rituximab

LMD, leptomeningeal disease. Frequently the IT chemotherapy drugs are given in sequence depending on the initial response and patient's tolerance. Some physicians combine drugs in hopes of improving efficacy although clinical trial data for this approach is not available.

DVT/PE	Cardiac tamponade
Nausea/vomiting	Infection
Depression	Decreased appetite
Fatigue	Abnormal lab values

NEURO-ONCOLOGY PROCEDURES

This section reviews the most common procedures performed in neuro-oncology clinics. These include LP, Ommaya tap, Ommaya IT delivery (single and dual agent), IT chemotherapy delivery via LP, and VP shunt and VNS interrogation and reprogramming. We provided the most common indications/contraindications and an abbreviated procedural stepwise guide based on our clinical practice, supplies used, typical orders placed, and important points to remember related to each procedure. These are practice standards in our clinics and might vary between institutions.

a. Lumbar Puncture

i. Indications and Contraindications
  1. Indications: Suspected leptomeningeal metastases, suspected infection (i.e., meningitis), suspected subarachnoid hemorrhage (SAH), suspected inflammatory and demyelinating conditions, therapeutic relief of pseudotumor cerebri, to support diagnosis of normal pressure hydrocephalus
  2. Absolute contraindications: Significant midline shift, posterior fossa mass, loss of suprachiasmatic and basilar cisterns, loss of superior cerebellar cistern, or loss of the quadrigeminal plate cistern
  3. Relative contraindications: Increased intracranial pressure (ICP), coagulopathy, brain abscess
ii. Steps of the Technique and Common Supplies
  1. Supplies: Sterile dressing, lidocaine 1% without epinephrine, syringes, needles for injections, spinal needle (20- or 22-gauge), three-way stopcock, manometer, test tubes (all these can be found in a standard lumbar puncture kit)
  2. Steps:
    a. Review indications and contraindications, allergies, medications (anti-coagulants, anti-platelet agents); perform time-out procedure with licensed providers; check chart for consent; review any recent brain/spinal imaging; explain the procedure to the patient and possible adverse effects
    b. Perform brief neurologic exam and check vital signs
    c. Position the patient in lateral decubitus position or seated position bent over a table (this is provider preference)
    d. Locate the line crossing L3–L4 space by finding the posterior superior iliac crests and moving the thumbs in medially toward the spine— mark this area with a marker
    e. Set up the lumbar kit using sterile technique
    f. Clean the previously identified area with antiseptic and apply sterile fenestrated drape
    g. Draw up local anesthetic and anesthetize the skin first by creating a skin wheal using the 25-gauge needle, then change to the 20-gauge needle to anesthetize the deeper tissues, making sure to aspirate intermittently to confirm needle is not in a blood vessel. Repeat as needed to ensure patient is anesthetized in all areas where your needle may be entering.
    h. Then, using the 20- or 22-gauge spinal needle— insert the needle (bevel up if lateral decubitus or facing out if sitting position) angling toward the umbilicus. Slowly advance the needle, removing the stylet every 1–2 cm to check for CSF flow. If no flow, replace stylet and advance or withdraw needle a few millimeters and repeat the process until CSF is identified.
    i. Check opening pressure if required—attach manometer and ask the patient to straighten the legs for accurate reading.
    j. Collect CSF into collection tubes to send for testing.
    k. After CSF is collected, check closing pressure (if desired) then replace the stylet and slowly remove the spinal needle.
    l. Clean off skin using alcohol swabs, apply dressing, and place patient in supine position.
    m. Patient should lie supine for 30–45 minutes after procedure and should try to stay flat for the rest of the day.
    n. Check the vital signs and review possible side effects again before discharging the patient.
iii. Orders, Billing, and Coding
  1. Routine: Glucose, protein, cell count w/differential, Gram-stain, bacterial cultures
  2. Special: Cytology, flow cytometry, viral and fungal studies, Epstein-Barr virus (EBV) PCR, IgH gene-rearrangement studies (lymphoma), circulating tumor cells, and ctDNA using special assays (breast and lung cancer)
  3. Serum: EBV PCR
  4. CPT code 62270: Spinal puncture, lumbar, diagnostic
iv. Common Pitfalls or Important Related Points
  1. Most common complication is post-lumbar puncture headache that is usually relieved by lying flat, caffeine, or use of analgesics. If headaches persist despite conservative treatment, the patient might qualify for an epidural blood patch, which is typically done by an anesthesiologist.
  2. Anticoagulation is not an absolute contraindication; however, depending on which medication the patient is on, therapy might need to be held for a period of 1–7 days prior to the procedure.
    a. Warfarin (Coumadin): 5–7 days

b. Enoxaparin (Lovenox): 12–24 hours
c. New oral anticoagulants (Eliquis, Xarelto): 48–96 hours
d. Aspirin/nonsteroidal anti-inflammatory drugs (NSAIDs): Haven't been shown to have an increased risk for bleeding, but are typically held 5–10 days prior to the procedure
e. Patient's primary provider or prescribing physician for the preceding medications should be made aware to determine the risk for stopping these medications for the allotted time.

The most common complication of a lumbar puncture is a headache (known as post-LP headache) that is usually relieved by lying flat, caffeine, or use of analgesics.

b. **Ommaya Tap**
i. Indications and Contraindications
1. Indications: Leptomeningeal metastases, suspected infection, assessment of treatment response, temporary drainage of CSF when symptomatic hydrocephalus develops
2. Contraindications: No absolute (avoid tapping Ommaya when active skin infection is present)
ii. Steps of the Technique and Common Supplies
1. Supplies: Sterile dressing, alcohol wipes, Chloroprep and/or iodine, hair shaver, fenestrated drape, 24- or 25¾-gauge butterfly needle with tubing, three-way stopcock, test tubes, 10 mL Luer-lock syringes, gauze pads, adhesive bandage (use of standard LP kit might be helpful as it provides many of the needed supplies and sterile field)
2. Steps:
a. Review patient allergies, perform time-out for procedure, check for consent (see the steps for lumbar puncture).
b. Have patient lay supine on the exam table.
i. The head of the table may be raised slightly to make the patient more comfortable as needed.
ii. In some cases, the procedure can be done with patient sitting upright (see common pitfalls, later, for more on this).
c. Using non-sterile technique, prime Ommaya by pressing down in the center of the reservoir to ensure that the reservoir is working correctly.
i. You should be able to visualize normal depression and bounce-back of the Ommaya reservoir dome (this may vary depending on the model and size of the reservoir).
d. Shave the hair with electric shaver if needed.
e. Clean skin with alcohol wipes.
f. Set up supplies (lumbar or Ommaya kit) and use sterile technique.
i. Attach butterfly needle tubing to 3-way stopcock and attach the 10 mL Luer-lock syringes for CSF collection.

g. Clean skin with sterile iodine or chloro-prep as alternative.
h. Apply fenestrated drape (optional)—make sure patient's face is visible and they can breathe freely.
i. Using 24- or 25¾-gauge butterfly needle, puncture the center of the Ommaya reservoir dome at a 45–90-degree angle (avoid reaching the base) but make sure the needle sits firmly in the reservoir.
j. Slowly withdraw CSF using the 10 mL syringes attached to the stopcock, turning the valve in the necessary directions. After desired amount of CSF is collected, remove needle, and apply dressing to skin.
k. Transfer CSF from the syringes into the collection tubes to be sent off for testing.
l. Post-procedure monitoring is typically not necessary for a tap only.
iii. Orders, Billing, and Coding
1. CSF orders are the same as noted for the LP.
2. CPT (billing) procedure code 61020 or 61070: Removal of CSF from brain/shunt
iv. Common Pitfalls or Important Related Points
1. If there is difficulty withdrawing CSF from the Ommaya reservoir, the following should be considered:
a. What position is the patient in?
i. If sitting or more upright, consider having patient supine or vice versa to improve return of CSF.
b. Is there a recent head CT? Does the patient have slit-like ventricles?
i. Repeat head CT without contrast if needed.
c. Consider pumping the shunt again.
d. Consult neurosurgery for reservoir evaluation/adjustment.
2. Anticoagulation and moderate thrombocytopenia are not absolute contraindications, but these patients are at higher risk for bleeding (potential injury to the choroid plexus), and the fluid extraction should be done using a smaller syringe (5 cc) and very low rate; in addition, note that upon removal of needle bleeding time will be prolonged.
a. Apply light pressure with gauze until hemostasis is achieved.
b. Consider adding PT/INR as a pre-lab for the procedure.

c. **Ommaya IT Chemotherapy with Single Agent +/– Tap**
i. Indications and Contraindications
1. Indications: Leptomeningeal metastases, central nervous system (CNS) prophylaxis in lymphoma and leukemia patients who have a high risk for spread to CNS
2. Contraindications: Current infection or signs of infection, severe thrombocytopenia or

neutropenia, concomitant treatment with systemic CNS-penetrating drugs (use caution)

ii. Steps of the Technique and Common Supplies
  1. Supplies are the same as for the Ommaya tap.
  2. Steps are similar to the Ommaya tap (notable differences below).
  3. Order and complete pre-treatment labs.
    a. Complete blood count with differential (CBC/diff), comprehensive metabolic panel (CMP), and chemotherapy drug level if indicated (usually for use of methotrexate)
    b. Consider PT/INR if on anticoagulation
  4. Premedicate with an antinausea medication and steroid about 10–15 minutes before the procedure.
    a. Examples: Ondansetron 8 mg and dexamethasone 4 mg
  5. Signed off chemotherapy by 2 licensed professionals (follow your institution's protocol).
    a. Most commonly a registered nurse and APP or physician
  6. After CSF is collected, disconnect one of the 10 mL syringes from the 3-way stopcock and replace with the 10 mL syringe containing intrathecal chemotherapy agent (volume may vary by the type of the drug and dose: usually 2–5 cc).
  7. Slowly administer chemotherapy: general rule for the rate of administration is 1 cc/minute.
  8. Flush the tubing by administering 3–4 cc of the autologous CSF or preservative-free normal saline Withdraw needle, apply hemostasis if needed, apply adhesive bandage.
  9. Transfer CSF to collection tubes (if sending for testing) or discard if no testing needed.
  10. Discard any supplies that encountered chemotherapy into the appropriate chemotherapy receptacle (follow your institution's guidelines).

iii. Orders, Billing, and Coding
  1. Same as LP and Ommaya tap.
  2. CPT code 96542: Chemotherapy injection

iv. Common Pitfalls or Important Related Points
  1. Never instill a higher volume of CSF than what is withdrawn from the reservoir/cistern.
    a. For example, if there is a planned delivery of 10 mL chemotherapy, then at least 10 mL of CSF should be removed prior to procedure (more if there is a plan to flush with CSF).
  2. Ensure that there is CSF remaining to flush the remaining chemotherapy that is in the tubing (or use preservative-free normal saline).
  3. The patient should be monitored for about 10–15 minutes after each treatment to observe for any side effects.
  4. Common side effects of IT chemotherapy include immediate or subacute complications such as nausea, vomiting, headache, fever, stiff neck, and dizziness. Patients remain at risk for developing chemical meningitis for 24–48 hours after IT chemotherapy. Other symptoms

associated with IT chemotherapy may include malaise, seizures, abnormal MRI brain imaging (leukoencephalopathy, usually asymptomatic), and cognitive changes

d. Ommaya IT Chemotherapy with Dual Agents +/− Tap

i. Indications and Contraindications
  1. Indications: Same as Ommaya IT with single agent. Dual IT chemotherapy is more commonly indicated in breast cancer patients.
  2. Contraindications are the same as single-therapy IT.

ii. Steps of the Technique and Common Supplies
  1. Same as single therapy.
  2. After the first chemotherapy is injected, remove the empty syringe and attach the second 10 mL syringe with the second chemotherapy medication.

iii. Orders, Billing, and Coding
  1. Same as single therapy.

iv. Common Pitfalls or Important Related Points
  1. All IT therapies must be IT-grade approved by pharmacy.
  2. Common intrathecal therapies used are methotrexate, topotecan, trastuzumab, cytarabine, thiotepa, and etoposide.
  3. Other IT-infused therapies have included dexamethasone and rituximab.
  4. If/when giving dual chemotherapies, administer clear-colored therapies first and follow with tinted (colored) therapies second to observe final clearance of the line with final flushing.

e. IT Chemotherapy via Lumbar Cistern

i. Indications and Contraindications
  1. Same as those for IT chemotherapy.
  2. These are typically patients who require a designated number of IT treatments with contraindications for or otherwise do not have Ommaya reservoirs.

ii. Steps of the Technique and Common Supplies
  1. Same as LP procedure with the addition of administration of chemotherapy agents. Once the subarachnoid space is reached and CSF flow established, collect the desired amount of CSF (the minimum volume collected must be equal or greater to the volume of chemotherapy to be injected plus the flush). Connect the syringe containing chemotherapy directly to the spinal needle (being careful not to move it) or via tubing provided in the LP tray. Using tubing decreases the chances of spinal needle movement (less stiff connection) and provides visual control of chemotherapy flow. Please make sure to prepare a separate syringe with preservative-free normal saline for the flush after chemotherapy is administered. Using autologous CSF in this setting is less practical as it will require transferring the CSF from the collection tubes into the syringe and will prolong the procedure for the patient.

2. Pre-labs need to include PT/INR.
3. If patient is on anticoagulation, it will need to be held prior to the procedure as noted earlier in a previous section; review platelet count and follow guidelines for LP in the setting of thrombocytopenia

iii. Orders, Billing, and Coding
1. Same as above.

iv. Common Pitfalls or Important Related Points
1. Access via LP isn't guaranteed each time, and the patient may not be able to tolerate the number of procedures needed for treatment regimen. As with a lumbar puncture, patient should lie flat for 30–45 minutes after procedure and should try to stay flat for the rest of the day; use of reverse Trendelenburg position is desirable (if tolerated) to facilitate distribution of chemotherapy.

f. VP Shunt Interrogation and Reprogramming

i. Indications and Contraindications
1. Indications: Programmable shunts need to be interrogated after MRIs to ensure the settings are the same as pre-MRI. Programmable shunts may need to be adjusted based on clinical symptoms (i.e., over-shunting or under-shunting).
2. Contraindications: None

ii. Steps of the Technique and Common Supplies
1. Steps and supplies will vary based on manufacturer, model, and generation of the shunt.
2. Typically done by neurosurgery.

iii. Common Pitfalls or Important Related Points
1. Some VP shunts are not typically impacted by the MRI magnet and usually do not need to be interrogated or adjusted after MRI. These include Aesculapm, Prograv, and Codman Certas models.
2. VP that commonly require interrogation and reprogramming/adjustment after MRI include Medtronic Strata and Codman Hakim.
3. Signs/symptoms of shunt malfunction: Headaches, vomiting, lethargy, seizures, swelling or erythema around the shunt tract, periods of confusion.
4. If concern for shunt malfunction: X-ray shunt series and CT head without contrast are typically ordered.

g. VNS Interrogation and Reprogramming

i. Indications and Contraindications
1. Indications: Change settings (increase or decrease), check the battery

ii. Steps of the Technique and Common Supplies
1. Supplies: VNS interrogation device for the model
   a. Most commonly includes a programming wand and a programming computer
2. Steps: will vary based on patient needs and model of device. A set of general guidelines for changing settings is available via www.vnstherapy.com.

iii. Common Pitfalls or Important Related Points
1. VNS device can't tell the provider if the patient had a seizure.

2. VNS is MRI brain-compatible, but must be turned off prior to MRI and then turned back on.
3. VNS/leads are not compatible for a thoracic MRI.
4. If there is less than 15% battery power left on the device, seizure frequency may increase.
5. When is a VNS considered for a patient?
   a. When patient has refractory epilepsy and doesn't have any other treatment options.

OTHER APP ROLES WITHIN NEURO-ONCOLOGY CLINICS

Here we provide a summary of additional alternative roles of the APP in neuro-oncology clinics which add value to the multidisciplinary care of these cancer patients. These roles include leading fast-track clinics, in-patient and emergency department consultation services, and survivorship/health literacy programs. We have outlined some of the key points related to these additional roles. Effective utilization of our APP partner relationships is critical to patient outcomes and practice success.

Follow-Up/Fast-Track Clinics

Well-Check and Lab Follow-Up

- Address any abnormal lab values that need intervention and tolerance of new therapies

Mid-Radiation Therapy Visits

- Assess tolerance of the therapy

- Follow-up planning for MRIs and start of adjuvant therapies/devices

- Patient education

72-Hour Walk-In Clinic Slots

- The goal is to limit patient visits to the emergency department (ED).

- Types of patients suitable for these slots are those with non-emergent but serious reported symptoms.

Cancer Neurology Patients

- Cancer patients with neurology concerns that are either believed to be secondary to the cancer or to cancer therapies

  - Chemotherapy-induced neuropathy, cognitive changes, tremor, seizures, gait/balance disturbance, headache, vision changes, stroke, abnormal MRI, insomnia, tremors, insomnia, sexual dysfunction, psychosis/mood disturbance, peri-operative neurologic clearance, paraneoplastic syndrome, and evaluation for CNS neoplastic prophylaxis

Hospital Discharge Clinics

- Patients seen in a 3- to 10-day time frame after discharge.

  - Some may be transitioned to the multidisciplinary clinics versus general neurology clinics

- APPs at Geisinger maintain a 20% (0.2 clinical FTE) general neurology clinic to remain familiar with general neurology standards of care and maintain communication with other neurology partners.

IN-PATIENT AND ED CONSULTS (TO ASSIST WITH CARE TRANSITIONS)

Transition to Floor

- Common conditions: New brain tumor diagnosis with edema, midline shift, vasogenic edema, seizures (new or uncontrolled), or new neurological deficits

Transition to Ambulatory Clinics

- Multidisciplinary clinic (at Geisinger and Banner Health these clinics include a medical/neuro-oncologist, neurosurgeon, and a radiation oncologist in the same visit)

  - New brain tumor diagnoses (2-week post-surgery): Introduction to the team, diagnostic education, and charting the treatment course.

  - Post-radiation or post-chemoradiation follow-up with brain imaging

  - Progressed tumors for treatment discussion

- Ommaya clinic

- General/other subspecialty neurology clinics (These are common in neuro-oncology)

  - New stroke, refractory seizures, refractory headaches, movement disorders, cognitive changes, and neuromuscular

SURVIVORSHIP PROGRAMS AND PATIENT EDUCATION

Patient Caregiver and Remembrance Ceremonies

- Support groups for brain tumor patients

- Celebration of life ceremonies for the families, caregivers, and other patient providers for those patients who died while under the care of the cancer clinics

  Education Sessions

- Patient health literacy: MRI/brain tumor modeling

- Review MRIs with patient and explain findings

- Use of 3D brain tumor models to help patients better understand tumor imaging

- Educational chemotherapy and treatment calendars

  - Providing patients with information on the chemotherapy, side effects, and schedule

  - Providing calendars for patients to keep track of when they are to get lab work and their chemotherapy days

- Seizure control/education
  - Most commonly prescribed antiepileptic drugs (AEDs) in neuro-oncology are levetiracetam (Keppra) and lacosamide (Vimpat) but often other therapies are used for refractory or otherwise unsuitable patients on these AEDs

- Discuss common side effects and teratogenicity

- Choice of AEDs in brain tumor patients is driven by goal for reduced drug-to-drug interaction and less hematological side effects (such as bone marrow suppression). Cost and dosing schedule are also a consideration in cancer patients.

  vi. Factors that increase the risk of having a seizure (infection, dehydration, alcohol use, lack of sleep, skipping meals, psychological or physical stress, taking medication incorrectly/inappropriately, drug-to-drug interactions, genetic predisposition, and dietary changes)

  vii. Examples of drug-to-drug interactions

    1. Efficacy of oral contraceptives: Carbamazepine, phenytoin, topiramate, lamotrigine, oxcarbazepine can cause reduced efficacy of oral contraception

    2. Anticoagulation: Carbamazepine and barbiturates can increase the metabolism of warfarin whereas phenytoin and valproic acid can decrease the metabolism and cause increased levels of warfarin

    3. Antidepressants: Serum drug level concentration of antidepressant can be decreased by the enzyme inducing AEDs and lower seizure threshold therefore potentiating seizures (trazodone, Wellbutrin, etc.).

FLASHCARD

What are the absolute contraindications for a lumbar puncture?	Midline shift, posterior fossa mass, loss of suprachiasmatic/basilar cisterns, loss of superior cerebellar cistern or loss of the quadrigeminal plate cistern, severe coagulopathy
What are the relative contraindications for a lumbar puncture?	Increased intracranial pressure, coagulopathy, brain abscess
Common indications for a lumbar puncture in neuro-oncology are:	Suspicion for neoplastic leptomeningeal dissemination, CNS infection/inflammatory conditions, and normal-pressure hydrocephalus
Treatment of post LP headaches typically includes:	Lying supine, caffeine, and/or non-narcotic analgesics
Ommaya reservoir placement helps to do what?	Easily administer IT chemotherapy and limits need for multiple lumbar punctures
Multiple LP procedures in the same patient risks what outcomes?	Fistula formation, CSF leak, scaring, pain, and infection at the site or in the CSF
The most common cancer types that lead to development of leptomeningeal disease are:	Breast cancer, lung cancer, and melanoma (less commonly are GU/GI and hematological cancers)
The most commonly utilized IT chemotherapy is:	Methotrexate
The most common side effects of IT chemotherapy are:	Headache, nausea/vomiting, seizure, fever, stiff neck, fatigue, MRI changes, and cognitive decline
Commonly prescribed AEDs in neuro-oncology	Levetiracetam and lacosamide

_____ are AEDs that increase and _____ are AEDs that decrease the clearance/metabolism of other drugs

Inducers

Inhibitors

What factors increase risk for seizure in patients with epilepsy?

Infection, dehydration, alcohol use, lack of sleep, skipping meals, psychological or physical stress, medication non-adherence, drug-drug interactions

QUESTIONS

1. What is the most common side effect of a lumbar puncture?
   a. Bleeding
   b. Headache
   c. Vision changes
   d. Local infection

2. Which lumbar space is most commonly accessed during lumbar puncture?
   a. L1–L2
   b. L2–L3
   c. L3–L4
   d. S1–S2

3. When there is a concern for ventriculoperitoneal (VP) shunt malfunction, which orders should be placed?
   a. CT head without contrast
   b. X-ray shunt series
   c. Peritoneal ultrasound
   d. Both a and b

4. Which of the following are signs/symptoms of VP shunt malfunction?
   a. Headaches
   b. Nausea or vomiting
   c. Lethargy
   d. Edema surrounding the shunt tract
   e. All of the above

5. Which of the following is a common indication for intrathecal chemotherapy?
   a. Leptomeningeal metastasis
   b. Brain metastasis
   c. CNS neoplastic prophylaxis
   d. Both a and c

6. Which of the following should be considered in a patient with persisting post-LP headache despite conservative therapy?
   a. Epidural blood patch
   b. IV fluid administration
   c. 48-hour continuous supine positioning
   d. Steroid therapy

7. Which of the following is a contraindication to the administration of intrathecal chemotherapy?
   a. Patient has concern for acute infection
   b. Low serum chemotherapy drug levels
   c. Patient is on anticoagulation
   d. Both a and b

8. Which of the following is an absolute contraindication to lumbar puncture?
   a. Brain imaging concerning for herniation
   b. History of deep venous thrombus
   c. Brain abscess
   d. Age older than 85

9. What is a relative contraindication to lumbar puncture?
   a. Fever
   b. Back pain
   c. History of coagulopathy
   d. History of knee surgery

10. How is the opening pressure most accurately obtained in a lumbar puncture?
    a. Have the patient cough.
    b. Have the patient in the lateral decubitus position.
    c. Have the patient bring their knees as close as possible to their chest.
    d. Keep them in the upright seated position.

11. Which of the following statements is true about APPs?
    a. APPs cannot prescribe medications.
    b. APPs can perform procedures prior to being privileged with permission from the supervising physician.
    c. APPs cannot order blood products or supportive therapies.
    d. APPs can work up to the capacity of their supervising physician with some limitations that typically vary from state to state.

12. Which of the following is a common medication administered intrathecally?
    a. Methotrexate
    b. Levetiracetam
    c. Lacosamide
    d. None of the above

13. The volume of CSF to be withdrawn intrathecally should be twice the volume of chemotherapy being delivered.
    a. True
    b. False

14. While collecting CSF from the Ommaya reservoir, you begin to feel resistance and notice a lack of CSF return and the Ommaya dome is depressed. Which of the following should be considered?
    a. The patient's position on the procedure table
    b. Patient's postoperative head CT demonstrates slit-like ventricles
    c. Need for repeat head CT without contrast
    d. Need to consult neurosurgery for adjustment
    e. All the above

15. What is a pitfall to administering chemotherapy via the lumbar cistern?
    a. Increased nausea and vomiting with LP procedure
    b. Only one chemotherapy is approved for administration via the lumbar cistern
    c. Multiple lumbar punctures increase the risk for fistulas and CSF leaks
    d. Patients must remain in the left lateral decubitus position for 45 minutes after LP procedure

ANSWERS

1. b
2. c
3. d
4. e
5. d
6. a
7. a
8. a
9. c
10. b
11. d
12. a
13. b
14. e
15. c

REFERENCES

1. Sarzynski E, Barry H. Current evidence and controversies: Advanced practice providers in healthcare. *Am J Manag Care.* 2019;25(8):366–368.
2. Leese EN, Weeder JL, Manikowski JJ, et al. PA- and NP-led Ommaya clinics to manage leptomeningeal carcinomatosis. *JAAPA.* 2021;34(12):35–41.
3. Clarke JL. Leptomeningeal metastasis from systemic cancer. *Continuum Lifelong Learning Neurol.* 2012;18(2):328–342.
4. Wang N, Bertalan MS, Brastianos PK. Leptomeningeal metastasis from systemic cancer: Review and update on management. *Cancer.* 2018;124:21–35.
5. Groves MD, Glantz MJ, Chamberlain MC, et al. A multicenter phase II trial of intrathecal topotecan in patients with meningeal malignancies. *Neuro-Oncology.* 2008;10(2):208–215.
6. Byrnes, DM, Vargas, F, Dermarkarian, C, et al. Complications of intrathecal chemotherapy in Suadults: Single-institution experience in 109 consecutive patients. *J Oncol.* 2019, 4047617.

SUGGESTED READING

1. Johnson KS, Sexton DJ. Lumbar puncture: Technique, indications, contraindications and complications in adults. *UpToDate.* 2018. https://www.uptodate.com/contents/lumbar-puncture-technique-indications-contraindications-and-complications-in-adults
2. Shlamovitz GZ, Shah NR. Lumbar puncture. Medscape. 2018. https://emedicine.medscape.com/article/80773-technique
3. CPT Code Lookup and Search. 2020. https://coder.aapc.com/cpt-codes/
4. Bateman BT, Cole NL, Sun-Edelstein C, Lay C. Post dural puncture headache. *UpToDate.* 2020. https://www.uptodate.com/contents/post-dural-puncture-headache?topicRef=4832source=see_link
5. Intrathecal Chemotherapy (IT Chemo). November 18, 2019. https://www.oncolink.org/cancer-treatment/cancer-medications/overview/intrathecal-chemotherapy-it-chemo
6. Shunt Malfunction Signs. June 2018. https://www.cincinnatichildrens.org/health/s/shunt-malfunction
7. Resources. VNS Therapy. 2020. https://vnstherapy.com/healthcare-professionals/
8. Shafer PO, Dean PM. Placement, programming and safety of vagus nerve stimulation (VNS). March 12, 2018. https://www.epilepsy.com/learn/treating-seizures-and-epilepsy/devices/vagus-nerve-stimulation/placement-programming-and
9. Gallagher P, Leach JP, Grant R. Time to focus on brain tumor-related epilepsy trials. *Neuro-Oncology Pract.* 2014;1(3):123–133. https://doi.org/10.1093/nop/npu010
10. Perucca E. Clinically relevant drug interactions with antiepileptic drugs. *Br J Clin Pharmacol.* 2006;61(3):246–255. https://doi.org/10.1111/j.1365-2125.2005.02529.x

VALERIA INTERNÒ, ROBERTA RUDÀ, AND RICCARDO SOFFIETTI

INTRODUCTION

The "silver tsunami" defines the socio-health phenomenon of progressive aging in the worldwide population because of a significant increase of life expectancy. People older than 65 years are commonly considered of advanced age and divided into two groups: early-elderly (from 66 to 75 years) and late-elderly (older than 76 years). In clinical practice, early-elderly patients with good performance status could be considered and treated as middle-aged patients, but this assumption is only based on clinicians' experience in absence of standardized guidelines.[1]

As a consequence of the "silver tsunami," the incidence of brain tumors in the elderly has increased in the past few decades, forcing neuro-oncologists to investigate and define appropriate therapeutic strategies in this population to avoid inappropriate undertreatment. In the past, elderly patients were commonly considered too frail to be treated with aggressive and active therapeutic strategies such as surgery, radiotherapy (RT), and chemotherapy.[2]

> The incidence of brain tumors in the elderly has increased in the past few decades, forcing neuro-oncologists to investigate and define new, appropriate therapeutic strategies in this population.

Treating neuro-oncologic diseases in elderly patients represents a challenge mainly due to comorbidities that increase the amount of treatment-related adverse effects. As a result, the identification of goals of care and the presence of social support serve an important role in the decision-making process.[3] With regard to the aforementioned demographic shift and good performance status of many elderly patients, advanced age may not be the only reason to avoid active therapeutic strategies.[4] On the other hand, these patients frequently suffer from neurocognitive impairment, affective or mood disorders, seizures, thromboembolic complications, and fatigue that can be difficult to adequately manage. In recent years many neuro-oncology trials have focused on the elderly population to identify adequate treatment strategies and/or the optimal supportive care for symptom control, improvement of quality of life, and reduction of mortality.[5]

GLIOMAS IN ELDERLY PATIENTS

HIGH-GRADE GLIOMAS

Glioblastoma multiforme (GBM) is the most common type of high-grade glioma (HGG) in elderly people, with a median age at diagnosis of 64 years. As a consequence of increased average life expectancy, the age of GBM patients is anticipated to continue to rise. The incidence rate of GBM among elderly patients is 17.5 per 100,000 person-year and a risk of 3–4 times compared with young adults[6,7] (Figure 30.1).

Advanced age is considered a negative prognostic factor for GBM, with a median survival in this population of less than 1 year compared to more than 15 months for the younger population.[8]

The assessment of standardized scales tailored to the elderly population can facilitate clinicians in discriminating fit from unfit patients. A comprehensive geriatric assessment (CGA) should be adopted by clinicians for oncologic elderly patients to help guide treatment decisions. In 2015, the American Society of Clinical Oncology (ASCO) published geriatric oncology guidelines to predict adverse outcomes, suggesting that every patient should undergo an assessment of physiological function, comorbidities, falls, depression, cognition, and nutrition. Clinicians may use different methods to evaluate these patient characteristics, such as an assessment of instrumental activities of daily living (IADLs) for function, a thorough history or validated tools to assess comorbidity and fall risk, the Geriatric Depression Scale (GDS) for depression, the Mini-Cog or Blessed Orientation-Memory-Concentration test (BOMC) for cognition, and an assessment of unintentional weight loss to evaluate nutrition. Short tools, such as the Geriatric-8 or Vulnerable Elders Survey-13 (VES-13), can help clinicians to predict mortality.[9]

> A comprehensive geriatric assessment (CGA) should be adopted by clinicians for oncologic elderly patients to help guide treatment decisions.

In 2011, Owusu and colleagues evaluated the efficacy of Eastern Cooperative Oncology Group Performance Status (ECOG-PS) and Karnofsky Index of Performance Status (KPS) scales to identify abnormalities on CGA and compared these instruments with the VES-13. They found that elderly

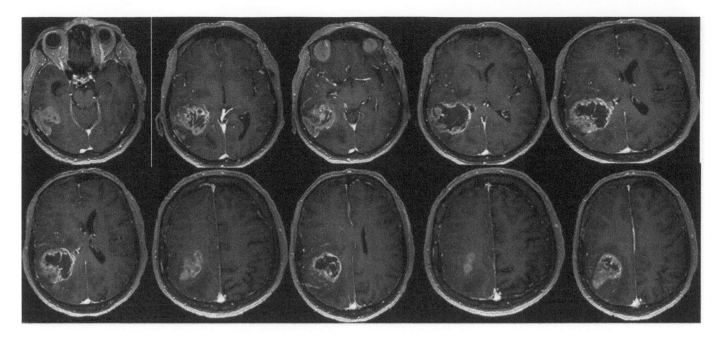

Figure 30.1 MRI of a 75-year-old patient with glioblastoma showing typical features such as central necrosis.

oncologic patients with a VES-13 score of 3 or greater, ECOG-PS score of 1 or greater, or a KPS score of 80% or less have alterations in the CGA and should be referred to a geriatric-oncologist for a full CGA to intervene in geriatric problems that may otherwise remain undetected and negatively impact outcome.[10]

Other factors that are common among elderly GBM patients can contribute to a worse outcome. The prognostic impact of TP53 mutations, epidermal growth factor receptor (EGFR) amplification, CDKN2A/p16 alterations, and loss of chromosome 1p are age-dependent.[11] In particular, TP53 mutations and CDKN2A alterations are negative prognostic factors for elderly patients, while EGFR amplifications and loss of chromosome 1p have a good prognostic effect.[3] Interestingly, TP53 and EGFR alterations have an opposite prognostic value in comparison to younger population.[12,13] TERT promoter mutations, which can interfere with intracellular telomerase function, have a prognostic impact that depends on IDH mutational status. TERT promoter mutations are more common in the elderly and have a negative impact on survival in isocitrate dehydrogenase (IDH) wildtype tumors, which are common in the elderly.[14]

> TP53 mutations and CDKN2A alterations are negative prognostic factors for elderly patients with GBM, while EGFR amplifications and loss of chromosome 1p have a better prognostic value.

Based on gene expression signatures, GBMs are subdivided into four distinct subgroups: classical, mesenchymal, neural, and proneural. The proneural signature confers significantly longer survival compared with the other subtypes, but elderly patients rarely exhibit the proneural gene expression signature.[15,16]

TREATMENT STRATEGIES FOR ELDERLY GBM PATIENTS

The standard treatment for GBM includes surgical resection (as complete as possible), followed by adjuvant therapy with radiation (RT) (60 Gy in 30 daily fractions over 6 weeks) and chemotherapy with temozolomide (TMZ), an oral DNA alkylating agent, delivered concomitantly with RT and adjuvantly in cycles of 5 days per month up to 6–12 months or until radiological progression or unacceptable toxicity.[17] In fit patients, use of tumor-treating fields in the adjuvant setting could also be considered.

The extent of resection (EOR) at time of initial diagnosis strongly correlates with overall survival (OS) in GBM patients.[18] A retrospective German study analyzed prognostic factors in 103 elderly patients with GBM and concluded that the most important predictor of outcome was the EOR, with an OS of 2.2, 7.0, or 13.9 months for patients who underwent biopsy, partial resection, or gross total resection (GTR), respectively.[19] Similar results were reported by the Neurooncology Working Group of the German Cancer Society (NOA-08 trial) that revaluated a phase III trial with a similar population and concluded that EOR was the sole independent prognostic factor for survival.[20]

However, resection could expose elderly GBM patients, especially those with comorbidities, to life-threatening complications and, as a consequence, elderly GBM patients are often excluded from aggressive surgery in favor of a diagnostic stereotactic biopsy. In 2007, Martinez and colleagues evaluated the prognostic value of GTR based on age in 138 consecutive patients with malignant gliomas, of whom half were younger and half were older than 65 years of age. Elderly patients had a larger burden of comorbidities which, unexpectedly, did not influence post-surgical outcome. GTR was significantly associated with longer survival compared to biopsy and subtotal resection (STR) in both elderly and younger patients. Notably, the authors did not find a higher incidence of surgical complications in the elderly population, except for psychosomatic syndrome. Based on these data, when anatomically feasible and in the presence of good performance status, GTR should be attempted in elderly patients suspected of having a GBM.[21]

> When anatomically feasible and in the presence of a good performance status, GTR should be attempted in elderly patients suspected of having a GBM.

After surgery, neuro-oncologists must define optimal adjuvant therapy. The benefit of RT is well established, but the optimal schedule for elderly patients is still unclear.[5]

A study randomized GBM patients aged 70 or older to receive either best supportive care alone or post-surgical RT (50 Gy in fractions of 1.8 Gy fractions); this study reported a prolongation of progression-free survival (14.9 weeks vs. 5.4 weeks) and OS (29.1 weeks vs. 16.9 weeks) in the RT group, without any severe adverse events.[22] Another trial compared the efficacy of hypofractionated RT (40 Gy total dose over 3 weeks) with that of standard fractionation treatment (60 Gy over 6 weeks) in elderly patients with a KPS of greater than 50 after surgery and did not show a significant difference in outcome or adverse events between the two arms, with a median OS of 5–6 months.[23]

The post-surgical role of chemotherapy alone in GBM elderly patients was explored in a prospective, single-arm study by Association des Neuro-oncologues d'Expression Francaise (ANOCEF). This study showed that median OS (6.25 months) for patients who received chemotherapy was better than that reported in historic controls who received supportive care only (3.5 months). Moreover, the authors observed that patients who had O^6-methylguanine DNA methyltransferase (MGMT) methylated tumors had a significantly longer survival compared to those who had unmethylated tumors (7.75 vs. 4.5 months, respectively).[24]

Some studies compared the safety and efficacy of RT versus chemotherapy. The phase III Nordic trial included elderly patients with ECOG PS 0-2 who were randomized to receive either standard radiation (60 Gy in 30 fractions) or hypofractionated radiation (34 Gy in 10 fractions) or monthly TMZ for 6 cycles.[25] Median OS was 6 months for patients who received standard RT alone, while longer survival was seen in patients who received either hypofractionated RT (7.5 months) or TMZ (8.3 months). Patients with MGMT promoter methylation had a significantly longer median OS with TMZ (9.7 months) than those who did not have this genetic alteration (6.8 months). With respect to quality of life, patients in the TMZ group reported better scores on quality of life metrics than patients in the other treatment arms.

The phase III German trial (NOA-08) investigated the impact of chemotherapy versus radiation in 373 elderly patients with GBM (89%) or anaplastic astrocytoma (11%) and KPS of 60 or greater.[20] Patients received TMZ alone in a dose-intensified regimen of 100 mg/m² given on days 1–7 every other week or RT (60 Gy given in 30 fractions). TMZ was not inferior to RT, with a median survival of 8.6 versus 9.6 months, respectively. In this trial, as in the NORDIC trial, MGMT-methylated tumors had a longer PFS when receiving TMZ as compared to RT (8.4 months vs. 4.9 months) while patients with unmethylated tumors did not derive any benefit from TMZ (PFS 3.3 months for TMZ vs. 4.6 months for RT).

The safety and efficacy of concomitant and adjuvant radiochemotherapy in elderly GBM patients has been historically questioned due to the age cutoff of 70 years in the landmark registration trial EORTC 26981, which demonstrated the efficacy of radiochemotherapy in GBM. A post-hoc analysis of the study data showed that patients from 65 to 70 years old did not derive a statistically significant benefit by adding chemotherapy to RT.[17] Thus, it is still unclear whether people older than 70 years benefit from combination chemoradiation therapy.

Studies have suggested a role for RT with concomitant and adjuvant TMZ in elderly patients with GBM. A single-arm phase II trial suggested efficacy and a tolerable safety profile of chemoradiotherapy for elderly people with newly diagnosed GBM.[26] This has been confirmed by a phase III randomized trial (EORTC 26062/22061) that reported a superior efficacy of an hypofractionated RT with concomitant/adjuvant TMZ over hypofractionated RT alone in terms of prolonged OS (9.3 vs. 7.6 months) without worsening quality of life.[27]

> A phase III randomized trial in elderly patients with GBM reported a superior efficacy of hypofractionated RT with concomitant/adjuvant TMZ over hypofractionated RT alone in terms of prolonged OS without worsening quality of life.

These results are particularly interesting when analyzed by MGMT promoter methylation status: in the RT-alone group, MGMT methylation was not a predictive factor. The greatest benefit was observed in MGMT-methylated GBM patients, with a nearly doubled survival when treated with chemoradiotherapy (mOS 13.5 months) in comparison RT alone (mOS 7.7 months). However, a modest survival advantage (p = 0.05) was evident even in GBM patients without methylation of MGMT promoter when receiving the combined treatment.

Based on these data, select elderly GBM patients with good prognostic factors, such as extensive resection and good performance status, can benefit from standard combination chemoradiotherapy. Combination chemoradiotherapy for treatment of GBM in elderly patients with good performance status is also supported by the results of a meta-analysis which demonstrated that radiochemotherapy prolonged OS in this patient population, with a reduction in the risk of death compared to RT alone.[28]

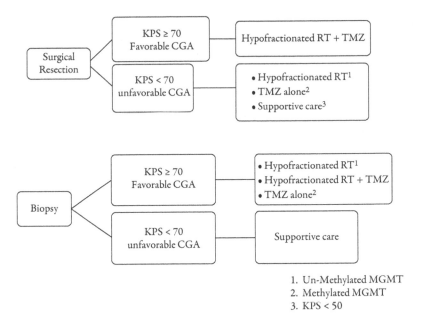

1. Un-Methylated MGMT
2. Methylated MGMT
3. KPS < 50

Figure 30.2 Proposed decision tree guiding treatment of glioblastoma patients older than 70 years.

A recent large multicenter retrospective Italian study analyzed the effectiveness and safety of standard versus short course RT when combined with concomitant TMZ in elderly patients with GBM. Patients with high performance status receiving the concomitant standard fractionation RT had a better outcome compared to hypofractionated regimens, with a more favorable toxicity profile.[29]

In terms of daily clinical practice (Figure 30.2), radiochemotherapy is appropriate standard treatment after surgery for elderly patients (>70 years) who are "fit" (good performance status, substantial tumor resection, limited volume of brain to be treated by RT, and lack of significant comorbidities). In case of "non-fit" patients, TMZ alone could be proposed to MGMT-methylated patients, while hypofractionated RT could be proposed for MGMT-unmethylated patients. Supportive care alone could be reserved for patients with poor performance status (Karnofsky <50).[30]

LOW-GRADE GLIOMAS

Low-grade gliomas (LGG; World Health Organization [WHO] grade 2) represent a heterogeneous group of gliomas with distinct histopathological and molecular characteristics that make them less aggressive and that have better outcomes than HGG.[31] LGG are more commonly diagnosed at a younger age, localized in the cerebral hemispheres (90% of cases), and do not take contrast enhancement on magnetic resonance imaging (MRI) in 75% of cases.[32] Older age (>40 years), larger tumor size, astrocytoma histology, tumor crossing midline, and partial surgical resection are negative prognostic factors. Patients with at least two of the aforementioned factors are considered "high-risk" and are treated with more aggressive post-surgical treatment strategies, such as RT and/or chemotherapy.[33,34]

Due to the low incidence of LGGs, there are little available data on treatment strategies of LGGs in elderly patients, and, in clinical practice, these patients are considered high-risk largely based on age.

In 2009, Schomas and colleagues retrospectively analyzed a cohort of 32 patients aged at least 55 years with WHO grade 2 LGG treated at Mayo Clinic. The authors evaluated outcome and efficacy of different treatment strategies, with particular attention to timing of postoperative RT. In this cohort, only one patient underwent a GTR without further treatment, and the frequency of oligodendrogliomas (better prognosis than astrocytomas) was low (9%). The authors found that LGGs in patients older than 55 years have a poorer prognosis (median OS of 2.7 years) than that of younger patients (median OS of 13 years). Thus, due to the worse outcome of LGG in older patients, especially in case of residual tumor after surgery, an aggressive approach consisting of early use of adjuvant therapy is strongly considered.[32]

> Given worse outcomes of LGG in older patients, especially in cases of residual tumor after surgery, an aggressive approach consisting of an early use of adjuvant therapy should be strongly considered.

Kaloshi and colleagues, in 2009, retrospectively evaluated the clinico-radiological characteristics and outcomes of 62 elderly (>60 years) patients with LGG compared with those of a cohort of younger patients. Elderly patients more often suffered from clinical deficit and had a lower performance status, a larger tumor on MRI, and a lower rate of tumor resection. Survival was shorter for elderly patients with 40% at 5 years compared to nearly 80% for the younger counterpart.[35]

Another retrospective study reviewed 20 patients aged 60 years or older treated at the University of Virginia[36] and found that median OS was 27.3 months and 6-, 12-, 24-, and 60-month OS were 75%, 70%, 55%, and 39%, respectively. This could suggest that in older patients with LGG, those who survive beyond the first 6 months could show longer PFS and OS similar to younger patients.

Overall, the great challenge for the future is to define histopathological, molecular, and clinical characteristics that subdivide elderly LGG patients into specific prognostic subgroups and then develop individualized treatment strategies based on patient risk stratification.

PRIMARY CENTRAL NERVOUS SYSTEM LYMPHOMAS

Primary central nervous system lymphomas (PCNSL) are a subtype of non-Hodgkin lymphomas, mostly of B-cell origin, confined to the CNS (Figure 30.3). The incidence of PCNSL in immunocompetent patients has been increasing in the past 30 years.[37] Patients older than 60 years account for almost 50% of patients with PCNSL, and, although the majority are able to tolerate aggressive therapeutic strategies, they have a worse prognosis and often suffer more from side effects of treatment in comparison to their younger counterparts. Thus, treatment decisions for the elderly with PCNSL need to be tailored to the individual, based on careful clinico-radiological evaluation of individual patient characteristics.[38]

> Patients older than 60 years account for almost 50% of patients with PCNSL, and, although the majority are able to tolerate aggressive therapeutic strategies, they have a worse prognosis and often suffer more from side effects of treatment in comparison to their younger counterparts.

The worse prognosis of PCNSL in elderly patients could be partly related to specific biological characteristics of the tumor, which may contribute to resistance to treatment. Recent studies have reported that the frequency of MYD88 in elderly PCNSL patients is higher compared to DLBCL (38–86% versus 15–30%), and this mutation may indicate poor prognosis in comparison to the wildtype counterpart (OS 11.4 vs. 56.2 months).[39]

PCNSL can be very responsive to steroids, with partial or complete tumor regression. Thus, in the clinico-radiological suspicion of a PCNSL (e.g., progressive cognitive deterioration with multiple homogeneously enhancing lesions in basal ganglia or corpus callosum) steroids should be avoided before biopsy is performed due to the risk of non-diagnostic histological findings. Tumor resection is not therapeutically beneficial in patients with PCNSL. Treatment of PCNSL has significantly changed during the past several decades (Table 30.1). A once common initial treatment for newly diagnosed PCNSL in elderly patients was whole-brain RT (WBRT) that induced a high rate of complete or partial responses and a median OS of 7.6 months. However, WBRT caused significant neurotoxicity (neurocognitive dysfunctions until dementia, leukoencephalopathy on MRI, with ataxia and urinary incontinence) in 19–83% of patients older than 60 years.[40,41]

In attempt to reduce neurotoxicity, Abrey and colleagues conducted a trial evaluating the efficacy of high-dose methotrexate (MTX) chemotherapy alone versus combination RT and high-dose MTX.[40] The authors reported that patients had a similar median OS with or without the RT (32 vs. 33 months), but neurotoxicity was significantly more common in patients who received RT, which held true among the elderly patients included in the trial. With the same aim of reducing

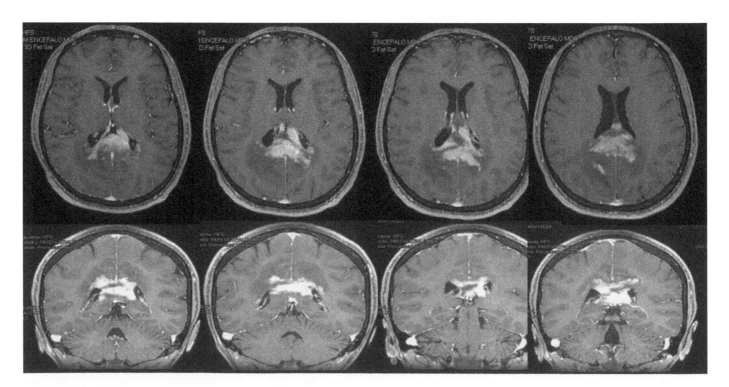

Figure 30.3 MRI of an 80-year-old woman with primary central nervous system lymphoma (PCNSL) showing homogeneously enhancing lesion involving corpus callosum.

STUDY	NO.	MEDIAN AGE (YRS)	REGIMEN	RR (%)	MPFS (MONTHS)	MOS (MONTHS)	NEUROTOXICITY (%)
Nelson et al., 1992	27	>60	WBRT (40 Gy) plus boost to tumor (20 Gy)	NA	NA	7.6	NA
Roth et al., 1998	12	>70	MTX (4 g/m²), ifosfamide plus WBRT (45 Gy)	75	24.1	29.3	NA
Abrey et al., 2000	12	67	MTX (3.5 g/m²) plus IT MTX, PCB, VCR plus WBRT (45 Gy)	NA	NA	32	83
Hoang-xuan et al., 2003	50	72	MTX, CCNU, procarbazine, prednisolone. MTX and IT cytarabine	48	10.6	14.3	NA
Gavrilovic et al., 2006	12	>60	MTX (3.5 g/m²) plus IT MTX, PCB, VCR plus WBRT (45 Gy)	-	NR	29	75
Omuro et al., 2007	23	68	MTX, TMZ	55	8	35	NA
Illerhaus et al., 2009	30	70	MTX, CCNU, procarbazine	68	5.9	15.4	NA
Fritsch et al., 2011	28	76	MTX, CCNU, procarbazine, rituximab	82	16	17.5	NA
Roth et al., 2012	126	73	MTX, ifosfamide, +/− WBRT	44	4	12.5	NA
Omuro et al., 2013	95	73	MTX, PCB, VCR and cytarabine Vs. MTX and TMZ	88 65	9.5 6.1	31 14	NA NA

RR, response rate; mPFS, median progression-free survival; mOS, median overall survival; NA, not available; IT, intrathecally administered; MTX, methotrexate; PCB, procarbazine; VCR, vincristine; WBRT, whole-brain radiotherapy.

neurotoxicity, the use of reduced doses of WBRT or local RT have been investigated to decrease neurologic side effects while maintaining efficacy.[42–44] A phase II Radiation Therapy Oncology Group (RTOG) multicenter trial compared the efficacy and safety of a hyperfractionated schedule of WBRT (36 Gy in 30 treatments) with standard course WBRT (45 Gy in 25 treatments) in PCNSL patients: both regimens achieved similar disease control, but the hyperfractionated regimen resulted in a delay (though not avoidance) of neurotoxicity.[42,43]

The adverse effects of RT in elderly patients resulted in the standard current practice of avoiding RT and administering chemotherapy alone as the first-line treatment for PCNSL patients older than 65 years. Many studies have shown the efficacy of a MTX-based regimen, achieving 30–79% of complete responses and OS of 14–50 months regardless of age.[45] MTX, when administered to elderly patients, often requires dose adjustments due to altered renal function. However, MTX dose adjustments do not reduce the efficacy of treatment when adjusted for renal function: two retrospective studies on PCNSL patients older than 70 treated with MTX adjusted for creatinine clearance showed 60% of complete responses and a mOS of 37 months.[46,47]

> MTX, when administered to elderly patients, often requires dose adjustments (reductions) due to altered renal function; however, these dose adjustments do not reduce the efficacy of treatment.

The necessity of MTX dose reductions in many elderly patients led to the evaluation of the safety and efficacy of other chemotherapy agents used in combination with MTX.[48] In one randomized phase II trial, the addition of cytarabine to MTX was studied. Complete remission rate was 18% in patients receiving MTX alone and 46% in patients receiving the combination. The dose intensity of MTX in this study was lower, as it was administered every 3 weeks instead of the usual 2 weeks.[48]

MTX in combination with procarbazine and vincristine in elderly patients (even older than 80 years) has shown encouraging tumor responses and outcomes, with an objective response rate of 62% and a median OS of 7.9 months.[49]

WBRT has also commonly been used as a consolidation treatment strategy after MTX-based therapy. The G-PCNSL-SG-1 trial demonstrated that the omission of WBRT does not negatively influence the OS of patients. In particular, the authors conducted a post-hoc analysis and divided the population into two groups by age, with a cutoff of 70 years. In the 126 patients older than 70, an acceptable profile of toxicity was shown with MTX, a lower response rate to chemotherapy, a lower efficacy of WBRT, and a higher risk of neurotoxicity in older compared to younger patients.

OS, PFS, and duration of complete response (CR) were significantly different between the two groups, with worse results in elderly patients. Overall, PCNSL should be considered as biologically different and more aggressive in elderly patients.[50]

Unfortunately, some elderly PCNSL patients cannot receive MTX due to severe comorbidities (creatinine clearance <50 mL/min), and the first-line treatment strategy remains unsolved. Kurzwelly and colleagues, in 2010, retrospectively analyzed 17 elderly patients who received TMZ as first-line therapy for PCNSL due to contraindications to MTX. Eight patients had a CR (47%), 1 a PR (6%), and other 8 showed progressive disease (PD) (47%). Five of 17 patients (29%) maintain a response for more than 12 months, and mOS was 21 months. Patients with MGMT methylation had a greater benefit in terms of mOS (21 months) compared to those with unmethylated MGMT patients (mOS 9 months). As a result, TMZ appears to be a safe and efficacious first-line treatment for PCNSL elderly patients who cannot receive MTX.[51]

Novel treatment approaches have focused on the role of other chemotherapeutic agents or targeted drugs. Given the positivity for CD20 antigen in nearly 95% of patients with PCNSL, some studies have investigated the role of rituximab, a chimeric monoclonal antibody against the CD20 antigen. Although rituximab has poor penetration of the blood–brain barrier, some authors have reported a modest efficacy in the treatment of PCNSL in elderly patients[52]: in particular, the association with MTX-based regimens achieved a CR rate of 64% and a 3-year OS of 31%. Patients older than 80 years do not have benefit from this treatment.[53]

Once PCNSL relapses there are few available treatments as salvage. The utilization of rituximab in association with TMZ appears to be safe and efficacious, with a mOS of 14 months and a mPFS of 7 months.[54] Conflicting results were obtained by Nayak and colleagues, in 2013, who conducted a phase II trial evaluating the safety and efficacy of rituximab and TMZ in older patients (median age 63 years): mPFS was 7 weeks and the trial was prematurely closed after an interim analysis.[55]

In conclusion, PCNSL in elderly patients seems to be more aggressive and less responsive to standard treatment. Once relapsed, there are few therapeutic options. Future trials in this population of patients hopefully will improve our understanding of the optimal treatment. For more information regarding treatment of PCNSL, see Chapter 11.

CONCLUSION

The incidence of brain tumors in elderly patients has increased over the past few decades. New treatment strategies, guided by patient's comorbidities, performance status, and molecular characteristics of the tumor, have been studied and developed. Several important clinical trials in elderly patients with malignant glioma have been conducted and are now informing decision-making in daily clinical practice. Patients older than 60 years are now accounting for almost 50% of PCNSL. While PCNSL in the elderly maybe more aggressive and less responsive to standard therapy, these patients can be treated with high-dose MTX-based regimens using appropriate dose reduction paradigms, thus allowing for deferred RT and decreasing the risk of neurocognitive changes.

FLASHCARD

What are the main challenges in treatment of glioma in elderly patients?

1. Multiple comorbidities
2. Inability to undergo more extensive resection
3. Inability to tolerate more aggressive therapy
4. Overall low performance status

Negative molecular prognostic factors in older patients with GBM include:

1. IDH-wildtype
2. Lack of MGMT methylation
3. TP53 mutations
4. CDKN2A alterations

How do you assess patient's "fitness" for oncologic therapy?

By using standardized scales such as comprehensive geriatric assessment (CGA)

When should gross total resection be attempted in an elderly patient with glioma?

When the resection is anatomically feasible and the patient has good performance status and absence of comorbidities

Is advanced age alone an absolute contraindication to aggressive therapy for glioma?

No

A recent phase III study in elderly patients with GBM showed that:

Hypofractionated RT with concomitant/adjuvant TMZ was superior to hypofractionated RT alone in terms of prolonged overall survival and without worsening quality of life

Low-grade gliomas in elderly patients have what characteristics?

They are more aggressive and early use of adjuvant treatment is recommended in fit individuals

Possible therapy options for "non-fit" GBM patients could be:

1. Temozolomide alone for patients with MGMT promoter methylation
2. Hypofractionated radiotherapy alone for patients with lack of the MGMT methylation
3. Supportive care/hospice

Newly diagnosed primary CNS lymphoma in elderly patients is best treated with:	High-dose methotrexate-based regimen with appropriate dose adjustments
Should WBRT be given to all elderly patients with PCNSL who achieved complete response with chemotherapy?	No. WBRT should be deferred to decrease the risk of neurotoxicity
List chemotherapy drugs studied in PCNLS in elderly patients (other than MTX):	Temozolomide Rituximab
List newer agents being investigated in PCNSL:	Ibrutinib Lenalidomide
MTX dose adjustments (reductions) in elderly patients with PCNSL typically result in what outcome?	Preserved efficacy and improved safety of treatment

QUESTIONS

1. Does gross total resection (GTR) improve survival in glioblastoma (GBM) of the elderly?
   a. Yes
   b. No
   c. Yes, only in neurologically intact people
   d. Yes, in patients without significant comorbidities

2. Which is the optimal treatment for "fit" patients with glioblastoma in the elderly?
   a. Radiotherapy with concomitant and adjuvant temozolomide
   b. Radiotherapy and adjuvant temozolomide
   c. Temozolomide alone
   d. Radiotherapy alone

3. Which are the reasonable choices for radiotherapy in newly diagnosed glioblastoma of the elderly?
   a. Hypofractionated radiotherapy
   b. Standard fractionated radiotherapy
   c. Radiosurgery
   d. Both a and b

4. What is the value of MGMT promoter methylation in glioblastoma of the elderly?
   a. Prognostic
   b. Predictive of response to chemotherapy
   c. Predictive of response to radiotherapy
   d. Predictive of response to radiochemotherapy

5. Supportive care alone in glioblastoma of the elderly should be prescribed to
   a. Patients with comorbidities
   b. Patients with poor performance status (Karnofsky ≤50)
   c. Patients with MGMT unmethylated tumors
   d. Patients with biopsy alone

6. Radiotherapy alone in glioblastoma of the elderly should be preferentially prescribed to
   a. Patients with unmethylated MGMT
   b. Patients with methylated MGMT
   c. Patients with lower performance status (Karnofsky 60–70) and comorbidities
   d. Patients with lower performance status (Karnofsky 60–70), comorbidities, and MGMT unmethylated tumors

7. Chemotherapy alone in glioblastoma of the elderly should be preferentially prescribed to
   a. Patients with MGMT unmethylated tumors
   b. Patients with MGMT methylated tumors
   c. Patients with lower performance status (Karnofsky 60–70) and comorbidities
   d. Patients with lower performance status (Karnofsky 60–70), comorbidities, and MGMT methylated tumors

8. Low-grade gliomas in elderly
   a. Are uncommon
   b. Can behave more aggressively
   c. Are the most common glioma type
   d. Both a and b

9. Elderly patients with low-grade gliomas are characterized by
   a. Progressive neurological deficits
   b. Larger tumor size on MRI
   c. Lower rate of complete resection
   d. All of the above

10. Following incomplete resection, elderly patients with low-grade glioma should receive:
    a. The same treatment as younger patients if they can tolerate it
    b. Radiotherapy alone
    c. Chemotherapy alone
    d. Palliative care

11. Overall, the prognosis of low-grade gliomas in elderly compared to younger patients
    a. Is better
    b. Is poorer
    c. Is the same
    d. Depends on individual prognostic factors

12. Which factors in PCNSL of elderly are associated with a risk of poor prognosis?
    a. Progressive neurological deficit
    b. Cerebrospinal fluid (CSF) involvement
    c. Multiple comorbidities
    d. All of the above

13. What is the optimal treatment of PCNSL in the elderly?
    a. Methotrexate-based up-front chemotherapy and consolidation WBRT regardless of response to chemotherapy
    b. Up-front methotrexate-based chemotherapy without consolidation WBRT in complete responders to chemotherapy
    c. WBRT alone
    d. WBRT followed by methotrexate-based chemotherapy

14. What is the optimal chemotherapy regimen in PCNSL of the elderly?
    a. Still unclear
    b. Methotrexate alone
    c. Methotrexate + rituximab
    d. Methotrexate + systemic poly-chemotherapy

15. The risk of neurocognitive deficits in elderly patients with PCSNL is higher with
    a. WBRT alone
    b. Methotrexate alone
    c. Methotrexate followed by WBRT
    d. Methotrexate + rituximab

ANSWERS

1. d
2. a
3. a
4. b
5. b
6. d
7. d
8. d
9. d
10. a
11. d
12. d
13. b
14. a
15. c

REFERENCES

1. Singh S, Bajorek B. Defining "elderly" in clinical practice guidelines for pharmacotherapy. *Pharm Pract (Granada)*. 2014 Oct;12(4):489.
2. Delafuente JC. The silver tsunami is coming: Will pharmacy be swept away with the tide? *Am J Pharm Educ*. 2009;73:1.
3. Gállego Pérez-Larraya, Delattre JY. Management of elderly patients with gliomas. *Oncologist*. 2014 Dec;19(12):1258–1267.
4. Lombardi G, Bergo E, Caccese M. Validation of the comprehensive geriatric assessment as a predictor of mortality in elderly glioblastoma patients. *Cancers (Basel)*. 2019 Oct 9;11(10):1–12.
5. Pruitt AA. Medical management of patients with brain tumors. *Curr Treat Options Neurol*. 2011;13:413–426.
6. Vuorinen V, Hinkka S, Farkkila M, Jaaskelainen J. Debulking or biopsy of malignant glioma in elderly people: A randomised study. *Acta Neurochir (Wien)*. 2003;145:5–10.
7. Dolecek TA, Propp JM, Stroup NE, Kruchko C. CBTRUS statistical report: Primary brain and central nervous system tumors diagnosed in the United States in 2005–2009. *Neuro-Oncol*. 2012 Nov;14(Suppl 5):v1–v49.
8. Lorimer CF, Saran F, Chalmers AJ, Brock J. Glioblastoma in the elderly: How do we choose who to treat? *J Geriatr Oncol*. 2016 Nov;7(6):453–456.
9. Mohile SG, Dale W, Somerfield MR. Practical assessment and management of vulnerabilities in older patients receiving chemotherapy: ASCO Guideline for Geriatric Oncology. *J Clin Oncol*. 2018 Aug 1;36(22):2326–2347.
10. Owusu C, Koroukian SM, Schluchter M, et al. Screening older cancer patients for a comprehensive geriatric assessment: A comparison of three instruments. *Geriatr Oncol*. 2011 Apr;2(2):121–129.
11. Batchelor TT, Betensky RA, Esposito JM. Age-dependent prognostic effects of genetic alterations in glioblastoma. *Clin Cancer Res*. 2004 Jan 1;10(1 Pt 1):228–233.
12. Simmons ML, Lamborn KR, Takahashi M. Analysis of complex relationships between age, p53, epidermal growth factor receptor, and survival in glioblastoma patients. *Cancer Res*. 2001 Feb 1;61(3):1122–1128.
13. Kleinschmidt-DeMasters BK, Lillehei KO, Varella-Garcia M. Glioblastomas in the older old. *Arch Pathol Lab Med*. 2005 May;129(5):624–631.
14. Arita H, Yamasaki K, Matsushita Y, et al. A combination of TERT promoter mutation and MGMT methylation status predicts clinically relevant subgroups of newly diagnosed glioblastomas. *Acta Neuropathol Commun*. 2016 Aug 8;4(1):79.
15. Lee Y, Scheck AC, Cloughesy TF, et al. Gene expression analysis of glioblastomas identifies the major molecular basis for the prognostic benefit of younger age. *BMC Med Genomics*. 2008;1:52.
16. Hegi M, Stupp R. In search of molecular markers of glioma in elderly patients. *Nat Rev Neurol*. 2013;9:424–425.
17. Stupp R, Mason WP, van den Bent MJ, et al. Radiotherapy plus concomitant and adjuvant temozolomide for glioblastoma. *N Engl J Med*. 2005 Mar 10;352(10):987–996.
18. Marko NF, Weil RJ, Schroeder JL, et al. Extent of resection of glioblastoma revisited: Personalized survival modeling facilitates more accurate survival prediction and supports a maximum-safe-resection approach to surgery. *J Clin Oncol*. 2014 Mar 10;32(8):774–782.
19. Ewelt C, Goeppert M, Rapp M, et al. Glioblastoma multiforme of the elderly: The prognostic effect of resection on survival. *J Neurooncol*. 2011 Jul;103(3):611–618.
20. Wick W, Platten M, Meisner C, et al. Temozolomide chemotherapy alone versus radiotherapy alone for malignant astrocytoma in the elderly: The NOA-08 randomised, phase 3 trial. NOA-08 Study Group of Neuro-oncology Working Group (NOA) of German Cancer Society. *Lancet Oncol*. 2012 Jul;13(7):707–715.
21. Kellermann SG, Hamisch CA, Rueß D, et al. Stereotactic biopsy in elderly patients: Risk assessment and impact on treatment decision. *J Neurooncol*. 2017 Sep;134(2):303–307.
22. Keime-Guibert F, Chinot O, Taillandier L, et al. Radiotherapy for glioblastoma in the elderly. Association of French-Speaking Neuro-Oncologists. *N Engl J Med*. 2007 Apr 12;356(15):1527–1535.
23. Roa W, Brasher PM, Bauman G, et al. Abbreviated course of radiation therapy in older patients with glioblastoma multiforme: A prospective randomized clinical trial. *J Clin Oncol*. 2004 May 1;22(9):1583–1588.
24. Gállego Pérez-Larraya J, Ducray F, et al. Temozolomide in elderly patients with newly diagnosed glioblastoma and poor performance status: An ANOCEF phase II trial. *J Clin Oncol*. 2011 Aug 1;29(22):3050–3055.
25. Malmström A, Grønberg BH, Marosi C, et al. Temozolomide versus standard 6-week radiotherapy versus hypofractionated radiotherapy in patients older than 60 years with glioblastoma: The Nordic randomised, phase 3 trial. Nordic Clinical Brain Tumour Study Group (NCBTSG). *Lancet Oncol*. 2012 Sep;13(9):916–926.
26. Minniti G, Lanzetta G, Scaringi C, et al. Phase II study of short-course radiotherapy plus concomitant and adjuvant temozolomide in elderly patients with glioblastoma. *Int J Radiat Oncol Biol Phys*. 2012 May 1;83(1):93–99.
27. Perry JR, Laperriere N, O'Callaghan CJ, et al. Short-course radiation plus temozolomide in elderly patients with glioblastoma. *N Engl J Med*. 2017 Mar 16;376(11):1027–1037.
28. Yin AA, Cai S, Dong Y, et al. A meta-analysis of temozolomide versus radiotherapy in elderly glioblastoma patients. *J Neurooncol*. 2014 Jan;116(2):315–324.
29. Lombardi G, Pace A, Pasqualetti, et al. Predictors of survival and effect of short (40 Gy) or standard-course (60 Gy) irradiation plus concomitant temozolomide in elderly patients with glioblastoma: A multicenter retrospective study of AINO (Italian Association of Neuro-Oncology). *J Neurooncol*. 2015 Nov;125(2):359–367.
30. Hanna C, Lawrie TA, Rogozińska E, et al. Treatment of newly diagnosed glioblastoma in the elderly: A network meta-analysis. *Cochrane Database Syst Rev*. 2020;(3):CD013261.
31. Kumthekar P, Patel V, Bridge C, et al. Prognosis of older patients with low-grade glioma: A retrospective study. *Integr Cancer Sci Therap*. 2017;4:5. doi:10.15761/icst.1000255
32. Schomas DA, Issa Laack NN, Rao R, et al. Intracranial low-grade gliomas in adults: 30-Year experience with long-term follow-up at Mayo Clinic. *Neuro-Oncology*. 2009;11(4):437–445.
33. Shaw E, Arusell R, Scheithauer B, et al. Prospective randomized trial of low- versus high-dose radiation therapy in adults with supratentorial low-grade glioma: Initial report of a North Central Cancer Treatment Group/ Radiation Therapy Oncology Group/Eastern Cooperative Oncology Group study. *J Clin Oncol*. 2002 May 1;20(9):2267–2276.
34. Daniels TB, Brown PD, et al. Validation of EORTC Prognostic Factors for Adults With Low-Grade Glioma: A Report Using Intergroup 86-72-51 Oral presentation at the 48th Annual Meeting of the American Society for Therapeutic Radiology and Oncology. Philadelphia, PA, Nov 8, 2006, and the 11th Annual Meeting of Society for Neuro-Oncology, Orlando, FL, Nov 19, 2006.
35. Kaloshi G, Psimaras D, Mokhtari K, et al. Supratentorial low-grade gliomas in older patients. *Neurology*. 2009 Dec 15;73(24):2093–2098. doi:10.1212/WNL.0b013e3181c6781e. PMID: 19907009.

36. Pouratian N, Mut M, Jagannathan J, et al. Low-grade gliomas in older patients: A retrospective analysis of prognostic factors. *J Neurooncol.* 2008;90:341.

37. Haldorsen IS, O'Neill BP. Epidemiology of primary central nervous system lymphoma. In Batchelor T, DeAngelis LM, eds. *Lymphoma and Leukemia of the Nervous System.* New York: Springer; 2012:89–97.

38. Roth P, Hoang-Xuan K. Challenges in the treatment of elderly patients with primary central nervous system lymphoma. *Curr Opin Neurol.* 2014 Dec;27(6):697–701.

39. Takano S, Hattori K, Ishikawa E, et al. MyD88 mutation in elderly predicts poor prognosis in primary central nervous system lymphoma: Multi-institutional analysis. *World Neurosurg.* 2018 Apr;112:e69–e73.

40. Omuro AM, Ben-Porat LS, Panageas KS, et al. Delayed neurotoxicity in primary central nervous system lymphoma. *Arch Neurol.* 2005 Oct;62(10):1595–600.

41. Correa DD1, Shi W, Abrey LE, et al. Cognitive functions in primary CNS lymphoma after single or combined modality regimens. *Neuro-Oncol.* 2012 Jan;14(1):101–108.

42. DeAngelis LM, Seiferheld W, Schold SC, et al. Combination chemotherapy and radiotherapy for primary central nervous system lymphoma: Radiation Therapy Oncology Group Study 93-10. *J Clin Oncol.* 2002 Dec 15;20(24):4643–4638.

43. Fisher B1, Seiferheld W, Schultz C, et al. Secondary analysis of Radiation Therapy Oncology Group study (RTOG) 9310: An intergroup phase II combined modality treatment of primary central nervous system lymphoma. *J Neurooncol.* 2005 Sep;74(2):201–205.

44. Shah GD, Yahalom J, Correa DD, et al. Combined immunochemotherapy with reduced whole-brain radiotherapy for newly diagnosed primary CNS lymphoma. *J Clin Oncol.* 2007 Oct 20;25(30):4730–4735.

45. Herrlinger U, Schabet M, Brugger W, et al. German Cancer Society Neuro-Oncology Working Group NOA-03 multicenter trial of single-agent high-dose methotrexate for primary central nervous system lymphoma. *Ann Neurol.* 2002;51:247–252.

46. Ng S, Rosenthal MA, Ashley D, Cher L. High-dose methotrexate for primary CNS lymphoma in the elderly. *Neuro-Oncol.* 2000;2(1):40–44. doi:10.1093/neuonc/2.1.40

47. Zhu JJ, Gerstner ER, et al. High-dose methotrexate for elderly patients with primary CNS lymphoma. *Neuro-Oncol.* Apr 2009;11(2):211–215.

48. Ferreri AJ, Reni M, Foppoli M, et al. High-dose cytarabine plus high-dose methotrexate versus high-dose methotrexate alone in patients with primary CNS lymphoma: A randomised phase 2 trial. *Lancet.* 2009 Oct 31;374(9700):1512–1520. doi:10.1016/S0140-6736(09)61416-1

49. Welch MR, Omuro A, Deangelis LM. Outcomes of the oldest patients with primary CNS lymphoma treated at Memorial Sloan-Kettering Cancer Center. *Neuro-Oncol.* 2012 Oct;14(10):1304–1311.

50. Roth P, Martus P, Kiewe P, et al. Outcome of elderly patients with primary CNS lymphoma in the G-PCNSL-SG-1 trial. *Neurology.* 2012 Aug 28;79(9):890–896. doi:10.1212/WNL.0b013e318266fcb2

51. Kurzwelly D, Glas M, Roth P, et al. Primary CNS lymphoma in the elderly: Temozolomide therapy and MGMT status. *J Neurooncol.* 2010 May;97(3):389–392.

52. Ruhstaller TW, Amsler U, Cerny T. Rituximab: Active treatment of central nervous system involvement by non-Hodgkin's lymphoma? *Ann Oncol.* 2000 Mar;11(3):374–375.

53. Fritsch K, Kasenda B, Hader C, et al. Immunochemotherapy with rituximab, methotrexate, procarbazine, and lomustine for primary CNS lymphoma (PCNSL) in the elderly. *Ann Oncol.* 2011 Sep;22(9):2080–2085.

54. Enting RH1, Demopoulos A, DeAngelis LM, Abrey LE. Salvage therapy for primary CNS lymphoma with a combination of rituximab and temozolomide. *Neurology.* 2004 Sep 14;63(5):901–903.

55. Nayak L, Abrey LE, Drappatz J. Multicenter phase II study of rituximab and temozolomide in recurrent primary central nervous system lymphoma. *Leuk Lymphoma.* 2013 Jan;54(1):58–61.

31 | PALLIATIVE CARE, REHABILITATION, AND SUPPORTIVE CARE IN NEURO-ONCOLOGY

JAMAL MOHAMUD AND KATHRYN S. NEVEL

INTRODUCTION

Neuro-oncological conditions include a wide array of disease processes involving central nervous system (CNS) neoplastic lesions arising from primary or metastatic sources. Current epidemiological data note greater than 50,000 new yearly primary CNS neoplastic diagnoses within the United States, with an incidence rate of nearly 29 cases per 100,000 persons worldwide.[1-3] These conditions carry a varying degree of mortality and associated symptoms. General survivorship rates differ dramatically in CNS tumor subtypes, with median survival between 12 and 20.9 months among patients with glioblastoma,[4,5] less than 6 months in multilesion CNS metastatic disease,[6] and as little as 1–2 months in instances of leptomeningeal disease without treatment.[7] Individuals with newly diagnosed neuro-oncological conditions face a myriad of difficult choices in terms of treatment, management, and acceptance due to an understanding that the diagnosis itself usually carries a poor prognosis with limited survivability.[8] As such, this chapter focuses on the role of palliative care in the overall treatment of patients with these conditions, the common symptoms and challenges they face throughout their illness, and end-of-life care.

> Individuals with newly diagnosed neuro-oncological conditions face a myriad of difficult choices in terms of treatment, management, and acceptance due to an understanding that the diagnosis itself usually carries a poor prognosis with limited survivability.

PALLIATIVE CARE

The role of palliative care in neuro-oncology includes patient–provider discussions on disease prognosis, establishing patient goals of care including end-of-life (EOL) care, and mitigation of symptoms affecting patients to improve quality of life without improper prolongation of suffering in patients with severe, debilitating life-limiting conditions. Advance planning in EOL care should be introduced early in the disease course and management of patients with brain tumors, and proactive discussions with all involved parties has been shown to lead to better EOL care among patients.[9-11] This is of vital importance because these patients are more susceptible to cognitive impairment and delirium that results in decreased decision-making capacity toward the end of life and may ultimately limit their ability to participate in decisions about their care.[12] Regrettably, a significant number of these patients fail to receive any form of palliative care, education, or referral until significantly late in the disease course, often in the final days to weeks of their life.[13,14] Failure to initiate palliative care measures early on allows for greater risk of suffering due to unmanaged or undermanaged progression of symptom burden, unnecessary or unwanted inpatient hospitalization/s, and diminished quality of life.[15]

> Advance planning in EOL care should be introduced early in the disease course and management of patients with brain tumors, and proactive discussions with all involved parties has been shown to lead to better EOL care among patients.

A comprehensive palliative care team consists of a multidisciplinary collection of physician and non-physician specialists and, depending on patient needs, can include the primary provider (neurologist, oncologist, neuro-oncologist), other members of the treatment team (surgical, radiation, chemotherapy), pain management specialists, social workers and psychiatrists, physical and occupational therapists, dieticians, councillors, spiritual care specialists, and palliative care and home hospice providers.[15] This can occur in the inpatient hospital environment, the ambulatory outpatient clinic, or even in the patient's own home.[16] Palliative care should be differentiated from *hospice care*, which is defined as care following the cessation of life-extending treatment and can be provided when expected survival is less than 6 months.[17] Conversely, palliative care can start at any point from the onset of any chronic illness diagnosis, can cover the entire trajectory of the disease course, and does not exclude anti-tumor treatment.[18] The difference between hospice care and palliative care is often a source of confusion for both patients and their caregivers, as well as for some providers, which unfortunately can lead to decreased acceptance.

> Palliative care can start at any point from the onset of any chronic illness diagnosis, can cover the entire trajectory of the disease course, and does not exclude anti-tumor treatment.

One barrier to the use of palliative care appears to be from providers' own apprehension to initiate EOL discussions due to concerns of adversely impacting hopefulness or indicating a failure in therapy that would preclude further treatment. In a series of studies surveying neuro-oncology specialists managing a wide array of neoplastic conditions, nearly 30–45% of providers had expressed significant reservations in beginning EOL discussions with patients early on in their treatment course.[19] Furthermore, only 60% of providers indicated that they had referred patients to some form of palliative care, with 20% referring patients only once symptom burden became severe in the final weeks of life. However, a majority of brain tumor patients indicated greater satisfaction and lessened bereavement by family upon death when provided with comprehensive palliative care and advance care planning discussions early on in therapy.[20,21]

> A majority of brain tumor patients indicated greater satisfaction and lessened family bereavement upon death when provided with comprehensive palliative care and advance care planning discussions early on in therapy.

Patients, family members, and caregivers often experience significant psychosocial stressors throughout the patient's medical course on top of the physical and cognitive disabling sequelae associated with their disease process.[22] This includes psychological, social, familial, and financial hardships.[23] This is further compounded by behavioral changes and neurocognitive decline in patients which limits their ability to manage these situations and can lead to poorer outcomes in recovery and maintaining an optimal quality of life toward the EOL phase.[24] Organizational support systems both at the macro and micro levels have been shown to dramatically reduce instances of caregiver burnout, increase treatment compliance, and support a dignified death.[20,25,26] Addressing patient, caregiver, and provider misconceptions regarding palliative care and advance care planning may lead to greater utilization of palliative care practices, which in turn improve patient and caregiver quality of life.

SUPPORTIVE CARE OF SELECTED SYMPTOMS IN NEURO-ONCOLOGY

EPILEPSY

The prevalence of seizures in patients with primary intracranial neoplasms is elevated in comparison to similar disease-free population cohorts, and risk increases in patients with concomitant histories of epilepsy or episodes of status epilepticus.[27] Frequency and severity of seizures in patients with CNS neoplasms can vary based on tumor type and location, tumor markers, stage of therapy, or associated medical history.[28] Current literature indicates seizures occur in as many as 10% of patients with CNS lymphomas, 35% of patients with metastatic tumors, and 30–55% of patients with gliomas.[29] Patients are often on some form of steroid therapy which decreases intracerebral swelling and can reduce risk of seizure but can also increase risk of metabolic and electrolyte imbalances or CNS infections, which may potentially further predispose patients to epileptic events.[30] Seizures have significant impact on quality of life in this patient population, as epileptic events are the most frequent cause of inpatient admission for patients with CNS neoplasms.[31]

> Current literature indicates seizures occur in as many as 10% of patients with CNS lymphomas, 35% of patients with metastatic tumors, and 30–55% of patients with gliomas.

Current guidelines from the American Society of Clinical Oncology (ASCO) recommend against the use of anti-epileptic drugs (AEDs) for routine use of seizure prophylaxis in patients with metastatic CNS lesions. In patients with seizures with cerebral edema and mass effect, ASCO favors the administration of appropriate AEDs in addition to corticosteroids, namely dexamethasone, with dosages of 4–16 mg/day depending on severity.[32] Status epilepticus should be managed similarly to non-neoplastic patients, with prompt abortive therapies and, if needed, inpatient hospitalization. Evaluation with imaging in patients with worsening seizure frequency is indicated to rule out intracerebral hemorrhage or significant tumor progression. Similar management among patients with primary CNS neoplasms is generally accepted. It is common for patients with primary and metastatic lesions to be placed on prophylactic AED for 1–2 weeks after intracranial surgery for tumor resection, but these medications should be tapered off and not continued indefinitely as prophylaxis in a patient who has never had a seizure.

> In patients with seizures with cerebral edema and mass effect, ASCO favors the administration of appropriate AEDs in addition to corticosteroids, namely dexamethasone, with dosages of 4–16 mg/day depending on severity.

As patients near the EOL phase of the disease process, seizure frequency typically increases secondary to increasing tumor size and cerebral edema. Worsening dysphagia, limiting oral administration of antiepileptic medications, can also result in subtherapeutic levels of AED, resulting in increased seizure frequency.[27] Many antiepileptic medications are available or can be compounded into liquid formulations that may be easier for some patients to swallow, depending on their degree of dysphagia. Non-oral options for AED medications include intranasal, buccal, and rectal administration of agents such as midazolam, clonazepam, and diazepam.[33-35] Subcutaneous versions of phenobarbital and levetiracetam are also suitable alternatives but often difficult to obtain because they may not be kept on formulary. As seizures often increase in the final weeks of life, in general we do not recommend stopping AEDs at EOL. The decision to discontinue seizure medications due to concerns for side effects should only be considered in patients with presumed low risk of seizures (which is rare) and should be made in conjunction with the patient, caregiver, and palliative management team.

HEADACHE

Headache is a common complaint of patients with CNS neoplasms, occurring in up to 90% of patients, and it is often an early presenting symptom in undiagnosed patients.[36] The underlying causal factor of headache in brain tumor patients is often multifactorial and may be related to the tumor itself, edema, the associated therapy, and/or triggering of a primary headache syndrome. Elevation of intracranial pressure secondary to tumor burden or intracerebral edema, as well as localized meningeal inflammation, can lead to headaches.[37] Treatment-related factors include post-surgical scarring, radiation, and chemotherapy-related side effects. These headaches can manifest as a broad constellation of primary headache types including tension, migraine, and cluster symptoms, and they can occur with or without aura or associated nausea.

The management of tumor-related headache depends on underlying etiology. In patients with an associated mass effect or signs of increased intracranial pressure secondary to cerebral edema, corticosteroids should be administered. Dexamethasone is the preferred agent given its efficacy, longer half-life, and more limited mineralocorticoid activity.[38] Dosage should be titrated for maximal efficacy while minimizing associated side effects such as hyperglycemia, steroid-induced myopathy, and immunosuppression-related infections, which are often related to the dosage and duration of steroid use and may increase mortality in the EOL phase. Often proton pump inhibitors or histamine-2 blockers are prescribed when high-dose steroid therapy is prescribed to reduce the likelihood of gastritis and gastric ulceration, and antibiotic prophylaxis for Pneumocystis jiroveci should be prescribed depending on the steroid dose and expected duration.[39]

Dexamethasone dosage should be titrated for maximal efficacy while minimizing drug side effects such as hyperglycemia, steroid induced myopathy, and immunosuppression-related infections, which are often related to the dosage and duration of steroid use and may increase mortality and decrease quality of life in the EOL phase.

In patients with headaches in the absence of cerebral edema, a conservative approach toward pain management is indicated which mirrors standard therapy in non-oncology patients. Relatively infrequent mild to moderate headaches can be managed with non-steroidal anti-inflammatory drugs and over-the-counter analgesics.[40] Prolonged headaches with durations greater than 48 hours or occurring for a majority of days within a week should be treated as chronic and managed with both acute abortive therapies as well as daily prophylactic treatment to reduce symptom frequency. Consultation with headache and pain management specialist should be considered in severe non-relapsing migraine for possible procedural therapies including sensory nerve ablations, regional nerve blocks, and botulinum toxin injections. The use of opioids is indicated for severe and refractory headaches. The benefits of opioid-induced pain relief should be weighed against risks of worsening encephalopathy, autonomic instability, and respiratory depression.

NAUSEA

Nausea and vomiting are also common presenting symptoms that can lead to discovery of neuro-oncological lesions. Nausea can persist throughout the treatment phase of cancer therapy due to side effects of chemotherapy and radiation. Chemoreceptor triggers within the ventral tegmental region within the brainstem are particularly sensitive to chemotherapeutics. Increased intracranial pressure and/or localized cerebral edema can result in compression of vestibular and cerebellar regions of the nervous system that produces nausea and vomiting. Following the 2017 updated ASCO guidelines, management of nausea in patients with malignancies can include a 5-HT$_3$ receptor antagonist (ondansetron/palonosetron/dolasetron), corticosteroids (dexamethasone), or dopamine receptor antagonists (metoclopramide, olanzapine).[41] Sometimes benzodiazepines, such as lorazepam, are used to treat and prevent nausea, but their use must be weighed against the potential CNS depressive effects of this medication class. The role of newer antiemetic agents such as NK1-receptor antagonists (aprepitant/fosaprepitant) or CB1/CB2 receptor compounds (dronabinol) is not as well understood in the setting of CNS lesion-induced nausea, and further evaluation is required before formal recommendations on their use can be made. Worsening and refractory nausea despite escalating antinausea therapy should be further evaluated with imaging as a possible warning sign of disease progression.

The 2017 ASCO guidelines recommends that management of nausea in patients with malignancies can include a 5-HT$_3$ receptor antagonist (ondansetron/palonosetron/dolasetron), corticosteroids (dexamethasone), or dopamine receptor antagonists (metoclopramide, olanzapine).

FATIGUE

The overall mechanisms leading to fatigue in the setting of cancer and treatment is still poorly understood, although fatigue is reported in 25–90% of patients.[42] Current hypotheses include tumor- and treatment-related trauma inducing pro-inflammatory changes and cytokine release, disruption of auto-regulatory circadian sleep–wake rhythms, alteration in neuroendocrine functions which can be related to direct tumor invasion or chronic steroid use, neurological impairment from the tumor leading to physical inactivity, and cognitive decline.[43,44] Management strategies include both pharmacological and non-pharmacological therapies that, when used in combination, can improve quality of life metrics.[45] Pharmacotherapy with dopamine reuptake inhibitors has previously demonstrated improvements in alertness in limited cases for general cancer patients.[46,47] However, when examined more narrowly, individual agents such as modafinil failed to show superiority to placebo in improving fatigue in CNS cancer patients.[48] In a study of modafinil versus placebo in patients with primary brain tumors, no significant difference was found in validated fatigue and self-perceived cognitive functioning assessment scale scores. Further pharmacotherapy studies are needed to best elucidate targets of therapy for patients with brain tumors who have significant fatigue.

Conversely, studies have shown clinically significant improvement in self-reported fatigue symptoms in cancer patients who engage in physical therapy and exercise regimens, but study in the CNS malignancy population is lacking.[49] Comorbid conditions such as depression, hypothyroidism, chronic anemia, and metabolic and nutritional abnormalities such as B_{12} deficiencies can exacerbate cancer-related fatigue and should be evaluated for and addressed. Medication-induced fatigue should also be considered, as well as adrenal insufficiency in patients discontinuing long-term steroid therapy. Last, it is important to differentiate worsening fatigue from alterations in patient mentation, such as encephalopathy or worsening delirium, as both can occur at the EOL phase.[31]

> Comorbid conditions such as depression, hypothyroidism, chronic anemia, and metabolic and nutritional abnormalities such as B_{12} deficiencies can exacerbate cancer related fatigue and should be evaluated for and addressed.

DELIRIUM

Delirium and neurocognitive deterioration are common eventual complications in patient with neuro-oncological conditions, and these are noted to occur in as many as 70% of patients with primary brain tumors in the final weeks of life. This may manifest as somnolence, confusion, behavioral disturbances, impaired verbal fluency, and hyper-/hypomotor activity.[28] Treatment for altered mental status remains the same in brain tumor and non-oncological patients and includes correcting metabolic imbalances, removal of offending medications when possible, and minimizing environmental disturbances. These interventions have been shown to reverse delirium in about half of cases. Specific pharmacological therapies for the management of cognitive impairment are poorly studied in brain tumor patients and are not recommended, but some antipsychotic medications are used occasionally in cases of severe, agitated delirium.[50]

REHABILITATION IN NEURO-ONCOLOGY

As a direct consequence of tumor burden and tumor treatment interventions which often include surgery, radiation, and systemic chemotherapy, patients are prone to develop significant neuro-physical and cognitive deficits. While these impairments can vary, common neurological deficits include weakness (78% of cases), cognitive decline (80% of cases), and sensory impairment (50% of cases); a majority of patients develop multiple deficits.[51,52] A multidisciplinary rehabilitation approach that best identifies functional loss and targets acute therapy while maximizing long-term quality of life has been shown to have great benefit to non-CNS cancer patients. Unfortunately, compared to our understanding of rehabilitation in the setting of traumatic brain injury (TBI) or stroke, the role of neuro-rehabilitation in patients with CNS neoplasms is poorly understood and requires further investigation. The efficacy of rehabilitation appears to depend on factors such as the patient's age, disease burden, treatment, prognosis, pre-existing level of debility, and social support system.[53] These factors must be carefully considered when developing an individualized rehabilitation treatment plan for a patient with a neuro-oncologic condition.

EXERCISE

The benefits of exercise have been well-document throughout cancer literature, and exercise has been consistently shown to improve the overall functional outcomes in the general cancer patient population.[54,55] Specifically, increased daily activity in the immediate post-therapy phase of treatments has been associated with significant improvements in patient cardiopulmonary function, oxygen capacity, and reduction of muscle wasting.[56,57] This resulted in improvements in both long-term functional independence, quality of life metrics, and overall mortality in cancer patients who engaged in physical activity when compared to control populations.[58]

> Limited studies have suggested improvement in disability in glioma patients who are able to tolerate increased physical activity.

It would seem logical that physical activity would be especially beneficial in patients with CNS neoplasms, particularly given the compounded risk of generalized weakness and myopathy due to the chronic long-term use of corticosteroids that are often prescribed for management of intracerebral edema.[59] While limited studies have suggested improvement in disability in glioma patients who are able to tolerate increased physical activity,[60] larger long-term studies examining the possible benefits of exercise in glioma populations are still ongoing.[61]

REHABILITATION

Inpatient rehabilitation for patients with CNS malignancy is most common in the immediate post-surgical period and shortly after the completion of concurrent radiation and chemotherapy. A meta-analysis of 11 retrospective studies on the impact of rehab in brain tumor patients showed 36% of patients experienced a significant improvement in functional independence, with a median length of stay in rehab of 1.5 months.[62] Functional gains after inpatient rehabilitation in patients with primary CNS neoplasms in the postoperative period are similar compared to patients with other neurological conditions such as stroke or

TBI in a matched control study, so should be encouraged for all brain tumor patients who qualify.[63] However, as many as 35% of patients with neuro-oncologic conditions re-enter acute rehabilitation during their disease course, often due to functional decline related to the tumor or its treatment.[64] Likelihood of improvement with rehab in part depends on tumor type, size, and location; patients with meningioma appear to have the greatest gains, while patients with glioblastoma are less likely to experience significant functional improvement.[63]

> As many as 35% of patients with neuro-oncologic conditions re-enter acute rehabilitation during their disease course, often due to functional decline related to the tumor or its treatment.

Vocational studies have shown that individuals with CNS neoplasms have greater difficulty maintaining employment than patients with other cancer subtypes.[65,66] This is often due to the functional limitations caused by neurocognitive and physical impairment and side effects and the time requirements of tumor treatment. Unemployment leads to financial difficulty, which can impact treatment and monitoring compliance for these patients. The role of occupational therapy is of significant benefit in this population, leading to a better likelihood of a return to activities of daily living and higher levels of satisfaction toward the EOL phase.[67] Whether occupational therapy improves likelihood of return to work is unclear, however, and difficult to study due to variability in patient occupations, local work requirements, and workplace flexibility. Current examination of the long-term effect of this therapy is ongoing and requires further investigation.

Cancer-related dysphagia and aphasia account for significant symptom burden in patients with intracranial neoplasms.[68] Failure to address this early on may increase dysphagia-associated injury/illness and dependence on external feeding mechanisms.[69] Early assessment and treatment with speech therapy has been shown to decrease poor outcome and mortality in non-CNS cancer patients with associated speech and swallowing difficulties.[70] Though the current the literature primarily evaluates its role in post- stroke and non-CNS cancer patients, it is reasonable to extend these findings to CNS neoplastic-induced causes of oral pharyngeal dysfunction and the benefit of speech therapy in their management.

END-OF-LIFE CARE

Patients within 3 months of death enter into what is referred to as the "end-of-life phase" of their disease.[71] This period presents with its own multitude of symptoms and special considerations for disease and symptom management. The focus of providers during this period should be to reduce distress; identify, honor, and respect patient preferences and choices; and ensure patients the opportunity for a dignified death. A "dignified death" is defined as one which occurs in accordance with a patient's preferred wishes and beliefs, treatment decisions are congruent with goals of care, and transpires within the preferred setting of the patient and their family.[72,73] A key factor

in providing EOL care is the presence of an advance care directive, which should clearly communicate patient wishes on which actions or levels of intervention they would want toward EOL.[74] An advance care directive should be established early on in the disease course because these patients are more susceptible to neurologic impairments as their disease progresses, which may limit their ability to communicate and their decision-making capacity.

> Patients within 3 months of death enter into what is referred to as the "end-of-life phase" of their disease.

Dysphagia is one of the most common and severely limiting symptoms in EOL, occurring in up to 85% of cases toward the final weeks of life.[75] Consequences of dysphagia include nutritional insufficiency, dehydration, failure to thrive, and aspiration-induced respiratory compromise.[76] Medication compliance can be impacted due to loss of oral access, prompting symptom exacerbation which increases hospitalization rates and medical complications. Thus, alternate routes of essential medications (buccal, rectal, intravenous, or intranasal) must be planned for in patients nearing the EOL phase to avoid pain, nausea, seizures, and other common distressing symptoms.

In cases of severe malnutrition secondary to dysphagia, enteral nutritional supplementation is sometimes pursued early on in the disease course as a means to prolong survival. Patients with CNS malignancies have a greater risk of having a structural, permanent etiology to their dysphagia and, as such, are unlikely to return to nutritional independence once tube feeding is initiated.[77] Based on study from other cancer types, potential reasonable candidates for initiating artificial nutrition include malnourished patients with otherwise good functional status who are receiving anti-cancer therapy, but who are unable to tolerate oral intake for adequate nutrition for greater than 1–2 weeks with reasonable likelihood of regaining nutritional independence, with a goal of maintaining a body mass index (BMI) of greater than 18.5 kg/m^2.[78] In one study of head and neck cancer patients, the method of enteral feeding (nasogastric tube vs. percutaneous endoscopic gastrostomy) had no effect on the patient's level of satisfaction, were equally distressing, and resulted in greater dissatisfaction at the EOL when compared to continued oral intake (often called "feed for comfort") in patients with dysphagia.[79] In general, enteral feeding is uncommonly initiated among patients with advanced-stage disease in or nearing the EOL phase. In advanced terminal disease in patients with enteral feeding already established, there is little known benefit to quality of life in continuing enteral feeding. Decisions to discontinue enteral feeding in such cases must be made in conjunction with patients' advance care directives.

> Patients with CNS malignancies have greater risk of a structural, permanent etiology of their dysphagia and, as such, are unlikely to return to nutritional independence once tube feeding is initiated.

During the EOL phase, patients often lose the ability to communicate their desired wishes for their ongoing medical care, and decisions often fall to the discretion of the caregiver(s) and/or provider. It is essential that patients and their caregivers define future goals of care during advance care planning, early on in their treatment and with their physician, to proactively address expected complications in care. Decisions in disease-related illness treatment and comfort measures should remain congruent with pre-stated goals of care. Inappropriate escalation of treatment may cause undue harm to patients, such as repeated inpatient admission for symptom management, prolonged and futile cancer treatment, and a lack of access to timely hospice medical care.[20] This has been shown to decrease patient and caregiver satisfaction of care in the final days and postmortem period.[80]

> It is essential that patients and their caregivers define future goals of care during advance care planning, early on in their treatment and with their physician, to proactively address expected complications in care.

CONCLUSION

The topic of palliative care in the setting of a patient with neuro-oncologic conditions is multifaceted, requiring the input of multiple parties including the patient, the caregiver or support team, the physician and treatment team, and rehabilitation services. It is beneficial to initiate the conversation surrounding palliative care and EOL goals early in the disease course, in order to maintain clear conversations on patient goals prior to the decline and loss of decision-making capacity. Supportive care and management of the patient's disease-specific symptoms becomes increasingly more important as the disease burden develops and worsens over time and as it limits the patient's ability to actively engage in their own care. Headaches, nausea, seizures, and fatigue are all common symptoms throughout the disease process that can be best managed with a multitude of pharmacological and non-pharmacological interventions (Table 31.1). Patients with CNS neoplasms are at a greater risk for developing long-term disability due to either the disease burden of the tumor itself or from the neurotoxic effects of aggressive chemotherapy,

TABLE 31.1 Symptom management and therapies in patients with central nervous system (CNS) malignancies, including the end-of-life (EOL) phase

SYMPTOM	MANAGEMENT
Epilepsy	Continue home AED regimen Dexamethasone for breakthrough seizures in patients with cerebral edema, with dosage dependent on severity[32] *Non-oral options for AED medications* – Intranasal midazolam – Buccal clonazepam – Rectal diazepam[33–35]
Headache	*Secondary to mass effect/increased ICP/cerebral edema* – Corticosteroids (dexamethasone)[38] *Headaches in the absence of cerebral edema* – Non-steroidal anti-inflammatory drugs – Over-the-counter analgesics[40] *Prolonged (>48 hours) or frequent (more than 2 per week) headache:* – Acute abortive therapies – Daily prophylactics – Procedural therapies: Sensory nerve ablations, regional nerve blocks, botulinum toxin *Severe and refractory headaches* – Opioid analgesics
Nausea	5-HT$_3$ receptor antagonist (ondansetron/palonosetron/dolasetron) Dopamine receptor antagonists (metoclopramide, olanzapine)[41] Corticosteroids (dexamethasone) *Newer antiemetic agents* – NK1-receptor antagonists (aprepitant/fosaprepitant) – CB1/CB2 receptor compounds (dronabinol)
Fatigue	*Pharmacological* Dopamine reuptake inhibitors can be considered[46,47] *Non-pharmacological therapies* Address comorbid conditions: Depression, hypothyroidism, chronic anemia, metabolic/nutritional abnormalities Medication-induced fatigue (evaluate potential contributing medications)
Delirium	Correction of metabolic imbalances Removal of offending medications Minimization environmental disturbance Specific anti-delirium pharmacological therapies are not recommended, but such medications can be used in cases of agitated delirium[50]

radiation therapy, and surgical resection. Rehabilitation plays a significant role in the overall treatment of patients with brain tumors. In small, limited studies, patients who undergo aggressive inpatient rehabilitation immediately along with psychosocial support groups after therapy have been shown to have improved quality of life metrics and better overall function within the acute period when compared to non-rehabilitation cohorts. However, current literature is limited and often does not include neuro-oncologic disease-specific outcomes in response to rehabilitation; this warrants further investigation. As patients enter into the EOL phase, the goals of their care should be oriented toward reducing symptoms while maximizing quality of life with loved ones, ultimately moving toward a dignified death.

What are the goals of palliative care in brain cancer patients?	Improvement of quality of life, reduction of symptom burden, and prevention of suffering
Providers as part of the palliative care team can include:	Neuro-oncologist, palliative care specialist, physical medicine and rehab, other members of rehabilitation team, social work, case management, pain management, and others
It is important for the provider to establish this with the patient early in the disease course, so that as disease progresses and the patient may be unable to participate in decision-making discussions, wishes are already discussed and known	Goals of care/treatment and advance care planning, including advance directive and health care proxy, and wishes in EOL phase
These two often are mistaken as being the same thing by patients and occasionally by some medical professionals	Hospice and palliative care
What is the most common event requiring acute level care, hospital admission, and management in patients with brain tumors?	Seizures
In addition to antiepileptics, this class of medications should be given to patients with brain tumors with edema and breakthrough seizures.	Corticosteroids
What class of drugs can be considered for pharmacotherapy management of fatigue, although not yet shown to be definitely efficacious in patients with brain tumors?	Dopamine reuptake inhibitors
What percentage of patients go to inpatient rehab more than once due to functional decline?	Up to 35%
The end-of-life phase occurs during what time frame in a patient's disease course?	Within 3 months of death

QUESTIONS

1. A 48-year-old patient presents with a new diagnosis of a glioblastoma. At what point should an advance goals and directives discussion occur between the patient, caregiver, and physician?
   a. At 12 months into the patient's diagnosis
   b. At time of second progression
   c. When patient is in the end-of-life phase
   d. Early in diagnosis and treatment discussions

2. What team members can be part of the palliative care team caring for a patient?
   a. Neuro-oncology physician
   b. Physical therapist
   c. Palliative care physician
   d. Social worker
   e. Both a and c
   f. All of the above

3. Fatigue is common in patients with neuro-oncologic conditions
   a. True
   b. False

4. When evaluating new-onset moderate to severe headaches with nausea and vomiting in a patient with glioblastoma, what should be some initial steps in management and evaluation? (Last MRI was 1 month prior and was stable)
   a. Tell patient to take ibuprofen and call back later in the day to report if symptoms improved
   b. Coordinate expedited, updated CNS imaging/MRI while managing acute pain
   c. Start on steroids and wait for scheduled follow-up in 1 month

5. Pharmacotherapy with dopamine reuptake inhibitors has been definitively shown to improve fatigue in patients with CNS cancers.
   a. True
   b. False, but may provide improvement in alertness in general cancer patients

6. A 58-year-old man presents to the emergency department with new-onset seizures with no prior history of epilepsy in the setting of a glioma post-surgical resection and on cycle 1 of adjuvant temozolomide therapy. MRI 2 days ago was stable. The epileptic event resolves following abortive therapy, and the patient is at baseline. CT head shows stable edema around residual tumor, which also appears stable, and no hemorrhage. What would be appropriate management?
   a. Discharge home with no change to medications and instructions to follow up in clinic
   b. Discharge home with new script for anti-epileptic medication
   c. Discharge home with new script for dexamethasone
   d. Both b and c

7. A patient with glioblastoma and tumor-related epilepsy is nearing the EOL phase and having difficulty swallowing. The patient normally takes Keppra. What is a reasonable therapeutic option for the patient to manage seizures?
   a. Oral lacosamide
   b. Intramuscular phenytoin
   c. Rectal diazepam
   d. IV lamotrigine

8. A 65-year-old woman with HER2$^+$ breast cancer and metastatic brain lesions has completed WBRT and adjuvant chemotherapy and is status post-treatment. Current imaging shows no improvement of her disease course, and she has begun to develop severe cachexia secondary to dysphagia. Initiating temporary enteral feeding in patient may lead to greater likelihood of loss of independent feeding in the future.
   a. True
   b. False

9. In the general cancer population, exercise has been shown to have what benefits?
   a. Increased likelihood of functional independence
   b. Improved quality of life metrics
   c. Decreased overall mortality
   d. All of the above

10. A patient is nearing the EOL phase of their care and is no longer capable of making independent decisions for their care moving forward. The caregiver present states that they would like to pursue therapy incongruent with the patients advance directives made earlier in their disease course. What is the best way to avoid conflict between caregiver and patient expectations?
    a. Discuss with caregiver and patient, and refer to the patient's pre-stated advance care directives
    b. Defer to caregiver in EOL decisions as patient no longer has capacity
    c. Rely solely on physician discussion
    d. None of the above

ANSWERS

1. c
2. f
3. a
4. b
5. b
6. d
7. c
8. a
9. d
10. a

REFERENCES

1. de Robles P, Fiest KM, Frolkis AD, et al. The worldwide incidence and prevalence of primary brain tumors: A systematic review and meta-analysis. *Neuro Oncol.* 2015;17(6):776–783.
2. Ostrom QT, Gittleman H, Truitt G, et al. CBTRUS statistical report: Primary brain and other central nervous system tumors diagnosed in the United States in 2011–2015. *Neuro Oncol.* 2018;20(suppl_4):iv1–iv86.
3. Cagney DN, Martin AM, Catalano PJ, et al. Incidence and prognosis of patients with brain metastases at diagnosis of systemic malignancy: A population-based study. *Neuro Oncol.* 2017;19(11):1511–1521.
4. Wen PY, Kesari S. Malignant gliomas in adults. *N Engl J Med.* 2008;359(5):492–507.
5. Stupp R, Taillibert S, Kanner A, et al. Effect of tumor-treating fields plus maintenance temozolomide vs maintenance temozolomide alone on survival in patients with glioblastoma: A randomized clinical trial. *JAMA.* 2017;318(23):2306–2316.
6. Vargo MM. Brain tumors and metastases. *Phys Med Rehabil Clin N Am.* 2017;28(1):115–141.
7. Wang N, Bertalan MS, Brastianos PK. Leptomeningeal metastasis from systemic cancer: Review and update on management. *Cancer.* 2018;124(1):21–35.
8. Perkins A, Liu G. Primary brain tumors in adults: Diagnosis and treatment. *Am Fam Physician.* 2016;93(3):211–217.
9. Walbert T. Palliative care, end-of-life care, and advance care planning in neuro-oncology. *Continuum (Minneap Minn).* 2017;23(6, Neuro-oncology):1709–1726.
10. Philip J, Collins A, Brand C, et al. A proposed framework of supportive and palliative care for people with high-grade glioma. *Neuro Oncol.* 2018;20(3):391–399.
11. Golla H, Nettekoven C, Bausewein C, et al. Effect of early palliative care for patients with glioblastoma (EPCOG): A randomised phase III clinical trial protocol. *BMJ Open.* 2020;10(1):e034378.
12. Walbert T, Khan M. End-of-life symptoms and care in patients with primary malignant brain tumors: A systematic literature review. *J Neurooncol.* 2014;117(2):217–224.
13. Walbert T. Integration of palliative care into the neuro-oncology practice: Patterns in the United States. *Neurooncol Pract.* 2014;1(1):3–7.
14. Diamond EL, Russell D, Kryza-Lacombe M, et al. Rates and risks for late referral to hospice in patients with primary malignant brain tumors. *Neuro Oncol.* 2016;18(1):78–86.
15. Faithfull S, Cook K, Lucas C. Palliative care of patients with a primary malignant brain tumour: Case review of service use and support provided. *Palliat Med.* 2005;19(7):545–550.
16. Pompili A, Telera S, Villani V, Pace A. Home palliative care and end of life issues in glioblastoma multiforme: Results and comments from a homogeneous cohort of patients. *Neurosurg Focus.* 2014;37(6):E5.
17. Pace A, Villani V. Palliative and supportive care of patients with intracranial glioma. *Prog Neurol Surg.* 2018;31:229–237.
18. Ferrell BR, Temel JS, Temin S, Smith TJ. Integration of palliative care into standard oncology care: ASCO clinical practice guideline update summary. *J Oncol Pract.* 2017;13(2):119–121.
19. Walbert T, Glantz M, Schultz L, Puduvalli VK. Impact of provider level, training and gender on the utilization of palliative care and hospice in neuro-oncology: A North-American survey. *J Neurooncol.* 2016;126(2):337–345.
20. Andreassen P, Neergaard MA, Brogaard T, et al. The diverse impact of advance care planning: A long-term follow-up study on patients' and relatives' experiences. *BMJ Support Palliat Care.* 2017;7(3):335–340.
21. Parker SM, Clayton JM, Hancock K, et al. A systematic review of prognostic/end-of-life communication with adults in the advanced stages of a life-limiting illness: Patient/caregiver preferences for the content, style, and timing of information. *J Pain Symptom Manage.* 2007;34(1):81–93.
22. Catt S, Chalmers A, Fallowfield L. Psychosocial and supportive-care needs in high-grade glioma. *Lancet Oncol.* 2008;9(9):884–891.
23. Cubis L, Ownsworth T, Pinkham MB, Chambers S. The social trajectory of brain tumor: A qualitative metasynthesis. *Disabil Rehabil.* 2018;40(16):1857–1869.
24. Vanbutsele G, Van Belle S, Surmont V, et al. The effect of early and systematic integration of palliative care in oncology on quality of life and health care use near the end of life: A randomised controlled trial. *Eur J Cancer.* 2020;124:186–193.
25. Glajchen M. The emerging role and needs of family caregivers in cancer care. *J Support Oncol.* 2004;2(2):145–155.
26. Schubart JR, Kinzie MB, Farace E. Caring for the brain tumor patient: Family caregiver burden and unmet needs. *Neuro Oncol.* 2008;10(1):61–72.
27. Koekkoek JAF, Dirven L, Reijneveld JC, et al. Epilepsy in the end of life phase of brain tumor patients: A systematic review. *Neurooncol Pract.* 2014;1(3):134–140.
28. Pace A, Di Lorenzo C, Guariglia L, et al. End of life issues in brain tumor patients. *J Neurooncol.* 2009;91(1):39–43.
29. van Breemen MS, Wilms EB, Vecht CJ. Epilepsy in patients with brain tumours: Epidemiology, mechanisms, and management. *Lancet Neurol.* 2007;6(5):421–430.
30. Daly FN, Schiff D. Supportive management of patients with brain tumors. *Expert Rev Neurother.* 2007;7(10):1327–1336.
31. Oberndorfer S, Lindeck-Pozza E, Lahrmann H, et al. The end-of-life hospital setting in patients with glioblastoma. *J Palliat Med.* 2008;11(1):26–30.
32. Chang SM, Messersmith H, Ahluwalia M, et al. Anticonvulsant prophylaxis and steroid use in adults with metastatic brain tumors: ASCO and SNO endorsement of the Congress of Neurological Surgeons guidelines. *J Clin Oncol.* 2019;37(13):1130–1135.
33. Anderson GD, Saneto RP. Current oral and non-oral routes of antiepileptic drug delivery. *Adv Drug Deliv Rev.* 2012;64(10):911–918.
34. Armijo JA, Herranz JL, Pena Pardo MA, Adin J. Intranasal and buccal midazolam in the treatment of acute seizures. *Rev Neurol.* 2004;38(5):458–468.
35. Mula M. The safety and tolerability of intranasal midazolam in epilepsy. *Expert Rev Neurother.* 2014;14(7):735–740.
36. Nelson S, Taylor LP. Headaches in brain tumor patients: Primary or secondary? *Headache.* 2014;54(4):776–785.
37. Taylor LP. Mechanism of brain tumor headache. *Headache.* 2014;54(4):772–775.
38. Stewart-Amidei C. Managing symptoms and side effects during brain tumor illness. *Expert Rev Neurother.* 2005;5(6 Suppl):S71–76.
39. Tosetti C, Nanni I. Use of proton pump inhibitors in general practice. *World J Gastrointest Pharmacol Ther.* 2017;8(3):180–185.
40. Hadidchi S, Surento W, Lerner A, et al. Headache and brain tumor. *Neuroimaging Clin N Am.* 2019;29(2):291–300.
41. Hesketh PJ, Kris MG, Basch E, et al. Antiemetics: American Society of Clinical Oncology clinical practice guideline update. *J Clin Oncol.* 2017;35(28):3240–3261.
42. Grant R, Brown PD. Fatigue randomized controlled trials-how tired is "too tired" in patients undergoing glioma treatment? *Neuro Oncol.* 2016;18(6):759–760.
43. Armstrong TS, Gilbert MR. Practical strategies for management of fatigue and sleep disorders in people with brain tumors. *Neuro Oncol.* 2012;14 Suppl 4:iv65–72.
44. Pace A, Dirven L, Koekkoek JAF, et al. European Association for Neuro-Oncology (EANO) guidelines for palliative care in adults with glioma. *Lancet Oncol.* 2017;18(6):e330–e340.
45. de Raaf PJ, van der Rijt CC. Can you help me feel less exhausted all the time? *J Clin Oncol.* 2013;31(25):3056–3060.
46. Lee EQ, Muzikansky A, Drappatz J, et al. A randomized, placebo-controlled pilot trial of armodafinil for fatigue in patients with gliomas undergoing radiotherapy. *Neuro Oncol.* 2016;18(6):849–854.
47. Page BR, Shaw EG, Lu L, et al. Phase II double-blind placebo-controlled randomized study of armodafinil for brain radiation-induced fatigue. *Neuro Oncol.* 2015;17(10):1393–1401.
48. Boele FW, Douw L, de Groot M, et al. The effect of modafinil on fatigue, cognitive functioning, and mood in primary brain tumor patients: A multicenter randomized controlled trial. *Neuro Oncol.* 2013;15(10):1420–1428.
49. Escalante CP. Treatment of cancer-related fatigue: An update. *Support Care Cancer.* 2003;11(2):79–83.
50. Shaw EG, Rosdhal R, D'Agostino RB, Jr., et al. Phase II study of donepezil in irradiated brain tumor patients: Effect on cognitive function, mood, and quality of life. *J Clin Oncol.* 2006;24(9):1415–1420.
51. Burg MA, Adorno G, Lopez ED, et al. Current unmet needs of cancer survivors: Analysis of open-ended responses to the American Cancer Society Study of Cancer Survivors II. *Cancer.* 2015;121(4):623–630.
52. Vargo M. Brain tumor rehabilitation. *Am J Phys Med Rehabil.* 2011;90(5 Suppl 1):S50–62.
53. Mukand JA, Blackinton DD, Crincoli MG, et al. Incidence of neurologic deficits and rehabilitation of patients with brain tumors. *Am J Phys Med Rehabil.* 2001;80(5):346–350.
54. Stout NL, Baima J, Swisher AK, et al. A systematic review of exercise systematic reviews in the cancer literature (2005–2017). *Pm R.* 2017;9(9s2):S347–s384.
55. Schwartz AL, de Heer HD, Bea JW. Initiating exercise interventions to promote wellness in cancer patients and survivors. *Oncology (Williston Park).* 2017;31(10):711–717.

56. Gutin PH. Corticosteroid therapy in patients with brain tumors. *Natl Cancer Inst Monogr.* 1977;46:151–156.
57. Hempen C, Weiss E, Hess CF. Dexamethasone treatment in patients with brain metastases and primary brain tumors: Do the benefits outweigh the side-effects? *Support Care Cancer.* 2002;10(4):322–328.
58. Cormie P, Zopf EM, Zhang X, Schmitz KH. The impact of exercise on cancer mortality, recurrence, and treatment-related adverse effects. *Epidemiol Rev.* 2017;39(1):71–92.
59. Cormie P, Nowak AK, Chambers SK, et al. The potential role of exercise in neuro-oncology. *Front Oncol.* 2015;5:85.
60. Khan F, Amatya B, Ng L, et al. Multidisciplinary rehabilitation after primary brain tumour treatment. *Cochrane Database Syst Rev.* 2015(8):Cd009509.
61. Cordier D, Gerber M, Brand S. Effects of two types of exercise training on psychological well-being, sleep, quality of life and physical fitness in patients with high-grade glioma (WHO III and IV): Study protocol for a randomized controlled trial. *Cancer Commun (Lond).* 2019;39(1):46.
62. Formica V, Del Monte G, Giacchetti I, et al. Rehabilitation in neuro-oncology: A meta-analysis of published data and a mono-institutional experience. *Integr Cancer Ther.* 2011;10(2):119–126.
63. Bartolo M, Zucchella C, Pace A, et al. Early rehabilitation after surgery improves functional outcome in inpatients with brain tumours. *J Neurooncol.* 2012;107(3):537–544.
64. Alam E, Wilson RD, Vargo MM. Inpatient cancer rehabilitation: A retrospective comparison of transfer back to acute care between patients with neoplasm and other rehabilitation patients. *Arch Phys Med Rehabil.* 2008;89(7):1284–1289.
65. Taskila-Brandt T, Martikainen R, Virtanen SV, et al. The impact of education and occupation on the employment status of cancer survivors. *Eur J Cancer.* 2004;40(16):2488–2493.
66. Schultz PN, Beck ML, Stava C, Sellin RV. Cancer survivors. Work related issues. *Aaohn j.* 2002;50(5):220–226.
67. Taskila T, Lindbohm ML. Factors affecting cancer survivors' employment and work ability. *Acta Oncol.* 2007;46(4):446–451.
68. van der Bogt RD, Vermeulen BD, Reijm AN, et al. Palliation of dysphagia. *Best Pract Res Clin Gastroenterol.* 2018;36-37:97–103.
69. Thomas R, O'Connor AM, Ashley S. Speech and language disorders in patients with high grade glioma and its influence on prognosis. *J Neurooncol.* 1995;23(3):265–270.
70. Greco E, Simic T, Ringash J, et al. Dysphagia treatment for patients with head and neck cancer undergoing radiation therapy: A meta-analysis review. *Int J Radiat Oncol Biol Phys.* 2018;101(2):421–444.
71. Sizoo EM, Pasman HR, Dirven L, et al. The end-of-life phase of high-grade glioma patients: A systematic review. *Support Care Cancer.* 2014;22(3):847–857.
72. Mummudi N, Jalali R. Palliative care and quality of life in neuro-oncology. *F1000Prime Rep.* 2014;6:71–71.
73. Sizoo EM, Taphoorn MJ, Uitdehaag B, et al. The end-of-life phase of high-grade glioma patients: Dying with dignity? *Oncologist.* 2013;18(2):198–203.
74. Leeper H, Milbury K. Survivorship care planning and implementation in neuro-oncology. *Neuro Oncol.* 2018;20(Suppl_7):vii40–vii46.
75. Koekkoek JA, Dirven L, Sizoo EM, et al. Symptoms and medication management in the end of life phase of high-grade glioma patients. *J Neurooncol.* 2014;120(3):589–595.
76. Newton HB, Newton C, Pearl D, Davidson T. Swallowing assessment in primary brain tumor patients with dysphagia. *Neurology.* 1994;44(10):1927–1932.
77. Bossola M. Nutritional interventions in head and neck cancer patients undergoing chemoradiotherapy: A narrative review. *Nutrients.* 2015;7(1):265–276.
78. de Las Peñas R, Majem M, Perez-Altozano J, et al. SEOM clinical guidelines on nutrition in cancer patients (2018). *Clin Transl Oncol.* 2019;21(1):87–93.
79. Ehrsson YT, Sundberg K, Laurell G, Langius-Eklöf A. Head and neck cancer patients' perceptions of quality of life and how it is affected by the disease and enteral tube feeding during treatment. *Ups J Med Sci.* 2015;120(4):280–289.
80. Renovanz M, Hechtner M, Janko M, et al. Factors associated with supportive care needs in glioma patients in the neuro-oncological outpatient setting. *J Neurooncol.* 2017;133(3):653–662.

32 | THE NEURO-ONCOLOGY OF WOMEN (NOW)

NA TOSHA N. GATSON, KERIANNE R. TAYLOR, MARIA L. BOCCIA, AND TERRI L. WOODARD

INTRODUCTION

The study of the neuro-biological and psychosocial impact of brain tumors in women, paired with the academic movement to encourage female focused clinical and translational brain tumor research is referred to as "The Neuro-Oncology of Women (NOW)."
—Dr. Na Tosha N. Gatson (2018)

The neuro-oncology of women (NOW) comprises a wide variety of issues relevant to women with brain tumors because they experience a range of endogenous and exogenous hormonal changes (including fertility preservation treatments, pregnancy, lactation, and pregnancy prevention) over the course of their lives from puberty to the postmenopausal period. It encompasses important psychosocial issues that impact quality of life, sex and sexuality, relationships, sex-discrepant responses to therapy, and issues in trans-health (such as in cross-sex hormone exposure in gender affirmation). While not all of these points can be addressed in this chapter, there is a growing demand to better understand these issues from an ethical and scientific evidence-based approach. Brain tumors and brain tumor therapies can influence sexual desire, sexual function, intimacy in relationships, and, ultimately, quality of life (QoL).[1-4] Providers are responsible for addressing these psychosocial issues just as readily as they deal with issues of reproductive planning and prevention in these patients. The manner in which we communicate the available knowledge in the field is critical to guide patients in making informed treatment decisions and to prepare for potential life changes.

Women harbor the majority of intracranial tumors (malignant or benign), so it should follow that the evidence in the field with reference to women's neuro-oncology also be abundant. This is not the case. Understanding how various tumors respond to endogenous and exogenous/iatrogenic hormones, menstrual cycles, pregnancy, and the post-pregnancy period is not well-studied and less well-incorporated into practice guidelines.

With respect to sexuality and sexual function in cancer patients, most research pertains to breast and prostate cancer.[1-4] Sexual function–related research in patients with brain tumors has been predominantly focused on pituitary tumors.[5-7] Interestingly, the most prevalent research regarding the impact of sexual function on QoL in pituitary adenomas addresses male sexual function with an emphasis on erectile dysfunction.[8]

Fertility preservation is also an important but understudied issue in brain tumor patients. Each year, approximately 70,000 adolescents and young adults (AYA) between the ages of 15 and 39 will be diagnosed with cancer.[9] Brain tumors are the third most common cancer overall in this age group, and an estimated 11,700 new cases of AYA brain tumors will be diagnosed this year.[9] The most common tumor types in this age group are pituitary tumors, meningiomas, and nerve sheath tumors.[9] Fortunately, the 5-year relative survival rate for AYA patients diagnosed with a primary brain tumor is 90.4%, making survivorship issues such as fertility of the utmost importance.[9]

This chapter provides an overview of key guidelines and considerations for imaging, neurosurgery and anesthesia, radiation therapy, and chemotherapy during pregnancy in women with central nervous system (CNS) tumors. We also discuss high-yield points about common primary intracranial tumors in women and women's sexuality, as well as share pearls on fertility maintenance in brain cancer. The objective of this chapter is to increase provider and caregiver awareness of the key issues and gaps in the field as it pertains to the neuro-oncology of women.

IMAGING GUIDELINES AND CONSIDERATIONS FOR CNS TUMORS DURING PREGNANCY

General guidelines exist for tumor imaging modalities and the use of imaging contrast in pregnant women with brain tumors as part of the American College of Obstetricians and Gynecologists (ACOG) and the American College of Radiology (ACR).[10,11] The ACOG and ACR note that noncontrast magnetic resonance imaging (MRI) studies do not pose a significant risk to the mother or fetus when using less than a 3 Tesla magnet.[10,11] Unfortunately, the use of non-contrasted imaging studies could limit accurate identification of the tumor margins and impact surgical and radiation planning. MRI gadolinium contrast readily crosses the placenta into the fetus; therefore, this use should be reserved for cases where the diagnostic benefit to the mother is expected to outweigh the unknown

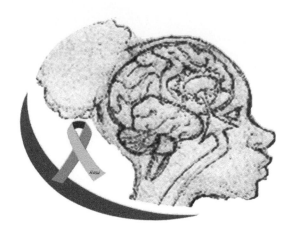

Figure 32.1 Adapted logo for the Neuro-Oncology of Women (NOW). Arrow depicting peripheral circulating factors impact on brain tumors. The peach and gray ribbon represents NOW.

risk to the fetus.[10,12] Computed tomography (CT) imaging involves exposure to ionizing radiation and therefore should be considered in acute cases when the benefit to the mother outweighs any risk to the fetus.[10,12]

> MRI gadolinium contrast readily crosses the placenta into the fetus; therefore, this use should be reserved for cases where the diagnostic benefit to the mother is expected to outweigh the unknown risk to the fetus.

NEUROSURGICAL AND ANESTHESIA CONSIDERATIONS FOR CNS TUMORS DURING PREGNANCY

Considerations for neurosurgical interventions depend on tumor malignant status, location, fetal gestational age, and patient clinical status.[13,14] In stable pregnant patients, surgical intervention is elective; however, for these patients, surgery is encouraged after delivery.[14,15] Acute situations or aggressive tumors potentially require a more aggressive approach. In cases of unstable patients with progression and viable fetuses (beyond 24 weeks gestation), neurosurgical intervention should be considered.[14,15] Although surgery can be undertaken in pregnant patients, pregnancy termination should be discussed with patients when aggressive disease requires immediate surgery and fetal gestational age is pre-viable.[14,15] If delaying surgery to the postpartum period is not recommended, neurosurgical procedures are preferable in the second trimester of pregnancy for optimal hemodynamic responsiveness.[14,16] Ultimately, pregnant patients with brain tumors require an individualized approach to their care under the guidance of a multidisciplinary team.[15]

> If delaying surgery to the postpartum period is not recommended, neurosurgical procedures are preferable in the second trimester of pregnancy for optimal hemodynamic responsiveness.

Physiological and pharmacodynamic changes of pregnancy have an impact on anesthetic management. In pregnant patients, proper neurosurgical positioning is important to prevent disruption of placental blood perfusion and excessive fetal drug exposure.[14] Further anesthetic considerations are made in these patients as the various physiological changes of pregnancy affect maternal vascular resistance, minute ventilation, oxygen consumption, and lung volumes, among other parameters.[17] Management of intracranial pressures is of major concern during neurosurgical procedures in pregnant women, and anesthesiologists must maintain strict control of the arterial carbon dioxide tension.[17,18] Importantly, there is no established general anesthetic of choice for use during pregnancy as none of the currently used agents has evidence for teratogenicity in humans and none has been demonstrated to be more safe or efficacious in this setting.[18]

> There is no established preferred general anesthetic for use during pregnancy.

RADIATION GUIDELINES AND CONSIDERATIONS FOR CNS TUMORS DURING PREGNANCY

Considerations for radiation therapy in pregnant patients include decision-making that weighs the risk against the benefit to the maternal host as opposed to those that are known to the developing fetus. The risk to the fetus is based on a calculated (phantom measurement) fetal dose due to radiation scatter during cranial irradiation.[15] Congenital malformations and neurocognitive delays have been associated with fetal radiation dosages greater than 10 cGy.[19] Importantly, the risk in pregnancy with use of stereotactic radiosurgery is similar to that of standard involved-field/external beam radiation.[19]

> Congenital malformations and neurocognitive delays have been associated with fetal radiation exposure dosages greater than 10 cGy.

CHEMOTHERAPEUTIC RECOMMENDATIONS AND CONSIDERATIONS FOR PRIMARY CNS TUMORS DURING PREGNANCY

Considerations for use of chemotherapy during pregnancy is largely debated in neuro-oncology. This is due to the fact that pregnancy concurrent with primary brain tumors is infrequent and has not led to any level I or level II evidence for guideline development.[15] Systemic chemotherapy during pregnancy could result in congenital malformations, spontaneous abortion, still birth, or other toxicities to the developing fetus, and this is especially concerning for exposure during the first trimester.[15,20] While it is ideal to postpone chemotherapy until after delivery, there are situations where chemotherapeutic intervention is required sooner. In these cases, patients are faced with decisions such as termination of pregnancy, pregnancy maintenance with education around the potential risks, or abstaining from chemotherapy use with education around the risk of tumor progression.

If chemotherapy is required, the second trimester is more ideal than the first trimester, as this time point approximates completion of organogenesis.[16] Temozolomide (TMZ) is an oral alkylating agent and is the first-line treatment of choice for high-grade astrocytoma.[21] While TMZ has been demonstrated to cause embryo lethality and fetal malformations in animal studies, there are no controlled studies in humans.[22] While TMZ is not recommended during pregnancy, there are anecdotal accounts of early-pregnancy TMZ exposure and case reports of first-trimester exposure with resultant healthy term newborns.[22] Procarbazine, commonly used to treat oligodendroglioma, has been proved to cross the placenta and is a potent carcinogen and teratogen.[16] The most recent recommendation for women (and men) with brain tumors is to discontinue chemotherapies 4–6 months prior to conception.[16,22]

> If chemotherapy is required during pregnancy, the second trimester is more ideal than the first trimester, as this time point approximates completion of organogenesis.

COMMON PRIMARY INTRACRANIAL TUMORS IN WOMEN

The Central Brain Tumor Registry of the United States (CBTRUS) estimates more than 84,170 new cases of primary CNS tumors will be diagnosed in the United States in 2021; 56–60% of these cases will be women.[9] The most common primary CNS tumors affecting women include meningiomas, pituitary adenomas, and gliomas. Interestingly, most of these tumors have reported evidence of hormone or pregnancy responsiveness.[23–26] Some hormone-dependent tumors express sex-specific hormone receptors and bind to circulating hormones, potentially driving tumor oncogenicity, while others might respond to various host microenvironmental changes which are less well understood.[23–26]

> CBTRUS estimates more than 84,170 new cases of primary CNS tumors will be diagnosed in the United States in 2021; 56–60% of these cases will be women.

MENINGIOMAS

TUMOR OVERVIEW

Meningiomas are typically slow-growing benign tumors that arise from the arachnoid cap cells of the meninges. Meningioma is the most common benign intracranial tumor, representing 38.3% of all cases.[9] They can range from benign (WHO grade 1) and atypical (WHO grade 2) to malignant (WHO grade 3). The prognosis for meningioma is typically good; however, there can be complications due to tumor location, and some pathologic findings increase the risk for recurrence and impact patient survival.[27–29] Many studies have been aimed at characterizing the putative tumor-specific factors involved in meningioma aggressive behavior, and there is consensus around associating risk for recurrence with high cellular proliferation indices.[28,29] A recent article by Nagahama et al. suggests that p53-positive tumor status was additive to a high proliferation index for risk of recurrence. Nevertheless, there is not enough evidence to support the development of a definitive guideline for sex hormone avoidance in patients with meningiomas.[30]

> Meningioma is the most common benign intracranial tumor, representing 38.3% of all cases.

OVERALL SEX DISCREPANCY

There is a clear sex dimorphism in meningiomas: women are twice as likely to have meningiomas as are males.[9] In 2006, Korhonen et al. reported that this discrepancy cannot be readily explained by differential expression of hormone receptors.[31] Interestingly, the discrepancy is not present prior to age 14.[32]

AGE RISK

Between the third and fifth decades of life, a woman's risk for meningioma increases to nearly three times that of her male counterpart.[32] The overall risk for meningioma increases, without respect for sex, after age 65.[32]

> Between the third and fifth decades of life, a woman's risk for meningioma increases to nearly three times that of her male counterpart.

EVIDENCE FOR HORMONE OR PREGNANCY DEPENDENCE

Most low-grade meningiomas express hormone receptors for progesterone (80–88%), potentially portending less aggressive tumor behavior, and another 30–40% are estrogen-positive.[31,33–35] Androgens and growth hormone receptors can be found in less than 10–39% of tumors and potentially portends a more aggressive tumor behavior.[35–38] Unfortunately, most hormone-targeted interventional studies in meningioma have been inconclusive to support this as a treatment approach.[38,39] Furthermore, there is limited evidence to support guidelines that discuss any potential risk for use of hormone replacement therapy (HRT) in patients with meningiomas.[40,41]

While it is debated whether sex-specific hormone receptor expression influences the noted sex discrepancy, it remains to be clearly defined how the expression of these hormone receptors influences tumor aggressive behavior.[31,41] Furthermore, there is evidence for increased meningioma aggressiveness during pregnancy and during the luteal phase of the menstrual cycle.[36,42] This is thought to be due to the circulating hormone's influence on cellular proliferation.[36,42] Another study supports the assertion that multiparous and postmenopausal women also have a notably higher risk for new diagnosis and progression of meningiomas.[40]

PITUITARY ADENOMAS

TUMOR OVERVIEW

Pituitary adenomas account for approximately 17.5% of all intracranial tumors.[9,43] These tumors are typically categorized based on their biological function: benign adenoma (most common), invasive adenoma (~35%), and carcinoma (~0.15%); however, further classification is based on histology and radiographic size plus radioanatomical findings.[43] Indicators of disease often include vision changes, headaches, and abnormal endocrine function.[43-45] These tumors often lead to abnormal secretion of hormones such as growth hormone, prolactin, corticotropin, or thyrotropin and potentially cause clinical syndromes that affect fertility. Unfortunately, these tumors typically occur in women during the primary reproductive years.[44,45]

OVERALL SEX DISCREPANCY AND ISSUES OF FERTILITY AND PREGNANCY

Females are disproportionately overrepresented in pituitary tumors, with the highest incidence across most of the reproductive period (ages 15–39-years).[46] Prolactinomas are the most common type of functioning pituitary tumor and are 4.5 times more likely to occur in females compared to males.[44,47] These tumors frequently cause disruption of the gonadal axis and might result in infertility.[47] However, treatment with bromocriptine (dopamine agonist of choice during pregnancy due to its shorter half-life) could improve fertility.[47] Patients who become pregnant with a history of pituitary tumors are initially treated with medical therapies if observation is not indicated; however, some resistant cases must be treated surgically.[47] During pregnancy, periodic clinical evaluations promote early detection of tumor growth, and sellar imaging for symptomatic cases is recommended to promote best clinical decision-making.[47]

> Prolactinomas are the most common type of functioning pituitary tumor.

> During pregnancy, periodic clinical evaluations promote early detection of tumor growth, and sellar imaging for symptomatic cases is recommended to promote best clinical decision-making.

EVIDENCE FOR HORMONE OR PREGNANCY DEPENDENCE

It is well-established that the pituitary gland is affected by pregnancy, parity, parturition, lactation, use of exogenous hormones, and other hormonal factors.[48-50] However, over the past four decades, studies using sequential cranial MR assessments have debated which specific factors best correlate with changes in the total pituitary volume or the glandular dimensions.[48-50] Ultimately, providers should inquire about reproductive planning and hormonal treatments in patients with pituitary tumors.[47]

GLIOMAS

TUMOR OVERVIEW

Gliomas are CNS tumors that develop from the neuronal supportive glial cells (astrocytes, oligodendrocytes, and ependymal cells). Gliomas are the most common form of primary brain tumor, comprising 80% of all primary malignant CNS tumors.[9,51] These tumors range in aggressiveness from WHO grade 1 to WHO grades 3 or 4 and can severely impact patient survival and QoL. The most aggressive glioma, glioblastoma (GBM) WHO grade 4, is the most common of these tumors in adults and has a median overall survival (mOS) of less than 16 months after standard maximal resection and radiation and chemotherapy with TMZ.[21] Median survival for GBM has improved with the use of tumor-treating field devices when added in the adjuvant setting.[52] GBMs make up 15% of all primary brain tumors and are 50% of all malignant primary brain tumors.[9]

OVERALL SEX AND SURVIVAL DISCREPANCIES AND AGE RISK

GBMs have a slight male predominance (1.6:1) and a peak incidence in patients older than 75 years; however, non-GBM gliomas occur in males and females at a similar rate and have a peak incidence between 35 and 44 years.[9,53] The median age at diagnosis was not significantly different between males and females for both GBM and non-GBM diagnoses.[53]

> GBMs have a slight male predominance (1.6:1) and a peak incidence in patients older than 75 years; however, non-GBM gliomas occur in males and females at a similar rate and have a peak incidence between 35 and 44 years.

Females have consistently demonstrated an overall survival advantage over males in GBM (mOS in mos, 20.1 vs. 17.8 mos) respectively, but there is no observed survival advantage in non-GBM cases.[53] Younger GBM patients (younger than 55 years) also demonstrate a female survival advantage (mOS 24.3 mos) compared to males (mOS 22.5 mos).[53] In non-GBM cases, oligodendroglioma/mixed glioma and astrocytoma demonstrated no sex differences in mOS.[53]

EVIDENCE FOR HORMONE OR PREGNANCY DEPENDENCE

Pregnancy concurrent with all cancers is estimated at 1 cancer per 1,000 pregnancies and is most common in cancers that are most frequently diagnosed in women.[54] Glioma in pregnancy is a rare occurrence but is likely underreported. In gliomas, the second and third trimesters of pregnancy have been associated with increased tumor aggressiveness.[16,26,55-57] Often, women with existing WHO grade 2 or higher and subsequent pregnancy experience tumor progression during mid- to late gestation.[16,26] Patients with WHO grade 1 tumors were not found to have progression during pregnancy.[26]

> The second and third trimesters of pregnancy have been associated with increased aggressiveness of gliomas.

In summary, there is a demonstrated need for more contemporary studies concerning common primary intracranial tumors that occur over various hormonal and reproductive phases in women. These studies should help drive guideline development and inform providers about tumor surveillance strategies and clinical recommendations in women with CNS tumors.

BRAIN TUMORS AND WOMEN'S SEXUALITY

While understanding how tumor behavior is influenced during various phases of a woman's life is very important, it is similarly important to understand how tumors and treatment of tumors can modify human behavior. This section deals with sexuality and sexual function.

Cancer research on sexual function disproportionately focuses on breast and prostate cancers.[1-4] Studies on sexual dysfunction in brain tumor patients typically addresses sex hormone dysregulation, as in the case of pituitary tumors.[5-7] Pituitary tumors have also been the primary research focus for the impact of sexual function on QoL. Interestingly, these tumors occur more commonly in women, but the preponderance of data focus on functional aspects such as erectile dysfunction.

Sexual function in the broader sexuality literature tends to be holistic and includes consideration of relationship intimacy and pleasure. In contrast, the emphasis in cancer care literature on restoring/maintaining the capacity for sexual intercourse is reductionist in this context.[58] Noticeably absent from this literature is patient perspectives on sexuality and the impact of changes in their sexual experience on QoL.

> Noticeably absent from literature on sexuality in cancer patients is patient perspectives on sexuality and the impact of changes in their sexual experience on QoL.

Self-esteem, body image, and sexual satisfaction have clear associations in studies of healthy women.[59] These same issues in women with cancer are of particular interest and might be multifactorial. The diagnosis and treatment of cancer can lead to both physical and psychological traumas in women and subsequently affect processes that are associated with QoL, such as sexuality.

SEXUALITY IN WOMEN WITH LOW-GRADE GLIOMAS

Although sexuality is a significant area within QoL research, studies on QoL in brain tumor patients have paid little attention to sexuality. Questionnaires assessing QoL typically limit assessment of sexuality to a single question of sexual satisfaction and tend to overlook function, body image, and self-esteem.[60] Interestingly, in a number of studies which were not intended to assess sexual function

in postoperative low-grade glioma patients, more than half of the patients reported sexual dysfunction.[60,61] In these cases, there was a high concordance rate with worse QoL and higher levels of depression and anxiety.[60,61] Despite a noted high rate of sexual dysfunction reported, only 15% of patients received any information about possible sexual side effects prior to surgery, and very few explicitly requested such information.[60] Surbeck et al. keenly noted specific sex-discrepant outcomes based on the location of the resection and peri-operative therapies. Both males and females with right-sided resections experienced difficulty with reaching orgasm as compared to having left-sided resections; however, these same males who remained on postoperative antiepileptics had more complaints of sexual dysfunction overall.[60] Women with temporal lobe resections maintained sexual drive and arousal as compared to males with temporal lobe resections.[60] New efforts are under way to mandate inclusion of adverse cancer impact on relationships and sexual function.[62] More studies in this area are needed to make definitive associations and actionable guidelines.

> Studies have found sex-discrepant outcomes based on the location of the brain tumor resection.

SEXUALITY IN WOMEN WITH PITUITARY TUMORS

Females are more likely than their male counterparts to be diagnosed with pituitary tumors and to report associated infertility.[63,64] Pituitary tumors present with high rates of hormone disruption and are often accompanied by amenorrhea and loss of sexual desire, as well as infertility.[65,66] Lundberg et al., in 1991, also reported problems with lubrication and orgasm in two-thirds of the women studied and found that tumor growth was correlated with sexual function.[65]

> Pituitary tumors present with high rates of hormone disruption and are often accompanied by amenorrhea and loss of sexual desire, as well as infertility.

While multiple treatment modalities can be used to help restore hormonal function or limit tumor recurrence, some approaches come with significant risks for complications. For example, particular hormone derangements can impair sexual function. One study reported that radiotherapy results in hormone deficiencies in more than 50% of patients[67] and appeared to be related to the total dose of radiation utilized and the length of follow-up.[68,69] Surgical interventions are also reported to impair sexual function.[70] Acquati et al. directly compared sexual function across treatment types and found that medical therapy resulted in the highest rates of restored sexual function, and the converse was true for radiotherapy. This study led to the recommendation that radiotherapy be reserved for otherwise refractory tumors.[71]

ASSESSMENT OF QOL AND SEXUAL FUNCTION IN BRAIN TUMOR PATIENTS

One assessment tool used in brain cancer patients is the Functional Assessment of Cancer Therapy (FACT)–Brain (FACT-Br),[72] which is an extension of the FACT–General (FACT-G)[73] for brain tumor patients. The FACT-Br has multiple scales designed to assess QoL along a number of domains. These include physical, social, emotional, and functional dimensions of well-being. The FACT-Br has one question regarding sexuality, "Am I satisfied with my sex life?" However, it is the only question within the entire battery that allows for the participant to *skip the question if they prefer not to answer it*. Boccia et al. found that one-quarter of the women opted to skip this question.[74] Still, readers must be keen when reviewing how specific assessment instruments are delivered, as some might report on dysfunction but remain vague in their method.[75]

Boccia et al. recently reported on QoL and sexual function in women with brain tumors. In this study, women were given the FACT-Br QoL questionnaire and the Female Sexual Function Index (FSFI).[74] The FSFI was developed to assess individual aspects of female sexual function, including desire, arousal, lubrication, orgasm, satisfaction, and pain. In addition, information about the tumor location and postoperative treatment course (radiation and/or chemotherapy) was collected. GBM was the most common brain tumor diagnosis in this cohort, and frontal lobe tumors were the most common tumor location. There were significantly more reports of sexual dysfunction in this study, with 66% of sexually active women meeting criteria for elevated FSFI. QoL measures were correlated with sexual dysfunction (Figure 32.2). In particular, sexual desire was correlated with QoL, and the patient's social well-being QoL assessments were correlated with FSFI subscales.[74] Thus, QoL in these patients is closely related to issues around sexuality and sexual function.

> QoL in patients with brain tumors is closely related to issues around sexuality and sexual function.

Clear and direct physician–patient communication is essential for patient satisfaction and participation in treatment planning. This can be difficult because there are barriers to effective communication on both sides of this dialogue when the issue of sexuality is the primary topic. Physicians reported difficulty in discussing sexuality with their patients for fear of offending the patient, a notion that sexuality is not sufficiently important, a personal discomfort with sexuality, a lack of time in the encounter to prioritize this discussion, and value judgments about what constitutes "normal" and "healthy" sexual expression.[76] Perceptions of adequate training in this area are a significant predictor of willingness to initiate these conversations with patients.[76]

> Physicians reported difficulty in discussing sexuality with their patients.

TREATING SEXUAL DYSFUNCTION IN BRAIN TUMOR PATIENTS

Because the literature is sparse regarding sexual dysfunction in women with brain tumors, it follows that the evidence for treating female sexual dysfunction is also inadequate. However, some recent developments in the pharmacological treatment of sexual dysfunction in women suggests interventions more directly addressing sexual dysfunction in these patients is possible. For example, low desire is the most common type of sexual dysfunction in women and can be treated with sex therapy and/or the recently approved medications flibanserin[77] or bremelanotide.[78] Little is known about how these centrally acting therapies will impact brain tumors or brain tumor therapy.

> Low desire is the most common type of sexual dysfunction in women.

Sexuality is a vital part of QoL, with the potential to impact patient satisfaction and influence their treatment decision-making. There remains a knowledge gap about how we can best survey, inform patients, inquire, and treat sexuality issues in women with brain tumors. Even among the studies reviewed in this chapter, there is a lack of consensus around the best utilization of available assessment tools and best approaches to standardized clinical research. Notably absent from the literature are patient perspectives and patient-reported outcomes as well as the number of QoL studies that appropriately included sexuality as a reliable measure.[79] The gap in researching and discussing sexuality impacts our ability to address another important topic: preservation of fertility in our female patients with brain tumors.

In summary, sexuality in brain tumor patients is still understudied. From this review, it is obvious that the issues of

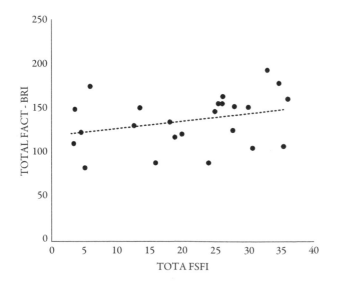

Figure 32.2 Relationship between total sexual function and total quality of life (QoL) scores. Pearson correlation (24 df) = +.54, p = .006.

sexuality are complicated by multiple factors such as hormones and tumor types and location which directly affect the QoL of our patients. To better address this, more research with a special focus on sexuality in brain tumor and its impact on patient QoL will be needed. In addition, brain tumor practitioners will need to aggressively address sexuality issues as a routine part of brain tumor care and education.

CONSIDERATIONS IN PRESERVING FERTILITY IN GIRLS AND WOMEN WITH BRAIN TUMORS

Brain tumors are the third most common cancer overall between the ages of 15- and 39-years-old with nearly 12,000 new cases in the US in 2021.[9] Importantly, these patients typically experience an approximate 90% 5-year relative survival rate making survivorship and QOL of utmost importance when considering treatment and management approaches in this age group.[9]

Many people in this age group have not initiated or completed their family building plans. Survivors report that fertility is an important issue for them and many express a desire to have children in the future.[80] Cancer-related infertility has proved a significant cause of distress that may persist post-treatment and well into survivorship.[81] It is imperative that healthcare providers who care for people with cancer discuss fertility risk and options for fertility preservation prior to treatment. The American Society for Clinical Oncology (ASCO) developed a clinical guideline on fertility preservation in 2006 and the most recent update states that

> As part of education and informed consent before cancer therapy, health care providers should address the possibility of infertility with patients treated during their reproductive years and be prepared to discuss possible fertility preservation options and/or to refer all potential patients to appropriate reproductive specialists.[82]

Although patients may be focused initially on their cancer diagnosis, physician guidelines encourage providers to advise patients regarding potential threats to fertility as early as possible in the treatment process to allow for the widest array of options for fertility preservation.[82,83] Letourneau et al. noted the importance of pre-treatment fertility counseling stating, "In addition to being a part of informed consent, fertility preservation counseling has been shown to reduce long-term regret and improve quality of life, even if not pursued."[84]

> "In addition to being a part of informed consent, fertility preservation counseling has been shown to reduce long-term regret and improve quality of life, even if not pursued."

Cancer treatment can impact fertility in many ways. Surgery and radiation can alter or destroy hypothalamic and/or pituitary function and disrupt the hypothalamic-pituitary-gonadal axis, resulting in hypogonadism. Radiation to or near the gonads could damage them, leading to gonadal failure or hypertrophic hypogonadism. Finally, chemotherapy can also have a direct impact on gonadal function that can be temporary or permanent. The risk of infertility depends on the type of chemotherapy (especially alkylating agents), the dose, and patient age (especially for women).

> Oocyte (egg) and embryo cryopreservation is considered standard of care fertility preservation in women.

Several options for fertility preservation exist. For women (Table 32.1), oocyte (egg) and embryo cryopreservation is considered standard of care. Both involve stimulating the ovary with gonadotropins over the course of approximately 9–12 days to recruit multiple follicles from which oocytes can be retrieved transvaginally. Once the oocytes are retrieved, they can be cryopreserved or inseminated to form embryos which are grown out in embryo culture for several days and then cryopreserved.[85,86] Freezing eggs or embryos allows the possibility of using preimplantation genetic testing (PGT) to test embryos for aneuploidy (PGT-A) or gene mutations that can cause future disease (PGT-M).[85,86] To meet the unique needs of patients with cancer, several modifications have been developed. If there are significant time constraints, random-start protocols may be used to start the ovarian stimulation process right away instead of waiting for a woman to start menses.[85] If a patient has an estrogen-dependent tumor, such as a meningioma, an aromatase inhibitor can be used to prevent estrogen from reaching super-physiologic levels.[86] In all cases, collaboration and communication between the oncologist and reproductive medicine is necessary to streamline and optimize patient outcomes.

> If there are significant time constraints, random-start protocols may be used to start the ovarian stimulation process right away instead of waiting for a woman to start menses.

Ovarian tissue cryopreservation (OTC) is a fertility preservation option that is no longer considered experimental but is not widely available. For OTC, ovarian tissue is laparoscopically removed and cryopreserved. If a woman has premature ovarian insufficiency or failure after treatment, her ovarian tissue can be thawed and surgically placed back into the body, and, after a short period of time, it may start to function. One concern about OTC is that there is a possibility of reseeding the body with malignant cells, especially with hematologic cancers. OTC is the only fertility preservation option that is available to prepubertal girls.[87]

> In ovarian tissue cryopreservation, ovarian tissue is laparoscopically removed and cryopreserved.

TABLE 32.1 Fertility preservation options for women and girls with cancer

	OOCYTE CRYOPRESERVATION	EMBRYO CRYOPRESERVATION	OVARIAN TISSUE CRYOPRESERVATION	OVARIAN SUPPRESSION
Effectiveness	4–14% live birth rate per oocyte (depending on age)	3.1–47.6% live birth per embryo transfer (depending on age)	>130 live births worldwide	Uncertain
Appropriate for	Women Postpubertal girls	Women who are partnered Women who desire to use donor sperm	Women Prepubertal girls	Women Post-pubertal girls
Process	Daily injections Outpatient surgical procedure (transvaginal oocyte retrieval) Oocytes are cryopreserved for future use	Daily injections Outpatient surgical procedure (transvaginal oocyte retrieval) Oocytes are inseminated with sperm to create embryos that are cryopreserved for future use	Short surgical procedure where an ovary or part of an ovary is removed and cryopreserved for future use	Injection every 1–3 months while receiving chemotherapy
Costs	+++	++++	+++	+
Risks	Infection Bleeding Ovarian hyperstimulation syndrome (OHSS)	Infection Bleeding Ovarian hyperstimulation syndrome (OHSS)	Risk of cancer reoccurrence if reimplanted tissue contains cancer cells	Decreased bone density
Side effects	Bloating, cramping, mood swings	Bloating, cramping, mood swings	Surgical pain and recovery	Hot flashes, vaginal dryness, mood swings
Time required	Approximately 2 weeks	Approximately 2 weeks	Variable; days	Variable; days Best administered several days before starting chemotherapy
Important considerations	Requires frequent monitoring Provides reproductive autonomy	Requires frequent monitoring Gives opportunity for preimplantation genetic testing	Difficult to find places that provide ovarian tissue cryopreservation services May be able to make mature oocytes from the cryopreserved tissue in the future	Often covered by insurance for menstrual suppression

Ovarian suppression (OS) for fertility preservation is considered experimental. For this method, women are given a GnRH agonist to downregulate the ovary and make it quiescent during chemotherapy administration.[88] The data on the efficacy of OS are mixed, and use of OS is controversial.[88,89] The GnRH agonists are typically administered as a subcutaneous injection every month or every 3 months while the patient receives chemotherapy. Potential side effects include hot flashes, mood changes, and decreased bone mass; in addition, there is a concern that it lowers the seizure threshold, so OS may not be appropriate for some women with brain cancer.[90]

Similarly, for men (Table 32.2), the standard of care for fertility preservation is sperm cryopreservation (sperm banking). Sperm banking should always be performed prior to treatment initiation. Once a man gives a sample, it is analyzed to determine the total motile sperm count before being frozen into vials. The amount of sperm frozen determines what options a patient has for further use (such as whether his sperm can be used for intrauterine inseminations or for in vitro fertilization). Even if a sample has low numbers, it is still beneficial to freeze it because very little sperm is needed for IVF. For prepubertal boys, testicular tissue cryopreservation (TTC) is the

only viable method of fertility preservation that is available, and it is considered experimental.[87] For TTC, a small sample of testicular tissue is surgically removed and cryopreserved. To the best of our knowledge, as of 2021, no live human births have resulted from cryopreserved testicular tissue.

For prepubertal boys, testicular tissue cryopreservation (TTC) is the only viable method of fertility preservation that is available, and it is considered experimental.

To the best of our knowledge as of 2021, no live human births have resulted from cryopreserved testicular tissue.

Once a patient has completed treatment, fertility testing (ovarian reserve testing for women and a semen analysis for men) can be offered to assess reproductive status. Generally, in cancer medicine, it is recommended to wait at least 1 year off chemotherapy before trying to conceive[87]; however, this time range is shortened to 4–6 months when referencing brain tumor patients.[16,22] During that time, effective contraception

TABLE 32.2 Fertility preservation options for men and boys with cancer

	SPERM CRYOPRESERVATION	TESTICULAR TISSUE CRYOPRESERVATION
Effectiveness	Highly effect	No human births using this method
Appropriate for	Men Postpubertal boys	Prepubertal boys
Process	An ejaculated specimen is provided and then analyzed and cryopreserved for future use	A short surgical procedure is performed where a small piece of testicular tissue is removed (biopsy)
Costs	+	++
Risks	None	Infection, bleeding, discomfort
Side effects	None	None
Time Required	Days (sometime same day)	Days
Important Considerations	Sperm may need to be retrieved surgically if a male is unable to ejaculate sperm Several samples may be desired to increase options for how it is used	Experimental status Difficult to find places that provide testicular tissue cryopreservation services May be able to make mature sperm cells from the cryopreserved tissue in the future

should be utilized to avoid unintended pregnancy. This wait time is clearly more problematic for patients with malignant brain tumors and is typically emphasized for cancer patients with a longer median survival time.

Some patients will be able to have children after cancer treatment even if they choose not to preserve fertility. If a patient has gonadal failure or infertility, there are additional options available to building families such as third-party reproduction (i.e., the use of donor eggs, donor sperm, or donor embryos) and adoption. Some women may choose to use a gestational carrier if they are unable or unwilling to carry a pregnancy.

Pregnancy after brain cancer is possible.[91] Preconceptual counseling with a maternal-fetal medicine specialist is advised so that health conditions and medications are optimized. The timing of pregnancy requires thoughtful discussion between the patient and the oncology and reproductive medicine teams. While cancer survivors may be at increased risk for adverse obstetrical outcomes, including preterm delivery and low-birth-weight infants, many women will have normal, healthy pregnancies and deliveries.[92]

> Preconceptual counseling with a maternal-fetal medicine specialist is advised in brain tumor patients.

While fertility preservation counseling is a necessary component of comprehensive cancer care, there are several challenges and barriers to ensuring that patients receive these services. Time constraints, personal biases about who should be counseled, and misperceptions about safety may prevent providers from initiating these discussions.[93] In addition, many patients may lack geographical access to fertility clinics, and most do not have insurance coverage for fertility services.[94] Oncologists can partner with local fertility practices to improve access and help connect patient to resources that help

defray costs. Multidisciplinary collaboration can ensure that the fertility needs of patients are met, ultimately improving their survivorship experience.

In summary, it is imperative that patients who are at risk for cancer-related infertility are informed of their risk and the availability of fertility preservation strategies. Collaboration between oncologists and reproductive medicine specialists can facilitate access to fertility services and help cancer patients achieve their family building goals.

CONCLUSION

In 1986, the National Institutes of Health (NIH) began talks on developing a policy aimed to include women in clinical research.[95] This was further developed to include minorities as part of the NIH Revitalization Act of 1993 and signed into law.[95] It has been more than three and a half decades, and the field lacks research that significantly improves our understanding of the psychosocial, reproductive/hormonal, fertility, and survivorship areas that best support our female brain tumor patients over the course of their disease.

As women experience hormonal and other physiological changes over their life spans, the impact on brain tumors over this time period should be well understood. The very diagnosis of an intracranial tumor could change the course of a woman's reproductive choices. Furthermore, the treatments potentially disfigure and limit sexuality and self-esteem, as well as impact her fertility, and are of great consequence. Studies that evaluate the impact of diagnosis and treatment on female sexual confidence, pleasure, desire, and fertility are equally important as those that evaluate survival and tumor response to therapy.

Different hormonal stages occur across the female maturation process from early development, puberty, pregnancy, lactation, and years of pregnancy-avoidance through the peri- and postmenopausal periods. Also, there are various iatrogenic exposures to hormone therapies based on lifestyle preferences, health, and choices related to gender affirmation. These changes might lead to other health risks or even modify response to cancer therapies. Dedicated research is needed in neuro-oncology to also encourage guideline development and to bring awareness to these issues for best clinical practices.

Finally, recognizing and addressing issues of women's sexuality in neuro-oncology should be a routine part of the clinical discussion on patient follow-up. Sexuality in brain tumor patients remains understudied. Issues pertaining to sexuality are complicated by multiple factors such as hormones, tumor types, and tumor location, which directly affect our patients' QoL. More research with a special focus on sexuality in brain tumor and its impact on patient QoL is needed, and brain tumor practitioners need to aggressively address sexuality issues as part of routine brain tumor care and education.

REFERENCES

1. McInnis MK, Pukall CF. Sex after prostate cancer in gay and bisexual men: A review of the literature. *Sex Med Rev.* 2020;8(3):466–472.
2. Salakari M, Nurminen R, Sillanmäki L, et al. The importance of and satisfaction with sex life among breast cancer survivors in comparison with healthy female controls and women with mental depression or arterial hypertension: Results from the Finnish nationwide HeSSup cohort study. *Support Care Cancer.* 2020;28(8):3847–3854.
3. Salonia A, Adaikan G, Buvat J, et al. Sexual rehabilitation after treatment for prostate cancer-part 2: Recommendations from the fourth International Consultation for Sexual Medicine (ICSM 2015). *J Sex Med.* 2017;14(3):297–315.
4. von Hippel C, Rosenberg SM, Austin SB, et al. Identifying distinct trajectories of change in young breast cancer survivors' sexual functioning. *Psychooncology.* 2019;28(5):1033–1040.
5. Bouloux PM, Grossman A. Hyperprolactinaemia and sexual function in the male. *Br J Hosp Med.* 1987;37(6):503–510.
6. Corona G, Mannucci E, Jannini EA, et al. Hypoprolactinemia: A new clinical syndrome in patients with sexual dysfunction. *J Sex Med.* 2009;6(5):1457–1466.
7. Zhou WJ, Ma SC, Zhao M, et al. Risk factors and the prognosis of sexual dysfunction in male patients with pituitary adenomas: A multivariate analysis. *Asian J Androl.* 2018;20(1):43–49.
8. Donovan KA, Gonzalez BD, Nelson AM, et al. Effect of androgen deprivation therapy on sexual function and bother in men with prostate cancer: A controlled comparison. *Psychooncology.* 2018;27(1):316–324.
9. Ostrom QT, Patil N, Cioffi G, et al. CBTRUS statistical report: Primary brain and other central nervous system tumors diagnosed in the United States in 2013–2017. *Neuro Oncol.* 2020.
10. ACOG Committee Opinion No. 723: guidelines for diagnostic imaging during pregnancy and lactation.
11. Expert Panel on MR Safety, Emanuel Kanal, A James Barkovich, et al. Expert Panel on MR Safety. ACR guidance document on MR safe practices: 2013. *J Magn Reson Imaging.* 2013;37:501–530.
12. Kodzwa R. ACR manual on contrast media. *Radiol Technol.* 2019;91:97–100
13. Ng J, Kitchen N. Neurosurgery and pregnancy. *J Neurol Neurosurg Psychiatry.* 2008;79:745–752.
14. Lynch JC, Gouvêa F, Emmerich JC, et al. Management strategy for brain tumour diagnosed during pregnancy. *Br J Neurosurg.* 2011;25:225–230.
15. Rodrigues A, Waldrop A, Suharwardy S, et al. Management of brain tumors presenting in pregnancy: A cases series and systematic review. *AJOG MFM.* 2021;(3)1–11.
16. van Westrhenen A, Senders JT, Martin E, et al. Clinical challenges of glioma and pregnancy: A systematic review. *J Neurooncol.* 2018;139(1):1–11.
17. Wang LP, Paech MJ. Neuroanesthesia for the pregnant woman. *Anesth Analg.* 2008;107:193–200.
18. Reitman E, Flood P. Anaesthetic considerations for non-obstetric surgery during pregnancy. *Br J Anaesth.* 2011;107:i72–i78.
19. Pantelis E, Antypas C, Frassanito MC, et al. Radiation dose to the fetus during CyberKnife radiosurgery for a brain tumor in pregnancy. *Phys Med.* 2016;32:237–241.
20. Blumenthal DT, Parreño MG, Batten J, Chamberlain MC. Management of malignant gliomas during pregnancy: A case series. *Cancer.* 2008;113:3349–3354.
21. Stupp R, Mason WP, van den Bent MJ, et al. Radiotherapy plus concomitant and adjuvant temozolomide for glioblastoma. *N Engl J Med.* 2005;352:987–996.
22. Nolan B, Balakrishna M, George M. Exposure to temozolmide in the first trimester of pregnancy in a young woman with glioblastoma multiforme. *World J Oncol.* 2012;3(6):286–287. doi:10.4021/wjon570w
23. Kaaks R, Berrino F, Key T, et al. Serum sex steroids in premenopausal women and breast cancer risk within the European Prospective Investigation into Cancer and Nutrition (EPIC). *J Nat Cancer Inst.* 2005;97(10):755–765.
24. Zheng D, Williams C, Vold JA, et al. Regulation of sex hormone receptors in sexual dimorphism of human cancers. *Cancer Lett.* 2018;438:24–31.
25. Brinton LA, Key TJ, Kolonel LN, et al. Prediagnostic sex steroid hormones in relation to male breast cancer risk. *J Clin Oncol.* 2015;33(18):2041–2050.
26. Yust-Katz S, de Groot JF, Liu D, et al. Pregnancy and glial brain tumors. *Neuro-Oncology.* 2014;16(9):1289–1294.
27. Magill ST, Theodosopoulos PV, McDermott MW Resection of falx and parasagittal meningioma: Complication avoidance. *J Neuro-Oncol.* 2016;130(2):253–262. doi:10.1007/s11060-016-2283-x
28. Engenhart-Cabillic R, Farhoud A, Sure U, et al. Clinicopathologic features of aggressive meningioma emphasizing the role of radiotherapy in treatment. *Strahlentherapie und Onkologie : Organ der Deutschen Rontgengesellschaft.* 2006;182(11):641–646. https://doi.org/10.1007/s00066-006-1555-3
29. de Carvalho GTC, de Silva-Martiins WC, deMagãlhaes KCSF, et al. Recurrence/regrowth in grade I meningioma: How to predict? *Front Oncol.* 2020;10:1144. doi:10.3389/fonc.2020.01144
30. Nagahama A, Yashiro M, Kawashima T, et al. Combination of p53 and Ki67 as a promising predictor of postoperative recurrence of meningioma. *Anticancer Res.* 2021;41(1):203–210. doi:10.21873/anticanres.14766
31. Korhonen K, Salminen T, Raitanen J, et al. Female predominance in meningiomas cannot be explained by differences in progesterone, estrogen, or androgen receptor expression. *J Neuro-Oncol.* 2006;80(1):1–7.
32. Ostrom QT, Gittleman H, Xu J, et al. CBTRUS statistical report: Primary brain and other central nervous system tumors diagnosed in the united states in 2009–2013. *Neuro-Oncology.* 2016 Oct; 18(5):1–75.
33. Wolfsberger S, et al. Progesterone-receptor index in meningiomas: Correlation with clinico-pathological parameters and review of the literature. *Neurosurg Rev.* 2004;27(4):238–245.
34. Ji Y, Rankin C, Grunberg S, Sherrod AE, et al. Double-blind phase III randomized trial of the antiprogestin agent mifepristone in the treatment of unresectable meningioma: SWOG S9005. *J Clin Oncol.* 2015 Dec; 33(34):4093–4098.
35. Rubinstein AB, Loren D, Geier A, et al. Hormone receptors in initially excised versus recurrent intracranial meningiomas. *J Neurosurg.* 1994;81:184–187.
36. Carroll RS, Zhang J, Dashner K, et al. Androgen receptor expression in meningiomas. *J Neurosurg.* 1995;82:453–460.
37. Chamberlain MC, Barnholtz JS. Medical treatment of recurrent meningiomas. *Exp Rev Neurothera.* 2014 Jan;11(10):1425–1432.
38. Qi Z, Shao C, Huang Y, et al. Reproductive and exogenous hormone factors in relation to risk of meningioma in women: A meta-analysis. *PLoS ONE.* 2013;8(12):e83261.
39. Blitshteyn S, Cook JE, Jaeckle KA. Is there an association between meningioma and hormone replacement therapy? *J Clin Oncol.* 2008;26(2):279–282.
40. Shu X, et al. Association of hormone replacement therapy with increased risk of meningioma in women: A hospital-based multicenter study with propensity score matching. *Asia-Pacific J Clin Oncol.* 2019;15(5):e147–e153.
41. Deli T, et al. Hormone replacement therapy in cancer survivors: Review of the literature. *Pathol Oncol Res.* 2020;26(1):63–78.
42. Maxwell, M et al. Expression of androgen and progesterone receptors in primary human meningiomas. *J Neurosurg.* 1993;78(3):456–462. doi:10.3171/jns.1993.78.3.0456
43. Melmed S. Pituitary-tumor endocrinopathies. *N Engl J Med.* 2020;382(10):937–950. doi:10.1056/NEJMra1810772
44. Huang W, Molitch ME. Pituitary tumors in pregnancy. *Endocrinol Metabol Clin N Am.* 2019;48(3):569–581.
45. Molitc ME. Diagnosis and treatment of pituitary adenomas: A review. *JAMA.* 2017;317(5):516–524.
46. National Brain Tumor Society. Quick Brain Tumor Facts. Jan 10, 2021. https://braintumor.org/brain-tumor-information/brain-tumor-facts/#AYA-brain-tumors
47. Glezer A, Bronstein MD. Prolactinomas in pregnancy: Considerations before conception and during pregnancy. *Pituitary.* 2020;23(1):65–69. doi:10.1007/s11102-019-01010-5

48. Gonzalez JG, Elizondo G, Saldivar D, et al. Pituitary gland growth during normal pregnancy: An in vivo study using magnetic resonance imaging. *Am J Med.* 1988;85(2):217–220. doi:10.1016/s0002-9343(88)80346-2

49. Dinç H, Esen F, Demirci A, Sari A, Resit Gümele H. Pituitary dimensions and volume measurements in pregnancy and post partum. MR assessment. *Acta Radiologica (Stockholm, Sweden : 1987).* 1998;39(1):64–69. doi:10.1080/02841859809172152

50. Daghighi MH, Seifar F, Parviz A, et al. The effect of females' reproductive factors on pituitary gland size in women at reproductive age. *Medicina (Kaunas, Lithuania).* Jul 2019;55(7):367. doi:10.3390/medicina55070367

51. Omuro A, DeAngelis LM. Glioblastoma and other malignant gliomas: A clinical review. *JAMA.* 2013;310(17):1842–1850.

52. Stupp R, Taillibert S, Kanner A, et al. Effect of tumor-treating fields plus maintenance temozolomide vs maintenance temozolomide alone on survival in patients with glioblastoma: A randomized clinical trial. *JAMA.* 2017;318(23):2306–2316. doi:10.1001/jama.2017.18718

53. Gittleman H, Ostrom QT, Stetson LC, et al. Sex is an important prognostic factor for glioblastoma but not for nonglioblastoma. *Neuro-Oncol Pract.* 2019;6(6):451–462. https://doi.org/10.1093/nop/npz019

54. McCormick A, Peterson E. Cancer in pregnancy. *Obstet Gynecol Clin North Am.* 2018 Jun;45(2):187–200.

55. Peeters S, Pagès M, Gauchotte G, et al. Interactions between glioma and pregnancy: Insight from a 52-case multicenter series. *J Neurosurg.* 2017;128:1–11.

56. Pallud J, Duffau H, Razak RA, et al. Influence of pregnancy in the behavior of diffuse gliomas: Clinical cases of a French glioma study group. *J Neurol.* 2009;256(12):2014–2020.

57. Pallud J, Mandonnet E, Deroulers C, et al. Pregnancy increases the growth rates of World Health Organization Grade II Gliomas. *Ann Neurol.* 2010;67(3):398–404.

58. Hordern A. Intimacy and sexuality after cancer: A critical review of the literature. *Cancer Nurs.* 2008;31(2):E9–E17.

59. Heinrichs KD, MacKnee C, Auton-Cuff F, Domene JF. Factors affecting sexual-self esteem among young adult women in long-term heterosexual relationships. *Can J Hum Sex.* 2009;18(4):183–199.

60. Surbeck W, Herbert G, Duffau H. Sexuality after surgery for diffuse low-grade glioma. *Neuro Oncol.* 2015;17(4):574–579. doi:10.1093/neuonc/nou326

61. Finocchiaro CY, Petruzzi A, Fedeli G, et al. Hidden reality: Sexual sphere in brain tumor patients. *Psychol Health Med.* 2017;22(3):370–380. doi:10.1080/13548506.2016.1210176

62. Stricker CT, et al. Survivorship care planning after the institute of medicine recommendations: How are we faring? *J Cancer Survivorship Res Pract.* 2011;5:358–370. doi:10.1007/s11764-011-0196-4

63. Colao A, Sarno AD, Cappabianca P, et al. Gender differences in the prevalence, clinical features and response to cabergoline in hyperprolactinemia. *Eur J Endocrinol.* 2003;148(3):325–331.

64. Kann PH, Juratli N, Kabalan Y. Prolactinoma and hyperprolactinaemia: A transcultural comparative study between Germany as a western, liberal, industrialised country and Syria as an oriental society with a strong Islamic tradition. *Gynecol Endocrinol.* 2010;26(10):749–754. doi:10.3109/09513590.2010.487600

65. Lundberg PO, Hulter B. Sexual dysfunction in patients with hypothalamo-pituitary disorders. *Exp Clin Endocrinol.* 1991;98(2), 81–88. doi:10.1055/s-0029-1211104

66. Zaidi HA, Cote DJ, Castlen JP, et al. Time course of resolution of hyperprolactinemia after transsphenoidal surgery among patients presenting with pituitary stalk compression. *World Neurosurg.* 2017;97:2–7. doi:10.1016/j.wneu.2016.09.066

67. Auriemma RS, Grasso LF, Pivonello R, Colao A. The safety of treatments for prolactinomas. *Expert Opin Drug Saf.* 2016;15(4):503–512. doi:10.1517/14740338.2016.1151493

68. Darzy KH, Shalet SM. Hypopituitarism after cranial irradiation. *J Endocrinol Invest.* 2005;28(5 Suppl):78–87.

69. Darzy KH, Shalet SM. Hypopituitarism following Radiotherapy Revisited. *Endocr Dev.* 2009;15:1–24. doi:10.1159/000207607

70. Ritvonen E, Karppinen A, Sintonen H, et al. Normal long-term health-related quality of life can be achieved in patients with functional pituitary adenomas having surgery as primary treatment. *Clin Endocrinol (Oxf).* 2015;82(3):412–421. doi:10.1111/cen.12550

71. Acquati S, Pizzocaro A, Tomei G, et al. A comparative evaluation of effectiveness of medical and surgical therapy in patients with macroprolactinoma. *J Neurosurg Sci.* 2001;45(2):65–69.

72. Thavarajah N, Bedard G, Zhang L, et al. Psychometric validation of the functional assessment of cancer therapy–brain (FACT-Br) for assessing quality of life in patients with brain metastases. *Support Care Cancer.* 2014;22:1017–1028.

73. Weitzner MA, Meyers CA, Gelke CK, et al. The functional assessment of cancer therapy (FACT) Scale. *Cancer.* 1995;75:151–161.

74. Boccia ML, Anyanda EI, Fonkem E. A preliminary report on quality of life and sexual function in brain tumor patients. *J Sex Med.* 2021. doi:10.1016/j.jsxm.2021.01.171

75. Pinzone JJ, Katznelson L, Danila DC, et al. Primary medical therapy of micro- and macroprolactinomas in men. *J Clin Endocrinol Metab.* 2000;85(9):3053–3057. doi:10.1210/jcem.85.9.6798

76. Shindel AW, Parish SJ. Sexuality education in North American medical schools: Current status and future directions. *J Sex Med.* 2013;10(1):3–17; quiz 18. doi:10.1111/j.1743-6109.2012.02987.x

77. Simon JA, Thorp J, Millheiser L. Flibanserin for premenopausal hypoactive sexual desire disorder: Pooled analysis of clinical trials. *J Womens Health (Larchmt).* 2019;28(6):769–777. doi:10.1089/jwh.2018.7516

79. Brown PD, Ballman KV, Rummans TA, et al. Prospective study of quality of life in adults with newly diagnosed high-grade gliomas. *J Neurooncol.* 2006;76(3):283–291. doi:10.1007/s11060-005-7020-9

78. Mayer D, Lynch SE. Bremelanotide: New drug approved for treating hypoactive sexual desire disorder. *Ann Pharmacother.* 2020;54(7):684–690. doi:10.1177/1060028019899152

79. Brown PD, Ballman KV, Rummans TA, et al. Prospective study of quality of life in adults with newly diagnosed high-grade gliomas. *J Neurooncol.* 2006;76(3):283–291. doi:10.1007/s11060-005-7020-9

80. Schover LR, Rybicki LA, Martin BA, Bringelsen KA. Having children after cancer: A pilot survey of survivors' attitudes and experiences. *Cancer.* 1999 Aug 15;86(4):697–709.

81. Canada AL, Schover LR. The psychosocial impact of interrupted childbearing in long-term female cancer survivors. *Psychooncology.* 2012 Feb;21(2):134–143.

82. Lee SJ, Schover LR, Partridge AH, et al. American Society of Clinical Oncology. American Society of Clinical Oncology recommendations on fertility preservation in cancer patients. *J Clin Oncol.* 2006 Jun 20;24(18):2917–2931.

83. Oktay K, Harvey BE, Partridge AH, et al. Fertility Preservation in Patients With Cancer: ASCO Clinical Practice Guideline Update. *J Clin Oncol.* 2018 Jul 1;36(19):1994–2001.

84. Letourneau JM, Ebbel EE, Katz PP, et al. Pretreatment fertility counseling and fertility preservation improve quality of life in reproductive age women with cancer. *Cancer.* 2012 Mar 15;118(6):1710–1717.

85. Cakmak H, Rosen MP. Random-start ovarian stimulation in patients with cancer. *Curr Opin Obstet Gynecol.* 2015 Jun;27(3):215–221.

86. Ben-Haroush A, Ben-Aharon I, Lande Y, Fisch B. Use of aromatase inhibitors in IVF for fertility preservation of non-breast cancer patients: A case series. *Isr Med Assoc J.* 2018.

87. Wallace WH, Kelsey TW, Anderson RA. Fertility preservation in pre-pubertal girls with cancer: The role of ovarian tissue cryopreservation. *Fertil Steril.* 2016;105(1):6–12. Mar;20(3):145–146.

88. Chen H, Xiao L, Li J, et al. Adjuvant gonadotropin-releasing hormone analogues for the prevention of chemotherapy-induced premature ovarian failure in premenopausal women. *Cochrane Database Syst Rev.* 2019 Mar 3;3(3):CD008018.

89. Durrani S, Heena H. Controversies regarding ovarian suppression and infertility in early stage breast cancer. *Cancer Manag Res.* 2020;12:813–817.

90. De Sanctis V, et al. Long-term effects and significant adverse drug reactions (ADRs) associated with the use of gonadotropin-releasing hormone analogs (GnRHa) for central precocious puberty: A brief review of literature. *Acta Bio-Medica Atenei Parmensis.* 6 Sep 2019;90(3):345–359. doi:10.23750/abm.v90i3.8736

91. Peyser A, Bristow SL, Hershlag A. Two successful pregnancies following fertility preservation in a patient with anaplastic astrocytoma: A case report. *BMC Cancer.* 2018 May 9;18(1):544.

92. Signorello LB, Cohen SS, Bosetti C, et al. Female survivors of childhood cancer: Preterm birth and low birth weight among their children. *J Nat Cancer Instit.* 2006;98(20):1453–1461.

93. Covelli A, Facey M, Kennedy E, et al. Clinicians' perspectives on barriers to discussing infertility and fertility preservation with young women with cancer. *JAMA Netw Open.* 2019;2(11):e1914511.

94. Flink DM, Sheeder J, Kondapalli LA. A review of the oncology patient's challenges for utilizing fertility preservation services. *J Adolesc Young Adult Oncol.* 2017;6(1):31–44.

95. NIH Office of Research on Women's Health (ORWH). NIH inclusion outreach toolkit: How to engage, recruit, and retain women in clinical research. https://orwh.od.nih.gov/toolkit/recruitment/history.

Congenital malformations and neurocognitive delays have been associated with fetal radiation dosages greater than what level?	10 cGy
Meningiomas make up what percentage of all benign intracranial tumors?	Approximately 40% (38.3%)
Which intracranial tumor type should have more frequent routine clinical evaluations during pregnancy for early detection of tumor growth?	Pituitary adenoma
GBMs have a slight male predominance of_____ and a peak incidence in age over ___	(1.6:1) Male-to-female 75 years
Non-GBM gliomas are not sex-discrepant (1:1) males to females and have a peak incidence between the ages of:	35 and 44 years
Which tumor type has been the primary research focus for the impact of sexual function on quality of life (QoL)?	Pituitary tumors
Which symptoms commonly accompany pituitary tumors along with vision changes, headaches, and hormone disruption?	Amenorrhea Loss of sexual desire Infertility
What is the most common sexual dysfunction in women?	Low or loss of libido
If there are significant time constraints to treat a woman with brain tumor, _____start protocols may be used to start the ovarian stimulation process right away as opposed to awaiting start of menses	Random

To date, _____ live human births have resulted from cryopreserved testicular tissue	No
Physiological and pharmacodynamic changes of pregnancy have an impact on _____ and _____ management	Neurosurgical and Anesthetic
In pregnant patients, proper _____is important to prevent disruption of placental blood perfusion and excessive fetal drug exposure	Neurosurgical positioning
Prolactinomas are the most common type of _____ pituitary tumor and are ___ times more likely to occur in females	Functioning 4.5

QUESTIONS

1. Meningiomas are known to grow during which phase of the menstrual cycle?
   a. Ovulation phase
   b. Luteal phase
   c. Follicular phase
   d. Menstruation phase

2. Females account for what percentage of all intracranial tumors (benign and malignant)?
   a. 15–20%
   b. 25–30%
   c. 45–50%
   d. 55–60%

3. The most common type of hormone producing pituitary tumor is a _____ and is _____ times more likely to occur in females.
   a. Prolactinoma, 4–5
   b. Growth hormone producing adenoma, 1–2
   c. Null cell adenoma, 1–2
   d. Pituicytoma, 4–5

4. The National Institutes of Health (NIH) was founded in 1887; however, it was not until this Act was passed that the organization fully signed a policy into law which mandated the inclusion of women and other minorities in clinical research.
   a. Women's National Pan-Hellenic Act of 1913
   b. Organization on Women and Inclusion Act of 1964
   c. NIH Revitalization Act of 1993
   d. NIH Women's and Minorities Act of 2001

5. For women with gliomas who subsequently become pregnant, which time periods have been associated with increased tumor aggressiveness?
   a. At 1–2 months postpartum
   b. Second and third trimesters of pregnancy
   c. First and second trimesters of pregnancy
   d. There is no pregnancy association with glioma aggressive behavior

6. In review of the established radiology guidelines for brain tumor imaging using magnetic resonance (MR) in pregnant women, the following is true:
   a. All MR imaging is discouraged based on the risk to the mother.
   b. Use of contrasted MR is uniformly contraindicated despite any risk to the mother.
   c. Head CT is preferred over MR due to known risk for fetal deafness due to MR.
   d. None of the above.

7. As it pertains to brain tumors and sexuality, _____ is the most well researched tumor and studies primarily focus on _____.
   a. Glioma, lack of libido in females
   b. Glioma, hypogonadism in males
   c. Pituitary adenoma, painful intercourse in females
   d. Pituitary adenoma, lack of libido in males

8. A 2001 study compared sexual function across various treatment types in cancer patients and found which treatment approach resulted in the highest potential to restore sexual function?
   a. Surgery
   b. Medical therapy
   c. Radiation therapy
   d. None of the above

9. _____ is the most commonly reported sexual dysfunction in females with a history of cancer and _____.
   a. Performance anxiety; there are no available treatment options.
   b. Anorgasmia; flibanserin was recently approved to treat this condition.
   c. Loss of desire; it is unclear if approved therapies impact brain tumors.
   d. Decreased libido; sex therapy has not been found to be effective.

10. Major barriers that complicate a woman's ability to access fertility services include
    a. Geographical limits to established fertility clinics
    b. Lack of insurance coverage for fertility services
    c. Limited need in cancer as most women are post reproductive
    d. Both b and c
    e. Both a and b

11. Considerations for neurosurgery during pregnancy would include the following:
    a. First trimester is optimal for resection due to small size of the fetus.
    b. When necessary, the second trimester is the preferred neurosurgical time period.
    c. Patients are encouraged to terminate pregnancy if there is an urgent neurosurgical need.
    d. Biopsy is the primary neurosurgical option during early pregnancy.

12. Considerations for radiation therapy during pregnancy would include the following:
    a. There is no way to calculate fetal radiation doses due to scatter during brain irradiation.

b. Radiation therapy is absolutely contraindicated in pregnancy.
c. The recommendation is to use stereotactic radiation therapy to limit fetal risk.
d. Radiation therapy is recommended when the risk of not treating the tumor outweighs the known risk to the fetus.

13. Considerations for brain tumor surgery during pregnancy would include the following:
a. First trimester is optimal for resection due to small size of the fetus.
b. Second trimester is ideal neurosurgical time period when necessary.
c. Patients are encouraged to terminate pregnancy if there is an urgent neurosurgical need.
d. Biopsy is the primary neurosurgical option during early pregnancy.

14. Considerations for anesthesia during pregnancy would include the following:
a. There is no commonly used general anesthetic proved to be safer than another.
b. Monitoring intracranial pressures is only important in the first trimester of pregnancy.

c. Lung volumes and oxygenation are only impacted during the peripartum period.
d. Use of anesthesia during pregnancy has been determined to have teratogenic effects on the developing fetus.

ANSWERS

1. b
2. d
3. a
4. c
5. b
6. d
7. d
8. b
9. c
10. e
11. b
12. d
13. b
14. a

TEST EXAM NUMBER ONE

1. Which of the following central nervous system (CNS) tumors are most commonly seen with Turcot syndrome?
   a. Glioma
   b. Ependymoma
   c. Meningioma
   d. Medulloblastoma

2. The most frequently encountered toxicity with tumor treating fields (TTFields) is:
   a. Low grade (grade 1–2) skin toxicity
   b. High grade (grade 3–4) skin toxicity
   c. An electric-like sensation
   d. A heat sensation

3. Reasonable induction regimens in primary CNS lymphoma (PCNSL) include all of the following *except*
   a. High-dose methotrexate (HD-MTX) alone
   b. HD-MTX with rituximab and temozolomide (TMZ)
   c. HD-MTX with whole-brain radiotherapy (WBRT)
   d. HD-MTX, rituximab, procarbazine, and vincristine

4. A 65-year-old man presents with focal seizures involving the left upper extremity and left face. Magnetic resonance imaging (MRI) reveals a 2 cm enhancing mass in the right frontal lobe. Of note, he is a heavy smoker, and chest computed tomography (CT) shows large mass at the left lower lobe of his lungs. What is the most likely diagnosis?
   a. Glioblastoma (GBM)
   b. Lung cancer metastasis
   c. Anaplastic oligodendroglioma
   d. Melanoma metastases

5. Which of the following statements is true?
   a. Meningiomas represent the most common malignant brain tumors, with an incidence of 500,000 per year.
   b. Meningiomas represent the most common intracranial tumors, with an incidence of 20,000 per year.
   c. Meningiomas most commonly occur in children and are frequently associated with prior radiation exposure.
   d. The incidence of meningioma increases with age, and meningiomas tend to be more aggressive in older individuals.

6. The risk of long-term radiation toxicity depends on:
   a. Radiation dose
   b. Volume treated
   c. Fraction size
   d. All of the above

7. A prospective cohort trial assessed the contribution of mobile phone use to the development of gliomas. The 5-year relative risk for the heaviest mobile phone users (cumulative lifetime duration of calls ≥896 hours) compared to participants who were not regular mobile phone users was 1.4. The 95% confidence interval was 1.02–1.85. Which p-value is most consistent with these results?
   a. 0.03
   b. 0.06
   c. 0.09
   d. 0.11
   e. 0.25

8. Which of the following statements is false regarding pituitary tumors?
   a. Surgical resection is never indicated for prolactinomas.
   b. Surgical decompression improves visual acuity outcomes for patients with pituitary apoplexy.
   c. Surgical treatment is the first-line treatment for Cushing disease.
   d. Residual tumor within the cavernous sinus is common.

9. Which of the following pathologic features is found in nearly all ependymomas?
   a. Pseudorosettes
   b. True ependymal rosettes
   c. Rosenthal fibers
   d. Homer-Wright rosettes

10. A patient with history of medulloblastoma status post resection, radiation, and chemotherapy undergoes their routine surveillance imaging. Given the highly cellular nature of medulloblastoma, which MRI finding is most suggestive of recurrent disease?
    a. Contrast enhancement
    b. T2/fluid-attenuated inversion recovery (FLAIR) hyperintensity

c. T1 hyperintensity

d. Positivity on diffusion-weighted imaging

11. A 1-year-old girl undergoes gross total resection for a newly diagnosed lesion of the left frontal lobe. Pathology reveals GBM (World Health Organization [WHO] grade 4). What is the next best step in management?

a. Radiochemotherapy, including focal radiation therapy and TMZ

b. Radiochemotherapy, including craniospinal radiation therapy

c. Genomic testing and administration of molecular targeted therapy

d. Chemotherapy only

12. Which of the following is the correct mechanism of action for the agent listed?

a. Vincristine: Formation of DNA adducts

b. Cytarabine: Anti-folate

c. Erlotinib: Anti-vascular endothelial growth factor (VEGF) tyrosine kinase inhibitor

d. Lomustine: Alkylating agent

13. A 32-year-old man is brought to the hospital with 3 weeks of progressive confusion and abnormal behavior. He also developed dysphagia, dysarthria, and a decreased level of consciousness. Brain MRI shows increased T2 signal of the brainstem and medial temporal lobes bilaterally. Which of the following tests is most likely to identify an underlying malignancy?

a. CT scan of the chest

b. CT scan of the abdomen

c. Thyroid ultrasound

d. Testicular ultrasound

e. CT scan of the pelvis

14. The volume of cerebrospinal fluid (CSF) to be withdrawn intrathecally should be twice the volume of chemotherapy being delivered.

a. True

b. False

15. Which of the following tumors is statistically most likely to cause epilepsy?

a. Frontal lobe GBM

b. Frontal lobe grade 2 oligodendroglioma

c. Brainstem glioma

d. Occipital lobe isocitrate dehydrogenase (IDH)-WT astrocytoma

16. Radiotherapy alone in GBM of the elderly should be preferentially prescribed to:

a. Patients with unmethylated O^6-methylguanine DNA methyltransferase (MGMT)

b. Patients with methylated MGMT

c. Patients with lower performance status (Karnofsky 60–70) and comorbidities

d. Patients with lower performance status (Karnofsky 60–70), comorbidities, and MGMT unmethylated tumors

17. A 10-year-old boy with neurofibromatosis (NF1) was found to have a presumed focal area of signal intensity (FASI) in his temporal lobe on MRI brain during evaluation of a concussion. What is important to counsel the family?

a. He needs surgical excision of the lesion since it is likely a low-grade glioma.

b. He will likely develop epilepsy.

c. He is unlikely to have any clinical manifestations from this lesion.

d. The lesion is likely to develop into high-grade glioma in the future.

18. A 30-year-old woman with NF2 undergoes a spine MRI with the following finding. What is the most likely diagnosis?

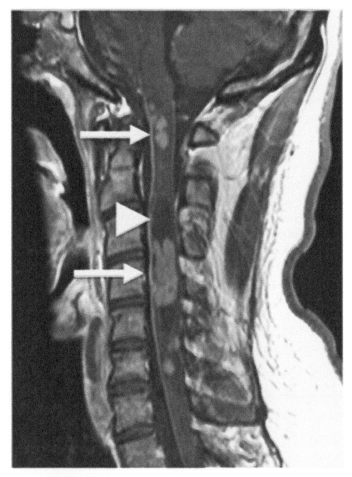

a. Meningioma

b. Ependymoma

c. Astrocytoma

d. Multiple schwannomas

19. A patient with GBM and tumor-related epilepsy is nearing the end-of-life phase and is having difficulty with swallowing. The patient normally takes levetiracetam. What is a reasonable therapeutic option for this patient to manage seizures?
    a. Oral lacosamide
    b. Intramuscular phenytoin
    c. IV lamotrigine
    d. Rectal diazepam

20. Which combination therapy has been proven to have high intracranial activity in BRAF-wildtype metastatic melanoma to the brain?
    a. Ipilimumab and nivolumab
    b. Pembrolizumab, pemetrexed, and carboplatin
    c. Dabrafenib and trametinib
    d. Lapatinib and capecitabine

21. Brain tumor patients who require anticoagulation due to venous thromboembolism (VTE) are preferably treated with:
    a. Warfarin
    b. Rivaroxaban
    c. Dabigatran
    d. Low-molecular-weight heparin (LMWH)
    e. Both LMWH and newer oral anticoagulants can be used

22. A 4-year-old boy is referred by his primary pediatrician because, on a well-child visit, he is noted to have a subtle cranial nerve VII palsy. A MRI brain demonstrates a focal, exophytic, contrast-enhancing mass in the pons. The pons appears to be pushed aside. What is the next step in management?
    a. Diagnosis is consistent with diffuse intrinsic pontine glioma (DIPG) and biopsy is not required
    b. Biopsy for suspected dorsally exophytic low-grade glioma
    c. MRI spine and lumbar puncture to stage the neuroaxis
    d. Focal radiation therapy to the pontine lesion

23. Tuberous sclerosis complex is associated with activation of which of the following intracellular signaling molecules?
    a. MAPK
    b. mTOR
    c. BRAF
    d. EGFR

24. Which tumor was removed from the WHO 2016 classification?
    a. Primitive neuroectodermal tumor (PNET)
    b. Diffuse midline glioma
    c. Ependymoma
    d. Germinoma

25. What is true in regard to the BRAF V600E mutation?
    a. It is mostly found in ganglioglioma.
    b. It is mostly found in pilocytic astrocytoma.

    c. It is commonly found in combination with H3K27M mutation low-grade gliomas.
    d. It has no clinical importance.

26. Each of the following factors may impede delivery of chemotherapeutic drugs to the CNS *except*:
    a. Drug efflux pumps
    b. High lipid solubility
    c. High protein binding of the drug
    d. Concurrent use of corticosteroids
    e. Concurrent use of hepatic enzyme inducing antiepileptic drugs

27. What was the median overall survival (OS) of GBM patients who were treated with the Stupp regimen followed by TTFields combined with adjuvant TMZ?
    a. 4 months
    b. 7 months
    c. 10 months
    d. 15 months
    e. 20 months

28. The incidence of status epilepticus is highest in:
    a. Low-grade glioma
    b. High-grade glioma
    c. Brain metastases
    d. Meningioma

29. Based on the Common Terminology Criteria for Adverse Events (CTCAE v. 5.0), neutropenic fever defined as
    a. ANC <500/mm^3 and a single temperature of >38.0°C (100.4°F)
    b. ANC <1000/mm^3 and a single temperature of >38.0°C (100.4°F)
    c. ANC <1000/mm^3 and a single temperature of >38.3°C (101°F)
    d. Sustained temperature of 38.3°C (101°F)

30. Adult ependymomas most commonly occur in the:
    a. Spine
    b. Lateral ventricles
    c. Third ventricle
    d. Fourth ventricle

31. PCNSLs in immunocompromised patients classically exhibit:
    a. No ring enhancement on MRI
    b. Overall irregular contrast enhancement on imaging
    c. Homogeneous contrast enhancement on imaging
    d. Decreased signal on diffusion-weighted imaging

32. Which of the following tumors is the least likely cause of CSF seeding/dissemination?
    a. Pineoblastoma
    b. Craniopharyngioma
    c. Ependymoma
    d. Medulloblastoma

33. Which of these statements is false about pseudoprogression?
    a. Pseudoprogression is associated with longer survival.
    b. Studies have shown that tumors with hypermethylated MGMT promoter status have up to 91% incidence of pseudoprogression.
    c. MRI perfusion maps commonly show increase in relative cerebral blood volume (rCBV) in pseudoprogression compared to the pre-treatment values.
    d. Imaging can demonstrate increasing size of enhancing components of the tumor.

34. Which of the following is a common indication for intrathecal chemotherapy?
    a. Leptomeningeal metastasis
    b. Brain metastasis
    c. CNS neoplastic prophylaxis
    d. Both a and c

35. The molecular analysis of a resected glioma reveals high mitotic index, IDH-1 mutation, and intact 1p/19q chromosomes. What is the pathologic diagnosis?
    a. WHO grade 2, IDH-1 mutated astrocytoma
    b. WHO grade 2, oligodendroglioma
    c. WHO grade 3, IDH-1 mutated astrocytoma
    d. WHO grade 3, oligodendroglioma

36. The current CODEL study aims to assess:
    a. The role of radiation therapy in treatment of oligodendrogliomas
    b. The role of radiation therapy in treatment of astrocytomas
    c. The role of TMZ versus procarbazine, lomustine and vincristine (PCV) in treatment of oligodendrogliomas
    d. The role of TMZ versus PCV in treatment of astrocytomas

37. Which of the following familial syndromes would not be expected to increase risk for glioma development?
    a. Li-Fraumeni
    b. NF1
    c. Multiple endocrine neoplasia (MEN) type 2a
    d. Lynch syndrome

38. Which of the following statements is false with regard to the prognosis of germ cell tumors?
    a. The 10-year OS of germinoma is about 95%.
    b. The 10-year OS of non-germinomatous germ cell tumor is about 50%.
    c. Germinoma often disseminates along the ventricles.
    d. Histology can change at second-look surgery when compared with the initial diagnosis.

39. What mutation in cranipharyngiomas shows promise for a chemotherapy target?
    a. PLD
    b. MEK
    c. BRAFV600E
    d. EGFR

40. A 58-year-old man presents to the emergency department with new-onset seizures with no prior history of epilepsy in the setting of a glioma postsurgical resection and on cycle 1 of adjuvant TMZ therapy. MRI 2 days ago was stable. The epileptic event resolves following abortive therapy, and the patient is at baseline. CT head shows stable edema around residual tumor, which also appears stable, and no hemorrhage. What would be appropriate management?
    a. Discharge home with no change to medications and instructions to follow-up in clinic.
    b. Discharge home with new script for antiepileptic medication.
    c. Discharge home with new script for dexamethasone.
    d. Both b and c

41. Patients with gangliogliomas most commonly present with the following symptom:
    a. Headache
    b. Seizure
    c. Stroke
    d. Hearing loss

42. The tumor depicted here has the following characteristics:
    a. It may have calcifications that are detectable on imaging.
    b. It is frequently associated with seizures.
    c. It has loss of ATRX expression.
    d. It responds well to mTOR inhibitors.
    e. Both a and b

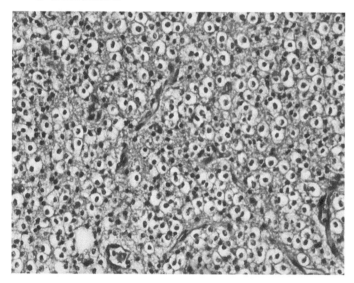

43. A 64-year-old right-handed man, previous smoker, is diagnosed with EGFR mutant non-small cell lung cancer (T2N1M1a). He is started on initial therapy with erlotinib, and his cancer remains stable for 6 months. On his next series of staging, however, he's found to have new metastases in his contralateral lung, liver, and abdominal lymph nodes. At his oncologist's office to discuss these results, he endorses also new posterior headaches waking him from sleep, associated with nausea and frequent vomiting. He's also been experiencing increasing gait difficulty. He is sent to the hospital for emergent non-contrast head CT, which demonstrates a space-occupying hypodensity in the left

cerebellum with surrounding edema, effacement of the fourth ventricle, and early mild hydrocephalus. What is the next best immediate step in his management?

a. Arrange for outpatient neurosurgical consultation.
b. Perform lumbar puncture to measure opening pressure and lower elevated pressure.
c. Bolus with dexamethasone 10 mg IV followed by standing 6 mg BID.
d. Both b and c

44. In adults, the most common type of intramedullary spinal cord tumor (IMSCT) is:
a. Ependymoma
b. Astrocytoma
c. Hemangioblastoma
d. Metastatic lesion

45. Risk factors for malignant transformation of peripheral nerve sheath tumors include the following *except*:
a. Prior radiation treatment
b. Presence of plexiform neurofibromas
c. Smoking
d. NF1 germline mutations

46. All of the following are histologic characteristics of schwannoma, except
a. Antoni A fibers
b. Verocay bodies
c. Spindle cells
d. Antoni B fibers

47. A 32-year-old man presents with headaches and subtle balance difficulties. His MRI is shown here. Risks and benefits of potential biopsy are discussed with the patient. If he ends up having a biopsy done, you are likely to see which of the following features in the pathology report?

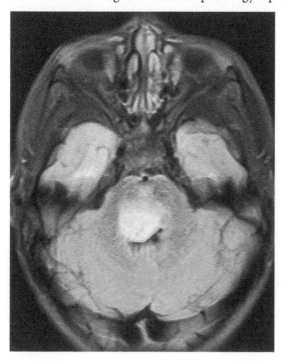

a. Rosenthal fibers
b. H3K27 mutation
c. 1p19q co-deletion
d. IDH-1 mutation
e. Microvascular proliferation and necrosis

48. Which chemotherapy has been shown to improve hearing and shrink vestibular schwannomas (VS) in NF2 patients?
a. Bevacizumab
b. Selumetinib
c. TMZ
d. Carboplatin/vincristine

49. Which of the following has become the gold standard approach for surgical intervention for pituitary pathologies?
a. Transcranial
b. Endonasal microscopic
c. Transsphenoidal endonasal endoscopic
d. Sublabial transsphenoidal

50. Which of the following statements is true with regards to the radiation treatment of germ cell tumors?
a. Radiation to the focal field of tumors is recommended for localized germinoma
b. Craniospinal irradiation is recommended for all germinomas
c. Radiation after resection of mature teratoma is not recommended
d. Germinomas located in the basal ganglia only require focal radiation

51. The risk of neurocognitive deficits in elderly patients with PCSNL is higher with:
a. WBRT alone
b. MTX alone
c. MTX followed by WBRT
d. MTX + rituximab

52. Which of the following factors would have the largest impact on prognosticating a patient's OS after a diagnosis of low-grade glioma?
a. IDH mutation status
b. Extent of resection
c. Completion of chemotherapy cycles
d. Total dose given for radiation therapy
e. None of above

53. Which of the following glioma findings is not associated with the diagnosis of molecular equivalent of GBM?
a. TERT promoter gene mutation
b. EGFR amplification
c. MT promotor unmethylation
d. Chromosome 7p gain, 10q loss

54. Which of these tumors commonly presents as an intraventricular mass attached to the wall of the

lateral ventricle or septum pellucidum with numerous intratumoral cystic areas?
a. Ependymoma
b. Choroid plexus papilloma
c. Central neurocytoma
d. Germinoma

55. A 70-year-old man with progressive GBM presents with acute abdominal pain. A kidney, ureter, bladder (KUB) study shows free air under the diaphragm. You don't have access to his medical records, the patient is confused, and family is not available. The surgeon consulting on the case asks you about possible treatments that the patient could have received recently and if there are any concerns about potential surgical intervention. You suspect:
a. Bowel perforation secondary to bevacizumab, and you tell the surgeon about potential postsurgical wound healing complications
b. Severe constipation from ondansetron; this is not a surgical case
c. Appendicitis unrelated to patient's primary diagnosis
d. Bowel perforation caused by TMZ, and you educate the surgeon about possible neutropenia

56. A 6-month-old boy is brought to the clinic for spells suspicious for infantile spasms. His medical record notes that he has had a heart murmur since birth. A dermatological exam shows three areas of hypopigmentation on his body that are each 1–2 cm in size. A brain MRI reveals four periventricular nodules that distort the normally smooth ventricular margins. What is this patient's most likely diagnosis?
a. Tuberous sclerosis complex
b. NF1
c. NF2
d. Turcot syndrome

57. Please choose the *false* statement:
a. Seizures are more common in patients with high-grade glioma than in patients with low-grade glioma.
b. Patients who harbor tumors with IDH1 mutations have higher risk for seizures.
c. Most patients with brain tumors and seizures should be treated with non-enzyme–inducing antiepileptic drugs.
d. There is no evidence that prophylactic use of an anticonvulsant should be recommended to all brain tumor patients.
e. The anticonvulsant most commonly used in neuro-oncology practice is levetiracetam.

58. In two large clinical trials (RTOG 0825 and AVAglio) in newly diagnosed GBM, bevacizumab was shown to:
a. Increase OS in patients with GBM
b. Increase progression-free survival (PFS) and OS in GBM
c. Improve overall response rate (ORR) and PFS in GBM
d. Have no effect on either OS or PFS in GBM
e. None of above

59. In a randomized trial for elderly patients with newly diagnosed GBM, the following regimen has been demonstrated to be superior to short-course radiation (40 Gy) monotherapy:
a. Radiation (40 Gy) + nivolumab
b. Radiation (60 gy) + with concurrent TMZ + adjuvant TMZ + adjuvant TTFields
c. Radiation (60 Gy) with concurrent TMZ + adjuvant TMZ
d. Radiation (40 Gy) with concurrent TMZ + adjuvant TMZ

60. Which of the following markers on malignant cells would not be in keeping with a diagnosis of diffuse large B-cell PCNSL?
a. CD4
b. CD19
c. CD20
d. CD79a

61. Intrathecal prophylaxis remains part of the routine care of patients with which of the following?
a. Follicular lymphoma
b. Chronic lymphocytic leukemia
c. Waldenstrom's macroglobulimia
d. Lymphoblastic lymphoma

62. A 36-year-old woman with a newly diagnosed sarcoma undergoes chemotherapy in the inpatient oncology unit. After the infusion of chemotherapy, she develops confusion, agitation, hallucinations, and seizures. What is likely responsible for this phenomenon?
a. Infusion of bevacizumab
b. Leptomeningeal disease
c. Infusion of ifosfamide
d. Depression

63. What infection is associated with limbic encephalitis for cancer patients during the first-month post stem cell transplantation?
a. HIV
b. Cytomegalovirus
c. Human herpesvirus 6
d. Varicella
e. Hepatitis B virus

64. Current potential medical treatment targets in meningiomas include all of the following, except:
a. AKT and SMO
b. SSTR2
c. Merlin
d. VEGF and VEGFR pathways

65. Which of the following is not associated with tectal plate lesions?
a. Obstructive hydrocephalus
b. Parinaud's syndrome
c. Foster-Kennedy syndrome
d. Glial pathology

66. An MRI scan shows a solid, hyperintense, elongated intradural lesion in the region of the cauda equina consistent with an ependymoma. The most likely pathology consistent with this lesion is:
    a. Subependymoma
    b. Myxopapillary ependymoma
    c. Classic ependymoma
    d. Anaplastic ependymoma

67. Which of the following CNS embryonal tumors has the highest incidence in children?
    a. Medulloblastoma
    b. Embryonal tumors with multilayered rosettes (ETMR)
    c. Atypical teratoid rhabdoid tumor (ATRT)
    d. Pineoblastoma

68. A 14-year-old girl presents with a 4-week history of progressively worsening right-sided facial weakness. She was initially diagnosed with Bell's palsy in the emergency room and received steroids with mild improvement. However, her symptoms have now progressed including a new right hemiparesis. MRI demonstrates a 4 × 3.5 cm mass within the left thalamic region with mild surrounding edema and patchy enhancement. Given the acute onset of symptoms and imaging appearance, you suspect a high-grade glioma. The most appropriate next step in management is:
    a. Craniospinal radiation therapy with focal boost
    b. Focal radiation therapy
    c. Biopsy or maximal safe resection if feasible
    d. Neoadjuvant chemotherapy
    e. Palliative care alone

69. An 11-year-old boy with familial NF1 recently had a disease surveillance MRI showing optic pathway enhancement without thickening of optic nerves. Ophthalmology evaluation does not identify any visual deficits, and patient is visually asymptomatic. What is the best management approach?
    a. Biopsy of tumor to obtain a pathological diagnosis
    b. Close ophthalmology follow-up with interval imaging
    c. Full-body MRI to identify other tumors
    d. Antiseizure medications due to history of NF1

70. Which of the following agents used in the treatment of CNS malignancies would be considered "targeted therapy"?
    a. TMZ
    b. Lomustine
    c. Nivolumab
    d. Bevacizumab
    e. MTX

71. Mr. Brown is a 61-year-old man with a right frontal GBM with symptomatic progressive disease associated with substantial vasogenic edema. For which of the following scenarios would bevacizumab be a reasonable option?
    a. Deep vein thrombosis (DVT) managed with inferior vena cava (IVC) filter due to contraindication for anticoagulation
    b. Petechial hemorrhage on MRI of the brain
    c. Transient ischemic attack (TIA) 3 weeks ago
    d. Poorly controlled hypertension
    e. At 2 weeks post op from appendectomy

72. Which of the following statements regarding the management of leptomeningeal disease is false?
    a. A phase III trial showed promising efficacy for intrathecal MTX for patients with leptomeningeal involvement from breast cancer.
    b. Prognosis is uniformly poor, and symptom management is the main goal of therapy.
    c. Penetration of intrathecal chemotherapy in bulky leptomeningeal disease is limited to a few millimeters.
    d. Intrathecal targeted therapies such as rituximab in lymphoma and trastuzumab in HER2/neu positive breast cancer may be of benefit, but additional data are needed.

73. A 25-year-old woman presented with 2 weeks of paranoia and abnormal behavior and required psychiatry hospitalization. MRI of the brain was unremarkable. Over the following week, she become less responsive, developed orofacial dyskinesias, and eventually required transfer to the ICU due to low level of consciousness, blood pressure variability, and respiratory failure. Which of the following antibodies are most likely to be associated with this syndrome?
    a. LGI-1
    b. Ma2
    c. NMDA-R
    d. P/Q VGCC
    e. PCA-1

74. A ring of enhancement or "flame sign" on T1 gadolinium-weighted MRI at the periphery of a IMSCT is suggestive of what pathology?
    a. Astrocytoma
    b. Ependymoma
    c. Hemangioblastoma
    d. Metastasis

75. Which of the following CNS tumors is seen most commonly in patients with Li-Fraumeni syndrome?
    a. Infiltrative astrocytoma
    b. Ependymoma
    c. Meningioma
    d. Medulloblastoma

76. The following are all risk factors for the development of post-transplant lymphoproliferative disorder *except*:
    a. Long duration of immunosuppressive treatment
    b. Positive EBV status

c. Solid organ transplant

d. Age >50

77. A 59-year-old woman with ovarian cancer develops oral dysesthesias during the first chemotherapy infusion. What is the likely causative agent?

a. Carboplatin

b. Cisplatin

c. Cyclophosphamide

d. Oxaliplatin

78. A 52-year-old woman was diagnosed with and underwent resection of a right parietal WHO grade 2 meningioma 6 years ago. She received radiation at time of tumor recurrence 4 years ago and has now undergone repeat subtotal resection with the same pathology. What are the two most reasonable treatment options that could be considered here?

a. Repeat surgery with goal of gross-total tumor resection

b. Re-irradiation, either by involved-field radiotherapy (IFRT) or by stereotactic radiosurgery (SRS)

c. Participation in a clinical trial, if eligible

d. Immunotherapy

e. Both b and c

79. Which of the following may be used to mitigate the neurocognitive effects of WBRT?

a. Memantine

b. Entacapone

c. Selegiline

d. Rivastigmine

80. There is evidence from a randomized controlled clinical trial that which of the following surgical interventions is associated with improved PFS for patients with malignant glioma?

a. The use of awake craniotomy

b. The use of neuronavigation

c. The use of intraoperative MRI

d. The use of 5-ALA

81. Based on the COG A9952 study, which evaluated treatment with carboplatin and vincristine (CV) versus treatment with thioguanine PCV (TPCV) in 274 children with low-grade gliomas, the following statements are true *except*:

a. All patients in this study had received radiation prior to chemotherapy.

b. The 5-year OS was comparable in both treatment groups.

c. Toxicity was worse in patients who received TPCV.

d. The 5-year EFS rate was not significantly different.

82. Which of the following tyrosine kinase inhibitors is correctly matched to its target mutation?

a. Erlotinib: Anaplastic lymphoma kinase (ALK)

b. Dabrafenib: B-raf (BRAF)

c. Olaparib: Epidermal growth factor receptor (EGFR)

d. Lorlatinib: Human epidermal growth factor receptor 2 (HER2)

83. A 32-year-old right-handed woman with metastatic breast cancer (ER+, PR−, HER2+) with osseous and lung metastases is currently receiving anastrozole, trastuzumab, and pertuzumab with stable systemic disease and a KPS of 90. She presents to the hospital with 2 weeks of intermittent confusion, language disturbances, and severe headaches. Her family states that at times "her speech is gibberish" for minutes at a time, and, after a period of fatigue, she returns to near baseline but with more mild word-finding difficulties. On exam, she appears uncomfortable and has paraphasic errors, right arm pronator drift, and subtle dysmetria in her left arm. MRI brain with and without gadolinium demonstrates four ring-enhancing lesions with vasogenic edema, the largest of which is 3.5 cm in the left temporal lobe. She has additional smaller (2–3 cm) metastases in the right frontal lobe, left occipital lobe, and left cerebellum. What is the best immediate next step in management?

a. Lumbar puncture to assess for leptomeningeal metastases

b. Start dexamethasone 4 mg BID and levetiracetam 500 mg BID

c. Send her home with outpatient follow-up with her medical oncologist

d. Consult radiation oncology for WBRT

84. Gangliocytomas are tumors that typically are found in the

a. Temporal lobe

b. Brainstem

c. Spinal cord

d. Cerebellum

85. Which is the optimal treatment of PCNSL in the elderly?

a. MTX-based upfront chemotherapy and consolidation WBRT regardless of response to chemotherapy

b. Upfront MTX-based chemotherapy without consolidation WBRT in complete responders to chemotherapy

c. WBRT alone

d. WBRT followed by MTX-based chemotherapy

86. Which of these tumors is associated with bony hyperostosis?

a. Meningioma

b. GBM

c. Pilocytic astrocytoma

d. Craniopharyngioma

87. The following is true of the Response Assessment n Neuro-Oncology (RANO) criteria for assessing GBM:

a. Progressive disease is defined as a 10% increase in volume of the enhancing lesion.

b. Progressive disease is defined as a ≥25% increase in cross-sectional area of the enhancing lesion.

c. Partial response is defined as a ≥25% decrease in cross-sectional area of the enhancing lesion.
d. Response assessments are independent of the steroid dosing.

88. A 70-year-old woman presents with altered mental status prompting the MRI scan shown here. The patient is placed on steroids, and her symptoms dramatically improve. Biopsy is performed, and it is nondiagnostic. What is the most likely diagnosis, and why was the biopsy nondiagnostic?

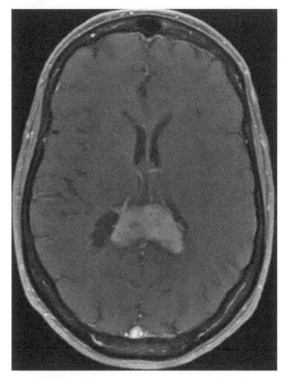

a. GBM; the surgeon missed the target lesion
b. Primary CNS Lymphoma (PCNSL); steroids decreased the ability to make the pathological diagnosis
c. Multiple sclerosis (MS); brain biopsies in MS are frequently nondiagnostic
d. GBM; steroids altered the tissue, making pathological diagnosis impossible

89. In the landmark study of *IDH* mutational status impact on prognosis by Yan et al. (2009), the median OS was:
a. 9 months in GBM *IDH* wildtype and 18 months in GBM *IDH* mutated
b. 12 months in GBM *IDH* wildtype and 24 months in GBM *IDH* mutated
c. 15 months in GBM *IDH* wildtype and 31 months in GBM *IDH* mutated
d. 24 months in GBM *IDH* wildtype and 38 months in GBM *IDH* mutated

90. The following therapeutic modality is *not* approved by the US Food and Drug Administration (FDA) for the treatment of newly diagnosed GBM:
a. Bevacizumab

b. TMZ
c. Carmustine (BCNU)-impregnated wafers
d. TTFields

91. All individuals with familial adenomatous polyposis syndrome (FAP) are at decreased risk of developing a brain tumor.
a. True
b. False

92. Which of the following is true regarding proton and photon therapy?
a. Protons have improved rates of tumor control.
b. Protons reduce low-dose exposure to normal tissues, thus decreasing side effects of treatment.
c. Protons and photons are equally available in radiation therapy centers around the United States.
d. Protons and photons have the same radiobiologic mechanism of causing cell damage.

93. Which of the following grading scales is used to assess meningioma resection?
a. Koo
b. Simpson
c. House-Brackman
d. Hunt and Hess

94. A patient presents with a left frontal mass. Histologically, it demonstrates rhabdoid components and a characteristic genetic alteration that confirms the diagnosis of ATRT. This alteration is in
a. SMARCD2 or SMARCB1
b. SMARCB1 or SMARCA4
c. SMARCA4 or SUFU
d. MYC or TYR

95. A 4-year-old boy with recurrent DIPG previously treated with standard definitive radiation therapy is scheduled to undergo focal salvage radiation. What factors put him at increased risk for symptomatic brainstem radionecrosis?
a. Young age
b. Tumor location in the posterior fossa
c. Radiation dose
d. All of the above

96. For a patient with NF2 and VS, it is best to:
a. Treat immediately with SRS, since response is very good and hearing can be saved
b. Operate immediately to save hearing
c. VS in NF2 patients tend to have the same biological behavior as in non-NF patients
d. Both b and c
e. None of the above

97. Which of the following is true regarding the use of alkylating agents?
a. For GBM patients on adjuvant TMZ, dose-intense treatment (e.g., given 21 of 28 days) improves outcomes when compared to standard dosing (i.e., 5 of 28 days).

b. The risk of pneumonitis represents a contraindication to TMZ for patients with severe chronic obstructive pulmonary disease (COPD).

c. Patients who receive procarbazine should avoid selective serotonin reuptake inhibitors (SSRIs) and foods high in tyramine.

d. Patients who develop neutropenia on TMZ should receive concurrent filgrastim (G-CSF [Neupogen]) with subsequent cycles of TMZ.

98. A 60-year-old man presents with 3 weeks of confusion, short-term memory difficulties, and seizures. MRI of the brain showed abnormal T2 signal of bilateral medial temporal lobes. Which of the following antibodies has the lowest probability of being associated with limbic encephalitis in this patient?
    a. LGI-1
    b. AMPA-R
    c. GABA type B
    d. ANNA-1
    e. Ma2

99. You are reviewing imaging of a GBM patient who recently underwent gross total resection. You see a thin rim of diffusion restriction at the margin of a resection cavity, and radiology report suggests acute stroke. Your next steps are:
    a. Call stroke code and evaluate the patient for anti-thrombotic therapy.
    b. Put the patient on low-dose aspirin.
    c. Call neurosurgery for urgent consult.
    d. Order follow up MRI in 2–4 weeks.

100. RTOG 0424 was a single-arm study of grade 2 gliomas evaluating RT + TMZ in grade 2 gliomas with three or more high-risk features (age ≥40, astrocytoma histology, bi-hemispheric tumor, preoperative tumor diameter >6 cm, preoperative neurologic function status >1). This study found:
    a. Median OS was 3.1 years
    b. Median OS was 8.2 years
    c. The majority of adverse effects were gastrointestinal
    d. 10-year OS was 2%

ANSWERS

1. d
2. a
3. c
4. b
5. b
6. d
7. a
8. a
9. a
10. d
11. d
12. d
13. d
14. b
15. b
16. d
17. c
18. b
19. d
20. a
21. e
22. b
23. b
24. a
25. a
26. b
27. e
28. b
29. c
30. a
31. b
32. b
33. c
34. d
35. c
36. c
37. c
38. b
39. c
40. d
41. b
42. e
43. c
44. a
45. c
46. c
47. b
48. a
49. c
50. c
51. c
52. a
53. c
54. c
55. a
56. a
57. a
58. c
59. d
60. a
61. d
62. c
63. c
64. c
65. c
66. b
67. a
68. c

69. b
70. d
71. b
72. a
73. c
74. d
75. a
76. d
77. d
78. e
79. a
80. d
81. a
82. b
83. b
84. d

85. b
86. a
87. b
88. b
89. c
90. a
91. b
92. b
93. b
94. b
95. d
96. e
97. c
98. a
99. d
100. b

TEST EXAM NUMBER TWO

1. What is the most common tumor associated with N-methyl-D-aspartic acid receptor (NMDAR) autoantibodies?
   a. Chondrosarcoma
   b. Rhabdomyosarcoma
   c. Ovarian teratoma
   d. Yolk sac tumor

2. What is a reasonable management option for a presumed World Health Organization (WHO) grade 1 meningioma?
   a. Observation
   b. Surgical resection
   c. SRS
   d. Any of the above

3. What is a widely practiced dose fractionation for whole-brain radiotherapy (WBRT)?
   a. 8 Gy/1 fraction
   b. 12 Gy/4 fractions
   c. 24 Gy/6 fractions
   d. 30 Gy/10 fractions

4. A 6-year-old girl presents with seizures. Magnetic resonance imaging (MRI) demonstrates a left temporal lesion which is highly infiltrative and heterogeneously contrast enhancing. Pathology demonstrates a high-grade neuroepithelial neoplasm with astrocytic components consistent with anaplastic pleomorphic xanthoastrocytoma WHO grade 3. Molecular testing will most likely demonstrate:
   a. *BRAF-KIAA1549* fusion
   b. *FGFR3-TACC3* fusion
   c. *BRAF V600E* mutation
   d. *QKI-RAF1* fusion

5. Identify the incorrect pair:
   a. Gorlin's syndrome—Ependymoma
   b. NF1—Optic pathway glioma
   c. Tuberous sclerosis—Subependymal giant cell astrocytoma
   d. Li-Fraumeni syndrome—Choroid plexus carcinoma

6. The best course of treatment for newly diagnosed suspected atypical teratoid rhabdoid tumor (ATRT) is:
   a. Follow-up only, prognosis is very good
   b. Maximal safe resection and adjuvant therapy using chemotherapy +/− radiotherapy (RT)
   c. Palliative care only, prognosis is dismal
   d. Biopsy only and immediate radiation therapy

7. In a patient with a radiosensitive tumor and unstable low-grade metastatic spinal cord compression without myelopathy, the optimal treatment modality is:
   a. External beam RT
   b. Stabilization followed by external beam RT
   c. Stereotactic radiosurgery (SRS)
   d. Stabilization followed by SRS
   e. Decompression followed by stabilization and SRS

8. Which of these statements is false about diffuse midline gliomas?
   a. Some of them were previously called diffuse intrinsic pontine gliomas (DIPG).
   b. They are H3 K27M-mutant.
   c. They are WHO grade 4 tumors.
   d. They usually show diffuse intense enhancement.

9. Current practice guidelines recommend WHO grade 3, isocitrate dehydrogenase (IDH)-1 mutated astrocytomas be treated with:
   a. Maximal resective surgery, high-dose RT, concomitant temozolomide (TMZ), adjuvant TMZ
   b. Maximal resective surgery, low-dose RT, concomitant TMZ, adjuvant TMZ
   c. Maximal resective surgery, high-dose RT
   d. Maximal resective surgery, low-dose RT
   e. None of above

10. What are the most common class of adverse events that should be monitored for when administering immune checkpoint inhibitor therapy?
   a. Bone marrow suppression
   b. Stevens-Johnson syndrome
   c. Venous thromboembolism
   d. Neurotoxicity
   e. Autoimmune reactions

11. A 22-year-old man of Asian descent presents with severe headaches, nausea, and diplopia. MRI shows an avidly enhancing lesion in the pineal area. Biopsy is done, and you review the slides with your pathologist who shows you the picture shown here. Based on your assessment you will recommend:
    a. Cerebrospinal fluid (CSF) testing for cytology, alpha-fetoprotein (AFP), and beta-human chorionic gonadotropin (HCG)
    b. Additional surgery to achieve gross total resection
    c. Bilateral orchiectomy
    d. Immediate start of WBRT
    e. Steroids and reassessment with MRI in 1–2 months

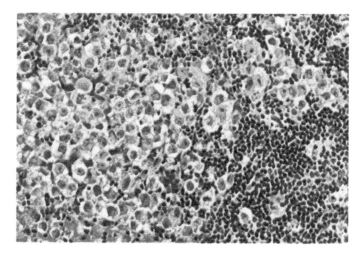

12. Malignant peripheral nerve sheath tumors (MPNSTs) may develop from all *except*
    a. Degeneration of schwannomas
    b. Degeneration of meningiomas
    c. Degeneration of neurofibromas
    d. They may arise *de novo*

13. Spinal cord ependymomas are associated with which syndrome?
    a. Neurofibromatosis type 1 (NF1)
    b. Neurofibromatosis type 2 (NF2)
    c. Down's syndrome
    d. Von-Hippel Lindau (VHL) syndrome

14. What is true about the development and workup of leptomeningeal metastases?
    a. CSF cytology is highly sensitive and specific, and so a negative result reliably rules out this diagnosis.
    b. History of cerebellar metastasis with resection places a patient at a higher risk of developing leptomeningeal metastases.
    c. Osimertinib has no proven efficacy for treating leptomeningeal disease.
    d. All of the above.

15. The most common genetic abnormality found in gangliogliomas is:
    a. IDH-mutation

16. b. O⁶-methylguanine DNA methyltransferase (MGMT) promoter methylation
    c. BRAF V600E mutation
    d. BRAF fusion mutation

16. A 65-year-old woman with HER2⁺ breast cancer status and metastatic brain lesions has completed WBRT and adjuvant chemotherapy and is status post treatment. Current imaging shows no improvement of her disease course, and she has begun to develop severe cachexia secondary to dysphagia. Initiating enteral feeding in this patient may increase the likelihood that she will lose independent feeding in the future.
    a. True
    b. False

17. Which of the following is *not* a common complication of radiation therapy in NF1 patients?
    a. Moyamoya syndrome
    b. Malignant transformation of tumors
    c. Pseudoprogression
    d. Endocrinopathies

18. A 65-year-old woman with anaplastic astrocytoma comes to emergency department (ED) with fever (102°F), chills, and shortness of breath. Her absolute neutrophil count is 500/mm3. You are reviewing her oncologic history. The drug that most likely led to her current condition is:
    a. Bevacizumab
    b. TMZ
    c. Lomustine
    d. Vincristine
    e. Levetiracetam

19. A 54-year-old man with history of small-cell lung cancer (SCLC) treated 2 years ago presents with 8 weeks of progressive numbness and sensory ataxia. He also has gastroparesis. He is found to have ANNA-1 antibodies. Which of the following is the most appropriate next step in the management of this patient?
    a. Screening for melanoma
    b. Symptomatic treatment for small fiber neuropathy secondary to chemotherapy
    c. Watchful waiting
    d. Testicular ultrasound
    e. The patient requires workup to rule out recurrent SCLC.

20. What is an advantage of the second-generation Optune system?
    a. Improved portability
    b. Improved efficacy
    c. Decreased time of use required to achieve similar results
    d. Fewer side effects
    e. Decreased cost

21. You are evaluating a 45-year-old immunocompetent man with the newly diagnosed brain lesion depicted here. Based

on the radiographic appearance of the lesion, match the correct pathological diagnosis with the most likely RT treatment that would be required following surgery.

   a. This is most likely glioblastoma (GBM), treat with XRT to 40 Gy over 3 weeks.

   b. This is most likely GBM, treat with XRT to 60 Gy over 6 weeks.

   c. This is most likely primary central nervous system lymphoma (PCNSL), treat with XRT to 75 Gy over 6 weeks.

   d. None of the above.

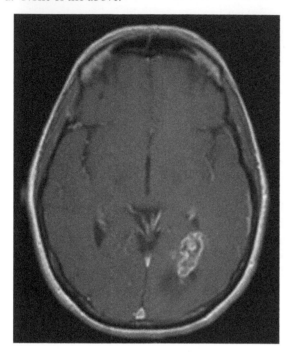

22. What is required to classify a tumor as a secondary to cranial radiation therapy?

   a. Short interval between radiation therapy and the development of secondary tumor

   b. Long interval between radiation therapy and the development of secondary tumor

   c. Concomitant chemotherapy

   d. Concomitant SRS with WBRT

23. A 65-year-old man with hypertension, hyperlipidemia, and diabetes presents with a new-onset seizure. On exam, he has postictal right hemiparesis from which he recovers quickly. MRI brain reveals a 4.5 × 3.9 cm homogeneously enhancing extra-axial mass lesion overlying the left frontal motor cortex with associated vasogenic edema. You are consulted for recommendations in regards to the next steps. What do you suggest?

   a. Seizure management per neurology recommendations and MRI brain and outpatient neuro-oncology follow-up in 1 month

   b. Systemic cancer workup including computed tomography (CT) chest, abdomen, pelvis, and oncology consultation

   c. Radiation oncology consultation for consideration of SRS

   d. Neurosurgery consult for tumor resection to establish diagnosis and tumor grade to inform further treatment recommendations

   e. Referral to palliative care for symptom management

24. All of the following are true regarding hemangioblastomas *except*

   a. Extracapsular resection is preferable to avoid significant blood loss.

   b. It is important to identify patients with pheochromocytoma preoperatively.

   c. Supratentorial hemangioblastomas are almost always associated with VHL syndrome.

   d. Early surgery is preferable once lesions are identified, especially in patients with VHL syndrome.

25. Radiation therapy is recommended in the management of ependymoma after which of the following scenarios?

   a. Gross total resection of a myxopapillary ependymoma

   b. Gross total resection of an anaplastic ependymoma

   c. Gross total resection of a posterior fossa Group B ependymoma

   d. Gross total resection of a classic ependymoma with YAP-1 fusion

   e. None of the above is correct

26. A 3-year-old girl presents with new-onset vomiting, convergence-retraction nystagmus, and upward gaze paralysis. You astutely recommend brain imaging. Which of the following embryonal tumors are you most concerned about?

   a. Medulloblastoma

   b. Embryonal tumors with multilayered rosettes (ETMR) of the frontal lobe

   c. Pineoblastoma

   d. ATRT of the posterior fossa

27. Diffusion-weighted imaging (DWI) MRI is used to identify

   a. Cerebral blood flow in a tumor relative to the water content of parenchymal tissue

   b. High tissue cellularity that may limit the movement of water

   c. Cerebral blood volume compared to net water content

   d. The amount of CSF diffusion through the arachnoid villi

28. Which of the following is true regarding the management of patients with anaplastic gliomas?

   a. Level I evidence demonstrates that the addition of chemotherapy with procarbazine (PCV) to RT offers a statistically significant overall survival benefit over RT alone among patients with oligodendrogliomas; similar trends were observed among patients with astrocytomas.

   b. TMZ demonstrated superior efficacy and side-effect profile compared to PCV in the adjuvant treatment of anaplastic glioma following surgery and radiation therapy in two recent phase III trials; these data led to its widespread adoption

c. The CATNON trial showed no benefit for the use of adjuvant TMZ in grade 3 astrocytomas.

d. Bevacizumab in combination with an alkylating agent adds a survival benefit compared to chemotherapy alone following resection of anaplastic oligodendrogliomas.

29. A 55-year-old man presents with subacute cerebellar degeneration. He is found to have PCA-Tr antibodies. Malignancy workup included CT with contrast of the chest, abdomen, and pelvis, which were unremarkable. Which of the following tests is indicated?

a. Positron emission tomography (PET)/CT to rule out Hodgkin lymphoma

b. Testicular ultrasound to rule out seminoma

c. Thyroid ultrasound to rule out thyroid cancer

d. Rectal ultrasound to rule out prostate adenocarcinoma

e. No further malignancy workup is necessary

30. Primary outpatient thromboprophylaxis is generally recommended in brain tumor patients in the following scenarios:

a. For all brain tumor patients

b. In the perioperative setting

c. During treatment with antiangiogenic therapy

d. During chemotherapy

31. Colloid cysts can result in sudden death from

a. Stroke

b. Elevated intracranial pressure

c. Acute obstructive hydrocephalus

d. Acute hemorrhage

32. After inserting the needle into the Ommaya reservoir and initiation of CSF withdrawal, you feel resistance with no further CSF return and notice the Ommaya appears depressed. Which of the following should be considered?

a. The patient's position on the procedure table may need to be adjusted.

b. Patient's postoperative head CT might have demonstrated slit-like ventricles.

c. The distal end of the catheter might be blocked by the choroid plexus.

d. Gentle pumping of the reservoir following needle removal might be considered.

e. All the above.

33. Supportive care only in GBM of the elderly should be prescribed for

a. Patients with hypertension

b. Patients with poor performance status (Karnofsky ≤50)

c. Patients with MGMT unmethylated tumors

d. Patients with biopsy alone

34. Which description is use cursive with regards to tumor markers for germ cell tumors?

a. AFP is elevated in embryonal carcinoma.

b. AFP is elevated in immature teratoma.

c. HCG is elevated in choriocarcinoma.

d. HCG is elevated in germinoma with syncytiotrophoblastic giant cells.

35. Which subtype of craniopharyngioma most commonly shows the mutation that may prove to be a chemotherapy target?

a. Adamantinomatous

b. Papillary

c. None of the above

d. Both a and b

36. A 20-year-old man presents with unilateral vestibular schwannoma and a family history of NF2. Which of the following would not be required for initial evaluation?

a. Genetic testing

b. MRI brain and spine

c. Ophthalmologic exam

d. Audiology testing

37. A 6-year-old boy is noted to have right sided sixth and seventh nerve palsies on a routine annual exam. Family further reports some ataxia, dysphagia, and clumsiness due to left sided weakness over the past 3–4 months. An MRI reveals an exophytic, contrast enhancing mass approximating the brainstem, not involving the basilar artery and pushing the pons to the side. What is the likely diagnosis?

a. High-grade astrocytoma

b. High-grade midline glioma

c. Pilocytic astrocytoma

d. Ependymoma

38. Which one of the tumors described below corresponds to WHO grade 2?

a. Infiltrating hemispheric glioma without microvascular proliferation or necrosis, harboring *IDH1* and *TERT* promoter hotspot mutations.

b. Infiltrating thalamic glioma without microvascular proliferation or necrosis, harboring H3 K27M mutation

c. Infiltrating hemispheric glioma without microvascular proliferation or necrosis, harboring *EGFR* amplification and *TERT* promoter mutation

d. Circumscribed hemispheric glioma without microvascular proliferation or necrosis, harboring *BRAF-KIAA1549* fusion

e. Infiltrating hemispheric glioma with numerous mitoses and microvascular proliferation, harboring *IDH1* mutation and 1p/19q codeletion.

39. You are seeing an 18-year-old patient with enlarged and painful right leg. During your exam you note prominent inguinal freckling. His MRI is shown here (Exhibit A).

Exhibit A

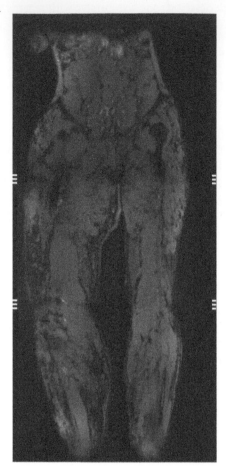

Based on your initial assessment, you suspect
   a. Plexiform neurofibroma in the setting of NF1
   b. Schwannomatosis
   c. Elephantiasis
   d. Osteosarcoma

40. The patient from question 39 undergoes a biopsy of the lesion in his right leg. Pathology slide (Exhibit B) shows fascicles of spindle cells (*arrow*) and areas of geographic necrosis (*arrows*). Based on the information you now have, you tell the patient:

Exhibit B

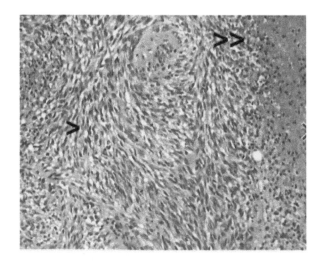

a. This is a benign lesion and no additional treatment is needed.
b. This is a malignant lesion and additional therapy will be necessary.
c. The biopsy is non-diagnostic.
d. You refer the patient to the orthopedic oncology.
e. Both b and d

41. Which of the following toxic effects are associated with the agent listed?
   a. Ibrutinib—Decreased wound healing
   b. Bevacizumab—Hypertension
   c. TMZ—Peripheral neuropathy
   d. Pemetrexed—Hemorrhagic cystitis
   e. Lomustine—Hypotension after rapid infusion

42. Among subependymal giant cell tumors, which of the following is true?
   a. Malignant transformation is common.
   b. Even after gross total resection, these tumors tend to recur.
   c. These tumors most commonly occur in the sixth to seventh decades of life.
   d. The mammalian target of rapamycin (mTOR) inhibitor everolimus is a primary treatment.

43. Which of the following CNS tumors is seen in patients with Gorlin syndrome?
   a. Glioma
   b. Ependymoma
   c. Meningioma
   d. Medulloblastoma

44. Glioblastoma
   a. Comprises 35% of all primary central nervous system (CNS) tumors
   b. Is the most common primary CNS tumor
   c. Comprises 15% of all primary CNS tumors
   d. Comprises 5% of infiltrating gliomas

45. In the EORTC 26981/22981 NCIC CE3 phase III trial, which established the benefit of TMZ added to RT in newly diagnosed GBM, the 2-year survival in patients treated with TMZ compared to those not treated with TMZ was:
   a. 90% vs. 10%
   b. 75% vs. 25%
   c. 25% vs. 10%
   d. 10% vs. 5%

46. A 70-year-old patient with a history of chronic lymphocytic leukemia (CLL) presents with a 2-week history of altered mental status. Which of the following would you consider for the initial workup of this patient?
   a. MRI brain with and without contrast
   b. MRI whole spine with and without contrast
   c. CSF studies with flow cytometry and cytology
   d. All of the above

47. A 67-year-old man presents for treatment for primary CNS lymphoma. He acutely develops confusion during MTX infusion. What is the next step in management?
a. Increase dose of MTX
b. Start dexamethasone
c. Administer methylene blue
d. Administer leucovorin

48. What is the origin of meningiomas?
a. Meningiomas originate from arachnoid cap cells, and pathogenesis is incompletely understood.
b. Meningiomas originate from the ependymal lining of the ventricles and disseminate via CSF spread.
c. Meningiomas originate from glioma stem cells, and the exact pathogenesis is unclear.
d. Meningiomas originate from arachnoid cap cells and pathogenesis is driven by alterations in merlin, which is encoded in the *NF2* gene.

49. Which of the following lesions is least accessible by an endoscopic endonasal approach?
a. Clival chordoma
b. Olfactory groove meningioma
c. Pituitary adenoma
d. Tectal plate glioma

50. RELA fusion is thought to activate which of the following signaling pathways?
a. RTK pathway
b. PI3K pathway
c. Sonic hedgehog pathway
d. NFKB pathway

51. A 4-year-old patient is found to have a calcified pineal mass with areas of restricted diffusion. Preliminary pathology suggests a small round blue cell tumor. AFP and beta-HCG (BhCG) are within normal limits. Based on these findings, you suspect
a. Pineal cyst
b. Germ cell tumor
c. Pineoblastoma
d. Medulloblastoma

52. A 44-year-old woman with history of breast cancer is involved in motor vehicle accident. She undergoes brain MRI to rule out acute injury. While reviewing the scan a few days later in clinic you notice the changes shown in Exhibit A. She mentions intermittent diplopia that has been bothering her for the past few weeks and potentially contributed to the accident. You recommend
a. MRI of the entire neuroaxis
b. CSF analysis
c. High-dose steroids
d. An angiogram
e. Both a and b

Exhibit A

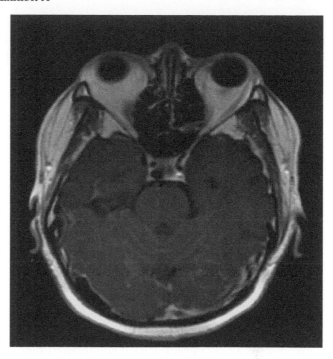

53. Presentation with multiple spinal meningiomas would be most likely with which condition:
a. Charcot-Marie-Tooth disease
b. VHL syndrome
c. Tay Sachs disease
d. NF2

54. Which is the optimal treatment for "fit" elderly patients with glioblastoma?
a. RT with concomitant and adjuvant TMZ
b. RT and adjuvant TMZ
c. TMZ alone
d. RT alone
e. None of the above

55. Selumetinib was approved in April 2020 for treatment of symptomatic plexiform neurofibromas in children older than age 2, largely based on SPRINT, the phase II trial which showed that
a. 72% of NF1 patients had a partial response, most responses were sustained for ≥6 months
b. 30% of NF1 patients had a partial response sustained for ≥6 months
c. Pain intensity and pain interference scores were not significantly changed
d. Strength and range of motion of affected muscle groups/joints were not significantly changed

56. What prospective phase II CNS lymphoma trial demonstrated that adding rituximab to high-dose methotrexate (HD-MTX) and cytarabine improved response rate?
a. IELSG32
b. EORTC 26033

c. NRG-BN001
d. Alliance A071401
e. RTOG 0825

57. CNS tumors may develop is roughly what percentage of patients with Li-Fraumeni syndrome?
   a. 25%
   b. 100%
   c. 1%
   d. 10%

58. EORTC 22033-26033 compared RT to TMZ in patients with low-grade gliomas. This study found that
   a. Progression-free survival (PFS) was better in the RT group among IDH-mutant, 1p19q co-deleted tumors (oligodendrogliomas)
   b. PFS was better in the TMZ group among IDH-wildtype tumors (IDH wildtype astrocytomas)
   c. Overall survival was better in the TMZ group among IDH-mutant, 1p19q co-deleted tumors (oligodendrogliomas)
   d. PFS survival was better in the RT group among IDH-mutant, 1p19q non-co-deleted tumors (IDH-mutant astrocytomas)

59. The pathogenesis of an acute systemic inflammatory syndrome characterized by multiorgan dysfunction and fever associated with chimeric antigen receptor (CAR)-T cell therapy is primarily driven by which of these groups of cytokines?
   a. Growth factor receptors
   b. Interleukin (IL)-6, IL-10, and interferon (IFN)-gamma
   c. IL-6, IL-12, JAK-2
   d. IL-1, IL-2, and IL-10

60. The following criteria are utilized to standardize imaging assessments in clinical trials for GBM:
   a. Response Assessment in Neuro-Oncology (RANO)
   b. Neurological Assessment in Neuro-Oncology (NANO)
   c. MacDonald criteria
   d. Karnofsky Performance Status (KPS)

61. Which of the following is the *least* helpful CSF test to pursue in the workup of possible PCNSL?
   a. CSF cytology
   b. MYD88 testing
   c. IgH rearrangement studies
   d. CSF lactate dehydrogenase

62. A 40-year-old man presented with new-onset seizures and was found to have a dural-based circumscribed tumor involving the left parietal-temporal convexity. Histopathologic examination revealed a hypercellular neoplasm composed of epithelioid cells arranged in a patternless growth pattern, in the background of thin-walled, branching vessels. Immunohistochemical stains for epithelial membrane antigen (EMA), S100, and glial fibrillary acidic protein (GFAP) are negative, and the lesion shows nuclear staining for STAT6 and INI1. What is the most likely diagnosis?
   a. Epithelioid sarcoma
   b. Rhabdoid meningioma
   c. Fibrous meningioma
   d. Solitary fibrous tumor
   e. Hemangioblastoma

63. During transventricular neuroendoscopy
   a. Complete tumor resection is never possible
   b. Hydrocephalus can be treated by third ventriculostomy
   c. Tumor resection or biopsy requires multiple port sites
   d. The third ventricle is entered directly, after traversing the white matter

64. A 2-year-old boy presents with nystagmus ongoing for 6 months. An MRI reveals a large optic pathway glioma which was partially resected. Diagnosis of pilocytic astrocytoma is made, and the tumor is positive for KIAA1549-BRAF fusion. He experienced tumor progression after 3 months of adjuvant treatment with carboplatin/vincristine. What is the next best treatment option?
   a. MEK inhibitor
   b. FGFR1 inhibitor
   c. mTOR inhibitor
   d. NTRK inhibitor

65. In addition to adequate anti-emetics, proper adjunctive measures for high-dose cytarabine must include
   a. PEG-filgrastim given on day 1.
   b. Filgrastim given on day 1.
   c. Dexamethasone 8 mg at the time of anti-emetics.
   d. Oral leucovorin rescue for 4 days.
   e. Dexamethasone eye drops for 4 days.

66. Which of the following paraneoplastic syndromes is paired with an incorrect antibody?
   a. Cerebellar degeneration—PCA-1
   b. Sensory neuronopathy—ANNA-1
   c. Limbic encephalitis—GABA-B receptor
   d. Brainstem encephalitis—Ma2
   e. Lambert-Eaton myasthenic syndrome—GAD65

67. Which one of the following statements is true regarding the use of chemotherapy in pediatric patients with high-grade gliomas?
   a. The COG study ACNS0126 was a single-arm phase II study that evaluated the use of single-agent TMZ concurrent with and following radiation and demonstrated improved outcomes for the combination when compared to historical results from the CCG-945 study. However, this remains to be confirmed in a randomized controlled study.

b. The COG study ACNS0423 was a single-arm phase II study that evaluated treatment consisting of radiation with concurrent single-agent TMZ followed by combinatorial alkylating chemotherapy with lomustine (CCNU) and TMZ. Compared to the ACNS0126 results, there was no improvement in OS or EFS and the combination of CCNU and TMZ was associated with increased myelotoxicity.

c. In COG study ACNS0126, patients with MGMT promoter hypermethylated tumors appeared to derive the strongest treatment benefit from TMZ.

d. The HERBY trial was a randomized phase II study that assigned patients to receive radiation and concurrent/adjuvant TMZ with or without bevacizumab

68. Among choroid plexus tumors, which of the following is true?
    a. Choroid plexus carcinomas appear more homogeneous on MRI than do choroid plexus papillomas.
    b. Atypical choroid plexus papillomas have lower probabilities of recurrence than choroid plexus papillomas.
    c. The imaging characteristics of choroid plexus papillomas and choroid plexus carcinomas are vastly different.
    d. Gross total resection of choroid plexus papilloma has a high probability of cure with a low probability of recurrence.

69. Which of these statements is use cursive about pseudoprogression?
    a. Pseudoprogression is associated with longer survival.
    b. Studies have shown that tumors with hypermethylated MGMT promoter status have up to 91% incidence of pseudoprogression.
    c. MRI perfusion maps commonly show increase in relative cerebral blood volume (rCBV) in pseudoprogression compared to the pre-treatment values.
    d. Imaging can demonstrate increasing size of enhancing components of the tumor.

70. What amount of prolactin is consistent with a secreting lactotroph pituitary adenoma?
    a. <100
    b. 100–150
    c. >200
    d. All of the above

71. Low-grade gliomas in elderly
    a. Are uncommon
    b. Can behave more aggressively
    c. Are the most common glioma type
    d. Both a and b

72. A phase II trial of selumetinib in pediatric patients with pilocytic astrocytomas harboring either KIAA1549-BRAF fusion or the BRAF^{V600E} mutation or with any neurofibromatosis type 1–associated low-grade glioma found that
    a. There were no partial responses, but 50% of patients had stable disease at 1 year
    b. 10% of patients with pilocytic astrocytomas with a BRAF mutation achieved a partial response
    c. 40% of patients with NF1-associated low-grade gliomas achieved a sustained partial response
    d. The most frequent grade 3 or 4 adverse event was diarrhea

73. Chemotherapy alone in glioblastoma of the elderly should be preferentially prescribed to
    a. Patients with unmethylated MGMT
    b. Patients with methylated MGMT
    c. Patients with lower performance status (Karnofsky 60–70) and comorbidities
    d. Patients with lower performance status (Karnofsky 60–70), comorbidities, and MGMT-methylated tumors

74. In the EORTC 22845 randomized trial to evaluate the long-term efficacy of early versus delayed RT with 54 Gy in low-grade gliomas, there was no significant difference in the median PFS.
    a. True
    b. False

75. What is the recommended WBRT dose and fractionation schedule for metastatic carcinomas in patients with poor prognostic indicators such as limited survival?
    a. 30 Gy in 10 fractions
    b. 20 Gy in 5 fractions
    c. 35 Gy in 5 fractions
    d. 20 Gy in 10 fractions

76. Which clinical trial demonstrated that there was no added benefit to a dose-intense schedule of adjuvant TMZ versus the 5/28-day regimen for initial treatment of GBM?
    a. RTOG 0825
    b. RTOG 9802
    c. EORTC 26951
    d. RTOG 0525
    e. NOA-08

77. Which of the following glioma subtypes was eliminated from the WHO 2016 classification scheme?
    a. Grade 1/grade 2 astrocytoma
    b. Grade 1/grade 2 oligodendroglioma
    c. Grade 1/grade 2 oligoastrocytoma
    d. Glioblastoma, IDH-mutant

78. A 12-year-old girl comes to you with chronic headaches. Her MRI (shown here) shows a lesion that will most likely have the following genetic alteration:
    a. MGMT methylation
    b. IDH-1 mutation

c. H3K27M mutation

d. Endothelial growth factor receptor (EGFR) amplification

e. Loss of ATRX

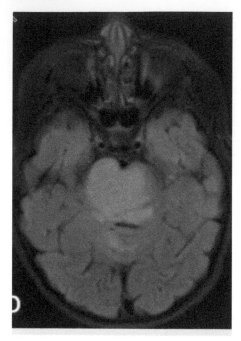

79. What is a pitfall to administering chemotherapy via the lumbar puncture (LP)?

a. Increased nausea and vomiting with LP procedure

b. Only one chemotherapy is approved for administration via the LP cistern

c. Multiple LPs increase the risk for fistula formation or CSF leak

d. Patients must remain in the left lateral decubitus position for 45 minutes after LP procedure

80. Which of these tumors commonly shows multicystic bubbly appearance on T2W MRI?

a. Dysembryoplastic neuroepithelial tumor (DNET)

b. Solitary fibrous tumor

c. Oligodendroglioma

d. Germinoma

81. Several agents used for systemic malignancies have shown activity in brain metastases. All of the following statements are true *except*

a. Ipilimumab, a CTLA4 inhibitor, can cause hypopituitarism.

b. Therapy with immune active agents such as nivolumab can result in pseudoprogression, which can include the appearance of new enhancement on imaging that can sometimes last for months.

c. Vemurafenib and dabrafenib are inhibitors of MGMT with activity in subsets of patients with melanoma.

d. Trametinib inhibits MEK, a component of the MAP kinase pathway.

82. Ms. Young was originally diagnosed with a left parietal glioblastoma with methylation of the MGMT promoter at the age of 65. She underwent surgical resection followed by radiation with concurrent and adjuvant TMZ, which she completed 3 months ago with no significant toxicities. MRI today demonstrates progressive disease at the surgical site. Consultation with a neurosurgeon and a radiation oncologist indicates that localized treatment for the recurrence is not technically feasible. There is mild peritumoral edema. The patient has good performance status and is interested in further therapy. If the patient is not eligible for a clinical trial, which of the following agents would be most appropriate in this setting?

a. Lomustine

b. Rechallenge with TMZ

c. Etoposide

d. Carboplatin

e. Bevacizumab

83. Diffusion-weighted imaging (DWI) MRI is not used to identify

a. Cerebral blood flow in a tumor relative to the water content of parenchymal tissue

b. High tissue cellularity that may limit the movement of water

c. Cerebral blood volume compared to net water content

d. a and c

84. What are the different molecular subtypes of medulloblastoma?

a. Atypical and malignant

b. WNT, SHH, and YAP1

c. WNT, SHH (TP53 mutant or wildtype), Group 3 and Group 4

d. Group A and Group B

85. A 12-year-old girl with a diagnosis of tuberous sclerosis recently started complaining of headaches associated with nausea and early morning vomiting. An MRI brain reveals a mass at the level of foramen of Monroe with evidence of obstructive hydrocephalus. What is the most likely diagnosis?

a. DNET

b. Primitive neuroepithelial tumor (PNET)

c. Subependymal giant cell astrocytoma (SEGA)

d. Benign hamartoma

e. Central neurocytoma

86. A 9-year-old boy presents with a posterior fossa mass and is found to have medulloblastoma. Family history is significant for multiple relatives with innumerable colonic polyps. You suspect a germline mutation in

a. RB1

b. APC

c. TP53

d. DICER1

87. Which of the following are contraindications to awake craniotomy with language mapping?
    a. Obesity
    b. Severe perioperative language deficits that are unresponsive to steroids
    c. Preoperative seizures
    d. Age <18 years

88. Which of the following is a potential long-term risk for pediatric patients who receive craniospinal irradiation?
    a. Meningioma resulting from radiation exposure
    b. Growth hormone deficiency
    c. Sleep–wake cycle disturbance
    d. Stroke within 20 years
    e. All of the above

89. A 36-year-old man presents with an intramedullary tumor involving T2 associated with syrinx. Biopsy of the tumor showed fibrillary acellular zones around vessels, surrounded by uniform cells with round nuclei. Tumor cells show cytoplasmic GFAP and dot-like EMA staining. The patient had a history of schwannoma resected from the left cerebellopontine angle 5 years ago. What is the most likely genetic alteration in this tumor?
    a. *NF1* mutation
    b. *NF2* mutation
    c. *SMARCB1* mutation
    d. *SMARCA4* mutation
    e. *TP53* mutation

90. What outcome did EORTC 22844 demonstrate for grade 2 gliomas?
    a. The addition of PCV chemotherapy to up-front radiation for high-risk grade 2 gliomas improved survival.
    b. Dose escalation from 50.4 to 64.8 Gy did not improve survival, and 92% of patients still had in-field tumor progression.
    c. Dose escalation from 45 to 59.4 Gy did not improve survival.
    d. There was no significant difference in PFS for patients with high-risk grade 2 glioma treated with dose-dense TMZ versus RT alone to 50.4 Gy.
    e. Although PFS improved, there was no difference in overall survival for patients treated with post-op RT versus observation (with RT at progression).

91. The following criteria/rating systems are utilized to standardize imaging assessments in brain cancer clinical trials:
    a. Response Assessment in Neuro-Oncology (RANO)
    b. Neurological Assessment in Neuro-Oncology (NANO)
    c. MacDonald criteria
    d. Karnofsky performance status (KPS)
    e. ECOG performance status

92. Which primary cancer is most commonly responsible for the development of leptomeningeal disease?
    a. Breast cancer
    b. Cervical cancer
    c. Ovarian cancer
    d. Uterine cancer

93. A 45-year-old patient with PCNSL has achieved complete response after HD-MTX-based induction and consolidative high-dose chemotherapy with autologous stem cell transplant. He is now 3 years post-treatment completion and has no evidence of disease recurrence. What is the ideal follow-up interval for this patient according to the International Primary CNS Lymphoma Collaborative Group (IPCG) consensus guidelines?
    a. Every 3 months
    b. Every 6 months
    c. Every year
    d. No follow-up needed as he is now 3 years post-treatment

94. The use of a dose-dense (75 mg/m² for 21/28 days in the adjuvant phase) regimen of TMZ when compared to "standard" dose TMZ (150–200 mg/m² for 5/28 days in the adjuvant phase) is associated with
    a. Improved overall survival
    b. Improved response rates
    c. Improved tolerability
    d. Increased rate of grade 3/4 toxicities

95. The dose map depicted here shows a radiation plan for a patient with a low-grade glioma. Based on your analysis of the plan, you can conclude the following:
    a. This treatment modality will eliminate exit dose, which can spare normal brain and the contralateral hippocampus.
    b. This plan will deliver very high exit dose and will increase the risk of neurotoxicity.
    c. This treatment modality should not be used for patients with low-grade glioma.
    d. This treatment modality has the highest energy at the entry of the beam.

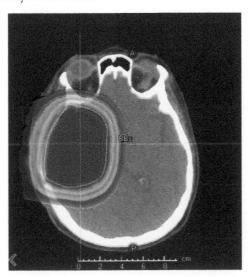

96. A 24-year-old man presented with seizures and was found to have a circumscribed, solid, and cystic right temporal lobe mass. Histopathological examination revealed scattered large cells with prominent nucleoli, abundant amphiphilic cytoplasm with Nissl substance in the background of uniform small cells with elongate nuclei, and long fibrillary processes associated with eosinophilic granular bodies. Large cells stain with synaptophysin and small cells stain with GFAP. Immunohistochemical stain against BRAF V600E mutant protein is also positive. What is the most likely diagnosis?
    a. Oligodendroglioma, IDH-mutant and 1p/19q-codeleted, WHO grade 2
    b. Pilocytic astrocytoma, WHO grade 1
    c. Ganglioglioma, WHO grade 1
    d. Diffuse astrocytoma, IDH-wildtype, WHO grade 2
    e. Central neurocytoma, WHO grade 2

97. A 52-year-old man with a recurrent WHO grade 2 meningioma presents for follow-up. The MRI demonstrates new tumor progression in the left frontal lobe resulting in new right hemiparesis. Surgical and radiation options have been exhausted. What medical treatment options may be considered based on the best available evidence?
    a. Somatostatin receptor 2 (STR2)-targeted therapy with radionuclides
    b. PD-L1-targeted therapy
    c. Vascular endothelial growth factor (VEGF)-targeted therapy with bevacizumab ± mTOR-targeted therapies with everolimus
    d. SSTR2-targeted therapy with somatostatin analogs ± mTOR-targeted therapies with everolimus

98. A 6-year-old girl presented with visual loss and was found to have an optic nerve mass. A physical examination revealed multiple palpable lesions on extremities and trunk as well as pigmented skin lesions. What is the most probable diagnosis of the mass on the optic nerve and the associated tumor syndrome in this patient?
    a. Subependymal giant cell astrocytoma—Tuberous sclerosis
    b. Schwannoma—NF2
    c. Pilocytic astrocytoma—NF1
    d. Ependymoma—Turcot syndrome type 1
    e. Anaplastic oligodendroglioma—Ehlers-Danlos syndrome

99. Which one of the following has not been identified as a neurological complication of nivolumab treatment?
    a. Moyamoya disease
    b. Guillain-Barré syndrome
    c. Myasthenia gravis
    d. Encephalitis

100. Evaluation of suspected PCNSL should always include all of the following *except*
    a. PET-CT (skull base to mid-thighs)
    b. Slit lamp examination
    c. CSF analysis
    d. Bone marrow biopsy
    e. MRI of the entire neuraxis

ANSWERS

1. c
2. d
3. d
4. c
5. a
6. b
7. b
8. d
9. a
10. e
11. a
12. b
13. b
14. b
15. c
16. a
17. c
18. c
19. e
20. a
21. b
22. b
23. d
24. d
25. b
26. c
27. b
28. a
29. a
30. b
31. c
32. e
33. b
34. a
35. b
36. a
37. c
38. a
39. a
40. e
41. b
42. d
43. d
44. c

45. c
46. a
47. d
48. a
49. d
50. d
51. c
52. e
53. d
54. a
55. a
56. a
57. d
58. d
59. b
60. a
61. d
62. d
63. b
64. a
65. e
66. e
67. d
68. d
69. c
70. c
71. d
72. c

73. d
74. b
75. b
76. d
77. c
78. c
79. c
80. a
81. c
82. a
83. d
84. c
85. c
86. b
87. b
88. e
89. b
90. c
91. a
92. a
93. b
94. d
95. a
96. b
97. c
98. c
99. a
100. d

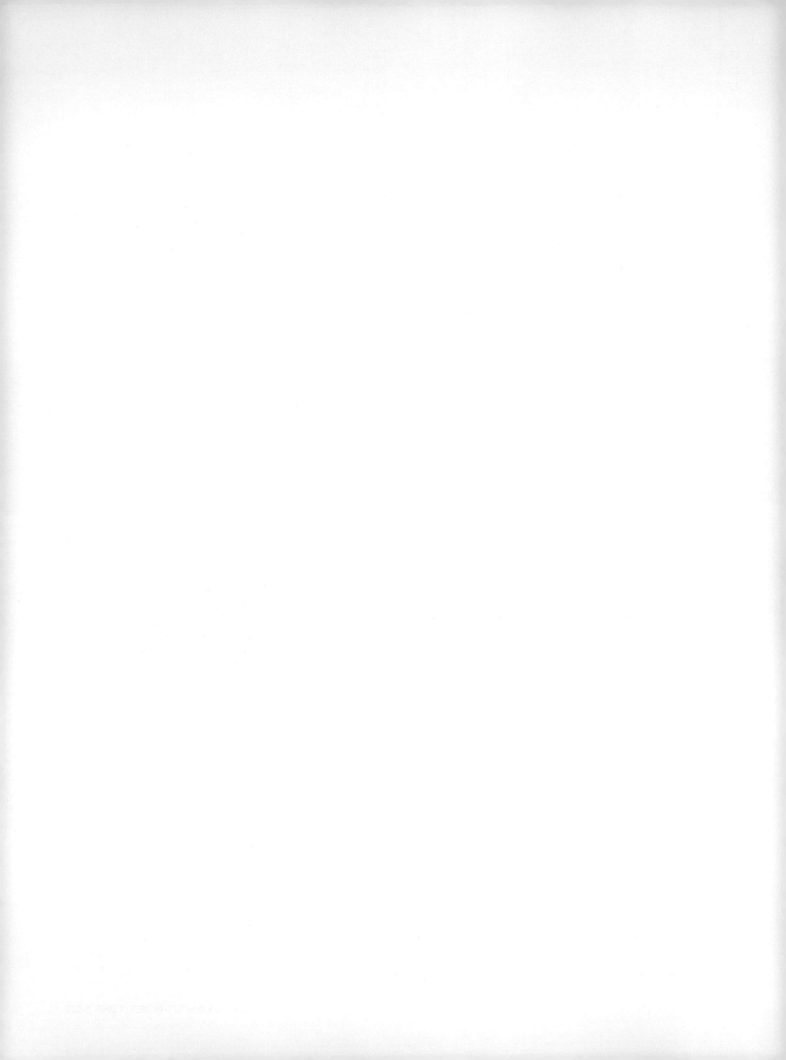

ABOUT THE EDITORS

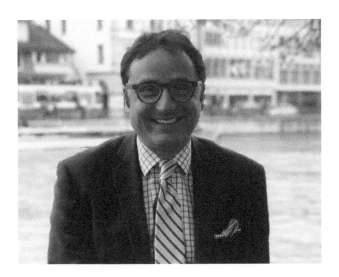

Maciej M. Mrugala. I am a neuro-oncologist at the Mayo Clinic Cancer Center in Phoenix, Arizona. I am a Professor of Medicine and Neurology and I direct a Comprehensive Neuro-Oncology Program and Neuro-Oncology Fellowship Program. I received my medical doctor degree from the Medical University of Warsaw, in Poland, and went on to train in neurology at the University of Massachusetts Medical School in Worcester, Massachusetts. In 2003, I earned a doctor of philosophy degree in neurobiology from the Copernicus University in Torun, Poland, for my work on neural stem cells and circadian system in mammals. My neuro-oncology training took me to Boston, where I completed a 3-year fellowship at Massachusetts General Hospital and Dana-Farber Cancer Institute, earning Master of Public Health at the Harvard School of Public Health along the way. I am board certified in neurology and neuro-oncology. In 2006, I joined Dr. Alexander Spence and the faculty of the Department of Neurology at the University of Washington (UW) and Fred Hutchinson Cancer Center in Seattle, Washington. My more than 10-year tenure in Seattle allowed me to help build and open Alvord Brain Tumor Center and culminated in earning the inaugural Alexander M. Spence Endowed Chair in Neuro-Oncology. I also created the neuro-oncology fellowship program at UW and led a busy clinical research program. In 2014, in collaboration with the Society for Neuro-Oncology (SNO), I started the Neuro-Oncology Review Course, organized in conjunction with the SNO annual meeting and endorsed by the American Academy of Neurology (AAN). Over the next several years, while working with the fantastic faculty from the best neuro-oncology programs in the United States, we created an educational offering that became a staple of the society meeting and is attended by more than

300 participants annually. The course organically led me to this project—the book you are holding in your hands. Through friendship and collaboration with my co-editors, members of the Neuro-Oncology Trainee Forum, we were able to gather top talent from around the globe and bring this compendium to you. I am grateful to my co-editors and colleagues for their support throughout this project. As the Immediate Past Chair of the Neuro-Oncology Section of the American Academy of Neurology, I could not be more proud that this book is crowning my term. Ultimately, this project was the seed of an idea to start the Foundation for Education and Research in Neuro-Oncology (FERN). I would like to dedicate this work to my parents, Ewa and Jan, who have always supported my academic endeavors. Words of immense gratitude for editorial assistance and critique throughout the project go to my colleague and friend Dr. Piotr Zlomanczuk.

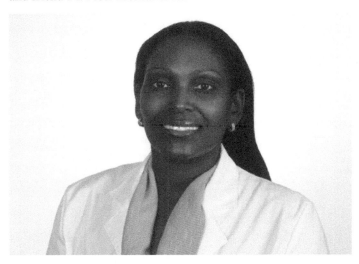

Na Tosha N. Gatson. I am the mother of four children ages 29, 27, 18, and 10 – and the Founder and CEO of Living Oncology. These are my greatest acheivements.

I am the Medical Director of Neuro-Oncology, leading a new multidisciplinary brain tumor program at Banner MD Anderson Cancer Center in Phoenix, AZ and I am involved trainee education as an Associate Professor of Medicine and Neurology at the University of Arizona College of Medicine and at the Geisinger Commonwealth School of Medicine. I completed my undergraduate pre-medicine studies at Indiana University before moving on to complete a combined MD/PhD training program, neurology residency, and an enfolded NIH/R25 neurosurgery research post-doctoral fellowship at The Ohio State University in Columbus, OH. My PhD was focused within molecular virology, immunology, and medical genetics with a major emphasis on neuro-immunology. Finally, I completed a 2-year neuro-oncology fellowship at the University of Texas MD Anderson Cancer Center in Houston, TX. My decision to lead a career in neuro-oncology was based on my mission to preserve the most basic elements of what it means to be human (thought, speech, movement, sensation, and emotion) - *adapted from the spirited words of neurologist, Dr. N. Mejia*. Brain cancer risks the slow deterioration of these human neurologic functions, and I endeavor to preserve, recover, and/or transition these abilities to allow for quality survival. My practice philosophy is based on extending not just the length of life, but also the quality of LIVING. Life is not short – *Life* (the time from our birth to our death) is the longest thing we will ever do. However, the time we have with our loved ones, in our careers, and enjoying the Earth with clarity of mind is relatively *short*. I consider this when designing patient treatment. Over years of practice, I have learned that neuro-oncologists suffer alongside their patients. So, I reject a practice which focuses on helping cancer patients *die* the best way possible. Instead, I endeavor to help my patients, and thereby myself, *live* the best way possible.

Academically, I enjoy population science and brain tumor imaging research as well as innovating in the neuro-oncology of women and trainee education. Excellence in these areas is important to my career satisfaction. Educating myself, my peers, and my colleagues is as important as how I deliver patient care. I served as lead editor on this project as part of my contribution to the field and in continuing my own professional development. I also maintain active leadership roles within the following organizations: American Brain Foundation, American Academy of Neurology, Society of Neuro-Oncology, NRG Oncology, Society of Clinical Neurology, National Medical Association, and the American Society of Clinical Oncology. Outside of my academic and career pursuits, I enjoy weightlifting, Qigong, motivational speaking, meditation, travel, the arts, and spending time with my family.

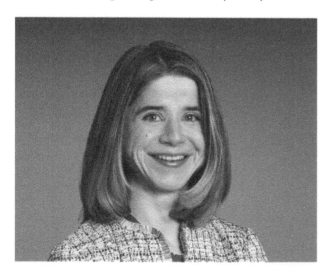

Sylvia C. Kurz. I am the Interim Director of Neuro-Oncology at the Brain and Spine Tumor Center/Perlmutter Cancer Center and an Assistant Professor of Neurology,

Hematology and Medical Oncology at New York University Langone Health.

After completing medical school at the Ludwig-Maximilans-University in Munich, Germany, I received my professional training at University Hospitals and Case Western Reserve University in Cleveland, Ohio, and at the Massachusetts General Hospital and the Dana-Farber Cancer Institute at Harvard University in Boston, Massachusetts. I am a neurologist certified by the American Board of Psychiatry and Neurology (ABPN) and a neuro-oncologist certified through the United Council of Neurological subspecialities (UCNS).

Besides being a passionate clinician, I am a translational and clinical investigator. In this role, I serve as a principal investigator on a number of investigator-initiated, cooperative group, and industry-sponsored trials.

Beyond that, I am an active member of the American Academy of Neurology (AAN) Neuro-Oncology section, and I am co-leading the working group Neuro-Oncology Trainee Forum (NOTF). The NOTF is aiming at providing hands-on guidance to early-career neuro-oncologists. The lack of a truly comprehensive study guide for residents, fellows, and junior faculty looking to take the board exams in neuro-oncology and medical oncology sparked the idea and laid the groundwork for the *Neuro-Oncology Compendium for the Boards and Clinical Practice*. I am glad it finally made it into a book! Editor's note:

Dr. Kurz is currently practicing in the Center for Interdisciplinary Neuro-Oncology at the University Hospital Tübingen.

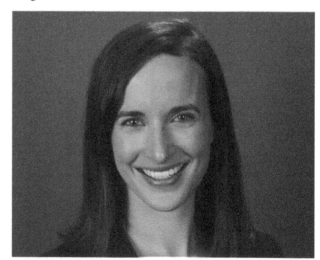

Kathryn S. Nevel. I am a neuro-oncologist and neurologist at Indiana University (IU) Health/IU School of Medicine. I completed medical school at IU in 2012, then completed my neurology residency at the University of Virginia in 2016, followed by a neuro-oncology fellowship at Memorial Sloan-Kettering in 2018. I have been on faculty at IU as an Assistant Professor of Clinical Neurology since completing my fellowship training. I am a clinician, an educator, and a principal investigator on several neuro-oncology trials with special research interests in neuro-oncology trainee education and patient quality of life. I am board certified in Neurology by the American Board of Psychiatry and Neurology (ABPN) and hold certification in Neuro-Oncology through the United Council of Neurological subspecialties (UCNS). I am an active member of the American Academy of Neurology, Society of Neuro-Oncology, American Neurological Association, and the American Society of Clinical Oncology.

Like several other editors of this book, I am a founding member of the NOTF. It has been an incredible experience to play a role in this compendium's development from a kernel of an idea shared during a NOTF phone meeting all the way to publication. I am honored to have worked on this book with my wonderful co-editors and colleagues, and I am thankful to my supportive husband and children (ages 6, 2, and 7 weeks) who are glad that the book is finally complete!

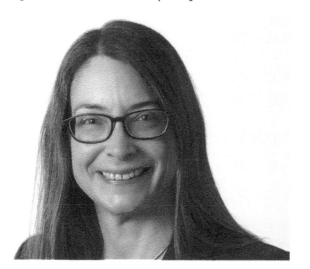

Jennifer L. Clarke. I am a neuro-oncologist at the University of California, San Francisco (UCSF), where I am a Professor of Clinical Neurology and Neurological Surgery in the UCSF Weill Institute of Neurosciences. I am also a member of the Neuro-oncology Program in the UCSF Helen Diller Family Comprehensive Cancer Center, where I serve as the Chair of the Protocol Review and Monitoring Committee. I completed medical school at UCSF in 2002, concurrently receiving a Master's degree in Public Health from the University of California at Berkeley in 2001. I then completed my neurology residency at UCSF, followed by neuro-oncology fellowship at Memorial Sloan-Kettering before joining the faculty at UCSF in 2008, where I am a clinician and clinical trialist as well as clinical researcher with specific research interests that include precision medicine and brain tumor epidemiology. I am both board-certified in Neurology by the American Board of Psychiatry and Neurology (ABPN) and certified in Neuro-Oncology by the United Council of Neurological Subspecialities (UCNS), and I am an active member in the American Society for Clinical Oncology, the Society for Neuro-oncology, and the American Academy of Neurology.

I have been a member of the Neuro-oncology Trainee Forum working group since its inception; it arose from the American Academy of Neurology's Neuro-oncology Section several years ago in an effort to better support trainees and junior faculty, and it has been a very rewarding effort to be part of. Out of that, in turn, came the recognition that a focused study guide for the neuro-oncology specialty exam did not exist, leading to the development of this book. I am thrilled to see it come to fruition!

INDEX